Anaesthesia A-Z

An Encyclopaedia of Principles and Practice

To Gill, Alison and Geraldine,
for their support, help and patience during the preparation of this book.

Anaesthesia A–Z

An Encyclopaedia of Principles and Practice

S.M. Yentis BSc, MBBS, FRCA

*Senior Registrar in Anaesthesia, Westminster and Charing Cross Hospitals,
London, UK*

N.P. Hirsch MBBS, FRCA

*Consultant Anaesthetist, The National Hospital for Neurology and Neurosurgery;
Honorary Lecturer, The Institute of Neurology, Queen Square, London, UK*

and

G.B. Smith BM, FRCA

*Consultant Anaesthetist and Head of Intensive Care Services,
Portsmouth Hospitals, UK*

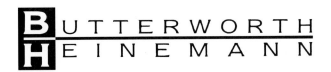

Butterworth-Heinemann Ltd
Linacre House, Jordan Hill, Oxford OX2 8DP

℞ A member of the Reed Elsevier group

OXFORD LONDON BOSTON
MUNICH NEW DELHI SINGAPORE SYDNEY
TOKYO TORONTO WELLINGTON

First published 1993

British Library Cataloguing in Publication Data

Yentis, Steven M.
    Anaesthesia A–Z: An Encyclopaedia of Principles
    and Practice
    I. Title
    617.9

ISBN 0 7506 0174 4

Composition by Scribe Design, Gillingham, Kent
Printed and bound in Great Britain by Bath Press Ltd, Avon

Preface

In recent times, the role of the anaesthetist has become increasingly diversified and now encompasses areas such as pain therapy and intensive care medicine as well as general anaesthetic practice. In consequence, the examination candidate for the Fellowship of the Royal College of Anaesthetists is required to have an extensive breadth of knowledge of these diverse specialities. As a result, there has been a great increase in the number of general and specialized anaesthetic texts. Inevitably it has become increasingly difficult to obtain the relevant facts in a concise form. The aim of this book is to provide, in a single volume, a source of readily-available information concerning aspects of physiology, pharmacology, anatomy, physics, statistics, history, clinical anaesthesia, equipment, intensive care, medicine and surgery. Unavoidably, there will be readers who will disagree with our selection of entries; however, considering the constraints of space, we have attempted to include those topics that the examination candidate is required to know or might find interesting.

Although the book is primarily aimed at the Part 3 Fellowship examination candidate, we hope that it will also be of use to candidates revising for the first two parts of the examination. Furthermore, we hope that those teaching examination candidates will find the book a useful source of information.

SMY
NPH
GBS

Acknowledgements

We are grateful to the publishers, editors and authors concerned for permission to reproduce or modify the following Figures and Tables:

Figure 2b: from Bowman WC (1990) *Pharmacology of Neuromuscular Function*, 2nd edn, Wright, Bristol
Figures 73, 74 and 86: from Soni N (1989) *Anaesthesia and Intensive Care*, Heinemann, Oxford.
Figure 77: from Samsoon GLT and Young JRB (1987) Difficult tracheal intubation: a retrospective study. *Anaesthesia*, **42**, 482–6
Figure 80: from Parbrook GD, Davis PD and Parbrook EO (1990) *Basic Physics and Measurement in Anaesthesia*, 3rd edn, Butterworth-Heinemann, Oxford
Figure 116: from Ross Russell RW and Wiles CM (1985) *Neurology*, Heinemann, Oxford
Figure 130: from Lentner C (ed.) (1981) *Geigy Scientific Tables*, 8th edn, vol. 1, Ciba-Geigy, Basle
Figure 138: from Howell RS (1980) Piped medical gas and vacuum systems. *Anaesthesia*, **35**, 676–98
Table 6: from Knaus WA, Draper EA, Wagner DP and Zimmerman JE (1985) APACHE II: a severity of disease classification system for acutely ill patients. *Crit Care Med*, **13**, 818–29

Explanatory notes

Arrangement of text. Entries are arranged alphabetically, with some related subjects grouped together to make coverage of one subject easier. For example, entries relating to tracheal intubation may be found under **I** as in **Intubation, awake**, **Intubation, blind nasal**, etc.

Cross-referencing. Bold type indicates a cross reference. An abbreviation highlighted in bold type refers to an entry in its fully-spelled form. For example, '...**ARDS** may occur....' refers to the entry **Adult respiratory distress syndrome**. Further instructions appear in italics.

References. Reference to a suitable article is provided at the foot of the entry where appropriate.

Proper Names. Where possible, a short biographical note is provided at the foot of the entry when a person is mentioned. Dates of birth and death are given, or the date of description if these dates are unknown. No dates are given for contemporary names. Where more than one eponymous entry occurs, e.g. **Haldane apparatus** and **Haldane effect**, details are given under the first entry.

The term 'anaesthetist' is used in the English sense, i.e. a medical practitioner who practises anaesthesia; the terms 'anesthesiologist' and 'anaesthesiologist' are not used.

Abbreviations

ACTH	adrenocorticotrophic hormone
ADP	adenosine diphosphate
AIDS	acquired immune deficiency syndrome
cAMP	cyclic adenosine monophosphate
APACHE	acute physiology and chronic health evaluation
ARDS	adult respiratory distress syndrome
ASA	American Society of Anesthesiologists
ASD	atrial septal defect
ATP	adenosine triphosphate
BP	blood pressure
CAT	computed axial tomography
$CMRO_2$	cerebral metabolic rate for oxygen
CNS	central nervous system
CO_2	carbon dioxide
COAD	chronic obstructive airways disease
CPAP	continuous positive airway pressure
CPR	cardiopulmonary resuscitation
CSF	cerebrospinal fluid
CVA	cerebrovascular accident
CVP	central venous pressure
CVS	cardiovascular system
CXR	chest X-ray
DIC	disseminated intravascular coagulation
DNA	deoxyribonucleic acid
2, 3-DPG	2, 3-diphosphoglycerate
DVT	deep vein thrombosis
ECF	extracellular fluid
ECG	electocardiography
EEG	electroencephalography
EMG	electromyography
ENT	ear, nose and throat
FEV_1	forced expiratory volume in 1 second
F_IO_2	fractional inspired concentration of oxygen
FRC	functional residual capacity
FVC	forced vital capacity
G	gauge
GABA	γ-aminobutyric acid
GFR	glomerular filtration rate
GIT	gastrointestinal tract
HCO_3^-	bicarbonate
HDU	high dependency unit
HIV	human immunodeficiency virus
5-HT	5-hydroxytryptamine

ICP	intracranial pressure
ICU	intensive care unit
IgA, IgG, etc.	immunoglobulin, A, G, etc.
im	intramuscular
IMV	intermittent mandatory ventilation
IPPV	intermittent positive pressure ventilation
iv	intravenous
IVRA	intravenous regional anaesthesia
JVP	jugular venous pressure
MAC	minimal alveolar concentration
MAP	mean arterial pressure
MH	malignant hyperthermia
MI	myocardial infarction
mw	molecular weight
NHS	National Health Service
N_2O	nitrous oxide
NSAID	non-steroidal anti-inflammatory drug
O_2	oxygen
PCO_2	partial pressure of carbon dioxide
PE	pulmonary embolus
PEEP	positive end-expiratory pressure
PO_2	partial pressure of oxygen
pr	per rectum
RNA	ribonucleic acid
RS	respiratory system
sc	subcutaneous
SVP	saturated vapour pressure
SVR	systemic vascular resistance
SVT	supraventricular tachycardia
TB	tuberculosis
TENS	transcutaneous electrical nerve stimulation
TIVA	total intravenous anaesthesia
TPN	total parenteral nutrition
TURP	transurethral resection of prostate
UK	United Kingdom
US(A)	United States (of America)
VF	ventricular fibrillation
$\dot{V}/\dot{Q}$	ventilation/perfusion
VSD	ventricular septal defect
VT	ventricular tachycardia

A

A–ado₂, *see Alveolar–arterial oxygen difference*

ABA, *see American Board of Anesthesiology*

Abbott, Gilbert, *see Morton, William*

Abdominal decompression. Technique in obstetric analgesia whereby negative pressure is applied to the abdomen in order to reduce labour pain and possibly shorten labour. Thought to act by making the uterus more spherical during contractions, thus contracting with less force. Now rarely used.
See also, Obstetric analgesia and anaesthesia

Abdominal field block. Technique using 100–200 ml **local anaesthetic agent**, involving infiltration of the skin, subcutaneous tissues, abdominal muscles and fascia. Provides analgesia of the abdominal wall and anterior peritoneum, but not of the viscera. Now rarely used. **Rectus sheath block, iliac crest block** and **inguinal field block** are more specific blocks.

ABO blood groups. Discovered in 1900 by Landsteiner in Vienna. Antigens may be present on red blood cells, with antibodies in the plasma (Table 1). The antibodies, mostly type-M **immunoglobulins**, develop within the first few months of life, presumably in response to naturally occurring antigens of similar structure to the blood antigens. Infusion of blood containing an ABO antigen into a patient who already has the corresponding antibody may lead to an adverse reaction; hence the description of group O individuals as universal donors, and of group AB individuals as universal recipients.
[Karl Landsteiner (1868–1943), Austrian-born US pathologist]
See also, Blood cross-matching; Blood groups; Blood transfusion

Table 1. Antigens and antibodies in ABO blood groups

Group	Incidence in UK (%)	Red cell antigen	Plasma antibody
A	42	A	Anti-B
B	8	B	Anti-A
AB	3	A and B	None
O	47	None	Anti-A and anti-B

Abuse of anaesthetic agents. May occur because of easy access to potent drugs by operating theatre staff. **Opioid analgesic drugs** are the most commonly abused

agents, but others include **benzodiazepines** and **inhalational anaesthetic agents**. Abuse may be suggested by behavioural or mood changes, or excessive and inappropriate requests for opioids. Main considerations include the safety of patients, counselling and psychiatric therapy for the abuser, and legal aspects of drug abuse. May be associated with **alcohol** abuse.
Farley WJ (1992) Can J Anaesth; 39: R11–3
See also, Sick doctor scheme

Accessory nerve block. Performed for spasm of trapezius and sternomastoid muscles (there is no sensory component to the nerve). 5–10 ml **local anaesthetic agent** is injected 2 cm below the mastoid process into the sternomastoid muscle, through which the nerve runs.

Accident, major. Practical hospital definition: any event involving casualties causing significant disruption of normal running of the hospital. Has also been defined according to the number of casualties. May refer to transport accidents, riots, terrorist activities, natural disasters, etc.
● Main problems:
 –large number of patients to be sorted (**triage**) for treatment and transfer, with their sudden arrival at hospital. Whether prehospital treatment is better than a 'scoop and run' policy is controversial. Adequate record-keeping is difficult, e.g. patient identification, assessment, treatment given, location, etc.
 –coordination of emergency services, with organization of staff and resources at the scene of the accident and receiving (designated) hospitals.
 –clearing of non-urgent cases from wards, ICU, operating theatre, etc.
 –communication between medical teams, hospitals, police, fire brigade, press and public.
 –sudden need for blood, blood products, and other support services, e.g. X-ray, etc.
 –dispersal of patients once initially treated; identification and holding of corpses.
● Major Accident plans of most hospitals are similar:
 –affected hospitals are informed, and main receiving hospitals designated. Use is made of nearby specialist centres, e.g. thoracic, neurosurgical, etc.
 –specific duties are assigned to each member of staff on duty, i.e. medical staff (including formation of a mobile team), nursing staff, telephone operators, porters, etc. Assignment of a team leader in each area is vital.
 –duties of anaesthetists include triage and treatment at the scene of the accident, resuscitation in the receiving area, anaesthesia for surgery, and organizing and managing admissions to ICU. Emergency boxes are

kept ready; contents include iv fluids, cannulae, self-inflating bag, tracheal intubation equipment, bandages, scissors and drugs. **Triservice apparatus** has been suggested as suitable for field anaesthesia, but most anaesthetists' experience of this is limited, and anaesthesia is rarely required before transfer to hospital.

Miles S (1990) BMJ; 301: 919–23
See also, Trauma

ACD, Acid–citrate–dextrose solution, *see Blood storage*

ACE, Angiotensin converting enzyme, *see Renin/angiotensin system*

ACE anaesthetic mixture. Mixture of alcohol, chloroform and diethyl ether, in a ratio of 1:2:3 parts, suggested in 1860 as an alternative to chloroform alone. Popular into the 1900s as a means of reducing total dose and side effects of any one of the three drugs.

ACE inhibitors, *see Angiotensin converting enzyme inhibitors*

Acetaminophen, *see Paracetamol*

Acetazolamide. Carbonic anhydrase inhibitor, which reduces **bicarbonate** formation and **hydrogen ion** excretion. Also a weak **diuretic**, but rarely used as such. Used to treat **glaucoma**, metabolic **alkalosis**, altitude sickness and childhood **epilepsy**.
• Dosage: 0.25–0.5 g orally/iv, once/twice daily.

Acetylcholine (ACh). **Neurotransmitter**, the acetyl ester of the base choline (Fig. 1). Synthesized from acetyl-coenzyme A and choline in **nerve** ending cytoplasm; the reaction is catalysed by choline acetyltransferase. Choline is actively transported into the nerve and acetyl-coenzyme A is formed in mitochondria. ACh is stored in vesicles.

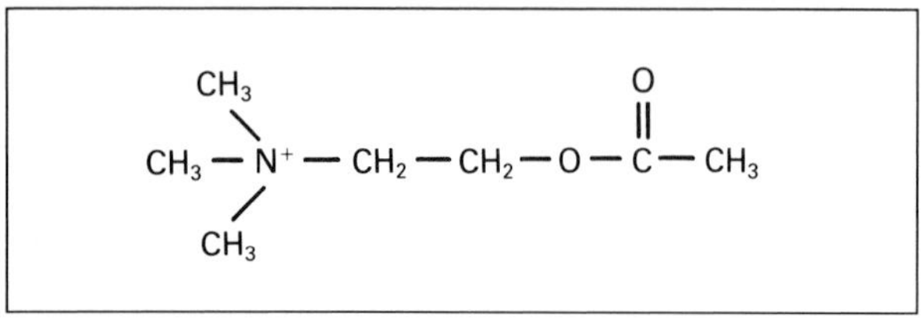

$$CH_3 - N^+ - CH_2 - CH_2 - O - \overset{\displaystyle O}{\overset{\displaystyle \|}{C}} - CH_3$$

with CH_3 groups above and below N^+

Figure 1 *Structure of acetylcholine*

• ACh is the transmitter at:
  –autonomic ganglia.
  –parasympathetic postganglionic nerve endings.
  –sympathetic postganglionic nerve endings at sweat glands and some muscle blood vessels.
  –the **neuromuscular junction**.
  –many parts of the CNS.
Has either muscarinic or nicotinic actions, depending on the **acetylcholine receptors** involved. ACh is hydrolysed to choline and acetate by **acetylcholinesterase** on the postsynaptic membrane. Other esterases also exist, e.g. plasma **cholinesterase**.

See also, Muscarine and muscarinic receptors; Neuromuscular transmission; Nicotine and nicotinic receptors; Parasympathetic nervous system; Sympathetic nervous system; Synaptic transmission

Acetylcholine receptors. Transmembrane proteins (mw 250 000) composed of protein subunits. Activation by **acetylcholine** (ACh) results in an **action potential**. ACh receptors may be muscarinic or nicotinic (Fig. 2a). Injected ACh first stimulates muscarinic receptors. As the dose is increased, nicotinic receptors are stimulated; i.e. parasympathetic stimulation and sweating precedes effects at ganglia and the **neuromuscular junction** (NMJ).

The structure of the postsynaptic (nicotinic) receptors at the NMJ has been identified largely through work on the electric eel, and it is thought that this corresponds to the structure of ACh receptors in general. Each receptor consists of five glycosylated protein subunits which project into the synaptic cleft. The subunits have been designated α (mw 40 000), β (mw 49 000), γ (mw 60 000) and δ (mw 67 000). The γ subunit is thought to be replaced by an ϵ subunit in mammals. The subunits span the postsynaptic **membrane** and form a cylinder around a central ion channel (Fig. 2b). The two α subunits of each receptor carry the binding sites for ACh. Occupation of these sites causes a configurational change of the subunits, thus

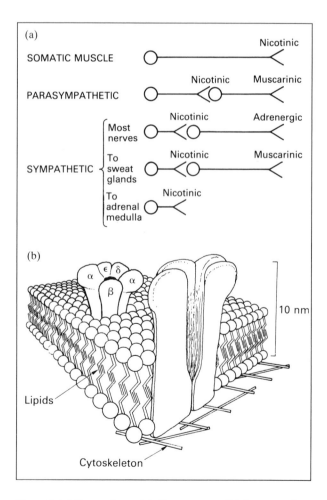

Figure 2 *(a) Types of acetylcholine receptors. (b) Structure of acetylcholine receptor*

opening the ion channel; cations (mainly sodium, potassium and calcium) flow through the channel according to their concentration gradients and thus generate an action potential. Non-depolarizing **neuromuscular blocking drugs** at normal doses reduce the number of receptors available to ACh. At higher doses they may also block the ion channel.

See also, Muscarine and muscarinic receptors; Neuromuscular transmission; Nicotine and nicotinic receptors; Parasympathetic nervous system; Sympathetic nervous system; Synaptic transmission

Acetylcholinesterase. **Enzyme** present in the postsynaptic membranes of cholinergic **synapses** and **neuromuscular junctions**. Also found in red blood cells and the placenta. Converts **acetylcholine** (ACh) into acetate and choline, thus terminating its action. The $N(CH_3)_3^+$ part of ACh binds to the anionic site of the enzyme, and the acetate end of ACh forms an intermediate bond at the esteratic site. Choline is liberated, and the intermediate substrate/enzyme complex is then hydrolysed to release acetate (Fig. 3).

See also, Acetylcholinesterase inhibitors; Neuromuscular transmission; Synaptic transmission

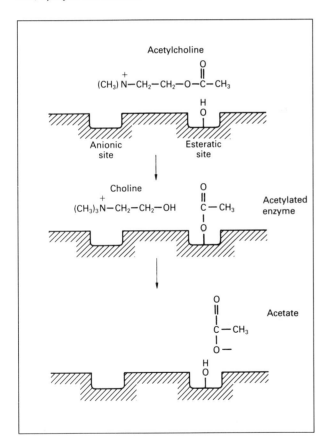

Figure 3 *Action of acetylcholinesterase*

Acetylcholinesterase inhibitors. Substances which increase **acetylcholine** (ACh) concentrations by inhibiting **acetylcholinesterase**. Used clinically for their action at the **neuromuscular junction** in **myasthenia gravis** and in the reversal of **non-depolarizing neuromuscular blockade**. Concurrent administration of an antimuscarinic agent, e.g. **atropine**, reduces unwanted effects of increased ACh concentrations at muscarinic receptors. Effects at ganglia are minimal at normal doses. Central effects may occur if the drug readily crosses the **blood–brain barrier**, e.g. **physostigmine** (used to treat the **central anticholinergic syndrome**).

Have also been used to treat tachyarrhythmias.

- Classification:
  - prosthetic: competitive inhibition at the anionic site of the enzyme prevents binding of ACh, e.g. **edrophonium, tetrahydroaminocrine**.
  - oxydiaphoretic: acts as a substrate for the enzyme; the reaction proceeds as far as the intermediate substrate/enzyme complex. Hydrolysis of the complex and thus reactivation of the enzyme is slow. Examples:
    - **neostigmine**, physostigmine (few hours)
    - **pyridostigmine** (several hours)
    - **distigmine** (up to a day).

  Organophosphorus compounds act as oxydiaphoretic inhibitors, but the substrate/enzyme complex is minimally hydrolysed; inhibition lasts for weeks until new enzyme is synthesized.

Acetylcholinesterase inhibitors augment **depolarizing neuromuscular blockade** and may cause depolarizing blockade in overdose. They may also cause bradycardia, hypotension, agitation, miosis, increased GIT activity, sweating and salivation.

See also, Neuromuscular transmission; Organophosphorus poisoning

Achalasia. Disorder of oesophageal motility caused by idiopathic degeneration of nerve cells in the myenteric plexus or vagal nuclei. Results in dysphagia and oesophageal dilatation. A similar condition may result from American trypanosomal infection (Chagas' disease). **Aspiration pneumonitis** or repeated chest infections may occur. Achalasia is treated by mechanical distension of the lower oesophagus or by surgery. Heller's myotomy (longitudinal myotomy leaving the mucosa intact) may be undertaken via abdominal or thoracic approaches. Preoperative respiratory assessment is essential. Patients are at high risk of aspirating oesophageal contents, and rapid sequence induction must be performed.

[Carlos Chagas (1879–1934), Brazilian physician; Ernst Heller (1877–1964), German surgeon]

See also, Aspiration of gastric contents; Induction, rapid sequence

Achondroplasia. Skeletal disorder, inherited as an autosomal dominant gene, although most cases arise by spontaneous mutation. Results in dwarfism, with normally sized trunk and shortened limbs. Flat face, bulging skull vault and spinal deformity may make tracheal intubation difficult, and the larynx may be smaller than normal. Obstructive **sleep apnoea** may occur. Foramen magnum and spinal canal stenoses may be present. The former may result in cord compression on neck extension; the latter may make central regional blockade difficult and reduce volume requirements for **extradural anaesthesia**.

Berkowitz ID, Raja SN, Bender KS, Kopits SE. (1990) Anesthesiology; 73: 739–59

Acid. Substance which yields **hydrogen ions** in solution.

Acidaemia. Lower than normal plasma **pH**.
See also, Acid–base balance; Acidosis

Acid–base balance. Maintenance of stable **pH** in body fluids is necessary for normal **enzyme** activity, ion distribution and protein structure. Normally, blood pH is maintained at 7.36–7.44 (36–44 nmol/l); intracellular pH changes with extracellular pH. During normal metabolism of neutral substances, organic acids are produced which generate **hydrogen ions** (H⁺).
● Maintenance of pH depends on:
   –**buffers** in tissues and blood, which minimize the increase of H⁺ concentration.
   –regulation by kidneys and lungs; the kidneys excrete about 60–80 mmol and the lungs about 15–20 000 mmol H⁺ per day.
Because of the relationship between CO_2, carbonic acid, **bicarbonate** (HCO_3^-) and H⁺, and the ability to excrete CO_2 rapidly from the lungs, respiratory function is important in acid-base balance:

$$H_2O + CO_2 \rightleftharpoons H_2CO_3 \rightleftharpoons HCO_3^- + H^+$$

Thus hyper- and hypoventilation cause **alkalosis** and **acidosis** respectively. Similarly, hyper- or hypoventilation may compensate for non-respiratory acidosis or alkalosis respectively, by returning pH towards normal.
   Sources of H⁺ excreted via the kidneys include sulphuric acid from metabolism of sulphur-containing proteins, and acetoacetic acid from fatty acid metabolism.
● The kidney can compensate for acid–base disturbances in three ways:
   –by regulating the amount of HCO_3^- reabsorbed. 80–90% of filtered HCO_3^- is reabsorbed in the proximal tubule:
     –filtered sodium ion is exchanged for H⁺ across the tubule cell membrane.
     –filtered HCO_3^- and excreted H⁺ form carbonic acid.
     –carbonic acid is converted to CO_2 and water by **carbonic anhydrase** on the cell membrane.
     –CO_2 and water reform carbonic acid (catalysed again by carbonic anhydrase) within the cell.
     –carbonic acid releases HCO_3^- and H⁺.
     –HCO_3^- passes into the blood; H⁺ is exchanged for sodium ion, etc.
   –by forming dihydrogen phosphate from monohydrogen phosphate in the distal tubule ($HPO_4^{2-} + H^+ \rightarrow H_2PO_4^-$). The H⁺ is supplied from carbonic acid, leaving HCO_3^- which passes into the blood.
   –by combination of ammonia, passing out of the cells, with H⁺, supplied as above. The resultant ammonium ions cannot pass back into the cells.
In acid–base disorders, the primary change determines whether a disturbance is respiratory or metabolic. The direction of change in H⁺ concentration determines acidosis or alkalosis. Renal or respiratory compensation attempts to restore normal pH, not reverse the primary change. For example, in the **Henderson–Hasselbalch equation**:

$$pH = pKa + \log \frac{[HCO_3^-],}{[CO_2]}$$

adjustment of the HCO_3^-/CO_2 concentration ratio restores pH towards its normal value, e.g.:

–primary change: increased CO_2: leads to decreased pH (respiratory acidosis).
–compensation: HCO_3^- retention by kidneys; increased ammonium secretion, etc.
Cohen RD (1991) Br J Anaesth; 67: 154–64
See also, Acid; Base; Blood gas tensions; Breathing, control of; Davenport diagram; Siggaard-Andersen nomogram

Acid–citrate–dextrose solution, *see Blood storage*

Acidosis. Condition in which **hydrogen ion** concentration is raised, or would be raised in the absence of compensatory mechanisms.
See also, Acid–base balance; Acidosis, metabolic; Acidosis, respiratory

Acidosis, metabolic. Acidosis due to metabolic causes, resulting in an inappropriately low **pH** for the measured arterial P_{CO_2}.
● Caused by:
   –increased **acid** production:
     –**ketone** bodies e.g. in **diabetes mellitus**.
     –**lactate** e.g. in **shock**, exercise.
   –acid ingestion: e.g. **salicylate poisoning**.
   –failure to excrete **hydrogen ion** (H⁺):
     –**renal failure**.
     –distal **renal tubular acidosis**.
     –**carbonic anhydrase inhibitors**.
   –loss of **bicarbonate**:
     –diarrhoea.
     –gastrointestinal fistulae.
     –proximal renal tubular acidosis.
     –ureteroenterostomy.
● Primary change: increased H⁺/decreased bicarbonate.
● Compensation:
   –**hyperventilation**.
   –increased renal H⁺ secretion.
● Effects:
   –hyperventilation (**Kussmaul breathing**).
   –confusion, weakness, coma.
   –cardiac depression.
   –**hyperkalaemia**.
● Treatment:
   –of underlying cause.
   –bicarbonate therapy is reserved for treatment of severe acidaemia (e.g. pH under 7.1) because of problems associated with its use.
   If bicarbonate is required, a formula for iv infusion is:

$$\frac{\text{base excess} \times \text{body weight (kg)}}{3} \text{ mmol}$$

   Half this amount is given initially.
   –other agents under investigation include sodium dichloroacetate, Carbicarb (sodium bicarbonate and carbonate in equimolar concentrations) and THAM (2-amino-2-hydroxymethyl-1,3–propanediol).
See also, Acid–base balance; Acidaemia; Anion gap

Acidosis, respiratory. Acidosis due to increased arterial P_{CO_2}. Caused by alveolar **hypoventilation**.
● Primary change: increased arterial P_{CO_2}.
● Compensation:
   –initial rise in plasma **bicarbonate** due to increased carbonic acid formation and dissociation.

–increased **acid** secretion/bicarbonate retention by the kidneys.

In acute **hypercapnia**, bicarbonate concentration increases by about 0.7 mmol/l per 1 kPa rise in arterial P_{CO_2}. In chronic hypercapnia it increases by 2.6 mmol/l per 1 kPa.

- Effects: those of hypercapnia.
- Treatment: of underlying cause.

See also, Acid–base balance; Acidaemia

Acquired immune deficiency syndrome (AIDS), *see Human immunodeficiency viral infection*

Acromegaly. Disease caused by excessive **growth hormone** secretion after puberty; usually caused by a pituitary adenoma but ectopic secretion may also occur.

- Features:
  - –enlarged jaw, tongue and larynx; widespread increase in soft tissue mass; enlarged feet and hands. Nerve entrapment may occur, e.g. carpal tunnel syndrome.
  - –respiratory obstruction, including **sleep apnoea**.
  - –tendency towards **diabetes mellitus**, **hypertension** and **cardiac failure** (may be due to **cardiomyopathy**). Thyroid and adrenal impairment may occur.

Apart from the above diseases, acromegaly may present difficulties with tracheal intubation and maintenance of the airway.

- Treatment:
  - –bromocriptine (dopamine agonist, reducing growth hormone release).
  - –radioactive yttrium-90 implantation.
  - –pituitary surgery, with hormone treatment as required.

Chan VWS, Tindall S (1988) Br J Anaesth; 60: 464–8

ACT, Activated clotting time, *see Coagulation studies*

ACTH, *see Adrenocorticotrophic hormone*

Actin. One of the protein components of **muscle** (mw 43 000). Present in all cells as microfilaments.

See also, Muscle contraction

Action potential. Sequential changes in transmembrane potential that result in the propagation of electrical impulses in excitable cells (Fig. 4a).

- Stages involved are summarized as follows:
  - –A: depolarization of the membrane by 15 mV (threshold level).
  - –B: rapid depolarization to +40 mV.
  - –C: repolarization, rapid at first then slow.
  - –D: hyperpolarization.
  - –E: return to the resting **membrane potential**.

Depolarization causes opening of sodium channels and entry of sodium ions into the cell, which causes further depolarization. Sodium permeability then falls. Potassium permeability increases slowly and helps bring about repolarization. Normal ion distribution is restored due to action of the **sodium/potassium pump**. The action potential is followed by a **refractory period**.

Action potentials in **nerve** and other cells involve similar changes; in cardiac muscle, however, a plateau follows depolarization, brought about by calcium entry. The refractory period is thus lengthened (Fig. 4b).

- There are five phases of the cardiac action potential:

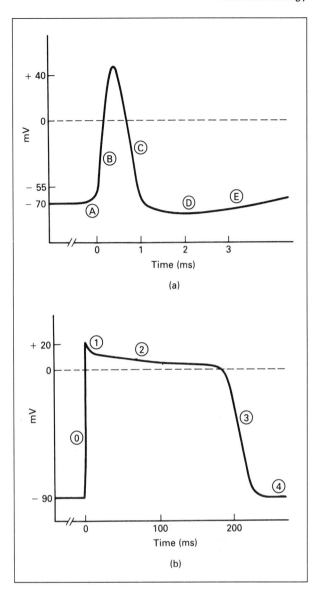

Figure 4 *(a) Action potential. (b) Cardiac action potential (see text)*

  - –phase 0: fast depolarization and sodium entry.
  - –phase 1: onset of repolarization.
  - –phase 2: plateau due to calcium entry.
  - –phase 3: repolarization.
  - –phase 4: resting membrane potential. In **pacemaker cells**, there is slow spontaneous depolarization, due to decreased potassium permeability, leading to initiation of impulses.

See also, Nerve conduction

Activated clotting time, *see Coagulation studies*

Activation energy. Energy required to initiate a chemical reaction. For ignition of explosive mixtures of anaesthetic agents the energy may be provided by sparks, e.g. from build up of static electricity or electrical equipment. Combustion of **cyclopropane** requires less activation energy than that of **diethyl ether**. Activation energy is less

for mixtures with O_2 than with air, and least for **stoichiometric mixtures** of reactants.
See also, Explosions and fires

Active transport. Energy-requiring transport of particles across cell **membranes**. Protein 'pumps' within the membranes utilize energy which is usually supplied by **ATP** metabolism, in order to move ions and molecules, often against concentration gradients. A typical example is the **sodium/potassium pump**.

Acupuncture. Use of fine **needles** (usually 30–33 G) to produce healing and pain relief. Originated in China thousands of years ago, and closely linked with the philosophy and practice of traditional Chinese medicine. Thus abnormalities in the flow of Qi (Chi: the life energy that circulates around the body along meridians, nourishing the internal organs) results in imbalance between Yin and Yang, the two polar opposites present in all aspects of the universe. Internal abnormalities may be diagnosed by pulse diagnosis (palpation of the radial arteries at different positions and depths). The appropriate organ is then treated by acupuncture at specific points on the skin, often along the meridian named after, and related to, that organ. Yin and Yang, and flow of Qi, are thus restored.

Modern Western acupuncture involves needle insertion at sites chosen for more 'scientific' reasons; e.g. around an affected area, at **trigger points** found nearby, or more proximally but within the appropriate **dermatome**. These may be combined with distant or local traditional points, although conclusive evidence for the existence of acupuncture points and meridians has never been shown. The needles may be left inserted and stimulated manually, electrically or thermally to increase intensity of stimulation. Pressure at acupuncture points (acupressure) may produce similar but less intense stimulation.
● Possible mechanisms:
 –local reflex pathways at spinal level.
 –closure of the 'gate' in the **gate control theory of pain**.
 –central release of **endorphins/enkephalins**, and possibly involvement of other **neurotransmitters**.
 –modulation of the 'memory' of pain.
Still used widely in China. Increasingly used in the West for chronic pain, musculoskeletal disorders, headache and migraine, and other disorders in which modern Western medicine has had little success, e.g. myalgic encephalomyelitis. Claims that acupuncture may be employed alone to provide analgesia for surgery are now viewed with scepticism, although it has been used to provide analgesia and reduce postoperative **vomiting**.
Filshie J, Morrison PJ (1988) Palliative Medicine; 2: 1–14

Acute physiology and chronic health evaluation, *see APACHE scoring system*

Acyclovir, *see Antiviral drugs*

Addiction, *see Drug addiction*

Addison's disease, *see Adrenocortical insufficiency*

Adenosine. Nucleoside, of importance in energy homeostasis at the cellular level. Reduces O_2 consumption, increases coronary blood flow, causes vasodilatation and slows atrioventricular conduction (possibly via increased potassium **conductance** and reduced calcium conductance). Possibly a CNS **neurotransmitter**.

Recently made available for treatment of **SVT** and diagnosis of other tachyarrhythmias by slowing atrioventricular conduction. Its short **half-life** (less than 20 s) and lack of negative inotropism make it an attractive alternative to **verapamil**.

Has also been used as a directly-acting **vasodilator drug** in **hypotensive anaesthesia.** Increases cardiac output, with stable heart rate. Its effects are rapidly reversible on stopping the infusion.
● Dosage:
 –SVT: 3 mg by rapid iv injection; if unsuccessful after 1–2 minutes this is followed by 6 mg and then 12 mg.
 –hypotensive anaesthesia: 50–300 µg/kg/min. **ATP** has also been used.
● Side effects are usually mild and include flushing, dyspnoea and nausea. Bronchoconstriction may occur in asthmatics. Bradycardia is resistant to atropine. Adenosine's action is prolonged in **dipyridamole** therapy and reduced by **theophyllines**.
Camm AJ, Garratt CJ (1991) New Engl J Med; 325: 1621–9

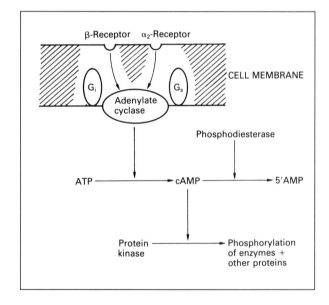

Figure 5 *cAMP involvement in transmembrane signalling. G_s stimulatory guanine nucleotide regulatory protein; G_i inhibitory guanine nucleotide regulatory protein*

Adenosine monophosphate, cyclic (cAMP). Cyclic adenosine 3', 5'-monophosphate, formed from **ATP** by the enzyme adenylate cyclase. Activation of surface receptors may cause a guanine nucleotide regulatory protein to interact with adenylate cyclase with resultant increases in intracellular cAMP levels (Fig. 5). Many substances act on surface receptors in this way, including **catecholamines** (β effects), **vasopressin**, **ACTH**, **histamine**, **glucagon**, parathyroid hormone and calcitonin.

Some substances inhibit adenylate cyclase via an inhibitory regulatory protein, e.g. **noradrenaline** at α_2-adrenergic receptors.

cAMP causes phosphorylation of proteins, particularly enzymes, by activating protein kinases. Phosphorylation changes enzyme activity and therefore cell metabolism; thus the intracellular concentration of cAMP determines cell activity, and cAMP acts as a 'second messenger'.

cAMP is inactivated by phosphodiesterase to 5'-AMP. **Phosphodiesterase inhibitors**, e.g. **aminophylline** and **enoximone**, increase cAMP levels.

Adenosine triphosphate and diphosphate (ATP and ADP). ATP is the most important high-energy phosphate compound. When hydrolysed to form ADP, it releases large amounts of **energy** which may be utilized in many cellular processes, e.g. **active transport**, **muscle contraction**, etc. Its phosphate bonds are formed using energy from catabolism; aerobic **glycolysis** generates 38 moles ATP per mole of glucose, and anaerobic glycolysis yields 2 moles ATP.

Other high-energy phosphate compounds include phosphorylcreatine (in muscle), ADP itself, and other nucleotides.
See also, Cytochrome oxidase system; Metabolism; Tricarboxylic acid cycle

Adenylate cyclase, *see Adenosine monophosphate, cyclic*

ADH, Antidiuretic hormone, *see Vasopressin*

Adiabatic change. Volume change of a gas in which there is no transfer of heat to or from the system. Sudden compression of a gas without removal of resultant heat causes a rise in temperature. This may occur in the gas already present in the valves and pipes of an **anaesthetic machine** when a cylinder is turned on (hence the danger of explosion if oil or grease are present). Sudden adiabatic expansion of a gas results in cooling, as in the **cryoprobe**.
See also, Isothermal change

Adjustable pressure-limiting valve. Valve which opens to allow passage of expired and surplus fresh gas from a breathing system, but closes to prevent indrawing of air. Ideally the opening pressure should be as low as possible to reduce resistance to expiration, but not so low as to allow the reservoir bag to empty through it. Most contain a thin disc held against its seating by a spring, as in the Heidbrink valve. Adjusting the tension in the spring, usually by screwing the valve top, alters the pressure at which the valve opens. The valve must be vertical in order to function correctly.

Modern valves, even when screwed fully down, will open at high pressures (60 cmH$_2$O). Most are now encased in a hood for **scavenging** of waste gases.
[Jay A Heidbrink (1875–1957), US anaesthetist]
See also, Anaesthetic breathing systems; Non-rebreathing valves

ADP, *see Adenosine triphosphate and diphosphate*

Adrenal gland. Situated on the upper pole of the **kidney**, each gland is composed of an outer cortex and an inner medulla. The cortex consists of the outer zona glomerulosa (secreting **aldosterone**), the middle zona fasciculata (secreting **glucocorticoids**) and inner zona reticularis (secreting sex hormones). Hypersecretion may result in **hyperaldosteronism**, **Cushing's syndrome** and viriliza-

tion/feminization, respectively. Hyposecretion causes **adrenocortical insufficiency**.

The adrenal medulla is thought to be derived from a sympathetic ganglion in which the postganglionic neurones have lost their axons, and secrete **catecholamines** into the bloodstream. Hypersecretion results in **phaeochromocytoma**.
See also, Sympathetic nervous system

Adrenaline. Catecholamine, acting as a hormone and **neurotransmitter** in the **sympathetic nervous system** and brainstem pathways. Synthesized and released from the **adrenal gland** medulla and central adrenergic neurones (*for structure, synthesis and metabolism, see Catecholamines*).

Stimulates both α- and β-**adrenergic receptors**; displays predominantly β-effects at low doses, α- at higher doses. Low dose infusion may lower BP by causing vasodilatation in muscle via β$_2$-receptors, despite increased cardiac output via β$_1$-receptors. Higher doses cause α-mediated vasoconstriction and increasd systolic BP, although diastolic pressure may still decrease.
● Clinical uses:
　–with **local anaesthetic agents**, as a vasoconstrictor.
　–in **anaphylactic reaction, cardiac arrest, bronchospasm**.
　–as an **inotropic drug**.
　–in **glaucoma** (reduces aqueous humour production).
Adrenaline may cause cardiac **arrhythmias**, especially in the presence of hypercapnia, hypoxia and certain drugs, e.g **halothane, cyclopropane** and **cocaine**. During halothane anaesthesia, suggested maximal dosage of adrenaline is 10 ml 1:100 000 solution (100 μg) in 10 minutes, or 30 ml (300 μg) in 1 hour. More dilute solutions should be used if possible. Adrenaline should not be used for ring blocks of digits or for penile nerve blocks, because of possible ischaemia to distal tissues.
● Dosage:
　–anaphylaxis: 0.1 mg iv (1 ml 1:10 000 solution), repeated as required. May be given im: 0.5–1.0 mg (0.5–1.0 ml 1:1000 solution).
　–cardiac arrest: 1 mg iv.
　–by infusion: 0.01– 0.15 μg/kg/min initially.
Subcutaneous injection in shocked patients results in unreliable absorption. Adrenaline may be administered via a tracheal tube in twice the iv dose.
See also, Tracheal administration of drugs

α-Adrenergic receptor agonists. Naturally-occurring **agonists** include **adrenaline** and **noradrenaline** which stimulate both α$_1$- and α$_2$-**adrenergic receptors**.

Methoxamine and **phenylephrine** are synthetic α$_1$–receptor agonists, used to cause vasoconstriction, e.g. to correct hypotension in **spinal anaesthesia**.
Clonidine acts on central α$_2$-receptors. Clonidine and other α$_2$-receptor agonists (e.g. **dexmedetomidine**) have been shown to reduce pain sensation and reduce requirements for general anaesthetics.
Prys-Roberts C (1991) Curr Opin Anaesth; 4: 111–21

β-Adrenergic receptor agonists. Agonists include **adrenaline** and **isoprenaline** which stimulate both β$_1$- and β$_2$-**adrenergic receptors**. **Dopamine** and **dobutamine** act mainly at β$_1$ receptors.
Salbutamol and **terbutaline** predominantly affect β$_2$-

receptors, and are used clinically to cause bronchodilatation in **asthma**, and as **tocolytic drugs** in premature labour. Some β_1–receptor effects are seen at high doses, e.g. tachycardia. They have been used in the treatment of **cardiac failure** and **cardiogenic shock**; stimulation of vascular β_2-receptors causes vasodilatation and reduced afterload.
Prys-Roberts C (1991) Curr Opin Anaesth; 4: 111–21

α-Adrenergic receptor antagonists (α-Blockers).
Usually refer to **antagonists** which act exclusively at α-**adrenergic receptors**.

• Drugs may be:
  –selective:
    –α_1-receptors: e.g. **prazosin, phenoxybenzamine, indoramin.**
    –α_2-receptors: **yohimbine.**
  –non-selective, e.g. **phentolamine.**
Labetalol is an antagonist at both α- and β-receptors. Other drugs may also act at α-receptors as part of a range of effects, e.g. **chlorpromazine, droperidol.**

Antagonism may be competitive, e.g. phentolamine, or non-competitive and therefore longer-lasting, e.g. phenoxybenzamine.

Used to lower BP and reduce **afterload** by causing vasodilatation. Compensatory tachycardia may occur.

• Side effects: postural hypotension, dizziness, tachycardia (less so with the selective α_1-antagonists, possibly because the negative feedback of noradrenaline at α_2-receptors is unaffected). **Tachyphylaxis** may occur.
Foex P (1984) Br J Anaesth; 56: 751–65

β-Adrenergic receptor antagonists (β-Blockers).
Competitive **antagonists** at β-**adrenergic receptors**.

• Actions:
  –reduce heart rate, force of contraction and myocardial O_2 consumption.
  –increase **coronary blood flow** by increasing diastolic filling time.
  –antiarrhythmic action results from β-receptor antagonism and possibly a membrane-stabilizing effect at high doses.
  –antihypertensive action (not fully understood but may involve reductions in cardiac output, central sympathetic activity, and renin levels).
  –some have partial agonist activity (**intrinsic sympathomimetic activity**), e.g. pindolol, acebutolol and oxprenolol.
  –practolol, atenolol and metoprolol are relatively cardioselective, but all will block β_2-receptors at high doses. Celiprolol has β_1-receptor antagonist and β_2-receptor agonist properties, thus causing peripheral vasodilatation in addition to cardiac effects.
  –labetalol has α- and β-receptor blocking properties.

• **Half-lives:**
  –**esmolol**, a new agent: a few minutes. Hydrolysed by esterases, e.g. in red blood cells.
  –metoprolol, oxprenolol, pindolol, **propranolol**, timolol: 2–4 hours.
  –atenolol, practolol, sotalol: 6–12 hours.
  –nadolol: 24 hours.
Most are readily absorbed by mouth, and undergo extensive **first-pass metabolism**. Practolol and sotolol are water soluble and largely excreted unchanged in the urine; propranolol and metoprolol are lipid soluble and almost completely metabolized in the liver.

Table 2. Dosage of β-adrenergic receptor antagonists

Drug	Oral	Intravenous
Atenolol	50–100 mg once/twice daily	2–10 mg
Esmolol	Not available	50–200 µg/kg/min
Labetalol	50–200 mg twice daily	Up to 200 mg; 5–10 mg increments are usually used peroperatively
Metoprolol	50–100 mg 2–3 times daily	1–10 mg
Propranolol	10–160 mg 2–4 times daily	1 mg increments up to 10 mg
Sotalol	80–120 mg once/twice daily	20–60 mg

• Uses:
  –**hypertension, ischaemic heart disease, MI, arrhythmias, hyperthyroidism,** anxiety, migraine prophylaxis.
  –during anaesthesia: to reduce the hypertensive response to laryngoscopy; to treat perioperative hypertension, tachycardias and **myocardial ischaemia**; in **hypotensive anaesthesia**.
Dosage of those available for iv use is shown in Table 2.

• Side effects:
  –**cardiac failure**, especially in combination with other negative inotropes.
  –**bronchospasm** and peripheral arterial insufficiency, via blockade of β_2-receptors.
  –reduced cardiovascular (β_1) and metabolic (β_2) response to **hypoglycaemia** in diabetics.
  –sleep disturbances: less likely with water-soluble drugs, e.g. atenolol, nadolol, sotalol.
  –oral practolol was withdrawn because of the oculomucocutaneous syndrome following its use. The iv preparation has been withdrawn for commercial reasons.
Foex P (1984) Br J Anaesth; 56: 751–65

Adrenergic receptors. Membrane proteins, activated by **adrenaline** and other **catecholamines**, and divided into α- and β-receptors. Further subdivided into β_1/β_2 and α_1/α_2-receptors (Table 3).

Their effects are mediated by '**second messengers**': α_1-receptor effects by increases in intracellular **calcium** ion concentration, α_2-receptor effects by reducing intracellular **cAMP**, and β_1- and β_2-receptor effects by increasing cAMP. There is evidence for mixed receptor populations at both pre- and postsynaptic membranes.
Prys-Roberts C (1991) Curr Opin Anaesth; 4: 111–21
See also, α-Adrenergic receptor agonists; β-Adrenergic receptor agonists; α-Adrenergic receptor antagonists; β-Adrenergic receptor antagonists; Sympathetic nervous system

Adrenocortical insufficiency. May be due to:
  –primary adrenal failure (Addison's disease) due to:
    –**autoimmune disease** (most common cause). May be associated with other autoimmune disease, e.g. diabetes, thyroid disease, pernicious anaemia, vitiligo.
    –TB, amyloidosis, metastatic infiltration, haemorrhage or infarction, e.g. in **shock**.

Table 3. Classification and actions of adrenergic receptors

Receptor type	Site	Effect of stimulation
α₁	Vascular smooth muscle	Contraction
	Bladder smooth muscle (sphincter)	Contraction
	Radial muscle of iris	Contraction
	Intestinal smooth muscle	Relaxation, but contraction of sphincters
	Uterus	Variable
	Salivary glands	Viscous secretion
	Liver	Glycogenolysis
	Pancreas	Decreased secretion of enzymes, insulin and glucagon
α₂	Presynaptic membranes of adrenergic synapses	Reduced release of noradrenaline
	Postsynaptic membranes	Smooth muscle contraction
	Platelets	Aggregation
β₁	Heart	Increased rate and force of contraction
	Adipose tissue	Breakdown of stored triglycerides to fatty acids
	Juxtaglomerular apparatus	Increased renin secretion
β₂	Vascular smooth muscle (muscle beds)	Relaxation
	Bronchial smooth muscle	Relaxation
	Intestinal smooth muscle	Relaxation
	Bladder sphincter	Relaxation
	Uterus	Variable; relaxes the pregnant uterus
	Salivary glands	Watery secretion
	Liver	Glycogenolysis
	Pancreas	Increased insulin and glucagon secretion

and aldosterone) or secondary (requiring cortisol only) disease.
[Thomas Addison (1793–1860), English physician]
Weatherill D, Spence AA (1984) Br J Anaesth; 56: 741–9

Adrenocorticotrophic hormone (Corticotrophin; ACTH). Polypeptide hormone (39 amino acids; mw 4500) secreted by the anterior **pituitary gland** in response to corticotrophin releasing factor secreted by the **hypothalamus**. Release of ACTH is increased by emotional and physical stress, including surgery. It increases steroid synthesis in the **adrenal glands**, particularly **glucocorticoids** but also **aldosterone**. ACTH production is inhibited by glucocorticoids (i.e. negative feedback). ACTH has been used in place of **steroid therapy** in an attempt to reduce adrenocortical suppression, and is used for diagnostic tests in endocrinology.
See also, Stress response to surgery

Adult respiratory distress syndrome (ARDS). First described in 1967 as non-cardiogenic **pulmonary oedema** secondary to conditions not necessarily affecting the lungs. Histological appearances are similar to respiratory distress syndrome of the newborn, hence its name. Overall mortality remains at 50–60%, but depends on the underlying cause; it is highest following **aspiration pneumonitis** or **septicaemia**. Residual pulmonary impairment is possible but rarely severe. May follow any major illness, sepsis, surgery or other physical injury. Results from increased pulmonary vascular permeability and lung water, but the mechanism is unclear. Pulmonary infiltration by neutrophils leads to interstitial fibrosis, possibly as a result of damage caused by **free radicals**. **Platelets**, eosinophils, **leukotrienes**, neutrophil enzymes and **complement** activation have also been implicated. The role of O_2 in tissue damage is uncertain.
- Features:
  - reduced respiratory **compliance** and increased work of breathing.
  - $\dot{V}/\dot{Q}$ mismatch and increased **shunt** result in **hypoxaemia** despite increased F_1O_2. Arterial PO_2 below 8 kPa (60 mmHg) with F_1O_2 0.6 has been suggested as one diagnostic criterion.
  - **pulmonary vascular resistance** may be raised.
  - bilateral patchy 'cotton wool' infiltrates, typically peripherally, on chest X-ray. An air bronchogram may be seen.
  - in uncomplicated ARDS, **pulmonary capillary wedge pressure** and plasma **oncotic pressure** are normal.
  - multiorgan failure may occur and is a common cause of death.
- Management is largely supportive:
  - general treatment: **nutrition**, **DVT** prophylaxis, prevention of infection, etc.
  - **O_2 therapy**, trying to keep F_1O_2 below 0.6. **CPAP** is often helpful. **IPPV** may be required. **PEEP** is often required, but airway pressures are often already high because of reduced compliance, increasing risk of **barotrauma** and impaired cardiac output. CO_2 elimination may require increasing minute volumes; allowing the CO_2 to rise by keeping minute volume and thus airway pressures low (permissive hypercapnia) may reduce the incidence of barotrauma. **Inverse ratio ventilation**, **airway pressure release ventilation** and **high frequency ventilation** have been used, but

- secondary adrenal failure due to:
  - **steroid therapy** withdrawal.
  - **ACTH** deficiency, e.g. due to surgery, head injury, tumours, infarction.
- Features:
  - chronic: weight loss, vomiting, diarrhoea, malaise, postural hypotension, increased risk of infection. Dark pigmentation in scars and skin creases occur in primary disease. Acute insufficiency (crises) may develop following stress, e.g. infection, surgery, or any critical illness.
  - acute: hypotension and electrolyte abnormalities (**hyponatraemia**, **hyperkalaemia**, hypochloraemia, **hypercalcaemia** and **hypoglycaemia**).
Diagnosed by measurement of plasma cortisol and ACTH levels, including demonstration of an impaired cortisol response following tetracosactrin (synthetic ACTH terminal portion).
- Treatment:
  - **CPR**, (iv fluids, O_2, etc.).
  - steroid therapy, e.g. iv hydrocortisone 100 mg 6-hourly initially. Replacement therapy is required, depending on whether primary (requiring cortisol

their role is still uncertain. **Extracorporeal membrane oxygenation** and **extracorporeal CO$_2$ removal** have been used with varying success.

–fluid restriction is usually instituted to reduce lung water. **Diuretics** have been used, with careful monitoring of renal function.

–**vasodilator drugs** have been used to decrease pulmonary vascular resistance, e.g. **prostacyclin**.

–fears over leakage of **colloids** into pulmonary interstitial spaces, with subsequent exacerbation of oedema, are balanced by possible advantages of colloids in maintaining oncotic pressure.

–**steroid therapy** is controversial; no benefit has yet been shown.

–free radical scavengers, antiprostaglandins and antiproteinases have been investigated.

Weiner-Kronish JP, Gropper MA, Matthay MA (1990) Br J Anaesth; 65: 107–29

Adverse drug reactions. Undesired drug effects, usually divided into:

–predictable, dose related side effects, e.g. hypotension following **thiopentone**.

–unpredictable, usually less common reactions. These are unrelated to known pharmacological properties of a drug (i.e. not due to common side effects or overdose), usually involving the immune system in some way (but not always, e.g. **MH**).

Suspected adverse reactions are voluntarily reported to the **Committee on Safety of Medicines** on yellow cards, introduced in 1964. Specific yellow cards for reporting anaesthetic drug reactions were introduced in 1988, to encourage reporting of serious reactions to established drugs and any reaction to new drugs. Anaesthetists give many different drugs iv to large numbers of patients, and therefore reactions are often seen. Reactions may be more likely if drugs are given quickly and in combination.

● Mechanisms:

–on first exposure:

–direct **histamine** release, e.g. **tubocurarine**, **atracurium**, thiopentone, **Althesin**.

–alternative pathway **complement** activation, e.g. Althesin.

–apparently on first exposure: prior sensitization by other e.g. environmental antigens may cause crossover sensitivity to subsequently administered drugs; e.g. reactions to **dextrans** may involve prior exposure to bacterial antigens.

–requiring prior exposure:

–**anaphylactic reaction**, e.g. to thiopentone.

–classical pathway complement activation, e.g. Althesin. Other drugs dissolved in **Cremophor EL** may crossreact.

Features range from mild skin rash to anaphylaxis. First exposure reactions tend to be milder and more frequent than those requiring prior exposure.

● Incidence of reactions to iv agents:

–thiopentone   1:14 000–1:35 000
–methohexitone   1:7000–1:23 000
–propranidid   1:200–1:1700
–Althesin   1:400–1:2000

● Management: as for anaphylaxis. Sequential blood samples (for histamine, complement and immunoglobulin levels, and differential white cell count) should be taken at 0, 6, 12 and 24 hours if a drug reaction is

suspected. The role of skin testing, antibody screening and in vitro tests, e.g. basophil studies, is controversial, partly because of cross-sensitivity between agents.

Moudgil GC (1986) Can Anaesth Soc J; 33: 400–14

AF, *see Atrial fibrillation*

Affinity. Extent to which a drug binds to a receptor. A drug with high affinity binds more strongly than one with lower affinity, whatever its **intrinsic activity**.

Afterload. Ventricular wall tension required to eject **stroke volume** during systole.

● For the left ventricle, afterload is increased by:

–an anatomical obstruction, e.g. **aortic stenosis**.
–raised **SVR** .
–decreased elasticity of the aorta and large blood vessels.
–increased ventricular volume (greater tension is needed to produce the necessary pressure [**Laplace's law**]).

Increased afterload results in increased myocardial work and O$_2$ consumption, and decreased stroke volume. Reduction of afterload may be achieved with **vasodilator drugs**.

See also, Preload

Agonist. Substance which binds to a receptor to cause a response within the cell. It has high **affinity** for the receptor and high **intrinsic activity**.

A partial agonist binds to the receptor, but causes less response; it may have high affinity, but it has less intrinsic activity. It may therefore act as a competitive **antagonist** in the presence of a pure agonist.

An agonist–antagonist causes agonism at certain receptors and antagonism at others.

See also, Dose-response curves; Receptor theory

AGSS, Anaesthetic gas scavenging system, *see Scavenging*

AIDS, Acquired immunodeficiency syndrome, *see Human immunodeficiency viral infection*

Air. Dry natural air contains by volume:

Nitrogen	78.03%	Hydrogen	0.001%
O$_2$	20.99%	**Helium**	0.0005%
Argon	0.93%	Krypton	0.0001%
CO$_2$	0.03%	**Xenon**	0.000008%
Neon	0.0015%		

'Medical' air may be supplied by a compressor or in **cylinders**. The latter (containing air at 137 bar) are grey with black and white shoulders. Piped air is normally at 4 bar.

Air embolism. Introduction of air bubbles into the circulation, usually into veins. May occur when venous pressure is lower than atmospheric pressure. It may occur during any surgery when an open vein is raised above the heart; it is particularly likely in **neurosurgery** with the patient in the sitting position since the dural sinuses do not collapse. May also occur during **central venous cannulation** (minimized by tilting the patient head-down). Procedures involving insufflation or injection of gas, e.g. **laparoscopy** or **extradural anaesthesia** using loss of resistance to air, may also lead to embolism. **N$_2$O** diffuses into bubbles, increasing their volume and exacerbating their effects.

Air in the heart is compressed with each beat and not expelled, causing interruption of blood flow. Pulmonary vessels may become obstructed. Small bubbles may have little effect. Paradoxical air emboli pass to the systemic circulation via the pulmonary vascular bed or cardiac septal defects (a probe-patent foramen ovale exists in 20–30% of patients at autopsy). The bubbles may obstruct the coronary or cerebral vessels.

- Clinical features:
  - reduced cardiac output.
  - tachycardia.
  - cyanosis.
  - bronchospasm and pulmonary oedema may occur.
  - tinkling sounds on auscultation, e.g. with an oesophageal/praecordial stethoscope; large amounts of air may cause a 'mill-wheel' murmur. Embolism may be detected by a praecordial probe utilizing the **Doppler effect**.
  - sudden reduction of end-tidal CO_2 due to increased **dead space** and decreased cardiac output.
  - raised pulmonary artery pressure.
  - signs of right-sided strain on the ECG; ventricular ectopics or fibrillation may occur.
- Treatment:
  - to prevent further embolism:
    - seal veins.
    - flood the wound with fluid.
    - increase venous pressure:
      - head-down tilt.
      - iv fluids.
      - jugular venous compression may be applied in the sitting position. **PEEP** and the **antigravity suit** have been advocated for prevention of air embolism in neurosurgery.
  - stop N_2O.
  - remove air from the right atrium or ventricle via a central line.
  - the head down, left lateral position is said to increase the likelihood of air remaining in the right atrium.
  - hyperbaric O_2 has been used.

Airway. The upper airway is comprised of mouth, **nose**, **pharynx** and **larynx**. Maintenance of the airway in the unconscious or anaesthetized patient is achieved by combined flexion of the neck and extension at the atlanto-occipital joint (the 'sniffing position'), and lifting the angles of the mandible forward. The **tongue** is lifted forward by the genioglossus muscle which is attached to the back of the point of the jaw; the hyoid bone and larynx are pulled forward by the hyoglossus, mylohyoid, geniohyoid and digastric muscles. Upward pressure on the soft tissues of the floor of the mouth may cause obstruction, particularly in children, and should be avoided. In the lateral (**recovery**) position, the tongue and jaw fall forward under gravity, improving the airway. **Airway obstruction** during anaesthesia has traditionally been attributed to the tongue falling back against the posterior pharyngeal wall. Recent radiological and electromyographic studies suggest that obstruction by the soft palate or epiglottis secondary to reduced local muscle activity may also be responsible.

Drummond GB (1991) Br J Anaesth; 66: 153–6

See also, Airways; Tracheobronchial tree

Airway obstruction. Obstruction may occur at the mouth, pharynx, larynx, trachea and large bronchi. It may be caused by the tongue falling backwards, **laryngospasm**, strictures, tumours and soft tissue swellings, oedema, infection (e.g. **diphtheria**, **epiglottitis**) and **foreign objects**, including teeth and anaesthetic equipment. Hypotonia of the muscles involved in upper **airway** maintenance is common during anaesthesia. During IPPV, mechanical obstruction may occur at any point along the breathing system.

Airway obstruction results in **hypoventilation** and increased work of breathing. It may present as an acute medical emergency requiring immediate management.

- Features:
  - spontaneous ventilation:
    - dyspnoea, noisy respiration, **stridor**.
    - use of accessory muscles of respiration, with tracheal tug, supraclavicular and intercostal indrawing, and paradoxical 'see-saw' movement of abdomen and chest.
    - tachypnoea, tachycardia and other features of **hypoxaemia**, **hypercapnia** and **respiratory failure**.
    - **pulmonary oedema** may occur if negative intrathoracic pressures are excessive.
    - during anaesthesia, poor movement of the reservoir bag may occur.
  - IPPV:
    - increased **airway pressures** with reduced chest movement; noisy respiration or wheeze.
    - features of hypoxaemia and hypercapnia may be present.
- Management:
  - **O_2 therapy** (increased F_IO_2 during anaesthesia).
  - spontaneous ventilation:
    - general measures in unconscious/anaesthetized patients:
      - positioning in the lateral position if practical.
      - correct positioning of the head, elevation of the jaw, and use of oropharyngeal or nasopharyngeal **airways**. Tracheal intubation may be required as below.
    - specific treatment, e.g.:
      - **antibacterial drugs** for infection.
      - plasma for **hereditary angioneurotic oedema**.
      - nebulized **adrenaline** for **croup**.
      - **Heimlich maneouvre** for removing inhaled objects. Small children can be held upside down and slapped on the back.
    - increasing **gas flow**: helium–O_2 mixtures.
    - bypassing the obstruction: tracheal intubation, **tracheostomy** or **cricothyrotomy**. The former may be difficult if the anatomy is distorted.
  - IPPV:
    - causes of increased airway pressure and hypoventilation other than obstruction due to equipment (e.g. **bronchospasm**, **pneumothorax**, inadequate neuromuscular blockade and coughing) should be considered.
    - whilst ventilating by hand, all tubing should be checked for kinks. A suction catheter will not pass down the **tracheal tube** if the latter is obstructed, e.g. by kinks, mucus, herniated cuff, etc. If auscultation of the chest does not suggest bronchospasm or pneumothorax, the cuff should be deflated and the tracheal tube pulled back slightly. If ventilation

does not improve, the tube should be removed and ventilation attempted by facepiece.

- Anaesthesia for patients with airway obstruction:
  - –preoperatively:
    - –**preoperative assessment** for the above features and management as above.
    - –useful pre-induction investigations include:
      - –radiography, including tomograms, **thoracic inlet** views and **CAT scanning**.
      - –arterial blood gas analysis.
      - –**flow–volume loops**.
    - –**premedication** may aid smooth **induction of anaesthesia** but excessive sedation should be avoided.
  - –peroperatively:
    - –anaesthesia should be induced with facilities for resuscitation and tracheostomy/cricothyrotomy available.
    - –patients with upper airway obstruction usually adopt the optimal head and neck position for maximal air movement; muscle relaxation caused by iv induction may therefore lead to sudden complete obstruction. It may be impossible to ventilate the patient by facepiece, and tracheal intubation may be difficult or impossible. **IV anaesthetic agents** should therefore be avoided. Similarly, **neuromuscular blocking drugs** should not be used until the airway has been secured. Inhalational induction, classically with **halothane** and N_2O/O_2 (or O_2 alone if obstruction is severe), should be employed. Deep anaesthesia is achieved slowly; if obstruction worsens, anaesthesia is allowed to lighten. Full **monitoring** is mandatory.
    - –tracheal intubation is performed without paralysis; **lignocaine** spray may be useful.
    - –alternatively, awake intubation may be performed, possibly with a flexible endoscope. Tracheostomy using local anaesthesia is another option.

Classical management of patients with large airway compression, e.g. by mediastinal tumours, also employs inhalational induction and anaesthesia. This avoids acute exacerbation of airway obstruction caused by sudden muscle relaxation.

In the **recovery room** or casualty department, all unconscious patients should be positioned in the **recovery** position, to protect them from aspiration and airway obstruction.

See also, Intubation, awake; Intubation, difficult

Airway pressure. Pressure within the breathing system and tracheobronchial tree. Useful as an indicator of mechanical obstruction to expiration during spontaneous ventilation. During IPPV, airway pressures may indicate disconnection, level of **PEEP**, mechanical obstruction, decreased lung **compliance** or increased **airway resistance**, and the risk of **barotrauma**. The pressure measured at the mouth may considerably exceed alveolar pressure during positive pressure breaths, especially if airway resistance and gas flow rates are high. During expiration, mouth pressure falls to zero, but alveolar pressure may lag behind. In some **ventilators** airway pressure is measured in the expiratory limb of the breathing system.

Airway pressure release ventilation (APRV). **CPAP** with intermittent release to ambient pressure (or a lower level of CPAP) causing expiration. Spontaneous ventilation may continue between APRV breaths. Allows reduction of mean **airway pressure**, and has been used to support respiration in **ARDS**. **Weaning** is achieved by reducing the frequency of CPAP release until the patient is breathing spontaneously with CPAP maintained.
Bray JG, Cane RD (1992) Curr Opin Anaesth; 5: 855–8

Airway resistance.

$$\text{Resistance} = \frac{\text{Driving pressure.}}{\text{Gas flow}}$$

Driving pressure is the difference between alveolar and mouth pressures, and may be measured using the **body plethysmograph**. Alternatively, gas flow may be halted repeatedly for a tenth of a second at a time with a shutter; during the brief period of no flow, alveolar pressure may be measured at the mouth. Gas flow can be measured with a **pneumotachygraph**.

Most of the resistance resides in the large and medium-sized bronchi; severe damage to the small airways may occur before a measurable increase in resistance.

At low lung volumes, the radial traction produced by lung parenchyma surrounding the airways, and which holds them open, is reduced; thus airway calibre is reduced, and resistance increased. During forced expiration, some airways may close, causing air trapping. Bronchoconstriction, and increased density or viscosity of the inspired gas increase resistance (density because flow is not purely laminar in the airways). Resistance is increased in chronic bronchitis due to airway narrowing and bronchoconstriction. In emphysema the airways close because of lung parenchymal destruction.

Airway resistance increases during anaesthesia; this may be caused by bronchospasm, reduction in **FRC** and lung volume, or by the tubes and connections of the breathing system.

See also, Closing capacity; Compliance

Airways. Devices placed in the upper **airway** (but not into the larynx); used to:
  - –relieve **airway obstruction**.
  - –prevent biting and occlusion of the **tracheal tube**.
  - –support the tracheal tube.
  - –allow suction.

Thus usually employed during anaesthesia and in unconscious patients.

- Types:
  - –oropharyngeal: **Guedel**'s airway is most commonly used. Modifications include a side port for attachment to a fresh gas source (**Waters**' airway), caps with side ports, and split airways to allow insertion of a flexible endoscope. Oropharyngeal airways are the commonest cause of damage to **teeth** in anaesthetized patients. The **laryngeal mask** represents a new concept in airway management.
  - –nasopharyngeal: usually smooth non-cuffed tubes with a flange to prevent pushing them completely into the nose.

    Avoid risk to capped teeth, but may cause epistaxis. Cuffed nasal airways may be held in place by the inflated cuff, and allow attachment to a breathing system.

Insertion of an airway may cause gagging, coughing and laryngospasm unless the patient is comatose or adequately anaesthetized; these may also occur on waking.

Other devices have been designed specifically for **expired air ventilation** in **CPR**, e.g. **oesophageal obturators and airways**, airways incorporating one-way valves, etc.

Albumin. Protein (mw 69 000), the major constituent of **plasma** protein (normal plasma levels: 35–50 g/l). Important in the maintenance of plasma **oncotic pressure**, as a **buffer**, and in the transport of various molecules such as bilirubin, hormones, fatty acids, etc., and drugs. It is synthesized by the liver and removed from the plasma into the interstitial fluid. It may then pass via lymphatics back to the plasma, or into cells to be metabolized. Albumin depletion occurs in severe illness, infection, trauma, etc. Available for transfusion as 4.5% and 20% solutions.

McClelland DBL (1990) Br Med J; 300: 35–7
See also, Blood products; Protein binding

Albuterol, *see Salbutamol*

Alcohol. May precipitate or complicate acute illness or injury, e.g. **trauma**, GIT bleeding.
- Effects:
  - –acute:
    - –depressed consciousness, making assessment of **head injury** difficult. Effects of depressant drugs are potentiated, e.g. barbiturates, opioids, etc. Patients may be uncooperative.
    - –vasodilatation, tachycardia, **arrhythmias**.
    - –vomiting, reduced **lower oesophageal sphincter** pressure, gastric irritation.
    - –**hypoglycaemia**, metabolic **acidosis**.
  - –chronic:
    - –cerebral/cerebellar degeneration, peripheral neuropathy, psychiatric disturbances (Wernicke's encephalopathy, Korsakoff's psychosis).
    - –withdrawal may lead to tremor, anxiety, hallucinations (**delerium tremens**) or **convulsions**.
    - –gastritis, peptic ulcer, oesophageal varices.
    - –**pancreatitis**.
    - –fatty liver, hepatic **enzyme induction**, cirrhosis causing **hepatic failure**, coagulopathy.
    - –**malnutrition, immunodeficiency**.
    - –myopathy, **cardiomyopathy**.
- Metabolism:
  - –mostly to acetaldehyde by cytoplasmic dehydrogenase in the liver, with some microsomal oxidation. Dehydrogenated further to acetylcoenzyme A and thence to CO_2 and water via the **tricarboxylic acid cycle**. 5% is excreted unchanged.
  - –rate of metabolism is 10 ml/h (**Michaelis–Menten kinetics**).
  - –produces 130 kJ/g (7 kcal/g); it has been used as an iv energy source.

Resistance to anaesthetic agents is common in alcoholics, possibly due to cross-tolerance and enzyme induction. Effects of withdrawal typically start within the first day or two, and are classically treated with **chlormethiazole**, although other sedative drugs may be used.

Alcohol abuse is not uncommon among doctors, including anaesthetists (*see Sick doctor scheme*).

Alcohol injection may be used for treatment of intractable **pain** or **trigeminal neuralgia**.

[Karl Wernicke (1848–1904), German neurologist; Sergei Korsakoff (1853–1900), Russian neurologist and psychologist]

Edwards, R (1985) Br Med J; 291: 423–4

Alcuronium chloride. Non-depolarizing **neuromuscular blocking drug**, introduced in 1961. Initial dose: 0.2–0.3 mg/kg; onset is within 3–5 minutes; lasts for 20–40 minutes. Supplementary dose: 0.05–0.1 mg/kg. May cause **histamine** release, but less so than **tubocurarine**. Transient hypotension may follow injection. Anaphylaxis has been reported. Excreted mainly in the urine.

Aldosterone. Steroid hormone secreted by the adrenal cortex in response to reduced renal blood flow (via **renin/angiotensin system**), trauma and anxiety (via **ACTH** release), and **hyperkalaemia** and **hyponatraemia** (direct effect on the adrenal cortex). Increases sodium reabsorption from urine, sweat and saliva. Acts on the sodium/potassium pump via intracellular messenger RNA production. Net effects: sodium and water are retained, with potassium and hydrogen ions lost in exchange for sodium ions.

Hyperaldosteronism results in **hypertension** and **hypokalaemia**. In cardiac failure and cirrhosis, aldosterone levels may be raised, although the mechanism is unclear.

Aldosterone antagonists, e.g. **spironolactone** and potassium canrenoate, cause sodium loss and potassium retention.

Weatherill D, Spence AA (1984) Br J Anaesth; 56: 741–9

Alfentanil hydrochloride. Opioid analgesic drug derived from **fentanyl**, with 1/5–1/10 of the latter's potency. Developed in 1976. Onset of action is within 1 minute. More extensively protein-bound than fentanyl. Its **volume of distribution** is 1/4 that of fentanyl, resulting in higher plasma levels; despite a lower **clearance** this results in a shorter elimination **half-life** (about 90 minutes) and duration of action. Has minimal cardiovascular effects, although bradycardia and hypotension may occur. Other effects are similar to those of fentanyl. Cleared by the liver. Excretion is delayed in patients with liver disease and in the elderly. Has been used by infusion because of its short half-life and duration of action.
- Dosage:
  - –for spontaneously breathing patients, up to 500 µg initially, followed by increments of 250 µg. Slow injection reduces the incidence of apnoea.
  - –30–50 µg/kg to obtund the hypertensive response to tracheal intubation. Up to 125 µg/kg is used in **cardiac surgery**.
  - –for infusion, a loading dose of 50–100 µg/kg, followed by 0.5–1 µg/kg/min. Higher rates have been used in **TIVA**. The infusion is discontinued 10–30 minutes before surgery ends. Also used for **sedation** in ICU at 30–60 µg/kg/h initially.

Alkalaemia. Greater than normal plasma **pH**.
See also, Acid–base balance; Alkalosis

Alkalosis. Condition in which **hydrogen ion** concentration is reduced, or would be reduced in the absence of compensatory mechanisms.
See also, Acid–base balance; Alkalosis, metabolic; Alkalosis, respiratory

Alkalosis, metabolic. Inappropriately high **pH** for the measured arterial P_{CO_2}.
- Caused by:
  - acid loss, e.g. vomiting, nasogastric aspiration.
  - base ingestion:
    - **bicarbonate** (usually iatrogenic).
    - citrate from **blood transfusion**.
    - milk–alkali syndrome.
    - forced alkaline diuresis.
  - potassium/chloride depletion leading to acid urine production.
- Primary change: increased bicarbonate/decreased hydrogen ion.
- Compensation:
  - hypoventilation.
  - decreased renal acid secretion.
- Effects:
  - confusion.
  - parasthesiae/**tetany** (reduced free ionized calcium concentration due to altered protein binding).
- Treatment:
  - correction of ECF and potassium depletion.
  - rarely, acid therapy, e.g. ammonium chloride or hydrochloric acid: deficit = **base excess** × body weight (kg) mmol.

See also, Acid–base balance

Alkalosis, respiratory. Alkalosis due to decreased arterial P_{CO_2}. Caused by alveolar **hyperventilation**, e.g. fear, pain, hypoxia, or during IPPV.
- Primary change: decreased arterial P_{CO_2}.
- Compensation:
  - initial fall in plasma **bicarbonate** due to decreased carbonic acid formation and dissociation.
  - decreased acid secretion/increased bicarbonate excretion by the kidneys.
    In acute **hypocapnia**, bicarbonate concentration falls by about 1.3 mmol/l per 1 kPa fall in arterial P_{CO_2}. In chronic hypocapnia the fall per 1 kPa is 4.0 mmol/l.
- Effects: those of hypocapnia.
- Treatment: of underlying cause.

See also, Acid–base balance

Alkylating drugs, *see Antimitotic drugs*

Allen's test. Originally described for assessing arterial flow to the hand in thromboangiitis obliterans. Modified for assessment of ulnar artery flow prior to radial **arterial cannulation**. The ulnar and radial arteries are compressed at the wrist, and the patient asked to clench tightly and open the hand, causing blanching. Pressure over the ulnar artery is released; the colour of the palm normally takes less than 5–10 seconds to return to normal, with over 15 seconds considered abnormal. A similar maneouvre may be performed with the radial artery before ulnar artery cannulation. Although widely performed, it is inaccurate in predicting risk from ischaemic damage.
[EV Allen (1892–1943), US physician]

Allergic reactions, *see Adverse drug reactions*

Allodynia. Pain from a stimulus that is not normally painful.

Alpha-adrenergic..., *see α-Adrenergic...*

Alprostadil, *see Prostaglandins*

Althesin. IV anaesthetic agent introduced in 1971, composed of two steroids, alphaxalone 9 mg/ml and alphadolone 3 mg/ml. Withdrawn in 1984 because of a high incidence of **adverse drug reactions**, mostly minor but occasionally severe. These were thought to be due to **Cremophor EL**, the solubilizing agent. Previously widely used because of its rapid onset and short duration of action.

Altitude, high. Problems include:
- lack of O_2: e.g. atmospheric pressure at 18 000 ft (5486 m) is half that at sea level. F_IO_2 is constant, but P_{O_2} is lowered. This effect is offset initially by the shape of the **oxyhaemoglobin dissociation curve**, which maintains haemoglobin saturation above 90% up to 10 000 ft. Compensatory changes due to hypoxia include hyperventilation, polycythaemia, increased **2,3-DPG**, proliferation of peripheral capillaries, and alterations in intracellular oxidative enzymes. **Alkalaemia** is reduced after a few days, via increased renal bicarbonate loss. CSF pH is returned towards normal. Pulmonary vasoconstriction may result in right heart strain. Acute mountain sickness is thought to be related to acute hypoxia and alkalosis; it consists of headache, malaise, nausea, diarrhoea, and may lead to pulmonary or cerebral oedema.
- low temperatures, e.g. ambient temperature is –20°C at 18 000 ft.
- expansion of gas-containing cavities, e.g. inner ear.
- **decompression sickness**.
- anaesthetic apparatus at high altitude:
  - **vaporizers**: **SVP** is unaffected by atmospheric pressure, thus the partial pressure of volatile agent in the vaporizer is the same as at sea level. Because atmospheric pressure is reduced, the delivered concentration is increased from that marked on the dial, but since anaesthetic action depends on alveolar partial pressure, not concentration, the same settings may be used as at sea level. However, reduced temperature may alter vaporization.
  - **flowmeters**: since atmospheric pressure is reduced, a given amount of gas occupies a greater volume than at sea level; i.e. has reduced density. Thus a greater volume is required to pass through a Rotameter flowmeter to maintain the bobbin at a certain height, because it is the number of gas molecules hitting the bobbin that support it. The flowmeters therefore under-read at high altitudes. However, since the clinical effects depend on the number of molecules, not volume of gas, the flowmeters may be used as normal.

James MFM, White JF (1984) Anesth Analg; 63: 1097–1105

Altitude, low. Problems are related to high pressure:
- those of hyperbaric O_2 (*see Oxygen, hyperbaric*).
- **inert gas narcosis**.
- neurological impairment, e.g. tremor, disorientation.
- pressure reversal of anaesthesia.
- effects on equipment:
  - implosion of glass ampoules, etc.
  - deflation of air-filled tracheal tube cuffs, etc.

–functioning of **vaporizers** and **flowmeters** is normal as above.

Cox J, Robinson DJ (1980) Br J Hosp Med; 23: 144–51

Alveolar air equation. In its simplified form:

$$\text{alveolar } PO_2 = F_IO_2 \, (P_B - P_AH_2O) - \frac{P_ACO_2}{R}$$

$$\text{or } P_IO_2 - \frac{P_ACO_2}{R}$$

where P_B = ambient barometric pressure.

P_AH_2O = alveolar partial pressure of water (normally 6.3 kPa [47 mmHg]).

P_ACO_2 = alveolar PCO_2; approximately equals arterial PCO_2.

R = **respiratory exchange ratio**, normally 0.8.

P_IO_2 = inspired PO_2.

Useful for estimating alveolar PO_2, e.g. when determining **alveolar-arterial O₂ difference**, **shunt** fractions, etc. The equation also illustrates how **hypercapnia** may lower P_AO_2. Another form of the equation allows for differences between inspired and expired gas volumes, and is unaffected by inert gas exchange:

$$\text{alveolar } PO_2 = P_IO_2 - P_ACO_2 \left(\frac{P_IO_2 - P_EO_2}{P_ECO_2} \right)$$

where P_EO_2 = mixed expired PO_2

P_ECO_2 = mixed expired PCO_2

Alveolar–arterial oxygen difference (A–ado₂). Alveolar PO_2 minus arterial PO_2. Useful as a measure of $\dot{V}/\dot{Q}$ **mismatch** and **shunt**. Alveolar PO_2 is estimated using the **alveolar air equation**; arterial PO_2 is measured directly. The small shunt and $\dot{V}/\dot{Q}$ mismatch in normal subjects results in a normal A–ado₂ of less than 2.0 kPa (15 mmHg) breathing air; this may reach 4.0 kPa (30 mmHg) in the elderly. It increases when breathing high O₂ concentrations because the shunt component is not corrected; i.e. normally up to 15 kPa (115 mmHg) breathing 100% O₂.

Alveolar gases. Normal alveolar gas partial pressures and intravascular gas tensions are shown in Table 4. End-tidal gas approximates to alveolar gas in normal subjects and may be monitored, e.g. during anaesthesia.

See also, End-tidal gas sampling

Table 4. Normal respiratory gas partial pressures and tensions in kPa(mmHg)

	Inspired	Alveolar	Arterial	Venous	Expired
O₂	21 (160)	14 (106)	13.3 (100)	5.3 (40)	15 (105)
CO₂	0.03 (0.2)	5.3 (40)	5.3 (40)	6.1 (46)	4 (30)
Nitrogen	80 (600)	74 (560)	74 (560)	74 (560)	75 (570)
H₂O	Variable	6.3 (47)	6.3 (47)	6.3 (47)	6.3 (47)

Alveolar gas transfer. Depends on:

–**alveolar ventilation**.

–**diffusion** across alveolar membrane, fluid interface and capillary endothelium (normally less than 0.5 μm).

–**solubility** of gases in blood.

–**cardiac output**.

For gases transferred from the bloodstream to the alveolus, e.g. CO₂, and anaesthetic vapours during recovery, the same factors apply, but in reverse order.

With normal cardiac output, blood cells take about 0.75 seconds to pass through pulmonary capillaries. O₂ transfer is usually complete within 0.25 seconds; part of the time is taken for the reaction with **haemoglobin**. CO₂ diffuses 20 times more quickly through tissue layers; transfer is also complete within 0.25 seconds. Transfer of highly soluble gases, e.g. carbon monoxide, is limited by diffusion between alveolus and capillary, since large volumes can be taken up by the blood once they reach it. Transfer of insoluble gases, e.g. N₂O, is limited by blood flow from alveoli, since capillary blood is rapidly saturated.

See also, Carbon dioxide transport; Diffusing capacity; Oxygen transport

Alveolar hypoventilation syndrome (Pickwickian syndrome, after a character from Dickens' *Pickwick Papers*). **Obesity**, somnolence and CO₂ retention due to abnormal respiratory control. **Airway obstruction** during sleep may lead to **sleep apnoea**, **hypoxaemia**, **hypercapnia**, **arrhythmias** and **pulmonary hypertension**. Excessive daytime sleepiness is typical; **Cheyne–Stokes respiration** may occur. Cyanosis and plethora are common, due to **polycythaemia** secondary to hypoxia. Right ventricular failure and respiratory failure may occur. Sudden nocturnal death is common.

General and anaesthetic management is as for obesity and **cor pulmonale**. F_IO_2 should be increased cautiously to avoid depression of hypoxic ventilatory drive. **CPAP** may be useful. Respiratory depressant drugs should also be used cautiously; postoperative respiratory failure may occur.

[Charles Dickens (1812–1870), English author]

Alveolar ventilation. Volume of gas entering the alveoli per minute; normally about 4–4.5 l/min. Equals (**tidal volume** minus **dead space**) × respiratory rate; thus rapid small breaths result in a much smaller alveolar ventilation than slow deep breaths, even though **minute ventilation** remains constant. In the upright position, apical alveoli receive less ventilation than basal ones, because the former are already expanded by gravity and are thus less able to expand further on inspiration. Since all the exhaled CO₂ comes from the alveoli, the amount exhaled in a minute equals alveolar ventilation × alveolar concentration of CO₂. Thus alveolar (and hence arterial) CO₂ concentration is inversely proportional to alveolar ventilation, at any fixed rate of CO₂ production.

See also, Ventilation/perfusion mismatch

Alveolus. Terminal part of the respiratory tree; the site of gas exchange. About 3×10^8 exist in both **lungs**, with estimated total surface area 70–80 m². Their walls are comprised of a capillary meshwork covered in cytoplasmic extensions of type I pneumocytes. Traditionally thought to conform to the bubble model; i.e. spherical in structure with a thin water lining, with **surfactant** molecules preventing collapse. Electron microscopy, and experimental and mathematical models, have led to alternate theories, e.g. pooling of water at septal corners with dry areas of surfactant in between, and surface tension helping return water to interstitial fluid.

Ambu-bag, *see Self-inflating bags*

Ambu-E valve, *see Non-rebreathing valves*

American Board of Anesthesiology (ABA). Recognized as an independent Board by the American Board of Medical Specialties in 1941, having been an affiliate of the American Board of Surgery since 1938. Issues the Diploma of the ABA.

American Society of Anesthesiologists (ASA). Formed from the American Society of Anesthetists in 1945, to distinguish 'anesthesiologists' from 'anesthetists'. The American Society of Anesthetists had been formed in 1936 from the New York Society of Anesthetists, which until 1911 had been the Long Island Society of Anesthetists, founded in 1905. The ASA is concerned with improving the standards, education and audit of anaesthesia, and publishes the journal **Anesthesiology**.

Amethocaine hydrochloride. Ester **local anaesthetic agent**, introduced in 1931. Widely used in the USA as tetracaine for **spinal anaesthesia**; in the UK, used only for surface anaesthesia, e.g. in ophthalmology. More potent and longer lasting than **lignocaine**, but more toxic. Toxicity resembles that of **cocaine**. Rapidly absorbed from mucous membranes. Hydrolysed completely by plasma **cholinesterase**. Administration: 0.5–1% solution for spinal anaesthesia; 0.4–0.5% for **extradural anaesthesia**; 0.1–0.2% solution for infiltration, usually with adrenaline; 0.5–1% solutions for surface analgesia. Previously available as lozenges. Maximal safe dose: 1.5 mg/kg.

Amino acids. Organic acid components of **proteins**; they produce polypeptide chains by forming peptide bonds between the amino group of one and the carboxyl group of another, with the elimination of water.

Amino acids from the breakdown of ingested and endogenous proteins form an amino acid pool from which new proteins are synthesized. Amino acids are involved in **carbohydrate** and **fat** metabolism; amino groups may be removed or transferred to other molecules (deamination and transamination respectively). Deamination results in the liberation of ammonia, which may be excreted as urea, or taken up by other amino acids to form amides.

Eight dietary amino acids are essential for life in humans: valine, leucine, isoleucine, threonine, methionine, phenylalanine, tryptophan and lysine. Arginine and histidine are required for normal growth. Other amino acids may be synthesized from carbohydrate and fat breakdown products.
See also, Nitrogen balance

γ-Aminobutyric acid (GABA). Inhibitory **neurotransmitter** found in many parts of the brain. Binds to specific GABA receptors, causing opening of chloride channels and chloride entry into cells. The GABA receptor complex is closely associated with receptor sites for picrotoxin, which closes the chloride channels, and **benzodiazepines**, which augment the opening induced by GABA. Many **anticonvulsant drugs** facilitate the action of GABA,

suggesting its role in the regulation of central activity and **epilepsy**. GABA may also be involved in presynaptic inhibition at many central **synapses**. The significance of a second GABA receptor, activation of which increases potassium **conductance**, is uncertain.

Aminophylline. Phosphodiesterase inhibitor, a mixture of **theophylline** and ethylenediamine. Much more soluble than theophylline alone, hence its use iv. Used as a **bronchodilator drug**, and as an **inotropic drug** especially in paediatrics.
Causes bronchodilatation, increased diaphragmatic contractility, vasodilatation, increased cardiac output (direct effect on the heart), diuresis (direct effect on the kidney), and CNS stimulation.
- Dosage:
  –100–500 mg 6–12 hourly, orally (depending on the preparation), usually as slow-release preparations. Rectal preparations are no longer used, as they were associated with proctitis and unpredictable response.
  –for emergency iv use, injection of 5–7 mg/kg over 30 minutes may be followed by an infusion of 0.5 mg/kg/h (up to 1 mg/kg/h in smokers), with ECG monitoring. Dosage should be reduced in cardiac and hepatic failure, and during therapy with **cimetidine**, erythromycin and ciprofloxacin.
- Side effects: arrhythmias, agitation and convulsions, GIT disturbances.
Care should be taken when patients already on oral treatment are given iv aminophylline, since the drug has a low **therapeutic ratio**. Plasma levels should be measured; therapeutic range is 10–20 mg/l.

Aminopyridine. Originally 4–aminopyridine, a drug which may be used to reverse **non-depolarizing neuromuscular blockade**, and to treat **myasthenic syndrome**. Does not inhibit **acetylcholinesterase**, but acts presynaptically to increase **acetycholine** release, thereby increasing the force of **muscle contraction**. It also enters the brain and may cause convulsions. Replaced by 3,4–diaminopyridine, which does not cross the **blood–brain barrier**.

Amiodarone hydrochloride. Class III **antiarrhythmic drug**, used for treating supraventricular and ventricular **arrhythmias**. Acts by prolonging the cardiac **action potential** and **refractory period**. Causes minimal myocardial depression. **Half-life** is over 4 weeks. Acts rapidly following iv administration.
- Dosage:
  –200 mg orally, thrice daily for one week, reducing to once daily for maintenance.
  –as an iv infusion: 5 mg/kg over 20–120 minutes followed by up to 15 mg/kg/24 h, with ECG monitoring. Bradycardia may occur. May cause inflammation of peripheral veins. The dose should be reduced after 1–2 days.
- Prolonged administration results commonly in corneal microdeposits (reversible, and rarely affecting vision), and may cause photosensitivity, peripheral neuropathy, hyper- or hypothyroidism, hepatitis and pulmonary fibrosis.
Teesdale S, Downar E (1990) Can J Anaesth; 37: 151–5

Amnesia. Impairment of **memory**. May occur with intracranial pathology, dementia, metabolic disturbances,

alcohol abuse and psychological disturbances. May be caused by **head injury** and drugs. Patients who recover from critical illness may have poor recall of events afterwards.

Retrograde amnesia (between the causative agent/event and the last memory beforehand) is common after head injury. Anterograde amnesia (loss of memory for the period following the causative agent/event) may occur after head injury, and is common after administration of certain drugs, typically **benzodiazepines** and **hyoscine**. **Awareness** during anaesthesia, with amnesia preventing subsequent recall, may be more common than previously thought.

Amniotic fluid embolism. Condition occurring typically in multiparous women, during or following forceful labour. May cause coughing, shivering, cyanosis, vomiting, **convulsions** and **shock**, leading to **DIC** and **ARDS**. **Hypoxaemia** and pulmonary vasoconstriction may occur; chest X-ray may be normal. Amniotic fluid components may be recovered from central venous blood. Treatment is supportive. Although rare, it carries a high mortality (up to 80%), and thus remains a major cause of maternal death.
Sperry K (1986) JAMA 255: 2183–6

Ampere. SI **unit** of **current**. Defined as the current flowing in two straight parallel wires of infinite length, 1 metre apart in a vacuum, which will produce a force of 2 $\times$ 10^{-7} newtons per metre length on each of the wires.
[Andre Ampère (1775–1836), French physicist]

Amphetamines. Group of drugs related to **adrenaline**, causing stimulation of the central and **sympathetic nervous systems**. Commonly abused, they cause addiction and are controlled drugs. Used in narcolepsy. May increase **MAC** of **inhalational anaesthetic agents**. Overdosage may cause hyperactivity, hypertension, hallucinations and hyperthermia. Treatment includes **chlorpromazine** and **β-adrenergic receptor antagonists**. Forced acid diuresis increases their excretion.

Amrinone lactate. Phosphodiesterase inhibitor, used as an **inotropic drug**. Active iv and orally. Increases cardiac output and reduces SVR via inhibition of cardiac and vascular muscle phosphodiesterase. MAP and heart rate are unaltered. **Half-life** is 3–6 hours.
- Dosage: 0.5–1.0 mg/kg iv, followed by 2–10 µg/kg/min.
- May cause GIT side effects and thrombocytopenia; **milrinone**, a more potent derivative, has fewer side effects.

Anaemia. Reduced **haemoglobin** concentration; usually defined as less than 13 g/dl for males, 12 g/dl for females. In children, the figure varies; 18 g/dl (1–2 weeks of age); 11 g/dl (6 months–6 years); 12 g/dl (6–12 years).
- Caused by:
  - reduced production:
    - deficiency of iron, **vitamin** B$_{12}$, folate.
    - chronic disease, e.g. **malignancy**, infection.
    - endocrine disease, e.g. **hypothyroidism**, hypoadrenalism.
    - bone marrow infiltration, e.g. leukaemia, myelofibrosis.
    - aplastic anaemia, including drug-induced, e.g. chloramphenicol.
    - reduced **erythropoietin** secretion, e.g. **renal failure**.
    - abnormal red cells/haemoglobin, e.g. sideroblastic anaemia, **thalassaemia**.
  - increased **haemolysis**.
  - **haemorrhage**:
    - acute.
    - chronic.
- Investigated by measuring the size and haemoglobin content of **erythrocytes**:
  - hypochromic, microcytic: e.g. thalassaemia, iron deficiency including chronic haemorrhage, chronic disease.
  - normochromic, macrocytic: vitamin B$_{12}$ or folate deficiency, alcoholism.
  - normochromic, normocytic: chronic disease, e.g infection, malignancy, renal failure, endocrine disease; aplastic anaemia, bone marrow disease or infiltration.
  Other investigations include examination of blood film (e.g. for sickle cells, parasites, reticulocytes suggesting increased breakdown or haemorrhage, etc.), measurement of platelets and white cells, bone marrow aspiration and further blood tests, e.g. iron, vitamin B$_{12}$, etc.
- Effects:
  - reduced O$_2$ carrying capacity of blood: fatigue, dyspnoea on exertion, angina.
  - increased cardiac output, to maintain **O$_2$ flux**: palpatations, tachycardia, systolic murmurs, cardiac failure. Reduced **viscosity** increases **flow** but turbulence is more likely.
  - increased **2,3–DPG**.
  - maintenance of blood volume by **haemodilution**.

Unexpected anaemia should be investigated before routine surgery. Traditional minimal 'safe' haemoglobin concentration for anaesthesia is 10 g/dl, unless surgery is urgent; below this level, reduced O$_2$ carriage outweighs the advantage of reduced blood viscosity and increased flow. Many would dispute this value as too high; 8 g/dl has been suggested. Reduction of cardiac output during anaesthesia is particularly hazardous. F_IO_2 of 0.5 is often advocated to reduce risk of peroperative hypoxia by increasing the O$_2$ reserve within the lungs.

Transfused stored blood takes up to 24 hours to reach its full O$_2$ carrying capacity; ideally transfusion should occur at least 1 day preoperatively. Slow transfusion also minimizes the risk of fluid overload in chronic anaemia.

Anaesthesia. Journal of the **Association of Anaesthetists of Great Britain and Ireland**, first published in 1946.

Anaesthesia (from Greek: an + aisthesis; without feeling). Term suggested by Oliver Wendell **Holmes** in 1846 to describe the state of sleep produced by ether; the word had been used previously to describe lack of feeling, e.g. due to peripheral neuropathy. He introduced derived words, e.g. 'anaesthetic agent'.

Anaesthesia, balanced, *see Balanced anaesthesia*

Anaesthesia, depth of. Anaesthesia is generally accepted as being a continuum in which increasing depth of anaesthesia results in loss of consciousness, recall, and somatic and autonomic reflexes. Some would argue that, whilst these are the effects of anaesthetic drugs in increasing dosage, 'anaesthesia' itself occurs at a particular undefined point, and is therefore either present or absent.

Anaesthesia dolorosa

Assessment is important in order to avoid inadequate anaesthesia with **awareness** and troublesome reflexes, or overdose.

- Methods of assessment:
  - clinical:
    - stages of anaesthesia (see *Anaesthesia, stages of*).
    - signs of light anaesthesia:
      - lacrimation.
      - tachycardia.
      - hypertension.
      - sweating.
      - reactive dilated pupils.
      - movement, laryngospasm, etc.

      These signs may be altered by anaesthetic drugs themselves, and by others, e.g. opioids, **atropine, neuromuscular blocking drugs**.
    - **isolated forearm technique**.
  - EEG:
    - conventional EEG: bulky and difficult to interpret. Poor correlation between different anaesthetic agents.
    - **cerebral function monitor** and **analysing monitor**: easier to use and read, but less informative than conventional EEG.
    - **power spectral analysis**: graphic display of complicated data; easier to interpret than conventional EEG. Apparatus is very expensive.
  - **evoked potentials**: similar effects are produced by different anaesthetic agents.
  - **oesophageal contractility**: affected by smooth muscle relaxants and ganglion blocking drugs, also by disease, e.g. **achalasia**.
  - EMG: particularly of the frontalis muscle. Requires separate monitoring of peripheral neuromuscular blockade in addition.

Plourde G (1991) Can J Anaesth; 38: 270–4

Anaesthesia dolorosa. Pain in an anaesthetic area, typically following destructive treatment of **trigeminal neuralgia**. Unpleasant symptoms, ranging from paraesthesiae to severe pain, develop in the area of the face rendered anaesthetic, and may be more distressing than the original symptoms. Anaesthesia dolorosa may develop many months after the lesion, and is often refractory to further treatment, including surgery.

Anaesthesia, history of.
- Early attempts at pain relief:
  - **opium** used for many centuries, especially in the Far East. First injected iv in the 1660s.
  - use of other plants and derivatives for many centuries, e.g. **cocaine (cocada), mandragora, alcohol**.
  - **acupuncture**.
  - unconsciousness produced by carotid compression.
  - analgesia produced by cold (**refrigeration anaesthesia**), compression and ischaemia: 1500–1600s.
  - **mesmerism**: 1700–1800s.
- General anaesthesia:
  - effects of **diethyl ether** on animals described by **Paracelsus**: 1540.
  - understanding of basic physiology, especially respiratory and cardiovascular, and isolation of many gases, e.g. O_2, CO_2, N_2O: 1600–1700s.
  - N_2O suggested for analgesia by **Davy** in 1799.
  - CO_2 inhalation to produce insensibility described by **Hickman** in 1824.

- use of **diethyl ether** for anaesthesia by **Long, Clarke**: 1842.
- use of N_2O for anaesthesia by **Wells, Colton**: 1844.
- first public demonstration of ether anaesthesia in Boston by **Morton**: October 16th 1846 (see *Bigelow; Holmes; Warren*).
- first UK use in **Dumfries** and London: December 19th 1846 (see *Boott*). Used in London by Squire 2 days later (see *Liston*).
- **chloroform** introduced by **Simpson**: 1847.
- first death: **Greener**: 1848.
- development in UK led by **Snow**, then **Clover**.
- **rectal administration** of anaesthetic drugs described.
- iv anaesthesia produced with **chloral hydrate** by **Oré**: 1872.
- ether versus chloroform: the former was favoured in England and northern USA, the latter in Scotland and southern USA. Other agents introduced (see *Inhalational anaesthetic agents*). **Boyle** machine described 1917.
- iv anaesthesia popularized by Weese, **Lundy** and **Waters**: 1930s (see *Intravenous anaesthetic agents*). Neuromuscular blockade introduced by **Griffith**: 1942. **Halothane** introduced 1956.
- UK pioneers: **Hewitt, Macewen, Magill, Rowbotham, Macintosh** (first UK professor), **Hewer, Organe**.
- USA pioneers: Waters (first university professor), **Guedel, Mckesson, Crile, McMechan**, Lundy.
- UK: **Association of Anaesthetists** founded 1932; **DA** examination 1935; **Faculty of Anaesthetists** 1948; **FFARCS** examination 1953; **College of Anaesthetists** 1988.
- USA: **American Society of Anaesthesiologists** founded 1945.
- **World Federation of Societies of Anaesthesiologists** founded 1955.

- Local anaesthesia:
  - cocaine isolated 1860.
  - topical anaesthesia produced by **Koller**: 1884.
  - **spinal anaesthesia** by **Corning**: 1885; **Bier**: 1898.
  - **extradural anaesthesia** 1901.
  - pioneers: **Braun, Lawen, Labat**.

[Helmut Weese (1897–1954), German pharmacologist]
See also, Cardiopulmonary resuscitation; Intermittent positive pressure ventilation; Intubation, tracheal; Local anaesthetic agents

Anaesthesia, mechanism of. The precise mechanism is unknown, but theories are as follows:
- gross level:
  - **ascending reticular activating system** is thought to be the most likely site, but cerebral cortex, olfactory cortex, hippocampus and **limbic system** are probably involved.
  - **spinal cord** is also affected by anaesthetics.
  - synaptic sites are thought to be more important than axonal sites, since the former are blocked more easily than the latter at clinically effective concentrations of anaesthetic agent. Agents are thought to modify presynaptic release of neurotransmitter, and/or postsynaptic binding. They may modulate overall synaptic function by delaying certain impulses only, or by a global effect. Reduced excitation is thought to be mainly responsible, but increased inhibitory activity has also been shown.

18

–cellular level: **membranes** are thought to be the likeliest site of action, although anaesthetics have been shown to interact with microtubules and other cytoplasmic structures.

–potency of volatile agents is related to their lipid solubility (**Meyer–Overton rule**), hence the suggestion of membrane lipids as the target site. However, this does not explain the **cutoff effect**, nor the lack of potentiation of anaesthetics by heat.

–membrane or other proteins may be affected by anaesthetics. Interaction with certain proteins has also been shown to be related to potency. Specific molecule systems may be involved; i.e. an 'anaesthetic receptor' site may exist. Other receptor systems may also be affected, e.g. the opioid system.

–membrane expansion by anaesthetics to beyond a critical volume has been postulated, supported by pressure reversal of anaesthesia in tadpoles and some other animal experiments. The multisite expansion hypothesis has been suggested to account for differences between different agents and experimental conditions; it proposes that different agents act at various sites within the membrane to cause membrane expansion and alter fluidity. The function of membrane pumps and configuration of ionic channels are thus altered.

–other theories, now thought to be less important:

–**clathrate** theory (water hydrates of anaesthetic agents).

–Ferguson's thermodynamic activity theory: related activity to the chemical composition of the agent concerned, by determining the energy contained within the chemical bonds of its molecules. Related to lipid solubity and other physical properties.

–**Bernard** suggested that anaesthetics caused intracellular protein coagulation.

[J Ferguson (described 1949), English scientist]
Pocock G, Richards CD (1991) Br J Anaesth; 66: 116–28

Anaesthesia, one lung, *see One-lung anaesthesia*

Anaesthesia, stages of. In 1847, **Snow** described five stages of narcotism, although a less detailed classification had already been described. The classic description of anaesthetic stages was by **Guedel** in 1937 in unpremedicated patients, breathing **diethyl ether** in air:

–stage 1 (analgesia):
–normal reflexes.
–ends with loss of the eyelash reflex and unconsciousness.
–stage 2 (excitement):
–irregular breathing, struggling.
–dilated pupils.
–vomiting, coughing and laryngospasm may occur.
–ends with the onset of automatic breathing and loss of the eyelid reflex.
–stage 3 (surgical anaesthesia):
–plane I:
–until eyes centrally placed with loss of conjunctival reflex.
–swallowing and vomiting depressed.
–pupils normal/small.
–lacrimation increased.
–plane II:

–until onset of intercostal paralysis.
–regular deep breathing.
–loss of corneal reflex.
–pupils becoming larger.
–lacrimation increased.
–plane III:
–until complete intercostal paralysis.
–shallow breathing.
–light reflex depressed.
–laryngeal reflexes depressed.
–lacrimation depressed.
–plane IV:
–until diaphragmatic paralysis.
–carinal reflexes depressed.
–stage 4 (overdose):
–apnoea.
–dilated pupils.

With modern agents and techniques, the stages often occur too rapidly to be easily distinguished.

The stages may be seen in reverse order on emergence from anaesthesia.
See also, Anaesthesia, depth of

Anaesthesia, total intravenous, *see Total intravenous anaesthesia*

Anaesthetic accidents, *see Anaesthetic morbidity and mortality*

Anaesthetic agents, *see Inhalational anaesthetic agents; Intravenous anaesthetic agents; Local anaesthetic agents*

Anaesthetic breathing systems.

• Definitions:
–open: unrestricted ambient air as the fresh gas supply.
–semi-open: as above, but some restriction to air supply, e.g. enclosed mask.
–closed: totally closed circle system.
–semi-closed: air intake prevented but venting of excess gases allowed. Classified by Mapleson into five groups, A to E, in 1954; a sixth was added later (Fig. 6).

• Mapleson's classification (excludes **open drop techniques, circle systems**, and use of **non-rebreathing valves**):
–Mapleson A (**Magill** attachment):
–efficient for spontaneous ventilation, because exhaled dead space gas is reused at the next inspiration, and exhaled alveolar gas passes out through the valve. Thus fresh gas flow (FGF) theoretically may equal alveolar minute volume (70 ml/kg/min).
–inefficient for IPPV, because some fresh gas is lost through the valve when the bag is squeezed, and exhaled alveolar gas may be retained in the system and rebreathed. High gas flows are therefore needed (2–3 × minute volume).
–Mapleson B and C: rarely used, other than for resuscitation. Inefficient; thus 2–3 × minute volume is required.
–Mapleson D:
–inefficient for spontaneous ventilation, because exhaled gas passes into the reservoir bag with fresh gas, and may be rebreathed unless FGF is high. Suggested values for FGF range from 150–250 ml/kg/min; resistance to breathing may be a problem at high FGF.

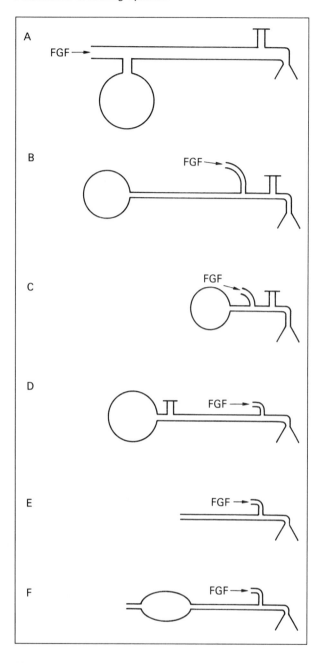

Figure 6 *Classification of anaesthetic breathing systems (see text)*

–efficient for IPPV; exhaled dead space gas passes into the bag and is re-used but when alveolar gas reaches the bag, the bag is full of fresh gas and dead space gas; alveolar gas is thus voided through the valve. Theoretically, 70 ml/kg/min will maintain normocapnia.

–Mapleson E (Ayre's T-piece): used for children, because of its low resistance to breathing. To prevent breathing of atmospheric air, the reservoir limb should exceed tidal volume. A FGF of 2–3 × minute volume is required to prevent rebreathing. May be used for IPPV by intermittent occlusion of the reservoir limb outlet.

–Mapleson F (Jackson Rees Modification): adapted from Ayre's T-piece. The bag allows easier control of ventilation, and its movement demonstrates breathing during spontaneous ventilation. Suggested FGF: 2–3 × minute volume for spontaneous ventilation. For IPPV, 200 ml/kg has been suggested, although more complicated formulae exist.

- Modifications include:
  –coaxial versions of the A and D systems (Lack and Bain respectively); the valve is accessible to the anaesthetist for adjustment and **scavenging**, and the tubing is longer and lighter.
  –Humphrey ADE system: valve and bag are at the machine end, with a lever incorporated within the valve block; may be converted into type A, D or E systems depending on requirements.

British and International Standard taper sizes of breathing system connections are 15 mm for tracheal tube **connectors** and paediatric components, and 22 mm for adult components. Some components have external tapers of 22 mm, and internal tapers of 15 mm. Some paediatric equipment has 8.5 mm diameter fittings, although not standard. Upstream parts of connections are traditionally 'male', and fit into the 'female' downstream parts.

[William W Mapleson, Cardiff physicist; Philip Ayre (1902–1980), Newcastle anaesthetist; Gordon Jackson Rees, Liverpool anaesthetist; D Humphrey, South African physiologist and anaesthetist]

Conway CM (1985) Br J Anaesth; 57: 649–57

See also, Adjustable pressure-limiting valve; Catheter mounts; Coaxial anaesthetic breathing systems; Facepieces; Reservoir bags; Tracheal tubes; Valveless anaesthetic breathing systems

Anaesthetic machines. Term commonly refers to machines providing continous flow of anaesthetic gases (c.f. **intermittent flow anaesthetic machines**). The original **Boyle** machine was developed in 1917 at St Bartholomew's Hospital, although similar apparatus was already being used in America and France.

- Usual system:
  –**piped gas supply** or **cylinders**.
  –pressure gauges may indicate pipeline, cylinder or regulated (reduced) pressure (*see Pressure measurement*).
  –**pressure regulators** provide constant gas pressure, usually about 400 kPa (4 bar) in the UK. Pipelines are already at this pressure.
  –**flowmeters**, usually **Rotameters**.
  –**vaporizers**.
  –pressure relief valve downstream from the vaporizers protects the flowmeters from excessive pressure; it opens at about 38–40 kPa. May be combined with a non-return valve.
  –O_2 flush; bypasses flowmeters and vaporizers, delivering at least 35 l/min.
  –**O_2 failure warning device**.
  –**ventilators**, **monitoring** equipment, **suction equipment**, and various **anaesthetic breathing systems** may be incorporated. Some machines contain microprocessors for digitalized control of functions, e.g. gas flow.
- Modern safety features reduce the risk of:
  –delivering hypoxic gas mixtures:
    –to avoid incorrect gas delivery:
      –**pin index system** for cylinders and non-interchangeable connectors for piped gas outlet.

–colour coding of pipelines and cylinders.

–O_2 analyser.

–O_2 flowmeter control is bigger and has a different profile to others; it is positioned in the same place on all machines (i.e. on the left in the UK; on the right in the USA).

–interconnection of N_2O and O_2 Rotameters, so that less than 25% O_2 cannot be 'dialed up', e.g. **Quantiflex apparatus** and newer machines.

–to avoid O_2 leak: O_2 flowmeter feeds downstream from the others; thus a cracked CO_2 Rotameter leaks N_2O in preference to O_2.

–to avoid risk of O_2 delivery failure:

  –O_2 pressure gauge.

  –O_2 failure warning device; preferably switching off other gas flows and allowing air to be breathed.

  –O_2 analyser.

–delivering excessive CO_2 (e.g. caused by the CO_2 flowmeter opened fully, with the bobbin hidden at the top of the flowmeter tube):

  –maximal possible CO_2 flow is limited, e.g. to 500 ml/min.

  –bobbin is clearly visible throughout the length of the Rotameter tube.

  –CO_2 cylinder is connected to the machine only when specifically required.

–delivering excessive pressures:

  –**adjustable pressure limiting valve** on breathing systems: modern ones produce maximal pressures of 70 cmH$_2$O when fully closed. Many ventilators also have cut-off maximal pressures.

  –distensible **reservoir bag**; maximal pressure attainable is about 60 cmH$_2$O. Pressure reaches a plateau as the bag distends, falling slightly (**Laplace's law**) before bursting.

• Other safety features:

  –switches to prevent **soda lime** being used with **trichloroethylene**.

  –**key filling system** for vaporizers.

  –negative and positive pressure relief valves within **scavenging** systems.

  –**antistatic precautions**.

Thompson PW, Wilkinson DJ (1985) Br J Anaesth; 57: 640–8

See also, Checking of anaesthetic equipment

Anaesthetic morbidity and mortality.
Complications during and following anaesthesia are difficult to quantify, since many may be related to surgery or other factors. Many are avoidable, and may be more disturbing to the patient than the surgery itself.

• Examples:

  –nausea and **vomiting**.

  –**sore throat**.

  –headache: often related to perioperative dehydration and starvation. **Postspinal headache**.

  –damage to **teeth**, mouth, eye, etc.

  –backache: especially after lithotomy position. Reduced by lumbar pillows.

  –muscle pains following **suxamethonium**.

  –thrombophlebitis/pain at injection or infusion sites.

  –extravasation of injectate/intra-arterial injection.

  –drowsiness, disorientation.

  –**blood transfusion** hazards.

  –**nerve injury** and damage due to careless **positioning of the patient**.

  –burns, e.g. from **diathermy**.

  –falls during transfer from/to trolleys, etc.

  –**awareness**.

  –tracheal intubation difficulties (*see Intubation, complications of*).

  –**adverse drug reactions**, e.g. **halothane hepatitis**, **MH**.

  –drug overdose.

  –renal impairment, e.g. following uncorrected hypotension.

  –cardiovascular complications: **MI**, **hypertension/hypotension**, **air embolism**, **arrhythmias**.

  –respiratory complications: **hypoventilation**, **atelectasis**, **chest infection**, **PE**, **pneumothorax**, **aspiration pneumonitis**, **airway obstruction**, **bronchospasm**.

  –psychological changes.

  –severe neurological complications: **CVA**, brain damage, spinal cord infarction; they often follow severe hypotension/cardiac arrest/hypoxia.

  –death.

• Mortality may be related to anaesthesia, surgery, or the medical condition of the patient. Mortality studies in the UK, USA, Canada, Scandinavia, Europe, and Australia have all implicated similar factors:

  –preoperatively:

    –inadequate assessment.

    –hypovolaemia and inadequate resuscitation.

  –peroperatively:

    –aspiration.

    –inadequate **monitoring**.

    –intubation difficulties.

    –delivery of hypoxic gas mixtures and equipment failure.

    –inexperience/inadequate supervision.

  –postoperatively:

    –inadequate observation.

    –hypoventilation due to respiratory depression, residual neuromuscular blockade, and respiratory obstruction.

• Morbidity and mortality are thus reduced by:

  –thorough **preoperative assessment** and adequate resuscitation.

  –**checking of anaesthetic equipment** and drugs.

  –adequate monitoring.

  –anticipation of likely problems.

  –attention to detail.

  –adequate **recovery** facilities.

  –adequate supervision/assistance.

Clear **record-keeping** assists retrospective analysis of complications and future anaesthetic management.

Postgraduate Educational Issue (1987) Br J Anaesth; 59; 813–927

See also, Audit; Confidential Enquiries into Maternal Deaths, Report on; Confidential Enquiry into Perioperative Deaths

Anaesthetic rooms (Induction rooms).
Usual in the UK but not used in many other countries.

• Advantages:

  –quiet area for induction of anaesthesia.

  –less frightening for the patient than lying on the operating table.

  –anaesthetists' domain; i.e. without pressure from surgeons, etc.

  –store for anaesthetic drugs, equipment, etc.

–increased throughput of the operating suite, if another anaesthetist is available to start whilst previous cases are being completed in theatre.

● Disadvantages:
–expensive duplication of equipment is required, e.g. anaesthetic machine, monitoring, etc.
–monitoring is disconnected during transfer of the patient.
–transfer and positioning for surgery is more hazardous with the patient anaesthetized than when awake.
–equipment, iv fluids, drugs, etc. may not be immediately available in the operating theatre.

The above disadvantages lead many anaesthetists to induce anaesthesia in the operating theatre for high risk patients. Continued existence of anaesthetic rooms is controversial. Holding areas capable of processing many patients at once (allowing premedication and performance of regional blocks), have been suggested as an alternative.
Meyer-Witting M, Wilkinson DJ (1992) Anaesthesia; 47: 1021–2

Analeptic drugs. Drugs causing stimulation of the CNS as their most prominent action (many other drugs also have stimulant properties, e.g. **aminophylline**).
● Mechanism of action:
–block inhibition, e.g. strychnine (via **glycine** antagonism), picrotoxin (via **GABA** antagonism).
–increase excitation, e.g. **doxapram**, **nikethamide**.
Doxapram and nikethamide increase respiration via stimulation of peripheral chemoreceptors. All the analeptics may cause cardiovascular stimulation, and convulsions at sufficient doses.

Analgesia. Lack of sensation of **pain** from a normally painful stimulus.
See also, Analgesic drugs

Analgesic drugs. May be divided into:
–opioid analgesic drugs.
–inhibitors of **prostaglandin** synthesis.
–**NSAIDs**.
–**paracetamol**.
–others:
–**inhalational anaesthetic agents** e.g. **N₂O**, **trichloroethylene**.
–**ketamine**.
–**nefopam, ethoheptazine**.
–**local anaesthetic agents**.
–adjuncts: i.e. reduce **pain** or pain sensation by alternate means: e.g. **antidepressant drugs, steroid therapy, carbamazepine**, muscle relaxants e.g. **diazepam**, etc. Used widely in chronic **pain management**. **Caffeine** is often included in oral analgesic preparations.

Analgesic drugs are distinguished from anaesthetic agents by their ability to reduce pain sensation without inducing sleep; thus N₂O is a good analgesic but a poor anaesthetic, and halothane has poor analgesic properties but is a potent anaesthetic. In practice the distinction is not precise, as analgesic drugs, e.g. opiates, will cause unconsciousness at high doses, and anaesthetic drugs, e.g. halothane, will abolish pain sensation at deep planes of anaesthesia.

Anaphylactic reaction. Type I immune reaction, resulting from an antigen–antibody reaction on the surface of **mast cells**. Crosslinking of two immunoglobulin type-E (reagin) molecules by the antigen results in the release of **histamine** and other vasoactive substances, e.g. **kinins, 5–HT** and **leukotrienes**. Type-G immunoglobulin may also be involved. True anaphylaxis requires previous exposure to the antigen responsible, sometimes many exposures; e.g. anaphylaxis to thiopentone classically occurs after more than ten exposures.

In the most severe form, there may be urticaria, angiooedema, bronchospasm, and cardiovascular collapse due to vasodilatation, increased vascular permeability and myocardial depression. There may also be coagulation abnormalities.

● Treatment:
–**CPR**, especially iv fluids and O₂ administration.
–iv **adrenaline** 1:10 000 in 1 ml increments.
–**antihistamine drugs** and hydrocortisone may also be used.

Bochner BS, Lichtenstein LM (1991) New Engl J Med; 324: 1785–90
See also, Adverse drug reactions

Anaphylactoid reaction. Although clinically similar to an **anaphylactic reaction**, anaphylactoid reactions do not involve immunoglobulin crosslinkage. Underlying mechanisms include the release of vasoactive substances, e.g. **histamine**, by:
–direct histamine release from mast cells. **Neuromuscular blocking drugs** are common causes, especially **tubocurarine**.
–**complement** activation, either via classical or alternative pathways. **Althesin** may cause either.

Direct histamine release and alternative pathway complement activation do not require prior exposure to the causative agent, whereas true anaphylaxis does.
Fisher M, Baldo BA (1992) Curr Opin Anaesth; 5: 488–91
See also, Adverse drug reactions

Aneroid gauge, *see Pressure measurement*

Anesthesia and Analgesia. Oldest current journal of anaesthesia, first published in 1922 as *Current Researches in Anesthesia and Analgesia* (the journal of the National Anesthesia Research Society, which became the International Anesthesia Research Society in 1925).

Anesthesiology. Journal of the **American Society of Anesthesiologists**, first published in 1940.

Anesthesiology. American term describing the practice of anaesthesia by trained physicians (anesthesiologists) as opposed to others who might administer anaesthetics (e.g. nurse anesthetists). Formally accepted as a speciality by the American Medical Association in 1940. In the UK, the term 'anaesthetist' implies medical qualification.

Angina, *see Ischaemic heart disease; Myocardial ischaemia*

Angiotensin converting enzyme inhibitors (ACE inhibitors). Originally isolated from snake venom. **Captopril** and **enalapril** are used in the treatment of **hypertension** and **cardiac failure**, not usually as first-line drugs. They block the action of angiotensin converting enzyme; apart from converting angiotensin I to angiotensin II, this enzyme breaks down **bradykinin**, a naturally occurring

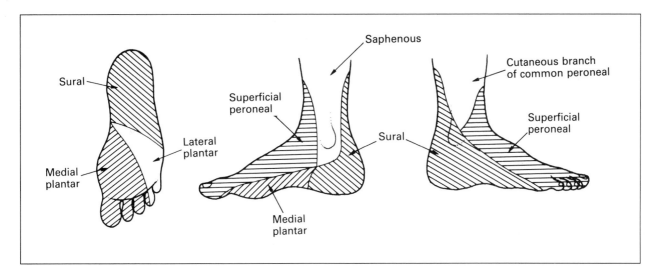

Figure 7 *Cutaneous innervation of the ankle and foot*

vasodilator. The ACE inhibitors cause vasodilatation and a drop in BP, which may be profound after the first dose. Side effects include hypotension, rashes, leucopenia, renal damage, loss of taste, and cough. Severe hypotension may follow induction of anaesthesia or peroperative haemorrhage, especially if the patient is fluid and/or sodium depleted.
Mirenda JV, Grissom TE (1991) Anesth Analg; 72: 667–83
See also, Renin/angiotensin system

Angiotensins, *see Renin/angiotensin system*

Anion gap. Difference between measured cation and anion concentration in the plasma. Sodium plus potassium concentrations normally exceed chloride plus bicarbonate concentrations by 12–18 mmol/l. Anionic proteins, phosphate, and sulphate make up the difference. Of use in the differential diagnosis of metabolic **acidosis**; anionic gap increases when organic anions accumulate, e.g. in **lactic acidosis, ketoacidosis**, uraemia. It does not increase in acidosis due to loss of bicarbonate or intake of hydrochloric acid.

Ankle, nerve blocks. Useful for surgery distal to the ankle.
• Nerves to be blocked are as follows (Fig. 7):
  –tibial nerve (L5–S3): lies posterior to the posterior tibial artery, between flexor digitorum longus and flexor hallucis longus tendons. Divides into lateral and medial plantar nerves behind the medial malleolus. Supplies the anterior and medial parts of the sole of the foot. A needle is inserted lateral to the posterior tibial artery at the level of the medial malleolus, or medial to the Achilles tendon if the artery cannot be felt. It is passed anteriorly and 5–10 ml **local anaesthetic agent** injected as it is withdrawn.
  –sural nerve (L5–S2): formed from branches of the tibial and common peroneal nerves. Accompanies the short saphenous vein behind the lateral malleolus and supplies the posterior part of the sole, the back of the lower leg, the heel and lateral side of the foot. Subcu-

taneous infiltration is performed from the Achilles tendon to the lateral malleolus, using 5–10 ml solution.
  –deep and superficial peroneal nerves (both L4–S2); the deep peroneal nerve supplies the area between the first and second toes. It lies between anterior tibial (medially) and extensor hallucis longus (laterally) tendons, lateral to the anterior tibial artery. A needle is inserted between these tendons; a click may be felt as it penetrates the extensor retinaculum. 5 ml solution is injected. The superficial peroneal nerve is blocked by subcutaneous infiltration from the lateral malleolus to the front of the tibia. It supplies the dorsum of the foot.
  –saphenous nerve (L3–4): the terminal branch of the femoral nerve; blocked by subcutaneous infiltration above and anterior to the medial malleolus. It supplies the medial side of the ankle joint.

Ankylosing spondylitis. Disease characterized by inflammation and fusion of the sacroiliac joints and lumbar vertebrae; may also involve the thoracic and cervical spine. Commonest in males, with a high proportion carrying tissue type antigen HLA B27.
• Features:
  –backache and stiffness. Spinal cord compression may occur; atlantoaxial subluxation or cervical fracture may also occur. **Spinal/extradural anaesthesia** may be difficult.
  –restricted ventilation if thoracic spine or costovertebral joints are severely affected; increased diaphragmatic movement usually preserves good lung function. **Pulmonary fibrosis** is rare.
  –tracheal intubation may be difficult due to a stiff or rigid neck, or **temporomandibular joint** involvement.
  –aortitis may occur (in less than 5% of chronic sufferers), causing **aortic regurgitation**. **Cardiomyopathy** and conduction defects are rare.
  –amyloidosis may occur.
Sinclair JR, Mason RA (1984) Anaesthesia; 39: 3–11

Anorexia nervosa. Psychiatric condition, most common in young women. Characterized by loss of weight, distortion of body image and amenorrhoea; the last results from weight loss, and psychological and endocrine factors.

- Anaesthetic considerations:
  - electrolyte disturbances, especially **hypokalaemia**, are associated with laxative abuse or self-induced vomiting.
  - tendency towards hypothermia, hypotension and bradycardia.
  - reduced lean body mass.
  - **anaemia**.
  - rare complications: myopathy, **cardiomyopathy**, peripheral neuritis, hepatic impairment, gastric dilatation.

Treatment includes behavioural and psychotherapy; **chlorpromazine** has been used in addition.

Anrep effect. Intrinsic regulatory mechanism of the heart in response to acute increases in **afterload**. Initial reduction in stroke volume and increase in left ventricular diastolic pressure are followed by restoration to near original values.

[Gleb V Anrep (1891–1955), Russian-born Egyptian physiologist]

Antacids. Used to relieve pain in **peptic ulcer disease**, **hiatus hernia** and **gastro-oesophageal reflux** by increasing gastric pH. Used preoperatively in patients at high risk from **aspiration of gastric contents**, e.g. in obstetrics. Many preparations are available; **sodium citrate** and **magnesium trisilicate** are most commonly used in anaesthetic practice. Chronic overuse of antacids may result in **alkalosis**, **hypercalcaemia** (calcium salts), constipation (aluminium salts) and diarrhoea (magnesium salts).

Antagonist. Substance that opposes the action of an **agonist**.

- Antagonism may be:
  - competitive: the substance reversibly binds to a receptor, and causes no direct response within the cell (i.e. has no **intrinsic activity**), but may cause a response by displacing an agonist, e.g. **naloxone**.
  - non-competitive: as above but with irreversible binding, e.g. **phenoxybenzamine**.
  - physiological: opposing actions are produced by binding at different receptors, e.g. **histamine** and **adrenaline** causing bronchoconstriction and bronchodilatation, respectively.

See also, Dose–response curves; Receptor theory

Antanalgesia. Increased sensitivity to painful stimuli caused by small doses of depressant drugs, e.g. **thiopentone**. Thought to result from suppression of the inhibitory action of the **ascending reticular activating system**, allowing increased cortical responsiveness (decreased pain threshold). Larger doses depress the activating system and induce sleep. Antanalgesia may also occur as blood drug levels fall, e.g. causing postoperative restlessness when barbiturates or **trimeprazine** are used as premedication, especially in children.

Antecubital fossa (Cubital fossa). Triangular fossa, anterior to the elbow joint (Fig. 8).

- Borders:
  - proximal: a line between the humeral epicondyles.

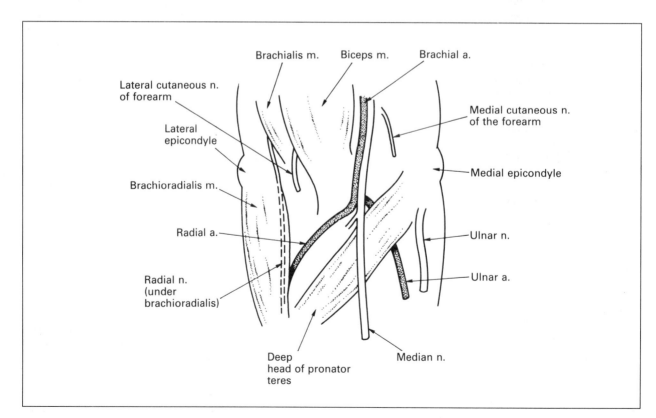

Figure 8 *Anatomy of the antecubital fossa*

–lateral: brachioradialis muscle.
–medial: pronator teres
–floor: supinator and brachialis muscles, with the joint capsule behind.
–roof: deep fascia with the median cubital vein and median cutaneous nerve on top.
• Contents from medial to lateral (embedded in fat):
–**median nerve**.
–brachial artery, dividing into **radial** and **ulnar arteries**.
–biceps tendon.
–posterior interosseus and **radial nerves**.
The bicipital aponeurosis lies between the superficial veins and deeper structures, protecting the latter during venepuncture. Damage may still be caused to nerves and arteries during this procedure; anomalous branches are relatively common. Accidental intra-arterial injection of drugs is a particular hazard.
See also, Venous drainage of arm

Anterior spinal artery syndrome. Infarction of the **spinal cord** due to anterior spinal artery insufficiency. May follow profound **hypotension**, e.g. in **spinal** or **extradural anaesthesia**. May also occur after aortic surgery. Results in lower **motor neurone** paralysis at the level of the lesion, and spastic paraplegia with reduced pain and temperature sensation below the level. Because the posterior spinal arteries supply the dorsal columns and posterior horns, joint position sense and vibration sensation are preserved.

Antiarrhythmic drugs. Classified by Vaughan Williams into four classes, depending on their effects on the **action potential** *in vitro* (Table 5). It has been suggested that **cardiac glycosides** represent a fifth class. More usefully classified for clinical purposes according to their site of action:
–atrioventricular node: **calcium channel blocking drugs**, **digoxin**, **β-adrenergic receptor antagonists** (used for supraventricular arrhythmias).
–atria, ventricles and accessory pathways: **quinidine**, **procainamide**, **disopyramide**, **amiodarone** (used for supraventricular and ventricular arrhythmias).
–ventricles only: **lignocaine**, **mexiletine**, **tocainide**, **phenytoin** (used for ventricular arrhythmias).
[EM Vaughan Williams, English pharmacologist]
Feneck RO (1990) Curr Opin Anaesth; 3: 110–6
See also, individual arrhythmias

Antibacterial drugs. Drugs used to kill bacteria (bactericidal) or inhibit bacterial replication (bacteriostatic). Antibiotics are synthesized by micro-organisms and kill or inhibit other micro-organisms. Drugs synthesized *in vitro*, e.g. sulphonamides, are not antibiotics.
• Main groups:
–β-lactams: bacteriocidal; act by inhibiting cell wall synthesis. Include:
–penicillins:
–active against Gram-negative and -positive cocci, actinomycosis, and organisms causing anthrax, gas-gangrene, syphilis and diphtheria. Ampicillin and amoxycillin have a wide spectrum, especially against Gram-negative organisms. Others, e.g. piperacillin, are also active against pseudomonas. Some penicillins are broken down by β-lactamase produced by staphylococci; Augmentin (amoxycillin plus clavulanic acid) and flucloxacillin are resistant to β-lactamase.
–enter the brain poorly unless the meninges are inflamed.
–side effects: allergy, haemolytic anaemia, encephalopathy. Many contain sodium or potassium; i.e. may represent large electrolyte loads.
–excreted mainly via urine but also in bile. Probenecid delays renal excretion.
–cephalosporins:
–broad spectrum of activity. Second generation drugs, e.g. cefuroxime, are more resistant to β-lactamase. Third generation drugs, e.g. cefotaxime and caftazidime, have greater activity against Gram-negative organisms than second generation drugs but are less active against Gram-positive bacteria. Ceftazidime has good activity against pseudomonas.
–side effects: allergy (occurs in 10% of penicillin-sensitive patients), renal toxicity, interaction with **coagulation factors**.
–excreted in urine.
–other β-lactams:
–aztreonam: active against Gram-negative organisms but poorly active against Gram-positive ones.
–imipenem: active against most aerobic and anaerobic Gram-positive and negative organisms. Given with cilastatin, which inhibits its renal breakdown.
–macrolides: bacteriostatic; act by inhibiting protein synthesis. Erythromycin is the most widely used:
–activity is similar to that of penicillin; thus used in penicillin-sensitive patients. Also active against mycoplasma, legionella and staphylococcus.

Table 5. Classification of antiarrhythmic drugs

Class	Action	Examples
I	Slow depolarization rate by inhibiting sodium influx	
a	Prolong action potential	Quinidine Procainamide Disopyramide
b	Shorten action potential	Lignocaine Mexiletine Tocainamide Phenytoin
c	No effect on action potential	Flecainide Propafenone Encainide
II	Diminish effect of catecholamines	β-adrenergic receptor antagonists Bretylium
III	Prolong action potential, without affecting depolarization rate	Amiodarone Sotalol Bretylium
IV	Inhibit calcium influx	Calcium channel blocking drugs

–painful on injection; therefore given by infusion. Causes nausea and vomiting. The estolate form may cause jaundice.

–excreted in urine and bile.

–aminoglycosides: bacteriocidal; inhibit protein synthesis.

  –broad spectrum of activity, including activity against staphylococcus and pseudomonas.

  –gentamicin and netilmicin are mainly used against Gram-negative organisms. Streptomycin is used to treat **TB**.

  –side effects: ototoxicity (especially in combination with other ototoxic drugs, e.g. **frusemide**), nephrotoxicity. They may impair neuromuscular transmission; **non-depolarizing neuromuscular blockade** may be prolonged. Blood levels should be measured.

  –excreted in urine

–tetracyclines: bacteriostatic ; inhibit protein synthesis.

  –broad spectrum of activity, but many staphylococci, streptococci and pseudomonas species are resistant. Active against mycoplasma, chlamydia and brucella.

  –may exacerbate **renal failure**.

  –excreted in urine.

–sulphonamides and trimethoprim: each alone is bacteriostatic; the combination is bacteriocidal. Impair folate metabolism. Use has decreased as bacterial resistance has increased.

  –broad spectrum of activity, but inactive against pseudomonas. Co-trimoxazole (sulphamethoxazole and trimethoprim 5:1) is active against haemophilus and pneumocystis.

  –side effects: hypersensitivity, erythema multiforme, renal impairment, bone marrow suppression.

  –excreted in urine.

–4–quinolones: bacteriocidal; impair nucleic acid replication.

  –nalidixic acid: used for Gram-negative urinary tract infections.

  –ciprofloxacin:

    –active against many Gram-positive and -negative organisms, especially the latter (including salmonella, shigella, campylobacter, neisseria and pseudomonas). Usually reserved for infections resistant to other agents.

    –side effects: GIT upsets, convulsions, rash, hepatic impairment; increased **theophylline** levels.

–others include:

  –metronidazole: bacteriostatic; impairs nucleic acid synthesis.

    –active against anaerobic organisms, including protozoa.

    –may cause **peripheral neuropathy** following prolonged therapy. An 'Antabuse' reaction may follow alcohol intake.

    –excreted in urine.

  –chloramphenicol: bacteriostatic; inhibits protein synthesis.

    –broad spectrum of activity, but inactive against pseudomonas.

    –toxicity restricts its use to salmonella and severe haemophilus infections, e.g. **meningitis**.

    –side effects: bone marrow depression (rarely aplasia), peripheral and optic neuritis, cardiovascular collapse in neonates ('grey baby syndrome').

    –excreted in urine.

  –vancomycin: bacteriocidal.

    –especially active against Gram-positive cocci, including multiresistant staphylococci.

    –side effects: hypersensitivity, renal impairment, ototoxicity, hypotension.

–those used in TB.

[Hans Gram (1853–1938), Danish physician]

Finch R (1988) Br Med J; 296: 261–4

See also, Antifungal drugs; Antiviral drugs

Antibiotics, *see Antibacterial drugs*

Antibodies, *see Immunoglobulins*

Anticholinergic drugs. Strictly, should include all drugs impairing cholinergic transmission, although the term usually refers to **antagonists** of **acetylcholine** at muscarinic receptors. Antagonists at nicotinic receptors are classified as either **ganglion blocking drugs** or **neuromuscular blocking drugs**. Effects include tachycardia, bronchodilatation, mydriasis, reduced gland secretion, smooth muscle relaxation, and sedation or restlessness.

● In anaesthesia, the most commonly used agents are **atropine**, **hyoscine** and **glycopyrronium**. Comparison of actions:

  –atropine:

    –central excitation.

    –greater action than hyoscine on the heart, bronchial smooth muscle and GIT.

  –hyoscine:

    –central depression; amnesia (may cause excitement in the elderly).

    –greater action than atropine on the pupil and sweat, salivary and bronchial glands.

  –glycopyrronium:

    –minimal central effects (quaternary ammonium ion; crosses the **blood–brain barrier** less readily than atropine and hyoscine, both tertiary ions).

    –similar peripheral actions to atropine, but with greater antisialogogue effect and less effect on the heart. Less antiemetic action than hyoscine and atropine.

    –longer duration of action.

● Other uses of anticholinergic drugs include:

  –antispasmodic effect (on bowel and bladder), e.g. propantheline.

  –ulcer healing, e.g. pirenzepine.

  –bronchodilatation, e.g. **ipratropium**.

  –mydriasis and cycloplegia (dilatation of pupil and paralysis of accommodation), e.g. atropine.

Anticholinergic **antiparkinsonian drugs**, e.g. benztropine, are used for their central effects.

Mirakhur RK (1988) Can J Anaesth; 35: 443–7

See also, Acetylcholine receptors; Central anticholinergic syndrome; Muscarine and muscarinic receptors; Nicotine and nicotinic receptors

Anticholinesterases, *see Acetylcholinesterase inhibitors*

Anticoagulant drugs. Mechanisms of action:

–prevent synthesis of **coagulation** factors, e.g. **warfarin**.

4

–inhibit existing factors, e.g. **heparin**.
–inhibit **platelet** aggregation, i.e. **antiplatelet drugs**.
–break down circulating fibrinogen, e.g. ancrod (snake venom derivative; not commonly used).

Fibrinolytic drugs break down thrombus once formed. Warfarin and heparin are more effective at preventing venous thrombus than arterial thrombus, as the former contains relatively more fibrin. Antiplatelet drugs are more effective in arterial blood, where thrombus contains many platelets and little fibrin. Patients recieving warfarin or heparin should have their clotting investigated preoperatively.

Stow PJ, Burrows FA (1987) Can J Anaesth; 34: 632–49

Anticonvulsant drugs. Postulated mechanism of action is via activation of the **GABA** receptor complex. Activation is enhanced by:
–**benzodiazepines**, via a specific receptor.
–**phenytoin** and **barbiturates**, via blockade of the picrotoxin receptor (picrotoxin, an **analeptic drug**, antagonizes the action of GABA by acting on an adjacent receptor).
–vigabatrin, via direct GABA receptor agonism or inhibition of GABA breakdown.

Diazepam is most commonly used for emergency treatment of **convulsions**. **Thiopentone** is also used, especially perioperatively.
● For treatment of **epilepsy**, certain drugs are more likely to succeed:
–grand mal: phenytoin, **phenobarbitone**, primidone, **carbamazepine**.
–petit mal: ethosuximide, **clonazepam**, **sodium valproate**.
–focal epilepsy: as for grand mal.

Patients on anticonvulsant therapy should continue medication up to surgery, and recommence treatment as soon as possible postoperatively. If oral therapy is delayed postoperatively, parenteral administration may be substituted. Phenobarbitone and phenytoin cause hepatic **enzyme induction** and increase certain drug metabolism.

See also, Status epilepticus

Antidepressant drugs. Most increase central amine concentrations (e.g. **dopamine, noradrenaline, 5–HT**), supporting the theory that depression results from amine deficiency. Further evidence is that central depletion (e.g. by **reserpine)** may cause depression.
● May be classified thus:
–**tricyclic antidepressant drugs** and related substances; block noradrenaline uptake from synapses.
–**monoamine oxidase inhibitors** (MAOIs); prevent catecholamine breakdown.
–others, e.g. **lithium**. Mechanism of action is unknown.

Perioperative problems arising from concurrent antidepressant therapy may occur, particularly with MAOIs.

Antidiuretic hormone, *see Vasopressin*

Antiemetic drugs. Most act on the vomiting centre directly, e.g. **antihistamine** and **anticholinergic drugs**, or on the **chemoreceptor trigger zone** (CTZ), e.g. **phenothiazines, butyrophenones** and **metoclopramide**. The latter group are **dopamine receptor** antagonists. In addition, metoclopramide increases **lower oesophageal sphincter** tone and gastric emptying by a peripheral action.

Metoclopramide in very high dosage is thought to act via central **5-HT** receptors; a specific 5-HT$_3$-receptor antagonist, **ondansetron**, is now available.

Dopamine antagonists are suitable for treatment of **vomiting** associated with **morphine**, which stimulates the CTZ. Increased vestibular stimulation of the vomiting centre, e.g. in motion sickness, is best treated with drugs acting on the vomiting centre, e.g. **hyoscine**. Sedation is a common side effect, particularly of antihistamines, anticholinergic drugs and phenothiazines. In addition, phenothiazines may cause hypotension, and all dopamine antagonists may cause **dystonic reactions**.

Rowbotham DJ (1992) Br J Anaesth; 69: 46S–59S

Antiendotoxin antibodies. Monoclonal human antibodies which bind to many **endotoxins** and Gram-negative bacteria isolates. May reduce mortality from Gram-negative **septicaemia**, especially **septic shock**, by up to 40%. They are given iv in one dose (100 mg over 15–30 minutes), as early as possible in septicaemia. Ineffective in patients without bacteraemia, and extremely expensive (over £2000 per dose); thus strict protocols have been suggested to maximize cost-effectiveness. Withdrawn in 1993 as they may increase mortality in patients without Gram-negative sepsis.

Warren HS, Danner RL, Munford RS (1992) New Engl J Med; 326: 1153–7

Antifibrinolytic drugs. Aminocaproic acid and **tranexamic acid** inhibit plasminogen activation and thus reduce **fibrinolysis**. Sometimes used to reduce bleeding after prostatectomy and dental extraction.

See also, Coagulation

Antifungal drugs. Heterogeneous group of drugs, including:
–amphotericin: penetrates tissues poorly. Given iv. Side effects include GIT disturbances, renal toxicity, hypokalaemia, hypomagnesaemia, hypotension, blood dyscrasias and convulsions.
–flucytosine: given iv or orally. May cause GIT disturbances and blood dyscrasias.
–griseofulvin: given orally. May cause headache, hepatic impairment, and reduced activity of **warfarin**.
–miconazole and fluconazole: may be given iv or orally. Side effects include GIT disturbances and rash. Parenteral miconazole preparations contain **Cremaphor EL**. Itraconazole is given orally and is active against Aspergillus; it undergoes significant **first-pass metabolism** and should not be given in liver disease.
–nystatin: given topically only.

Davey PG (1991) Br Med J; 300: 793–8

Antigen. Substance which may provoke an immune response, then react with the cells or antibodies produced. Usually a protein or carbohydrate molecule. Some substances (called haptens), too small to provoke immune reactions alone, may combine with host molecules, e.g. proteins, to form a larger antigenic combination.

Antigravity suit. Garment used to apply pressure to the lower half of the body, in order to increase blood volume in the upper half and prevent hypotension, e.g. in the sitting position in **neurosurgery**. Systolic BP and CVP are increased; the latter may aid prevention of **air embolism**.

Modern suits are inflated pneumatically around the legs and abdomen, to a pressure of 2–8 kPa.

Military antishock trousers (MAST) have been used in **trauma** to produce similar effects. They also splint broken bones and apply pressure to bleeding points.

Broderick PM, Ingram GS (1988) Anaesthesia; 43: 762–5

Antihistamine drugs. Refers to H_1 **histamine receptor antagonists**.

● Uses:
 –treatment of allergic disorders, e.g. hay fever and urticaria, e.g. **chlorpheniramine**.
 –**premedication**, e.g. **promethazine** and **trimeprazine**.

They have anticholinergic effects (e.g. dry mouth, blurring of vision, urinary retention) and sedative properties, and are **antiemetic drugs** acting on the vomiting centre. Newer drugs, e.g. terfenadine, cross the **blood–brain barrier** to a lesser extent, causing less sedation.

See also, H_2 receptor antagonists

Antihypertensive drugs. Drugs used to reduce BP may act at different sites (Fig. 9):
 –**diuretics**: reduce **ECF** volume initially and also cause vasodilatation (1).
 –**vasodilator drugs**: act on the vascular smooth muscle (2), either directly, e.g. **hydralazine**, **sodium nitroprusside**, or indirectly, e.g. **α-adrenergic receptor antagonists**, **calcium channel blocking drugs**. **Angiotensin converting enzyme inhibitors** also decrease water and sodium retention.
 –**β-adrenergic receptor antagonists**: lower cardiac output (3).
 –adrenergic neurone blocking drugs (4): e.g. **guanethidine** depletes nerve endings of noradrenaline, preventing its release. **Reserpine** prevents storage and release of noradrenaline. **α-Methyl-*p*-tyrosine** inhibits dopa formation from tyrosine.
 –**ganglion blocking drugs** (5).

–centrally-acting drugs (6): reduce sympathetic activity, e.g. reserpine, **α-methyldopa**, **clonidine**.

In addition, anaesthetic agents and techniques may reduce BP; e.g. **halothane** depresses **baroreceptor** activity (7) and also reduces sympathetic activity and cardiac output; **spinal** and **extradural anaesthesia** block sympathetic outflow (8).

In the treatment of **hypertension**, thiazide diuretics, β-adrenergic receptor antagonists and oral vasodilators (except for α-adrenergic receptor antagonists) are used most commonly. Ganglion blockers, adrenergic neurone blocking drugs and the centrally-acting drugs are seldom used, because of their side effects.

In the treatment of a **hypertensive crisis**, vasodilator drugs are often given iv.

Antihypertensive drugs should be continued up to surgery, and recommenced as soon as possible postoperatively.

See also, Hypotensive anaesthesia

Antimitotic drugs. Used in the treatment of **malignancy**. All may cause nausea and vomiting, and bone marrow suppression. Some have side effects of particular anaesthetic relevance:
 –alkylating agents: cyclophosphamide may prolong the effect of **suxamethonium**; busulphan may cause **pulmonary fibrosis**.
 –vinca alkaloids: vincristine and vinblastine may cause **autonomic neuropathy** and **peripheral neuropathy**.
 –antibiotics: doxorubicin may cause **cardiomyopathy**; bleomycin may cause pulmonary fibrosis.
 –others: cisplatin may cause nephrotoxicity, ototoxicity and peripheral neuropathy; procarbazine has **monoamine oxidase inhibitor** effects.

O_2 therapy has been implicated in exacerbating the pulmonary fibrosis caused by antimitotic drugs.

Antiparkinsonian drugs. Treatment of **Parkinson's disease** is directed towards increasing central dopaminergic activity, or decreasing cholinergic activity:
 –increasing **dopamine**:
  –levodopa: crosses the **blood–brain barrier** and is converted to dopamine by dopa decarboxylase. Decarboxylase inhibitors (carbidopa, benserazide) which do not cross the blood–brain barrier prevent peripheral dopamine formation, thus reducing the dose of levodopa required and incidence of side effects. Levodopa is most effective for bradykinesia. Its use may be limited by nausea and vomiting, dystonic movements, postural hypotension and psychiatric disturbances. Improvement is usually only temporary and may exhibit 'on–off' effectiveness.
  –bromocriptine, lysuride and pergolide: dopamine agonists.
  –amantadine: increases release of endogenous dopamine.
  –selegiline: **monoamine oxidase inhibitor** type B.
  –**amphetamines** have been used.
 –**anticholinergic drugs**, e.g. **atropine**, benztropine, benzhexol, procyclidine: most effective for rigidity, tremor, and treatment of drug-induced parkinsonism. For acute drug-induced **dystonic reactions**, benztropine 1–2 mg or procyclidine 5–10 mg may be given iv.

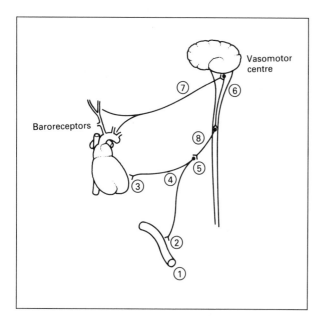

Figure 9 *Sites of action of antihypertensive drugs (see text)*

There is a higher risk of intraoperative arrhythmias and labile BP in patients taking these drugs.
Stewart DA, MacPhee GJA (1991) Hosp Update; 17: 900–11

Antiplatelet drugs. Reduce **platelet** adhesion and aggregation. Low-dose **salicylates**, e.g. **aspirin**, and other **NSAIDs** irreversibly inhibit platelet cyclo-oxygenase and **thomboxane** A_2 production. **Dipyridamole** acts by increasing intraplatelet **cAMP** levels. **Dextran** also has an antiplatelet action. Low-dose aspirin and dipyridamole are prescribed to improve arterial blood supply in peripheral vascular disease and cerebrovascular disease. Aspirin has been shown to be beneficial in preventing mortality in **ischaemic heart disease**. Dextran infusion has been used to prevent postoperative **DVT** and **PE**. **Prostacyclin** has been used to prevent platelet aggregation.
See also, Anticoagulant drugs; Coagulation

Antistatic precautions. Employed in operating suites, to prevent build-up of static electricity with possible sparks, **explosions and fires**. Surfaces and materials should have relatively low electrical resistance, to allow leakage of charge to earth, but not so low as to allow **electrocution and electical burns**.
● Precautions include:
  –avoidance of wool, nylon, silk, etc., which may generate static charge. Cotton blankets and clothing are suitable (resistance is very low in moist atmospheres).
  –antistatic rubber (containing carbon) for tubing, etc. Coloured black with yellow labels for identification. Resistance is 100 000–10 000 000 ohms/cm.
  –terazzo floor (stone pieces embedded in cement and polished): resistance should be 20 000–5 000 000 ohms between two points 60 cm apart.
  –trolleys and other equipment have conducting wheels; staff wear antistatic footwear.
Sparks are more likely in cold dry atmospheres, therefore relative **humidity** should exceed 50% and temperature exceed 20°C.
  The requirement for expensive antistatic flooring and other precautions has been questioned, since the use of flammable agents is declining.

Antiviral drugs. Heterogeneous group of drugs with generally non-specific actions. Parenteral use is usually reserved for severe life-threatening systemic infections, especially in the immunocompromised patient. Available drugs include:
  –acyclovir: purine nucleoside analogue; after phosphorylation, it inhibits viral DNA polymerase. Phosphorylated by, and therefore active against, herpes simplex and varicella zoster viruses. Early initiation of treatment is important. May be useful in **HIV infection**. May be given topically, orally or iv; side effects include GIT upset, rashes, and deteriorating renal and liver function.
  –phosphonoformate and ganciclovir: both drugs inhibit DNA polymerase and are active against cytomegalovirus. Side effects are common, including neutropenia, vomiting and hepatic impairment. Ganciclovir is similar to acyclovir but much more toxic; thus reserved for severe cytomegalovirus infection.
  –zidovudine (azidothymidine: AZT): thymidine deriv-

ative; inhibits DNA synthesis via incorporation into DNA. Given orally in HIV infection; prolongs life but bone marrow depression and nausea are common.
  –interferons: produced by infected cells, preventing viral growth and stimulating body defences. Still being evaluated.
  –amantadine: also used in **Parkinson's disease**. Affects the virus wall. Has been used to prevent influenza, and to treat shingles.
  –ribavirin: nucleoside; inhibits DNA synthesis. Has been used to treat respiratory syncytial viral infection and Lassa fever. Side effects are rare.
Davey PG (1991) BMJ; 300: 793–8

Antoine equation. Describes the theoretical variation of **SVP** with temperature. Empirically relates SVP to three constants, derived from experimental data for each substance.
[C Antoine (described 1888), French scientist]

Aortic aneurysm, abdominal. Anaesthetic considerations for elective repair:
  –**preoperative assessment** is particularly directed to the effects of widespread **atherosclerosis**, i.e. affecting coronary, renal, cerebral and peripheral arteries. **Hypertension** is also common.
  –peroperatively:
    –monitoring: ECG; direct arterial, central venous and possibly pulmonary artery pressure measurement; temperature; **urine** output. **Capnography**, pulse **oximetry** and arterial blood gas analysis are necessary.
    –at least two large bore iv cannulae.
    –warming blanket and warming of iv fluids. **Humidification** of inspired gases.
    –cardiovascular responses:
      –hypertension during tracheal intubation.
      –increased **afterload** caused by aortic crossclamping. Hypertension and left ventricular failure may occur. Anticipatory use of **vasodilator drugs** may help to reduce hypertension and left ventricular strain.
      –reduction of afterload, return of vasodilator metabolites from lower part of the body, and possible haemorrhage following aortic unclamping (declamping syndrome). **Myocardial contractility** is reduced by the acidotic venous return. Anticipatory volume loading prior to unclamping, with termination of vasodilator therapy before slow controlled release of the clamp, may reduce hypotension. **Bicarbonate** therapy is guided by arterial acid–base analysis; it often not required if clamping time is less than 1–1.5 hours.
  –blood loss and effects of massive **blood transfusion**.
  –postoperative visceral dysfunction:
    –**renal failure** may follow aortic surgery; it is more likely to occur after suprarenal crossclamping. **Mannitol** or renal dosage of **dopamine** are often given before aortic clamping, to encourage diuresis.
    –GIT ischaemia and infarction may occur if the mesenteric arterial supply is interrupted.
  Attempts to reduce the effects of renal and GIT

ischaemia have also included **hypothermia** and use of metabolic precursors e.g. **inosine**.

–postoperatively: ICU or HDU. Elective IPPV may be required.

• For **emergency surgery**, the following are important:

–preinduction monitoring and insertion of lines.

–preparation and towelling of the patient before induction.

–availability of blood, O negative if necessary.

–rapid sequence induction. **Etomidate** or **ketamine** are usually used.

Severe hypotension may occur when the abdominal muscles relax after induction. Prognosis is generally poor.

Cunningham AJ (1992) Curr Opin Anaesth; 5: 34–48

See also, Aortic aneurysm, thoracic; Blood transfusion, massive; Induction, rapid sequence

Aortic aneurysm, thoracic. Usually results from dissection; classified according to site:

–type I: starts in the ascending aorta, extending proximally to the aortic valve and distally around the aortic arch (least common).

–type II: limited to the ascending aorta.

–type III: starts near the left subclavian artery, extending along the descending aorta.

Surgical approach is via left thoracotomy; **one-lung anaesthesia** facilitates surgery. Concurrent aortic valve replacement may be required. General anaesthetic management is as for abdominal aneurysm repair. Cardiovascular instability may be more dramatic because of the proximity of the aortic clamp to the heart, and the reduction of venous return and cardiac output during surgical maneouvres. Complications include haemorrhage and infarction of spinal cord, liver, gut, kidneys and heart. Operative techniques may include atriofemoral **cardiopulmonary bypass**, or use of a shunt across the clamped aortic section.

Shenaq SA (1992) Curr Opin Anaesth; 5: 62–7

See also, Aortic aneurysm, abdominal

Aortic bodies. Peripheral **chemoreceptors** near the aortic arch. Similar in structure and function to the **carotid bodies**. Afferents pass to the medulla via the vagus.

Aortic coarctation, *see Coarctation of aorta*

Aortic counter-pulsation balloon pump, *see Intra-aortic counter-pulsation balloon pump*

Aortic dissection. Passage of blood into the aortic wall, usually involving the media of the vessel. Degeneration of this layer is usually caused by **atherosclerosis**, and usually occurs in the ascending aorta. Often associated with **hypertension**. Dissection may involve branches of the aorta, including the coronary arteries. Additionally, rupture into pericardium, pleural cavity, mediastinum or abdomen may occur.

• Features:

–severe tearing central chest pain; may mimic **MI**. May radiate to the back or abdomen.

–signs of **aortic regurgitation**.

–signs of **haemorrhage** or **cardiac tamponade**.

–progressive loss of radial pulses and **CVA** may indicate extension along the aortic arch. Coronary artery involvement may cause MI. Renal vessels may be involved.

–**chest X-ray** may reveal a widened mediastinum or **pleural effusion**. **Echocardiography**, **CAT scanning** and aortography may be used in diagnosis.

• Management:

–analgesia.

–control of BP, e.g. using **vasodilator drugs**.

–surgery is increasingly employed, especially if the aortic valve is involved, dissection progresses or rupture occurs. Management: as for thoracic aortic aneurysm.

Asfoura JY, Vidt DG (1991) Chest; 99: 724–9

See also, Aortic aneurysm, thoracic

Aortic regurgitation. Retrograde flow of blood through the aortic valve during diastole. Causes left ventricular hypertrophy and dilatation, with greatly increased stroke volume. Later, compliance decreases and end-diastolic pressure increases, with ventricular failure.

• Caused by:

–**rheumatic fever**; the mitral valve is usually involved too.

–**aortic dissection**.

–**endocarditis** (especially acute regurgitation).

–**Marfan's syndrome**.

–congenital (associated with **aortic stenosis**).

–**chest trauma, ankylosing spondylitis, syphilis**.

• Features:

–collapsing **pulse** with widened pulse pressure (water-hammer).

–early diastolic murmur, high pitched and blowing. Loudest in expiration and with the patient leaning forward, and heard at the left sternal edge, sometimes at the apex. The 3rd **heart sound** may be present. A thrill is absent. An aortic ejection murmur is usually present, radiating to the neck; a mid-diastolic mitral murmur may be present due to obstruction by aortic backflow (Austin Flint murmur).

–left ventricular failure.

–angina is usually late.

–investigations: **ECG** may show left ventricular hypertrophy; **chest X-ray** may show ventricular enlargement/failure. **Echocardiography** and **cardiac catheterization** are also useful.

• Anaesthetic management:

–antibiotic prophylaxis as for **congenital heart disease**.

–general principles: as for **cardiac surgery/ischaemic heart disease**. **Myocardial ischaemia** and left ventricular failure may occur.

–the following should be avoided:

–bradycardia: increases time for regurgitation.

–peripheral vasoconstriction and increased diastolic pressure: increases afterload and therefore regurgitation. Peripheral vasodilatation reduces regurgitation and increases forward flow.

–**cardioplegia** solution is infused directly into the coronary arteries during cardiac surgery, since if injected into the aortic root it will enter the ventricle.

–**left ventricular end-diastolic pressure** may be much greater than measured **pulmonary capillary wedge pressure**, if the mitral valve is closed early by the regurgitant backflow.

–postoperative hypertension may occur.

[Austin Flint (1812–1886), US physician]

See also, Heart murmurs; Preoperative assessment; Valvular heart disease

Aortic stenosis. Narrowed aortic valve with obstruction to the left ventricular outflow, resulting in a pressure gradient between the left ventricle and aortic root. Initially, left ventricular hypertrophy and increased force of contraction maintain **stroke volume**. Compliance is decreased. **Coronary blood flow** is decreased due to increased **left ventricular end diastolic pressure** and involvement of the coronary sinuses, whilst left ventricular work increases. Ultimately, contractility falls, with left ventricular dilatation and reduced cardiac output.

- Caused by:
  - –rheumatic fever: may present at any age (usually also involves the mitral valve).
  - –congenital bicuspid valve: usually presents in middle age.
  - –degenerative calcification: usually in the elderly.
- Features:
  - –angina, syncope, left ventricular failure.
  - –sudden death.
  - –low volume slow-rising pulse with reduced pulse pressure (plateau pulse). **AF** usually signifies coexistant mitral disease.
  - –ejection systolic murmur, radiating to the neck. Loudest in the aortic area, with the patient sitting forward in expiration. The second **heart sound** is quiet, with reversed splitting if stenosis is severe (due to delayed left ventricular emptying). A thrill, 4th sound and ejection click may be present.
  - –investigations: **ECG** may show left ventricular hypertrophy; **chest X-ray** may show ventricular enlargement/failure, possibly with calcification and post stenotic dilatation. **Echocardiography** and **cardiac catheterization** are also useful.
- Anaesthetic management:
  - –antibiotic prophylaxis as for **congenital heart disease**.
  - –general principles: as for **cardiac surgery/ischaemic heart disease**. **Myocardial ischaemia**, ventricular arrhythmias and left ventricular failure may occur.
  - –the following should be avoided:
    - –loss of sinus rhythm: atrial contraction is vital to maintain adequate ventricular filling.
    - –peripheral vasodilatation: cardiac output is fixed, therefore BP may fall dramatically causing myocardial ischaemia.
    - –excessive peripheral vasoconstriction: further reduces left ventricular outflow.
    - –tachycardia: ventricular filling is impaired and coronary blood flow reduced.
    - –myocardial depression.
  - –postoperative hypertension may occur.

See also, Heart murmurs; Preoperative assessment; Valvular heart disease

Aortocaval compression (Supine hypotension syndrome). Compression of the great vessels against the vertebral bodies by the gravid uterus in the supine position in late **pregnancy**. Vena caval compression reduces venous return and cardiac output with a compensatory increase in SVR; this may be symptomless ('concealed'), or associated with hypotension, bradycardia or syncope ('revealed'). Reduced placental blood flow may result from the reduced cardiac output, vasoconstriction and compression of the aorta. During uterine contractions, the compression may worsen (**Poseiro effect**). Reduced cardiac output is more likely to occur if vasoconstrictor reflexes are impaired, e.g. during regional or general anaesthesia. May be reduced by tilting the mother to one side e.g. with a wedge. Up to 45° tilt may be required. Left lateral tilt is usually preferable.

See also, Obstetric analgesia and anaesthesia

Aortovelography. Use of a **Doppler** ultrasound probe in the suprasternal notch to measure blood velocity and acceleration in the ascending aorta. Used for **cardiac output measurement**, but inaccurate.

APACHE scoring system (Acute physiology and chronic health evaluation). Used on **ICU** to assess the severity of illness in individual patients and to allow stratification of patient groups in order to compare different therapies. APACHE I (introduced in 1981) assessed 34 physiological measurements, but was replaced in 1985 by APACHE II, which assessed 12. 11 of these physiological variables are each allocated points from 0 to 4 according to their deviation from the normal range. The sum of these variables is added to a numerical assessment of neurological function (15 minus **Glasgow Coma Scale**) to make up the Acute Physiology Score (APS), which is added in turn to numerical assessments of chronic health and age to produce the APACHE II score, out of a maximum of 71 (Table 6). APACHE II has been validated in many large centres and has been shown to be a reliable method for estimating group outcome amongst ICU patients. Scores may be weighted according to illness to give a mortality prediction for a particular patient. Originally, the worst result during the first 24 hours of admission to ICU was recorded. Survival rates of 50% have been reported for an admission score of about 25 points, with 80% mortality for scores above 35 points. More recently, repeated assessments have been used to chart patients' progress. Methods of improving the predictive power of APACHE II have been studied (APACHE III).

Supplement (1989) Crit Care Med; 17: S169–221
See also, Mortality/survival prediction on intensive care unit

Apgar scoring system. Widely used method of evaluating the condition of the **neonate**. Points are awarded up to a maximum total of 10 according to clinical findings (Table 7). Assessments are commonly performed at 1 and 5 minutes after birth, but may be repeated as necessary. Colour may be omitted from the observed signs to give a maximum score of 8 (Apgar minus colour score).
[Virginia Apgar (1909–1975), US anaesthetist]

Apneustic centre, *see Breathing, control of*

Apnoea. Absence of breathing. Causes are as for **hypoventilation**. Results in **hypercapnia** and **hypoxaemia**. The rate of onset and severity of hypoxaemia are related to the F_IO_2, **FRC** and O_2 consumption. Thus **preoxygenation** delays the onset of hypoxaemia following apnoea. In **pregnancy**, hypoxaemia develops more quickly, due to reduced FRC and increased O_2 consumption.

Alveolar PCO_2 rises at about 0.5 kPa/min (3.8 mmHg/min) when CO_2 production is normal.

In paediatrics, prematurity is a major cause of recurrent apnoea. In newborn animals, induced hypoxaemia results in vigorous efforts to breathe, followed by primary apnoea and bradycardia, then secondary (terminal) apnoea after a few

Table 6. APACHE II scoring system

Physiological variable	High abnormal range				0	Low abnormal range			
	+4	+3	+2	+1	0	+1	+2	+3	+4
Temperature – rectal (°C)	≥41°	39°–40.9°		38.5°–38.9°	36°–38.4°	34°–35.9°	32°–33.9°	30°–31.9°	≤29.9°
Mean arterial pressure (mmHg)	≥160	130–159	110–129		70–109		50–69		≤49
Heart rate (ventricular response)	≥180	140–179	110–139		70–109		55–69	40–54	≤39
Respiratory rate – (non-ventilated or ventilated)	≥50	35–49		25–34	12–24	10–11	6–9		≤5
Oxygenation: A-aDo₂ or Pao₂ (kPa(mmHg)) (a) Flo₂≥0.5 record A-aDo₂	>67 (>500)	47–66.9 (350–499)	27–46.9 (200–349)		<27 (<200)				
(b) Flo₂<0.5 record only Pao₂					>9.3 (>70)	8.1–9.3 (61–70)		7.3–8.0 (55–60)	<7.3 (<55)
Arterial pH	≥7.7	7.6–7.69		7.5–7.59	7.33–7.49		7.25–7.32	7.15–7.24	<7.15
Serum sodium (mmol/l)	≥180	160–179	155–159	150–154	130–149		120–129	111–119	≤110
Serum potassium (mmol/l)	≥7	6–6.9		5.5–5.9	3.5–5.4	3–3.4	2.5–2.9		<2.5
Serum creatinine (mmol/l (mg/100 ml)) (Double point score for *acute* renal failure)	>301 (≥3.5)	170–300 (2–3.4)	130–169 (1.5–1.9)		50–129 (0.6–1.4)		<50 (<0.6)		
Haematocrit (%)	≥60		50–59.9	46–49.9	30–45.9		20–29.9		<20
White blood count (total/mm³) (in 1000s)	≥40		20–39.9	15–19.9	3–14.9		1–2.9		<1
Glasgow Coma Score (GCS) Score = 15 minus actual GCS									
[A] Total Acute Phsiology Score (APS) Sum of the 12 individual variable points									
Serum HCO, (venous mmol/l) (Not preferred, use if no ABGs)	≥52	41–51.9		32–40.9	22–31.9		18–21.9	15–17.9	<15

[B] AGE POINTS

Assign points to age as follows:

AGE (years)	Points
≤44	0
45–54	2
55–64	3
65–74	5
≥75	6

[C] CHRONIC HEALTH POINTS

If the patient has a histor of severe organ system insufficiency or is immunocompromised assign points as follows:

(a) for non-operative or emergency postoperative patients – 5 points

or

(b) for elective postoperative patients – 2 points

DEFINITIONS

Organ insufficiency or immunocompromised state must have been evident *prior* to this hospital admission and conform to the following criteria:

LIVER Biopsy proven cirrhosis and documented portal hypetension; episodes of past upper GI bleeding attributed to portal hypertension, or prior episodes of hepatic failure/encephalopathy/coma

CARDIOVASCULAR New York Heart Association Class IV (inability to perform physical activity)

RESPIRATORY: Chronic restrictive, obstructive, or vascular disease resulting in severe exercise restriction, i.e. unable to climb stairs or perform household duties, or documented chronic hypoxia, hypercapna, secondary polycythaemia, severe pulmonary hypertension (>40 mmHg), or respiratory dependency

RENAL: Receiving chronic dialysis

IMMUNOCOMPROMISED: The patient has received therapy that suppresses resistance to infection, e.g. immunosuppression, chemotherapy, radiation, long-term or recent high dose steroids, or has a disease that is sufficiently advanced to suppress resistance to infection, e.g. leukaemia, lymphoma, AIDS

APACHE II SCORE

Sum of [A] + [B] + [C]

[A] APS points

[B] Age points

[C] Chronic Health points

Total APACHE II

---

gasps. During primary apnoea, gasping and possibly spontaneous respiration may be induced by stimulation; the **gasp reflex** is also active. During secondary apnoea, active resuscitation and oxygenation is required to restore breathing.

See also, Cardiopulmonary resuscitation, neonatal; Sleep apnoea

Apnoeic oxygenation. Method of delivering O_2 to the lungs by insufflation during apnoea. A catheter is passed into the trachea, its tip lying at the carina. O_2 passed through it at 4–6 l/min reaches the alveoli mainly by mass diffusion, with O_2 utilized faster than CO_2 is produced. The technique does not remove CO_2, which rises at a rate of approximately 0.5 kPa/min (3.8 mmHg/min) at normal rates of CO_2 production. **Hypercapnia** may therefore occur during prolonged procedures.

May be used to maintain oxygenation e.g. during **bronchoscopy**, or during the diagnosis of **brainstem death**.

See also, Insufflation techniques

Table 7. Apgar scoring system

Sign	Score 0	Score 1	Score 2
Heart rate	Absent	<100	>100
Respiratory effort	Absent	Weak cry	Strong cry
Muscle tone	Limp	Poor tone	Good tone
Reflex irritability	No response	Some movement	Strong withdrawal
Colour	Blue, pale	Pink body, blue extremities	Pink

Apomorphine. Alkaloid derived from **morphine**, with powerful **dopamine** agonist action. Causes intense stimulation of the **chemoreceptor trigger zone** resulting in **vomiting**. Has been used as an **emetic drug** to empty the stomach, e.g. preoperatively, but rarely used now because of its inefficiency and unpleasantness. 3–5 mg is diluted in 10 ml saline; 1 ml increments are given iv until vomiting occurs. **Atropine** reduces accompanying salivation.

Aprotinin. Proteolytic enzyme inhibitor. Inhibits:
 –plasmin (at low dose, causing reduced **fibrinolysis**).
 –**kallikrein** (at higher dose, causing reduced **coagulation**).
 –trypsin.
Intermediate doses cause reduced **platelet** aggregation. Has been used to reduce peroperative blood loss, e.g. in **TURP** and **cardiac surgery**. Its usefulness in acute **pancreatitis** is doubtful.
- Dosage: 500 000–1 000 000 Kallikrein Inactivator Units (KIU), given slowly iv; 50 000–200 000 KIU may be given hourly if haemorrhage continues. 2 000 000 KIU followed by 500 000 KIU/h has been used in cardiac surgery.
Hypersensitivity reactions may occur.
Boscoe MJ, Hunt BJ (1992) Br J Clin Pract; 46:9–12

APRV, *see Airway pressure release ventilation*

Apudomas. Tumours of *a*mine *p*recursor *u*ptake and *d*ecarboxylation (APUD) cells. APUD cells are present in the anterior **pituitary gland**, **thyroid gland**, **adrenal gland** medulla, GIT, pancreatic islets, **carotid body** and **lung**. Originally thought to arise from neural crest tissue; now thought to be derived from endoderm. They have similar structural and biochemical properties, secreting polypeptides and amines. They may secrete hormones which cause systemic disturbances, e.g. **insulin**, **glucagon**, **catecholamines**, **5–HT**, **somatostatin**, gastrin and **vasoactive intestinal peptide**.
See also, Carcinoid syndrome; Multiple endocrine adenomatosis; Phaeochromocytoma

Arachidonic acid. Essential fatty acid synthesized from phospholipids and metabolized by lipoxygenase and cyclo-oxygenase to **leukotrienes** and endoperoxides respectively (Fig. 10). Endoperoxides form **prostaglandins**, **prostacyclin** and **thromboxanes** via separate pathways. The pathways are inhibited by **steroid therapy** and **NSAIDs** as shown.
Holtzman MJ (1992) Am Rev Resp Dis; 43: 188–203

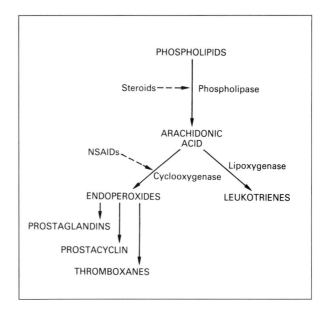

Figure 10 *Arachidonic acid pathways;* - - ► *indicates inhibition*

Arachnoiditis. Inflammation of the arachnoid and pial **meninges**. Has occurred after **spinal** and **extradural anaesthesia**; antiseptic solutions and preservatives in drug solutions (e.g. sodium bisulphite) have been implicated. Also occurs after radiotherapy, trauma and myelography with oil-based contrast media. May occur months or years after the insult. Progressive fibrosis may cause spinal canal narrowing, ischaemia and permanent nerve damage. The cauda equina is usually affected, with pain, muscle weakness, and loss of sphincter control. May rarely spread cranially. Response to treatment is generally poor.

ARAS, *see Ascending reticular activating system*

ARDS, *see Adult respiratory distress syndrome*

Arginine vasopressin, *see Vasopressin*

Arm–brain circulation time. Time taken for a substance injected into an arm vein (traditionally antecubital) to reach the brain. If a bile salt is injected, the time until arrival of the bitter taste at the tongue may be measured (normally 10–20 s; this may be greatly prolonged when cardiac output is reduced). Useful conceptually when comparing different **iv induction agents**; thus **thiopentone** acts 'within one arm–brain circulation time', whereas **midazolam** takes longer.

Arrhythmias. Disturbances in normal sinus rhythm.
- Classification:
 –disorders of impulse formation:
 –supraventricular:
 –**sinus arrhythmia**, **bradycardia**, and **tachycardia**.
 –**SVT** .
 –**sick sinus syndrome**.
 –**AF**, **atrial flutter**, **atrial ectopic beats**.
 –**junctional arrhythmias**.
 –**VF**, **ventricular tachycardia**, **ventricular ectopic beats**.

–disorders of impulse conduction:
  –slowed/blocked conduction (e.g. **heart block**).
  –abnormal pathway of conduction (e.g. **Wolff–Parkinson–White syndrome**).

During anaesthesia, ECG monitoring is mandatory. Bradycardia, junctional rhythm and ventricular ectopic beats (including bigemini) are common, but usually not serious.

- Arrhythmias are more likely with:
  –**hypoxaemia** and **hypercapnia**.
  –deep inhalational anaesthesia, especially with agents that sensitize the myocardium to **catecholamines**, e.g. **halothane** and **cyclopropane**.
  –surgical stimulation and light anaesthesia. Particularly common during **dental surgery** and visceral manipulation.
  –electrolyte imbalance, especially of **potassium**.
  –pre-existing cardiac disease.
  –use of **adrenaline** or **cocaine** as vasopressors.
  –**central venous/pulmonary artery catheterization**.

Arterial blood pressure. The pulsatile ejection of the **stroke volume** gives rise to the **arterial wave form**, from which systolic, diastolic and **mean arterial pressures** may be determined.

MAP = **cardiac output** × **SVR**

Thus arterial pressure may vary with changes in cardiac output (stroke volume × **heart rate**) and vascular resistance.

- Control of BP:
  –short term:
    –intrinsic regulatory properties of the heart: **Anrep effect**, **Bowditch effect**, **Starling's law**.
    –autonomic pathways involving **baroreceptors**, **vasomotor centre** and **cardioinhibitory centre**.
    –hormonal mechanisms:
      –**renin/angiotensin system**.
      –**vasopressin**.
      –**adrenaline** and **noradrenaline** as part of the sympathetic response.
  –intermediate/long term: renin/angiotensin system, **aldosterone**, vasopressin, **atrial natriuretic peptide**.

See also, Arterial blood pressure measurement; Diastolic blood pressure; Hypertension

Arterial blood pressure measurement. First attempted by Hales in 1733, who inserted pipes several feet long into the arteries of animals. The BP cuff was introduced by Riva-Rocci in 1896. Measurement and recording of BP was introduced into anaesthetic practice by **Cushing** in 1901.

- May be direct or indirect:
  –direct:
    –gives a continuous reading; i.e. changes may be noticed rapidly.
    –provides additional information from the shape of the **arterial waveform**.
    –requires **arterial cannulation**.
    –requires calibration and zeroing of the **monitoring system**.
    –**resonance** and **damping** may cause inaccuracy.
  –indirect:
    –palpation (unreliable).
    –mercury or aneroid manometer attached to a cuff: the brachial artery is palpated and the cuff inflated

until the pulsation disappears; the pressure is now above systolic. Cuff pressure is released, and pressure measured by detecting pulsation by using the **Korotkoff sounds**, a **pulse detector** or **Doppler** probe. The cuff width must be 20% greater than the arm's diameter; narrower cuffs will over-read. Error may arise between different observers.
    –**oscillotonometer**.
    –automatic measuring devices which use the same cuff for inflation and detection of movement of the arterial walls. Consecutive pulsations are compared, and complex circuitry prevents error from patient movement, etc. Systolic and MAP are usually measured and diastolic pressure calculated. Tend to overread when pressures are high, and underread when low.
    –Finapres device: a cuff is inflated around a finger, and its pressure varied continuously to keep its volume constant, using infrared photometry to measure volume. Cuff pressure is proportional to finger arterial pressure; a continuous display of the arterial pressure waveform is obtained.
    –continuous arterial tonometry: a pressure transducer is positioned over the radial artery, compressing it against the radius. The transducer output voltage is proportional to the arterial BP, which is displayed as a continuous trace. Periodic calibration is performed using an automatic oscillometric cuff on the arm.

[Stephen Hales (1677–1761), English curate and naturalist; Scipione Riva-Rocci (1863–1937), Italian physician]
Gardner RM (1990) Curr Anaesth and Crit Care; 1: 239–46
See also, Pressure measurement

Arterial cannulation. Used for direct **arterial BP measurement**, and to allow repeated arterial blood gas analysis. Peripheral cannulation, e.g. of radial and dorsalis pedis arteries, produces higher peak systolic pressure than more central cannulation, but is usually preferred because of reduced complication rates. **Allen's test** is often performed before radial artery catheterization, but is of doubtful value. Continuous slow flushing with heparinized saline (3–4 ml/h) reduces blockage and is preferable to intermittent injection. Flushing with excessive volumes of solution may introduce air into the carotid circulation, especially in children.

- System consists of:
  –cannula: ischaemia, emboli and tissue necrosis are uncommon if a 20–22 G parallel-sided Teflon cannula is used, and removed within 24–48 hours.
  –connecting catheter: short and stiff to reduce **resonance**.
  –**transducer** placed level with the heart. Requires calibration and zeroing.
  –electrical monitor and connections. An adequate frequency response of less than 40 Hz is required.

Bubbles, clots and kinks may cause **damping**.
Intravascular transducers may be placed within large arteries, but are expensive and not routinely used.

Arterial gas tensions, *see Blood gas tensions*

Arterial waveform. The shape of the pressure wave recorded directly from the aorta differs from that recorded from smaller arteries; the peak systolic pressure and **pulse pressure** increase, and the dicrotic notch becomes more apparent, peripherally (Fig. 11a). The aorta and large arteries are distended by the **stroke volume** during its ejection; during diastole, elastic recoil maintains diastolic blood flow (Windkessel effect). Smaller vessels are less compliant and therefore less distensible; thus the pressure peaks are higher and travel faster peripherally. In the elderly, decreased aortic compliance results in higher peak pressures.

- Abnormal waveforms (Fig. 11b):
  - anacrotic: **aortic stenosis**.
  - collapsing:
    - hyperdynamic circulation, e.g. **pregnancy**, fever, **anaemia**, **hyperthyroidism**, arteriovenous fistula.
    - **aortic regurgitation**.
  - bisferiens: aortic stenosis + aortic regurgitation.
  - alternans: left ventricular failure.
  - excessive **damping**: e.g. air bubble.
  - excessive **resonance**: e.g. catheter too long or flexible.
- Information that may be derived from the normal waveform:
  - arterial BP.
  - stroke volume and **cardiac output**, from the area under the systolic part of the waveform.
  - **myocardial contractility**, as indicated by rate of pressure change per unit time (dP/dt).
  - outflow resistance; estimated by the slope of the diastolic decay. A slow fall may occur in vasoconstriction, a rapid fall in vasodilatation.
  - **hypovolaemia** is suggested by a low dicrotic notch, narrow width of the waveform and large falls in peak pressure with IPPV breaths.

[Windkessel, German; wind-chamber]

See also, Arterial blood pressure; Cardiac cycle; Mean arterial pressure

Arteriovenous oxygen difference. Difference between arterial and mixed venous O_2 content, normally 5 ml $O_2/100$ ml blood. Increased with low cardiac ouput or exercise. Decreased with peripheral arteriovenous shunting, or when tissue O_2 extraction is impaired, e.g. sepsis or **cyanide poisoning**.

See also, Oxygen transport

Arthritis, *see Connective tissue diseases; Rheumatoid arthritis*

Artificial heart, *see Heart, artificial*

Artificial hibernation, *see Lytic cocktail*

Artificial ventilation, *see Expired air ventilation; Intermittent positive pressure ventilation*

ASA physical status. Classification system adopted by the **American Society of Anesthesiologists** for assessing preoperative physical status.

- There are five categories:
  - I: healthy patient.
  - II: mild systemic disease; no functional limitation.
  - III: moderate systemic disease; definite functional limitation.
  - IV: severe systemic disease that is a constant threat to life.

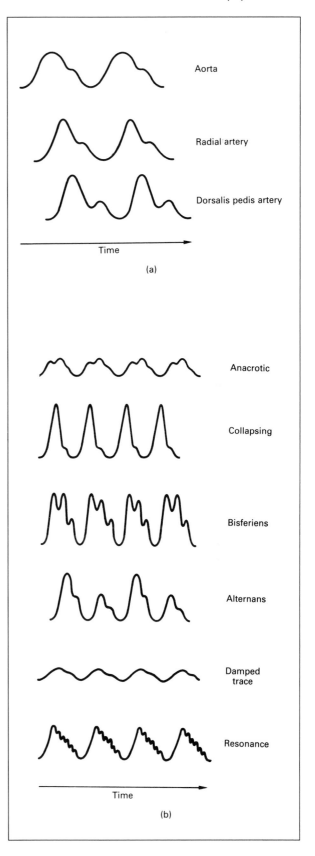

Figure 11 *(a) Arterial tracing from different sites. (b) Abnormal arterial waveforms*

V: moribund patient; unlikely to survive 24 hours with or without operation.

Addition of the postscript E indicates emergency surgery. Extremes of age, **smoking** and late **pregnancy** are sometimes taken as criteria for category II.

Although not a sensitive predictor of anaesthetic mortality, there is reasonable correlation with overall outcome. Widely used in **clinical trials** to standardize fitness of patients.

See also, Preoperative assessment

Ascending reticular activating system (ARAS). Ascending neural system which affects cerebral cortical activity; it extends from the medulla to the midbrain. Its main pathway is the central tegmental tract, conveying impulses to the hypothalamus and thalamus and then to the cortex. Any lesion interrupting the ARAS tends to cause **coma**. Because of close proximity to other brainstem nuclei, lesions often cause cardiovascular or respiratory disturbances. Anaesthetic agents are thought to produce their effect by blocking impulses from the ARAS.

Aspiration of gastric contents. Potentially a risk in all unconscious and anaesthetized patients, as **lower oesophageal sphincter** tone decreases and laryngeal reflexes are depressed. In all but extreme emergencies, patients are starved of food for 4–6 hours before anaesthesia, although recent evidence suggests that total fluid restriction may be unnecessary. After **trauma**, **gastric emptying** may be delayed for several hours, especially in children. Aspiration may follow passive regurgitation of **gastric contents** or vomiting.

- Factors predisposing to aspiration:
  - full stomach:
    - not starved.
    - gastrointestinal obstruction.
    - gastrointestinal bleeding.
    - ileus.
    - trauma/shock/anxiety/pain.
    - **hiatus hernia**.
    - drugs, e.g. **opioid analgesic drugs**.
    - **pregnancy**.
  - ineffecent lower oesophageal sphincter:
    - hiatus hernia.
    - drugs, e.g. opioids, **atropine**.
    - pregnancy with heartburn.
    - presence of a nasogastric tube.
  - raised intra-abdominal pressure:
    - pregnancy.
    - lithotomy position.
    - obesity.
  - oesophagus not empty:
    - **achalasia**.
    - strictures.
  - pharyngeal pouch.
  - ineffective laryngeal reflexes
    - general anaesthesia/**sedation**.
    - **topical anaesthesia**.
    - neurological disease.
- Measures to reduce risk:
  - starvation.
  - empty stomach:
    - via nasogastric tube.
    - **metoclopramide/cisapride**.
    - **apomorphine**-induced vomiting.
  - increase lower oesophageal sphincter tone, e.g. with metaclopramide, cisapride, **prochlorperazine**.
  - rapid sequence induction of anaesthesia.
  - induction in the lateral or sitting position.
  - reduction of the severity of **aspiration pneumonitis**: e.g. **H₂ receptor antagonists**, **antacids**, **omeprazole**.
- If aspiration occurs:
  - the patient should be placed in the head-down lateral position.
  - material is aspirated from the pharynx and larynx, and O_2 administered.
  - tracheal intubation may be necessary to protect the airway, and to allow tracheobronchial suction.
  - further management is as for aspiration pneumonitis.

See also, Induction, rapid sequence

Aspiration pneumonitis (Mendelson's syndrome). Inflammatory reaction of lung parenchyma following **aspiration of gastric contents**, originally described in obstetric patients. A 'critical' volume of 25 ml of aspirate, of pH 2.5, has been suggested to be required to produce the syndrome, although these figures have been disputed since they are based on animal studies. The more acidic the inhaled material, the less volume is required to produce pneumonitis.

Particulate **antacids**, e.g. **magnesium trisilicate**, may themselves be associated with pnemonitis if aspirated.

Pneumonitis occurs within hours of aspiration, with dyspnoea, tachypnoea, tachycardia, hypoxia and bronchospasm, with or without pyrexia. Crepitations and wheezes may be heard on chest auscultation. Irregular fluffy densities may appear on the **chest X-ray** from 8 to 24 hours. Movement of fluid into the lungs results in **hypovolaemia** and **hypotension**. The syndrome is often considered part of the **ARDS** spectrum. Differential diagnosis includes **cardiac failure**, **septicaemia**, **PE**, **amniotic fluid embolism** and **fat embolism**.

Treatment is mainly supportive with **O₂ therapy**, **bronchodilator drugs**, and removal of aspirate and secretions by **physiotherapy** and suction. **Bronchoscopy** may be required. Secondary infection may occur, and prophylactic antibiotics are often given. Use of steroids is declining. **IPPV** and **PEEP** may be required in severe cases. Mortality is high.

[Curtis L Mendelson, US obstetrician]

Aspirin. Acetylsalicylic acid, synthesized in the early 1900s in Germany. Commonest **salicylate** in use. Uses, effects, pharmacokinetics, etc. as for salicylates. Used in low dosage as an **antiplatelet drug**.

- Dosage: 300–900 mg orally 4–6 hourly, up to a maximum of 4 g daily.
  30–40 mg/day for antiplatelet effects.

See also, Salicylate poisoning

Assisted respiration. Positive pressure ventilation supplementing each spontaneous breath made by the patient. May be useful during transient **hypoventilation** caused by respiratory depressant drugs in spontaneously breathing anaesthetized patients. Also used in ICU, e.g. in **weaning from ventilators**.

- Different modes:
  - assist mode ventilation: delivery of positive pressure breaths triggered by inspiratory effort.

–assist-control mode ventilation: assist mode ventilation against a background of regular IPPV.
–**inspiratory pressure support**: inspiration continues to a preset inspiratory flow rate.

Association of Anaesthetists of Great Britain and Ireland. Founded in 1932 to represent anaesthetists' interests and to establish a diploma in anaesthetics (**DA examination**). Prior to this, the London Society of Anaesthetists (founded 1893) had formed the Anaesthetic Section of the Royal Society of Medicine in 1908, its purpose to advance the science and art of anaesthesia. Has 4300 members in the UK.
Helliwell PJ (1982) Anaesthesia; 37: 913–23

Asthma. Reversible airways obstruction, resulting from bronchoconstriction, bronchial mucosal oedema and mucus plugging. Causes **hypoxaemia**, air trapping, and increased work of breathing. Factors triggering 'attacks' include allergens, exercise, infections and emotional upsets. Patients' bronchi show increased sensitivity to triggering agents, constricting when normal bronchi may not. During anaesthesia, surgical stimulation or stimulation of the pharynx or larynx may cause **bronchospasm**.
- Chronic drug treatment:
  –**β_2-adrenergic receptor agonists**, e.g. **salbutamol**.
  –**aminophylline** and related drugs.
  –**steroid therapy**.
  –**cromoglycate**.
  –**anticholinergic drugs**, e.g. **ipratropium**.
- Acute severe asthma:
  –signs of a severe attack:
    –inability to talk.
    –tachycardia > 110/min.
    –tachypnoea > 25/min.
    –**pulsus paradoxus** > 10 mmHg.
    –**peak expiratory flow rate** (PEFR) < 40% of predicted normal.
  –signs of life-threatening attack:
    –silent chest on auscultation.
    –cyanosis.
    –bradycardia.
    –exhausted, confused or unconscious patient.
  –arterial blood gas measurement: hypoxaemia, largely from $\dot{V}/\dot{Q}$ **mismatch**, may be severe. It may worsen following bronchodilator treatment due to increased **dead space** and $\dot{V}/\dot{Q}$ mismatch. Arterial P_{CO_2} is usually reduced because of hyperventilation, but may rise in severe cases, indicating requirement for IPPV.
  –other problems: **pneumothorax,** infection, **dehydration. Hypokalaemia** is common due to **steroid therapy, catecholamine** administration, and respiratory **alkalosis**.
  –management:
    –humidified O_2 with high $F_{I}O_2$ is required.
    –nebulized salbutamol 2.5–5 mg or **terbutaline** 5–10 mg 4 hourly. IV salbutamol 250 µg may be given, followed by 5–20 µg/min.
    –nebulized ipratropium 0.1–0.5 mg may alternate with the above drugs.
    –aminophylline 3–6 mg/kg iv, followed by 0.5 mg/kg/h (with caution if the patient is already taking **theophyllines**).
    –steroids; e.g. hydrocortisone 100–200 mg 4 hourly iv, or by infusion.

–**diethyl ether, halothane, ketamine** and **adrenaline** have been used in resistant cases.
–IPPV:
    –intubation may provoke cardiac arrhythmias in severe hypoxia/hypercapnia.
    –**sedation** and muscle relaxation are required to aid IPPV.
    –high inflation pressures are required with risk of **barotrauma** and decreased cardiac output. **PEEP** exacerbates this and should be avoided if possible.
    –a flow generator **ventilator** is required, to ensure adequate **tidal volumes**.
    –adequate ventilation may be difficult; P_{CO_2} often remains high. Slow inspiratory flow rates and prolonged expiration may improve gas exchange.
–antibiotics, **physiotherapy**, iv rehydration.
–**bronchopulmonary lavage** has been used.
- Anaesthetic management of patients with asthma:
  –preoperatively:
    –**preoperative assessment** is directed towards respiratory function, frequency and severity of attacks, and drug therapy (including steroids).
    –investigations: **chest X-ray**; PEFR/spirometry (especially pre- and post-bronchodilator); arterial blood gas analysis.
    –**premedication**: although many **opioid analgesic drugs** may release **histamine**, they are commonly prescribed, particularly **pethidine. Antihistamines** are often used. **Anticholinergic drugs** may reduce parasympathetically induced bronchospasm, but excessive drying of secretions may be disadvantageous.
    –nebulized bronchodilators may be given with premedication. Preoperative physiotherapy may also be useful. Steroid cover may be required.
  –peroperatively:
    –regional anaesthesia is often suitable.
    –**thiopentone** has been implicated as causing bronchospasm, although this is controversial. **Etomidate** and ketamine are suitable alternatives. Halothane and other volatile agents cause bronchodilatation. **Tubocurarine** and **atracurium** may cause histamine release, whilst **vecuronium, pancuronium** and **fentanyl** do not.
    –tracheal intubation and the presence of a tracheal tube may cause bronchospasm. This may be reduced by spraying the larynx and trachea with **lignocaine**. IV lignocaine, 1–2 mg/kg, has been used to reduce the incidence of bronchospasm on intubation and extubation. Alternatively, techniques avoiding tracheal intubation may be employed.
    –**β-adrenergic receptor antagonists** should be avoided.
    –dehydration should be avoided.
McFadden ER, Gilbert IA (1992) N Engl J Med; 27: 1928–37
See also, Bronchodilator drugs

Astrup method. Used for the analysis of blood acid–base status. The **pH** of a blood sample is measured, and the sample equilibrated with two gases of different CO_2 concentration, usually 4% and 8%. pH is measured after each equilibration, and the standard **bicarbonate** and **base**

excess calculated. The original CO$_2$ tension is calculated from the pH of the original sample, using the **Siggaard-Andersen nomogram**.
[Poul Astrup, Danish chemist]

Asystole. Absent cardiac electrical activity. Common in **cardiac arrest** due to hypoxia or exsanguination, especially in children. Must be distinguished from accidental ECG disconnection. Management: as in **CPR**.

Atelectasis. Absence of gas from part of, or all of, the **lung**. Caused by inadequate aeration of alveoli, with subsequent absorption of gas. The latter occurs because the total partial pressure of dissolved gases in venous blood is less than atmospheric pressure; gas trapped behind obstructed airways, e.g. by secretions, is therefore slowly absorbed. **Nitrogen**, being relatively insoluble in blood, tends to splint alveoli when breathing air. Absorption atelectasis may follow high F_1O_2, since O$_2$ is readily absorbed into the blood. Atelectasis has been shown by CAT scanning to occur in dependent parts of the lung during anaesthesia in normal patients, contributing to impaired gas exchange. It may persist postoperatively, particularly in patients with poor lung function and sputum retention, and when chest movement is reduced, e.g. by pain after upper abdominal surgery. **Hypoxaemia**, tachypnoea and tachycardia result, with reduced air entry to the affected area of lung, which may then become infected. Treatment of atelectasis includes **physiotherapy**, **humidification** and **bronchoscopy** when indicated.

Atenolol, *see β-Adrenergic receptor antagonists*

Atherosclerosis. Disease involving the intima of medium and large arteries, resulting in fat accumulation and fibrous plaques which narrow the vessel lumen. Further stenosis may follow thrombosis and haemorrhage. Associated with **ischaemic heart disease**, cerebrovascular disease, and peripheral arterial insufficiency, especially in the legs. Thus patients for vascular surgery are likely to have other manifestations of the disease.

A rigid arterial tree results in a high systolic arterial BP with normal diastolic pressure, a common finding in the elderly, since virtually all elderly patients have some atherosclerosis. Antihypertensive treatment is not usually required in these patients.

Atmosphere. Unit of **pressure**. One atmosphere equals 760 mmHg (101.33 kPa), the average barometric pressure at sea level.

Atopy. Tendency to **asthma**, hay fever, eczema and other allergic conditions, including **adverse drug reactions**. Sufferers are sensitive to antigens which usually cause no reaction in normal subjects. May be familial. IgE levels may be raised. Drugs associated with **histamine** release should be avoided.

ATP, *see Adenosine triphosphate and diphosphate*

ATPD and ATPS. Ambient temperature and pressure, dry; and ambient temperature and pressure, saturated with water vapour. Used for standardizing gas volume measurements.

Atracurium besylate. Non-depolarizing **neuromuscular blocking drug**, first used in 1980. A bisquaternary nitrogenous plant derivative. Initial dose: 0.3–0.6 mg/kg. Intubation is possible approximately 90 seconds after a dose of 0.5 mg/kg. Effects last 20–30 minutes. Supplementary dose: 0.1–0.2 mg/kg. Has been given by iv infusion at 0.3–0.6 mg/kg/h. May cause **histamine** release, usually mild but severe reactions have been reported. At body temperature and pH, undergoes spontaneous **Hofmann elimination** to **laudanosine**. Up to 50% ester hydrolysis also occurs. Often considered the drug of choice in renal or hepatic impairment. Its cardiostability, low risk of accumulation and spontaneous reversal are also advantages. Stored at 2–8°C; at room temperature, activity decreases by only a few per cent per month.

Atrial ectopic beats. Impulses arising from abnormal pacemaker sites within the atria. The **P waves** are usually abnormal, and arise early in the **cardiac cycle**. They are usually conducted to the ventricles in the normal way, producing normal **QRS complexes** (Fig. 12). Very early

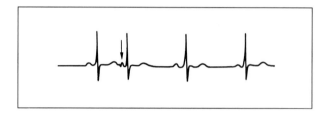

Figure 12 *Example of an atrial ectopic beat (arrowed)*

ectopics may produce abnormal QRS complexes, because the ventricular conducting system may still be refractory when the ectopic impulse reaches it. The resultant QRS may then be mistaken for a **ventricular ectopic beat**. Several ectopic sites may give rise to the 'wandering pacemaker', producing differently-shaped P waves with differing PR intervals. Rarely require treatment.
See also, Arrhythmias; Electrocardiography

Atrial fibrillation (AF). Lack of coordinated atrial contraction, resulting in impulses from many different parts of the atria reaching the atrioventricular (AV) node in quick succession, only some of which are transmitted. Ventricular response may be fast, resulting in inadequate ventricular filling, and reduced stroke volume and cardiac output. **Cardiac failure**, hypotension and systemic emboli from intra-atrial thrombus may occur.
● Features:
  –irregularly irregular pulse.
  –no **P waves** on the **ECG** (Fig. 13).
● Caused by:
  –**ischaemic heart disease** (most common cause), including acute **MI**.
  –mitral valve disease.
  –**hyperthyroidism**.
  –**PE**.
  –**cardiomyopathy**.
  –thoracic surgery/central venous cannulation.
  –acute **hypovolaemia**.

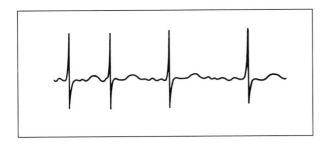

Figure 13 *Atrial fibrillation*

- Treatment:
  –drug therapy is aimed at reducing AV node conduction and ventricular rate. **Sinus rhythm** may be restored. Examples include **digoxin** (usually drug of choice), **β-adrenergic receptor antagonists**, **verapamil**, **amiodarone** and **disopyramide**.
  –**cardioversion**.

See also, Arrhythmias

Atrial flutter. **Arrhythmia** resulting from rapid atrial discharge (usually 300/min). Commonly occurs with 4:1 or 2:1 atrioventricular block; i.e. with ventricular rates 75/min or 150/min respectively.
- Features:
  –usually regular pulse.
  –saw-tooth flutter (F) waves on the **ECG** (Fig. 14); with 2:1 block the second flutter wave of each pair

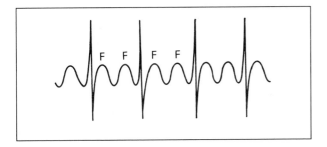

Figure 14 *Atrial flutter (F = flutter waves)*

may be hidden in the QRS or T waves, leading to the incorrect diagnosis of **sinus tachycardia**. **Carotid sinus massage** may slow the ventricular rate enough to reveal rapid flutter waves.
- Causes: as for **AF**.
- Treatment:
  –aimed at restoring sinus rhythm: **cardioversion**, rapid atrial pacing, and drug therapy as for AF.
  –**digoxin** may convert flutter to AF.

See also, Cardiac pacing

Atrial natriuretic peptide. Hormone isolated from the atria, also found in renal and nervous tissue. Released by atrial stretching, e.g. in fluid overload.
- Actions:
  –increases **GFR**, and urinary sodium and water excretion.

–relaxes vascular smooth muscle; renal vessels are more sensitive than others.
–inhibits plasma renin activity and **aldosterone** release. Levels may be raised in **cardiac failure** and essential **hypertension**, although its precise role is unclear.
Epstein FH (1986) New Engl J Med; 314: 828–34

Atrial septal defect (ASD). Accounts for up to 15% of **congenital heart disease**.
- Normal septal development is as follows:
  –the septum primum grows down from the top of the heart, separating the right and left halves of the common atrium.
  –the foramen secundum appears in its upper part.
  –the septum secundum grows down to the right of the septum primum, usually just covering the foramen secundum.
  –the foramen ovale is formed from the foramen secundum and overlapping septum secundum.
- Features of ASD:
  –pulmonary flow murmur with or without a tricuspid murmur, increasing on inspiration. Fixed splitting of the second **heart sound**.
  –right ventricular hypertrophy, right **bundle branch block** and right axis deviation may be present.
  –**pulmonary hypertension**.

Over 90% of defects are secundum ASDs; they may present in later life with pulmonary hypertension, right-sided cardiac failure, **Eisenmenger's syndrome** and **AF**. Suturing of the defect is usually quick if a patch is not required.

Ostium primum defects may involve the atrioventricular valves; they often present early. Repair is more complicated. Valve regurgitation and conduction defects may follow surgery.
- Anaesthetic management: as for congenital heart disease and **cardiac surgery**.

See also, Heart murmurs; Preoperative assessment

Atrial stretch receptors, *see Baroreceptors*

Atrioventricular block, *see Heart block*

Atrioventricular dissociation. Unrelated ventricular and atrial activity. The term is usually reserved for when the ventricular rate exceeds the atrial rate, to distinguish it from complete **heart block** (in which the reverse occurs). Ventricular activity may arise from the atrioventricular node or an ectopic pacemaker. It may occur during bradycardia as an escape mechanism, and during anaesthesia. On the **ECG**, **P waves** and **QRS complexes** are unrelated, the former more widely spaced than the latter (Fig. 15). Rarely clinically significant.

See also, Arrhythmias

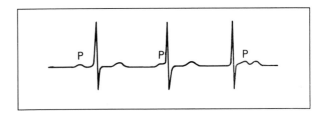

Figure 15 *Atrioventricular dissociation*

Atrioventricular node, *see Heart, conducting system*

Atropine sulphate. Anticholinergic drug, an ester of tropic acid and tropine. Found in the deadly nightshade. Used to reduce muscarinic effects of **acetylcholinesterase inhibitors,** for **premedication,** and in the treatment of bradycardia and **asystole.** Has also been used to reduce GIT motility, and as a mydriatic.
- Effects:
    - CVS:
        - tachycardia (may cause bradycardia initially; thought to be due to central vagal stimulation). BP rises only if initially low due to bradycardia.
        - cutaneous vasodilatation (cause unknown).
    - CNS:
        - excitement, hallucinations and hyperthermia, especially in children.
        - antiparkinsonian effect.
    - RS:
        - bronchodilatation and increased dead space.
        - reduced secretions.
    - GIT:
        - reduced salivation.
        - reduced motility.
        - reduced secretion.
        - reduced **lower oesophageal sphincter** tone.
    - others:
        - reduced sweating.
        - mydriasis and cycloplegia.
        - reduced bladder and ureteric tone.
- Standard doses:
    - 0.1–0.6 mg increments iv for bradycardia.
    - 0.3–0.6 mg im as premedication; 0.01–0.02 mg/kg for children.
    - 0.01–0.02 mg/kg when given with acetylcholinesterase inhibitors.
    - 1–2 mg during **CPR.**

2–3 mg is required to block the **vagus** completely.

May be administered via the tracheal tube in twice the iv dose.

Atropine should be avoided in pyrexial patients, particularly children.

Applied directly to the eye, it may provoke closed-angle **glaucoma** in susceptible patients, the iris obstructing drainage of aqueous humour when the pupil is dilated.

See also, Anticholinergic drugs, for comparison with hyoscine and glycopyrronium; Tracheal administration of drugs

Audioanaesthesia (White sound). Multifrequency sound, played to patients through headphones in order to reduce pain, e.g. in obstetrics. The volume is increased during contractions, with or without soft music in between. Has been employed to reduce **awareness** during **Caesarian section.** Now rarely used.

See also, Obstetric analgesia and anaesthesia

Audit. Medical audit is a systematic approach to peer review of medical care in order to identify and bring about potential improvements. Primarily a clinical activity, it overlaps the areas of general and resource management, including budget control. Audit has increased in recent years, especially relating to the cost implications of medical care. Anaesthetic applications include monitoring of:

- organization of anaesthetic departments (rotas, staffing, teaching, etc.).
- management of patients (drug usage, clinical policies, etc.).

Methods include analysis of currently-held data (e.g. anaesthetic **record-keeping**) or specific studies into particular aspects of care (e.g. **Confidential Enquiry into Perioperative Deaths** and **Confidential Enquiries into Maternal Deaths**).

Shaw CD, Costain DW (1989) BMJ; 299: 498–9

Auriculotemporal nerve block, *see Mandibular nerve blocks*

Auscultatory gap. During auscultatory **arterial BP measurement,** the **Korotkoff sounds** may disappear at a point below systolic pressure, to reappear at a lower pressure before disappearing again at diastolic pressure. The significance is unknown, but it emphasizes the importance of palpating the artery before auscultation, in order to ensure that the absence of sounds is because the pressure is above systolic, and not within the 'silent' gap.

Australia antigen, *see Hepatitis*

Autoimmune disease. Characterized by activation of the immune system, directed against host tissue. May involve antibody production, attacking intracellular, extracellular or cell membrane **antigens.** Pathogenesis is not fully understood, but involves imbalance of suppressor and helper T lymphocyte cell function. May affect specific organs, e.g. **adrenocortical insufficiency,** or many tissues, e.g. **connective tissue diseases.**
- May follow triggering agents, e.g.:
    - drugs: SLE-like syndrome after **procainamide** or **hydralazine** therapy, haemolytic anaemia after α-**methyldopa** therapy.
    - infection: **haemolysis** following mycoplasma pneumonia, **rheumatic fever** following streptococcal infection. Viral infections are often implicated.

Genetic factors are also important, hence the association between certain diseases and HLA types, e.g. **myasthenia gravis,** thyroid disease, pernicious anaemia and vitiligo. More than one of these diseases may occur in the same patient, suggesting common mechanisms. Testing for autoantibodies may be useful in the diagnosis and treatment of these conditions.

Autologous blood transfusion, *see Blood transfusion, autologous*

Autonomic hyperreflexia. Increased sensitivity of sympathetic reflexes in patients with **spinal cord injury** above T5/6. Cutaneous or visceral stimuli below the level of the lesion may result in mass discharge of sympathetic nerves, causing sweating, vasoconstriction and hypertension, with high levels of circulating **catecholamines.** **Baroreceptor** stimulation results in compensatory bradycardia. Distension of hollow viscera, especially of the bladder, is a potent stimulus. It may also occur during abdominal surgery and labour. Onset of susceptibility is usually within a few weeks of injury.

In anaesthesia, both general and regional techniques have been used; **spinal anaesthesia** has been suggested as the technique of choice, if appropriate. Control of hyper-

tension has been successfully achieved with **vasodilator drugs**. Hypotension may also occur.
See also, Paraplegia

Autonomic nervous system. System which regulates non-voluntary bodily functions, by means of reflex pathways. Efferent nerves contain medullated fibres which leave the brain and spinal cord to synapse with non-medullated fibres in peripheral ganglia. Closely related to the CNS, both anatomically and functionally; thus sensory input may affect autonomic activity and also consciousness and voluntary behaviour, e.g. pain, temperature sensation, etc.
- Divided into the **parasympathetic** and **sympathetic nervous systems**, on the basis of anatomical, pharmacological and functional differences (Fig. 16):
  - parasympathetic:
    - output in cranial and sacral nerves; ganglia near to target organs.
    - **acetylcholine** released as a transmitter at pre- and post- ganglionic nerve endings.
    - increases GIT activity, and reduces arousal and cardiovascular activity.
  - sympathetic:
    - output in thoracic and lumbar segments of the spinal cord; ganglia form the sympathetic trunk.
    - acetylcholine released at preganglionic nerve endings, **adrenaline** and **noradrenaline** (in general) at postganglionic nerve endings.
    - increases arousal and cardiovascular activity ('fight or flight' reaction), reduces visceral activity.
Some organs receive only sympathetic innervation (e.g. piloerector muscles, adipose tissue, **juxtaglomerular apparatus**), others only parasympathetic innervation (e.g. lacrimal glands); most are under dual control.

Autonomic neuropathy. May be:
- central:
  - primary, e.g. progressive autonomic failure (Shy–Drager syndrome).
  - secondary to **CVA**, infection, drugs, etc.
- peripheral, e.g. due to **diabetes mellitus**, amyloidosis, **autoimmune diseases**, **porphyria**.
Results in postural hypotension, cardiac conduction defects, bladder dysfunction and GIT disturbances including delayed gastric emptying. Diabetics with autonomic neuropathy have increased risk of perioperative cardiac or respiratory arrest.
- Useful bedside tests of autonomic function include:
  - pulse and BP measurement lying and standing; a postural drop of over 30 mmHg indicates autonomic dysfunction.
  - **Valsalva manoeuvre**.
  - effect of breathing on pulse rate (normally slows on expiration).
  - sustained hand grip (normal response: tachycardia and over 15 mmHg increase in diastolic BP).
ECG is useful for the latter two tests. Other tests include observation of sweating and pupillary responses, and catecholamine studies.
Patients with autonomic neuropathy are at risk of developing severe hypotension during anaesthesia, particularly with **spinal** or **extradural anaesthesia**, and **IPPV**. They may also show reduced response to **hypoglycaemia**. There may be increased risk of **aspiration of gastric contents**.

[George Shy (1919–1967) and Glenn Drager (1917–1967), US neurologists]
Sweeney BP, Jones S, Langford RM (1985) Anaesthesia; 40: 783–6
See also, Peripheral neuropathy

Autoregulation. The regulation of tissue **blood flow** by the tissues themselves, e.g. kidney, brain and heart.
- Several theories exist:
  - myogenic theory: postulates that muscle in the vessel wall contracts as intraluminal pressure increases, thus maintaining wall tension by reducing radius, in accordance with **Laplace's Law**.
  - metabolic theory: argues that vasodilator substances accumulate in the tissues at low blood flow; the resultant vasodilatation results in increased flow and the vasodilator metabolites are washed away.
  - tissue theory: states that as blood flow increases, the vessels are compressed by the increased amount of interstitial fluid that has accumulated.
Usually occurs at MAP of 60–160 mmHg in normotensive subjects; it may be impaired by volatile anaesthetic agents and **vasodilator drugs**.
See also, Systemic vascular resistance

Autotransfusion, *see Blood transfusion, autologous*

Average, *see Mean*

Avogadro's hypothesis. At constant temperature and pressure, equal volumes of all ideal gases contain the same number of molecules. One **mole** of a substance at standard temperature and pressure contains 6.023×10^{23} particles (Avogadro's number), and one mole of a gas occupies 22.4 litres.
[Count Amedeo Avogadro (1776–1856), Italian scientist]

AVP, Arginine vasopressin, *see Vasopressin*

Awareness. Ability to recall events occurring during general anaesthesia. Particularly a problem when **neuromuscular blocking drugs** are used with 'light anaesthesia'. Ranges from being wide awake but paralysed, to showing evidence of being awake peroperatively but without conscious recall (wakefulness; amnesic wakefulness). Signs of light anaesthesia (tachycardia, sweating, hypertension, large pupils, lacrimation) may not be present.
 Dreams, often vivid and unpleasant, may represent a subconscious form of awareness. Postoperative interview or hypnosis may reveal recall of pain, events, comments or specific messages played to patients. The significance of non-conscious recall is unknown; beneficial effects of encouraging messages during surgery have been reported. It may be **memory** of awareness, rather than the awareness itself, which is affected by anaesthesia.
- Associated with:
  - administration of low doses of anaesthetic agents, e.g. in **Caesarean section** or anaesthesia for moribund patients, especially when **premedication** is omitted.
  - delay in reaching adequate blood levels of inhalational agents, e.g. during nitrogen washout in low flow breathing systems.
  - reliance on iv agents given by bolus without inhalational agents, leading to awareness between doses;

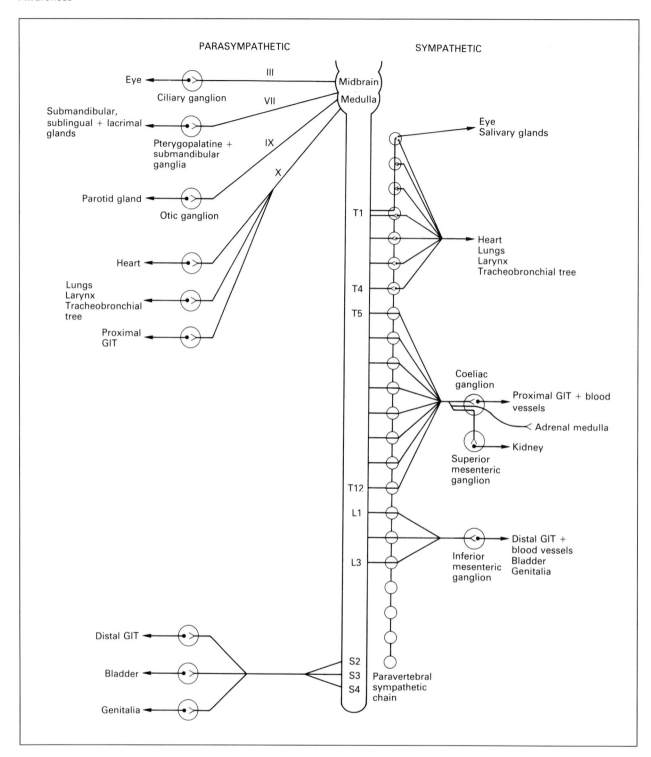

Figure 16 *Autonomic nervous system*

e.g. during **bronchoscopy**, or repeated attempts at difficult intubation.

–equipment failure.

Use of high dose opioid drugs may not prevent awareness, although the patient may not feel pain.

May be reduced by adequate **checking of equipment**, the use of amnesic drugs, e.g. **hyoscine** or **benzodiazepines**, and the addition of a small amount of volatile agent to inspired gases.

Ghoneim MM, Block RI (1992) Anesthesiology; 76: 279–305
See also, Anaesthesia, depth of; Isolated forearm technique; Traumatic neurotic syndrome

Ayre's T-piece, *see Anaesthetic breathing systems*

Azeotrope. Mixture of two or more liquids whose components cannot be separated by distillation. The boiling point of each is altered by the presence of the other substance, thus the components share the same boiling point, and the vapour contains the components in the same proportions as in the liquid mixture. Halothane and ether form an azeotrope, when mixed in the ratio of 2:1 by volume.

Azumolene sodium. Analogue of **dantrolene**, currently under investigation. More water-soluble than dantrolene, thus requiring a smaller volume of administration.

B

Backward failure, *see Cardiac failure*

Bacterial contamination of anaesthetic equipment, *see Contamination of anaesthetic equipment*

Bain breathing system, *see Coaxial anaesthetic breathing systems*

Bainbridge reflex. Reflex tachycardia following an increase in venous pressure, e.g. following rapid infusion of fluid. Does not occur in transplanted hearts, suggesting true reflex pathways. Of unknown significance
[Francis Bainbridge (1874–1921), English physiologist]

Balanced anaesthesia. Concept of using combinations of drugs and techniques (e.g. general and regional anaesthesia) to provide adequate analgesia, anaesthesia and muscle relaxation (triad of anaesthesia). Each drug reduces the requirement for the others, thereby reducing side effects due to any single agent, and also allowing faster recovery. Arose from **Crile's** description of anociassociation in 1911, and **Lundy's** refinement in 1926.

Ballistocardiography. Detection of body motion resulting from movement of blood within the body with each heartbeat. Used to measure **cardiac output** and **stroke volume**, and in the investigation of cardiac disease, but technically difficult to perform accurately.

Balloon pump, *see Intra-aortic counter-pulsation balloon pump*

Bar. Unit of **pressure**. Although not an SI unit, commonly used when referring to the pressures at which anaesthetic gases are delivered from **cylinders** and **piped gas supplies**.

$$1 \text{ bar} = 10^5 \text{ N/m}^2 \text{ (Pa)} = 10^6 \text{ dyne/cm}^2 = \text{approx. 1 atm.}$$

Baralyme. Calcium hydroxide 80% and barium octohydrate 20%. Used to absorb CO_2. Although less efficient than **soda lime**, it produces less heat and is more stable in dry atmospheres. Used in spacecraft.

Barbiturate poisoning. Causes CNS depression with **hypoventilation, hypotension, hypothermia** and **coma**. Skin blisters and muscle necrosis may also occur.
- Treatment:
    –general measures as for **poisoning and overdose**.
    –of the above complications.
    –forced alkaline diuresis, **dialysis** or **haemoperfusion** may be indicated.
Now rare, with the declining use of **barbiturates**.
See also, Forced diuresis

Barbiturates. Drugs derived from barbituric acid, itself derived from urea and malonic acid and first sythesized in 1864. The first sedative barbiturate, diethyl barbituric acid, was synthesized in 1903. Many others have been developed since, including **phenobarbitone** in 1912, hexobarbitone in 1932 (the first widely used iv barbiturate), **thiopentone** in 1934, and **methohexitone** in 1957.
- Substitutions at certain positions of the molecule confer hypnotic or other properties to the compound (Fig. 17).

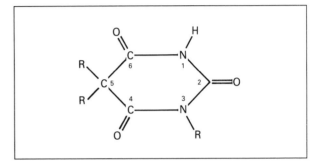

Figure 17 *Structure of the barbiturate ring*

Chemical classification:
   –oxybarbiturates: as shown. Slow onset and prolonged action, e.g. phenobarbitone.
   –thiobarbiturates: sulphur atom at position 2. Rapid onset, smooth action, and rapid recovery, e.g. thiopentone.
   –methylbarbiturates: methyl group at position 1. Rapid onset and recovery, with excitatory phenomena, e.g. methohexitone.
   –methylthiobarbiturates: both substitutions. Very rapid, but too high an incidence of excitatory phenomena to be useful clinically.
Long side groups are associated with greater potency and convulsant properties. Phenyl groups confer anticonvulsant action.
- Divided clinically into:
   –long acting, e.g. phenobarbitone.
   –medium acting, e.g. amylobarbitone.
   –very short acting, e.g. thiopentone.
Speed of onset of action reflects lipid solubility, and thus brain penetration. The actions of long and medium acting drugs are terminated by metabolism; the shorter duration of action of thiopentone and methohexitone is due to redistribution within the body.
- Actions:
   –general CNS depression, especially cerebral cortex and **ascending reticular activating system**.
   –central respiratory depression (dose related).
   –**antanalgesia**.

–reduction of rapid eye movement **sleep** (with rebound increase after cessation of chronic use).

–anticonvulsant or convulsant properties according to structure.

–cardiovascular depression. Central depression is usually mild; the hypotension seen after thiopentone is largely due to direct myocardial depression and venodilatation.

–hypothermia.

Hepatic metabolism is followed by renal excretion. Cause hepatic **enzyme induction**.

Contraindicated in **porphyria**.

Used mainly for **induction of anaesthesia**, and as **anticonvulsant drugs**. Have been largely replaced by **benzodiazepines** for use as sedatives and hypnotics, as the latter drugs are safer.

See also, Barbiturate poisoning

Barker, Arthur E (1850–1916). English Professor of Surgery at University of London. Helped popularize **spinal anaesthesia** in the UK. In 1907, became the first to use hyperbaric solutions of **local anaesthetic agents**, combined with alterations in the patient's posture, to vary the height of block achieved. Used specially prepared solutions of **stovaine** (combined with 5% glucose) from Paris.

Baroreceptor reflex (Pressoreceptor, Carotid sinus or Depressor reflex). Reflex involved in the short-term control of **arterial BP**. Increased BP stimulates **baroreceptors** in the **carotid sinus** and aortic arch, increasing afferent discharge which is inhibitory to the **vasomotor centre** and excitatory to the **cardioinhibitory centre** in the medulla. Vasomotor inhibition (reduced sympathetic activity) and increased cardioinhibitory activity (vagal stimulation) results in a lowering of BP. The opposite changes occur following a fall in BP, with sympathetic stimulation and parasympathetic inhibition. Resultant peripheral vasoconstriction occurs mainly in non-vital vascular beds, e.g. skin, muscle, GIT.

The reflex is reset within 30 minutes if the change in BP is sustained. It may be depressed by certain drugs, e.g. **halothane** and possibly **propofol**.

Baroreceptors. Stretch receptors in the walls of blood vessels and heart chambers. Respond to distension caused by increased pressure, and are involved in control of **arterial BP**.

- Exist in many sites:
  - **carotid sinus** and aortic arch:
    - at normal BP, discharge slowly. Rate of discharge is increased by a rise in BP, and by increased rate of rise.
    - send afferent impulses via the carotid sinus nerve (branch of glossopharyngeal nerve) and vagus (afferents from aortic arch) to the **vasomotor centre** and **cardioinhibitory centre** in the medulla. Raised BP invokes the **baroreceptor reflex**.
  - atrial stretch receptors:
    - found in both atria.
    - some discharge during atrial systole, causing tachycardia; these may be involved in the **Bainbridge reflex**. Others discharge during diastolic distension (more so when venous return is increased or during **IPPV**). Discharge results in reduced sympathetic

activity, and increased urine flow via inhibition of **vasopressin** release.

- ventricular stretch receptors: stimulation causes reduced sympathetic activity in animals, but the clinical significance is doubtful. May also respond to chemical stimulation (**Bezold–Jarisch reflex**).
- pulmonary stretch receptors:
  - stimulation results in bradycardia and hypotension, but to a lesser extent than systemic baroreceptor stimulation. Respiratory rate is reduced.
  - exact site is unknown.

Other baroreceptors may be present in the mesentery, affecting local blood flow.

Barotrauma. Physical injury caused by excessive pressure; the term usually refers to **pneumothorax**, pneumomediastinum, pneumoperitoneum or subcutaneous emphysema resulting from passage of air from the tracheobronchial tree and alveoli into adjacent tissues. Risk of barotrauma is increased by raised mean airway pressure, e.g. with **IPPV** and **PEEP** (especially if excessive tidal volume or air flow is delivered, or if the patient 'fights the ventilator'). **High frequency ventilation** may reduce the risk. Diseased lungs with reduced **compliance** are more at risk of developing barotrauma, e.g. in **asthma**, **ARDS**. Evidence of pulmonary interstitial emphysema may be seen on the chest X-ray (perivascular air, hilar air streaks and subpleural air cysts) before development of severe pneumothorax. In all cases, N_2O will aggravate the problem.

Risk of barotrauma during anaesthesia is reduced by various pressure-limiting features of **anaesthetic machines** and breathing systems.

Haake R, Schlichtig R, Ulstad DR, Henschen RR (1987) Chest; 91: 608–13

See also, Emphysema, subcutaneous

Basal metabolic rate (BMR). Amount of **energy** liberated by **catabolism** of food per unit time, under standardized conditions (i.e. a relaxed subject at comfortable temperature, 12–14 hours after a meal, corrected for age, sex and surface area).

- Determined by measuring:
  - heat produced by the subject enclosed in an insulated room, the outside walls of which are maintained at constant temperature. The heat produced raises the temperature of water passing through coils in the ceiling, allowing calculation of BMR.
  - O_2 consumption: the subject breathes via a sealed circuit (containing a CO_2 absorber) from an O_2 filled **spirometer**. As O_2 is consumed, the volume inside the spirometer falls, and a graph of volume against time is obtained. O_2 consumption per unit time is corrected to standard temperature and pressure. Average energy liberated per litre of O_2 consumed = 20.1 kJ (4.82 Cal; some variation occurs with different food sources); thus BMR may be calculated.

Normal BMR (adult male) is 197 kJ/m²/h (40 Cal/m²/h). BMR values are often expressed as percentages above or below normal values obtained from charts or tables.

- Metabolic rate is increased by :
  - circulating catecholamines, e.g. due to stress.
  - muscle activity.
  - raised temperature.

–**hyperthyroidism**.
–pregnancy.
–recent feeding (**specific dynamic action** of foods).
–age and sex (higher in males and children).
Measurement of metabolic rate under basal conditions eliminates many of these variables.
See also, Metabolism

Basal narcosis, *see Rectal administration of anaesthetic agents*

Base. Substance which can accept **hydrogen ions**, thereby reducing hydrogen ion concentration.

Base excess/deficit. Amount of **acid** or **base** (in mmol) required to restore 1 litre of blood to normal **pH** at $P\text{CO}_2$ of 5.3 kPa (40 mmHg) and at body temperature. By convention, its value is negative in **acidosis** and positive in **alkalosis**. May be read from the **Siggaard-Andersen nomogram**. Useful as an indication of severity of the metabolic component of acid–base disturbance, and in the calculation of the appropriate dose of acid or base in its treatment. For example, in acidosis,

total **bicarbonate** deficit (mmol) =

base deficit (mmol/l) × 'treatable' fluid compartment (l); estimated to be 30% of body weight, comprised of ECF and exchangeable intracellular fluid

$$= \text{base deficit} \times \frac{\text{body weight}}{3}$$

Because of problems associated with bicarbonate administration, half the calculated deficit is given initially.
See also, Acid–base balance; Blood gas tensions

Batson's plexus. Valveless extradural venous plexus composed of anterior and posterior longitudinal veins, communicating at each vertebral level with venous rings which pass transversely around the dural sac. Also communicates with basivertebral veins passing from the middle of the posterior surface of each vertebral body, and with sacral, lumbar, thoracic and cervical veins. It thus connects pelvic veins with intracranial veins. Provides an alternative route for venous blood to reach the heart from the legs. Originally described to explain a route for metastatic spread of tumours. Distends when vena caval venous return is obstructed, e.g. in pregnancy, thus reducing the space available for local anaesthetic solution in **extradural anaesthesia**.
[Oscar V Batson (1894–1979), US otolarygnologist]
See also, Extradural space

Becquerel. SI **unit** of radioactivity. One becquerel = amount of radioactivity produced when one nucleus disintegrates per second.
[Antoine Becquerel (1852–1908), French physicist]

Beer–Lambert law. Combination of two separate laws describing absorption of monochromatic light by a transparent substance through which it passes:
–Beer's law: intensity of transmitted light decreases exponentially as concentration of substance increases.

–Lambert's law: intensity of transmitted light decreases exponentially as distance travelled through the substance increases.
Forms the basis for spectrophotometric techniques, e.g. enzyme assays, **oximetry**.
[August Beer (1825–1863) and Johann Lambert (1728–1777), German physicists]

Bell–Magendie law. The dorsal roots of the **spinal cord** are sensory, the ventral roots motor.
[Sir Charles Bell (1774–1842), Scottish surgeon; François Magendie (1783–1855), French physiologist]

Bellows. Used in **CPR** and animal experiments for several centuries. Modern devices allow manual controlled ventilation, and are either applied directly to the patient's face or used in **draw-over techniques**.
● Examples:
–Cardiff bellows: mainly used for resuscitation. Design:
–concertina bellows with a facepiece at one end.
–**non-rebreathing valve** between the bellows and facepiece.
–one-way valve at the other end of the bellows which prevents air or O_2 leaks during compression, whilst allowing fresh gas entry during expansion.
–Oxford bellows: useful for draw-over anaesthesia. Design:
–concertina bellows mounted on a block containing one-way valves.
–held open by an internal spring, but may be manually compressed. Expansion draws in air or O_2 through a side port.
–unidirectional gas flow is ensured by the one-way valves, one on either side of the bellows. A non-rebreathing valve is required between the bellows and patient.
In earlier models, an O_2 inlet opened directly into the closed bellows system. This could allow build-up of excessive pressure, with risk of **barotrauma**.

Bends, *see Decompression sickness*

Benzodiazepines. Group of drugs with sedative, anxiolytic and anticonvulsant properties. Also cause **amnesia** and muscle relaxation. Act by enhancing **GABA**-mediated inhibition in the brain and spinal cord, especially the **limbic system** and **ascending reticular activating system**. Thought to activate specific receptors forming part of the GABA receptor complex, enhancing the increase in chloride ion conductance caused by GABA itself.
● Anaesthetic uses:
–**premedication**, e.g. **diazepam, temazepam, lorazepam**.
–**sedation**, e.g . diazepam, **midazolam**.
–as **anticonvulsant drugs**, e.g. diazepam.
–**induction of anaesthesia**, e.g. midazolam.
● **Half-life**:
–midazolam 1–3 h.
–oxazepam 3–8 h.
–temazepam 6–8 h.
–lorazepam 12 h.
–diazepam 24–48 h.
Metabolism often produces active products with long half-lives, e.g. diazepam to temazepam and nordiazepam (the

latter has a half-life of up to 900 hours and is itself metabolized to oxazepam). In chronic use, benzodiazepines have largely replaced **barbiturates** as hypnotics and anxiolytics, since they cause fewer and less serious side effects. Overdosage is also less dangerous, usually requiring supportive treatment only. Hepatic **enzyme induction** is rare. A chronic dependance state may occur, with withdrawal featuring tremor, anxiety and confusion.
Flumazanil is a specific benzodiazepine antagonist.

Bernard, Claude (1813–1878). French physiologist, whose many contributions to modern physiology include demonstrating that the liver could synthesize glucose, proving that pancreatic secretions could digest food, discovering vasomotor nerves, and investigating the effects of **curare** at the neuromuscular junction. Also suggested the concept of 'internal environment' (*milieu interieur*) and **homeostasis**.
Lee JA (1978) Anaesthesia; 33: 741–7

Bernoulli effect. Reduction of pressure when a **fluid** accelerates through a constriction. As velocity increases during passage through the constriction, kinetic **energy** increases. Total energy remains the same, therefore potential energy (hence pressure) falls. Beyond the constriction, the pressure rises again. A second fluid may be entrained through a side-arm into the area of lower pressure, causing mixing of the two fluids (**Venturi** principle).
[Daniel Bernoulli (1700–1782), Swiss mathematician]

Bert effect. Convulsions caused by acute O_2 **toxicity**, seen with hyperbaric O_2 **therapy** (3 atm).
[Paul Bert (1833–1896), French physiologist]
See also, Oxygen therapy, hyperbaric

Beta-adrenergic..., *see β-Adrenergic...*

Bethanidine sulphate. Antihypertensive drug which prevents release of **noradrenaline** from adrenergic nerve endings. Similar in actions to **guanethidine**, but shorter-acting. Administered orally (from 10 mg 8 hourly). Commonly causes postural hypotension, therefore rarely used.

Bezold–Jarisch reflex. Bradycardia and hypotension following stimulation of ventricular receptors by ischaemia or drugs, e.g. nicotine and veratridine. Ventricular stretch receptors may be responsible. Pulmonary receptor stimulation produces apnoea. Although of disputed clinical significance, a possible protective role (to prevent ventricular overload) has been suggested. The reflex may be activated during **MI**.
[Albert von Bezold (1836–1868), German physiologist; Adolf Jarisch (1850–1902), Austrian dermatologist]

Bicarbonate. Anion present in plasma at a concentration of 24–33 mmol/l, formed from dissociation of carbonic acid. Intimately involved with **acid-base balance**, as part of the major plasma **buffer** system. Filtered in the kidneys and reabsorbed to a variable extent, according to acid-base status. 80% of filtered bicarbonate is reabsorbed in the proximal tubule via formation of carbonic acid, which in turn forms CO_2 and water aided by **carbonic anhydrase**. The bicarbonate ion itself does not pass easily across cell membranes.

- Sodium bicarbonate may be administered iv to raise blood **pH** in severe **acidosis**, but with potentially undesirable effects:
  – increases formation of CO_2, which passes readily into cells (unlike bicarbonate), worsening intracellular acidosis.
  – increased blood pH shifts the **oxyhaemoglobin dissociation curve** to the left, with increased affinity of **haemoglobin** for O_2 and impaired O_2 delivery to the tissues.
  – solutions contain 1 mmol sodium ions per mmol bicarbonate ions, representing a significant sodium load.
  – 8.4% solution is hypertonic: increased plasma osmolality may cause arterial vasodilatation and hypotension.
  – severe tissue necrosis may follow extravasation.
  For these reasons, treatment is usually reserved for pH below 7.1–7.2.

- Dose: $\dfrac{\text{base deficit} \times \text{body weight (kg)}}{3}$ mmol

  Half of this dose is given initially.
  Presented as 8.4% and 1.26% solutions (1000 mmol/l and 150 mmol/l respectively).
  Arieff AI (1991) Br J Anaesth; 67: 165–77
  See also, Base excess/deficit

Bier, Karl August (1861–1949). Renowned German surgeon, Professor in Bonn and then Berlin. Introduced **spinal anaesthesia** using **cocaine**, describing its use on himself, his assistant and a series of patients, in 1899. Gave a classic description of the **postspinal headache** he later suffered, and suggested CSF leakage during the injection as a possible cause. Also introduced **IVRA**, using **procaine**, in 1908. As consulting surgeon during World War I, he introduced the German steel helmet.

Bier's block, *see Intravenous regional anaesthesia*

Bigelow, Henry Jacob (1818–1890). US surgeon at the Massachusetts General Hospital, Boston, he published the first account of **Morton's** use of **diethyl ether** anaesthesia for surgery. Described several operations and the intraoperative events that occurred during them. Later as a Professor, he became renowned for many contributions to surgery, including inventing a urological evacuator.

Biguanides. Hypoglycaemic drugs, used to treat non-insulin dependent **diabetes mellitus**. Act by decreasing gluconeogenesis and by increasing **glucose** utilization peripherally. Require some pancreatic islet cell function to be effective. May cause **lactic acidosis**, especially in renal or hepatic impairment. Lactic acidosis is particularly likely with phenformin, which is now unavailable in the UK. Metformin, the remaining biguanide, is often used in conjunction with a **sulphonylurea**.

Binding of drugs, *see Pharmacokinetics; Protein-binding*

Bioavailability. Extent and rate of uptake of active drug by the body. Expressed as a percentage, assuming iv injection provides 100% bioavailability. For an orally administered dose, it equals the area under the resultant concentration against time curve divided by that for an iv dose. Low values of bioavailability occur with poorly absorbed drugs, or those that undergo extensive **first-pass metabolism**. Various formulations of the same drug may have different bioavailability. 'Bioinequivalence' is a statistically significant difference in bioavailability, whereas 'therapeutic inequivalence' is a clinically important difference, e.g. as may occur with different preparations of **digoxin**.

See also, Pharmacokinetics

Biofeedback. Technique whereby bodily processes normally under involuntary control, e.g. heart rate, are displayed to the subject, enabling voluntary control to be learnt. Has been used to aid relaxation, and in chronic **pain management** when increased muscle tension is present, using the **EMG** as the displayed signal.

Biotransformation, *see Pharmacokinetics*

BIPAP, Bi-level positive airway pressure, *see Nasal positive pressure ventilation*

Bleeding time, *see Coagulation studies*

Blood. Cell formation occurs in the liver, spleen and bone marrow prior to birth, after which it occurs in bone marrow only. In adults, active bone marrow is confined to vertebrae, ribs, sternum, ilia and humeral and femoral heads. Stem cells differentiate into mature cellular components over many cell divisions. Primary stem cells may give rise to the lymphocyte series of stem cells or to secondary stem cells. The secondary stem cells may give rise to the **erythrocyte**, granulocyte, monocyte or megakaryocyte series of stem cells (the latter forming **platelets**).

See also, Blood volume; Leucocytes; Plasma

Blood, artificial. Man-made solutions capable of gas transport and O_2 delivery to the tissues. **Haemoglobin** solutions are hyperosmotic and are quickly broken down in the blood. Free haemoglobin solutions may cause renal failure. Perfluorocarbon solutions (e.g. Fluosol DA20) carry dissolved O_2 in an amount directly proportion to its partial pressure, and have been used to supplement O_2 delivery in organ ischaemia due to shock, arterial (including coronary) insufficiency and haemorrhage. Even with high F_1O_2, O_2 content is less than that of haemoglobin. Accumulation in the reticulo-endothelial system is of unknown significance.

Urbaniak SJ (1991) BMJ; 303: 1348–50

Blood–brain barrier. Physiological boundary between the bloodstream and CNS, preventing transfer of substances from plasma to brain. The original concept was suggested by the lack of staining of brain tissue by aniline dyes given systemically. Ill-defined anatomically, it arises from the poor permeability of brain capillaries. **Active transport** may still occur. Certain areas of the brain lie outside the barrier, e.g. the **hypothalamus** and areas lining the third and fourth ventricles (including the **chemoreceptor trigger zone**).

The ability of chemicals to cross the barrier is proportional to their lipid solubility, and inversely proportional to molecular size and charge. Water, O_2 and CO_2 cross freely; charged ions and larger molecules take longer to cross unless lipid soluble. All substances eventually penetrate the brain; the rate of penetration is important clinically. Some drugs only cross the barrier in their unionized, non-protein bound form, i.e. a small proportion of the injected dose, e.g. **thiopentone**. **Neuromuscular blocking drugs** are charged, and cross to a very limited extent. **Glycopyrronium**, being charged, crosses to a lesser extent than **atropine**.

The effectiveness of the barrier in **neonates** is less than in adults, hence the increased passage of drugs, e.g. **opioid analgesic drugs**, and other substances, e.g. bile salts causing kernicterus. Meningitis may reduce the integrity of the barrier.

Blood cross-matching. Necessary to avoid reactions caused by transfusion of blood into a recipient whose plasma contains antibodies against the transfused blood. **ABO** and **Rhesus** are the most relevant **blood group** systems clinically, although others may be important. Antibodies may be naturally occurring, e.g. ABO system, or only acquired after exposure, e.g. Rhesus.

● General method:
  –if red cells have serum added which contains antibody against them, agglutination of the cells occurs.
  –serum of known identity is used to identify the recipient's blood group (ABO and Rhesus).
  –recipient's serum is screened for atypical antibodies against other groups.
  –recipient's serum is added to red cells from each donor unit (i.e. cross-match).

Full cross-matching takes up to an hour. Emergency ABO typing is quicker but may not prevent minor incompatibilities. Uncross-matched O Rhesus negative blood is reserved for life-threatening emergencies. Antibody screening with selection of appropriate donor blood without formal cross-matching has been suggested, being cheaper and time-saving.

UK colour coding for labelling of blood for transfusion was replaced by a black and white lettering system in 1992.

Contreras M, Mollison PL (1989) BMJ; 299: 1446–9

See also, Blood transfusion

Blood filters. Devices for removing microaggregates during **blood transfusion**. Platelet microaggregates form early in stored blood, with leucocytes and fibrin aggregates occurring after 7 days' storage. Pulmonary microembolism has been suggested as a cause of pulmonary dysfunction following transfusion.

● Types of filters:
  –screen filters: sieves with pores of a certain size.
  –depth filters: remove particles mainly by adsorption. Pore size varies, and effective filtration may be reduced by channel formation within the filter.
  –combination filters.

Most contain woven fibre meshes, e.g. of polyester or nylon.

Standard iv giving sets suitable for blood transfusion contain screen filters of 170 μm pore size. Filtration of microaggregates requires microfilters of 20–40 μm pore size. The general use of microfilters is controversial; by activating **complement** in transfused blood they may increase formation of microaggregates within the recipient's bloodstream. They add to expense, increase resistance

to flow and may cause **haemolysis**. They have, however, been shown to be of use in **extracorporeal circulation**.
Kapadia F, Valentine S, Smith GB (1992) Intensive Care Med; 18: 258–63

Blood flow. For any organ:

$$\text{Flow} = \frac{\text{perfusion pressure}}{\text{resistance}}$$

Perfusion pressure depends not only on arterial and venous pressures, but on local pressures within the **capillary circulation**.

- Resistance depends on:
  - vessel radius, controlled by humoral, neural and local mechanisms (**autoregulation**).
  - vessel length.
  - blood **viscosity**. Reduced peripherally due to plasma skimmimg, which results in blood with reduced **haematocrit** leaving vessels via side branches. Reduced in **anaemia**.

Flow is normally laminar; i.e. it roughly obeys the **Hagen–Poiseuille equation**, although blood vessels are not rigid, arterial flow is pulsatile and blood is not an ideal fluid. Turbulent flow may occur in constricted arteries and in hyperdynamic circulation, particularly in anaemia, when viscosity is reduced (*see Reynold's number*).

- Measurement:
  - direct measurement of blood from the arterial supply.
  - **electromagnetic flow measurement**.
  - **Doppler** measurement.
  - indirect methods:
    - **Fick principle**.
    - **dilution techniques**.
    - **plethysmography**.

Approximate blood flow to and O_2 consumption of various organs are shown in Table 8.

Table 8. Blood flow to and O_2 consumption of heart, brain and kidneys

Organ	Blood flow		O_2 consumption	
	(ml/min)	(ml/100 g tissue/min)	(ml/min)	(ml/100 g tissue/min)
Heart	250	80	30	10
Brain	700	50	50	3
Kidneys	1200	400	20	6

Blood/gas partition coefficients, *see Partition coefficients*

Blood gas tensions. Normal values:
- arterial blood:
  - O_2 13.3 kPa (100 mmHg)
  - CO_2 5.3 kPa (40 mmHg)
- **mixed venous blood**:
  - O_2 5.3 kPa (40 mmHg)
  - CO_2 6.1 kPa (46 mmHg)

Inaccuracy may result from excess **heparin** (acidic), bubbles within the syringe, inadvertent venous sampling (when arterial sampling is intended), and metabolism by blood cells. The latter is reduced by rapid analysis after taking the sample, or storage of the sample in ice.

O_2, CO_2 and pH electrodes require maintenance at 37°C.

Arterial blood gas analysis usually provides values for O_2 and CO_2 tensions, **bicarbonate** and **standard bicarbonate** concentrations, **pH** and **base excess**.

- Suggested plan for interpretation:
  - oxygenation:
    - knowledge of the F_IO_2 is required before interpretation is possible.
    - calculation of the alveolar PO_2 (from **alveolar gas equation**).
    - calculation of the **alveolar–arterial O_2 difference**.
  - **acid–base balance**:
    - identification of **acidaemia** or **alkalaemia**, representing **acidosis** or **alkalosis** respectively.
    - identification of a respiratory component by looking at the CO_2 tension.
    - identification of a metabolic component by looking at the base excess/deficit or standard bicarbonate (both are corrected to a normal CO_2 tension, thus eliminating respiratory factors).
    - knowledge of the clinical situation helps to decide whether the respiratory or metabolic component represents the primary change.

see Carbon dioxide measurement; Carbon dioxide transport; Oxygen measurement; Oxygen transport

Blood groups. Each individual's red cells bear certain antigens capable of producing an antibody response in another person. Some are only present on red cells, e.g. **Rhesus** antigens; others are also present on other tissue cells, e.g. **ABO** antigens. **Immunoglobulins** may occur naturally, e.g. ABO and Lewis, or following exposure to the antigen, e.g. Rhesus; they are usually IgG or IgM. Administration of blood cells to a recipient who has the corresponding antibody causes **haemolysis** and a severe reaction.

Minor blood groups may be important clinically following ABO typed uncross-matched **blood transfusion**, or multiple transfusions; an atypical antibody in a recipient makes the finding of suitable donor blood difficult. Minor groups include the Kell, Duffy, Lewis and Kidd systems. Many more have been described; the significance of such diversity is unclear.

See also, Blood cross-matching

Blood loss, peroperative. Methods of estimation:
- clinical judgement of the patient's volume status.
- observation of wound and swabs.
- weighing swabs and subtracting their dry weight.
- measuring sucker loss.
- washing of all swabs, drapes, etc. in a known volume of water and measuring haemoglobin concentration. Volume of blood lost may then be calculated. Measurement of potassium released from lysed cells has also been used.
- measurement of **blood volume**.

Weighing swabs may underestimate blood loss if fluid is lost by evaporation or soaked into drapes. Overestimation may occur if saline, etc., is weighed without correction.

Replacement with blood has been suggested if losses exceed 15–20% of blood volume in adults, or 10% in children, although greater losses may be allowed if the preoperative haemoglobin concentration is high. Until

blood transfusion becomes necessary, losses may be replaced with **colloid** or **crystalloid** solutions (the latter in about 2–3 times the volume of the former).
- Blood loss may be reduced by:
    - **hypotensive anaesthesia**.
    - **tourniquets**.
    - local infiltration with **vasopressor drugs**.
    - appropriate positioning, e.g. head-up for ENT surgery.
    - **spinal** and **extradural anaesthesia**.
- Bleeding may be increased by:
    - raised venous pressure :
        - raised intrathoracic pressure e.g. due to respiratory obstruction, coughing, straining.
        - fluid overload and cardiac failure.
        - inappropriate positioning.
        - venous obstruction.
    - **hypercapnia**.
    - **coagulation disorders**:
        - pre-existing.
        - massive blood transfusion.
        - incompatible blood transfusion.
        - **anticoagulant drugs**.
        - **DIC**.
    - hypertension.
    - poor surgical technique.

Rawle PR, Seeley HF (1987) Br J Hosp Med; 38: 554–7
See also, Haemorrhage

Blood patch, extradural. Injection of 10–20 ml autologous venous blood, immediately after removal from a peripheral vein under sterile conditions, into the **extradural space** for the relief of **postspinal headache** following dural puncture. Blood is thought to seal the dura, preventing further CSF leak. Should be avoided if the patient is febrile, in case of bacteraemia and subsequent extradural abscess. The sending of blood for culture at the time of patching has also been suggested, in case infection does occur. Flushing the extradural needle with saline as the needle is withdrawn may prevent a continuous clot from lying between the extradural space and skin, thus reducing risk of extradural contamination.

Spectacular results have been claimed for blood patching, even when performed up to several months after dural puncture. Relief of headache may occur immediately or within 24 hours. Prophylactic use has been less consistently successful. Complications are rare, and include bradycardia, back and neck ache, root pain, pyrexia, tinnitus and vertigo. Subsequent extradural anaesthesia is unaffected.

Blood pressure, *see Arterial blood pressure; Diastolic blood pressure; Mean blood pressure; Systolic blood pressure*

Blood products. Many products may be obtained from donated blood (Fig. 18), including:
- whole blood: shelf-life of 35 days. 70 ml citrate preservative solution is added to 420 ml blood. It is the source from which all other blood products are derived and is therefore a precious commodity. Consequently the use of whole blood for **blood transfusion** is restricted by most transfusion centres. Heparinized whole blood (lasts for 2 days) has been used for paediatric cardiac surgery.

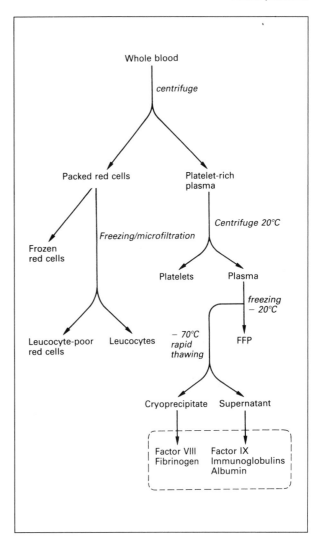

Figure 18 *Blood products available from whole blood. The products enclosed by the dotted line are obtained from pooled plasma*

- packed red cells (plasma reduced): haematocrit is approximately 0.6–0.7. Produced by removing 150–200 ml citrated plasma from a unit of whole blood.
- microaggregate free blood: leucocytes, platelets and debris removed (i.e. the 'buffy coat'). Used to prevent reactions to leucocyte and platelet antigens.
- leucocytes: separated from blood donated by patients whose leucocyte count has been increased by pretreatment with steroids, or those with chronic granulocytic leukaemia.
- frozen blood: used by the armed forces but too expensive and time-consuming for routine use. Glycerol is added to prevent haemolysis. Requires thawing and washing. May be stored for many years.
- SAG-M (saline–adenine–glucose–mannitol) suspended blood: citrated blood from which approximately 250 ml of plasma has been removed, and the red cells resuspended in 100 ml SAG-M solution. Haematocrit is about 0.6–0.7. Shelf-life is 35 days.

Suitable for use in most patients requiring blood transfusion, although plasma protein supplementation may be required earlier.

–platelets: last for 3–5 days. Transfusion is usually restricted to patients with a platelet count of 50 × 10^9/l or less, unless platelet function is abnormal. 6 units usually increase the platelet count by 20–30 × 10^9/l. Filtered by microfilters; ordinary iv giving sets are suitable. Require ABO cross-matching.

–fresh frozen plasma (FFP): lasts for a year. Requires thawing. Contains all the clotting factors. Also a source of plasma **cholinesterase**. Viral infection risk is as for whole blood.

–cryoprecipitate: obtained by rapidly thawing FFP. Frozen and stored at –20°C; thawed immediately before use. Rich in factor VIII and fibrinogen. Viral infection risk is as for whole blood.

–human albumin solution (HAS; previously called plasma protein fraction, PPF): shelf-life of about 2 years. Heat-treated to kill viruses. Contains virtually no clotting factors. Available as 4.5% and 20% (salt-poor albumin) solutions; both contain 140–150 mmol/l sodium but the latter contains less sodium per gram of albumin.

–fibrinogen. Rarely used. Concentrated from donor pools, therefore with higher risk of viral infections.

–factor VIII and IX concentrates. The former is now obtained by recombinant gene engineering, so the risk of viral infection is removed. Previously, the risk was as for fibrinogen.

Crosby ET (1992) Can J Anaesth; 39: 695–707
see also Blood storage

Blood storage. Viability of red cells is defined as at least 70% survival 24 hours post-transfusion.

- The following occur in stored blood:
  –reduced pH, as low as 6.7–7.0.
  –increased lactic acid.
  –increased potassium ion concentration, up to 30 mmol/l.
  –reduced **ATP** and glucose consumption.
  –shift to the left of **oxyhaemoglobin dissociation curve** (**Valtis-Kennedy effect**).
  –reduced **2,3–DPG** levels.
  –reduced viability of other blood constituents, e.g. **platelets** and **leucocytes**, and formation of microaggregates. **Coagulation factors** V and VIII are almost completely destroyed, XI is reduced, and IX and X are reduced after 7 days.

- Storage solutions:
  –ACD (acid–citrate–dextrose): trisodium citrate, citric acid and dextrose. Introduced in the 1940s. Red cell survival is 21 days. 2,3–DPG is greatly reduced after 7 days.
  –CPD (citrate–phosphate–dextrose): citrate, sodium dihydrogen phosphate and dextrose. Described in the late 1950s. Red cell survival: 28 days. 2,3–DPG is greatly reduced after 14 days.
  –CPD-A. Addition of adenine increases red cell ATP levels. Red cell survival: 35 days. 2,3–DPG is low after 14 days.
  –SAG-M (saline 140 mmol/l, adenine 1.5 mmol/l, glucose 50 mmol/l and mannitol 30 mmol/l). Used to resuspend concentrated red cells after removal of plasma from CPD anticoagulated blood, allowing a greater amount of plasma to be removed for other blood products. Has similar preserving properties to CPD-A. Mannitol prevents haemolysis. BAGPM (bicarbonate-added glucose–phosphate–mannitol) is similar.

Storage at 2–6°C is best for red cells but platelets and clotting factors are reduced. 22°C is best for platelets (survival time 3–5 days). Freezing of blood is expensive and time-consuming, but allows storage for many years. It requires two hours' thawing, and removal of glycerol (used to prevent haemolysis).

After rewarming and transfusion, potassium is taken up by red cells. 2,3–DPG levels are restored within 24 hours.

Plastic collection bags, permeable to CO_2 without altering the blood itself, were introduced in the 1960s. In the closed triple bag system, blood passes from the donor to the first collection bag, from which plasma and red cells are passed into separate bags if required. The closed system prevents exposure to air and infection.
See also, Blood products; Blood transfusion

Blood tests, preoperative, *see Investigations, preoperative*

Blood transfusion. Reports of transfusion between animals, and between animals and man, date from the seventeenth century. Transfusions between men were performed in the early nineteenth century. Adverse reactions in recipients, and clotting of blood, were major problems. **ABO blood groups** were discovered in 1900; improvements in **blood cross-matching** and anticoagulation followed.

In the UK, the National Blood Transfusion Service relies on voluntary donors, and is increasingly hard-pressed to meet demand for blood and **blood products**. Perioperative use accounts for about 50% of total blood usage.

- Complications of transfusion:
  –immunological:
    –reactions are associated with 2% of all transfusions.
    –immediate **haemolysis** (e.g. ABO incompatibility). Features include rapid onset of fever, back pain, skin rash, hypotension and dyspnoea. **DIC** and **renal failure** may occur. Hypotension and increased oozing of blood from wounds may be the only indication of incompatible transfusion in an anaesthetized patient. Immediate treatment is as for **anaphylactic reaction**, although the underlying mechanisms are different. Samples of recipient and donor blood should be taken for analysis. Mortality is up to 50%. Most cases arise from clerical errors (e.g. incorrect labelling or administration to the wrong patient).
    –delayed haemolysis (e.g. minor groups). Usually occurs 7–10 days after transfusion, with fever, anaemia and jaundice. Renal failure may occur.
    –reactions to platelets and leucocytes (HLA antigens). Slow onset of fever, dyspnoea and tachycardia; shock is rare.
    –reactions to donor plasma proteins (often immunoglobulin A). May cause anaphylactic reactions.
    –graft-versus-host reaction in immunosupressed patients.
    –febrile reactions of unknown aetiology, with or without urticaria.

–infusion of Rhesus positive blood into Rhesus negative women of child-bearing age may cause haemolytic disease of the newborn in future pregnancies.

–increased mortality has been reported in patients undergoing surgery for colonic cancer, who recieve peroperative transfusion. The mechanism is unknown but may be associated with a substance contained in plasma. Plasma reduced blood has been suggested as a better alternative to whole blood, if transfusion is absolutely neccessary in this group.

–infective:

–**hepatitis**. Donors are excluded for 1 year after hepatitis or jaundice. Donor blood is routinely screened for hepatitis B surface antigen. In the USA, 10% of transfusions have led to hepatitis (about 1% in the UK), 90% of which were thought to be non-A non-B (hepatitis C). Routine serological testing for hepatitis C was introduced in 1991. Hepatitis A is not tested for, as no carrier state exists. If post-transfusion hepatitis occurs, the donor may be traced and further investigated.

–**HIV infection**. At-risk groups are excluded from donating blood. Antibody testing of donor blood has been routine in the UK since 1985; a 1:73 000 incidence of HIV positive 'low-risk' donors has been found. Both cellular components and plasma may transmit HIV. HIV-2 screening began in 1990.

–human T cell leukaemia and lymphoma virus type I (HTLV-I) transmission may follow blood transfusion; screening is performed in the USA but not in the UK. Malignancy uncommonly follows infection.

–**malaria**. Donors are excluded within 6 months of visiting endemic areas. For the following 5 years, plasma only is collected, unless cleared by antibody testing.

–**syphilis**. Donors with past history are excluded. Blood is routinely screened.

–cytomegalovirus. Antibody testing is available for immunocompromised patients but not routine. About 55% of the population are CMV positive.

–glandular fever: donors are excluded for 2 years.

–brucellosis: donors with past history are excluded.

–bacterial contamination of donor units (rare) may result in fever and cardiovascular collapse. Gram-negative organisms are often responsible, e.g. Pseudomonas or coliforms. Platelet concentrates harbouring staphylococcus, yersinia and salmonella have been reported.

–metabolic:

–**hyperkalaemia**: rarely a problem, unless with rapid transfusion in hyperkalaemic patients, as potassium is rapidly taken up by red cells after infusion and warming.

–citrate toxicity: citrate is normally metabolized to bicarbonate within a few minutes. Rapid transfusion may cause **hypocalcaemia**, and **calcium** administration may be required. **Alkalosis** may follow citrate metabolism to bicarbonate.

–**acidosis** due to transfused blood is rarely a problem (see above).

–circulatory overload and cardiac failure. More likely in the elderly, and in the correction of chronic **anaemia**. Diuretics, e.g. **frusemide** 40 mg, may be given with transfusion.

–**hypothermia**. Rapid infusion of cold blood may cause cardiac arrest. All transfused blood should be warmed, especially when infused rapidly. Excessive heat may cause haemolysis.

–impaired O_2 delivery to tissues, due to the leftward shift of **oxyhaemoglobin dissociation curve** in stored blood which lasts up to 24 hours.

–impaired **coagulation** caused by dilution and/or consumption of circulating clotting factors and platelets. **DIC** is rare.

–microaggregates (*see Blood filters*).

–thrombophlebitis and extravasation.

–**air embolism**.

–iron overload (chronic transfusions).

Crosby ET (1992) Can J Anaesth; 39: 695–707 and 822–37

See also, Blood groups; Blood storage; Blood transfusion, massive; Intravenous fluid administration; Rhesus blood groups

Blood transfusion, autologous. Transfusion of blood into a patient, having been previously donated by the same patient. Avoids risks of transfusion reactions and infection, and is becoming more widespread.

● Different methods used:

–2–6 units are taken over a period of days or weeks before surgery. Concurrent oral iron therapy ensures an adequate bone-marrow response. **Erythropoeitin** has been used. Labelling of blood must be meticulous. Pretransfusion testing varies between centres, from ABO grouping to full cross-matching.

–perioperative **haemodilution**: simultaneous collection of blood and replacement of removed volume with colloid or crystalloid. The collected blood is available for transfusion when required.

–peri- or postoperative retransfusion of blood salvaged from the operation site during surgery. Washing and filtering removes debris and contaminants.

Turner DAB (1991) Br J Anaesth; 66: 281–4

See also, Blood transfusion

Blood transfusion, massive. Suggested definitions:

–transfusion of 10 units of blood within 6 hours.

–transfusion of 5 units of blood within 1 hour.

–replacement of blood volume with transfused blood within 24 hours.

● Adverse effects are those of **blood transfusion** generally; in particular:

–impaired O_2 delivery to tissues.

–impaired **coagulation**. Fresh frozen plasma and platelets should be given only when there is clinical and laboratory evidence of abnormal coagulation.

–**hypothermia**.

–**hypocalcaemia** (if rapid transfusion).

–**hyperkalaemia** may occur although this is rarely a problem; **hypokalaemia** may follow potassium uptake by red cells.

–metabolic **acidosis** may occur initially; **alkalosis** may follow as citrate is metabolized to bicarbonate.

–**hypovolaemia** or fluid overload.

–**ARDS** may follow many situations where large blood transfusions are required.

Donaldson MDJ, Seaman MJ, Park GR (1992) Br J Anaesth; 69: 621–30

See also, Blood products; Blood storage

Blood urea nitrogen (BUN). Nitrogen component of blood **urea**. Gives an indication of renal function in a similar way to urea measurement. Normally 1.5–3.3 mmol/l (10–20 mg/dl).

Blood volume. Measured by **dilution techniques**; plasma volume is found by injecting a known dose of marker (e.g. albumin labelled with dyes or radioactive iodine) into the blood and measuring plasma concentrations. Rapid exchange of albumin between plasma and interstitial fluid leads to slight overestimation using this method; larger molecules, e.g. immunoglobulin, may be used.

$$\text{Total blood volume} = \text{plasma volume} \times \frac{100}{100 - \textbf{haematocrit}}$$

Red cell volume may be found by labelling erythrocytes with radioactive markers, e.g. ^{51}Cr.

Total blood volume is approximately 70 ml/kg in adults, 80 ml/kg in children and 90 ml/kg in neonates (although the latter may vary widely, depending on how much blood is returned from the placenta at birth. The formula: [% haematocrit + 50] ml/kg has been suggested for neonates).
- Distribution (approximate):
  –60–70% venous
  –15% arterial
  –10% within the heart
  –5% capillary

Bloody tap, *see Extradural anaesthesia*

Blow-off valve, *see Adjustable pressure-limiting valve*

BMR, *see Basal metabolic rate*

Bodok seal. Metal-edged rubber bonded disk, used to prevent gas leaks from the **cylinder**/yoke interface on **anaesthetic machines**.

Body mass index, *see Obesity*

Body plethysmograph. Airtight box, large enough to enclose a human, used to study **lung volumes** and pressures. Once a subject is inside, air pressure and volume may be measured before and during respiration.
- May be used to measure:
  –**FRC:** the subject makes inspiratory effort against a shutter. Box volume is decreased due to lung expansion, and box pressure increased because of the decrease in volume. Applying **Boyle's law**

  original pressure × volume = new pressure × new volume

  where new volume = original volume - change in lung volume.
  Thus change in lung volume may be calculated. If airway pressures are also measured:

  original airway pressure × resting lung volume = new airway pressure × new lung volume

  where resting lung volume = FRC,
  and new volume = FRC + change in lung volume.
  Thus FRC may be calculated.
  –**airway resistance:**

$$= \frac{\text{alveolar pressure - mouth pressure}}{\text{air flow}}$$

The subject breathes the air in the box. Box volume is reduced by the change in alveolar volume during inspiration, measured as above. Lung volume may be measured at the same time, as above.

  lung volume × starting alveolar pressure = new lung volume × new alveolar pressure;
  where starting alveolar pressure = box pressure, and new lung volume = lung volume + alveolar volume.

Alveolar pressure may thus be calculated.
Mouth pressure = box pressure, and flow may be measured using a **pneumotachograph**.
  –pulmonary blood flow: the subject breathes from a bag containing N_2O and O_2 within the box. As the N_2O is taken up by the blood, the volume of the bag decreases. Since N_2O uptake is flow limited (*see Alveolar gas transfer*), uptake occurs in steps with each heartbeat. The decrease in bag size therefore occurs in steps, and is calculated by measuring bag pressure, and box volume and pressure. If the N_2O carrying capacity of blood is known, pulmonary blood flow may be calculated and displayed as a continuous trace showing pulsatile flow.

Body surface area, *see Surface area, body*

Bohr effect. Shift to the right of the **oxyhaemoglobin dissociation curve** associated with a rise in blood P_{CO_2}, mediated via a reduction in pH. Results in lower affinity of **haemoglobin** for O_2, favouring O_2 delivery to the tissues, where CO_2 levels are high.
- The double Bohr effect refers to pregnancy, when CO_2 passes from fetal to maternal blood at the placenta, causing the following changes:
  –maternal blood: CO_2 rises, i.e. shift of curve to right and reduced O_2 affinity.
  –fetal blood: CO_2 falls, i.e. shift of curve to left and increased O_2 affinity.
  The net effect is to favour O_2 transfer from maternal to fetal blood.
[Christian Bohr (1855–1911), Swedish physician]
See also, Oxygen transport

Bohr equation. Equation used to derive physiological **dead space**.

Expired CO_2 = inspired CO_2 + CO_2 given out by lungs,

Or, $F_E \times V_T = (F_I \times V_T) + (F_A \times V_A)$,

where F_E = fractional concentration of CO_2 in expired gas
  F_I = fractional concentration of CO_2 in inspired gas
  F_A = fractional concentration of CO_2 in alveolar gas
  V_T = tidal volume
  V_A = alveolar component of tidal volume

Since inspired CO_2 is negligible, it may be ignored:
i.e. $F_E \times V_T = F_A \times V_A$

But $V_A = V_T - V_D$, where V_D = dead space

Therefore $F_E \times V_T = F_A \times (V_T - V_D)$
$$= (F_A \times V_T) - (F_A \times V_D)$$

Or $F_A \times V_D = (F_A \times V_T) - (F_E \times V_T)$
$$= V_T (F_A - F_E)$$

Therefore $\dfrac{V_D}{V_T} = \dfrac{F_A - F_E}{F_A}$

Since partial pressure is proportional to concentration:

$$\frac{V_D}{V_T} = \frac{P_A CO_2 - P_E CO_2}{P_A CO_2}$$

where $P_A CO_2$ = alveolar partial pressure of CO_2
$P_E CO_2$ = mixed expired partial pressure of CO_2

Since alveolar $P CO_2$ approximately equals arterial $P CO_2$,

$$\frac{V_D}{V_T} = \frac{P_a CO_2 - P_E CO_2}{P_a CO_2}$$

where $P_a CO_2$ = arterial partial pressure of CO_2.
See also, Bohr effect

Boiling point (bp). Temperature of a substance at which its **SVP** equals external atmospheric pressure. Additional heat does not raise the temperature further, but provides the **latent heat** of vaporization necessary for the liquid to evaporate. If external pressure is raised, e.g. within a pressure cooker, bp is also raised; thus the maximal temperature attainable is raised, and food cooks more quickly.

Bone marrow harvest. Taking of bone marrow for transplantation, from either a healthy donor (allograft) or the patient-recipient prior to radio- or chemotherapy (autograft). Usually performed under general anaesthesia, especially in children, although local anaesthetic techniques may be used.
● Anaesthetic considerations:
  –preoperatively:
    –allografts: donors are usually fit.
    –autografts: usually performed for blood malignancy; i.e. patients may be anaemic, thrombocytopenic, etc. and prone to infections. Cardiovascular, respiratory, and renal function may be impaired. Drug treatment may include **antimitotic drugs** and **steroid therapy**.
  –peroperatively:
    –marrow is usually taken from the posterior and anterior iliac crests and sternum, requiring **positioning** first supine, then prone, although the lateral position may suffice. Tracheal intubation and IPPV is usually employed. Avoidance of **N₂O** has been suggested but this is controversial.
    –an iv cannula is mandatory, since large volume losses, initially from marrow cavity but eventually from the vascular compartment, must be replaced. Autologous **blood transfusion** is usually performed, especially for allografts. Non-autologous blood is irradiated prior to transfusion to kill any leucocytes present. The volume of marrow harvested is up to 20–30% of estimated blood volume, to provide the required leucocyte count.
    –**heparin** may be given to stop the marrow clotting; it may also protect against **fat embolism** which may occur during harvesting.

–postoperatively: large volumes of iv fluids are often required.

Boott, Francis (1792–1863). US-born London physician; qualified in Edinburgh. Read in a letter from **Bigelow**'s father about **Morton**'s demonstration of **diethyl ether**, and arranged a dental extraction by Robinson (who also administered the ether) on 19th December 1846 at his house in Gower St., London, now a nursing home and formerly location of part of the **FCAnaes examination**. Informed **Liston**, who operated using ether 2 days later.
[James Robinson (1813–1861), English dentist]

Bosun warning device, *see Oxygen failure warning devices*

Botulism. Disease caused by ingestion of exotoxins produced by the anaerobic Gram-positive bacillus *Clostridium botulinum*. The source is usually food, especially canned. Exotoxin binds irreversibly to nerve endings, preventing **acetylcholine** release. Affects the **neuromuscular junction**, autonomic ganglia and parasympathetic postganglionic fibres.
● Features occur within 12–72 hours:
  –nausea and vomiting.
  –symmetrical descending paralysis initially affecting **cranial nerves**, with diplopia, facial weakness, dysphagia, dysarthria, limb weakness, and respiratory difficulty.
  –autonomic disturbance: ileus, unresponsive pupils, dry mouth, urinary retention.
  –sensory deficit, mental disturbance, and fever do not occur.
Diagnosed by inoculation of the patient's serum into mice which have been treated or untreated with antitoxin. Different strains of toxin may be identified.
● Management:
  –supportive. IPPV may be necessary.
  –antitoxin to neutralize circulating exotoxin. Hypersensitivity may occur.
  –penicillin to kill live bacilli.
Complete recovery may take months.
  An infant form may also occur, in which colonization of the gut by the bacillus causes toxin production. Wound botulism is caused by colonization of open wounds and is very rare.

Bourdon gauge, *see Pressure measurement*

Bovie machine, *see Diathermy*

Bowditch effect. Intrinsic regulatory mechanism of cardiac muscle in response to increased rate of stimulation. As rate increases, contractility increases.
[Henry Bowditch (1840–1911), US physiologist]

Boyle, Henry Edmund Gaskin (1875–1941). English anaesthetist, best known for the **anaesthetic machine** named after him. Originally introduced in 1917, it consisted of N₂O and O₂ **cylinders**, pressure gauges, water-sight **flowmeters** and ether **vaporizer** ('Boyle's bottle') set in a wooden case. His name is also attached to the instrument used to maintain jaw opening during tonsillectomy (Boyle–Davis gag). Boyle practised at St Bartholomew's Hospital, London, was involved in the advancement and improve-

ment of anaesthesia in the UK, and performed much work into the use of N_2O, including under battle conditions.
[John S Davis (1824–1885), US surgeon]
Hadfield CF (1950) Br J Anaesth; 22: 107–17

Boyle's law. At constant temperature, the volume of a fixed mass of a perfect gas varies inversely with pressure.
[Robert Boyle (1627–1691), English chemist]
See also, Charles' law; Ideal gas law

Brachial plexus. Nerve plexus supplying the arm. Arises from the ventral rami of the lower cervical and first thoracic **spinal nerves**, and emerges between the scalene muscles in the neck. The plexus invaginates the scalene fascia and passes down over the first **rib** (Fig. 19a). It accompanies the subclavian artery (which becomes the axillary artery) within a perivascular sheath of connective tissue.
- Anatomy of the scalene muscles:
    –scalenus anterior arises from the anterior tubercles of the 3rd–6th cervical transverse processes, and inserts into the scalene tubercle on the first rib.
    –scalenus medius arises from the posterior tubercles of the 2nd–6th cervical transverse processes, and inserts into the first rib behind the groove for the subclavian artery.
    –scalenus posterior is the portion of the previous muscle attached to the second rib.
- The roots lie in the interscalene groove; the trunks cross the posterior triangle of the neck; the divisions lie behind the clavicle; the cords lie in the axilla. Branches arise at different levels (Fig. 19b):
    –roots: nerves to the rhomboids, scalene muscles and serratus anterior (long thoracic nerve), and a contribution to the **phrenic nerve** (C5).
    –trunks: nerve to subclavius, and the suprascapular nerve (to supraspinatus and infraspinatus).
    –cords:
        –lateral:
            –lateral pectoral nerve to pectoralis major.
            –musculocutaneous nerve: passes through the belly of coracobrachialis in the upper arm, supplying coracobrachialis, biceps and brachialis muscles and the elbow joint. Continues as the lateral cutaneous nerve of the forearm, supplying the radial surface of the forearm.
            –lateral part of the **median nerve**.
        –medial:
            –medial pectoral nerve to pectoralis major and minor.
            –medial cutaneous nerves of the arm and forearm: supply the medial aspect of the upper arm and forearm respectively.
            –**ulnar nerve**.
            –medial part of median nerve.
        –posterior:
            –subscapular nerves to subscapularis and teres major.
            –nerve to latissimus dorsi.
            –axillary nerve: passes posterior to the neck of the humerus. Supplies deltoid and teres minor and the shoulder joint, and continues as the upper lateral cutaneous nerve of the arm, supplying the skin of the outer shoulder.
            –**radial nerve**.

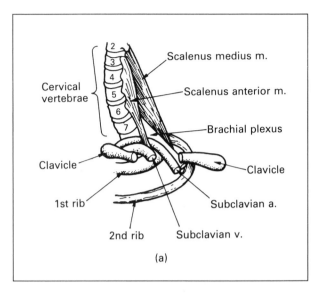

Figure 19 *(a) Relations of the upper brachial plexus. (b) Plan of the brachial plexus. (c) Cutaneous supply of the arm*

The plexus thus supplies the skin of the upper limb (Fig. 19c).
- Characteristic motor lesions of the plexus:
    –upper roots: 'waiter's tip' position; arm internally rotated and pronated, with wrist flexed (Erb's paralysis).
    –lower roots: claw hand (Klumpke's paralysis).
[Wilhelm Erb (1840–1921), German physician; Augusta Klumpke (1859–1927), French neurologist]
See also, Brachial plexus block; Dermatomes

Brachial plexus block. May be performed by injecting local anaesthetic solution into the fascial compartment surrounding the **brachial plexus** at several levels:
    –interscalene:
        –with the patient's head turned away from the side to be blocked, a needle is inserted in the interscalene groove, lateral to the sternomastoid, and level with the cricoid cartilage. It is directed towards the transverse process of C6 (medially, caudally and posteriorly). Accidental extradural, intrathecal or intravascular injections are more likely if the needle is directed cranially.
        –30–40 ml solution is injected when parasthesiae are produced or a click felt.
        –produces adequate block for shoulder manipulations.
        –**ulnar** nerve may be 'missed'.
        –complications include phrenic nerve block, recurrent laryngeal nerve block, **Horner's syndrome**, inadvertent extradural or spinal block, and injection into the vertebral artery. Bilateral blocks should be avoided.
    –supraclavicular:
        –with the patient's head turned away from the side to be blocked, a needle is inserted immediately posterior and lateral to the subclavian pulsation behind the mid-clavicle. It is directed caudally, medially and posteriorly to the upper surface of first rib, and 'walked' along the rib until parasthe-

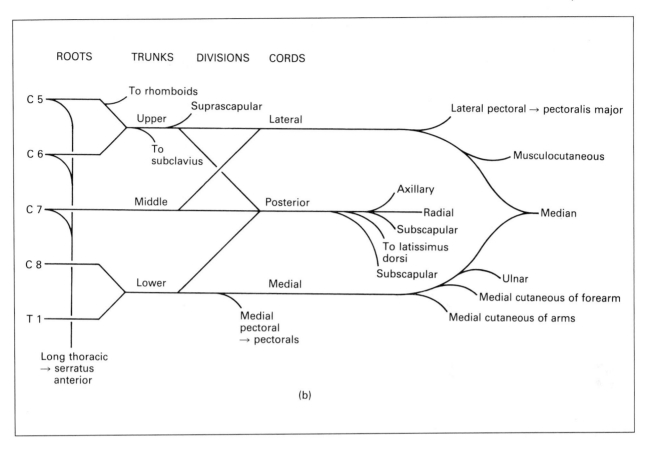

(b)

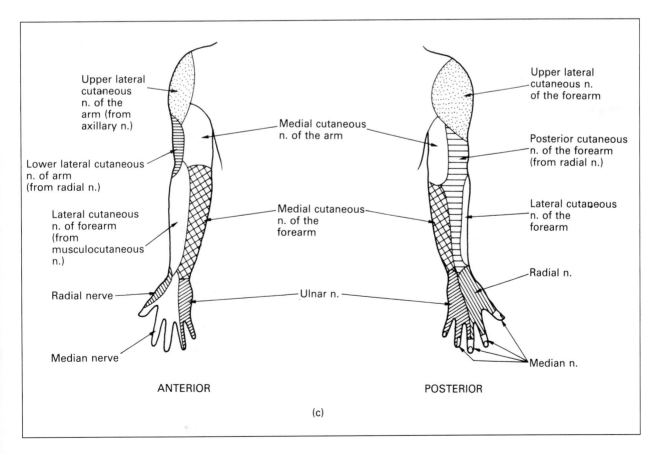

(c)

siae are produced; 8–10 ml solution are injected per division.

–**median** nerve may be 'missed'.

–complications: phrenic and recurrent laryngeal nerve blocks, Horner's syndrome, subclavian puncture, **pneumothorax**. Bilateral blocks should be avoided.

–subclavian perivascular:

–with the patient's head turned away from the side to be blocked, a needle is inserted in the interscalene groove, caudal to the level of the cricoid cartilage, and cranial and posterior to a finger palpating the subclavian artery. It is directed caudally only, until parasthesiae are produced in the arm/hand, not in the shoulder (which may be caused by stimulation of the suprascapular nerve).

–20–30 ml solution are injected.

–complications: as for supraclavicular block, but pneumothorax is less likely.

–axillary:

–with the patient's head turned away, the arm abducted to 90°, and the hand under the head, a needle is inserted just above the axillary artery pulsation, as high in the axilla as possible. A click is felt as the perivascular sheath is entered.

–25–50 ml solution is injected, with digital pressure or a tourniquet below the injection site to encourage upward spread of solution. Careful aspiration before application of digital pressure excludes placement of the needle in the axillary vein. The arm is returned to the patient's side after injection, to avoid compression of the proximal sheath by the humeral head, or before injection if a cannula technique is used.

–a cannula, e.g. iv type 18–20 G, may be inserted and used for repeated injection.

–may 'miss' the musculocutaneous and axillary nerves. The former may be blocked thus:

–upper arm: at the time of axillary block, 5–10 ml is injected above the perivascular sheath, into coracobrachialis muscle.

–elbow: 10 ml is injected in the groove between biceps tendon and brachioradialis in the **antecubital fossa**, and infiltrated subcutaneously around the lateral elbow.

–the intercostobrachial nerve, supplying the inner upper arm, may be blocked by superficial infiltration as the needle is withdrawn from the axillary block.

–fascial sheets within the neurovascular sheath may cause a 'patchy' block. Puncture both above and below the artery has been suggested as a remedy. Intentional transfixion of the artery has also been described: blood is aspirated as the needle is advanced through the artery; when aspiration ceases, solution is deposited posterior to the artery.

An infraclavicular approach has also been described.

• Suitable solutions:

–**prilocaine** or **lignocaine** 1–1.5% with adrenaline: onset within 20–30 minutes and lasts for 1.5–2 hours.

–**bupivacaine** 0.375–0.5%: onset up to an hour; lasts for up to 12 hours. Combination with 1% lignocaine speeds onset.

The area blocked is increased by using larger volumes of solution. Motor block is increased by increasing concentration, and intensity of block by increasing total dose. Although maximal safe doses have been exceeded without serious effects or high blood levels of agent, this cannot be recommended routinely. Systemic uptake of agent is greatest following interscalene block, and least following axillary block. Incidence of neurological damage is reduced by using short bevelled needles, and using a nerve stimulator rather than eliciting parasthesiae as the end-point for injection.

Brockway MS, Wildsmith JAW (1990) Br J Anaesth; 64: 224–31

Bradycardia, *see Heart block; Junctional arrhythmias; Sinus bradycardia*

Bradykinin, *see Kinins*

Brain. Intracranial part of the CNS. Forms from tubular neural tissue, developing into hindbrain, midbrain and forebrain:

–hindbrain:

–medulla: continuous with the **spinal cord**. Communicates with the cerebellum via the inferior cerebellar peduncle. Forms the posterior part of the fourth ventricle floor. Contains the decussation of pyramidal tracts, gracile and cuneate nuclei, nuclei of **cranial nerves** IX, X, XI and XII, and 'vital centres', e.g. for respiration and cardiovascular homeostasis.

–pons: communicates with the cerebellum via the middle cerebellar peduncle. Forms the anterior part of the fourth ventricle floor. Contains the nuclei of cranial nerves V, VI, VII and VIII, and pontine nuclei.

–cerebellum: occupies the posterior cranial fossa. Consists of grey cortex covering white matter. Communicates via the medulla, pons and midbrain with the thalamus, cerebral cortex and spinal cord. Regulates posture, coordination and muscle tone. Lesions cause ipsilateral effects.

–midbrain:

–communicates with the cerebellum via the superior cerebellar peduncle. Contains the pineal body and cranial nerve nuclei III and IV.

–forebrain:

–diencephalon: consists of the **hypothalamus** (floor of the third ventricle) with the **pituitary gland** below, and thalamus (lateral wall of the third ventricle). The thalamus integrates sensory pathways.

–basal ganglia: grey matter within cerebral hemispheres. The internal capsule, containing the major ascending and descending pathways to and from the cerebral cortex, passes between the basal ganglia. They receive and relay information concerned with fine motor control.

–cerebral cortex:

–frontal lobes: contain motor cortices, including areas for speech and eye movement; areas for intellectual and emotional functions lie anteriorly.

–parietal lobes: contain sensory cortices, and areas for association and integration of sensory input.

–temporal lobes: contain auditory cortices, and areas for integration and association of auditory input. Also contain the **limbic system**, possibly concerned with memory and mood.

–occipital lobes: contain the visual cortices, and areas for association and integration of visual sensory input.

See also, Brainstem; Cerebral circulation; Cerebrospinal fluid; Motor pathways; Sensory pathways

Brainstem. Composed of midbrain, pons and medulla. Contains neuron groups involved in the control of breathing, cardiovascular homeostasis, GIT function, balance and equilibrium, and eye movement. Also integrates ascending and descending pathways between the **spinal cord**, **cranial nerves**, cerebellum and higher centres, partly via the **ascending reticular activating system**.

See also, Brain; Brainstem death; Breathing, control of

Brainstem death. Irreversible absence of **brainstem** function despite artificial maintenance of circulation and gas exchange. Clinical experience has shown that once it is diagnosed, cardiac arrest is inevitable, usually within a few days. Guidelines have been established for the withdrawal of artificial support and, where appropriate, arrangement for **organ donation**, when recovery is impossible. These guidelines consist of certain preconditions and clinical criteria:

–unconscious patient with a known irreversible cause of coma.

–no possibility of drugs causing CNS depression or paralysis.

–no endocrine or metabolic disturbances causing CNS depression.

–no primary hypothermia; i.e. temperature >35°C.

–absent pupillary reflex to light.

–absent corneal reflex.

–absent oculovestibular reflex, i.e. no eye movement following injection of 20 ml icy water into the ear canal (normal response is nystagmus, with the fast component away from the ear tested). Each ear is tested in turn, having checked that the canal is not blocked.

–absent motor responses within cranial nerve distribution, to any peripheral stimuli.

–absent gag or cough reflex, including carinal reflex.

–absent respiratory efforts despite arterial $P\text{CO}_2$ of 6.6 kPa (50 mmHg), and adequate oxygenation (e.g. with **apnoeic oxygenation**). Blood gas tensions should be measured.

All the above requirements must be met for the diagnosis of brainstem death to be made. Testing should be independently performed by two doctors, one of whom is a consultant, the other a consultant or senior registrar. Although **EEG**, cerebral angiography and **oesophageal contractility** testing are performed in some centres, they are not required to make the diagnosis of brainstem death.

Persistent vegetative state associated with absent cortical function or cortical disconnection may occur with intact brainstem reflexes. Such patients may have spontaneous respiration and may live for years without recovery, and are not 'brainstem dead'.

Braun, Heinrich Friedrich Wilhelm (1862–1934). German surgeon; also practised and investigated anaesthesia. One of the pioneers of local anaesthesia, he described many local blocks, and published extensively on the subject. Introduced **adrenaline** to local anaesthetic solutions to prolong their action in 1902. Popularized **procaine** in 1905.

Breathing, control of. The exact origin of the signal for regular breathing is unknown. Brainstem centres involved in the control of breathing have been identified; their precise roles are unclear. There are three such centres:

–medullary centre:

–dorsal neurones cause diaphragmatic contraction via contralateral phrenic nerves; they also project to ventral neurones.

–ventral neurones cause contraction of ipsilateral accessory muscles (via vagus nerves) and intercostal muscles.

–apneustic centre in the lower pons: causes excitation of medullary inspiratory neurones. Surgical section above it causes prolonged inspiratory gasping. Vagal division in addition causes apneusis (breath held in inspiration).

–pneumotactic centre (nucleus parabrachialis) in the upper pons: curtails inspiration and regulates respiratory rate.

● The 'respiratory centre' comprised of these groups of neurones receives afferents from **chemoreceptors** and other structures:

–chemoreceptors :

–peripheral (**aortic** and **carotid bodies**): afferents pass via the vagus and glossopharyngeal nerves respectively. Stimulated by a fall in arterial $P\text{O}_2$, also by a rise in $P\text{CO}_2$ and hydrogen ion concentration. Their response to reduced O_2 increases markedly below 8–10 kPa (60–75 mmHg). The response to increased CO_2 is roughly linear.

–central: present on the ventral surface of the medulla, but separate from the respiratory centre. Stimulated by a rise in hydrogen ion concentration in CSF, due to increased $P\text{CO}_2$ or metabolic acidosis.

Hypoxaemia increases the sensitivity of the chemoreceptors to **hypercapnia**, and vice versa. Hypoxaemia causes direct depression of the respiratory centres, in addition to reflex stimulation. In chronic lung disease, the central chemoreceptors may not respond to increased CO_2 levels, either due to chemoreceptor 'resetting' or due to correction of CSF pH. Hypoxaemia then becomes the main drive to respiration (of importance in **O_2 therapy**).

–other structures:

–lungs:

–**pulmonary stretch receptors**, involved in the **Hering–Breuer** and **deflation reflexes**.

–**J receptors**, involved in dyspnoea due to pulmonary disease and pulmonary oedema.

–**pulmonary irritant receptors**, responding to noxious stimuli.

–proprioceptors in joints and muscles, thought to be important during exercise.

–**baroreceptors**; hypertension inhibits ventilation, but this is of little clinical significance.

–higher centres, responding to pain, fear, etc..

During anaesthesia, the responses to hypercapnia and hypoxaemia are depressed, the latter severely.

See also, Carbon dioxide response curve; Hypoventilation

Breathing, muscles of, *see Respiratory muscles*

Breathing systems, *see Anaesthetic breathing systems*

Breathing, work of. Equals the product of pressure change across the lung and volume of gas moved. During inspiration, most of the work of breathing is done to overcome elastic recoil of the thorax and lungs, and the resistance of the airways and non-elastic tissues (Fig. 20):

- –the area enclosed by the broken line represents work done to overcome elastic forces.
- –area A represents work done to overcome resistance during inspiration.
- –area B represents work done to overcome resistance during expiration.

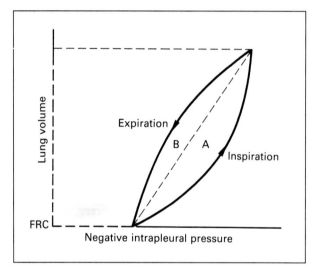

Figure 20 *Graph of intrapleural pressure against lung volume during breathing (see text)*

The greater the tidal volume or lung volume, the more work is required to overcome elastic recoil. The faster the flow rates, the greater the amount of work required to overcome resistance. Normally, energy is provided for expiration by potential energy stored in the stretched elastic tissues (i.e. area B lies within the broken line), but extra energy may be required in **airway obstruction**.

Total work of breathing is difficult to measure in spontaneous respiration. Volume may be measured with a **pneumotachograph**; oesophageal pressure, indicating **intrapleural pressure**, may be measured with an oesophageal balloon. Normally, the work of breathing accounts for less than 3% of the total body O_2 consumption at rest, but may be much higher in disease states, e.g. **COAD**, **cardiac failure**, and during exercise.

Expiratory valves in anaesthetic breathing systems increase work of expiration, particularly when not fully open. **Coaxial anaesthetic breathing systems** increase expiratory resistance, the Lack by virtue of its small calibre expiratory tube, and the Bain because of the high flow rate of fresh gas directed at the patient's mouth.

See also, Airway resistance; Compliance

Bretylium tosylate. Class II and III **antiarrhythmic drug**, originally introduced as an **antihypertensive drug**.

Reduces sympathetic drive to the heart and prolongs the **action potential**. Taken up by adrenergic nerve endings, causing release of **noradrenaline** followed by inhibition of release. Reserved for treatment of resistant ventricular arrythmias. Excreted largely unchanged in the urine.

- Dosage: 5–10 mg/kg slowly iv, followed by 5–10 mg/kg 6–8 hourly. May also be given im.

Initial hypertension may be followed by severe hypotension. May cause nausea and vomiting.

Brewer–Luckhardt reflex. Laryngospasm in response to remote stimulation, e.g. anal or cervical dilatation.
[Nathan Brewer and AB Luckhardt (described 1934), Chicago physiologists]

British Journal of Anaesthesia. Second oldest journal of anaesthesia (first published in 1923), and the first to be published monthly (in 1955). Previously unassociated with any association, institution or society, it became the official journal of the **College of Anaesthetists** in 1990.

Bromethol (Tribromethanol; Avertin). CBr_3CH_2OH. Sedative drug introduced in 1927 and no longer available. Given rectally to provide deep sedation or anaesthesia, particularly in children. May also be given iv. May cause cardiovascular and respiratory depression.

Bronchial blockers, *see Endobronchial blockers*

Bronchial carcinoma. Commonest cancer in Western men; the incidence is rapidly rising in women. Mostly associated with **smoking**, but also occurs following exposure to asbestos, and certain chemical and radioactive substances used in industry. Air pollution may also be a causative factor. Five-year survival is less than 10%.

- Types:
  - –squamous cell (35%): most present with bronchial obstruction. Better prognosis than the other common forms.
  - –small cell (24%): may arise from **APUD** cells, and secrete hormones. Extensive spread is usual at presentation. Extremely poor prognosis.
  - –adenocarcinoma (21%).
  - –large cell (19%): particularly related to smoking.
  - –others:
    - –bronchiolar alveolar, carcinoid: least related to smoking.
    - –carcinoma in situ.
    - –others.
- Features:
  - –local:
    - –haemoptysis, cough, dyspnoea.
    - –wheeze, stridor, chest discomfort.
    - –**chest infection, pleural effusion**.
  - –invasion of:
    - –mediastinum, chest wall, etc. May cause **superior vena caval obstruction**, dysphagia, cardiac **arrhythmias**, pericardial effusion, etc.
    - –vertebrae.
    - –recurrent laryngeal nerve, usually on the left.
    - –sympathetic trunk at C8/T1, causing **Horner's syndrome**.
    - –**brachial plexus** at lung apex, causing pain and wasting in the hand/arm (with Horner's syndrome,

± rib or vertebral erosion, ± superior vena caval obstruction, = Pancoast syndrome).
  –metastases: commonly lymph nodes, bone, liver, brain.
  –other features:
    –fatigue, anorexia, weight loss, anaemia.
    –hormone secretion, e.g. causing the **syndrome of inappropriate antidiuretic hormone secretion**, **Cushing's syndrome**, **hypercalcaemia** due to parathormone secretion, **carcinoid syndrome**. Most common with small cell tumours. Thyroid and sex hormone secretion may occur.
    –sensory or motor neuropathy; cerebellar atrophy.
    –**myasthenic syndrome**, muscle weakness, dermatomyositis.
    –finger clubbing and hypertrophic pulmonary osteoarthropathy.

May present for **bronchoscopy**, mediastinoscopy or **thoracic surgery**. Anaesthetic considerations are related to the above features and effects of smoking; thus **preoperative assessment** of respiratory, cardiovascular and neurological systems, and hormonal and metabolic status, is particularly important.

Radiotherapy is used mainly for palliative treatment of pain and obstructive lesions (e.g. superior vena caval obstruction) especially due to small cell carcinoma. Chemotherapy has also been used, particularly in small cell carcinoma.
[Henry Pancoast (1875–1939), US radiologist]

Bronchial tree, *see Tracheobronchial tree*

Bronchiectasis. Permanent abnormal bronchial dilatation, usually suppurative. May follow pneumonia, bronchial obstruction, chronic repeated chest infections, e.g. in **cystic fibrosis** and immunological impairment.
● Features:
  –haemoptysis.
  –chronic cough with purulent sputum.
  –chronic respiratory insufficiency, of restrictive and/or obstructive pattern.
  –empyema, abscesses, cor pulmonale, clubbing.
  –**chest X-ray**: increased lung markings, patchy shadowing, thick-walled dilated bronchi.
Treatment includes antibiotic therapy, **physiotherapy** and postural drainage, and lung resection if disease is localized.
● Anaesthetic management:
  –preoperatively:
    –early admission for **preoperative assessment**, medical treatment and physiotherapy.
    –chest X-ray, arterial blood gas analysis, **lung function tests** as appropriate.
  –peroperatively: soiling of the unaffected lung is reduced by appropriate positioning. Double-lumen **endobronchial tubes** may assist surgery and allow isolation and suction of copious secretions.
  –postoperatively: adequate analgesia and physiotherapy to reduce risk of respiratory complications.

Bronchodilator drugs. Drugs which increase bronchial diameter.
● Postulated mechanisms of action:
  –**β-adrenergic receptor agonists**, e.g. **salbutamol**:
    –inhibit degranulation of **mast cells**.
    –stimulate adenylate cyclase in smooth muscle cells, leading to increased **cAMP** levels, thus causing reduced intracellular **calcium** and relaxation.
  –**theophylline, aminophylline**:
    –**phosphodiesterase inhibitors** in smooth muscle cells, increasing cAMP levels.
    –possible effect via release of **catecholamines** via adenosine inhibition.
    –possible effect on **myosin** light chains, reducing contraction.
  –**anticholinergic drugs**, e.g. **ipratropium**:
    –block cholinergic receptors, decreasing intracellular guanine monophosphate (cGMP; opposes the bronchodilating action of cAMP).
    –possible effect via reduction in intracellular calcium.
  –**steroid therapy**:
    –anti-inflammatory action.
    –reduced capillary permeability.
    –possibly increase the effects of β-adrenergic receptor agonists .
Cromoglycate is not a bronchodilator, but helps prevent bronchoconstriction by inhibiting mast cell mediator release, via inhibition of calcium ion entry.
See also, Asthma; Bronchospasm

Bronchopleural fistula. Abnormal connection between the **tracheobronchial tree** and **pleura**. Most commonly occurs 2–10 days after pneumonectomy, although it may follow trauma, chronic infection and erosion by tumour.
● Features:
  –fever, productive cough, malaise.
  –X-ray evidence of infection in the remaining lung with fall in fluid level on the affected side.
● Problems caused:
  –source of (usually) infected material in one pleural cavity, with potential contamination of the normal lung through the fistula. Repeated spillage may cause pulmonary function impairment before corrective surgery.
  –IPPV may force fresh gas through the fistula, without inflating the remaining lung. Increased pressure in the affected pleura increases likelihood of contamination, and may impair cardiac output.
● Management:
  –chest drainage.
  –monitoring set up under local anaesthesia.
  –sitting the patient up, with affected side lowermost.
  –classical method for induction of anaesthesia: inhalational induction and intubation with a double-lumen **endobronchial tube**, with spontaneous ventilation. IPPV may be started once the affected side has been isolated. However, deep anaesthesia with volatile agents may cause profound cardiovascular effects, and coughing may increase contamination risk. Suggested alternatives include awake intubation under local anaesthesia, or preoxygenation, iv induction and intubation using **suxamethonium** (only advocated by, and for, experienced thoracic anaesthetists).
  –postoperatively, IPPV may be necessary. **High frequency ventilation** has been used.
See also, Thoracic surgery

Bronchopulmonary lavage. Performed in pulmonary alveolar proteinosis, to remove accumulated lipoproteinaceous material. Has also been used in **asthma** and **cystic fibrosis**. Usually performed under general anaesthesia, and involves instillation and drainage under gravity of 20–40 litres warm buffered saline (**heparin** may be added) through one lumen of a double lumen **endobronchial tube**, whilst ventilating via the other. The other lung is treated after a few days. Main problems are related to the pre-existing state of the patient, **one-lung anaesthesia**, and avoidance of soiling of the ventilated lung. **Cardiopulmonary bypass** has also been used. Lavage using small volumes is sometimes used to aid diagnosis of atypical chest infections, and is usually carried out via a flexible bronchoscope under local anaesthesia.

Bronchoscopy. Performed for diagnosis and management of bronchial disorders, e.g. tumours, infection, aspiration of sputum and aspirated material, etc. Fibreoptic bronchoscopy is commonly performed under local anaesthesia as for awake intubation; it may also be used during general anaesthesia to aid and check placement of **endobronchial tubes**, and on ICU. The fibreoptic bronchoscope may be passed through a rubber-sealed connector at the proximal end of a tracheal tube; ventilation then proceeds as usual. General anaesthesia is required most commonly for rigid bronchoscopy, and in children, e.g. for removal of foreign bodies.

- Anaesthetic management for rigid bronchoscopy:
  - preoperatively:
    - **preoperative assessment** is particularly directed at the respiratory and cardiovascular systems. Many patients will have **bronchial carcinoma** or other **smoking**-related diseases. Secretions may be improved by preoperative **physiotherapy**. Neck mobility and the teeth should be assessed.
    - **premedication** reduces **awareness**. The antisialogogue effects of **anticholinergic drugs** may be useful.
  - peroperatively:
    - iv **induction of anaesthesia** is usual. Inhalational induction may be indicated if **airway obstruction** is present, particularly in children. Neuromuscular blockade is commonly achieved with **suxamethonium** (intermittent doses or infusion), **atracurium** or **vecuronium**, because of their short duration of action.
    - spraying of the larynx with **lignocaine** may reduce peroperative and postoperative coughing and **laryngospasm**.
    - ventilation: several methods may be used:
      - **injector techniques**; air entrainment through the bronchoscope using intermittent blasts of O_2. Automatic jet ventilators have been used for long procedures.
      - IPPV via a side arm on the bronchoscope, the proximal end of which is occluded by a window or the operator's thumb.
      - deep anaesthesia with spontaneous ventilation. Often used in children, classically using **diethyl ether** but now **halothane**. Anaesthetic gases may be delivered via a side arm on the bronchoscope; before these 'ventilating bronchoscopes' became available, the patient breathed air and bronchoscopy was performed as anaesthesia lightened.
      - **insufflation techniques**, particularly **apnoeic oxygenation**. Suitable for short procedures only.
      - intermittent IPPV via a tracheal tube placed in the proximal end of the bronchoscope.
      - **high frequency ventilation** has been used.
    - **monitoring** as standard. Pulse **oximetry** is very useful, especially when intermittent IPPV is employed.
    - awareness is a particular problem, especially with jet ventilation using 100% O_2, or apnoeic oxygenation. Regular supplements or continuous infusion of **iv anaesthetic agents** reduce the incidence, as does premedication.
    - **recovery** should be in the lateral, head-down position, to encourage drainage of blood and secretions.

See also, Foreign body, inhaled; Intubation, awake

Bronchospasm. May occur during anaesthesia due to:
- surgical stimulation.
- presence of airway or tracheal tube.
- pharyngeal/laryngeal/bronchial secretions or blood.
- **aspiration of gastric contents**.
- **anaphylactic** or **anaphylactoid reaction**.
- **pulmonary oedema**.
- use of **β-adrenergic receptor antagonists**.

Particularly likely in patients with **asthma** or **COAD**, and if anaesthesia is inadequate.
- Features:
  - wheezing.
  - reduced movement of reservoir bag.
  - increased expiratory time.
  - increased airway pressures.
- Must be distinguished from:
  - **pneumothorax**.
  - mechanical obstruction.
  - **laryngospasm**.
  - pulmonary oedema.
- Treatment:
  - of primary cause.
  - increased F_1O_2.
  - increased inspired concentration of volatile **inhalational anaesthetic agent**.
  - **salbutamol** 250–500 µg sc/im or 250 µg iv. Delivery by nebulizer or aerosol may also be used but may be technically difficult.
  - **aminophylline** 3–6 mg/kg iv slowly, followed by 0.5 mg/kg/h infusion.
  - further management as for asthma.

Brown fat. Specialized adipose tissue used for heat generation because of its chemical makeup and structural composition. Of particular importance in **temperature regulation** in **neonates**. Laid down from about 22 weeks of gestation around the base of the neck, axillae, mediastinum and between the scapulae; gradually replaced by adult 'white' adipose tissue after birth, the process taking several years. Fat breakdown and thermogenesis is increased by α-adrenergic neurone activity.

BTPS. Body temperature and pressure, saturated with water vapour.

Buccal nerve block, *see Mandibular nerve blocks*

Buffer base. Blood anions which can act as **bases** and accept **hydrogen ions**. Mainly composed of **bicarbonate**,

haemoglobin and negatively charged proteins.
See also, Acid–base balance; buffers

Buffers. Substances which resist a change in **pH** by absorbing or releasing **hydrogen ions** when **acid** or **base** is added to the solution. In the body, buffering is one mechanism by which pH is kept relatively constant.

For the equation $HA \rightleftharpoons H^+ + A^-$, where HA = undissociated acid and A^- = anion, the equation shifts to the left if acid is added, and to the right if base is added; changes in H^+ concentration are thus minimized.

The **Henderson-Hasselbalch equation** enables analysis of pH changes:

$$pH = pK + \log \frac{[A^-]}{[HA]}$$

When pH equals **pK** of the buffer system, maximal buffering may occur, because HA and A^- exist in equal amounts.
- Body buffer systems:
  - –blood:
    - –carbonic acid/**bicarbonate**: $H_2CO_3 \rightleftharpoons H^+ + HCO_3^-$. The pK is 6.1; i.e. the system is not very efficient at body pH. However, CO_2 may be eliminated via the lungs, and bicarbonate regulated via the kidneys. These mechanisms, plus the large amount of plasma bicarbonate, make this the main buffer system in the blood.
    - –**haemoglobin**: dissociation of histidine residues gives haemoglobin six times the buffering capacity of plasma proteins. Deoxygenated haemoglobin is a better buffer than oxygenated haemoglobin (**Haldane effect**).
    - –plasma proteins: carboxyl and amino groups dissociate to form anions; this accounts for a small amount of buffer capacity.
    - –phosphate: $H_2PO_4^- \rightleftharpoons H^+ + HPO_4^{2-}$. Plays a small part in buffering in the ECF.
  - –intracellular:
    - –proteins.
    - –phosphate.

See also, Acid–base balance

Bumetanide. Diuretic, similar to **frusemide** in its actions, but with a faster onset and shorter duration of action. 1 mg is approximately equivalent to 40 mg frusemide. Diuresis begins within minutes of an iv dose and lasts for 2 hours. May also be given orally; usual starting dose: 1 mg.
- Side effects: as for frusemide; myalgia may also occur, especially with high doses.

BUN, *see Blood urea nitrogen*

Bundle branch block (BBB). Interruption of impulse propagation in the **heart conducting system** distal to the atrioventricular node. Causes are as for **heart block**.
- May involve right or left bundles:
  - –right BBB:
    - –common; usually clinically insignificant.
    - –**ECG** findings (Fig. 21a):
      - –QRS duration > 0.12 s.
      - –large S wave, lead I.
      - –RSR pattern, lead V_1.

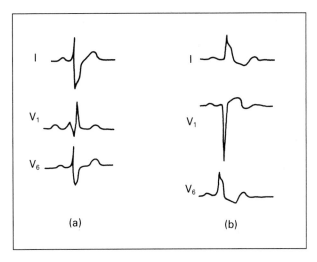

Figure 21 *ECG findings in bundle branch block: (a) right BBB; (b) left BBB*

  - –incomplete BBB may be due to an enlarged right ventricle, e.g. due to **cor pulmonale** or **ASD**.
  - –left BBB:
    - –represents more widespread disease, as the left bundle is a bigger and less discrete structure, consisting of anterior and posterior fascicles. If present preoperatively, it serves as an indicator of existing heart disease.
    - –ECG findings (Fig. 21b):
      - –QRS duration > 0.12 s.
      - –wide R waves, leads I and V_{4-6}.
    - –may be due to left ventricular hypertrophy, e.g. due to hypertension or valvular heart disease.
  - –hemiblock (involving individual fascicles of the left bundle):
    - –left anterior hemiblock:
      - –QRS may be normal or slightly widened.
      - –left axis deviation > 60°.
    - –left posterior hemiblock:
      - –less common, because the posterior fascicle is better perfused than the anterior.
      - –QRS normal or slightly widened.
      - –right axis deviation > 120°.
  - –bifascicular block:
    - –comprised of right BBB and one hemiblock:
      - –anterior:
        - –right BBB ECG pattern and left axis deviation.
        - –may lead to complete heart block later in life, but this is rare during anaesthesia.
      - –posterior:
        - –right BBB ECG pattern and right axis deviation.
        - –rare.
        - –at risk of developing complete heart block.
    - –bifascicular block plus prolonged P–R interval (i.e. partial trifascicular block) is particularly likely to progress to complete heart block.

BBB itself is not a contraindication to anaesthesia, but progression to complete heart block during anaesthesia remains the main risk. Temporary perioperative **cardiac pacing** should be considered if BBB is associated with either a history of syncope or a prologed P–R interval. Anaesthetic management is as for heart block.

Bungarotoxins. Snake venom neurotoxins. α-Bungarotoxin binds irreversibly to postsynaptic **acetylcholine receptors** at the **neuromuscular junction**; β-bungarotoxin acts presynaptically to block acetylcholine release. They have been used to study **neuromuscular transmission**.

Bupivacaine hydrochloride. Amide **local anaesthetic agent**, introduced in 1963. Of slower onset of action and longer duration than **lignocaine**, lasting 3–4 hours for extradural block and up to 12 hours for some nerve blocks, e.g. **brachial plexus**. The addition of **adrenaline** does not prolong the effect of bupivacaine as much as with lignocaine. 0.5% solution is equivalent to 2% lignocaine. Bupivacaine is extensively bound to tissue and plasma proteins. pK_a is 8.1. More cardiotoxic than lignocaine. Mainly metabolized by the liver, a small amount is excreted unchanged in the urine. Widely used for conduction, **spinal** and **extradural anaesthesia**. 0.25–0.5% solutions are used for most purposes. 0.75% produces more prolonged motor block when given epidurally; this concentration is contraindicated in obstetric practice because of toxicity. Contraindicated for use in **IVRA**. A hyperbaric 0.5% solution (with glucose 8%) exists for spinal administration. Maximal safe dose: 2 mg/kg; toxic plasma levels: > 2–4 μg/ml.
See also, individual blocks

Buprenorphine hydrochloride. Opioid analgesic drug derived from thebaine, with partial agonist properties. Synthesized in 1968. 0.4 mg is equivalent to 10 mg **morphine**; it has slower onset and its effects last longer (about 8 hours). May be given iv or im (0.3–0.6 mg), or sublingually (0.2–0.4 mg) 6–8 hourly. Respiratory depression does occur, but reaches a plateau which cannot be exceeded by increasing the dose. Respiratory depression is not readily reversed by **naloxone**. Carries a low risk of dependence.
See also, Opioid receptors

Burns. Burned patients may suffer from:
  –direct thermal injury to body and airway.
  –smoke inhalation, with e.g. **carbon monoxide** (CO) or **cyanide** (CN) **poisoning**.
  –extensive fluid loss into the dermis, into blisters and from skin surfaces.
• Management:
  –high F_IO_2 O_2 therapy. Tracheal intubation and IPPV are required in:
    –severe CO or CN poisoning.
    –upper **airway obstruction.** Obstruction due to oedema may develop over a few hours; thus tracheal intubation should be performed if burns to the airway are present. The latter may be indicated by burns or soot around the face and in the mouth, and are confirmed by fibreoptic bronchoscopy. Obstruction usually resolves within 2–4 days.
    –an unconscious patient.
    –respiratory failure.
  Measurement of blood gas tensions, carboxyhaemoglobin and possibly cyanide levels, should be performed. A chest X-ray is mandatory.
  –assessment of the extent of burns (**rule of nines**).
  –fluid replacement: many different regimens exist, using **colloid, crystalloid** or **hypertonic solutions**. Average total requirement: water (2–4 ml/kg/%

burn) and sodium 0.5 mmol/kg/% burn). Constant reassessment is the most important factor. Common UK regimen:
  –replacement volume (*V*) in ml:

$$V = \frac{\text{body weight (kg)} \times \text{\% surface area burnt}}{2}$$

  $3 \times V$ is infused in the first 12 hours from the time of burn;
  $2 \times V$ in the next 12 hours;
  $1 \times V$ in the next 12 hours.
  –choice of fluid: colloid (especially plasma) is thought to be best. Blood is given to keep **haematocrit** 35–45%. Rough guide: 1 unit per 10% burn, excluding the first 10%.
  Normal maintenance fluids are given in addition.
  –alternative regimen, using crystalloid:
    $2 \times$ weight $\times$ % burn in first 8 hours (ml);
    $2 \times$ weight $\times$ % burn in next 16 hours.
Frequent reassessment is crucial. Urine output should be maintained at 0.5–1 ml/kg/h with osmolality 600–1000 mosmol/kg (high due to high circulating levels of **vasopressin**). Low urine flow with high osmolality indicates under-replacement; high flow with low osmolality indicates over-replacement, in the absence of **renal failure**. The fluid regimen is altered as necessary.
  Oral rehydration is acceptable in burns of up to 10% (children) to 15% (adults). Oral rehydration fluid mixtures are suitable for children. For adults, water containing 75 mmol/l sodium chloride and 15 mmol/l sodium bicarbonate has been suggested, at 2–3 times normal water intake.
  –escharotomy (incision of contracted full-thickness burn which prevents ventilation or limb perfusion) may be necessary.
  –monitoring of:
    –urine output (via catheter if > 25% burn).
    –haematocrit and plasma electrolytes.
    –respiratory function.
    –CVP.
  –analgesia: opioid infusions are often required.
  –adequate **nutrition** (enteral if possible via a nasogastric tube).
  –prevention of **Curling ulcers** e.g. with **H₂ receptor antagonists**.
  –tetanus toxoid as necessary.
• Complications:
  –infection and **septicaemia**.
  –respiratory failure and **ARDS**.
  –renal failure, with **myoglobinuria** or haemoglobinuria. Suggested by low urine osmolarity and urine/blood urea ratio <10.
  –hypercatabolism.
Mortality is related to the extent and site of burns, and age, and is highest towards the extremes of age.
• Anaesthetic considerations in patients with burns:
  –patients often require repeat anaesthetics, e.g. for change of dressings, plastic surgery, etc.
  –difficult airway and/or intubation if burns exist around the head and neck, especially if contractures develop.
  –enhanced increase in plasma potassium may follow use of **suxamethonium**; cardiac arrest has been reported. Most likely 3–10 weeks after the burn, but it has been reported between 9 days and 2 months.

An increased number of extrajunctional **acetylcholine receptors** is thought to be responsible.

–increased requirement for non-depolarizing **neuromuscular blocking drugs**. The mechanism is unclear but may involve altered **pharmacokinetics**, e.g. changes in **protein binding**, **clearance**, **volume of distribution**. An alternative theory suggests the release of a specific yet undiscovered substance following burns, which reduces drug interaction with the neuromuscular junction, or affects the latter directly.

–limited venous access.
–hypermetabolism/catabolism.
–**heat loss** during prolonged surgery.
–extensive blood loss is possible.
–suggested techniques:
    –iv **opioid analgesic drugs**, with or without **butyrophenones**.
    –inhalational analgesia with **Entonox** or volatile agents.
    –**ketamine**.
    –standard general anaesthesia.

Deitch EA (1990) New Engl J Med; 323: 1249–53

Burns, during anaesthesia, *see Diathermy; Electrocution and electrical burns; Explosions and fires*

Burst suppression, *see Electroencephalography*

Butorphanol tartrate. Opioid analgesic drug with partial agonist properties, withdrawn in the UK in 1983. Similar in actions to **pentazocine**; **half-life** is about 3 hours. 2–3 mg is equivalent to 10 mg **morphine**. At higher doses, it produces less respiratory depression than morphine; it also requires more **naloxone** to reverse its effects.

See also, Opioid receptors

Butyrophenones. Group of centrally-acting drugs, originally described with **phenothiazines** as 'major tranquillizers' (a term no longer used). They produce a state of detachment from the environment and inhibit purposeful movement via **GABA** receptor binding. They may cause distressing inner restlessness which may be masked by outward calmness. They are powerful **antiemetic drugs**, acting as dopamine antagonists at the **chemoreceptor trigger zone**. Although some α-adrenergic blocking effect has been shown, cardiovascular effects are minimal. May cause extrapyramidal side effects, and the **neuroleptic malignant syndrome** especially after chronic usage. Used to treat psychoses (especially schizophrenia and mania), in **neuroleptanaesthesia** and as antiemetics. **Droperidol** has a faster onset of action and shorter **half-life** than haloperidol.

Bypass, cardiopulmonary, *see Cardiopulmonary bypass*

C

CABG, *see Coronary artery bypass graft*

Cachexia, *see Malnutrition*

Caesarean section. Particular anaesthetic considerations:
- –physiological changes accompanying **pregnancy**.
- –difficult tracheal intubation and **aspiration of gastric contents** associated with general anaesthesia comprise the major anaesthetic causes of maternal mortality. Mortality is higher for emergency Caesarean section (CS) than for elective CS.
- –**aortocaval compression** must be prevented by avoiding the supine position at all times.
- –uterine tone is decreased by volatile anaesthetic agents.
- –neonatal depression should be avoided, but maternal **awareness** may occur if depth of anaesthesia is inadequate.
- Preoperatively, the usual **preoperative assessment** should be made, with particular attention to:
  - –any predisposing cause for CS, e.g. **pre-eclampsia**, and other obstetric or medical conditions.
  - –whether CS is elective or emergency, and whether the fetus is distressed.
  - –assessment of the airway for possible difficulty in tracheal intubation.
  - –maternal wish for general or regional anaesthesia, and whether **extradural anaesthesia** has been provided in labour.
  - –assessment of the lumbar spine.

  The decision to employ regional or general anaesthesia results from consideration of the above points.
- Regimens used to reduce the risk of **aspiration pneumonitis**:
  - –no food by mouth. Many centres allow sips of water.
  - –**antacid** therapy: in some centres, antacids are administered at regular intervals to all women in labour; in others, antacids are given to those considered at risk of operative delivery, or when surgery is decided upon. The clear 0.3 M **sodium citrate** (30 ml) is preferred to the particulate **magnesium trisilicate** because of the latter's ability to cause chemical pneumonitis. Sodium citrate has a short duration of action, and should be given immediately before induction of anaesthesia, or institution of regional blockade.
  - –**H₂ receptor antagonists**. Many different regimens have been suggested, as for antacid therapy. Women receiving **pethidine** (causing reduced gastric emptying) are given **ranitidine** or **cimetidine** in some centres. For elective CS, ranitidine 150 mg orally is often given the night before, and 2 hours before surgery. For emergency CS, cimetidine 200 mg im has been suggested immediately the decision to operate

is made (cimetidine having a more rapid onset than ranitidine).
  - –emptying the stomach with **apomorphine** or a stomach tube is rarely performed because of its unpleasantness and ineffectiveness.
  - –**metocplopramide** is often given before CS, to increase **gastric emptying** and increase **lower oesophageal sphincter** tone.

Sedative **premedication** is usually avoided because of the risk of neonatal respiratory depression.
- Anaesthetic techniques:
  - –all types of anaesthesia:
    - –insertion of a large-bore iv cannula under local anaesthesia.
    - –cross-matched blood should always be available.
    - –skilled anaesthetic assistance should always be available, as should a range of laryngoscopes, blades, tubes, and resuscitative drugs and equipment.
    - –**monitoring** is instituted on arrival in the operating theatre.
    - –aortocaval compression is reduced by tilting the patient laterally during transport to theatre and surgery.
    - –**ergometrine** has been superseded by **oxytocin** (e.g. 5 units iv followed by 10–20 units added to 500 ml **crystalloid** over 2–4 hours) following delivery because of the former's side effects, particularly hypertension and vomiting.
    - –about 500 ml blood is expelled from the **uterus** into the circulation with delivery, and this helps offset the average blood loss at CS of 500–1500 ml (general anaesthesia) or 300–700 ml (regional anaesthesia).
  - –general anaesthesia (GA):
    - –**preoxygenation**, **cricoid pressure** and rapid sequence induction. An adequate 'sleep dose' of induction agent reduces risk of awareness; a 'maximal allowed dose' based on weight may be insufficient. Neonatal depression due to iv induction agents is minimal.
    - –failed intubation drill if required. Difficult intubation is more likely in obstetric patients than in the general population. Contributory factors include a full set of **teeth**, increased fat deposition, enlarged breasts, and the hand applying cricoid pressure hindering insertion of the laryngoscope blade into the mouth. Laryngeal oedema may be present in pre-eclampsia. **Apnoea** results in rapid **hypoxaemia** because of reduced **FRC** and increased O_2 demand.
    - –IPPV with 50% O_2 in **N_2O** is customary until delivery, but has recently been challenged; 33% O_2 may not be associated with neonatal hypoxaemia as originally thought.

–low concentrations of inhalational agents (up to 0.5% **halothane**, 1% **enflurane**, or 0.75% **isoflurane**) reduce the incidence of awareness without increasing uterine atony and bleeding, or neonatal depression. Placental blood flow is thought to be maintained by vasodilatation caused by the volatile agents, and high levels of vasoconstricting **catecholamines** associated with awareness are avoided. Delivery of higher concentrations of volatile agents in 66% N_2O has been suggested for the first 3–5 minutes whilst alveolar concentrations are low, to reduce awareness.

–normocapnia (4 kPa/30 mmHg) is now considered ideal; severe **hyperventilation** may be associated with fetal hypoxaemia and acidosis due to placental vasoconstriction, or due to reduced maternal venous return caused by excessive IPPV.

–all **neuromuscular blocking drugs** cross the **placenta** to a very small extent, **gallamine** more than others. Shorter-acting drugs e.g. **vecuronium** and **atracurium** are usually employed, since postoperative residual paralysis associated with longer-lasting drugs has been a significant factor in some maternal deaths.

–**opioid analgesic drugs** are withheld until delivery of the infant, to avoid neonatal respiratory depression.

–factors increasing the likelihood of awareness include lack of premedication, reduced concentrations of N_2O and volatile agents, and withholding of opioid analgesic drugs before delivery. Its incidence using low concentrations of volatile agents is less than 1%; up to 26% awareness was reported in early studies using 50% N_2O and no volatile agent.

–aspiration may also occur at the end of surgery and during recovery from anaesthesia (when the effect of sodium citrate may have worn off). Before tracheal extubation, the patient should be awake and on her side.

–advantages: usually quicker to perform in emergencies. May be used when regional techniques are contraindicated, e.g. in **coagulation disorders**. Safer in hypovolaemia.

–disadvantages: risk of aspiration, difficult intubation, awareness and neonatal depression. Hypotension and reduced cardiac output may result from anaesthetic drugs and IPPV. Blood loss is greater. The mother is more sleepy postoperatively.

–extradural anaesthesia (EA):
  –facilities for general anaesthesia should be available.
  –**bupivacaine** 0.5% is the most commonly used **local anaesthetic agent** in the UK; addition of adrenaline possibly produces better quality of block. **Lignocaine** 2% + adrenaline 1:200 000 has quicker onset of action. Mixtures of lignocaine and bupivacaine have been used. Adrenaline is usually avoided in pre-eclamptic patients because of the risk of increased placental vasoconstriction. 0.75% bupivacaine is associated with a high incidence of maternal toxic reactions, and has been withdrawn from obstetric use. **Chloroprocaine** is commonly used in the USA; onset is rapid but so is offset. **Etidocaine** has also been used.

–L2–3 or L3–4 interspace is usually chosen.

–on average, 8–24 ml solution is required for adequate blockade (from S5 to T5–6). Less is required when extradural analgesia has already been provided during labour. Smaller volumes are required for a specified level of block than in non-pregnant patients, as dilated extradural veins reduce the available volume in the **extradural space**.

–injection of solution in 5 ml increments at 5 minute intervals reduces the risk of hypotension and extensive blockade, e.g. due to accidental spinal injection, but increases preparatory time and total dose. Sequential positioning (e.g. on either side and sitting) between doses has been suggested as improving blockade but may not be necessary. Single injection of 20 ml is advocated by some as producing more rapid onset of blockade. A catheter technique is used most frequently, although injection through the extradural needle may be performed.

–opioids, e.g. **diamorphine** 2–4 mg and **fentanyl** 50–100 µg, have been given extradurally for per- and **postoperative analgesia**, but maternal respiratory depression has been reported.

–the incidence of hypotension is reduced by preloading with **iv fluid** (1–1.5 litres **crystalloid** is usually employed). The incidence varies with its definition but may be 20–30% even with preloading and if aortocaval compression is avoided. Treatment includes administration of **ephedrine,** e.g. 3–6 mg increments iv. Prophylactic use has been suggested, e.g. 15 mg im; it may also be added to the iv fluid. Other vasoconstrictors may greatly decrease placental blood flow. Adverse neonatal effects are thought to be minimal if hypotension lasts less than 1–2 minutes.

–nausea and vomiting may be caused by hypotension and/or bradycardia.

–O_2 should be administered by facemask, supplemented by up to 50% N_2O if necessary.

–during surgery many women feel pressure and movement, which may be unpleasant. Shoulder-tip pain may result from blood tracking up to the diaphragm. Small doses of iv opioid drugs may be required, given cautiously, if N_2O does not help.

–surgery must be gentle when performing CS under regional anaesthesia.

–advantages: the risks of GA are avoided. Onset of hypotension is usually slow and may be corrected before it becomes severe. The mother may be able to warn of aortocaval compression (e.g. feeling sick). Minimal neonatal depression occurs compared with GA. The mother is able to hold the baby soon after delivery and is not sleepy afterwards. Her partner is able to be present during the procedure. Extradural analgesia provided in labour can be extended for operative delivery. The catheter can be used for further 'top-up' during surgery if required, and for postoperative analgesia.

–disadvantages: risk of dural tap, total spinal blockade, toxic reaction to local anaesthetic agent, severe hypotension, etc. It may be slow to achieve adequate blockade with a chance of patchy block. Inability to move the legs may be disturbing.

–**spinal anaesthesia** (SA):
  –general considerations as for EA.
  –0.5% bupivacaine is used in the UK; plain bupivacaine (e.g. 3 ml) produces a more variable block than heavy bupivacaine (e.g. 1.8–2.8 ml). Heavy **amethocaine** 0.5% (1.2–1.6 ml) is commonly used in the USA.
  –injection is usually at the L3–4/L4–5 interspace.
  –blockade is less predictable than in non-pregnant patients, and hypotension and **postspinal headache** are more common. Some degree of headache may occur in up to 20% of patients, reduced to 2–10% if a fine **needle** is used, e.g. 25–29 G, with its bevel parallel to the fibres of the dura (i.e. longitudinal) on insertion. Non-cutting needles may reduce the incidence further. Postoperative confinement to bed is now thought not to affect the incidence of headache.
  –advantages: as for EA, but of quicker onset. Blockade is more intense and not patchy. Smaller doses of local anaesthetic drug are used.
  –disadvantages: single shot; i.e. may not last long enough if surgery is prolonged. Less predictable. Continuous spinal techniques allow more control over spread and duration but are technically more difficult. Risk of headache. Hypotension is of faster onset.

Combined spinal and extradural techniques have been performed in an attempt to combine the advantages of each, e.g. by inserting a long spinal needle through the extradural needle once the extradural space has been identified, with subarachnoid injection prior to insertion of the extradural catheter. Alternatively, separate extradural and spinal injections may be made at different sites.
For contraindications, techniques etc., see Extradural anaesthesia; Spinal anaesthesia

CS is possible using local anaesthetic infiltration of the abdominal wall with 0.5% lignocaine or prilocaine. Large volumes are required, with risk of toxicity. Infiltration of each layer is performed in stages. The procedure is lengthy and uncomfortable, but may be used as a last resort if other techniques are unavailable or unsuccessful. It may also be used to supplement inhalational anaesthesia following failed intubation.

[Julius Caesar (100–44 BC), Roman Emperor; said to have been born by the abdominal route; his name allegedly derived from *caedare*, to cut. An alternative suggestion is related to a law enforced under the Caesars concerning abdominal section following death in late pregnancy]
See also, Confidential Enquiries into Maternal Deaths, Report on; Fetus, effects of anaesthetic agents on; I–D interval; Induction, rapid sequence; Intubation, difficult; Intubation, failed; Obstetric analgesia and anaesthesia; U–D interval

Caffeine. Xanthine present in tea, coffee and certain soft drinks. Used as an adjunct to many oral **analgesic drug** preparations, although not analgesic itself. Causes CNS stimulation; traditionally thought to improve performance and mood, whilst reducing fatigue. Increases cerebral vascular resistance and decreases cerebral blood flow. **Half-life** is about 6 hours. Has been used iv and orally for treatment of **postspinal headache**.
- Dosage: up to 30 mg in compound oral preparations. 150–300 mg orally for postspinal headache; 250 mg iv (with 250 mg sodium benzoate).

- Side effects: as for **aminophylline**, especially CNS and cardiac stimulation.

Caisson disease, *see Decompression sickness*

Calcium. 99% of body calcium is contained in bone; plasma calcium consists of free ionized calcium (50%) and calcium bound to proteins and other ions. The free ionized form is involved as a **second messenger** in many intracellular responses to chemical and electrical stimuli, e.g. **neuromuscular transmission**, **muscle contraction**, cell division and movement, and certain oxidative pathways. Also involved in **coagulation**. Its actions are mediated via binding to intracellular proteins, e.g. calmodulin, causing configurational changes to proteins and enzyme activation. Intracellular calcium levels are much higher than extracellular, due to relative membrane impermeability and membrane pumps employing **active transport**. Calcium entry via specific channels leads to direct effects, e.g. **neurotransmitter** release in neurones, or further calcium release from intracellular organelles, e.g. in cardiac and skeletal **muscle**.

Ionized calcium increases with **acidosis**, and decreases with **alkalosis**. Thus for accurate measurement, blood should be taken without a tourniquet (which causes local acidosis), and without hyper-/hypoventilation. Ionized calcium is measured in some centres, but total plasma calcium is easier to measure; normal value is 2.12–2.65 mmol/l. Varies with the plasma protein level; corrected by adding 0.02 mmol/l calcium for each g/l albumin below 40 g/l, or subtracting for each g/l above 40 g/l.
- Regulation:
  –vitamin D: group of related sterols. Cholecalciferol is formed in the skin by the action of ultraviolet light, and is converted in the liver to 25–hydroxycholecalciferol (in turn converted to 1,25–dihydroxycholecalciferol in the proximal renal tubules). Formation is increased by parathyroid hormone and decreased by hyperphosphataemia. Actions:
    –increases intestinal calcium absorption.
    –increases renal calcium reabsorption.
    –mobilizes bone calcium and phosphate.
  –parathyroid hormone: secretion is increased by **hypocalcaemia** and **hypomagnesaemia**, and decreased by **hypercalcaemia** and **hypermagnesaemia**. Actions:
    –mobilizes bone calcium.
    –increases renal calcium reabsorption.
    –increases renal phosphate excretion.
    –increases formation of 1,25–dihydroxycholecalciferol.
  –calcitonin: secreted by the parafollicular cells of the **thyroid gland**. Secretion is increased by hypercalcaemia, **catecholamines** and gastrin. Actions:
    –inhibits mobilization of bone calcium.
    –increases renal calcium and phosphate excretion.

Calcium is used clinically to treat hypocalcaemia, e.g. during rapid **blood transfusion**. It is also used as an **inotropic drug**, e.g. during **cardiac surgery**. Its use during **CPR** is no longer recommended unless hypocalcaemia, **hyperkalaemia** or overdose of **calcium channel blocking drugs** are involved, because of adverse effects on ischaemic myocardium, and coronary and cerebral circulations.

Calcium chloride 10% contains 6.8 mmol/10 ml and 14.7% contains 10 mmol/10 ml; calcium gluconate 10%

contains 2.2–2.3 mmol/10 ml, depending on the formulation. 5–10 ml calcium chloride or 10–20 ml calcium gluconate are usually recommended by slow iv bolus. The chloride preparation is usually recommended for CPR, although equal rises in plasma calcium are produced by gluconate, if equal amounts of calcium are given. Arrhythmias and prolonged hypercalcaemia may follow the use of either.

Landers DF, Becker GL, Wong KC (1989) Anesth Analg; 69: 100–12

Calcium channel blocking drugs. Most common name for a group of drugs which interfere with slow channel **calcium** entry into cells; also called calcium ion antagonists. Thought to act by modifying calcium channels indirectly at different neighbouring sites, hence their wide variation in chemical structure. Particularly affect the muscle and conducting system of the heart, and vascular smooth muscle.

- Actions:
  - reduce myocardial contractility and O_2 consumption.
  - depress initiation and propagation of cardiac electrical impulses.
  - cause vasodilatation.
- The drugs include:
  - **verapamil**: acts mainly on the myocardium and conducting system; thus used to treat supraventricular arrhythmias, angina and hypertension. Severe myocardial depression may occur, especially in combination with **β-adrenergic receptor antagonists**.
  - **nifedipine**: acts mainly on coronary and systemic vascular muscle, with little myocardial depression. Used in angina and hypertension. Systemic vasodilatation may cause flushing and headache, especially for the first few days of treatment.
  - nicardipine: similar to nifedipine, but with less myocardial depression.
  - amlodipine: similar to nifedipine and nicardipine, but with longer duration of action and therefore taken once daily.
  - isradipine: similar to nifedipine but used for hypertension only.
  - diltiazem: causes less myocardial depression than verapamil. Used for angina. May cause bradycardia. A sustained-release formation is available for hypertension and angina.
  - **nimodipine**: particularly active on cerebral vascular smooth muscle, it has been used to relieve cerebral vasospasm following **subarachnoid haemorrhage**.

Additive effects might be expected between these drugs and **halothane**, **enflurane** and **isoflurane**, all of which decrease calcium entry into cells. Reduction in cardiac output, decreased atrioventricular conduction and vasodilatation may occur to different degrees, but severe interactions are rarely a problem in practice. **Non-depolarizing neuromuscular blockade** may be potentiated.

Jenkins LC, Scoates PJ (1985) Can Anaesth Soc J; 32: 436–47

Calorie. Unit of **energy**. Although not an SI unit, widely used, especially in relation to food-derived energy.
1 cal = energy required to heat 1 g water by 1°C.
1 kcal (1 Cal) = energy required to heat 1 kg water by 1°C,
= 1000 cal.
1 cal = 4.18 **joules**.

cAMP, *see Adenosine monophoshate, cyclic*

Campbell–Howell method, *see Carbon dioxide measurement*

Candela. SI **unit** of luminous intensity. Definition relates to the luminous intensity of a radiating black body at the freezing point of platinum.

Capacitance. Ability to retain electrical charge; defined as the charge stored by an object per voltage difference across it. Measured in farads (F).

A capacitor comprised of conductors separated by an insulator may be charged by a potential difference across it, but will not allow direct current to flow. Its stored charge may subsequently be discharged, e.g. in **defibrillation**. Repeated charging and discharging induced by an alternating current results in current flow across a capacitor.

[Michael Faraday (1791–1867), English chemist]

Capacitance vessels. Comprised of venae cavae and large veins; normally only partially distended, they may expand to accomodate a large volume of blood before venous pressure is increased. Innervated by the **sympathetic nervous system** in the same way as the arterial system (**resistance vessels**), they act as a blood reservoir. 60–70% of **blood volume** is within the veins normally.

Capacitor, *see Capacitance*

Capillary circulation. Contains 5% of circulating **blood volume**, which passes from arterioles to venules via capillaries, usually within 2 seconds. Controlled by local autoregulatory mechanisms, and possibly by autonomic neural reflexes. Molecules and ions which readily cross the capillary walls (mainly by **diffusion**) include water, O_2, CO_2, glucose and urea. Hydrostatic pressure falls from about 30 mmHg (arteriolar end) to 15 mmHg (venous end) within the capillary. Direction of fluid flow across capillary walls is determined by hydrostatic and osmotic pressure gradients (**Starling forces**).

Capnography, infra-red. Pictorial display of **CO$_2$** concentration measured by infra-red absorption. Capnometry refers to measurement only. The sample gas, usually end-tidal, is drawn into a chamber through which half of a split infra-red beam is passed. The other half passes through a reference chamber containing air. The amount of infra-red light absorbed by the sample gas depends on the amount of CO_2 present, and is determined by comparing the emergent beams from the sample and reference chambers. This is done with photoelectric cells behind each chamber, or by passing the beams through two further chambers containing CO_2, separated by a diaphragm. The heating effect of the infra-red light causes pressure to rise within these chambers; the difference in pressure between them depends on the amount of infra-red light absorbed by the CO_2 in the original sample gas.

Gases containing different atoms may be measured in this way. **N_2O** and volatile anaesthetic agents also absorb infra-red light, but at different wavelengths to CO_2. The technique may be used for multiple simultaneous **gas analysis**, as may photoacoustic spectroscopy, recently introduced. This relies on absorption of infra-red light of

different wavelengths by different molecules, with subsequent emission of sound at the wavelengths concerned for each molecule. Detection is with a microphone. The pictorial display provides more information than capnometry alone (*see Carbon dioxide, end-tidal*).
See also, Carbon dioxide measurment

Capsaicin. Naturally-occurring substance found in plants of the nightshade family. Decreases the activity of type C **pain** fibres by depleting them of **substance P** via reduction in its synthesis, storage and transport. Has been applied topically for temporary relief of pain associated with neuralgias, e.g. **postherpetic neuralgia**, and arthritis. Should be applied 6–8 hourly. Takes 1–4 weeks to produce its effect. Initial release of substance P may cause burning on application.

Captopril. Angiotensin converting enzyme inhibitor, used to treat **hypertension** and **cardiac failure**. Shorter acting than **enalapril**; onset is within 15 minutes with peak effect at 30–60 minutes. **Half-life** is 2 hours. Excreted renally; thus it should be avoided in renal impairment.
- Dosage: 12.5–50 mg 8–12 hourly.
- Side effects: severe hypotension after the first dose, cough, taste disturbances, rash, abdominal pain, agranulocytosis, neutropenia, hyperkalaemia, renal impairment. Severe hypotension may occur after induction of anaesthesia and in hypovolaemia.
Contraindicated in pregnancy and **porphyria**.

Carbamazepine. Anticonvulsant drug, used to treat all types of **epilepsy** except petit mal. Has fewer side effects than **phenytoin**, and has a greater **therapeutic index**. Also used for **pain management**, e.g. in **trigeminal neuralgia**, and in manic–depressive disease.
- Dosage: 100–200 mg increased to up to 1.6 g/day in divided doses.
  Plasma levels should be monitored (optimal levels 20–50 μmol/l).
- Side effects: dizziness, visual disturbances, GIT upset, rash, **hyponatraemia**. Blood dyscrasias may occur rarely. **Enzyme induction** may cause reduced effects of other drugs, e.g. **warfarin**.

Carbohydrates (Saccharides). Class of compounds with the general formula $C_n(H_2O)_n$, hence their name, although they are not true hydrates. n usually exceeds 3. Range in size; monosaccharides (simple sugars) are most common, where $n = 5$ or 6 (pentoses or hexoses, e.g. **glucose**, sucrose). Large polysaccharides include starch, cellulose and **glycogen**. Metabolites often contain phosphorus. Some polysaccharides are combined with proteins, e.g. mucopolysaccharides. Act as a source of **energy** in food, e.g.:

$$C_6H_{12}O_6 + 6O_2 \rightarrow 6CO_2 + 6H_2O + energy$$

1 g carbohydrate yields about 17 kJ energy (4 Cal).
- Ingested carbohydrates are broken down thus:
  –mouth: salivary amylase: starch → smaller units (n up to about 8).
  –small intestine:
  ––pancreatic amylase: starch as above.
  ––maltase: maltose → glucose.
  ––lactase: lactose → glucose + galactose.
  ––sucrase: sucrose → glucose + fructose.

Hexoses and pentoses absorbed from the GIT pass to the liver for energy production, storage molecule synthesis or alternate pathways.
See also, Metabolism

Carbon dioxide (CO_2). Gas produced by oxidation of carbon containing substances, including foodstuffs. Average rate of production under basal conditions in adults is about 200 ml/min, although it varies with the energy source (see Respiratory quotient).
- Partial pressures of CO_2:
  –inspired: 0.03 kPa (0.2 mmHg).
  –alveolar: 5.3 kPa (40 mmHg).
  –arterial: 5.3 kPa (40 mmHg).
  –venous: 6.1 kPa (46 mmHg).
  –expired: 4 kPa (30 mmHg).
Isolated in 1757 by Black. **CO_2 narcosis** was used for anaesthesia in animals by **Hickman** in 1824. Used to stimulate respiration during anaesthesia from the early 1900s, to maintain ventilation and speed uptake of volatile agents during induction; also used to assist blind nasal tracheal intubation. Administration is now generally considered hazardous because of the adverse effects of **hypercapnia**; avoidance of its accidental administration during anaesthesia by removing **cylinders** from **anaesthetic machines** altogether has been suggested. Still used by some anaesthetists to restore normocapnia at the end of peroperative IPPV. Manufactured by heating calcium or magnesium carbonate, producing CO_2 and calcium/magnesium oxide.
- Properties:
  –colourless gas, 1.5 times denser than air.
  –**mw** 44.
  –**boiling point** –79°C.
  –**critical temperature** –31°C.
  –non-flammable and non-explosive.
  –supplied in grey cylinders; pressure is 50 bar at 15°C, about 57 bar at room temperature.
- Effects: as for hypercapnia.
[Joseph Black (1728–1799), Scottish chemist]
See also, Acid–base balance; Alveolar gas transfer; Carbon dioxide absorption, in anaesthetic breathing systems; Carbon dioxide dissociation curve; Carbon dioxide, end-tidal; Carbon dioxide measurement; Carbon dioxide response curve; Carbon dioxide transport

Carbon dioxide absorption, in anaesthetic breathing systems. Investigated and described by **Waters** in the early 1920s, although used earlier. Exhaled gases are passed over **soda lime** or a similar material, e.g. **baralyme**, and reused. In totally closed systems, only basal O_2 requirements need be supplied; absorption may also be used with low fresh gas flows and a leak through an expiratory valve.
- Advantages:
  –less inhalational agent required, i.e. cheaper.
  –less pollution.
  –warms and humidifies inhaled gases.
- Disadvantages:
  –high flows are required initially, to ensure nitrogen washout. If N_2O is also used, risk of hypoxic gas mixtures makes an O_2 analyser mandatory.
  –failure of CO_2 absorption may be due to exhaustion of soda lime or inefficient equipment; thus **capnography** is required.

–resistance and **dead space** may be high with some systems, and inhalation of dust is possible.

–**trichloroethylene** is incompatible with soda lime.
- Methods:
  –Waters' cannister: cylindrical drum, 8 × 12 cm, containing 1 lb (0.45 kg) soda lime. Reservoir bag at one end, facepiece with fresh gas supply and expiratory valve at the other; exhaled gases pass to and fro through it. Most efficient when tidal volume equals the contained air space (400–450 ml). Smaller cannisters are used for children. Dead space equals the volume between the patient and soda lime; it increases during use as the soda lime nearest the patient is exhausted. Efficiency is also reduced by channelling of exhaled gases through gaps in the soda lime if loosely packed and allowed to settle. Also heavy and bulky to use.
  –**circle systems**: becoming more popular as concern about pollution and cost of inhalational agents increases. Soda lime cannisters are held vertically, reducing the risk of channelling.

Carbon dioxide dissociation curve. Graph of blood CO_2 content against its PCO_2 (Fig. 22). The curve is much steeper than the **oxyhaemoglobin dissociation curve**, and more linear. Different curves are obtained for oxygenated and deoxygenated blood, the latter able to carry more CO_2 (**Haldane effect**).

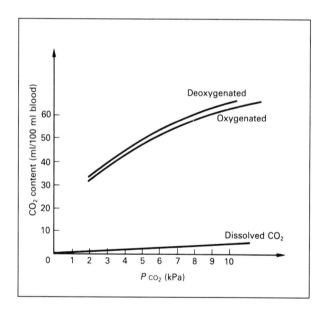

Figure 22 *Carbon dioxide dissociation curve*

Carbon dioxide, end-tidal (P_ECO_2). Partial pressure of **CO₂** measured in the final portion of exhaled gas. Approximates to alveolar $PCCO_2$ in normal anaesthetized subjects; the difference is about 0.4–0.7 kPa (3–5 mmHg). The difference increases in **$\dot{V}/\dot{Q}$ mismatch** and increased CO_2 production. May be monitored continuously during anaesthesia (often measured and displayed as CO_2 concentration in end-tidal gas), e.g. using infra-red **capnography** or **mass spectrometry**.
- Measurement is useful for assessing adequacy of ventilation, and allows normo- or hypocapnia to be produced

as required during IPPV. Measurement also aids detection of:
  –oesophageal intubation, since CO_2 is only present in the oesophagus and stomach in small amounts, if at all.
  –**PE** (including **fat** or **air embolism**): P_ECO_2 falls due to increased alveolar **dead space** and reduced **cardiac output**.
  –rebreathing.
  –disconnection.
  –**MH**: P_ECO_2 rises as muscle metabolism increases.
- Display of a continuous trace is more useful than values alone (Fig. 23).

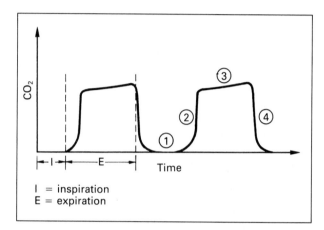

I = inspiration
E = expiration

Figure 23 *Normal trace of end-tidal PCO_2. I, inspiration; E, expiration*

–phase 1: zero baseline during inspiration; a raised baseline indicates rebreathing.
–phase 2: dead space gas (containing no CO_2) is followed by alveolar gas, represented by a sudden rise to a plateau. Excessive sloping of the upstroke may indicate obstruction to expiration.
–phase 3: near-horizontal plateau indicates mixing of alveolar gas. A steep upwards slope indicates obstruction to expiration or unequal mixing, e.g. **COAD**.
–phase 4: rapid fall to zero at the onset of inspiration.
–additional features may be present:
  –superimposed regular oscillations corresponding to the heart beat.
  –small waves representing spontaneous breaths between ventilator breaths, e.g. if neuromuscular blockade is insufficient.

Bhavani-Shankar K, Moseley H, Kumar AY, Delph Y (1992) Can J Anaesth; 39: 617–32
See also, Carbon dioxide measurement; End-tidal gas sampling

Carbon dioxide measurement. Estimation of arterial PCO_2:
  –direct: Severinghaus CO_2 electrode: glass pH electrode separated from arterial blood sample by a thin membrane. CO_2 diffuses into bicarbonate solution surrounding the glass electrode, lowering pH. pH is measured and displayed in terms of PCO_2. Kept at 37°C, and calibrated with known mixtures of CO_2/O_2 before use. Samples are stored in ice or analysed immediately, to reduce inaccuracy due to blood cell metabolism.

–indirect:
  –from gas:
    –to obtain gas for analysis:
      –**end-tidal gas sampling** (end-tidal $P\text{CO}_2$ approximates to alveolar $P\text{CO}_2$ which approximates to arterial $P\text{CO}_2$).
      –rebreathing technique of Campbell and Howell: rebreathing from a 2 litre bag containing 50% O_2 for 90 seconds, then a further 30 seconds after 3 minutes' rest. Bag $P\text{CO}_2$ then approximates to mixed venous $P\text{CO}_2$. Arterial $P\text{CO}_2$ is normally 0.8 kPa (6 mmHg) less than mixed venous $P\text{CO}_2$.
    –subsequent **gas analysis**:
      –chemical: formation of non-gaseous compounds, with reduction of overall volume of the gas mixture (**Haldane apparatus**).
      –physical: **capnography** and **mass spectrometer** are most widely used. **Interferometer**, **gas chromatography**, etc. may also be used.
  –from blood/tissues:
    –transcutaneous electrode: requires heating of the skin; relatively inaccurate.
    –measurement of venous $P\text{CO}_2$ and capillary $P\text{CO}_2$: inaccurate and unreliable.
    –**Siggaard-Anderson nomogram**: equilibration of the blood sample with gases of known CO_2.
    –**van Slyke apparatus**: liberation of gas from blood sample with subsequent chemical analysis.
    –fibreoptic sensors: under development.
[John W Severinghaus, San Fransisco anaesthetist; EJ Moran Campbell, English-born Canadian physiologist; John BL Howell, Southampton physician]

Carbon dioxide narcosis. Loss of consciousness caused by severe **hypercapnia**, i.e. arterial $P\text{CO}_2$ exceeding approximately 25 kPa (200 mmHg). Thought to be due to a profound fall in pH of CSF (under 6.9). Increasing central depression is seen at arterial $P\text{CO}_2$ greater than 13 kPa (100 mmHg), and CSF pH under 7.1. Other features of hypercapnia may be present.

Used by **Hickman** in 1824 to enable painless surgery on animals.

Carbon dioxide response curve. Obtained by measuring **minute ventilation** at different arterial CO_2 tensions. Rebreathing from a 6 litre bag containing 50% O_2 and 7% CO_2 may be used, measuring minute ventilation and bag $P\text{CO}_2$ periodically. This is easier than increasing inspired CO_2 levels and measuring the response after equilibration at each new level. The curve may be used to indicate depression of respiratory drive (Fig. 24); increased threshold is represented by a shift of the curve to the right (1), and decreased sensitivity by depression of the slope (2). Both may follow administration of opioid and other depressant drugs, and in chronic hypercapnia; the opposite occurs in **hypoxaemia**.
See also, Breathing, control of

Carbon dioxide transport. In arterial blood, approximately 50 ml CO_2 is carried per 100 ml blood, as:
  –**bicarbonate**: 45 ml.
  –carbonic acid: 2.5 ml.
  –carbamino compounds with proteins, mainly **haemoglobin**: 2.5 ml.

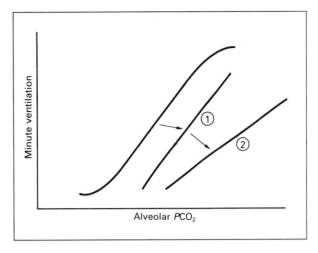

Figure 24 *Carbon dioxide response curve (see text)*

In venous blood, 54 ml is carried per 100 ml blood, as:
  –bicarbonate: 47.5 ml.
  –carbonic acid: 3.0 ml.
  –carbamino compounds: 3.5 ml.
CO_2 is rapidly converted by **carbonic anhydrase** in red cells to carbonic acid, which dissociates to bicarbonate and **hydrogen ions**. The former passes into plasma in exchange for chloride ions (**chloride shift**); the latter are buffered mainly by haemoglobin. Haemoglobin's buffering ability increases as it becomes deoxygenated, as does its ability to form carbamino groups (**Haldane effect**).
See also, Acid–base balance; Buffers

Carbon monoxide diffusing capacity, *see Diffusing capacity*

Carbon monoxide poisoning. May result from inhalation of fumes from car exhausts, fires, heating systems, coal gas supplies, etc. Carbon monoxide (CO) binds to haemoglobin with 200–250 times the affinity of O_2, forming carboxyhaemoglobin, which dissociates very slowly. The amount of carboxyhaemoglobin formed depends on inspired CO concentration and duration of exposure.

● Effects:
  –reduced capacity for O_2 transport.
  –**oxyhaemoglobin dissociation curve** shifted to the left.
  –inhibition of the cellular **cytochrome oxidase system**; tissue toxicity is proportional to the length of exposure.
  –**aortic** and **carotid bodies** do not detect hypoxia, since the arterial $P\text{O}_2$ is unaffected.
● Features:
  –non-specific if chronic, e.g. headache, weakness, dizziness, GIT disturbances, etc.
  –if acute: as above, with convulsions and coma if severe.
  –the 'cherry red' colour of carboxyhaemoglobin may be apparent.
  –neurological and psychiatric symptoms may follow recovery.
  –**O_2 saturation** measured by pulse **oximetry** may be misleading because carboxyhaemoglobin is interpreted as oxygenated haemoglobin.

- Treatment:
  - O_2 **therapy**: speeds carboxyaemoglobin dissociation. Tracheal intubation and **IPPV** may be necessary. Elimination **half-life** of carbon monoxide is reduced from 4 hours to under 1 hour with 100% O_2; it is reduced further to under 30 minutes with hyperbaric O_2 at 2.5–3 atm. At this pressure, dissolved O_2 alone satisfies tissue O_2 requirements. Hyperbaric O_2 has been suggested if the patient is unconscious or at carboxyhaemoglobin levels above 40%.
  - carboxyhaemoglobin levels correlate poorly with severity of symptoms, because of variable effects of tissue toxicity. Values often quoted:
    - 0.3–2%: normal non-smokers (some CO from pollution, some formed endogenously).
    - 5–6%: normal smokers.
    - 10–30%: mild symptoms common.
    - above 60%: severe symptoms common.

Broome JR, Pearson RR (1988) Br J Hosp Med; 39: 298–305

Carbon monoxide transfer factor, see *Diffusing capacity*

Carbonic anhydrase. Zinc-containing **enzyme** catalysing the reaction of CO_2 and water to form carbonic acid, which rapidly dissociates to **bicarbonate** and **hydrogen ions**. Absent from plasma, but present in high concentrations in:
- red blood cells: important in buffering, **CO_2 transport** and **O_2 transport**.
- renal tubular cells: important for maintaining **acid-base balance**.
- gastric mucosa: important in hydrochloric acid production.
- ciliary body: involved in aqueous humour formation.

Inhibited by **acetazolamide** and sulphonamides.

Carboxyhaemoglobin, see *Carbon monoxide poisoning*

Carcinogenicity of anaesthetic agents, see *Environmental safety of anaesthetists; Fetus, effects of anaesthetic agents on*

Carcinoid syndrome. Results from secretion of vasoactive and other substances from certain tumours, usually the terminal ileum of the GIT (85%). Secreted compounds are metabolized by the liver so that symptoms are absent until hepatic metastases are present. Tumours may also arise in the lung and gonads.
- Features:
  - flushing, mainly of the head and neck. May be associated with vasodilatation, hypotension, wheezing, skin wheals and sweating.
  - diarrhoea, perhaps with nausea and vomiting. Typically episodic, along with flushing. Weight loss is common.
  - endocardial fibrosis involving the tricuspid and pulmonary valves may cause right-sided **cardiac failure**.

Symptoms are traditionally ascribed to secretion of **5-HT** (diarrhoea) and **bradykinin** (flushing), but many more substances have been implicated, e.g. **substance P**, **prostaglandins**, **histamine** and **vasoactive intestinal hormone**. Diagnosis includes measurement of urinary 5-hydroxyindole acetic acid, a breakdown product of 5-HT.
- Anaesthetic management:
  - perioperative treatment with various drugs has been used to reduce hyper-/hypotensive episodes and bronchospasm:
    - methysergide, **ketanserin** (5-HT antagonists).
    - **aprotinin** (**kallikrein** inhibitor).
    - **antihistamines**.
    - **somatostatin** and octreotide, its analogue (prevents release of mediators).
  - invasive cardiovascular monitoring and careful fluid balance.
  - use of cardiostable drugs where possible; avoidance of drugs causing histamine release.
  - drugs should be prepared for bronchospasm and hyper-/hypotension.
  - admission to HDU/ICU postoperatively.

Roy RC, Carter RF, Wright PD (1987) Anaesthesia; 42: 627–32

Cardiac arrest. Sudden circulatory standstill. Common cause of death in cardiovascular disease, especially **ischaemic heart disease**. May also be caused by **PE**, electrolyte disturbances, e.g. of **potassium** or **calcium**, **hypoxaemia**, **hypercapnia**, **hypotension**, vagal reflexes, **hypothermia**, **anaphylactic reaction**, **electrocution**, drugs, e.g. **adrenaline**, and instrumentation of the heart, e.g. percutaneous cannulation.
- Features: unconsciousness within 15–30 seconds, apnoea or gasping respiration, pallor, cyanosis, absent pulses. Pupillary dilatation is variable.
- May be due to:
  - **VF**; usually associated with **myocardial ischaemia**. The most common ECG finding (about 60%), with the best prognosis.
  - **asystole**: occurs in about 30%. More likely in exsanguination and hypoxia, especially in children. May also follow vagally-mediated bradycardia.
  - **electromechanical dissociation**. May occur in widespread myocardial damage. The least common ECG finding, with the worst prognosis, unless due to mechanical causes of circulatory collapse, e.g. PE, **cardiac tamponade**, **pneumothorax**, etc.

Asystole and electromechanical dissociation may convert to VF, which eventually converts to asystole if untreated.

Only 15–20% of patients leave hospital after cardiac arrest. Up to 30–40% survival is thought to be possible if prompt **CPR** is instituted. Permanent brain damage is thought to occur within 4–5 minutes unless CPR is instituted. The prognosis is better if the patient regains consciousness within 10 minutes of the circulation restarting.

See also, *Cerebral ischaemia*

Cardiac asthma. Acute **pulmonary oedema** resembling **asthma**. Both may feature dyspnoea, decreased lung compliance and widespread rhonchi, although pulmonary oedema is suggested by pink frothy sputum. Increased airway resistance may result from true bronchospasm, or from bronchial oedema.

Cardiac catheterization. Passage of a catheter into the heart chambers for measurement of intracardiac pressures and O_2 saturations, or for injection of **radiological contrast media** for radiological imaging (angiocardiography). Used to investigate **ischaemic heart disease**, **valvular heart disease** and **congenital heart disease**; also used for treatment of lesions, e.g. balloon valvotomy, atrial septostomy (e.g. in **transposition of the great arteries**), **percutaneous transluminal coronary angioplasty**.

- Technique:
  - commonly performed under local anaesthesia except in small children, in whom general anaesthesia is required.
  - access is via a peripheral vein or artery, e.g. femoral or brachial vessels, using either a cut-down technique or percutaneous guidewire (**Seldinger technique**).
  - the right side of the heart is approached as for **pulmonary artery catheterization**.
  - the left side of the heart is approached retrogradely under X-ray control, via a peripheral artery or from the right side through the atrial septum or a defect thereof.
- Information gained:
  - pressure values, waveforms and gradients between chambers.
  - saturation values; greater than expected values on the right side indicate a left-to-right **shunt**.
  - **cardiac output** may be measured using the **Fick principle**.
  - angiocardiography: cardiac function may be assessed on cine film, or the coronary vessels filled with dye to assess patency.

Approximate normal pressures and measurements are shown in Table 9.

Table 9. Normal pressures and O_2 saturations obtained during cardiac catheterization

Site	Pressure (mmHg)	Saturation (%)
Right atrium	1–4	75
Right ventricle	25/4	75
Pulmonary artery	25/12	75
Left atrium	2–10	97
Left ventricle	120/10	97
Aorta	120/70	97

Cardiac cycle. Sequence of events occurring during cardiac activity; usually refers to changes in vascular pressures (especially **arterial BP**), **heart** chamber pressures, **ECG** and **phonocardiography** tracings during normal **sinus rhythm** (Fig. 25).

- Divided into five phases:
  - phase 1: atrial contraction: responsible for about 30% of ventricular filling. Some blood regurgitates into the venae cavae and pulmonary veins.
  - phase 2: isometric ventricular contraction: lasts from the closing of the tricuspid and mitral valves until ventricular pressures exceed aortic and pulmonary artery pressures, and the aortic and pulmonary valves open.
  - phase 3: ventricular ejection: most rapid at the start of systole. Lasts until the aortic and pulmonary valves close.
  - phase 4: isometric ventricular relaxation: last until the tricuspid and mitral valves open.

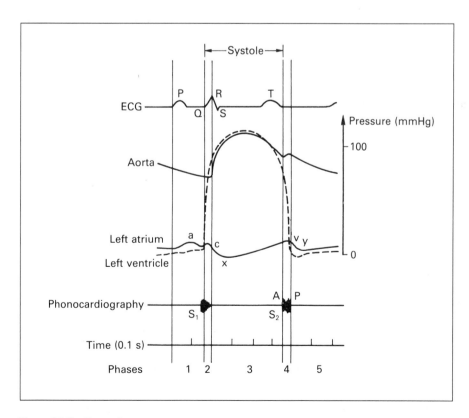

Figure 25 *Cardiac cycle*

–phase 5: passive ventricular filling: most rapid at the start of diastole.

See also, Arterial waveform; Pulse; Stroke volume; Venous waveform

Cardiac enzymes. **Enzymes** normally within cardiac cells; released into the blood when **MI** occurs, thus aiding diagnosis:
- –creatine kinase (CK or CPK):
  - –normally <190 iu/l.
  - –rises 4–6 hours after MI, peaks at 12 hours, falls at 2–3 days.
  - –also present in skeletal muscle.
- –aspartate aminotransferase (AST):
  - –normally <35 iu/l.
  - –rises after 12 hours, peaks at 1–2 days.
- –lactic dehydrogenase (LDH):
  - –normally <300 iu/l (depends on the assay).
  - –rises after 12 hours, peaks at 2–3 days, falls after 5–7 days.
  - –also present in red blood cells.

Isoenzymes specific to myocardial muscle exist for CK and LDH; testing may identify the source of origin where doubt exists, e.g. a rise in CK may also follow skeletal muscle injury.

Cardiac failure. Usually defined as inability of the heart to produce sufficient output for the body's requirements and venous return. The diagnosis is clinical, ranging from mild symptoms on exertion only, to **cardiogenic shock**. Several terms have been used to describe different forms of cardiac failure:
- –left or right ventricular failure (the most commonly used classification). The left ventricle is usually affected by general disease because its workload is much greater than that of the right.
- –forward or backward failure: the former refers to failure with reduced **cardiac output**; the latter refers to increased filling pressures with oedema, etc.
- –congestive cardiac failure: the term sometimes refers to backward failure, but is often reserved for left-sided failure leading to right-sided failure.
- –high output failure: associated with increased **preload** and increased cardiac output.
- Caused by:
  - –increased workload:
    - –preload:
      - –**aortic/mitral regurgitation**.
      - –**ASD/VSD**.
      - –severe **anaemia**, fluid overload, **hyperthyroidism**.
    - –afterload:
      - –**hypertension**.
      - –pulmonary/**aortic stenosis**, hypertrophic obstructive **cardiomyopathy**.
      - –**pulmonary hypertension**, **PE**.
  - –reduced force of contraction:
    - –**MI, ischaemic heart disease**.
    - –cardiomyopathy.
    - –**arrhythmias**.
    - –myocarditis.
  - –reduced filling:
    - –tricuspid/**mitral stenosis**.
    - –**cardiac tamponade**, constrictive **pericarditis** (right side).

–reduced ventricular compliance, e.g. amyloid infiltration.
- Effects:
  - –ventricular end-diastolic pressure increases, leading to compensatory mechanisms:
    - –ventricular hypertrophy.
    - –increased myocardial contractility (**Starling's law**).
    - –neuroendocrine response: mainly increased sympathetic activity, with tachycardia, vasoconstriction and increased force of contraction. **Aldosterone, renin/angiotensin** and **vasopressin** activity are increased, especially in chronic failure, but mechanisms are unclear. Salt and water retention result.
  - –ventricular compliance is reduced, leading to increased atrial pressure and atrial hypertrophy. Eventually, ventricular dilatation occurs, with higher wall tension required to produce a given pressure (**Laplace's law**).
  - –**coronary blood flow** is reduced by tachycardia, raised end-diastolic pressure, and increased muscle mass.
  - –left-sided failure may lead to **pulmonary oedema, pulmonary hypertension**, $\dot{V}/\dot{Q}$ mismatch, increased lung **compliance** and right-sided failure.
  - –right ventricular failure: **CVP** and **JVP** increase, with peripheral oedema and hepatic engorgement.
  - –reduced peripheral blood flow leads to increased O_2 uptake and reduction of mixed venous PO_2.
  - –sodium and water retention exacerbates oedema.
- Features:
  - –reduced cardiac output may result in hypotension, confusion and coma.
  - –left-sided failure:
    - –dyspnoea, typically worse on lying flat (orthopnoea) and sometimes waking the patient at night (paroxysmal nocturnal dyspnoea).
    - –peripheral shutdown, basal crepitations, left ventricular hypertrophy. Extra **heart sounds** e.g. gallop rhythm and **heart murmurs** may be present. **Cheyne-Stokes respiration** may accompany low output.
    - –acute pulmonary oedema.
  - –right-sided failure:
    - –raised JVP.
    - –dependent oedema, e.g. ankles if ambulant, sacrum if bedbound.
    - –hepatomegaly/ascites; the liver may be tender.
    - –right ventricular hypertrophy.
  - –**chest X-ray** may reveal cardiomegaly, upper lobe blood diversion, fluid in the pulmonary fissures, **Kerley lines**, **pleural effusion** and pulmonary oedema. **ECG** may reveal ventricular hypertrophy and strain, arrhythmias, etc.
- Management:
  - –general: of underlying cause, rest, sodium restriction (controversial), O_2 therapy if acute.
  - –**digoxin**: use (especially prolonged) is controversial.
  - –**diuretics**: reduce SVR, blood volume and oedema.
  - –**vasodilator drugs**: reduce preload and afterload.
  - –**inotropic drugs**: oral drugs are mostly disappointing. The most effective drugs are administered by iv infusion.
  - –emergency treatment: as for pulmonary oedema and cardiogenic shock.
- Response to treatment (Fig. 26):
  - –1: inotropic drugs/arterial vasodilators.

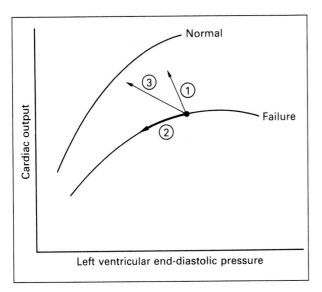

Figure 26 *Response to treatment of cardiac failure illustrated by Starling's curve (see text)*

–2: diuretics/venous vasodilators.
–3:
  –drug combinations, e.g. inotropes + vasodilators; often produce the greatest improvement.
  –intra-aortic counter-pulsation balloon pump.
- Anaesthetic considerations:
  –cardiac failure is consistently associated with increased perioperative morbidity and mortality; it should therefore be treated preoperatively whenever possible.
  –treatment as above. Electrolyte disturbances and digoxin toxicity may occur.
  –anaesthetic drugs should be given in small doses and slowly, because:
    –arm–brain circulation time is increased.
    –increased proportion of cardiac output goes to vital organs, e.g. brain and heart; thus greater effects are seen on these organs than in normal cardiac output states.
  –danger of myocardial depression, hypoxia, arrhythmias.
  –use of extradural/spinal anaesthesia is controversial; the benefit of reduction of SVR may be offset by the risk of hypotension. Perioperative risk is not diminished.
  –general anaesthetic management is as for the underlying condition.
Singer M (1993) Care of the Critically Ill; 9: 11–6

Cardiac glycosides. Drugs derived from plant extracts, used to treat supraventricular **arrhythmias** and **cardiac failure** (their use in the latter is controversial, since short-term benefit may not persist). Their actions are thought to be partly due to inhibition of the **sodium/potassium pump**, although increased **calcium** mobilization may also be involved. The drugs have long **half-lives** (e.g. **ouabain** 20 hours; **digoxin** 36 hours; digitoxin 4 days), large **volumes of distribution** (e.g. digoxin 700 litres) and low **therapeutic index**.
- Actions:
  – increase **myocardial contractility** and **stroke volume** (direct effect).

–decrease atrioventricular conduction, sinus node discharge, and thus heart rate (indirect effect via the vagus, and direct effect).
- Side effects: as for digoxin. They are increased by **hypokalaemia**, **hypercalcaemia** and **hypomagnesaemia**. Toxicity is also more likely in **renal failure** and pulmonary disease.
Digoxin is most widely used. Ouabain is more rapidly acting.

Cardiac index (CI). **Cardiac output** corrected for body size, expressed in terms of body **surface area**:

$$CI = \frac{\text{cardiac output (l/min).}}{\text{surface area (m}^2)}$$

Normal value is 2.5–4.2 l/min/m².

Cardiac massage. Periodic compression of the heart or chest in order to maintain **cardiac output**, e.g. during **CPR**. Both open (internal) and closed (external) cardiac massage were developed in the late 1800s. The latter became more popular in the 1960s following clear demonstration of its value in dogs and man, and was subsequently adopted by the American Heart Association and Resuscitation Council (UK) as method of choice.
- Closed cardiac massage:
  –with the patient supine on a rigid surface, the heel of one hand is placed on the lower third of the sternum, 1–2 finger's breadths cranial to the notch between the xiphisternum and ribcage (excessive trauma may result if compression is applied to the xiphisternum or ribs). The other hand is placed on the first, with fingers clear of the chest. With elbows straight and shoulders vertically above the hands, regular compressions are applied, with ratio of compression:relaxation 50:50 to 60:40. The sternum should be depressed 3.5–5 cm at each compression, at a rate of 80/min.
  –efficacy is assessed by feeling the femoral or carotid pulse, although palpable peak pressures may not reflect blood flow. End-tidal CO_2 measurement has been used to assess adequacy of massage; an increase reflects improved cardiac output.
  –may produce up to 30% of normal carotid and cerebral blood flows and cardiac output. Coronary flow is low during cardiac massage.
  –theories of mechanism (both may occur):
    –cardiac pump (as originally suggested): the heart is squeezed between sternum and vertebrae during compressions, expelling blood from the ventricles. During relaxation, blood is drawn into the chest by negative intrathoracic pressure, and the ventricles fill from the atria ('thoracic diastole'). Thought to be more important in children and when the heart is large.
    –thoracic pump: the theory arose from arterial and cardiac chamber pressure measurements during CPR, and from the phenomenon of **cough-CPR**. Positive intrathoracic pressure pushes blood out of heart and chest during compressions; reverse flow is prevented by cardiac and venous valves, and collapse of the thin-walled veins. During relaxation, blood is drawn into the chest by negative intrathoracic pressure.
    Intrathoracic pressures may be maximalized by synchronizing compressions with IPPV breaths,

with or without abdominal binding or compression ('new' CPR). Although arterial pressure, cerebral and carotid flows may increase, coronary blood flow and outcome are not improved. An automatic chest compressor ('chest thumper') may be used. A manual plunger device has recently been described, which increases venous return during relaxation by actively pulling the chest wall outwards.

–a modified technique is used in children (*see Cardiopulmonary resuscitation, paediatric*).

- Open cardiac massage:
  –increasingly used, because blood flows and cardiac output are greater than with closed massage. Also, direct vision and palpation are useful in assessing cardiac rhythm and filling, and **defibrillation** and intracardiac injection are easier.
  –skin and muscle are incised in an arc under the left nipple in the 4th or 5th intercostal space, stopping 2–3 cm from the sternum to avoid the internal thoracic artery. Pericardium is exposed using blunt dissection and pulling the ribs apart. The heart is squeezed from the patient's left side using the left hand, with fingers anteriorly over the right ventricle and thumb posteriorly over the left ventricle. Compressions are initially 60/min, adjusted according to cardiac filling. The descending aorta may be compressed with the other hand. The pericardium is opened for defibrillation or intracardiac injection. Because of the emergency nature of the procedure and the low risk of infection, sterile precautions are usually waived.
  –may also be performed per abdomen through the intact diaphragm; the heart is compressed against the sternum.
  –usually reserved for trauma, peroperative use, intra-abdominal or thoracic haemorrhage, massive PE, hypothermia, chest deformity, and ineffective closed massage.

Peters J, Ihle P (1990) Intensive Care Med; 16: 11–19 and 20–7

Cardiac output (CO). Volume of blood pumped by the heart per minute. Equals **stroke volume** (litres) × **heart rate** (beats/min). Normally about 5 l/min (0.7 litres × 70 beats/min) in a fit 70 kg man at rest; may increase up to 30 l/min, e.g. on vigorous exercise. Often corrected for body **surface area** (**cardiac index**).

Of central importance in maintaining **arterial BP** (equals cardiac output × **SVR**) and **O₂ delivery** to the tissues (**O₂ flux**).

Affected by metabolic rate (e.g. increased in **pregnancy**, **septicaemia**, **hyperthyroidism** and exercise), drugs, and many other physiological and pathological processes which affect heart rate, **preload**, **myocardial contractility** and **afterload**.

- Distribution of normal CO (approximate values):
  –heart: 5%.
  –brain: 14%.
  –muscle: 20%.
  –kidneys: 22%.
  –liver: 25%.
  –rest: 14%.

(*for comparisons of blood flow and oxygen consumption, see Blood flow*)

- Effects of **iv anaesthetic agents** on CO:
  –reduced by **thiopentone** > **methohexitone** > **etomidate**, mostly via decreased contractility. **Propofol** reduces CO via vasodilatation and bradycardia.

–increased by **ketamine**.

- Effects of **inhalational anaesthetic agents** on CO:
  –reduced by **enflurane** > **halothane** > **isoflurane** > **N₂O**. Proposed mechanisms include direct myocardial depression (via reduced concentration or modified activity of intracellular **calcium** ions during systole), inhibition of central or peripheral **sympathetic nervous system** outflow, and altered baroreceptor activity.
  –maintained by **diethyl ether** via sympathetic stimulation despite a direct myocardial depressant effect.
  –variable effects of **cyclopropane** due to its variable actions on the autonomic nervous system, despite a direct myocardial depressant effect.

Pinsky MR (1990) Intensive Care Med; 16: 415–7
See also, Cardiac output measurement

Cardiac output measurement. Methods which have been used include:

- **Fick principle**: most commonly O₂ consumption is measured. Requires samples of mixed venous and arterial blood. Alternatively, CO₂ production may be measured, deriving arterial $P\text{CO}_2$ from end-tidal expired partial pressure. Mixed venous $P\text{CO}_2$ may be derived from analysis of expired gas collected in a closed rebreathing bag, using a **mass spectrometer**. Both methods are lengthy, complicated and not suitable for routine use.
- **dilution techniques**, using dye or cold saline as indicators. For dye dilution, a known amount of dye is injected into the pulmonary artery, and its concentration measured peripherally using a photoelectric spectrometer. Indocyanine green is used because of its low toxicity, short **half-life** and absorption characteristics (i.e. unaffected by changes in O₂ saturation). Semilogarithmic replotting of the data curve is required, with extrapolation of the straight line obtained to correct for recirculation of the dye (Fig. 27). **Cardiac output** is calculated from the injected dose, the area under the curve within the extrapolated line and its duration. Curves of short duration are produced by high cardiac output; curves of long duration are produced by low cardiac output. Data from repeated injections may be affected by previous ones.

  Thermodilution techniques allow repeated estimations, and are suitable for use in ICU. 5–10 ml cold dextrose or saline is injected through the proximal port of a pulmonary artery catheter, with temperature changes measured by a thermistor at the catheter tip. A bedside computer is commonly used to calculate cardiac output, based on at least three measurements. Injection is usually performed at end expiration. Data are usually presented as a temperature drop against time, to produce similar curves as in dye techniques but without the secondary peak.
- **impedance plethysmography**: thought to be useful in estimating changes in individual subjects, but not useful for absolute measurements.
- **aortovelography** and **ballistocardiography**: inaccurate.
- **echocardiography** using the **Doppler effect**: the velocity of blood in the ascending aorta is measured, from which is derived the length of a column of blood passing through the aorta in unit time. This is multi-

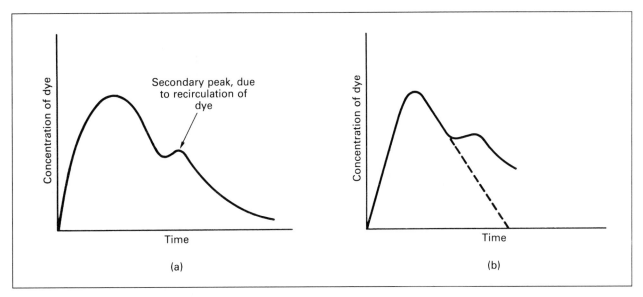

Figure 27 *Dilution technique for measuring cardiac output: (a) ordinary plot; (b) semilogarithmic plot*

plied by the cross-sectional area of the aorta to give stroke volume. The equipment required is expensive.
–**electromagnetic flow measurement** may be achieved during surgery by placing a probe around the root of the aorta, but its use is obviously limited.
–**cardiac catheterization** and angiography allows estimation of left ventricular volume and **ejection fraction**, as does **radioisotope** scanning.
–two-dimensional echocardiography can be used to measure the movement of the anterior and posterior ventricular walls, and ejection fraction. Derivation of stroke volume relies on the shape of the ventricular cavity being ellipsoid, which may not always be the case. Three-dimensional echocardiography may produce better results.
Taylor SH, Silke B (1988) Br J Anaesth; 60: 90S-8S

Cardiac pacing. Repetitive electrical stimulation of cardiac activity, used to treat brady- or tachyarrhythmias.
● Types of pacemakers:
  –temporary:
    –transvenous; i.e. pacing wire passed via a central vein to the right ventricle under X-ray control. Usually bipolar, i.e. with two electrodes at the end of the wire; current passes from the distal to the proximal electrode, stimulating adjacent myocardium. Wires may be rigid, or flexible and balloon tipped. Technique of insertion: as for **central venous cannulation**; the procedure may be technically difficult.
       Indications include acute **MI** (inferior MI often requires temporary pacing; anterior often requires permanent pacing). Preoperative use should be considered in:
      –**heart block**: 3rd degree, sometimes 2nd degree (e.g. if Mobitz type II, associated with symptoms, or intended surgery is extensive).
      –**bundle branch block**, e.g. bifascicular with symptoms or P-R prolongation.
      –bradyarrhythmias.
    Technique of pacing:

–bradyarrhythmias: once the wire is in place, the minimal stimulating current is determined (usually about 1–2 mA) and the pacing output set 2–3 times higher, using VVI (see below). Failure to pace may result from disconnections, oversensing or failure to capture. The pacing box should be converted to V00 and the wire repositioned if neccessary. Dual chamber pacing may be achieved using a special atrial wire in addition to the ventricular one.
–tachyarrhythmias, e.g. **SVT, atrial flutter**: A00 pacing is used, stimulating via a right atrial lead. The rate is slowly increased from 60/min to the spontaneous rate, held for 30 seconds, and pacing stopped. If unsuccessful, pacing at 400–800/min may be used to provoke **AF**, which usually reverts spontaneously to sinus rhythm. **VT** may be treated by slow ventricular V00 pacing, atrial pacing, or ventricular pacing at 10–30% faster rate than spontaneous for 5–10 beats only (burst pacing), with **defibrillation** available. Advantages over **cardioversion** include avoidance of anaesthesia and the adverse effects of electrical shock, easier repetition if unsuccessful, and availability of pacing if bradycardia or asystole occur.
–The pacing wire may conduct small currents directly to the heart with risk of **electrocution** (microshock); the metal contacts should therefore be insulated.
–transcutaneous pacing has also been used, using large surface area skin electrodes (e.g. one over the cardiac apex, one over the right scapula) and pulse duration of up to 50 ms to reduce cutaneous nerve and muscle stimulation. Avoids complications of transvenous pacing, and quicker to perform.
–transoesophageal pacing has also been used but is less reliable.
–permanent: a pulse generator is implanted subcutaneously. Electrodes are usually unipolar; i.e. one intracardiac electrode, with current returning to the

pacemaker via the body. The heart electrode is usually endocardial, passed via a central vein; epicardial electrodes have been used.

Indicated if an arrhythmia is associated with syncope, dizziness, cardiac failure, etc., e.g. in **sick sinus syndrome**, heart block or post-MI. Prophylactic use is controversial.

Table 10. Generic pacemaker code

Position 1: chamber paced	Position 2: chamber sensed	Position 3: response
0 = None	0 = None	0 = None
A = Atrium	A = Atrium	T = Triggered
V = Ventricle	V = Ventricle	I = Inhibited
D = Dual	D = Dual	D = Dual
		R = Reverse

A generic pacemaker code identifies function (Table 10). Thus VVI denotes ventricular pacing, with inhibition of pacing should any spontaneous ventricular complex occur (e.g. in temporary transvenous pacing). DDD denotes pacing and sensing of both chambers, with inhibition or triggering to maintain sequential atrial and ventricular contraction, allowing spontaneous activity should it occur. Two newer positions have been added: position 4 defines programmability of rate modulation (none/simple and multiple programmability/communicating/rate response), and position 5 defines available functions for use in tachycardias (none/pacing/shock/pacing + shock). Rate-responsive devices respond to physiological parameters normally associated with changes in heart rate (e.g. body movement, **Q–T interval**, respiration, temperature, pH, myocardial contractility, haemoglobin saturation) by increasing the pacing rate.

- Anaesthesia for patients with pacemakers:
  - preoperatively:
    - **preoperative assessment** is particularly directed towards the CVS.
    - pacemaker type and indication are ascertained. Pacemakers are usually checked regularly.
    - ECG:
      - if pacing spikes occur before all or most beats, heart rate is pacemaker-dependent.
      - demand pacemakers may be converted to fixed rate by placing a magnet over the pulse generator; the ECG is observed for pacing spikes.
    - CXR: pulse generator and number of leads may be identified.
    - the rate–response function may be switched off with a specific programming device.
  - peroperatively:
    - potential electrical interference or pacemaker damage by **diathermy** is more likely if the latter is applied near the device. Sensing may be triggered, with resultant chamber inhibition, or arrhythmias induced. Diathermy may also reprogramme the pacemaker to a different mode, possibly more likely to occur if a magnet is used peroperatively.
    - if avoidance of diathermy is not possible, risks are reduced by using bipolar diathermy, or placing the

plate distant from the pacemaker if unipolar diathermy is used. Current should not be applied across the chest, and its strength and duration of use should be minimal.
    - **isoprenaline** should be available in case pacemaker failure occurs.
    - alteration of pacemaker sensitivity by **halothane** has been described in older pacemaker models.
  - postoperative pacemaker checking may be required.

Bloomfield P, Bowler GMR (1989) Anaesthesia; 44: 42–6

Cardiac risk index (Goldman cardiac risk index). Scoring system for preoperative identification of patients at risk from major perioperative cardiovascular complications. Derived retrospectively in 1977 from data from 1001 patients undergoing non-cardiac surgery; analysis identified nine variables correlating with increased risk:
  - third **heart sound**/elevated **JVP**: 11 points.
  - **MI** within 6 months: 10 points.
  - **ventricular ectopic beats** > 5/min: 7 points.
  - rhythm other than sinus: 7 points.
  - age > 70 years: 5 points.
  - emergency operation: 4 points.
  - severe **aortic stenosis**: 3 points.
  - poor medical condition of patient: 3 points.
  - abdominal or thoracic operation: 3 points.

Patients with scores above 25 points had 56% incidence of death, with 22% incidence of severe cardiovascular complications. Corresponding figures for scores below 26 points were 4% and 17% respectively, with 0.2% and 0.7% for scores less than 6.

Confirmed by other studies as having high specificity but low sensitivity; i.e. high scoring patients are high-risk, but not all high-risk patients are identified.

[Lee B Goldman, Boston cardiologist]

Goldman L, Caldera DL, Nussbaum SR et al (1977) New Engl J Med 297: 845–50

See also, Ischaemic heart disease; Preoperative assessment

Cardiac surgery. First performed in the late 1800s/early 1900s but limited by the effects of circulatory interruption. Use of **hypothermia** increased the range of surgery possible, but 'open' heart surgery, i.e. employing **cardiopulmonary bypass** (CPB) was not developed until the 1950s.

- Indications:
  - **ischaemic heart disease**, i.e. **coronary artery bypass graft**.
  - **congenital heart disease**, e.g. **VSD**, **ASD**, **Fallot's tetralogy**, others.
  - acquired valve disease.
  - others (e.g. **PE**, **heart transplantation** and **trauma**) are less common.

Indications for 'closed' procedures include patent **ductus arteriosus**, aortic **coarctation**, thoracic **aortic aneurysm**, shunt procedures in congenital heart disease, **cardiac tamponade**, constrictive **pericarditis**, and valve stenoses (uncommon). Percutaneous balloon techniques are also employed, e.g. **percutaneous transluminal coronary angioplasty** and balloon septostomy, e.g. in **transposition of the great arteries**. Pacemaker insertion is usually performed under local anaesthesia.

- **Preoperative assessment** and management:
  - as for ischaemic and congenital heart disease. **Cardiac risk index** is widely quoted in assessing risk. **Cardiac**

failure is particularly important. Respiratory and cerebrovascular disease is common. Investigations include assessment of renal function, often liver function tests and coagulation studies. **Chest X-ray**, **ECG, cardiac catheterization** studies and **echocardiography** are usual.

–most cardiovascular drugs are continued. **Digoxin** is often started 1–2 days preoperatively, to reduce incidence of postoperative **arrhythmias**. **Anticoagulant drugs** are stopped or continued according to the risk of thromboembolism and surgeon's preference. **Antiplatelet drugs** are usually stopped 1 week preoperatively.

–**premedication** is traditionally heavy since anxiety is usually marked. An opioid/**hyoscine** mixture is often used, sometimes with **benzodiazepines**. Premedication is often omitted in emergency surgery. **Glyceryl trinitrate** patch or **β-adrenergic receptor antagonists** are often used. Antibiotic prophylaxis usually includes flucloxacillin and an aminoglycoside.

● Induction and maintenance of anaesthesia:

–**preoxygenation** is usually employed.

–venous and **arterial cannulation** is usually performed under local anaesthesia. **Central venous cannulation** may often be reserved until the patient is asleep.

–iv induction employs standard agents in small doses, as for ischaemic heart disease. **Ketamine** is usually avoided. Benzodiazepines have been used. Tracheal intubation and IPPV follows, using standard **neuromuscular blocking drugs**. **Pancuronium** is often used as BP is maintained, despite possible tachycardia.

–high doses of **opioid analgesic drugs** have been used, e.g. **morphine** up to 10 mg/kg, **fentanyl** up to 100 µg/kg and **sufentanil** up to 30 µg/kg.

  –Advantages:
    –obtund the hypertensive response to intubation.
    –cardiostable without requiring high doses of volatile agents.
    –provide analgesia.
  –Disadvantages:
    –may cause muscle rigidity (mechanism is unclear, but it responds to neuromuscular blockade).
    –prolonged postoperative IPPV may be required.
    –may not prevent **awareness**.
    –bradycardia may occur.

Alfentanil is often used to obtund the hypertensive response to intubation without causing prolonged postoperative respiratory depression, e.g. up to 125 µg/kg.

–**N₂O** is often avoided because of cardiac depression, especially in combination with high-dose opioids. It may also increase SVR and increase size of air bubbles. Volatile **inhalational anaesthetic agents** are used in low concentrations. The choice of agent is controversial, because of myocardial depression, heart rate changes and other effects. **Isoflurane** is implicated in causing **coronary steal**, but causes least myocardial depression and sensitization to catecholamines.

–**TIVA** has been used, including **neuroleptanaesthesia**.

● **Monitoring**:
  –ECG.
  –direct arterial BP measurement.
  –**central venous cannulation**: two lines are often used: one for **CVP** measurement, one for drug infusion. Multilumen catheters are increasingly used.

–**pulmonary artery catheterization** is controversial. **Cardiac output measurement** is used more frequently in the USA then in the UK. Left-sided pressures may be measured directly via a needle during surgery.

–oesophageal stethoscope, echocardiography and **Doppler** probe have been used, especially in the USA, to assess peroperative myocardial workload and **myocardial ischaemia**.

–**temperature measurement** (core and peripheral).

–the place of routine **EEG** and its derivatives is controversial.

–electrolyte and blood gas analysis should be readily available. Activated clotting time (ACT) may be determined in the operating theatre (*see Coagulation studies*).

–a urinary catheter is usual unless surgery is staightforward and short.

● Pre-CPB management:

–as for any operation.

–1–2 units of blood are often taken from the patient (for later retransfusion) and replaced with colloid.

–stimulation during opening of the chest and removal of vein grafts from the legs may cause hypertension.

–after baseline ACT measurement, **heparin** 2–3 mg/kg (90 mg/m² surface area) is injected iv through a tested line (sometimes injected by the surgeon). **Prostacyclin** has been used but is expensive and its role is uncertain. When ACT is 3–4 times normal i.e. about 400 seconds, cannulation for CPB is performed.

● Management during CPB:

–circulation is gradually taken over by the pump.

–drugs are diluted by the crystalloid prime, thus iv boluses are often required e.g. opioid, benzodiazepine, induction agent, neuromuscular blocking drug. Infusions may also be used, or drugs may be added to the CPB circuit. Inhalational agents may be fed to the oxygenator.

–**haemodilution** occurs.

–the place of **cerebral protection** is uncertain.

–core temperature is lowered to 28–30°C; the aorta is cross-clamped and **cardioplegia** used, lowering heart temperature to 10–15°C. A total ischaemia time of about 1 hour is considered acceptable. Core temperatures of 15–20°C are occasionally used without CPB or with low flows.

–IPPV is stopped; continuous positive pressure is applied to maintain some lung expansion. Air is thought to be better than 100% O₂ because of increased **atelectasis** with the latter; N₂O is avoided because of the risk of **air embolism**.

–optimal perfusion pressure is controversial; 30–50 mmHg is generally thought to be the minimum. CPB details are also controversial, e.g. type of oxygentor, pulsatile/non-pulsatile flow.

–SVR usually decreases in the first 15 minutes; **vasopressor drugs** are sometimes given, e.g. **methoxamine, metaraminol, phenylephrine**. SVR then slowly increases, due to increased **catecholamines, renin/ angiotensin system** activity, and **vasopressin** secretion. **Vasodilator drugs** are often given if MAP exceeds 80–100 mmHg, e.g. **sodium nitroprusside**, glyeryl trinitrate, **pentolinium**.

–ACT is checked every 30 minutes, with further heparin given if necessary, e.g. 1/4 - 1/2 initial dose. **Potassium** is added as required according to plasma levels. Arterial blood gases analysis is performed at 37°C in most machines; values have been traditionally corrected to body temperature to account for increased solubility of CO_2 at low temperatures, but this is now considered unnecessary. **Bicarbonate** is usually not administered unless **base excess** exceeds 7–8. Blood is transfused to keep the **haematocrit** above 0.2–0.3.

–after repair of the lesion, the cross-clamp is removed and rewarming undertaken. Cardiac activity is usually spontaneous, usually VF but sometimes sinus rhythm. Internal **defibrillation** is performed at 30–32°C, and normal Po_2, pH and electrolyte concentration. 20–50 J is usually used. **Cardiac pacing** is sometimes required; epicardial wires may be inserted prophylactically for postoperative use.

–CPB blood flow is gradually decreased as cardiac output increases. Drug boluses are given iv as before. Manual IPPV helps expel air from the pulmonary vessels. 100% O_2 or an O_2/air mixture is usually employed.

● Post-CPB and postoperative care:
   –left atrial pressure is optimized to 8–12 mmHg; vasodilators are used to accomodate CPB fluid volume.
   –a low output state may occur, especially if ventricular function was poor preoperatively and ischaemia time was prolonged. It may be improved by:
      –**inotropic drugs**: **calcium** is often used as a temporary measure. Others include **dopamine, dobutamine, adrenaline** and **isoprenaline**, more recently **enoximone, milrinone** and **dopexamine**. The choice is according to individual patient and drug characteristics, and personal preference.
      –vasodilators as above (often combined with inotropes).
      –correction of potassium/acid-base imbalance.
      –**intra-aortic counter-pulsation balloon pump** is occasionally required.
   –heparin is reversed with **protamine**, injected slowly to reduce side effects, especially in pulmonary hypertension. 1 mg/mg heparin is usually used, although less may be required.
   –hypertension is common if left ventricular function is good, especially in aortic valve disease. Vasodilators may be required.
   –temperature may fall as core heat is transferred to the periphery.
   –arrhythmias and heart block may occur.
   –pericardial and pleural drains are inserted before sternal closure.
   –transfer to ICU must be carefully managed because of the potential dangers from interrupted monitoring and infusions, and movement.
   –postoperative management is related to:
      –bleeding: may be surgical, or caused by consumption or dilution of **platelet** and **coagulation factors** during CPB, the effects of massive **blood transfusion**, or inadequate reversal of heparin. Perioperative **aprotinin, antifibrinolytic drugs** and **desmopressin** have been used to reduce blood requirements.
      –treatment of hyper-/hypotension and arrhythmias.
      –low output state as above. Cardiac tamponade may require drainage on ICU.

–maintenance of fluid balance and urine output. The crystalloid load from CPB usually causes diuresis but **pulmonary oedema** may occur, especially if cardiac output is low.
–rewarming; central/peripheral temperature difference is a useful indication.
–maintenance of electrolyte, acid-base and blood gas balance. Hypokalaemia is common.
–IPPV is usually continued for a few hours, sometimes overnight. Opioid/benzodiazepine boluses are commonly used for **sedation**. Immediate extubation after surgery is occasionally performed. Usual criteria for **weaning** include cardiovascular and respiratory stability, adequate warming and perfusion, good urine output, minimal blood loss and good orientation and arousal. Impaired gas exchange may be associated with pre-existing lung disease, atelectasis, and CPB-related factors, e.g. embolization with bubbles and platelet aggregates, complement activation, etc., especially if CPB was prolonged.
–CNS changes: CVA occurs in less than 2% of patients undergoing open-heart surgery, but subtle changes are found in up to 60%, thought to be related to embolization (e.g. with bubbles, aggregates, etc. during CPB) and/or inadequate perfusion. Effects may possibly be reduced by filtering the arterial inflow line.

Cardiac tamponade. Compression of the heart by fluid (e.g. blood) within the pericardium, restricting ventricular filling and reducing **stroke volume** and **cardiac output**. Myocardial O_2 supply is reduced by hypotension, increased end-diastolic pressure, tachycardia and compression of epicardial vessels. Tamponade should be differentiated from **pneumothorax** and **cardiac failure**.

● Features:
   –dyspnoea, restlessness, oliguria, hypotension, peripheral vasoconstriction. **JVP, CVP** and **left atrial pressure** are raised, and **pulsus paradoxus** is present. Jugular venous distension may occur during inspiration or when pressure is applied over the liver (Kussmaul's sign). Cardiovascular collapse and death may occur, especially if acute (e.g. following **chest trauma**).
   –**ECG** complexes may be small, and the heart shadow globular and enlarged on the **chest X-ray**. Confirmed by **echocardiography**.

● Immediate management is pericardial aspiration:
   –a long 18–22 G needle attached to a syringe is introduced between the xiphisternum and the left costal margin, and directed towards the left shoulder at 35–40° to the skin. Aspiration is performed as the right ventricle is approached, until pericardial fluid is obtained. A three-way tap is used. Pericardial blood does not clot, whereas intracardiac blood does.
   –an ECG chest lead may be attached to the needle; S–T elevation and ventricular ectopics may indicate contact with the ventricle.
   –trauma to myocardium and coronary vessels is reduced by inserting a plastic iv cannula over the needle into the pericardial space.
   –alternate approaches:
      –in the 5th intercostal space just lateral to the left sternal edge (approaches the left ventricle).

–one intercostal space lower, and 1–2 cm lateral to the apex beat, directed towards the right shoulder (approaches the apex).

Subsequent surgery may be required.

- Anaesthetic considerations: drugs or manoeuvres which reduce **venous return**, **heart rate** or **myocardial contractility** should be avoided, especially with coexistent **hypovolaemia**. **IPPV** should be performed cautiously.

[Adolf Kussmaul (1822–1909), German physician]

Lake CL (1983) Anesth Analg; 62: 431–43

See also, Cardiac surgery

Cardiogenic shock. Shock associated with primary cardiac pump failure. Most commonly caused by acute **MI**, but it may also follow **cardiac surgery** and **chest trauma**. Usually defined according to impaired myocardial muscle contraction; shock due to **PE**, **cardiac tamponade** and **arrhythmias** is sometimes included in the definition. Heart rate and SVR are usually increased to compensate for hypotension, exacerbating myocardial O_2 supply/demand imbalance. **Acidosis** resulting from poor perfusion further impairs **myocardial contractility**.

- Features:
  - –as for shock.
  - –increased left ventricular filling pressures and **pulmonary oedema** are usual. However, relative **hypovolaemia** may be present due to redistribution of fluid to lungs, previous fluid restriction, diuretic therapy and sweating. Right-sided failure may occur, e.g. in right ventricular infarction.
- Management:
  - –supportive as for MI/shock including O_2 administration.
  - –optimizing of left ventricular filling pressure; **pulmonary artery capillary wedge pressure** (PCWP) is a more useful guide than **CVP**, unless failure is predominantly right-sided. A PCWP of 18–22 mmHg is thought to be optimal for the failing heart, even though this is higher than normal. **Colloid** is usually employed if PCWP is low, **inotropic** and **vasodilator drugs** if PCWP is high.
  - –**intra-aortic counter-pulsation balloon pump** and cardiac surgery may be required.

Prognosis is generally poor, especially after MI.

Rae AP, Hutton I (1986) Br J Anaesth; 58: 151–68

See also, Cardiac failure

Cardioinhibitory centre (Cardioinhibitory area). Comprised of the nucleus ambiguus and adjacent neurones in the ventral medulla, with some input from the dorsal motor nucleus and nucleus of the tractus solitarius. Produces vagal 'tone', increased by **baroreceptor** discharge. Also receives afferents from higher centres. Impulses pass to the **vasomotor centre**, inhibiting it, and via the **vagus nerve**. Thus involved centrally in controlling **arterial BP**.

Cardiomyopathy. Disease of myocardium. Suggested definitions include:

- –myocardial disease of unknown aetiology.
- –myocardial disease not due to respiratory, coronary, or congenital heart disease, hypertension or rheumatic fever.

- May be:
  - –dilated (congestive):

- –reduced contractility and **ejection fraction**, with ventricular dilatation.
- –causes **cardiac failure**, **arrhythmias**, angina and systemic embolism from mural thrombus.
- –prognosis is poor; death is usually within a few years of cardiac failure.
- –a similar pattern may occur with **alcohol** abuse, viral infection, **pregnancy**, **antimitotic drugs**, **connective tissue diseases**, and metabolic and infiltrative disorders, e.g. **sarcoidosis**.
- –treatment includes **digoxin**, **diuretics**, **antiarrhythmic drugs**, **vasodilator drugs** and **anticoagulant drugs**.
- –anaesthetic management: as for **ischaemic heart disease**. Myocardial depression, **hypovolaemia** and increased SVR are particularly hazardous.
  - –hypertrophic (obstructive; HOCM):
    - –familial disorder, with left ventricular hypertrophy especially affecting the upper interventricular septum, causing left ventricular outflow obstruction.
    - –causes arrhythmias, syncope, angina and cardiac failure. Infective **endocarditis** may occur.
    - –treatment includes diuretics, antiarrhythmics and **β-adrenergic receptor antagonists**; the last reduce force and rate of contraction, reducing outflow obstruction. Conversely, digoxin should be avoided. Anticoagulants are often used in arrhythmias. Surgery has been used to relieve obstruction.
    - –anaesthetic management includes antibiotic prophylaxis as for **congenital heart disease**. The following especially should be avoided: increased sympathetic activity with increased contractility and tachycardia, arrhythmias, hypovolaemia and reduced SVR.
  - –restrictive:
    - –very rare; due to fibrosis or infiltration.
    - –effects and management are as for constrictive **pericarditis**.

ECG is usually non-specific, showing arrhythmias, **bundle branch block**, ventricular hypertrophy and ischaemia. **Chest X-ray** may show cardiac enlargement and pulmonary oedema. **Echocardiography**, **cardiac catheterization** and **nuclear cardiology** may be useful.

Goodwin JF (1989) Drugs; 38: 988–99

Cardioplegia. Intentional cardiac arrest caused by coronary perfusion with cold electrolyte solution, to allow **cardiac surgery**. After establishment of **cardiopulmonary bypass**, a cannula is inserted into the ascending aorta and connected to a bag of solution (traditionally at 4°C) having excluded air bubbles. After aortic cross-clamping distal to the cannula, the solution is passed under 200–300 mmHg pressure into the aortic root, closing the aortic valve and perfusing the coronary arteries. In aortic valve disease, individual coronary artery cannulation may be required. Severe coronary stenosis may require further injection of solution through the bypass graft. Asystole usually occurs after 100–200 ml, but 1 litre is used (20 ml/kg in children) in order to cool the heart to 10–12°C. Further infusion may be required in prolonged surgery. Iced saline is placed around the heart to maintain hypothermia.

- Solutions used may contain:
  - –NaCl 110–140 mmol/l: prevents excess water accumulation. May increase calcium entry if sodium concentration is too high.

–KCl 10–20 mmol/l: causes depolarization and cardiac arrest in diastole, reducing myocardial O_2 demand. Higher concentrations may cause arterial spasm.

–$MgCl_2$ 16 mmol/l and $CaCl_2$ 1.2–2.2 mmol/l: reduce automatic rhythmogenicity and protect against potassium-induced damage post-bypass. Excessive calcium may cause persistent myocardial contraction (stone heart). Magnesium reduces calcium entry.

–$NaHCO_3$ 0–10 mmol/l.

–procaine 0–1 mmol/l: stabilizes the membrane, reducing arrhythmias post-bypass.

–other additives are more controversial, and include:
  –buffers, e.g. histidine and tromethamine: help maintain normal intracellular pH and encourage ATP generation.
  –metabolic substrates, e.g. glucose and amino acids: increase ATP generation.
  –**mannitol**: reduces water accumulation and may improve cardiac function.
  –**free radical** scavengers.
  –steroids.
  –**calcium channel blocking drugs**.

• Other controversies:
  –use of blood instead of crystalloid: optimal osmotic, buffer and metabolic make-up but increased viscosity.
  –oxygenation of the solution.
  –use of warm solution: may cause better myocardial relaxation, with reduced membrane and protein damage associated with low temperatures.
  –continuous versus intermittent injection.

Usual solution pH is 5.5–7.8 and osmolality 285–300 mosm/Kg.

Noble WH, Lichtenstein SV, Mazar CD (1991) Can J Anaesth; 38: 1–6

Cardiopulmonary bypass (CPB). Developed largely by Gibbon in the 1950s from animal experiments performed in 1937. Haemolysis was caused by initial disc/bubble oxygenators; improved membrane oxygenators were developed in the late 1950s. Used in **cardiac surgery**; similar techniques are used for **extracorporeal membrane oxygenation** and **extracorporeal CO_2 removal** in **respiratory failure**.

• Principles:
  –venous drainage: under gravity via a right atrial cannula or separate superior/inferior vena caval cannulae if the right atrium is opened. Blood also drains via right atrial and left heart suckers/vents to avoid pooling of blood in the operative field. Blood passes through a filter and defoaming chamber, which may be combined with a reservoir and/or oxygenator.
  –oxygenator: flat screens and rotating discs were originally used. The main types are now:
    –bubble oxygenators: tiny bubbles provide a large surface area for gas exchange. Thorough defoaming is required. Thought to increase the risk of microscopic air emboli, blood component damage and consumption of coagulation factors.
    –membrane oxygenators: hollow capillary fibres through which blood passes, with gas exchange across their walls. Flat membrane oxygenators are also available. Increasing in popularity, since adverse effects are less likely. Have been used for

several days without requiring replacement. Can also be used for concurrent ultrafiltration.

Most incorporate temperature exchangers. CO_2 and O_2 are supplied independently to the oxygenator as required, e.g. 2.5% CO_2 in O_2.

  –pumps: usually rotating roller pumps using wide tubing. Rotating chambers are also used, reducing damage to blood components. Flow is traditionally non-pulsatile but pulsatile flow may provide better organ perfusion, with lower **vasopressin** and angiotensin levels; however, the equipment required is more complex and expensive. Pulsations may be synchronized with the ECG if the heart is pumping. Flows used vary between centres but are usually 1.0–2.4 l/min/m² surface area (up to 80 ml/min/kg). Lower flows are required with hypothermia.
  –arterial return: via ascending aorta (rarely, femoral artery) using a short wide cannula to reduce resistance and avoid accidental cannulation of aortic branches. The return is filtered to remove platelet aggregates, fibrin, debris, etc. 150–300 µm filters are standard; microemboli may be reduced by smaller filters but increased risk of **complement** activation has been suggested.

• Use:
  –disposable systems are usually employed.
  –the system is primed with 1.5–2.5 litres **crystalloid** usually, although **colloid** may be used, and rarely blood. **Heparin** 20 mg/l may be added. The tubing is checked for bubbles before use; flushing the system with CO_2 before priming has been suggested, to reduce bubble formation.
  –anticoagulation, introduction and termination of CPB: as for cardiac surgery.

• Complications:
  –technical, e.g. leaks, bubbles, disconnections, obstruction, coagulation, power failure, etc. Vascular damage may occur during cannulation.
  –embolization with clot, debris, bubbles, defoaming agent, etc. Bubbles may enter via the heart cavity during surgery, especially at end of bypass. Subtle neurological changes are thought to be related to microembolization.
  –related to surgery or anticoagulation.

[John H Gibbon (1903–1974), US surgeon]
Girling DK (1990) Hosp Update; 16: 799–804 and 875–83

Cardiopulmonary resuscitation (CPR). Over many centuries, numerous techniques have been tried in order to restore life; early attempts included use of heat, smoke, cold water, beating, and suspension from ropes.

• Artificial ventilation was developed within the last 400 years:
  –use of bellows via the mouth or nose is attributed to **Paracelsus** in the early 1500s. Used via tracheal tubes in the 1700s, e.g. by **Kite**.
  –postural techniques, e.g. compressing the chest and abdomen from behind with the victim prone, moving the arms, or using tilting boards, etc.: used from the 1850s.
  –**expired air ventilation**: developed in the 1700s, although reported earlier.

• **Cardiac massage**, external and internal, was first attempted in the late 1800s; external massage was popularized in the early 1960s.

- **Defibrillation** was investigated in animals in the 1700s/1800s; internal defibrillation was performed in man in the 1940s and external defibrillation in the 1950s.
- CPR is divided into:
  - basic life support: traditionally without any equipment, and therefore suitable for 'lay person resuscitation'. Increasingly includes the use of simple equipment e.g. **airways, facepieces, self-inflating bags, oesophageal obturators**, etc.
  - advanced life support: as above, plus use of specialized equipment, techniques, drugs, monitoring, etc.; usually confined to hospitals.
- Recommendations of the European Resuscitation Council (1992):
  - basic life support:
    - assess; e.g. shaking the victim, asking if all right, etc., and checking the carotid pulse and breathing. Help should be summoned.
    - 'ABC' of resuscitation:
      - **Airway**: chin lift, head tilt and jaw thrust are employed. Food, dentures, etc. are removed from the airway. Specialist equipment is used if available.
      - Breathing: expired air ventilation: two slow breaths over 1–2 seconds; rapid breaths are more likely to inflate the stomach. **Cricoid pressure** should be applied if additional help is available. Risk of **HIV infection, hepatitis**, etc. is considered negligible. Inflating equipment and 100% O_2 should be used if available. The victim is placed in the **recovery** postion if breathing spontaneously.
      - Circulation: external bleeding should be stopped and the feet raised. External cardiac massage is insituted at 80/min.
    - ratio for cardiac massage:breaths of 15:2 for a single operator and 5:1 for two operators.
    - the recovery position is used when stable unless **spinal cord injury** is suspected.
    - all medical and paramedical personnel should be able to administer basic life support (ideally every member of the public). Ability of hospital staff has been consistently shown to be poor. Regular training sessions are thought to be necessary, using training mannikins.
  - advanced life support:
    - drugs are given iv, preferably via a central vein. **Tracheal administration of drugs** is possible, using 2–3 iv doses of **atropine** and **adrenaline**. CPR should not be interrupted for more than 10 seconds.
    - action depends on the initial ECG trace in **cardiac arrest**:
      - VF:
        - praecordial thump.
        - 200 J defibrillation.
        - 200 J defibrillation.
        - 360 J defibrillation.
        - adrenaline 1 mg (10 ml of 1:10 000).
        - 10 compression/ventilation sequences.
        - 360 J defibrillation × 3 as required.
        - further adrenaline/repeated defibrillation cycles as required (approximately every 2–3 minutes).
        - after 3 adrenaline/defibrillation cycles, **bicarbonate** and **antiarrhythmic drugs** (e.g. **amiodarone, bretylium** and **lignocaine**) should be considered.
      - **asystole**:
        - praecordial thump.
        - correct connection of the ECG should be checked.
        - defibrillation if VF cannot be excluded.
        - adrenaline 1 mg.
        - 10 compression/ventilation sequences.
        - atropine 3 mg (× 1 only).
        - repeated cycles as required.
        - cardiac pacing should be considered if electrical activity is evident.
        - adrenaline 5 mg should be considered after 3 cycles if no response is obtained.
      - **electromechanical dissociation**:
        - **pneumothorax, hypovolaemia, cardiac tamponade, PE**, drug overdose, **hypothermia** and electrolyte imbalance should be considered and treated as appropriate.
        - adrenaline 1 mg.
        - 10 compression/ventilation sequences.
        - repeated cycles as required.
        - pressor agents, **calcium**, bicarbonate and adrenaline 5 mg should be considered.
    - when CPR is prolonged:
      - bicarbonate 50 mmol should be considered, repeated according to blood gas analysis.
      - recovery may follow 1–2 hours of CPR.
    - post-arrest care:
      - checking of arterial blood gases, electrolytes and chest X-ray.
      - transfer to ICU. Cardiorespiratory support as required. Multi-organ failure may occur.

  Similar guidelines are recommended in the USA.
- Special situations:
  - **trauma, airway obstruction, near-drowning, electrocution, anaphylactic reaction**.
  - paediatric CPR (*see Cardiopulmonary resuscitation, paediatric*).
- Recent changes to recommendations:
  - lignocaine has been replaced by adrenaline as the first drug in VF, since the former may reduce the chance of success of defibrillation. Adrenaline is thought to maintain cerebral perfusion during prolonged CPR.
  - bicarbonate is not recommended routinely, because of its adverse effects, e.g. exacerbating intracellular acidosis.
  - calcium is not recommended routinely, because it reduces coronary and cerebral blood flow.
  - intracardiac injection is no longer recommended, because of risk of trauma.
  - isoprenaline is no longer recommended in asystole.
  - high dose adrenaline and atropine introduced.
- Controversies:
  - the place of **cerebral protection**. IPPV and hypocapnia are usually continued for 24 hours. Other measures, e.g. steroid/barbiturate therapy, hypothermia, mannitol, calcium channel blockers and free radical scavengers, are not recommended at present.
  - internal (open) cardiac massage is thought to be more efficient by some; increased use has been suggested, especially in trauma, chest deformity,

hypothermia, intrathoracic bleeding or tamponade, and failure of external massage.

–'new' CPR (chest compression coinciding with IPPV). Increases intrathoracic pressure, cardiac output and carotid blood flow, supporting the thoracic pump theory of cardiac massage. However, survival not shown to be increased. Mechanical compressors are used.

–use of abdominal compression to increase venous return.

–**hyperglycaemia** is thought to worsen the effects of cerebral hypoxia. Avoidance of glucose solutions during CPR has been suggested.

–when to stop CPR.

–when CPR should not be instituted, e.g. terminally ill, elderly patients, etc. 'Not for resuscitation' policies have been suggested as routine.

Complications include trauma to abdominal organs, ribs, etc., and those associated with tracheal intubation/attempted intubation, vascular access, etc.

Holmberg S, Handley A, Bahr J et al (1992) Resuscitation; 24: 103–21

See also, Brainstem death; Cardiopulmonary resuscitation, neonatal; Cough-CPR

Cardiopulmonary resuscitation, neonatal.
Prompt resuscitation is important in order to prevent permanent mental or physical handicap. Neonatal **cardiac arrest** is almost always caused by **hypoxaemia** and thus prompt management of **apnoea** and airway obstruction is vital.

• Equipment required includes:
  –a tilting resuscitation surface, with radiant heater, clock and ECG monitor.
  –**suction apparatus**.
  –O_2 with funnel and **facepieces**.
  –**self-inflating bag** (volume 250 ml, with pressure relief valve set at 30–35 cmH_2O).
  –pharyngeal **airways** (sizes 000, 00 and 0).
  –**tracheal tubes**: shouldered (Cole) tubes are often used, but straight-sided ones are preferable since the former may cause greater trauma to the larynx in addition to increasing resistance to flow. Suitable sizes:
    –2.0–2.5 mm tubes for babies under 750 g weight or 26 weeks' gestation.
    –2.5–3.0 mm for 750–2000 g or 26–34 weeks.
    –3.0–3.5 mm for over 2000 g or 34 weeks.
  –**laryngoscope**, usually with straight blade (size 0–1).
  –iv cannulae including umbilical venous and arterial catheters.

Requirement for resuscitation may be anticipated from the course of pregnancy and labour, and assessment of **fetal wellbeing**. The **Apgar score** may also be useful.

• Basic principles are as for adult **CPR**. Practical points:
  –drying and wrapping the baby, and use of radiant heaters and warm towels, reduce heat loss.
  –gentle oropharyngeal suction may be required, although it may provoke bradycardia if too vigorous. Tracheal suction should precede IPPV if meconium aspiration is suspected.
  –tactile stimulation or blowing of O_2 on the face via the funnel may provoke breathing and activity.
  –administration of 100% O_2 if breathing is inadequate. If IPPV is required, the first inspiration should last for 3–5 seconds, to aid lung expansion. Subsequent inspirations of 0.5–1.0 seconds are suitable. Airway

pressures should not exceed 30–35 cmH_2O. Tracheal intubation may be required.

–if the mother has received opioids during labour, **naloxone** may be required: 10 µg/kg im, iv or sc repeated every 2–3 minutes or 60 µg/kg im as a single injection.

–heart rates below 100/min should be managed initially by IPPV with O_2. **Cardiac massage** should be instituted for rates below 60/min (*see Cardiopulmonary resuscitation, paediatric*).

–**hypoglycaemia** and **acidosis** are common.

Drugs are rarely required but may be given via a peripheral or umbilical venous catheter. Drugs used are as for paediatric CPR. **Bicarbonate** should be diluted to reduce the osmotic load (may otherwise cause intraventricular haemorrhages).

Congenital abnormalities e.g. **diaphragmatic hernia**, **tracheo-oesophageal fistula**, etc., should be remembered.

[Frank Cole (described 1945), US anaesthetist]

Guay J (1991) Can J Anaesth; 38: R83–8

Cardiopulmonary resuscitation, paediatric.
The same principles apply as for adult **CPR**, but primary cardiac disease is uncommon. **Sinus bradycardia** progressing to **asystole** is more common, especially if due to **hypoxaemia** or **haemorrhage**. Thus **cardiac arrest** is often secondary to respiratory arrest or exsanguination, and usually represents a severe insult.

• Practical points:
  –**cardiac massage**: compression interval and relaxation interval are equal. Assessed by feeling the carotid or brachial pulse.
    –under 1 year: two fingers are placed on the mid-sternum, or both thumbs with the hands encircling the chest. Compression rate should exceed 100/min, depressing the sternum by 1.5–2.5 cm.
    –under 8 years: three fingers or the heel of one hand are placed over the lower sternum. A rate of 80–100/min is used, depressing the sternum by 2.5–3 cm.
  –ventilation should proceed at the same ratio to cardiac massage as in adults, but with both at faster rates. **Expired air ventilation**: under 1 year: mouth-to-mouth and nose; up to 8 years: mouth-to-mouth or as for under 1 year.

• Special situations:
  –**airway obstruction**: **Heimlich manoeuvre** is more likely to damage the liver than in adults.
  –neonatal resuscitation (see Cardiopulmonary resuscitation, neonatal).
  –**electrocution**, **near-drowning**, **trauma**.

• Drugs: indications are as for adults, although **glucose** and **bicarbonate** are required more often. Doses:
  –**adrenaline**: 10 µg/kg iv or tracheal (0.1 ml/kg 1:10 000 solution).
  –**atropine**: 0.02 mg/kg iv or tracheal, up to 0.6 mg.
  –**bicarbonate**: 1 mmol/kg iv (1 ml/kg 8.4% solution).
  –**calcium** chloride: 0.2 mmol/kg iv (0.3 ml/kg 10% solution).
  –glucose 10%: 1 g/kg iv (10 ml/kg).
  –**lignocaine**: 1 mg/kg iv or tracheal.
  –**diazepam**:
    –0.25 mg/kg iv, up to 10 mg.
    –0.5 mg/kg pr, up to 10 mg, if < 20 kg.
  –**salbutamol**: 5 µg/kg iv.

- DC shock: 2 J/kg.
- Fluid bolus in hypovolaemia: 10 ml/kg initially.

Bray RJ (1985) Br J Hosp Med; 34: 72–81

See also, Paediatric anaesthesia

Cardioversion. Restoration of sinus rhythm by application of synchronized DC current across the chest. Current delivery is synchronized to occur with the **R wave** of the **ECG**, since delivery during ventricular repolarization may produce **VF** (**R on T phenomenon**).

- Used for:
  - **AF**, particularly of recent onset.
  - **atrial flutter**; usually successful with low energy.
  - **VT**, usually successful with low energy.
  - **SVT**.

Energy levels of 20–200 J are usually used.

Digoxin-induced arrhythmias may convert to serious ventricular arrhythmias; therefore digoxin is usually withheld for at least 24 hours.

In chronic atrial arrhythmias, anticoagulation is often administered to reduce risk of systemic embolization. Preparation of the patient, drugs and equipment, and monitoring should be as for any anaesthetic. The procedure is painful, therefore requiring brief sedation/anaesthesia. A single iv agent is commonly used, e.g. **thiopentone**, **methohexitone**, **etomidate**, **propofol** or **diazepam**. Etomidate causes least myocardial depression and is perhaps preferable. Further injections may be required if repeated shocks are delivered. 100% O_2 is breathed via a facepiece.

See also, Defibrillation

Carfentanil. Opioid analgesic drug, developed in 1974. Over 8700 times as potent as **morphine**, and used to immobilize large animals.

Carotid arteries. Anatomy is as follows (*see Fig. 97; Neck, cross-sectional anatomy*):

- common carotids:
  - right: arises from the brachiocephalic artery behind the sternoclavicular joint.
  - left: arises from the aortic arch medial to the left lung, vagus and phrenic nerves, then passing behind the sternoclavicular joint.
  - ascend in the neck within the carotid sheath.
  - divide level with C4 into internal and external carotids.
- internal carotid:
  - bears the **carotid sinus** at its origin.
  - runs firstly lateral, then behind and medial to the external carotid, with the internal jugular vein laterally and vagus and sympathetic chain posteriorly.
  - passes medial to the parotid gland, styloid process, glossopharyngeal nerve and pharyngeal branches of the vagus (with the external carotid lateral to these structures).
  - passes through the carotid canal at the base of the skull, with the internal jugular now lying posteriorly. After a tortuous path through the canal, it divides into the middle and anterior cerebral arteries.
- external carotid :
  - lies first deep, then lateral to the internal carotid, with the internal jugular posteriorly.
  - enters the parotid gland, ending behind the neck of the mandible.
    - branches, from below upwards:
      - ascending pharyngeal.
      - superior thyroid.
      - lingual.
      - facial.
      - occipital.
      - posterior auricular.
      - superficial temporal.
      - maxillary.

See also, Carotid body; Cerebral circulation; Skull

Carotid artery surgery. Usually performed for endarterectomy, to reduce risk of **CVA** in patients with carotid stenosis. Indications for surgery are controversial because of the risk of death associated with the operation (up to 7%, mostly from MI or CVA).

- Anaesthetic considerations:
  - preoperatively: poor condition of patients: **atherosclerosis** often affects coronary and renal, as well as cerebral, vessels. **Smoking, diabetes mellitus** and **hypertension** are common.
  - peroperatively:
    - **positioning of the patient** and restricted access: the eyes must be protected, and the tracheal tube guarded against kinking. **Lignocaine** spray to the vocal cords reduces stimulation during initial positioning.
    - several techniques have been tried to maintain **cerebral blood flow** and limit ischaemia during surgery:
      - **hypothermia**.
      - **cerebral protection**, e.g. using **barbiturates**. Glucose infusions have been implicated as exacerbating cerebral ischaemic damage, and are avoided.
      - **hypoventilation**, increasing cerebral blood flow via **hypercapnia**; **cerebral steal** may occur.
      - **vasopressor drugs** to maintain intraoperative BP, e.g. **phenylephrine**.
      - carotid shunting, bypassing the clamped section of artery.

Choice of technique is controversial but most now advocate normocapnia and normotension; hypotension is definitely to be avoided.

Arterial pressure is measured distal to the atheroma, before and after carotid clamping. A shunt is usually inserted if the pressure after clamping (stump pressure; provides some indication of collateral flow) is less than 30–50% of the preclamp value.

  - the following may be used to detect **cerebral ischaemia**: EEG, **cerebral function monitor**, or measurement of **evoked potentials** and cerebral blood flow.
  - **cervical plexus block** allows surgery to be performed on an awake patient; if ischaemic symptoms occur following carotid artery clamping, general anaesthesia with shunt insertion may be performed.
  - direct arterial BP monitoring is mandatory, with avoidance of hypotension at all times.
  - **capnography** allows adjustment of IPPV to normocapnia and aids detection of **air embolism**.
  - manipulation of the **carotid sinus** may lead to bradycardia and hypotension. Infiltration of lignocaine around the sinus prevents this.

–postoperatively:
  –assessment of neurological function.
  –control of BP: hypertension may occur, hypotension less commonly; the latter is often associated with bradycardia.

Cunningham AJ (1992) Curr Opin Anaesth; 5: 34–48

Carotid body. Small (2–3 mg) structure situated above the carotid bifurcation on each side; involved in the chemical control of breathing. Contains:
  –glomus cells (type I cells): thought to be inhibitory **neurones**. Contain **dopamine**.
  –glial cells (type II cells).
  –nerve endings: thought to be the **chemoreceptors** themselves.

Afferents pass via the glossopharyngeal nerve to the **brainstem** regulatory centres.

Rate of discharge is increased by reduced O_2 delivery (e.g. reduced arterial P_{O_2} or reduced cardiac output) or by impaired utilization of O_2 (e.g. due to **cyanide poisoning**). Below arterial P_{O_2} of 13.3 kPa (100 mmHg), rate of discharge rises greatly for any further decrease. Response time is rapid enough to cause fluctuations in discharge rate with breathing. Discharge rate is also increased by a rise in arterial P_{CO_2}, or fall in arterial pH.

Each carotid body receives 0.04 ml blood/min, equivalent to 2 l/100 g tissue/min (the highest blood flow per 100 g tissue in the body). Because of such high blood flow, dissolved O_2 alone is enough to provide the requirement for O_2; thus discharge is not increased by **anaemia** or **carbon monoxide poisoning**, where O_2 carriage by haemoglobin is reduced but arterial P_{O_2} is not.

See also, Breathing, control of

Carotid sinus. Dilatation of the internal carotid artery, just above the carotid bifurcation. **Baroreceptors** present in the walls respond to increased distension caused by raised **arterial BP** by increasing the rate of discharge via the carotid sinus nerve, a branch of the glossopharyngeal nerve. Resultant inhibition of the **vasomotor centre** and stimulation of the **cardioinhibitory centre** causes reduction in sympathetic tone and increase in vagal tone respectively. BP and heart rate therefore fall. The baroreceptors also respond to the rate of increase of BP. Similar baroreceptors exist in the walls of the aortic arch.

See also, Carotid sinus massage

Carotid sinus massage. Manual stimulation of the **carotid sinus** baroreceptors, causing reflex inhibition of the **vasomotor centre** and activation of the **cardioinhibitory centre**. Depression of sinoatrial (SA) and atrioventricular (AV) nodes results in bradycardia and may reduce myocardial contractility.

The sinus should be gently massaged below the angle of the jaw, where the carotid pulse is palpable. Concurrent ECG recording should be available. Only one side (the right is usually more effective) should be massaged at one time and for no longer than five seconds, or excessive reduction in **cerebral blood flow** may occur. It should be performed with care in patients with evidence of cerebrovascular disease. May restore sinus rhythm in **SVT**, and may aid diagnosis of other arrhythmias by slowing the ventricular rate, e.g. **AF** and **atrial flutter**. In **sinus tachycardia**, it causes gradual slowing of rate with speeding up when massage is stopped. May also demon-

strate SA and AV node disease by causing severe bradycardia or sinus arrest.

Syncope, transient ischaemic attacks and **CVA**, **asystole** and **VT** are rare complications.

CAT scanning, *see Computed axial tomography*

Catabolism. Breakdown of molecules into smaller ones, usually associated with **energy** production.
• Includes:
  –digestion of foodstuffs as in **metabolism of carbohydrate**, **fat** and **protein**.
  –breakdown of body stores, e.g. in **malnutrition**, severe illness and the **stress response to surgery**. These may occur in combination on ICU because of:
    –inadequate **nutrition**, e.g. nil by mouth, ileus, fluid restriction, etc.
    –increased energy and O_2 consumption associated with injury, especially multiple **trauma**, **burns**, and **septicaemia**.
  Includes breakdown of:
  –protein: causes increased urinary urea excretion and may contribute to reduced plasma **albumin**. Nitrogen loss may exceed 20–30 g/day, i.e. up to 5 kg body weight/week (mainly lost from muscle). **Amino acids** produced are used for synthesis of **glucose**, acute phase reactants and cell components.
  –fat: triglycerides from adipose tissue are broken down to fatty acids (used as an energy source) and glycerol (used to synthesize glucose).
  –carbohydrates: **glycogen** is broken down to glucose.

See also, Nutrition, total parenteral

Catecholamines. Group of substances containing catechol (benzene ring with OH groups at positions 3 and 4) and amine portions; includes naturally-occurring (e.g. **dopamine**, **adrenaline**, **noradrenaline**) and synthetic (e.g. **dobutamine**, **isoprenaline**) compounds. Catecholamines act at **adrenergic receptors** in the CNS and **sympathetic nervous system**; although many other substances may produce similar effects, i.e. are **sympathomimetic drugs**, they may not be true catecholamines.

Synthesis of naturally-occurring catecholamines proceeds in many steps from the amino acid phenylalanine (Fig. 28a). Formation of dopamine occurs in the cytoplasm; it is then taken up by an active process into vesicles and converted to noradrenaline.

Catecholamines are metabolized via **catechol-*O*-methyl transferase** (COMT) and **monoamine oxidase** (MAO) (Fig. 28b).

See also, Inotropic drugs

Catechol-*O*-methyl transferase (COMT). **Enzyme** present in most tissues (especially liver and kidneys) but not in nerve endings; catalyses the transfer of a methyl group from adenosylmethionine, a **methionine** derivative, to the 3–hydroxy group of the catechol part of **catecholamines**. Involved in the metabolism of circulating catecholamines and their derivatives, whilst catecholamines at nerve endings are metabolized by **monoamine oxidase**.

Catheter mounts (Tracheal tube adaptors). Original term refers to adaptors connecting the fresh gas supply to a catheter passed through the larynx into the trachea (**insufflation technique**), before tracheal intubation

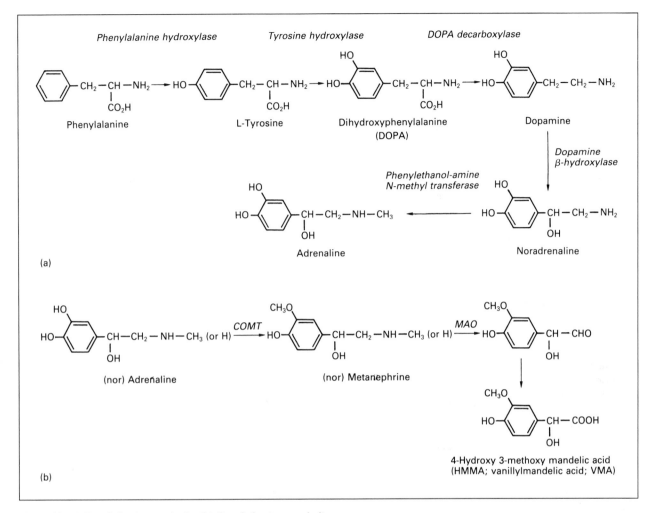

Figure 28 *(a) Catecholamine synthesis. (b) Catecholamine metabolism*

became popular. The term now refers to adaptors connecting the **tracheal tube** to the end of the **anaesthetic breathing system**. Various **connectors** fit between the distal end and the tracheal tube; the proximal end should be of standard 22 mm taper. Some contain heat–moisture exchangers.

Caudal analgesia. Produced by injection of **local anaesthetic agent** into the **sacral canal**, a continuation of the **extradural space**. First described independently by Cathelin and Sicard in 1901, predating lumbar **extradural anaesthesia**. Easily performed, but with a large failure rate due to variations in sacral anatomy. Produces block of the sacral and lumbar nerve roots; thus ideal for perineal surgery. Higher blocks require greater volumes of anaesthetic solution, but are more unpredictable. Useful as a supplement to general anaesthesia, and for provision of postoperative analgesia. Catheter insertion has been performed for continuous caudal block.

- Technique:
  - usually performed with the patient in the lateral position, with the knees drawn up to the chest. The prone and knee-elbow positions may also be used.
  - the sacral hiatus lies at the third point of an equilateral triangle formed with the two posterior superior iliac spines (each overlain by a skin dimple). The sacral cornua are palpable on either side of the hiatus.
  - using an aseptic technique, a needle is introduced in a slightly cranial direction through the hiatus. Ordinary iv needles and cannulae are commonly used, although specific caudal needles are available.
  - when the canal is entered (a click may be felt as the sacrococcygeal membrane is pierced), the needle is directed cranially, and advanced not more than 2 cm into the canal. The dura normally ends at S2, level with the posterior superior iliac spines, but may extend further.
  - after aspirating to confirm absence of blood or CSF, local anaesthetic is injected, feeling for accidental subcutaneous injection with the other hand. There should be little resistance to injection with a 19–21 G needle. If the patient is awake, pain is felt if the needle tip is under the periosteum of the anterior wall of the canal. Caudal needles may bear a sidehole to prevent this complication.
- Doses:
  - 20–30 ml 0.25–0.5% **bupivacaine**, or 1–2% **lignocaine** with adrenaline, in young adults, reduced in the elderly. The average volume of the sacral canal is 30–35 ml.

–0.5 ml/kg 0.25% bupivacaine has been used for sacrolumbar blockade in children; 1 ml/kg for upper abdominal blockade and 1.25 ml/kg for midthoracic blockade. 0.125% bupivacaine provides analgesia with less motor blockade.

Complications are as for extradural anaesthesia, but much less common. Insertion of the needle into the rectum, or presenting part of the fetus in obstetrics, has been reported.

[Fernand Cathelin (1873–1945), French surgeon; Jean-Athanase Sicard (1872–1929), French neurologist]

See also, Vertebral ligaments

Causalgia. Burning **pain** in the distribution of a partially damaged peripheral nerve, most commonly median, ulnar or sciatic. May occur within a month of injury, and may radiate beyond the nerve's normal cutaneous distribution. Exacerbated by cutaneous stimulation in the affected area, and often by emotional upset. Results from abnormal sweat and vasomotor sympathetic efferent pathways, possibly due to abnormal connections between efferent sympathetic fibres and somatic sensory fibres at the injury site. The skin of the affected limb is classically cold, moist and swollen, becoming atrophic later and leading to disuse and osteoporosis.

- Treatment:
  - **sympathetic nerve block**, e.g. **stellate ganglion, brachial plexus block, IVRA** with **guanethidine**.
  - regional sympathectomy.

The first technique may be repeated, e.g. on alternate days, for a week or two, to produce a more prolonged effect.

See also, Reflex sympathetic dystrophy

Caval compression, *see Aortocaval compression*

Cave of Retzius block, *see Retzius cave block*

CCF, Congestive cardiac failure, *see Cardiac failure*

CCT, Central conduction time, *see Evoked potentials*

CCU, *see Coronary care unit*

Central anticholinergic syndrome. Syndrome following the use of **anticholinergic drugs** (especially **hyoscine**), thought to be due to a decrease in inhibitory **acetylcholine** activity in the brain. Other drugs with anticholinergic activity may cause it, including **antihistamines, phenothiazines, antidepressant drugs, antiparkinsonian drugs** and **pethidine**. Has also been reported after volatile anaesthetic agents, **ketamine** and **benzodiazepines**. Reported incidence varies but has been up to 5–10% after general anaesthesia.

- Features:
  - confusion, agitation, restlessness, anxiety, amnesia, hallucinations.
  - speech disturbance, ataxia.
  - nausea, vomiting.
  - muscle incoordination.
  - convulsions, coma.
  - peripheral anticholinergic effects, e.g. tachycardia, dry mouth and skin, blurred vision, urinary retention.
- Treatment: **physostigmine** 0.04 mg/kg slowly iv. It usually acts within 5 minutes; features may recur after 1–2 hours.

Central conduction time, *see Evoked potentials*

Central pain. Diffuse continuous **pain**, usually burning and unilateral, with or without increased sensitivity and altered sensation. Due to CNS lesions, e.g. CVA, usually involving the thalamus (thalamic syndrome). Often associated with depression. Associated signs and distribution of pain are related to the site of lesion. May be helped by **phenothiazines, tricyclic antidepressant drugs** and **carbamazepine**.

Illis IS (1990) BMJ; 300: 1284–6

Central venous cannulation. Cannulation of a vein within the thorax via peripheral venepuncture.

- Performed for:
  - vascular access, e.g. for **dialysis**, TPN, infusion of irritant or potent drugs.
  - measurement of **CVP**.
  - **cardiac catheterization, pulmonary artery catheterization** and transvenous **cardiac pacing**.

The catheter tip should ideally lie in the superior vena cava above the pericardial reflection, to reduce risk of **arrhythmias**, and **cardiac tamponade** should erosion and bleeding occur.

- May be performed at different sites:
  - internal jugular vein:
    - easy to perform and reliable.
    - may cause **pneumothorax** or damage the common **carotid artery, brachial plexus, phrenic nerve**, thoracic duct (on left) or sympathetic chain.
    - uncomfortable for the patient.
  - subclavian vein:
    - more convenient and comfortable for long term use.
    - less chance of correct placement.
    - greater chance of pneumothorax or haemothorax.
    - may damage the subclavian artery; direct pressure cannot be applied to stop bleeding.
  - external jugular vein:
    - easy to perform since the vein is more superficial than the internal jugular or subclavian veins.
    - it may be difficult to thread the catheter through the junction with the subclavian vein. A J-shaped guide wire may help.
  - arm vein:
    - minimal risk of serious complications.
    - threading of a 'long line' is often difficult, especially via the cephalic vein because of valves at the junction with the axillary vein. Abduction of the arm may help.
    - 50% chance of correct placement.

Air embolism, subcutaneous emphysema and sepsis are risks of all techniques. Patients should be in the head-down position for jugular and subclavian cannulation to prevent air embolism. An aseptic technique is used. Introduction of a catheter into the heart may cause arrhythmias (therefore **ECG** monitoring is required) or cardiac perforation. Reintroduction of the needle into the cannula should never be performed whilst the tip is in the patient, as pieces of cannula are easily sheared off. Endocardial damage and central vein thrombosis may also occur, especially with pulmonary artery catheters and with prolonged placement.

Successful placement is suggested by easy aspiration of non-pulsatile blood, obtaining the **venous waveform**, and variation of measured pressure with respiration. Place-ment of the catheter in the right ventricle results in excessive swinging of central venous pressure with each heartbeat. Catheter position must be checked by X-ray, and pneumothorax excluded. Correct positioning may also be confirmed during insertion by filling the cannula with saline and connecting its proximal end to the left arm lead of the ECG. As the right atrium is approached, the **P waves** become increasingly peaked and tall, becoming biphasic as the atrium is entered.

Cannulation may also be carried out via the femoral or axillary veins, each vein lying medial to its respective artery.

See also, Central venous cannulation, long-term; Internal jugular venous cannulation; Subclavian venous cannulation

Central venous cannulation, long-term. Usually employed for long-term TPN, administration of drugs e.g. chemotherapy and antibiotics, and blood sampling. First developed in the 1970s. Silastic catheters (Hickman–Broviac) are usually inserted via the subclavian vein and tunnelled subcutaneously (emerging from the skin between the sternum and nipple). A Dacron cuff on the subcutaneous part incites an inflammatory reaction, providing fixation and a possible barrier to infection within 1–2 weeks. Single and double-lumen catheters are available.

Catheters are inserted under sterile conditions via a surgical cut-down procedure, or percutaneously using the **Seldinger technique**. In the latter, the catheter is passed into the vein through a sheath which is split and peeled away as the catheter is advanced.

Catheters may remain in place for years if required, with regular heparinized flushing and aseptic handling.

[John W Broviac, US physician; Robert O Hickman, US paediatrician]

See also, Central venous cannulation; Nutrition, total parenteral

Central venous pressure (CVP). Pressure within the right atrium and great veins of the thorax. Measured via

central venous cannulation, using a manometer or **transducer**. An estimate may be made by observing the distension of neck veins (**JVP**). CVP is usually measured with the patient lying flat, and expressed in cmH_2O above a point level with the right atrium, e.g. mid-axillary line. Normally 0–8 cmH_2O; 5–10 cmH_2O lower if the sternal angle is used as the reference point. By convention, it is measured at the end of expiration. The **venous waveform** may be seen on a pressure tracing, with the effects of ventilation superimposed (see below).

- Increased by:
  - raised intrathoracic pressure, e.g. **IPPV**, coughing. CVP normally rises in expiration during spontaneous ventilation.
  - impaired cardiac function, e.g. outlet obstruction, **cardiac failure**, **cardiac tamponade**. Primarily reflects right-sided function; thus CVP may be normal in the presence of left ventricular failure and **pulmonary oedema**, or raised in right-sided failure with normal left-sided function. With normal cardiac function, pressures on both sides move together. Left-sided function may be assessed by **pulmonary artery catheterization**.
  - circulatory overload.
  - venoconstriction.
  - **superior vena caval obstruction** (the normal venous waveform may be lost).
- Decreased by:
  - reduced **venous return**, e.g. due to **hypovolaemia**, venodilatation.
  - reduced intrathoracic pressure, e.g. in inspiration during spontaneous ventilation.

Useful in indicating right ventricular **preload** and cardiac function; e.g. a volume challenge of 200–300 ml saline causing a persistent rise in CVP of 2–5 cmH_2O suggests poor ventricular function in a normovolaemic patient. Also used to monitor **haemorrhage**, and in estimating the adequacy of volume replacement; e.g. hypovolaemia is suggested if a volume challenge of 300–500 ml saline

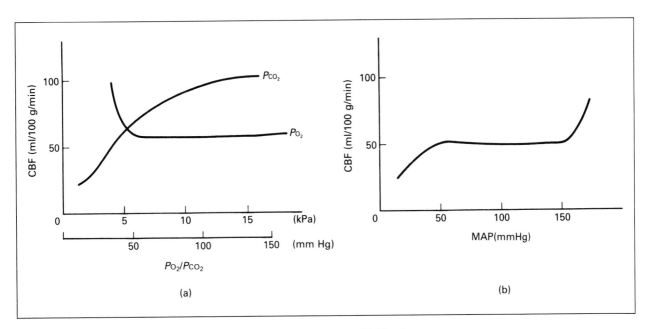

Figure 29 *Variation of cerebral blood flow with (a) arterial Po_2 and Pco_2; (b) blood pressure*

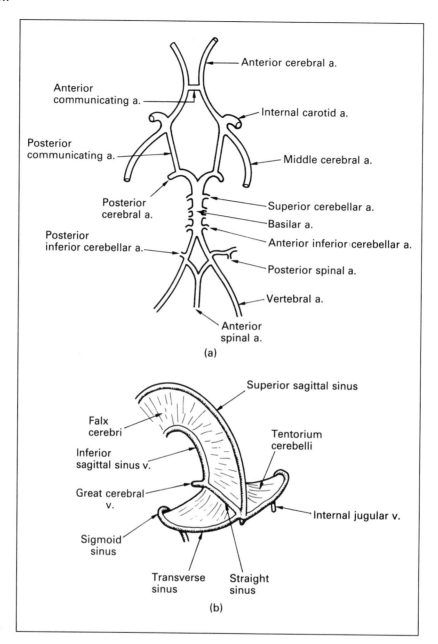

Figure 30 *Cerebral circulation: (a) arterial; (b) venous*

causes an increase in CVP that is not sustained for more than 10–15 minutes. Serial measurements are thus more informative than single readings.

Measurement is indicated in **shock**, hypovolaemia, acute cardiovascular disease and major surgery.
Mark JB (1991) J Cardiothor Vasc Anesth; 5: 163–73

Cerebral blood flow (CBF). Normally 14% of **cardiac ouput**, approximately 700 ml/minute (50 ml/100 g/min).
● Measurement:
  –applying the **Fick principle**, using N_2O (**Kety-Schmidt technique**). Values are obtained for the whole brain; regional variations in flow are not demonstrated.
  –detection of radioactivity over different parts of the head, following injection of dissolved radioactive xenon into a carotid artery. Regional differences are detected.
  –regional flow may be measured by **Doppler** probes placed extracranially.
● Affected by:
  –arterial $P\text{CO}_2$ (Fig. 29a): **hypercapnia** increases CBF via cerebral vasodilatation. **Hypocapnia** decreases CBF; reduction from 5.3 to 4 kPa (40 to 30 mmHg) reduces CBF by 30%. Reduction may not be sustained for more than 24–48 hours of hypocapnia.
  –arterial $P\text{O}_2$ (Fig. 29a): minimal effect until $P\text{O}_2$ falls below 6.7 kPa (50 mmHg).
  –**cerebral perfusion pressure** (Fig. 29b): **autoregulation** occurs between MAP of 60 and 130 mmHg (limits are raised in hypertensive subjects). Autoregulation may be impaired in diseased brains.

–drugs: all the volatile anaesthetic agents cause vasodilatation. Hyperventilation before introduction of the agent may reduce this effect; with **isoflurane**, hyperventilation following introduction is effective. **Ketamine** also increases CBF; **thiopentone, methohexitone, etomidate, benzodiazepines** and **propofol** reduce it. **Fentanyl** causes little change.
–**hypothermia**: reduces CBF.
–the role of vasoconstrictor sympathetic, and vasodilator parasympathetic fibres is unclear.

See also, Cerebral circulation; Cerebral ischaemia; Cerebral steal

Cerebral circulation.

- Arterial supply: ⅔ via the two internal **carotid arteries** and ⅓ via the two vertebral arteries. These arteries form the circle of Willis (Fig. 30a):
  –anterior cerebral artery: supplies superior and medial parts of the cerebral hemisphere.
  –posterior cerebral artery: supplies the occipital lobe and the medial side of the temporal lobe.
  –middle cerebral artery: supplies most of the lateral side of the hemisphere. Internal branches supply the internal capsule, through which most ascending and descending pathways pass. Commonly affected by **CVA**.
- Venous drainage (Fig. 30b):
  –deep structures drain via the internal cerebral vein on each side; these form the midline great cerebral vein which passes back to join the inferior sagittal sinus.
  –cerebral and cerebellar cortices drain via dural sinuses:
    –superior and inferior sagittal sinuses in the midline, between the layers of dura of the falx cerebri. The superior usually drains into the right transverse sinus; the inferior via the straight sinus into the left transverse sinus.
    –transverse sinuses within the tentorium cerebelli: pass via the sigmoid sinuses through the jugular foramina to become the internal **jugular veins**.
    –cavernous sinuses on either side of the pituitary fossa: receive blood from the eyes and nearby parts of the **brain**, draining into the transverse sinuses and internal jugular veins.

[Thomas Willis (1621–1675), English physician]

Cerebral function analysing monitor.
Development of the **cerebral function monitor** which provides information about the frequency distribution of the **EEG** signal as well as overall activity. Thus the relative proportions of the four standard EEG waveforms are presented. Said to be more useful than the cerebral function monitor, but suffers from similar drawbacks.

Maynard DE, Jenkinson JL (1984) Anaesthesia; 39: 678–90

Cerebral function monitor.
Device adapted from the conventional **EEG**, e.g. for use during anaesthesia. The signal from two parietal electrodes is filtered and amplified to produce a display of average peak voltage, charted on slow-moving paper. Thus monitors overall cerebral activity. Has been used to monitor depth of anaesthesia, but unreliable, especially using volatile anaesthetic agents. Used in **neurosurgery, cardiac surgery** and **carotid artery surgery**, where trends in activity may reflect changes in cerebral perfusion. Has also been used in ICU, e.g. for **head injury, poisoning and overdoses, status epilepticus**.

See also, Anaesthesia, depth of

Cerebral ischaemia. Inadequate blood supply to brain. May be:
–global:
  – complete, e.g. **cardiac arrest** or severely raised **ICP** with **hypotension**.
  –incomplete, e.g. hypotension and cerebrovascular disease.
–focal or regional, e.g. cerebrovascular disease, emboli, local lesions, e.g. tumours; may also be complete or incomplete.

- Effects of complete ischaemia:
  –energy stores decrease and waste products accumulate.
  –anaerobic metabolism increases, with greater **acidosis** if a **glucose** source is available.
  –protein synthesis is reduced and breakdown increased; impaired cell membrane pump activity results in leak of **potassium** out of cells, and chloride and **calcium** into cells.
  –**neurotransmitters** accumulate as their breakdown and uptake cease, e.g. **GABA** and **glutamate**.
  –**free radicals** are liberated.
  –recovery is thought to be impossible after about 4–5 minutes, although neuronal survival may be possible experimentally after 30–60 minutes.
  Reperfusion may be hindered by swelling, haemorrhage, etc.
- Effects of incomplete ischaemia:
  –reduced O_2 supply and waste product removal as above, but with continued glucose supply. Thus acidosis etc. is worse than if ischaemia is complete.
  –reduction in **cerebral blood flow** from the normal 50 ml/100 g/min causes the following:
    –30–40 ml/100 g/min: EEG slows.
    –20 ml/100 g/min: no spontaneous electrical activity. **Lactate** rises.
    –15 ml/100 g/min: **evoked potentials** disappear. pH increases. Ionic changes begin.
    –10 ml/100 g/min: water accumulates. Irreversible damage occurs.

Hypoxaemia with uninterrupted blood supply is better tolerated because of continued removal of waste products despite O_2 lack.

Damage is thought to result from increased intracellular calcium levels, free radicals, **arachidonic acid** metabolites, or lactic acid production. Investigated lines of treatment have been directed against these (**cerebral protection/resuscitation**). Effects depend on duration, site and cause of ischaemia, and patient factors, e.g. age, other disease, etc. Watershed areas between the main cerebral arteries are most at risk from ischaemia, especially in the elderly, if vessels are diseased, if blood **viscosity** is high, etc. Chronic ischaemia may cause transient ischaemic attack, **CVA** or dementia. During anaesthesia, excessive **hyperventilation** combined with hypotension may cause ischaemia.

See also, Brainstem death; Cerebral circulation; Cerebral metabolism; Cerebral steal

Cerebral metabolic rate for oxygen (CMRO₂).
Volume of O_2 consumed by the brain. Equals **cerebral blood flow** × arteriovenous O_2 content difference (*see Fick principle*). Normally about 50 ml/min (20% of total basal requirement), or 3.5 ml/100 g/min. Indicative of global **cerebral metabolism**, over 90% of which is aerobic; the relationship may not hold if O_2 or glucose supplies are reduced and alternate metabolic pathways employed.

Reduced by **hypothermia** (about 5% reduction per °C drop). Also reduced in old age and by certain drugs, e.g. **barbiturates**, **benzodiazepines**, volatile anaesthetic agents; increased by **ketamine** and possibly **N₂O**.

Cerebral metabolism. **Glucose** is the main substrate, although **ketone bodies**, **amino acids** and **fats** may be utilized, e.g. in starvation. 90–95% of **glycolysis** is aerobic, hence the requirement for a continuous supply of O_2. O_2 consumption is about 3.5 ml/100 g/min; CO_2 output is the same.

Cerebral metabolic rate for O_2 (CMRO₂) is used as a measure of global cerebral metabolism, and does not reflect regional variations; e.g. neuronal cells consume more O_2 than glial cells, grey matter more than white. Similar measurements may be made using glucose consumption (cerebral metabolic rate for glucose; normally about 4.5 mg/100 g/min) and lactate production (cerebral metabolic rate for lactate; normally about 2.3 mg/100 g/min).

Cerebral blood flow is closely related to metabolism according to one theory of **autoregulation**.

See also, Cerebral ischaemia

Cerebral oedema. Increased brain water content. May be:
- –vasogenic: increased vascular permeability and defective **blood–brain barrier**, e.g. associated with inflammatory conditions, tumours, trauma. Plasma protein and fluid penetrate the brain, tracking along fibre tracts. Exacerbated by raised hydrostatic pressures.
- –cytotoxic: cell damage due to **cerebral ischaemia**, **hypoxia**, encephalitis, toxins, metabolic disturbances, etc.; cells become depleted of **ATP** and accumulate water and sodium.
- –others:
  - –in **hydrocephalus** CSF may be forced from the ventricular system into white matter (interstitial oedema).
  - –in severe **hyponatraemia**, water enters the brain by **osmosis**.
- Effects:
  - –raised **ICP**, reduced **cerebral perfusion pressure**, compression of blood vessels and vital structures, papilloedema and **coning**.
  - –increased distance for O_2 diffusion from capillaries to cells.
  - –impaired consciousness, convulsions and coma.

Revealed by CAT scanning.
- Management:
  - –of primary cause.
  - –**IPPV**, with **hypocapnia** to arterial P_{CO_2} 3.5–4 kPA (27–30 mmHg). Fluid restriction to 1.5–2 l/day is usually instituted. Venous drainage is encouraged by head up posture, good sedation/paralysis and unobstructed jugular veins, as for ICP reduction. Measures are usually carried out for 24–48 hours after the insult.
  - –diuretics:
    - –**mannitol** 0.5–1 g/kg iv; relies on an intact blood-brain barrier. **Urea** is rarely used now.
    - –**frusemide** 10–40 mg.
  - –**steroid therapy** is used for oedema due to mass lesions, e.g. tumour or haematoma, but is ineffective in global oedema. Dexamethasone is usually employed, e.g. 4–8 mg iv 6–8 hourly.

Cerebral perfusion pressure (CPP). Difference between **MAP** and **ICP**; represents the pressure head available for **cerebral blood flow**. Normally 70–75 mmHg; critical level for **cerebral ischaemia** is thought to be 30–40 mmHg. In the presence of raised ICP, MAP increases in order to maintain CPP (**Cushing's reflex**).

Cerebral protection/resuscitation. Methods which attempt to reduce the effects of **cerebral ischaemia** and damage, e.g. during/after **CPR**, **carotid artery surgery**, **cardiac surgery**, **head injury** and intracranial haemorrhage. Protective measures are those taken before the insult; resuscitative measures are taken after, although both are similar.
- Possible techniques:
  - –general measures:
    - –maintaining normotension and oxygenation.
    - –maintaining metabolic stability and other organ function.
  - –increasing or maintaining cerebral perfusion:
    - –**nimodipine** in **subarachnoid haemorrhage**: thought to reduce vasospasm and maintain blood flow. Of uncertain benefit in other intracranial pathology.
    - –reduction of **ICP**, e.g. **hypocapnia** or **mannitol**.
    - –**haemodilution**. **Heparin** has been investigated.
  - –reducing **cerebral metabolic rate for O_2** (CMRO₂):
    - –**hypothermia**: used in cardiac surgery but little used otherwise.
    - –**barbiturates**: thought to be beneficial in transient incomplete ischaemia only, since some electrical activity is required for CMRO₂ reduction. Routine use is controversial, unless for sedation or treatment of convulsions. Profound hypotension is a major side-effect. **Phenytoin** has also been investigated.
    - –**isoflurane**: possibly beneficial in incomplete global ischaemia; **cerebral steal** is possible in focal ischaemia. **Halothane** may worsen local ischaemia.
  - –reducing cell damage:
    - –avoidance of **hyperglycaemia** (thought to exacerbate the effects of ischaemia).
    - –**free radical** scavengers.
    - –**glutamate** antagonists: glutamate is increased in ischaemia, and is thought to cause cell damage.

Rogers MC, Kirsch JR (1989) JAMA; 261: 3143–7

Cerebral steal. Diversion of blood flow away from abnormal areas of brain, e.g. tumours, infarcts and ischaemic areas, secondary to vasodilatation of normal cerebral blood vessels, e.g. due to **hypercapnia**. Vessels supplying the abnormal areas may already be maximally dilated; vasodilatation in normal areas may thus reduce blood flow in abnormal areas, with possibly deleterious effects. The reverse may occur in **hypocapnia**; thus general vasoconstriction may increase blood flow to abnormal areas (inverse steal).

Cerebrospinal fluid (CSF). Clear fluid bathing the CNS, providing support and protection against trauma, and helping to regulate **ICP**. Total volume is 100–150 ml, of which ⅓–½ is spinal.
- Production:
  - –by choroid plexuses in the 3rd, 4th and lateral ventricles at about 0.3 ml/min.
  - –formed by secretion, and filtration of plasma. Formation is largely independent of ICP, but removal increases with increasing pressure.

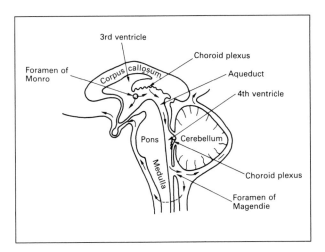

Figure 31 *Circulation of CSF*

- Circulation (Fig. 31):
  –from the lateral ventricles to the 3rd ventricle via the foramina of Monro, thence to the 4th ventricle via the aqueduct.
  –leaves the 4th ventricle via the foramina of Magendie (midline posteriorly) and Luschka (laterally) to pass down to the spinal cord or up over the cerebral hemispheres.
  –passes into dural venous sinuses via arachnoid villi, and possibly from spinal nerve cuffs into spinal veins.
- Normal constituents:
  –sodium: 135–145 mmol/l.
  –chloride: 115–125 mmol/l.
  –calcium: 1–1.5 mmol/l.
  –potassium: 2.5–3.5 mmol/l.
  –glucose: 2–5 mmol/l (if blood glucose normal).
  –pH: 7.3–7.5.
  –protein: 0.2–0.4 g/l.
  –urea: 1.5–6.0 mmol/l.
  –lymphocytes: $0–5 \times 10^6$/l.

[Alexander Monro (1733–1817), Scottish anatomist; Francois Magendie (1783–1855), French physiologist; Hubert von Luschka (1820–1875), German anatomist]
See also, Blood–brain barrier

Cerebrovascular accident (CVA; Stroke). Third commonest cause of death in the West.
- Caused by:
  –infarction (80–85%), e.g. caused by atheroma, embolism, arteritis/arterial spasm or hypotension. If symptoms resolve within 24 hours, defined as a transient ischaemic attack, although CAT scanning may reveal evidence of permanent damage. Multiple small emboli may cause dementia.
  –haemorrhage, e.g. from intracranial aneurysms, arteriovenous malformation, etc. May be associated with **hypertension** and abnormal cerebral vessel walls, also with **head injury**. **Subarachnoid haemorrhage** usually occurs from congenital aneurysms.
- Features:
  –impaired consciousness.
  –upper and lower **motor neurone** lesions; distribution depends on the site and extent of the lesion, e.g. lesions may cause contralateral hemiplegia/paresis, hemisen-

sory loss and homonymous hemianopia. Single limbs and the face may be affected. Speech disorders are common if the dominant hemisphere is affected.
- Treatment is mainly supportive, and directed at the predisposing cause if identified. CAT scanning is required to differentiate infarction from haemorrhage.
- Anaesthetic considerations:
  –assessment for predisposing conditions, e.g. hypertension, **coagulation disorders**, embolic conditions, **trauma**, arteritis due to **connective tissue diseases**, infections, etc.
  –immobility, contractures etc.: may affect drip sites, etc. Risk of **DVT**.
  –bulbar lesions and laryngeal incompetence, and autonomic disturbances.
  –communication difficulties.
  –massive hyperkalaemia after **suxamethonium** has been reported up to 6 months after CVA.
  –**hyperventilation** and reduction of **cerebral blood flow**, and hypotension, should be avoided during anaesthesia. End-tidal CO_2 monitoring is particularly useful. **Cerebral steal** may occur.
  –**confusion** is common postoperatively.

Risk of CVA during anaesthesia is increased in **cardiac surgery**, **carotid artery surgery** and **neurosurgery**.
Wong DHW (1991) Can J Anaesth; 38: 347–73 and 471–88
See also, Brain; Cerebral circulation; Cerebral ischaemia

Cervical plexus block. Provides analgesia of the upper cervical **dermatomes**; used for head and neck surgery and treatment of **pain**.
   The plexus is formed from the anterior branches of the upper four cervical nerves, lying between the anterior and posterior tubercles of the cervical vertebral transverse processes.
- Technique:
  –the patient is placed supine, looking away from the side to be blocked, with the neck partially extended. The transverse processes of C2–C4 are palpated posterior to a line between the mastoid process and transverse process of C6.
  –a fine needle is introduced perpendicular to the skin, 1–3 cm towards each transverse process in turn until contact is made or parasthesiae felt.
  –after careful aspiration 3–5 ml solution, e.g. 0.5% lignocaine with adrenaline, is injected at each level to block the deep branches. A further 3–5 ml is injected as the needle is withdrawn. The superficial branches are blocked by injecting 15–20 ml posterior to the middle of the sternomastoid muscle.

Complications include intravascular injection or puncture (e.g. vertebral artery), subarachnoid injection, sympathetic block, phrenic nerve block and recurrent laryngeal nerve block.

Cervical spine. Comprised of seven cervical **vertebrae**. Important in the positioning of the neck in **airway** management including tracheal intubation. Injury may often accompany **head injury**.
Crosby ET, Lui A (1990) Can J Anaesth; 37: 77–93
See also, Intubation, difficult; Spinal cord injury; Vertebral ligaments

CFAM, *see Cerebral function analysing monitor*

CFM, *see Cerebral function monitor*

cgs system of units. System based on the centimetre, gram and second; replaced in 1960 by the SI System based on the metre, kilogram and second.
See also, Units, SI

Charcoal, activated. Charcoal meeting certain adsorbance standards.
- Uses:
  - administered orally or via a nasogastric tube to reduce gastrointestinal absorption of certain toxic compounds (e.g. **barbiturates**, **tricyclic antidepressant drugs**) in the treatment of **poisoning and overdoses**. In addition to adsorbing toxins present in the stomach, it reduces blood levels by preventing enterohepatic circulation. Most effective when substances toxic in small amounts have been ingested, and within 4 hours of ingestion, although some benefit may occur many hours after ingestion. Adult dosage: 50–100 g 4 hourly, or 25 g 2 hourly.
  - during anaesthesia, waste gases have been passed through containers of activated charcoal (the Aldasorber) in an attempt to reduce pollution. Volatile anaesthetic agents are adsorbed, but not N_2O. The amount adsorbed is measured by weighing the container.
  - coated activated charcoal is used during **haemoperfusion**.

Vale JA, Proudfoot AT (1993) Br Med J; 306: 78–9

Charge. Quantity of electricity. Flow of charge constitutes a **current**. SI **unit** is the **coulomb**.

Charles' law. At constant pressure, the volume of a fixed mass of gas is proportional to its temperature.
[Jacques Charles (1746–1823), French chemist]
See also, Boyle's law; Ideal gas law

Chassaignac's tubercle. Transverse process of C6, against which the common **carotid artery** may be felt and compressed. Useful landmark for **stellate ganglion block**.
[Charles Chassaignac (1804–1879), French surgeon]

Checking of anaesthetic equipment. Should be performed before anaesthetizing any patient. Requirement for following a checklist is mandatory in the USA, Australia and Germany, and is strongly recommended in the UK.
- The following should be checked:
  - drugs, iv fluids, etc.
  - **tracheal tubes**, **cuffs**, introducers, etc., **laryngoscopes** (including spare), **suction apparatus**.
  - monitors.
  - **anaesthetic machine** (**Association of Anaesthetists** guidelines):
    - should be performed before every operating theatre session.
    - check and calibrate the O_2 analyser.
    - disconnect all pipelines.
    - **CO_2** and **cyclopropane cylinders** should only be present if specifically requested. Blanking plugs should be fitted to unused yokes.
    - open all **Rotameters**.
    - open the reserve O_2 cylinder; check the contents and ensure only the O_2 Rotameter rises. Repeat with other O_2 cylinders. Check the full range of the Rotameter and set at 5 l/min flow.

  - repeat with N_2O.
  - close the O_2 cylinder, ensuring that the gauge falls to zero and that the **O_2 failure warning device** and outlet cut-off are working.
  - connect the O_2 pipeline and check it is secure. Check the pipeline pressure.
  - close the N_2O cylinder and connect the pipeline as above.
  - check other cylinders if present.
  - close all Rotameters.
  - check the O_2 flush.
  - check the **vaporizer** fittings for leaks, and ensure the vaporizers are filled and able to be turned on. Vaporizers should not be swapped during use of the machine, since leaks from the vaporizer fittings may occur undetected.
  - obstruct the gas outlet, ensuring no leaks, and that the pressure relief valve opens (if fitted).
  - breathing system:
    - close the expiratory valve. Obstruct the distal end of the tubing to fill the reservoir bag; ensure no leaks.
    - open the valve, checking the bag empties.
    - **coaxial breathing systems**: as above, plus testing for correct attachment of the inner tubing of Bain system:
      - obstruct the distal end of the inner tube; the Rotameters should fall and pressure build up behind the obstruction.
      - close the expiratory valve and fill the bag by occluding the distal end of the outer tube. Use the O_2 flush with the tube now unobstructed: the reservoir bag should empty due to gas entrainment, unless the inner tube is detached (Pethick's test).
    - circle systems: check one-way valves, bag etc. Ensure the soda lime is properly packed and not expired.
    - **ventilator**: check on manual settings as above, and on automatic settings with the outlet obstructed. Check the disconnect alarm and that alternative means of IPPV are available.

[Simon L Pethick, Canadian anaesthetist]
Charlton JE (1990) Anaesthesia; 45: 425–6

Chelating agents. Compounds used in the treatment of heavy metal poisoning. Act by forming chelates, metal-containing ring structures, which are then eliminated.
- Examples (with the metals chelated):
  - dimercaprol (arsenic, mercury, gold).
  - sodium calciumedetate (lead, copper, radioactive metals).
  - penicillamine (copper, lead).
  - desferrioxamine (iron).

Chemoreceptor trigger zone (CTZ). Area situated in the area postrema of the medulla, on the lateral walls of the 4th ventricle. Lies outside the **blood–brain barrier**; chemoreceptor cells within it are thus directly exposed to blood-borne chemicals. Stimulated by **noradrenaline**, **dopamine**, **acetylcholine**, **5–HT** and **opioid receptor** agonists. Circulating emetics, e.g. **opioid analgesic drugs**, may cause **vomiting** by stimulating the CTZ, which sends efferents to the vomiting centre of the medulla. Some **antiemetic drugs**, e.g. **phenothiazines**, act by inhibiting **dopamine receptors** within the CTZ.

Chemoreceptors. Receptors responding to chemical stimulation, producing **action potentials** when triggered by certain (often specific) molecules. The precise linking mechanisms are generally unknown.
- Examples:
  - –taste and smell receptors.
  - –O_2, CO_2 and hydrogen ion receptors.
  - –**chemoreceptor trigger zone** cells.

See also, Aortic bodies; Breathing, control of; Carotid bodies

Chest drainage. Removal of air or liquid from the inter-pleural cavity, e.g. in the management of **pneumothorax**, haemothorax and pleural effusions.
- Effusions and small pneumothoraces are often drained by pleural tap. Technique:
  - –the patient is usually seated with shoulders flexed and arms resting on a pillow. A posterior approach is usually used.
  - –the needle or cannula is advanced above the upper edge of the **rib** (upper chest for pneumothorax; lower for effusion) to avoid the nerve and vessels in the **intercostal space**. Air entry is prevented by connecting the needle to a syringe at all times, and aspirating continuously during advancement.
  - –a three-way tap prevents air entry during aspiration.

  Wide-bore chest drains (pleural drains) are inserted for drainage of larger fluid collections and pneumothoraces. They may also be inserted prophylactically in patients with **rib fractures** about to undergo anaesthesia, especially involving **IPPV**. IV cannulae may be inserted for emergency treatment of tension pneumothorax.
- Insertion:
  - –the site chosen is usually between the 4th and 7th intercostal spaces, between the midaxillary and anterior axillary lines. Previous recommendations for use of the 2nd intercostal space anteriorly have lost popularity because a drain in this position tends to transfix the pectoral muscles and may interfere with ventilation. Patients may be sitting or supine.
  - –using aseptic technique, the skin and subcutaneous tissues are infiltrated with **local anaesthetic agent**, down to the periosteum of the upper surface of the chosen rib. The needle is advanced above the rib, continuing to inject local anaesthetic.
  - –the chest wall is incised about 2 cm below the proposed site of pleural incision, cutting down on to the rib below. Track dissection is achieved using artery forceps, through to the pleural cavity.
  - –the drain is inserted into the pleural cavity and slid over the trocar.
  - –the drain is connected to an underwater seal device (see below), observing the water level for swinging/bubbling with respiration. One-way flutter valves may also be used, e.g. Heimlich valve (flattened rubber tube within a clear plastic tubing).
  - –a purse-string suture is inserted around the puncture site to aid sealing after removal, and dressings are applied.
  - –plastic tubes are most commonly employed. Most tubes have side holes to aid drainage, and a radio-opaque longitudinal line. Sizes 20–28 FG (French Gauge: external circumference in mm; approximately ⅓ external diameter) are suitable for most adults.
  - –chest X-ray demonstrates the position and effect of the drain.

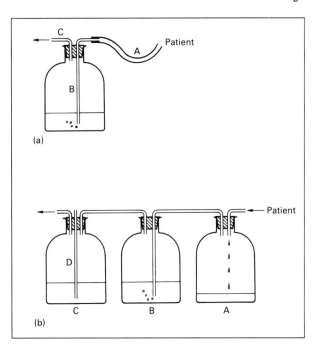

Figure 32 *Chest drainage systems: (a) one-bottle; (b) three-bottle*

  - –complications include haemorrhage, trauma to intrathoracic structures, vagally-mediated bradycardia during insertion, post-expansion pulmonary oedema, disconnection or blockage of the drain, and aspiration of air or water from the seal into the chest.
  - –the drain is usually removed 12–24 hours after cessation of air or fluid loss, often after a trial period of clamping. Chest X-ray is mandatory following removal.
- The underwater seal should have certain features (Fig. 32a):
  - –tube A must be wide to minimize resistance. Its volumetric capacity should exceed half of the patient's maximal inspiratory volume or water may be aspirated into the chest during inspiration.
  - –the volume of water above the end of tube B should exceed half of the patient's maximal inspiratory volume to prevent indrawing of air during inspiration.
  - –the end of tube B should not be more than 5 cm below the surface of the water, or its resistance may prevent air being blown off.
  - –the drain should always be at least 45 cm below the patient.
  - –tube A should be temporarily clamped when the underwater seal's integrity may be disrupted, e.g. during transfer from bed to trolley, etc.
  - –suction may be applied to tube C, although this is controversial. 10–20 cmH_2O suction is usually employed.
  - –a three-bottle system is often used, especially after cardiac or thoracic surgery (Fig. 32b). Bottle A acts as a fluid trap, e.g. for accurate measurement of blood. Bottle B provides the underwater seal. Bottle C allows suction; the height of the water level determines the amount of suction applied before air is drawn in through tube D as a safety suction-limiting device.

Kam AC, O'Brien M, Kam PCA (1993) Anaesthesia; 48: 154–61

Chest infection. Includes tracheitis, laryngotracheobronchitis (**croup**), acute bronchitis, bronchiolitis, acute exacerbations of **COAD** and **bronchiectasis** and pneumonia.

- Pneumonia may be:
  - primary: specific pathogens are usually involved:
    - bacteria, e.g. *Streptococcus pneumoniae* (causing classical lobar pneumonia), *Haemophilus influenzae*, *Mycobacterium **tuberculosis**, Klebsiella pneumoniae*.
    - viruses, e.g. influenza, parainfluenza, measles. Viral bronchitis is very common and rarely severe unless coexisting disease is present,
    - others (often classified as large viruses/small bacteria), e.g. Legionella, Mycoplasma, Rickettsia, Chlamydia.
    - fungi, e.g. Aspergillus.
  - opportunistic: occurs in **immunodeficiency**, e.g. infection with fungi, Pneumocystis (especially in **HIV infection**), and viruses, e.g. cytomegalovirus and herpes.
  - secondary: a respiratory tract abnormality allows usually less pathogenic organisms to spread, e.g. by aspiration from the GIT, upper airway, sinuses, etc. Thus bronchopneumonia may follow bronchial infection, causing patchy inflammation, collapse, consolidation and oedema. Commonly occurs in hospitalized patients, e.g. following anaesthesia, **atelectasis**, **aspiration of gastric contents** and **hypoventilation**. Gram-negative bacteria are commonly responsible, e.g. *Pseudomonas aeruginosa* and *Escherichia coli*.
- Features:
  - malaise, pyrexia, tachycardia, **septicaemia**. Legionnaire's disease may cause back pain and renal impairment.
  - cough, sputum, haemoptysis.
  - increased $\dot{V}/\dot{Q}$ **mismatch** and shunting causing **hypoxaemia** and tachypnoea.
  - clinical and radiological features of consolidation and collapse, possibly leading to **pleural effusion** and empyema. Severe pulmonary destruction and abscess formation (suppuration) may follow, especially in Staphylococcal infection.
  - may lead to **respiratory failure** or bronchiectasis.

Microbiological diagnosis may be made on sputum culture; treatment is started according to the most likely organism. Serology or bronchial biopsy/washings may be useful in atypical cases.

- Treatment:
  - antimicrobial drugs.
  - supportive therapy; i.e. **O_2 therapy**, **physiotherapy**, etc.
- Anaesthetic relevance:
  - **preoperative assessment** and treatment of chest disease.
  - prevention of aspiration and reduction of atelectasis.
  - postoperatively: physiotherapy, adequate analgesia and avoidance of hypoventilation are important, especially in pre-existing chest disease.
  - risk of **contamination of anaesthetic equipment** by infected cases.
  - treatment of respiratory failure on **ICU**, or development of infection in patients receiving IPPV. The latter is a common problem and is related to impaired host defences, instrumentation of the airway and colonization of the GIT with pathogenic organisms.

Selective decontamination of the digestive tract has been used to reduce the incidence of nosocomial infection (i.e. not present or incubating at the time of hospital admission) on ICU.

See also, Chest X-ray

Chest trauma. May be caused by road traffic accidents (RTA), falls, assaults including stabbings and shootings, and explosions. **Trauma** may be:
- penetrating: in stabbing injuries, trauma tends to be localized to the track of the implement. In gun-shot wounds, a small entry point may disguise major internal disruption (because of rapid dissipation of kinetic injury).
- non-penetrating:
  - blunt trauma, e.g. deceleration injury in RTAs. Damage is caused by direct impact (e.g. **rib fractures**, myocardial contusion) and shearing forces (e.g. aortic rupture, tracheobronchial tears).
  - blast injuries: sudden external chest and abdominal compression may cause alveolar and pulmonary vessel rupture, with oedema and haemorrhage. Further injury may result from flying objects, etc.
- Immediate life-threatening conditions:
  - severe **hypoventilation** caused by:
    - **airway obstruction** (especially likely with associated **head injury**).
    - **pneumothorax**/haemothorax.
    - **flail chest**.
  - reduced **cardiac output** caused by:
    - **hypovolaemia** caused by **haemorrhage**. Major vessel damage often accompanies fracture of the first two ribs. Aortic rupture usually occurs just beyond the left subclavian artery.
    - **cardiac tamponade**.
    - tension pneumothorax.
- Other conditions less immediately dangerous:
  - respiratory:
    - sternal/rib fractures.
    - tracheobronchial tears.
    - diaphragmatic rupture.
    - lung contusion.
    - **aspiration of gastric contents** (especially with head injury).
    - blast injury: symptoms may occur 2–3 days later. There may be associated **smoke inhalation**.
    $\dot{V}/\dot{Q}$ **mismatch** and **shunt** results in **hypoxaemia**. Ventilatory failure may also occur. Infection, **ARDS**, etc., may ensue.
  - cardiovascular:
    - myocardial contusion: may present as **arrhythmias**, **cardiac failure** or valve rupture.
    - damage to the coronary vessels and great vessels.
  - other injuries: head injury, vertebral and limb injuries, etc. Oesophageal rupture may occur, with risk of mediastinitis.
- Management:
  - immediate assessment and management of the above life-threatening conditions, i.e. sealing of any penetrating wound with dressings, etc., **O_2 therapy**, **iv fluid administration**. Airway patency and adequate respiratory movement should be checked. Chest percussion and auscultation may suggest pneumothorax or haemothorax. Heart sounds may be muffled in tamponade. **Pulsus paradoxus** may indicate tampon-

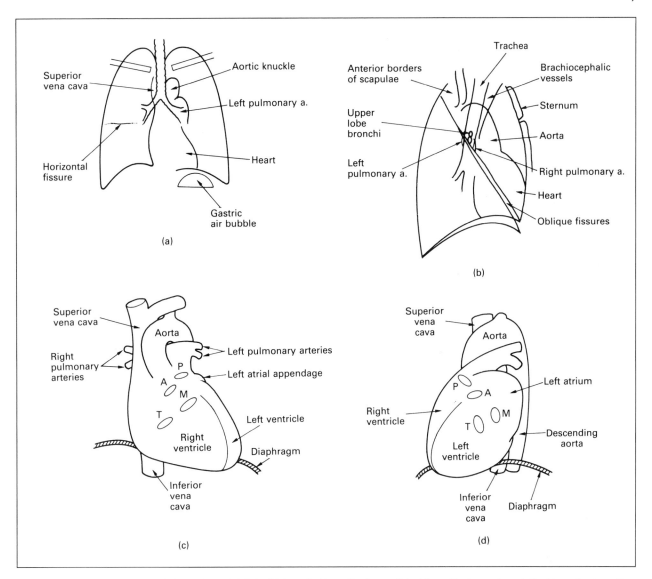

Figure 33 *Normal appearance of chest X-ray: (a) PA; (b) lateral; (c) mediastinum, PA; (d) mediastinum, lateral. Position of valves: P, pulmonary; A, aortic; M, mitral; T, tricuspid*

ade or tension pneumothorax, whilst unequal pulses may suggest **aortic dissection** or rupture. Hypotension may occur in hypovolaemia, tamponade, tension pneumothorax and myocardial contusion.

–subsequent assessment:

–**chest X-ray**: may reveal pneumothorax, surgical emphysema, fractures, evidence of aspiration, and widened mediastinum (may represent aortic rupture, especially if associated with left haemothorax, depressed left main bronchus and oesophageal displacement to the right). Lung contusion may appear as fluffy patchy shadowing within a few hours of injury.

–arterial blood gas analysis/pulse **oximetry** are especially useful.

–**ECG** as a baseline. Serial ECG and **cardiac enzyme** changes may occur in myocardial contusion.

–for other injuries.

–**chest drainage**/pericardial drainage as appropriate.

–methods of analgesia include iv **opioid analgesic drugs** in small doses (but with risk of respiratory and cerebral depression), **intercostal nerve block**, **interpleural analgesia**, and **extradural anaesthesia** with **local anaesthetic agent** or opioids.

–nasogastric tube to prevent gastric dilatation.

–surgery may be required for severe haemorrhage or trauma to the aorta, diaphragm, tracheobronchial tree, oesophagus, etc.

–**physiotherapy**/antibiotics. Lung contusion is exacerbated by overhydration, but hypovolaemia must be avoided.

Chest X-ray. Useful as an indication of structural abnormalities of cardiovascular and respiratory systems, but less informative about function. Often used as a screening test for unsuspected disease, e.g. preoperatively (*see Investigations, preoperative*).

• Plan for the interpretation of chest X-rays (Fig. 33):

–describe the film:
  –date, patient's name and nationality.
  –orientation: i.e. right/left marker. Posteroanterior (PA): the scapulae shadows are carried laterally. Anteroposterior (AP): usually portable films, i.e. the patient is too ill to leave the ward. Assume PA unless AP is written on the film.
–describe any obvious abnormality first, otherwise continue with the plan.
–heart shadow:
  –normal width is under 50% of thoracic diameter (PA film).
  –abnormal border: may be aneurysm, chamber dilatation or overlying lesion.
  –part of border indistinct: may represent lung collapse/consolidation.
  –calcified/prosthetic valves: the aortic valve lies above a line drawn from the anterior costophrenic angle to the hilum on the lateral X-ray; the mitral valve lies below.
–upper **mediastinum** (i.e. width, aortic shadow, hila):
  –hilar enlargement may be due to pulmonary vascular or lymph node enlargement, or overlying lesion. The left hilum is usually higher than the right by 1–2 cm.
  –the carina usually overlies T4–5 on inspiration.
–lung fields:
  –upper zone (above anterior part of 2nd rib).
  –midzone (between 2nd and 4th rib).
  –lower zone (below 4th rib).
  –compare each with the other side for translucency. Look for **pneumothorax**.
  –the anterior portions of the first eight ribs are visible with normal expansion.
  –the left hemidiaphragm is usually lower than the right by 2 cm.
  –if shadowing is seen, the lesion may lie in skin, bone, lung, etc.; i.e. one cannot determine the lesion's depth from the PA/AP film alone; this requires a lateral film.
  –lung consolidation:
    –no evidence of collapse.
    –the border of the shadow with neighbouring structures is lost, aiding identification of the affected lung portion; e.g. an indistinct heart border represents consolidation anteriorly, since the heart lies anteriorly in the chest. Thus in lower lobe consolidation (posterior in the chest) the heart border remains clear.
  –lung collapse: as for consolidation, with reduced expansion on the affected side, mediastinal shift or tracheal deviation. The collapsed portion of lung may be visible against neighbouring structures.
  –**pleural effusion**: seen as an opacity sloping upwards and outwards at the lung base; if horizontal, it represents a gas/fluid interface.
  –**Kerley's lines** may be present.
  –upper lobe blood diversion (representing dilatation of the pulmonary vessels) occurs in left ventricular failure and left-to-right cardiac **shunts**. Proximal dilatation with peripheral narrowing (pruning) may represent **pulmonary hypertension**.
–bones:
  –**ribs** (metastases, fractures, notching).
  –scapulae, **vertebrae**, humerus.

–soft tissues:
  –below **diaphragm**.
  –above clavicles; neck.
  –axillae.
  –breasts.
–central lines, tracheal tubes, etc.
Easily missed diagnoses to be remembered if unable to spot an abnormality include pneumothorax, dextrocardia and aortic coarctation.
Given-Wilson R, Karani J (1989) Hosp Update; 15: 177–92
See also, Thoracic inlet

Cheyne–Stokes respiration. Abnormal pattern of breathing characterized by alternating periods of **hyperventilation** and apnoea. Ventilation increases in depth and frequency to a peak, then decreases to apnoea. The cycle then repeats.
● Caused by:
  –central disturbance of control of breathing. **Hypoventilation** causes **hypercapnia**, which causes hyperventilation. Resultant **hypocapnia** causes apnoea until the arterial $P\text{CO}_2$ rises again. This pattern may occur in cerebral disease, **head injury** and **opioid poisoning**.
  –prolonged circulation between the lungs and brain. Hyperventilation continues until hypocapnia is registered by central **chemoreceptors**, although the CO_2 tension at the lungs is much lower. When the CO_2 content of blood arriving centrally is high enough to restart breathing, the CO_2 content of blood at the lungs is much higher, causing hyperventilation as it arrives at the chemoreceptors. This may occur with reduced cardiac output, e.g. in **cardiac failure**.
[John Cheyne (1777–1836), Scottish-born Irish physician; William Stokes (1804–78), Irish physician]
Tobin MJ, Snyder JV (1984) Crit Care Med; 12: 882–7
See also, Breathing, control of

Chi-square analysis, *see Statistical tests*

Chloral hydrate. Sedative **prodrug**, introduced in 1869. Metabolized to trichlorethanol, which has a **half-life** of 8–10 hours. Causes minimal cardiovascular or respiratory depression. Gastric irritation may occur; it is less frequent with triclofos or dichloralphenazone, both of which are also metabolized to trichlorethanol.
● Dosage: 25–50 mg/kg (children) orally/rectally.
  0.5–1 g (adults).

Chloride shift (Hamburger shift). Movement of chloride ions into red blood cells as O_2 is given up and exchanged for CO_2 in the tissues. CO_2 enters the cells, is converted to carbonic acid by **carbonic anhydrase**, and dissociates into **hydrogen ions** and **bicarbonate**. The former are buffered by the reduced haemoglobin; the latter passes into the plasma. Chloride ions enter the cells to maintain electrical equilibrium. The reverse occurs in the lungs.
[Hartog J Hamburger (1859–1924), Dutch physiologist]

Chlormethiazole edisylate. Sedative drug, structurally related to vitamin B_1. Used for **sedation** and as an **anticonvulsant drug**, e.g. in **pre-eclampsia**. Traditionally used to treat acute **alcohol** withdrawal.
● Dosage:
  –1–4 capsules (eqivalent to 5–20 ml elixir which contains 50 mg/ml) orally, 3–4 hourly.

−0.5–1 ml/min iv using 0.8% solution in 5% dextrose, after a 40–100 ml loading dose. 0.01 ml/kg/min is used in children.
- Side effects:
  - cardiovascular and respiratory depression with large iv doses. Unconsciousness may occur.
  - fluid overload, since the iv solution contains no electrolyte.
  - nasal irritation and thrombophlebitis when given iv.

Chloroform. $CHCl_3$. **Inhalational anaesthetic agent**; used in 1847 by **Simpson**, although it had been used earlier. Rapidly became more popular than **diethyl ether**, and was administered to Queen **Victoria** during childbirth. Sweet smelling and pleasant to inhale, with similar properties to **halothane** including non-flammability. Given by pouring on to a towel, especially in Scotland, or by inhalers, especially in London. Risk of sudden death, usually during induction, was attributed to respiratory depression in Scotland and cardiac standstill in England. The First and Second Hyderabad Commissions in 1888 and 1889 respectively, financed by the Nizam of Hyderabad (1866–1911), concluded that sudden death by respiratory depression preceded cardiac arrest. The reverse was generally accepted over 20 years later. **VF** occurred most commonly. Also caused severe **hepatic failure**. Gradually replaced by diethyl ether by the early/mid 1900s.
Payne JP (1981) Br J Anaesth; 53: 11S-15S
For physical properties, see Inhalational anaesthetic agents

Chloroprocaine hydrochloride. Ester **local anaesthetic agent**, introduced in 1952. Of short onset and duration of action, with low systemic toxicity and rapid offset (after approximately 45 minutes). Hydrolysed by plasma **cholinesterase**. Used for **extradural anaesthesia**, particularly for **Caesarean section** in the USA. Not available in the UK. Used in 2–3% solutions. Has been implicated in causing **arachnoiditis** and neurological deficits following accidental spinal injection (possibly related to its low pH or to accompanying preservatives) although this is controversial. Maximal safe dose is about 15 mg/kg.

Chlorpheniramine maleate. Antihistamine drug; competes with **histamine** at H_1 receptors. Used to treat allergic reactions, both mild, e.g. hay fever, and severe, e.g. **anaphylactic reaction**. Also used to treat generalized itching, e.g. in obstructive jaundice or after **spinal opioids**. Duration of action is up to 6 hours.
- Dosage:
  - 4 mg orally 4–6 hourly.
  - 10 mg im or iv by slow injection, up to 40 mg/day.
- Side effects:
  - drowsiness, anticholinergic effects.
  - hypotension and central nervous stimulation may follow iv injection.

Chlorpromazine hydrochloride. Phenothiazine, used as an antipsychotic and sedative drug, also in terminal disease and intractable hiccup. First used in the early 1950s, and called Largactil because of its large number of actions. Has been used before and during anaesthesia (e.g. **lytic cocktail**). Has powerful sedative and antiemetic properties, with anticholinergic, antidopaminergic and α-**adrenergic receptor** antagonist effects.

- Dosage: 25–50 mg orally or im, 8 hourly. May also be given iv, but well diluted to avoid thrombophlebitis. Hypotension may follow parenteral injection. May be given rectally as chlorpromazine base 100 mg.
- Side effects: as for phenothiazines.

Choanal atresia. Congenital blockage of one or both nasal passages. Incidence is 1:8000 births. If bilateral, it causes severe **airway obstruction** from birth, since **neonates** are obligatory nose breathers. Respiratory distress and **cyanosis** are characteristically reduced during crying, when mouth breathing occurs. May be demonstrated following attempted passage of a soft catheter through the nostrils. Other congenital defects and syndromes may be associated, e.g. **VSD**.
- Management:
  - oropharyngeal airway insertion, with secure taping to the face.
  - puncture of membrane/bone is usually performed within a few days, and plastic tubes inserted.
- Anaesthetic management: classically, awake tracheal intubation is performed following **preoxygenation**, using an oral tube and throat pack. Other considerations are as for any neonate. Extubation is performed awake.

Cholinergic crisis. Syndrome caused by relative overdosage of **acetylcholinesterase inhibitors** causing excess nicotinic (muscle weakness, fasciculation) and muscarinic (sweating, miosis, lacrimation, abdominal colic, etc.) stimulation by **acetylcholine**. May occur in **myasthenia gravis**, when differentiation from myasthenic crisis may be difficult. Administration of **edrophonium** 2 mg iv will improve myasthenic crises but worsen or have no effect on cholinergic crises. Usually treated by stopping acetylcholinesterase inhibitor therapy, giving **atropine**, and providing respiratory support if required.

Cholinergic receptors, *see Acetylcholine receptors*

Cholinesterase, plasma (Pseudocholinesterase). Circulating **enzyme** which hydrolyses **acetylcholine**, although most of the latter is hydrolysed by **acetylcholinesterase** at the **neuromuscular junction**. Also present in other tissues, e.g. brain, liver and kidneys. It also hydrolyses **suxamethonium**, removing choline groups to produce first succinylmonocholine and then succinic acid.
- Reduced enzyme activity causes prolonged paralysis after suxamethonium, and may be due to:
  - inherited atypical cholinesterase. Several autosomal recessive genes have been identified, using the degree of enzyme inhibition by various substances (e.g. dibucaine or fluoride) to describe the enzyme characteristics:
    - normal enzyme: 94% of the population are homozygotes. **Dibucaine number** (DN) is 75–85, and fluoride number (FN) 60.
    - atypical enzyme: 0.03% of the population are homozygotes, with DN 15–25 and FN 20.
    - silent gene: 0.001% of the population are homozygotes, with no plasma cholinesterase activity.
    - fluoride-resistant enzyme: 0.0001% of the population are homozygotes; DN is 65–75 but FN is 30.
  Paralysis may last 2–4 hours in homozygotes for silent and atypical genes, and 1–2 hours in homozygotes for the fluoride-resistant gene. In addition, heterozygotes

with one normal and one abnormal gene (5% of the population) with DN 40–60 may show prolonged paralysis of about 10–20 minutes. Most of these have the atypical gene. Combinations of abnormal genes comprise less than 0.01% of the population and also show slight or marked prolongation of paralysis.
   –acquired deficiency of cholinesterase, e.g. in **hepatic failure**, **hypoproteinaemia**, **pregnancy**, **malnutrition**, or following **plasmapheresis**.
   –inhibition of cholinesterase by drugs, e.g. **ecothiopate**, cyclophosphamide, **tetrahydroaminocrine**, **hexafluorenium** or phenelzine.
Plasma cholinesterase also hydrolyses other drugs, e.g. ester **local anaesthetic agents** and **propanidid**.
Whittaker M (1980) Anaesthesia; 35: 174–97

Chronic bronchitis, *see Chronic obstructive airways disease*

Chronic obstructive airways disease (COAD). Term encompassing chronic bronchitis and emphysema, which although different histologically, often coexist. The main features are lower airway obstruction, hyperinflated lungs and impaired gas exchange.
● Chronic bronchitis:
   –defined clinically by productive cough each morning for at least 3 months per year, for at least 2 successive years.
   –results from chronic bronchial irritation, e.g. by smoke, dust or fumes, causing:
      –mucosal hypersecretion.
      –mucosal oedema.
      –bronchoconstriction.
   –features: cough, dyspnoea, wheeze, tendency to develop **chest infection** causing acute exacerbations. Sufferers are typically described as 'blue bloaters' because of cyanosis and oedema.
   –**FEV$_1$**, expiratory flow rate and FEV/**FVC** are decreased, with increased **residual volume** and **FRC**, and $\dot{V}/\dot{Q}$ **mismatch**.
   –**hypoxaemia** and **hypercapnia** result, with possible loss of the central response to CO_2 (the mechanism is unclear). **Hypoxic pulmonary vasoconstriction** may lead to **pulmonary hypertension** with **cor pulmonale** and right ventricular failure.
● Emphysema:
   –defined histologically by dilated alveoli and/or respiratory bronchioles, often in upper areas of the lungs. Different patterns of dilatation are identified. Elastic recoil is reduced.
   –causes: as above, plus α_1–antitrypsin deficiency; the latter typically affects the lung bases.
   –features: dyspnoea. Air trapping and increased airflow resistance result from airway collapse during forceful expiration. Breath sounds are usually quiet. Sufferers are typically described as 'pink puffers' because of absent cyanosis and marked dyspnoea.
   –work of breathing is markedly increased, with hypocapnia (i.e. hyperventilation as opposed to hypoventilation as in chronic bronchitis), but only mild hypoxaemia.
   –FEV$_1$ is reduced and FRC increased as above.
Diffusing capacity is decreased in both conditions. **Respiratory muscle fatigue** may be a factor.
● Patients may present with **respiratory failure** requiring IPPV on ICU. Main considerations:

   –the decision to ventilate is sometimes hard, since **weaning from ventilators** is often difficult or even impossible. Useful information in making the decision concerning IPPV:
      –level of normal activity and lifestyle.
      –previous admissions, whether ventilated and ease of weaning.
      –whether the current crisis represents gradual decline or an acute treatable event, e.g. infection.
   –management is as for respiratory failure. **Doxapram** may be used in an attempt to prevent the requirement for IPPV: 1.5–4 mg/min according to response, with frequent arterial blood gas analysis. IPPV via a tightly-fitting mask is increasingly used for acute exacerbations of COAD.
● Anaesthetic management:
   –preoperatively:
      –**preoperative assessment** for exercise tolerance, bronchospasm, cor pulmonale and history of previous admissions. Patients are likely to be smokers; thus cardiovascular assessment including **ECG** is important. **Chest X-ray** may reveal a hyperexpanded chest, flattened diaphragm, narrow mediastinum, emphysematous bullae or infection. Arterial blood gas analysis and **lung function tests** may be useful.
      –improvement by **physiotherapy** and antibiotics if infection is present, and **bronchodilator drugs** if there is a reversible element to airway obstruction.
      –premedication: increased sensitivity to respiratory depressants, especially in chronic bronchitis, is rarely a problem. **Pethidine**, **promethazine** and **atropine** are often used; the latter may help prevent peroperative bronchospasm and reduce secretions, but may increase their tenacity.
   –peroperatively:
      –regional techniques are often suitable; problems may include inability to lie flat, possibility of coughing, and sensitivity to sedative drugs if used.
      –general anaesthesia:
         –inhalational techniques with a facepiece are suitable for short procedures, with minimal airway manipulation.
         –if tracheal intubation is undertaken, topical or iv **lignocaine** may be used to reduce irritation by the tracheal tube. Tracheal suction is often required. **Bronchospasm** and coughing may occur. Emphysematous bullae are at risk of expansion or rupture with IPPV and **N$_2$O**. **Capnography** allows maintenance of expired P_{CO_2} at the patient's normal (i.e. preoperative) level.
         –drugs causing **histamine** release are usually avoided.
   –postoperative problems include:
      –sputum retention, bronchospasm, **atelectasis** and infection. Physiotherapy and bronchodilator therapy are important. Respiratory failure may occur. Doxapram may be useful. Ventilation is often improved in the sitting position.
      –hypoventilation may be exacerbated by pain, depressant drugs and high F_1O_2. Adequate **postoperative analgesia** is vital; regional techniques are particularly useful, as excessive use of systemic opioids must be avoided. Parenteral opioids are

best given by infusion or small iv increments.
–patients with severe disease or those receiving
spinal opioids should be managed on ICU/HDU.
–elective IPPV may allow adequate gas exchange
whilst depressant anaesthetic drugs are cleared. It
also 'covers' the period of worst postoperative pain
and allows stabilization before weaning.

Churchill, Frederick, *see Liston, Robert*

Cigarette smoking, *see Smoking*

Ciliary activity. Continuous beating of the cilia of respiratory epithelial cells results in flow of thick mucus from
the nose to the pharynx, and from the bronchi to the
larynx. The mucus is then swallowed or expectorated. A
more watery mucus layer lies between the thick layer and
the epithelium, lubricating the cilia. Important in aiding
removal of foreign particles, microbes, etc. and clearing of
the airways. Reduced by **smoking**, extremes of temperature, volatile **inhalational anaesthetic agents**, **opioid
analgesic drugs** and prolonged exposure to high O_2 levels.
Prolonged inhalation of dry gases, anticholinergic drug
administration and volatile agents may impair mucus
production or flow.

Patients with inborn deficiency of cilia protein are
predisposed to **bronchiectasis**; if associated with decreased
spermatic activity, situs inversus and chronic sinusitis this
constitutes Kartagener's syndrome.
[Manes Kartagener (1897–1975), Swiss physician]

Cimetidine. H_2 receptor antagonist, of faster onset and
shorter-acting than **ranitidine**, lasting about 4 hours.
Half-life is 2 hours; up to 5 hours in **renal failure**.
● Dosage:
–400 mg orally, usually once/twice daily. Effective if
given 90 mins preoperatively.
–200 mg im or iv by infusion (may cause bradycardia
and hypotension after rapid iv injection).
● Side effects:
–Gynaecomastia, rarely impotence (binds to androgen
receptors).
–hepatic **enzyme inhibition** (binds to microsomal
cytochrome P_{450}). The actions of drugs such as
warfarin, **phenytoin** and **theophylline** may be
prolonged, and toxic effects seen.
–confusion, especially in the elderly and very ill.
–rarely, liver impairment and blood dyscrasias.

Cinchocaine hydrochloride. Amide **local anaesthetic
agent**, synthesized in 1925. Until recently, widely used in
the UK for **spinal anaesthesia**, in doses of 0.5–2.0 ml of
1:200 in 6% dextrose heavy solution. Now unavailable.
Has been used for **extradural anaesthesia** (1:600 solution),
infiltration and nerve blocks (1:1000–2000 with adrenaline), and surface analgesia, up to 2 mg/kg maximum. Of
slower onset and duration of action than **lignocaine**, and
more toxic.
Used to estimate plasma **cholinesterase activity
(dibucaine number)**.

Circle of Willis, *see Cerebral circulation*

Circle systems. CO_2 absorption with **soda lime** was used
by **Waters** in 1923, and a circle system employing valves by

Sword in 1926. Usage increased in 1930s with the introduction of **cyclopropane**, then declined. Interest has recently
resurged because of worries about cost and pollution.
● Advantages:
–cheap, since low gas flows are required.
–reduced risk of pollution, and of **explosions and fires**
with inflammable agents.
–warmth and humidity of expired gases are retained,
with further warming and humidification in the CO_2
absorber, although efficiency is reduced by passage
through lengths of tubing.
–spontaneous/controlled ventilation is easily
performed without changing the system.
–allows easy monitoring of O_2 uptake/CO_2 output.
● Disadvantages:
–higher resistance and thus work of breathing.
–bulky equipment.
–slow changes in anaesthetic concentrations at low gas
flows.
–an O_2 analyser is mandatory if N_2O is used, to avoid
hypoxic gas mixtures.
–more connections to come apart, valves to stick, etc.
● Systems used:
–resistance is reduced by using wide-bore tubing (may
be further reduced by circulating fans).
–consist of absorber, two one-way valves, **adjustable
pressure-limiting** (APL) **valve**, **reservoir bag**, tubing
to and from the patient and for fresh gas supply
(FGF). Efficiency is increased by placing:
–FGF downstream to APL valve (avoids venting of
fresh gas).
–bag and patient on opposite sides of the one-way
valves (maintains circulatory gas flow).
Examples of arrangements (Fig. 34): system A is
efficient for spontaneous ventilation and IPPV; **dead
space** gas is conserved beyond the APL valve during
expiration whilst alveolar gas is flushed by FGF via
the APL valve. System B is less efficient because the
APL valve is further away from the patient; dead
space and alveolar gases mix more before reaching it.
System B is more convenient practically, however,
since all components are away from the patient.
–ready-assembled circle systems are usually used now,
arranged as in system B within one housing (jumbo
absorber). The cannister is divided into two halves,
each containing about 1 kg soda lime; when one half
is exhausted the cannister is inverted. An on-off
switch allows the soda lime to be bypassed if
required.
● Use:
–if N_2O is used, build up of nitrogen in the system may
lead to a low F_1O_2. Nitrogen is removed first from the
lungs, then slowly from body tissues. A high FGF
(5–7 l/min) for 7–10 minutes is sufficient to remove
most body nitrogen; the remainder (approximately 1
litre) slowly accumulates within the system. High
flows are also required to prevent excessive dilution
of FGF by exhaled gas during initial uptake of FGF
gases. Hourly flushing with high flows has been
suggested. Re-flushing is required if the circle is
broken at any time. Increased N_2O concentration
within the system as its uptake decreases may also
contribute to low F_1O_2.
–if only O_2 is used, hypoxic mixtures do not occur, but
atelectasis and **O_2 toxicity** are more likely.

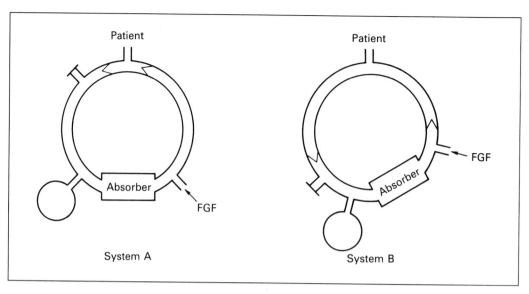

Figure 34 *Examples of circle systems (see text)*

–with high flow, the APL valve is open.
–low flow is defined as equal to or under 3 l/min FGF:
   –APL valve totally closed: FGF supplies basal requirements only, i.e. 220–250 ml/min O_2.
   –APL valve slightly open, i.e. allowing a small leak: 1–3 l/min is often used as a compromise between the closed and high flow systems.
–IPPV is achieved by hand or by attaching a suitable **ventilator** to the reservoir bag attachment by a length of tubing. Minute volume dividers are unsuitable unless specially adapted, since the ventilator output must be separate from the FGF delivered to the patient. The Penlon Nuffield ventilator is commonly used in the UK, driven by compressed O_2. Contamination of inspiratory gases by driving O_2 may occur if low FGFs are used and the tubing between the ventilator and circle is short.
–continuous **gas analysis** is particularly useful in monitoring gas concentrations. Ventilator/FGF settings are adjusted to produce suitable F_IO_2, N_2O and expired CO_2 concentrations. An O_2 analyser must be used if N_2O or low flows are used.
–**vaporizers**:
   –out of circle (VOC):
      –usual plenum vaporizers are used on the back bar of the anaesthetic machine.
      –the concentration of volatile agent within the circle is less than that delivered by the vaporizer, because of dilution by exhaled gas. The difference is highest initially, when uptake of agent is greatest, unless high FGFs are used.
   –in circle (VIC):
      –low resistance vaporizers are required, e.g. Goldman's. Delivered concentration is related to gas flow through the vaporizer.
      –as volatile agent is present in exhaled gas entering the vaporizer, high concentrations are possible. During spontaneous ventilation, respiratory depression increases as the concentration increases, reducing gas flow through the vaporizer. Thus dangerous levels of agent are not

reached. During IPPV, this feedback mechanism is absent; i.e. dangerous levels are attainable.
–volatile agent analysers are particularly useful to monitor concentrations.
–liquid anaesthetic may be injected directly into the tubing.
[Brian Sword (1889–1956), US anaesthetist]
Spence AA, Allison RH, Wishart HY (1981) Br J Anaesth; 53: 69S–73S

Cisapride. Drug which increases **lower oesophageal sphincter** pressure and increases **gastric emptying** and intestinal motility. Acts by increasing **acetylcholine** release in the myenteric plexus within the gut wall; has no antidopaminergic activity. Reverses **morphine**-induced gastric stasis. Used in oesophageal reflux and delayed upper GIT emptying. Has been used preoperatively to reduce the risk of regurgitation and **aspiration of gastric contents**.
● Dosage: 10 mg orally, 6–8 hourly.
● Side effects: headache, abdominal cramps, diarrhoea. Convulsions and extrapyramidal effects have been reported rarely.
Rowbotham DJ (1989) Br J Anaesth; 62: 121–3

Citrate and citrate solutions, *see Blood storage; Sodium citrate*

Clapeyron–Clausius equation. Describes the theoretical variation of **SVP** with temperature, depending on **latent heat** of vaporization (LH). Assumes LH is independent of temperature, and that the volume of liquid is negligible compared to that of the vapour.
[Benoit-Paul Clapeyron (1799–1864), French engineer; Rudolf Clausius (1822–88), German physicist]

Clark electrode, *see Oxygen measurement*

Clarke, William E. (1818–1878). US physician; used **diethyl ether** to allow dental extraction in January 1842 in New York, but only reported this after **Morton**'s demonstration in 1846.

Clathrates. Compounds formed by inclusion of molecules within a crystal lattice of a different substance. Formation of clathrates with water (gas hydrates) affecting brain cell membranes (as 'icebergs' within them) was suggested by Pauling and Miller in 1961 as a basis for the mechanism of action of **inhalational anaesthetic agents**. Now considered incorrect since:

- for some fluorocarbons, potency is not related to clathrate formation.
- some inhalational agents do not form clathrates at body temperature and pressure.
- effects of combining different agents are not accounted for.

[Linus Pauling and Stanley L Miller, US chemists]
See also, Anaesthesia, mechanism of

Clearance. Calculated figure, representing complete removal of a substance from plasma by passage through an organ, usually the kidney. Defined as the volume of plasma in ml completely cleared of substance per minute:

$$\text{clearance} = \frac{\text{amount of substance excreted in urine per unit time}}{\text{plasma concentration of substance}}$$

$$= \frac{\text{urinary concentration (mmol/l)} \times \text{urine volume (ml/min)}}{\text{plasma concentration (mmol/l)}}$$

The concept is useful in comparing excretion rates of different drugs; it is also used to determine **renal blood flow** and **GFR**. If clearance for a substance is less than GFR, there is incomplete removal by the kidney. If clearance exceeds GFR, the substance is secreted into the urine by tubular cells.

Clearance, creatinine, *see Creatinine clearance*

Clearance, free water. Volume of plasma cleared of excess water per minute. Equals urine volume (ml/min) minus osmotic **clearance** (ml/min). Normally negative, i.e. water is being conserved, and hypertonic urine produced. Positive in **water diuresis**.
See also, Clearance, osmotic

Clearance, osmotic. Estimation of renal solute excretion.

Equals
$$\frac{\text{urine osmolality (mosmol/l)} \times \text{urine volume (ml/min)}}{\text{plasma osmolality (mosmol/l)}}$$

If urine is hypotonic, urine volume exceeds osmotic **clearance**; if hypertonic, osmotic clearance is greater. The difference between them is free water clearance. Normally under 3 ml/min; increased by osmotic diuretics.
See also, Clearance, free water

Cleft lip and palate, *see Facial deformities, congenital*

Clinical trials. Performed to determine whether a treatment is useful, how it compares with other treatments, whether it affects different groups of patients differently, and how it is best given (e.g. drug dosage regimen, route, etc.).

- Setting up a trial:
  - aims of the trial are defined.
  - the number of patients is defined; ideally, the number is calculated by first defining the size of difference considered clinically important, and then the sample size required to enable such a difference to be revealed if present (i.e. **power** analysis). Groups should be of equal size if possible.
  - subjects:
    - patients with other diseases, those taking other drugs, etc. are excluded where possible.
    - controls:
      - pairs may be matched for age, sex, race, degree and duration of illness, etc., and one of each pair assigned to each treatment.
      - cross-over studies: patients act as their own controls by receiving first one treatment then another. The effect of the first treatment on the second must be excluded.
      - **randomization** into groups.
      - historical controls are avoided where possible.
      - treatment is compared with no treatment, placebo or existing treatment.
  - bias is further reduced by blindness:
    - single-blind (patient is unaware of treatment identity).
    - double-blind (doctor and patient are unaware).
  - variability is reduced by using the same location, time of day, medical/nursing staff, technique, etc., for all patients.
  - approval by an Ethical Review Committee: includes qualified and lay persons. Considers whether exposure of patients to the new treatment, denial of the old treatment to controls, or vice versa, is justified. No patient should be worse off than if the trial were not running.
  - informed **consent** is required from participating patients.
  - **data**:
    - what to measure; i.e. according to defined aims.
    - objective measurements are less prone to observer bias than subjective assessment.
    - how many measurements; e.g. measurement of too many variables increases the likelihood of at least one being significantly different due to chance alone.
    - which **statistical test** to use, and how to express results; e.g. use of the **null hypothesis** or **confidence intervals**.
  - end-point of the trial:
    - according to the numbers studied.
    - sequential analysis: the trial stops when results attain significance.

Various authors (1991) Prescribers' J; 31: 227–57
See also, Drug development; Statistics

Clonazepam. **Benzodiazepine**, used mainly to treat **epilepsy**. Has also been used in disorders of movement, e.g. dystonias, etc., and as an adjunct to **pain management**. Has similar effects to **diazepam**. 50% protein bound after iv injection. Metabolized in the liver and excreted in the urine. Elimination **half-life** is 24–48 hours.

- Dosage:
  - 1–8 mg/day orally in adults, depending on response.
  - 0.25–1 mg/day in infants.
  - 0.5–1 mg diluted in water for iv injection.
- Side effects include sedation (occasionally excitation), bronchial and salivary hypersecretion, and rarely hepatic impairment and blood dyscrasias.

Clonidine hydrochloride. α-Adrenergic receptor **agonist**, used as an **antihypertensive drug** and in the prophylaxis of migraine. Acts centrally by stimulating presynaptic α₂–**adrenergic receptors**, causing suppression of **catecholamine** release (i.e. activates a negative-feedback control system). May also stimulate inhibitory postsynaptic α₁–receptors, and may have some action peripherally. Its main effect is on **vasomotor centre** output. Also has an analgesic and sedative action, but the mechanism is unclear. Has been administered intrathecally and extradurally. When administered by mouth preoperatively, it reduces **MAC** of **inhalational anaesthetic agents**.

- Dosage:
  - 0.15–0.3 mg/day orally in divided doses, up to 1.2 mg.
  - 0.15–0.3 mg by slow iv injection. Effects occur within 10 minutes, and last 3–7 hours. Transient hypertension and bradycardia may occur.
- Side effects: sedation, dry mouth, depression, urinary retention. Increased sensitivity to parenteral catecholamines may occur; sudden withdrawal of clonidine may cause a severe hypertensive crisis.

Feldman S, Ooi R (1991) Anaesthesia; 46: 1003–4

Closing capacity. **Lung volume** at which airway closure occurs, mainly in the dependent parts of the lung. Equals closing volume plus **residual volume**. In fit young adults, closing capacity (CC) is considerably less than **FRC**; thus airway closure does not occur during normal quiet breathing. Airway closure occurring within FRC results in shunting.

- Measurement: inspiration of a bolus of marker gas, e.g. helium (He) at the end of maximal expiration (i.e. residual volume), followed by inspiration of air to total lung capacity (Fig. 35). Expired He concentration is measured during slow expiration: the same phases are seen as in **Fowler's method** (which may also be used to measure CC). Initially, **dead space** gas is exhaled, containing no He. Then, a mixture of **dead space** and alveolar gas, followed by alveolar gas. The He bolus entered the upper airways, because the lower ones were collapsed at residual volume. Thus at CC, there is a sharp rise in expired He concentration.
- Increased by:
  - age: CC = FRC in neonates and infants.
    CC = FRC in the supine position at 40 years.
    CC = FRC in the upright position at 65 years.

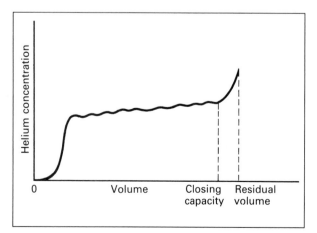

Figure 35 *Measurement of closing capacity*

- increased intrathoracic pressures, e.g. **asthma**.
- **smoking**.

CC may encroach upon a FRC reduced by **obesity**, the supine position, and anaesthesia. **PEEP** and **CPAP** may reduce airway closure.

Closing volume, *see Closing capacity*

Clover, Joseph Thomas (1825–1882). English anaesthetist; took over from **Snow** as anaesthesia's pioneer after the latter's death. A medical student at University College Hospital, London, said to have been present at **Liston**'s historic operation in 1846. Started his medical career in surgery and general practice. Devised inhalers for **chloroform** and later **diethyl ether** which delivered accurate concentrations of agent and were much copied by other practitioners. Also described the use of **N₂O**, alone or in combination with volatile agents. His apparatus included large capacity rubber bags, filled with N₂O or air and carried over the shoulder.

C$_m$, *see Minimal blocking concentration*

CMRO₂, *see Cerebral metabolic rate for oxygen*

COAD, *see Chronic obstructive airways disease*

Coagulation. Clot formation; follows vasospasm and platelet plug formation which cause temporary haemostasis.
- Normal sequence of events:
  - vasospasm, thought to be mediated by vasoconstrictor substances released from **platelets**, e.g. **5–HT** and **thromboxane**.
  - platelet plug: platelets are attracted by collagen exposed by damaged vascular endothelium. Adherence is followed by release of 5–HT and **ADP**, the latter causing further aggregation.
  - clot formation: the platelet plug is bound by resultant fibrin to form the definitive clot. Clot retraction is caused by platelet contractile microfilaments. The coagulation pathway involves many circulating factors in a cascade mechanism; each factor, when activated, activates the next in turn (Fig. 36). Most are produced by the liver. Nomenclature of factors is largely historical, according to the chronolgical order of discovery. The intrinsic pathway is initiated by exposure of blood to collagen, or *in vitro* by contact with glass e.g. test tubes. The extrinsic pathway is initiated by substances released from damaged tissues. Each may activate the common pathway, which culminates in formation of a tight fibrin clot.

Normally, the clotting mechanism is balanced by opposing reactions preventing coagulation, e.g. antithrombin III (formed from activated factor X) which inhibits active factors II, IX, X, XI and XII. **Prostacyclin** secreted by the vascular endothelium inhibits platelet aggregation.

Other pathways may be involved with the coagulation cascade, e.g. active factor XII leads to activation of **fibrinolysis** and **kinin** formation.

See also, Anticoagulant drugs; Coagulation disorders; Coagulation studies

Coagulation disorders. May result in impaired coagulation or hypercoagulability. The former is more common and may arise from defects in:

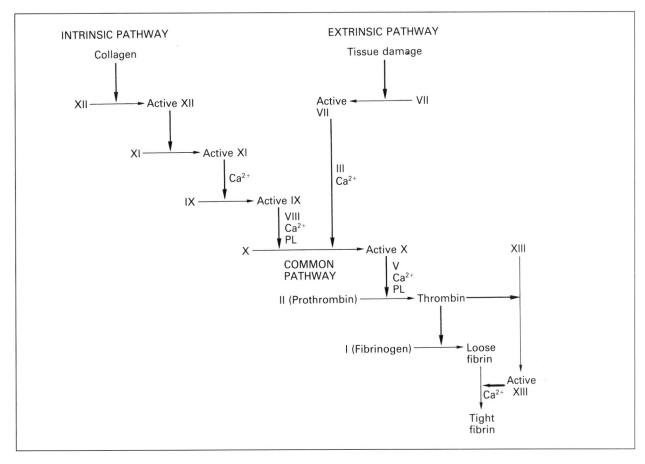

Figure 36 *Coagulation cascade. PL, phospholipid;* →, *'brings about'*; →, *'becomes'*

–blood vessels:
  –infection, e.g. meningococcal **meningitis, septi-caemia**.
  –metabolic disease, e.g. **hepatic failure, renal failure**, scurvy.
  –congenital, e.g. hereditary telangiectasia.
–**platelets**:
  –**thrombocytopenia**.
  –**DIC**.
  –impaired function, e.g. **antiplatelet drugs.**
–**coagulation**:
  –congenital, e.g. **haemophilia, von Willibrand's disease** (also associated with blood vessel and platelet defects).
  –**heparin, warfarin**, hepatic failure, **vitamin K** deficiency, DIC.
  –increased **fibrinolysis**.
Blood transfusion may be associated with dilution of platelets and coagulation factors by fluids and blood components deficient in them. Impaired organ function and possible DIC may contribute.
Diagnosed by the underlying problem, aided by **coagulation studies** (Table 11).
● Treatment:
  –of underlying disease.
  –replacement of defective circulatory components.
● Abnormal hypercoagulability may lead to recurrent **DVT** and PE. It may result from:

–primary disorders, e.g. antithrombin III deficiency, deficiencies of fibrinolytic components or factor XII, and presence of lupus anticoagulant (prolongs activated partial thromboplastin time, but causes hypercoagulability, possibly due to inhibition of **prostacyclin** production from vascular endothelium).
–secondary to **malignancy, pregnancy, diabetes mellitus**, platelet and vessel wall abnormalities, hyperviscosity and venous stasis.

Coagulation studies. May test different parts of the **coagulation** pathways:
–clotting factors: performed on fresh citrated plasma, with cells and platelets removed; physical activation of coagulation is avoided by using non-wettable plastic tubes. Normal plasma is used as a control.
  –prothrombin time (PT): tests the extrinsic and common pathways. Plasma then calcium is added to brain extract and phospholipid. Normal value is 11–15 seconds. International Normalized Ratio (INR; formerly British Ratio) is the ratio of sample time to a standard. A target ratio of 2–2.5 is used for prophylaxis of **DVT** with **warfarin**; 2–3 for treatment of DVT, **PE** and transient ischaemic attacks; 3–4.5 for prophylaxis of recurrent DVT or PE, and for patients with prosthetic heart valves and other arterial prostheses. A ratio of 1.5 is considered safe for surgery.

Table 11. Changes in prothrombin time (PT), activated partial thromboplastin time (APPT), thrombin time (TT), fibrin degradation products (FDPs), platelet count and fibrinogen levels in various coagulation disorders

Disorder	PT	APPT	TT	FDPs	Platelets	Fibrinogen
Thrombocytopenia	→	→	→	→	↓	→
DIC	↑	↑	↑	↑	↓	↓
Heparin therapy	↑	↑	↑	→	→*	→
Warfarin therapy	↑	↑	→	→	→	→
Hepatic failure	↑	↑	↑	→	→	↓
Massive blood transfusion	↑	↑	↑	→	↓	→
Primary fibrinolysis	↑	↑	↑	↑	→	↓

↑, Increase; ↓, decrease; →, no change.
*But thrombocytopenia may follow several days heparin therapy.
Note: DIC may complicate hepatic failure and massive blood transfusion.

–activated partial thromboplastin time (APTT; also partial thromboplastin time with kaolin, PTTK): tests the intrinsic and common pathways. Plasma, phospholipid and calcium are added to kaolin. Normal value is 35–40 seconds. A target ratio of 2–4 compared with normal plasma is used for treatment of DVT or PE with **heparin**. A ratio of 1.5 is considered safe for surgery.
–mixture tests: if PT or APTT is prolonged, the patient's plasma may be mixed with normal plasma and the test repeated. If the test is normal, factor deficiency is present; if still prolonged, the sample plasma contains an inhibitor, e.g. antibody.
–specific factor assays, e.g. factor VIII assay.
–reptilase time (RT): snake venom is added to plasma, converting fibrinogen to fibrin. Unaffected by heparin; thus if normal but the thrombin time is prolonged, presence of heparin is suggested.
–**platelets**:
–platelet count: normally 150–400 × 10^9/l.
–bleeding time: a standard incision is made on the forearm using a pricking device or template; a BP cuff is inflated around the upper arm to 40 mmHg. The incision is dabbed with filter paper every 30 seconds until the bleeding stops. Normal value is 2–9 minutes.
–**fibrinolysis**:
–thrombin time (TT): tests conversion of fibrinogen to fibrin. Exogenous thrombin is added to plasma. Normal value is 10–15 seconds. Inhibited by **fibrin degradation products** resulting from fibrinolysis. Also inhibited by heparin.
–fibrin degradation products (including the D-dimer portion).
–plasminogen assay.
–clot lysis times, e.g. euglobin, precipitated from plasma by adding acid. Contains fibrinogen, plasminogen and plasminogen activator. Addition of thrombin causes clot formation; subsequent lysis depends on the amount of plasminogen activating capacity present. Whole blood clot lysis and other variants are also used.
–whole blood clotting time: bedside test of intrinsic and common pathways (i.e. spontaneous coagulation occurring in a glass tube without external reactive substances, e.g. tissue fluid). 1 ml blood is added to each of three glass tubes, kept at body temperature.

The first is tilted every 15 seconds until clotted, then the second, third, etc. The time until the third is clotted is normally about 9–12 minutes.
–activated clotting time (ACT): bedside test; commonly used to monitor heparin anticoagulation during **cardiac surgery**. Similar to whole blood clotting time, but celite is added to the blood for quicker results. Automated devices are usually used to detect fibrin formation, with a small bar magnet within the test tube. The tube is placed within the device and rotated slowly; when fibrin forms in the tube, the magnet starts to rotate, thereby activating the detector. Normal value is 100–140 seconds. Values of 3–4 times the preheparin value are considered adequate during **extracorporeal circulation**.
–thromboelastography: measurement of the quality and speed of formation of clot. Used as a rapid indicator of coagulation status, e.g. during **liver transplantation**. Fibrin strands form between an oscillating container of fresh blood and a drum within it; the movements of the drum are recorded on to paper to produce a clotting profile whose shape represents the speed of coagulation and quality of clot.

Coanda effect. Development of reduced pressure between a fluid jet from a nozzle and an adjacent surface, resulting in adherence of the jet to the surface. Reduced pressure results from entrainment of surrounding molecules into the turbulent jet, with those next to the surface quickly 'used up'. If the jet has two surfaces to which it might adhere, it will attach to one only, without splitting. A small signal jet across the nozzle may switch the main jet from one surface to the other; this has formed the basis of control mechanisms in **fluidics**, e.g. control of ventilators.

Similar behaviour of fluids has been suggested to occur beyond constrictions in blood vessels, e.g. coronary arteries, contributing to ischaemia and infarction.

The effect was originally applied to the development of jet engines.
[Henri Coanda (1885–1972), Romanian engineer]

Coarctation of aorta. Accounts for 5–10% of **congenital heart disease**. More common in males. May be associated with **Turner's** and **Marfan's syndromes**. Acquired coarctation is rare and usually follows **chest trauma** or arteritis.

Over 95% are post-ductal, often presenting in later life. There may be associated cerebral aneurysms or a bicuspid aortic valve.

- Features:
  - **hypertension**, left ventricular hypertrophy and **cardiac failure**. BP is high in the arms, normal or low in the legs. **CVA** and **endocarditis** may occur.
  - weak femoral pulses, delayed compared with the radials.
  - systolic **heart murmur**; may be loudest posteriorly.
  - **ECG** findings include left ventricular hypertrophy.
  - characteristic **chest X-ray** findings:
    - double aortic knuckle ('3' sign).
    - small descending aorta.
    - rib notching; seen at the middle of the lower border of the ribs posteriorly; caused by enlarged collateral vessels.
    - left ventricular enlargement/failure.

The preductal form is more severe, usually presenting in infancy with cardiac failure. Often associated with cerebral aneurysms, bicuspid aortic valve, patent **ductus arteriosus**, **VSD**, and mitral and aortic abnormalities.

Repaired via left thoracotomy.

- Anaesthetic management is similar to that for thoracic **aortic aneurysm**, in particular:
  - preoperative treatment of hypertension and cardiac failure.
  - antibiotic prophylaxis as for congenital heart disease.
  - arterial BP should be monitored in the right arm as the left subclavian artery is usually clamped during resection.
  - complications include:
    - haemorrhage.
    - hypertension following aortic clamping, ischaemia to the spinal cord, bowel and kidneys, and acidosis and hypotension following unclamping.
  - hypertension may persist postoperatively and require treatment, especially in older patients.
  - simultaneous BP measurement in the arms and legs is often performed.

Fisher A, Benedict CR (1977) Anaesthesia; 32: 533–8
See also, Cardiac surgery

Coaxial anaesthetic breathing systems. Functionally, they are versions of Mapleson A (Lack) and D (Bain) systems, but more convenient to use:

- Lack (Fig. 37a): the expiratory valve is at the anaesthetic machine end (cf. **Magill** system). Thus easier to adjust and scavenge waste gases, especially when the patient's head is covered. The patient end is also lighter. The outer tube is wider than usual to accommodate the inner tube, itself as wide as possible to reduce resistance to expiration. The system is therefore bulky and relatively inflexible. It has greater resistance to expiration than the Magill system. Required fresh gas flows are as for the Magill system. Parallel versions are also available, in which the inner tube is replaced by a second external tube running alongside the main tube. Both tubes are wide-bore and thus of low resistance.
- Bain (Fig. 37b): lighter and longer than the standard systems, with the expiratory valve at the machine end, allowing easy adjustment and scavenging. Some resistance to expiration results from the flow of fresh gas directed at the patient's mouth from the inner

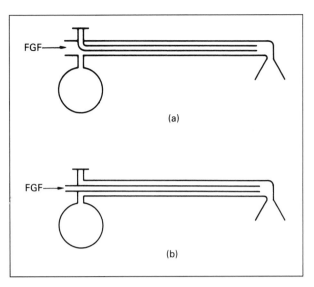

Figure 37 *Coaxial breathing systems: (a) Lack; (b) Bain*

tube. Ideal fresh gas flow rates for spontaneous ventilation are controversial, as high flows cause greater resistance. Suggested values range from 100 to 250 ml/kg. May be used for IPPV using a ventilator, e.g. Penlon Nuffield attached to the reservoir bag fitting (bag removed) by a length of tubing whose volume exceeds tidal volume. Disconnection of the inner tube from the fresh gas source (resulting in the whole length of tubing becoming dead space) must be excluded before use (*see Checking of anaesthetic equipment*).

[John A Lack, Salisbury anaesthetist; JA Bain, Canadian anaesthetist]
See also, Anaesthetic breathing systems

Cocada. Ball of coca leaves thought to be chewed by South American Incas to release free **cocaine** base. Dribbling of saliva on to wounds then allowed relatively painless surgery.

Cocaine/cocaine hydrochloride. Ester **local anaesthetic agent**, the first one discovered. An alkaloid originally extracted from the leaves and bark of South American coca plants. Used in 1884 for topical analgesia of the eye (by **Koller**), mandibular nerve block (by **Halstead** and Hall) and other uses including local infiltration. Now restricted to surface analgesia because of its toxicity. Commonly used as a 10% spray or paste to reduce bleeding caused by nasal intubation. Causes vasoconstriction by preventing uptake of **noradrenaline** by presynaptic nerve endings; also inhibits **monoamine oxidase**.

- Toxicity:
  - CNS stimulation: **convulsions** at high doses, followed by central depression and **apnoea**.
  - sympathetic stimulation: **arrhythmias**, tachycardia and hypertension may occur.
  - addiction may occur with chronic use. **Cardiomyopathy** and sudden death have been associated with chronic abuse.
- Maximal safe dose: 3 mg/kg.

Excreted mainly via the liver; a small amount is excreted unchanged in the urine.

[Richard J Hall (1856–1897), Irish-born US surgeon]
Fleming JA, Byck R, Barash PG (1990) Anesthesiology; 73: 518–31

'Cockpit drill', *see Checking of anaesthetic equipment*

Codeine phosphate. Naturally-occurring **opioid analgesic drug**, isolated in 1832; used to relieve mild to moderate **pain**. Also used in diarrhoea, and to suppress the cough reflex, e.g. in terminal care. Has similar effects to **morphine**, but with less potency and efficacy. Some metabolism to morphine may occur. Classically used as analgesic of choice in **head injury** and **neurosurgery**, since sedation, respiratory depression and pupillary constriction are said to be less than with other opioids, although this may reflect the small doses used. Partly excreted unchanged via the kidneys, and partly metabolized in the liver.
- Dosage: up to 60 mg orally or im; 1–1.5 mg/kg for children. Severe hypotension may follow iv use.

COELCB, *see Current-operated earth-leakage circuit breaker*

Coeliac plexus block. Sympathetic nerve block involving blockade of the coeliac plexuses, one lying on each side of L1. Through them pass afferent fibres from abdominal (but not pelvic) viscera.

Performed for relief of **pain** from non-pelvic intra-abdominal organs, especially due to pancreatic and gastric malignancies. Has also been used in acute/chronic pancreatitis (relaxes the sphincter of Oddi) and to provide intra-abdominal analgesia during surgery. Usually performed percutaneously with the patient prone, under X-ray control. CAT scanning has been used.
- Point of needle insertion: 5–10 cm from the midline, level with the spinous process of L1, below the 12th rib. A long (>10 cm) needle is inserted at 45° to the skin, directed medially and slightly cranially. It is passed until the needle tip lies anterior to the upper part of the body of L1. 15–25 ml **local anaesthetic agent** is injected on each side, e.g. **prilocaine** or **lignocaine** 0.5% with adrenaline, followed by 25 ml 50% alcohol if required, e.g. on the following day if the block is successful. Flushing with saline prevents alcohol deposition during needle withdrawal. Severe hypotension may result, even after unilateral block.
[Ruggero Oddi (1845–1906), Italian surgeon]
See also, Sympathetic nervous system

COLD, Chronic obstructive lung disease, *see Chronic obstructive airways disease*

College of Anaesthetists. Founded in 1988, in order to promote anaesthesia further as a separate speciality in the eyes of both the public and the medical profession. Replaced the **Faculty of Anaesthetists at the Royal College of Surgeons of England**; moved to new premises and was granted Royal status in 1992. Has 5500 Fellows. The ***British Journal of Anaesthesia*** has been its official journal since 1990.
Mushin W (1989) Anaesthesia; 44: 291–2
See also, Royal College of Anaesthetists

Colligative properties of solutions. Those properties varying with the amount, and not character, of solute particles present. Thus, as concentration increases:
- –freezing point decreases.
- –**osmotic pressure** increases.
- –boiling point increases.
- –vapour pressure of solvent decreases (**Raoult's law**).

Measurement of **osmolarity/osmolality** may utilize any of the above properties, since the changes produced by addition of solute are proportional to the amount added.

Colloid. Substance unable to pass through a semipermeable membrane, being a suspension of particles rather than a true solution (cf. **crystalloid**). The term is used to describe **iv fluids** which remain confined to the intravascular compartment, at least initially. More useful than crystalloids when replacing a vascular volume deficit, e.g. in **haemorrhage**, but of less use correcting specific water and electrolyte deficiencies, e.g. in **dehydration**. Also more expensive. Sometimes called plasma substitutes or **plasma expanders**, because the increase in plasma volume may be greater than the volume of colloid infused, due to their higher **osmolality** than plasma.
- Available products:
  - –**blood products**, e.g. blood, albumin, plasma: should be used for specific blood component deficiency only, since supplies are short, and risks of **blood transfusion** are present. Cost £30–50/500 ml.
  - –**hetastarch**. Plasma expansion lasts for over 24 hours. Incidence of severe reactions is about 1/16 000; cost is £15–20/500 ml. **Pentastarch** has also been developed: plasma expansion lasts for 18–24 hours. Adverse reactions and cost: as for hetastarch.
  - –**gelatin derivatives**. Effects last a few hours only. Severe reactions: 1/13 000 (succinylated), 1/2000 (urea linked; lower incidence with the newer formulation since 1981). Cost: £3–4/500 ml.
  - –**dextrans**. May affect renal function and coagulation. Severe reactions: 1/4500, reduced to 1/84 000 with hapten pretreatment. Cost: £4–5/500 ml.

See also, Colloid/crystalloid controversy

Colloid/crystalloid controversy. Arises from conflicting theoretical, experimental and clinical evidence concerning the use of iv **colloid** or **crystalloid** in **shock**, most work concerning **haemorrhage**.
- Arguments in favour of:
  - –colloid :
    - –more logical choice for intravascular volume replacement, since a greater proportion remains in the intravascular space for longer after infusion.
    - –less volume is required to restore cardiovascular parameters, e.g. BP, **CVP**, **pulmonary artery capillary wedge pressure**, etc. Thus initial resuscitation is more rapid.
    - –less peripheral/**pulmonary oedema** follows its use for the above reasons, and also because there is less reduction of plasma **oncotic pressure**.
  - –crystalloid :
    - –expands the intravascular compartment adequately if enough is used (2–4 times the colloid requirements).
    - –in haemorrhage, fluid moves from the interstitial space into the vascular compartment and **third space**; this **ECF** depletion is better replenished by crystalloid.

–if vascular permeability is increased, colloids will enter the interstitial space and increase interstitial oncotic pressure, thus exacerbating **oedema**. Crystalloids do not increase interstitial oncotic pressure to the same extent.

–peripheral oedema is usually not a problem.

–risk of allergic reactions to colloids.

–crystalloid is much cheaper than colloid.

- Difficulties in assessing fluid resuscitation:
  –infusion is usually guided by cardiovascular end-points but their relation to interstitial fluid, ECF etc. is unclear.
  –lung water may increase markedly before gas exchange is impaired.
  –other clinical processes may be involved, e.g. cardiovascular disease, impaired gas exchange and increased vascular permeability due to sepsis, **ARDS**, etc. The position is even less clear than in uncomplicated haemorrhage.

In the US, crystalloid e.g. **Hartmann's solution** is widely used for iv resuscitation, whereas colloids are more commonly used in the UK. Mixtures are favoured by many, guided by the nature of the deficit.
Vincent JL (1991) Br J Anaesth; 67: 185–93

Colloid oncotic pressure, *see Oncotic pressure*

Colton, Gardner Quincy (1814–1898). US lecturer and showman; studied medicine but never qualified. Demonstrated the exhilarating effects of **N₂O** inhalation for entertainment in 1844, inspiring **Wells** to suggest its use for dental analgesia. Said to have administered N₂O to Wells whilst the latter's tooth was painlessly removed. Left his lectures to prospect for gold, returning to N₂O and popularizing its reintroduction by founding the Colton Dental Association in 1863.
Smith GB, Hirsch NP (1991) Anesth Analg; 72: 382–91

Coma. State in which the patient is totally unaware of both self and external surroundings, and unable to respond meaningfully to external stimuli. Results from gross impairment of both cerebral hemispheres, and/or the **ascending reticular activating system**.

- Caused by:
  –focal brain dysfunction, e.g. tumour, vascular events, demyelination, infection, **head injury**.
  –diffuse brain dysfunction:
    –infection, e.g. **meningitis**, encephalitis.
    –**epilepsy**.
    –**hypoxia** and **hypercapnia**.
    –drugs, **poisoning and overdoses**.
    –metabolic/endocrine causes, e.g. **diabetic coma**, **hepatic** or **renal failure**, **hypothyroidism**, extreme electrolyte disturbance, e.g. **hyponatraemia**.
    –**hypotension**, **hypertensive crisis**.
    –head injury.
    –**subarachnoid haemorrhage**.
    –**hypothermia**, **hyperthermia**.

Assessment of the **pupils**, **doll's eye movements**, posture and motor responses (e.g. **decerebrate** and **decorticate postures**) and respiratory pattern are especially useful. Investigations are directed towards the above causes.

Initial management includes respiratory and cardiovascular support as for **CPR**. In addition, longer-term management includes attention to pressure areas, mouth, skin and eyes, physiotherapy, prophylaxis against **DVT**, **nutrition** and **fluid balance**, and urinary catheterization.
See also, Brainstem death; Coma scales

Coma scales. Scoring systems for assessing the degree of **coma** in unconscious patients and charting their progress; may also give an indication of outcome.

- Include general simple scales, e.g.:
  –1 = fully awake.
  –2 = conscious but drowsy.
  –3 = unconscious but responsive to pain with purposeful movement, e.g. flexion.
  –4 = unconscious; responds to pain with extension.
  –5 = unconscious with no response to pain.
- Other data, e.g. from eye reflexes, are ignored; hence more complex or specific scoring systems are used, e.g.:
  –**Glasgow Coma Scale**.
  –for specific conditions, e.g. **hepatic failure**, **subarachnoid haemorrhage**.

Committee on Safety of Medicines (CSM). Advisory body, originally set up as the Committee on Safety of Drugs in 1963 after the thalidomide disaster. Became the CSM in 1971 when the Medicines Act became law. Grants certificates to new drugs before **clinical trials** may proceed, and product licences (usually lasting 5 years) before marketing is allowed. Also monitors postmarketing safety.
See also, Adverse drug reactions; Drug development

Competition, drug, *see Antagonist; Dose–response curves*

Complement. Term describing a series of plasma proteins (labelled C1–C9), synthesized in the liver and involved in immunological and inflammatory reactions. Activation of the system causes a cascade, amplifying the initial stimulus.

- Pathways (Fig. 38):
  –classical (discovered first):
    –activated by immunological reactions, i.e. requires prior exposure to antigen, although it may follow prior exposure to a cross-reacting antigen.
    –antibody–antigen complex binds to C1.
    –via C4, C2 and C3, forming a complex which activates C5.
  –alternative:
    –activated by aggregated IgA, infections, or spontaneous reaction.
    –via other factors: B, D and H forming a complex activating C5.
    –may amplify itself or the classical pathway via C3b formation.
  –lytic:
    –activated by products of the above pathways, causing C5 to form C5a and C5b. The latter binds to the target membrane.
    –C5b binding in turn by C6, C7, C8 and C9.
    –the resultant complex causes membrane lysis.
- In addition, activated factors produced during all pathways may:
  –bind to **mast cells** and basophils, causing degranulation.
  –be chemotactic for phagocytes, aiding phagocytosis.

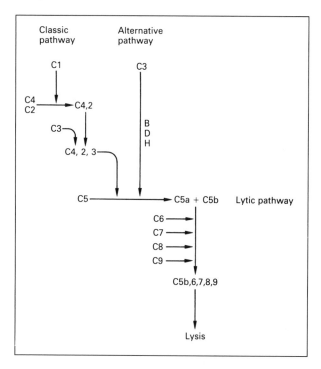

Figure 38 *Complement system*

–cause vasodilatation and increase capillary permeability. Complement activation may be involved in many disease processes. IgM and IgG both bind complement, and are involved in hypersensitivity reactions, e.g. **adverse drug reactions**. **Althesin** may cause either classical or alternative pathway activation. Assays for individual components may assist determination of the pathways involved; e.g. low levels of C4 indicate classical pathway activation, etc.
Williams LW, Burks AW, Steel RW (1988) Ann Allergy; 60: 293–300

Compliance. Volume change per unit pressure change; thus a measure of distensibility, e.g. of lungs, chest wall, heart, etc. For measurement of lung compliance, transmural pressure is required; i.e. the difference between alveolar and **intrapleural pressures**. The former is measured at the mouth during periods of no gas flow, e.g. with the lungs held partially inflated and a few seconds allowed for stabilization, or using a shutter at the mouth to interrupt flow momentarily. Intrapleural pressure is measured using a balloon positioned in the lower third of the oesophagus. The resulting pressure/volume curve is approximately linear at normal tidal volumes (Fig. 39). Different curves are measured during lung inflation and deflation (hysteresis); this is thought to represent the effects of **surface tension**.

Human lung compliance is about 1.5–2 l/kPa (150–200 ml/cmH$_2$O); reduced when supine because of decreased **FRC**. Chest wall compliance is thought to be similar, but measurement is difficult because of the effects of respiratory muscles. Total thoracic compliance requires measurement of alveolar and ambient pressure difference, and equals about 0.85 l/kPa (85 ml/cmH$_2$O).

- Compliance measurements are related thus:

$$\frac{1}{\text{total thoracic}} = \frac{1}{\text{chest wall}} + \frac{1}{\text{lung}}$$

- Lung compliance is divided into two components:
  –static; i.e. alveolar 'stretchability'; measured at steady state as above.
  –dynamic; related to **airway resistance** during equilibration of gases throughout the lung at end-inspiration or expiration.
  Time constant (resistance × compliance) is a reflection of combined static and dynamic compliance.

Compliance is related to body size; thus specific compliance is often referred to (compliance divided by FRC). It increases in old age and emphysema, due to destruction of elastic lung tissue. It is reduced in pulmonary fibrosis, vascular engorgement and oedema; dynamic compliance is decreased in chronic bronchitis. It is also reduced at the extremes of lung volume, as well as at the lung apices and bases in erect subjects.
See also, Breathing, work of

Complications of anaesthesia, *see Anaesthetic morbidity and mortality*

Compressed spectral array, *see Power spectrum analysis*

Computed axial tomography (CAT scanning; CT scanning). Imaging technique in which an X-ray source and detector are held opposite each other, with the patient midway between. The source and detector are rotated stepwise about the mid-point, thus scanning the patient from different angles. At each step, the amount of X-rays reaching the detector is measured, and the spatial arrangement of structures within the patient 'slice' computed and displayed on a screen. Used initially for brain scanning, now for all parts of the body. Used primarily for detection of malignancy, it has also been used to investigate **ischaemic heart disease**, to identify regions of **MI**, and for cinematographic angiography using contrast media.

Patients must remain still during scanning, and may require sedation or general anaesthesia, e.g. children and patients with **head injury**. Choice of techniques and drugs is dictated by the patient's condition; monitoring and maintenance of the airway are particular concerns. Management is similar to that for **radiotherapy**.
See also, Radiology, anaesthesia for

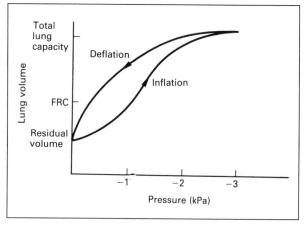

Figure 39 *Pressure/volume curve of lung*

Computers. Increasingly used in research and clinical settings, e.g.:
- data handling:
  - input of data by hand or directly from monitors, etc.
  - analysis and derivation of data, e.g. **ECG** analysis, **cerebral function monitoring**, **cardiac output measurement**.
  - display of information, e.g. on screen, paper, to disk, etc. Trends over different time scales, selection of data, etc., are easily produced.
  - statistical analysis and **audit**.
  - determining models, e.g. for **pharmacokinetics**, to predict drug behaviour.
- control systems:
  - gas flows, volatile agent injection into gas streams, etc.
  - closed loop systems: continuous feedback of information regarding a variable to the controlling device, which maintains steady state by adjusting an effector mechanism (e.g. computer-controlled infusion of **sodium nitroprusside** in the treatment of hypertension).
- decision making:
  - diagnostic.
  - teaching.
  - patient management, e.g. use of expert systems, risk analysis of treatment options, etc.

Zissos A, Strunin L (1985) Can Anaesth Soc J; 32: 374–84

COMT, *see Catechol-O-methyl transferase*

Concentration effect. Increased rate of uptake of **inhalational anaesthetic agent** as inspired concentration increases. The effect of lowering of alveolar concentration caused by absorption of agent from the alveoli is thus minimized.

Conductance. Reciprocal of **resistance**. For electrical circuits, the SI **unit** is the siemens. The term is often used to describe the permeability of cell **membranes** to various ions.
[Sir William Siemens (1823–1883), German-born English engineer]

Confidence intervals. Range of values derived from sample data, relating the data to the actual population. 95% confidence intervals contain the true (population) value with a **probability** (*P* value) of 0.05.
- When used to express the results of **statistical tests**, confidence intervals differ from **null hypothesis** testing thus:
  - null hypothesis testing indicates whether a difference in data is statistically significant (i.e. unlikely to be due to chance alone); the significance is expressed as a *P* value.
  - confidence intervals indicate the likely magnitude of such a difference, by giving a range within which the true value lies. By using the same units as the data, they allow estimations of clinical relevance to be made; for example, a statistically very significant result may be clinically irrelevant if the actual differences involved are very small.

Confidence intervals are wide if the sample size is small or **standard deviation** is large. If zero lies within the interval, this denotes that an increase or decrease may occur; a narrow band that does not include zero thus indicates a very significant result.
See also, Statistical significance

Confidential Enquiries into Maternal Deaths, Report on. Report into all maternal deaths in the UK (Scotland and Northern Ireland were excluded until 1985). Published three-yearly by the Department of Health, and first produced in 1952. Originally produced by the Royal College of Obstetricians and Gynaecologists in the 1930s. Analyses the causes of death during pregnancy and up to 42 days after delivery or termination; a newer section looks at late deaths (up to a year). Details of case reports are collected by District Medical Officers, who collect information from all involved medical staff, observing strict confidentiality. Regional and central assessors categorize the deaths according to cause. Anaesthesia has been a consistent cause of death, ranking third after hypertensive disease of pregnancy and **PE** in several previous reports, but sixth in the latest report after hypertensive disease, PE, ectopic pregnancy, **amniotic fluid embolism** and haemorrhage (Table 12).

Table 12. Report on Confidential Enquiries into Maternal Deaths

Period	No. deaths directly due to anaesthesia	Maternal deaths due to anaesthesia (%)	Deaths/million pregnancies due to anaesthesia
1970–72	37	10.8	12.8
1973–75	27	11.9	10.5
1976–78	27	12.4	12.1
1979–81	22	12.4	8.7
1982–84	18	13.0	7.2
1985–87	6	4.4	1.9

Improvements in anaesthetic mortality are thought to reflect better training and facilities, and are likely to be greater than suggested by the above figures, since the number of anaesthetic procedures performed has markedly increased. Most anaesthetic deaths involve inexperienced anaesthetists providing emergency anaesthesia for **Caesarean section**. Difficulty with tracheal intubation is the commonest factor, often associated with **aspiration of gastric contents**. In some cases, substandard care is provided, involving inadequate prevention of regurgitation (e.g. cricoid pressure not applied). Inadequate postoperative care has also been noted, including inadequate reversal of neuromuscular blockade associated with long acting neuromuscular blocking drugs, e.g. pancuronium. The need for proper training, facilities and help is repeatedly stressed.
- In the latest (1985–87) report:
  - 6 early plus 2 late deaths directly due to anaesthesia, 7 involving Caesarean section and 5 involving oesophageal intubation.
  - 1 aspiration of gastric contents.
  - 1 cardiovascular collapse following extradural anaesthesia in congenital heart disease.

Thomas TA (1991) Curr Opin Anaesth; 4: 325–8
See also, Audit; Obstetric analgesia and anaesthesia

Confidential Enquiry into Perioperative Deaths

(CEPOD). Study commissioned by the **Association of Anaesthetists of Great Britain and Ireland**, together with the Association of Surgeons of Great Britain and Ireland, and published in 1987.

- Main points:
  - the first UK study to involve both anaesthetists and surgeons.
  - analysed all NHS deaths in three Regions, occurring within 30 days of surgery during 1986, excluding obstetric and cardiac surgery.
  - 4034 deaths were reported, in over half a million operations (mortality rate 0.7%).
  - 2391 deaths had forms returned by both anaesthetists and surgeons.
  - most deaths occurred in elderly patients, due to progression of disease.
  - anaesthesia was partially responsible for 1 death per 1300 and totally responsible for 1 in 185 000.
  - surgery was partially responsible for 1 death per 660 and totally responsible for 1 in 2800.
  - many deaths involved junior anaesthetists and surgeons proceeding with cases without consultation with seniors. Time was not always allowed for adequate resuscitation, and surgery was not always appropriate or timely. Some surgeons operated outside their speciality.
  - joint anaesthetic and surgical morbidity/mortality studies were rare.

Recommendations were mainly directed towards the last two points.

A national version (NCEPOD) was started in 1988, aimed at investigating 6000 deaths per year (estimated as 1 in 5). Other medical bodies were also involved, and some independent hospitals were included. Its first year focused on children under 10 years. Most deaths occurred in children with severe congenital malformations, trauma or malignancy. General care was good. The need for specialist experience, and proper supervision and training, was reinforced.

The NCEPOD report for 1990 was published in 1992, and studied in detail more than 2000 out of the 18 817 deaths reported (excluding maternal deaths and those in children under 10). Forms were not completed in 20% of cases. The report drew similar conclusions to the 1987 report, with particular emphasis on deficiencies in **record-keeping**, inadequate provision of essential services such as ICUs, HDUs and recovery care, inadequate supervision of junior doctors and locums, and poor use of post-mortem examination. Cover of split sites was condemned, and a dedicated emergency operating theatre strongly suggested.
Graham SG (1992) Br J Anaesth; 69: 431–2

See also, Audit

Confusion, postoperative.
Common during emergence from anaesthesia, even in young fit patients.

- Possible causes include:
  - drugs: any, especially depressant drugs, **ketamine**, and those associated with the **central anticholinergic syndrome**.
  - **hypoxaemia, hypercapnia**.
  - **hypotension**.
  - restlessness due to pain or full bladder.
  - reduced **cerebral blood flow** resulting from peroperative **hyperventilation** (especially in the elderly) has been suggested as a cause.
  - metabolic disturbances, e.g. **hypoglycaemia, hypernatraemia, hyponatraemia, acidosis**, etc.
  - **alcohol** and **benzodiazepine** withdrawal.
  - **septicaemia**.
  - intracranial problems, e.g. raised **ICP, CVA**, post-ictal state, etc.
  - pre-existing confusion.

Confusion within a few days of surgery may be caused by any illness, e.g. sepsis, pulmonary disease, etc., especially in the elderly. Appropriate investigation, e.g. blood gas analysis, should be performed, rather than simply administering sedation, which may exacerbate the confusion. Many old patients are confused with a change of environment, i.e. hospitalization. Long-term decreases in intellectual function are thought to be possible, particularly in the elderly.

Congenital heart disease.
Incidence: up to 1% of live births; 15% survive to adulthood without treatment. May be associated with other congenital defects or syndromes.

- Simple classification:
  - acyanotic (no **shunt**):
    - **coarctation of aorta** (5–10%).
    - pulmonary and **aortic stenosis** (10–15% together).
  - potentially cyanotic, i.e. left to right shunt; may reverse if **pulmonary hypertension** develops (**Eisenmenger's syndrome**):
    - **ASD** (10–15%).
    - **VSD** (20–30%).
    - patent **ductus arteriosus** (10–15%).
  - cyanotic, due to:
    - right to left shunt:
      - **Fallot's tetralogy** (5–10%).
      - pulmonary atresia with septal defect.
      - **tricuspid valve lesions** including **Ebstein's anomaly**, with septal defect.
    - abnormal connections:
      - **transposition of the great arteries** (5%).
      - anomalous systemic or pulmonary venous drainage, the latter with right to left shunt.
    - mixing of systemic and pulmonary blood, e.g. single atrium or ventricle.

Common features include feeding difficulty, failure to thrive, **cyanosis, dyspnoea, heart murmurs** and **cardiac failure**. Patients may present soon after birth. Investigation includes **echocardiography** and **cardiac catheterization**. Increased risk of surgery within first year of life is offset by the high mortality without surgery. Palliative procedures are sometimes performed early, with later corrective surgery, e.g.:
  - pulmonary balloon valvuloplasty in pulmonary stenosis.
  - shunt procedures to increase pulmonary blood flow in severe right to left shunt, e.g Fallot's tetralogy. A prosthetic graft is inserted between the subclavian and pulmonary arteries (formerly involved direct anastamosis of the subclavian artery itself (Blalock-Taussig procedure)). Balloon atrial septostomy is sometimes performed in transposition of the great arteries, to allow oxygenated blood to pass from left to right sides of heart.
  - pulmonary banding to reduce pulmonary blood flow and prevent pulmonary hypertension in large left to right shunts.

Principles of anaesthesia are as for **cardiac surgery** and **paediatric anaesthesia**. Inhalational or iv techniques are suitable. Uptake of inhalational agents is slower when right to left shunts exist. **Ketamine** is preferred by some anaesthetists. Air bubbles in iv lines are particularly hazardous in right to left shunts, with risk of systemic embolism. Nasal tracheal tubes are preferred when postoperative IPPV is required.

- Antibiotic prophylaxis is given for invasive procedures in patients with congenital heart disease (or prosthetic heart valves) to prevent **endocarditis**; UK guidelines:
  - dental (local anaesthesia):
    - amoxycillin 3 g orally 1 hour preoperatively (erythromycin stearate 1.5 g instead, if allergic to penicillin, followed by 500 mg 6 hours later).
    - if previous endocarditis, treat as below.
  - dental (general anaesthesia):
    - amoxycillin 3 g orally 4 hours preoperatively, and 3 g as soon as possible postoperatively, or:
    - amoxycillin 1 g im before induction, and 500 mg orally 6 hours later.
    - if prosthetic valve or previous endocarditis: amoxycillin 1 g and gentamicin 1.5 mg/kg im before induction. Oral amoxycillin 500 mg 6 hours later (vancomycin 1 g iv over 1 hour, then gentamicin 1.5 mg/kg before induction, if allergic to penicillin),
  - genitourinary/colonic surgery: as for high risk dental.

[Alfred Blalock (1899–1964), US surgeon; Helen Taussig (1898–1986), US physician]
See also, Preoperative assessment; Pulmonary valve lesions; Valvular heart disease

Congestive cardiac failure, *see Cardiac failure*

Coning. Herniation of central **brain** structures caused by raised **ICP**. Often occurs acutely, e.g. due to rapidly expanding supratentorial lesions and **cerebral oedema**, or following lumbar puncture in their presence. **Brainstem** herniation is accompanied by disruption of its blood supply causing infarction and further swelling.
- Features:
  - initially **decorticate posture**, then **decerebrate posture**, eventually flaccid paralysis (i.e. flexor response of arms, then extensor response, then no response).
  - **pupils** become fixed and central.
  - **Cheyne–Stokes respiration** may progress to hyperventilation followed by gasping and apnoea.
  - hypertension and bradycardia (**Cushing's reflex**) may be followed by tachycardia, bradycardia or hypotension as the brainstem regulatory centres are compressed.

Conjoined twins. Incidence is about 1 in 200 000 births. Radiological assessment may require repeat anaesthesia. Each twin requires a separate anaesthetic team. Tracheal intubation and access may be difficult, depending on the site of union. If circulation is shared, induction of the first twin may be delayed, as anaesthetic drugs are taken up by the second twin. Induction of the second twin may thus be rapid. Blood loss at separation may be massive. Adrenal insufficiency may be present in one twin.
Roy M (1984) Anaesthesia; 39: 1225–8

Connective tissue diseases. Group of diseases sharing certain features, particularly inflammation of connective tissue and features of **autoimmune disease**. **Rheumatoid arthritis** is the most common, and is considered separately. Rheumatoid arthritis, systemic lupus erythematosus (SLE) and systemic sclerosis (SS) are more common in women. Polyarteritis nodosa (PN) is more common in men.
- Features may include the following:
  - autoimmune involvement: immunoglobulins may be directed against IgG (rheumatoid factors) and cell components, e.g. nuclear proteins, phospholipids, etc. Organ specific antibodies are also common, e.g. against thyroid and gastric parietal cells, smooth muscle and mitochondria. T and B cell dysfunction, immune complex deposition and **complement** activation may also occur. Diagnosis of specific disease is aided by the pattern of immune disturbance.
  - systemic involvement:
    - musculoskeletal: arthropathy, myopathy.
    - skin: rash, mouth ulcers. Thickening in SS, with characteristic pinched mouth.
    - renal: glomerulonephritis, vasculitis, nephrotic syndrome.
    - fever, malaise.
    - cardiovascular: **pericarditis**, myocarditis, conduction defects, vasculitis (affecting any organ). Raynaud's phenomenon (fingers turn white, then blue then red on exposure to cold, stress, vibration, etc.) is common. **Pulmonary hypertension** may occur.
    - haematological: **anaemia**, leucopenia, **thrombocytopenia**. Lupus anticoagulant may be present in SLE: it may prolong **coagulation**, especially the intrinsic pathway. Risk of bleeding is not increased if other factors and platelets are normal, but risk of thrombosis is increased, possibly via inhibition of **prostacyclin** production and **platelet** aggregation.
    - hepatosplenomegaly.
    - central and peripheral nervous involvement, e.g. central lesions, neuropathies and psychiatric disturbances (especially with SLE).
    - pulmonary: fibrosis, pleurisy, pleural effusions and pulmonary infiltrates. Haemorrhage with PN.
    - Sjögren's syndrome (reduced tear and saliva formation and secretion) may occur.
    - GIT: reduced oesophageal motility, oesophagitis and risk of regurgitation, especially in SS (CREST syndrome = calcinosis, Raynaud's phenomenon, (o)esophagitis, sclerodactyly, telectangasia).

Treatment includes **steroid therapy** and other **immunosuppressive drugs**. Antimalarials are used in SLE.
- Anaesthetic considerations:
  - careful **preoperative assessment** to identify the above features, complications and drugs, with appropriate management.
  - mouth opening may be difficult in SS.
  - general management: as for rheumatoid arthritis.

Other conditions without circulating rheumatoid factors may have systemic manifestations, e.g. **ankylosing spondylitis** and associated conditions. Arthritis may accompany inflammatory bowel disease and intestinal infection.
[Maurice Raynaud (1834–1881), French physician; Henrik Sjögren, Swedish ophthalmologist]

Connectors, tracheal tube. Adaptors for connecting **tracheal tubes** to **anaesthetic breathing systems** (Fig. 40). Modern connectors are plastic, and 15 mm in size distally.

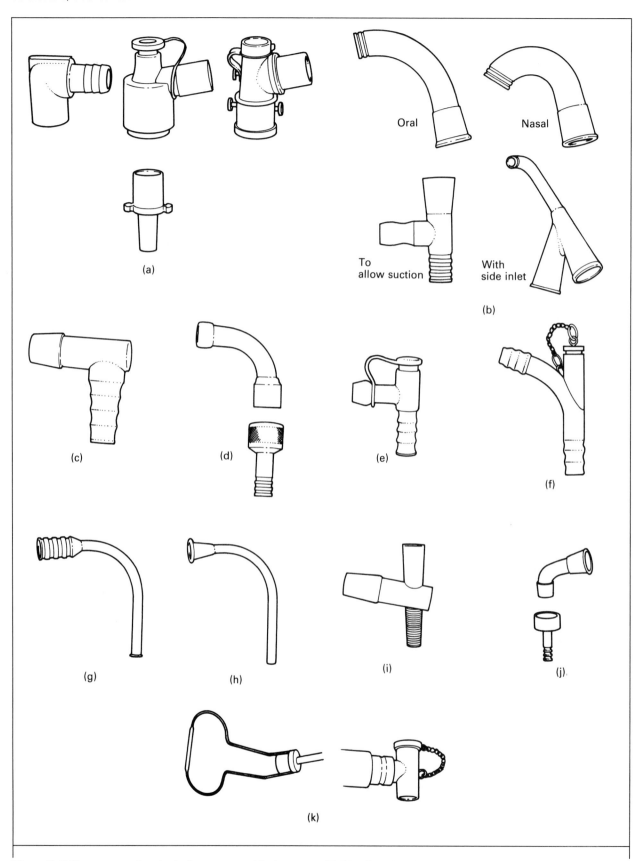

Figure 40 *Different types of tracheal tube connector: (a) plastic type; (b) Magill; (c) Rowbotham; (d) Nosworthy; (e) Cobb; (f) Rink; (g) Worcester; (h) Doughty; (i) Cardiff paediatric; (j) Knight paediatric; (k) Tunstall*

They fit to any standardized 15/22 mm equipment, e.g. directly to breathing tubing or to **catheter mounts**. They may connect directly or via angle pieces, which may swivel. Some incorporate a capped port for tracheo-bronchial suction, insertion of fibreoptic instruments, etc.

• Other types are less widely used now, and named after the anaesthetists who described them or where they were developed:

  –**Magill**: various types.
  –**Rowbotham**.
  –Nosworthy: pushed together and twisted to lock.
  –Cobb: allows tracheobronchial suction.
  –Rink: curved to reduce turbulence.
  –Worcester: for tonsillectomy.
  –Doughty: for tonsillectomy.
  –Cardiff paediatric: allows suction.
  –Knight paediatric: similar to Nosworthy's.
  –Tunstall: for infants: the wire portion is taped to the baby's forehead to allow fixation of nasal tubes, e.g. on ICU.

[WA Cobb (described 1943), London anaesthetist; Michael D Nosworthy, Ernest H Rink (1905–1959), Andrew G Doughty and Peter F Knight, London anaesthetists; Michael E Tunstall, Aberdeen anaesthetist]

Conn's syndrome, *see Hyperaldosteronism*

Consent for anaesthesia. Required before general and local anaesthetic techniques may be performed. Failure to obtain consent may result in charges of assault/battery; in addition, inadequate counselling whilst obtaining consent may result in charges of negligence. In the UK, doctors may use their discretion to explain risks and benefits as they feel appropriate for the patient concerned, as long as their decision is judged reasonable according to current medical opinion. In the USA, legally required 'Informed Consent' (i.e. full explanation of risks, benefits and alternatives) is judged according to what a reasonable patient would expect to have explained to him/her.

The patient should be over 16 years (in England) and 'of sound mind', i.e. unaffected by drugs, e.g. premedication. Emergency life-saving surgery, etc. may proceed without consent if the patient is unable to give it, assuming that an average reasonable adult would agree to the procedure. Consent in children is given by their parents or legal guardians, although this may be overruled by the courts. The 'emancipated minor' is a child under the age of majority who is able to understand and therefore make decisions about his/her treatment. Consent in mental illness may be given by the closest relative or an officer of the appropriate institution, rarely by the courts.

• Consent may be:
  –verbal or written. The latter serves as proof of consent afterwards, but is no 'stronger' than verbal consent, which should be witnessed if possible.
  –express or implied (i.e. by allowing treatment, insertion of a cannula, etc., the patient is demonstrating consent, without having specifically expressed it).

Consent forms are now standard for most types of surgery. A separate section for anaesthesia has been suggested, although the ability of junior surgeons (who usually obtain consent) to inform the patient adequately in this respect has led to some controversy. There is disagreement about the requirement for consent forms in other procedures; e.g. extradural analgesia in labour requires written consent only in some UK units.

Palmer RN (1988) Anaesthesia; 43: 265–6
See also, Medicolegal aspects of anaesthesia

Contamination of anaesthetic equipment. Although hospital acquired infection is common and sometimes fatal, the role of cross-infection involving anaesthetic equipment is uncertain. The incidence of postoperative respiratory infection is unaffected by the use of sterile disposable breathing systems and bacterial filters. Routine treatment of anaesthetic apparatus varies between hospitals, e.g. breathing systems cleaned or sterilized after each case, daily, weekly, etc. Disposable equipment is increasingly used for convenience and cheapness.

Particularly important in **ICU**, **immunodeficiency** states, and in high risk infectious cases, e.g. **HIV infection**, **hepatitis**, **chest infection**, **TB** (equipment is sterilized after use and other precautions taken, e.g. bacterial filters).

• Methods of killing contaminating organisms:
  –disinfection: kills most organisms but not spores, etc.
    –pasteurization: 20 minutes at 70°C;
        10 minutes at 80°C.
        5 minutes at 100°C.
    Rubber/plastic items may be distorted.
    –chemical agents:
      –formaldehyde, formalin.
      –alcohol 70%.
      –chlorhexidine 0.1–0.5%.
      –gluteraldehyde 2%: expensive and may irritate skin.
      –hypochlorite 10%: may corrode metal.
      –hydrogen peroxide, phenol.
    Must be followed by rinsing and thorough drying.
  –sterilization: kills all organisms and spores.
    –dry heat, e.g. 150°C for 30 minutes.
    –moist heat:
      –autoclave (most common method), e.g.:
        –30 minutes at 1 atm at 122°C;
        –10 minutes at 1.5 atm at 126°C;
        –3 minutes at 2 atm at 134°C.
      Steam is used to increase temperature. Indicator tape or tubes are used to confirm that the correct conditions are reached.
      –low temperature steam + formaldehyde.
    –ethylene oxide: expensive and flammable (the latter risk is reduced by adding 80–90% fluorohydrocarbons or CO_2). Toxic and taken up by plastics; up to 2 weeks elution time is suggested before use.
    –γ-irradiation: used commercially but expensive and inconvenient for most hospital use.

[Louis Pasteur (1822–1895), French bacteriologist]
Lumley J (1976) Br J Anaesth; 48: 3–8
See also, COSHH regulations

Continuous positive airway pressure (CPAP). Application of positive airway pressure throughout all phases of spontaneous ventilation. May be achieved with various systems, applied via a tightly-fitting mask or tracheal tube. In order to apply positive pressure throughout ventilation, a reservoir bag, or a fresh gas flow exceeding maximal inspiratory gas flow, must be provided. The latter may be achieved using a **Venturi** mixing device. Increases **FRC**, thereby reducing airway collapse and increasing arterial oxygenation. F_IO_2 may thus be reduced.

- Uses:
  - –to aid **weaning from ventilators**.
  - –to improve oxygenation during **one-lung anaesthesia**.
  - –in conditions of chronic airway collapse and hypoventilation, e.g. **alveolar hypoventilation syndrome**.
  - –in neonates, e.g. in **respiratory distress syndrome**, bronchomalacia and tracheomalacia, especially if associated with apnoeic episodes. May be applied via nasal cannulae.
- Complications: as for PEEP, but less severe. **Barotrauma** and reduction in cardiac output are more likely in neonates. Some patients cannot tolerate the sensation of CPAP.

Nasal CPAP, using a tightly-fitting nasal mask, has been used in obstructive **sleep apnoea**.

Duncan AW, Oh TE, Hillman DR (1986) Anaesth Intensive Care; 14: 236–50

Contraceptives, oral. Main anaesthetic considerations are related to the increased risk of perioperative **DVT**, especially with pills with a high oestrogen content (although less commonly used now). Other risk factors, e.g. **smoking**, **obesity**, etc., increase the risk further. Discontinuation of therapy before major or leg surgery is advocated by most practitioners; 1–3 months have been suggested. For urgent and emergency surgery, perioperative prophylactic sc **heparin** therapy is usually used. In view of the risk of pregnancy, sc heparin has been suggested as a routine alternative to drug discontinuation. The pill is restarted after the first period beyond a fortnight postoperatively. No extra precautions are thought to be necessary for minor surgery, e.g. dilatation and curettage, or with oestrogen-free therapy.

Whitehead EM, Whitehead MI (1991) Anaesthesia 46; 521–2

Contrast media, *see Radiological contrast media*

Controlled drugs, *see Misuse of Drugs Act*

Convulsions (Fits). Usually refer to clonic-tonic epileptic seizures. They increase cerebral and whole body O_2 demand and CO_2 production, whilst **airway obstruction** and chest wall rigidity may result in **hypoventilation**. Thus **hypoxaemia**, **acidosis**, **hypercapnia** and increased sympathetic activity may occur. Patients may also injure themselves. Fits may be generalized or focal. Anaesthetic involvement is usually necessary when they occur perioperatively, or in **status epilepticus**.

- Caused by:
  - –pre-existing **epilepsy** (i.e. a continuing susceptibiltiy to fits; may include other causes listed below).
  - –hypoxaemia.
  - –metabolic, e.g. **hypoglycaemia**, **hypocalcaemia**, **uraemia**.
  - –anaesthetic drugs:
    - –**diethyl ether**; convulsions classically occurred postoperatively in pyrexial children given anticholinergic premedication on hot days.
    - –**enflurane** especially following peroperative **hyperventilation** and **hypocapnia**.
    - –**ketamine**, **methohexitone** and **doxapram** in susceptible patients. **Propofol** has been implicated. Non-epileptogenic myoclonic activity may occur with **etomidate**; its role in causing convulsions has been disputed.
    - –**local anaesthetic drugs** in overdose.
    - –**pethidine** in very high dosage. Convulsions may also follow its interaction with **monoamine oxidase inhibitors**.
  - –other drugs, e.g. **alcohol**, **phenothiazines**, **tricyclic antidepressant drugs**. Several drugs in overdose.
  - –**fat embolism**, also clot or **air embolism**.
  - –**head injury**, **CVA**, cerebral infections, **meningitis**, **neurosurgery**, brain tumours and other cerebral disease.
  - –**eclampsia**.
  - –pyrexia in children.
  - –acute O_2 **toxicity** (**Bert effect**).
- Management:
  - –protection of the airway and maintenance of oxygenation, with positioning on the side if possible. Tracheal intubation and IPPV may be required, e.g. if large amounts of depressant drugs are needed.
  - –**anticonvulsant drugs**:
    - –**diazepam** 5 mg increments iv up to 20–30 mg; may be given rectally. **Midazolam** 5–15 mg im has been used as an alternative when iv cannulation is impossible.
    - –**phenytoin** iv, 13–15 mg/kg slowly, with ECG monitoring.
    - –**sodium valproate** iv, 5–10 mg/kg slowly.
    - –**chlormethiazole** iv, 40–100 ml 0.8% solution over 5 minutes, followed by 0.5–1.0 ml/min.
    - –**thiopentone** 2–3 mg/kg/h if convulsions persist. Very high doses may be required to achieve burst supression on the EEG. Recovery may be prolonged.
  - –other drugs include **clonezapam** 1 mg over 30 seconds iv, **paraldehyde** 5–10 ml im, and **magnesium sulphate** (in eclampsia).

See also, Status epilepticus

Cooley, Samuel, *see Wells*

COPD, Chronic obstructive pulmonary disease, *see Chronic obstructive airways disease*

Copper kettle, *see Vaporizers*

Cordotomy, anterolateral. Destruction of ascending spinothalamic tracts, classically in the cervical region (C1–2); used in chronic **pain management**. Usually performed percutaneously under X-ray control, using **sedation**. Electrical stimulation is used to confirm correct positioning of the needle before thermocoagulation.

Provides contralateral analgesia lasting up to 3 years; thus it is usually reserved for patients with a life expectancy below this, e.g. patients with malignancy. Descending respiratory fibres lie close to the sectioned fibres and therefore cordotomy is usually not performed in patients with respiratory disease. May damage pyramidal pathways, or cause **Horner's syndrome**, bladder disturbances and parasthesiae. Complications are more likely if cordotomy is bilateral.

See also, Sensory pathways

Corning, James Leonard (1855–1923). New York neurologist; first described (and coined the term) **spinal anaesthesia** in 1885. He had intended to observe the effects of **cocaine** on the spinal cord by injecting it into the interspinal space of a dog, believing erroneously that the interspinal blood vessels communicated with those of the cord. Hindquarter paralysis and anaesthesia followed. Repeated the experiment on a human, and subsequently suggested its use in the treatment of neurological disease. **Extradural anaesthesia** may have been produced in some of his studies. Published the first textbook on local anaesthesia in 1886.

Coronary angioplasty, *see Percutaneous transluminal coronary angioplasty*

Coronary artery bypass graft (CABG). Performed for **ischaemic heart disease** unresponsive to medical treatment (including unstable angina). Saphenous vein grafts were first performed in 1967. Sections of the long saphenous vein in the leg are removed, reversed (because of valves) and anastamosed between the aorta and coronary artery distal to its obstruction. Internal thoracic (internal mammary) artery grafting was first performed in man in the 1950s but discarded until its revival in the 1970s. Following dissection from the posterior surface of the anterior thoracic cage, the artery is anastomosed to the coronary artery. Results are better than saphenous vein grafting because prolonged patency is more likely, but the incidence of perioperative bleeding is greater.

- Life expectancy following CABG is improved in:
  - moderate/severe angina, triple vessel disease and impaired ventricular function.
  - double vessel disease including severe stenosis of the proximal left anterior descending artery.
  - severe stenosis of the left main stem coronary artery.
  Life expectancy is not improved in single vessel disease or if angina is not present.

Percutaneous transluminal coronary angioplasty is an alternative but emergency CABG may be required if unsuccessful.

Anaesthesia is as for ischaemic heart disease and **cardiac surgery**. Combinations of **aspirin**, **dipyridamole** and full anticoagulation are used postoperatively to maintain graft patency.

Mortality is under 1% for 1–2 grafts, but increases if more grafts are anastomosed. Mortality is greater in women.

Streisand JB, Wong KC (1988) Br J Anaesth; 61: 97–104

Coronary artery disease, *see Ischaemic heart disease*

Coronary blood flow. Normally approximately 5% of **cardiac output**, i.e. 250 ml/min or 80 ml/100 g/min. May increase up to five times in exercise. The inner 1 mm of the left ventricle obtains O_2 via diffusion from blood in the ventricular cavity; the remainder of the ventricle is supplied via epicardial vessels. The left coronary vessels are compressed by the contracting myocardium during systole; thus flow to the subendocardium occurs during diastole only. Superficial areas recieve more constant flow. Atrial and right ventricular flow occurs throught the **cardiac cycle**. The left ventricle is therefore most at risk from **myocardial ischaemia**.

- Left ventricular blood **flow** is related to:
  - difference between aortic end-diastolic pressure and **left ventricular end-diastolic pressure**.
  - duration of diastole (inversely related to **heart rate**).
  - patency/radius of the coronary arteries; related to:

- **autoregulation**: normally maintains blood flow, possibly via the action of adenine nucleotides, **potassium**, **hydrogen ions**, **prostaglandins**, lactic acid or CO_2 released from myocardial cells.
  - autonomic neural input: has little direct influence, being overridden by the effect on **SVR**, **myocardial contractility**, etc.
  - coronary stenosis/spasm and the state of collateral vessels (e.g. **coronary steal**).
  - drugs causing vasoconstriction/dilatation.
- blood **viscosity**.

The balance between flow and myocardial O_2 demand is important to prevent ischaemia. Reductions in flow may be minimized by controlling the above factors. Coronary perfusion pressure and duration of diastole may be assessed by the **diastolic pressure–time index**.

- Measurement:
  - **Fick principle** using N_2O or argon. Requires **coronary sinus catheterization**.
  - thermodilution techniques to estimate coronary sinus flow, thus providing an indication of left ventricular drainage.
  - **nuclear cardiology** may be used to indicate regional flow.

Sethna DH, Moffitt EA (1986) Anesth Analg; 65: 294–304 and 395–410

See also, Coronary circulation; Ischaemic heart disease; Myocardial metabolism

Coronary care unit (CCU). The first CCUs opened in 1961–63 and evolved from the concept that recovery from collapse following **MI** was possible with prompt **CPR**. Modern CCUs contain ECG monitoring, defibrillators, drugs and trained staff available 24 hours a day. They are used for surveillance and treatment of **arrhythmias** and **cardiac failure**, limitation of infarct size and restoration of blood flow in occluded coronary vessels using **fibrinolytic drugs**. Mortality from MI is thought to be reduced as a result. Now used also for patients without MI.

Anon (1988) Lancet; ii: 830–1

Coronary circulation.
- Arterial supply (Fig. 41a):
  - right coronary artery: arises from the anterior aortic sinus. Passes between the pulmonary trunk and right atrium, and runs in the right atrioventricular groove between the right atrium and ventricle. Descends the anterior surface of the heart, continuing inferiorly to anastamose with the left coronary artery. Supplies the right ventricle and sinoatrial node and, in 90% of the population, the atrioventricular node and posterior and inferior parts of the left ventricle.
  - left coronary artery: arises from the left posterior aortic sinus. Passes lateral to the pulmonary trunk and runs in the left atrioventricular groove. Supplies the anterior wall of the left ventricle and the interventricular septum via its left anterior descending branch, and the lateral wall of the left ventricle via its circumflex branch.
- Venous drainage (Fig. 41b):
  - ⅓ via small veins directly into the right atrium (venae cordis minimae (Thebesian veins) and anterior cardiac veins).
  - ⅔ via the coronary sinus, draining into the right atrium by the opening of the inferior vena cava.

[Adam Thebesius (1686–1732), German physician]

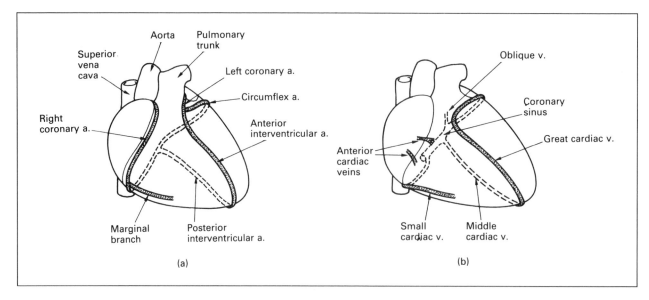

Figure 41 *Coronary circulation: (a) arterial; (b) venous*

Sethna DH, Moffitt EA (1986) Anesth Analg; 65: 294–305 and 395–410
See also, Coronary blood flow

Coronary sinus catheterization. Performed using fluoroscopy. May be used to determine:
- –coronary sinus blood flow, using a thermodilution technique.
- –**coronary blood flow**, using the **Fick principle**.
- –blood O_2 and **lactate** levels. The latter are raised in **myocardial ischaemia**, due to decreased uptake by myocardial tissue and increased production.

Coronary steal. Diversion of blood from poorly perfused areas of myocardium to those already adequately perfused. May be caused by vasodilator substances acting on small coronary arteries but not on larger epicardial vessels. Poorly perfused areas supplied by stenosed vessels may be dependent on collateral vessels for blood flow. Dilatation of normal small arteries increases flow to normal areas, but the stenosed vessels are unable to dilate sufficiently, resulting in steal. Antianginal drugs, e.g. nitrates, are thought to increase collateral flow by acting predominantly on the large epicardial vessels. **Adenosine, dipyridamole, papaverine** and **isoflurane** have all been shown to cause steal. The use of isoflurane in patients with **ischaemic heart disease** has therefore been questioned.
Becker LC (1987) Anesthesiology; 66: 259–61

Cor pulmonale. Right ventricular hypertrophy secondary to increased **pulmonary vascular resistance** due to chronic lung disease. **COAD** is the commonest cause, but any disease that causes chronic **hypoxaemia** (e.g. **pulmonary fibrosis**) may result in **hypoxic pulmonary vasoconstriction**, eventually with pulmonary vascular muscle hypertrophy and **pulmonary hypertension**. Right ventricular failure may ensue. **PE** is included in some definitions.
- Features:
  - –those of the underlying disease, including cyanosis and hypoxaemia.

- –those of right-sided **cardiac failure**: peripheral oedema, raised **JVP**, hepatomegaly, 3rd **heart sound**.
- –of pulmonary hypertension and underlying disease on **chest X-ray**. The **ECG** may show right ventricular hypertrophy and axis deviation, peaked **P waves** (P pulmonale), and **T wave** and **S–T segment** changes in the right chest leads.
- Anaesthetic management:
  - –as for COAD/underlying disease.
  - –as for **cardiac failure**.
  - –as for pulmonary hypertension.

Correlation, *see Statistical tests*

Corticosteroid therapy, *see Steroid therapy*

Corticotrophin, *see Adrenocorticotrophic hormone*

COSHH regulations (Control of Substances Hazardous to Health). Came into force in 1989 in Scotland, England and Wales, and in 1991 in Northern Ireland. Stipulate that employers must identify and control any substances which may be hazardous to health, e.g. chemicals and micro-organisms. Important guidance is given to allow employers to assess the risk to employees, eliminate or control the risk (e.g. with protective clothing, adequate ventilation), monitor the exposure and health of employees, and provide information and training. Employees must make full use of any control measure provided. Anaesthetic implications include concerns about the **environmental safety of anaesthetists, scavenging,** and **contamination of anaesthetic equipment**.
Tar-Ching AW (1989) BMJ; 299: 931–2

Cough. Reflex partially under voluntary control. A deep inspiration is followed by forceful expiration against a closed glottis which is suddenly opened to allow explosive exhalation. An intrathoracic pressure of up to 40 kPa may be produced, and the speed of exhaled air may exceed 900 km/h. Solid objects, liquids and mucus are thus expelled from the airways. Afferent pathways for coughing are from the mucosa of the **larynx**, trachea and large bronchi via the **vagus nerve** and medulla, and are stimulated by physical or chemical irritants.

- Factors associated with coughing during anaesthesia include:
  - –insertion of a pharyngeal **airway**, **tracheal tube**, etc. if depth of anaesthesia is inadequate.
  - –introduction of **inhalational anaesthetic agents** at too high a concentration.
  - –use of certain **iv anaesthetic agents**, e.g. **methohexitone**.
  - –presence/aspiration of blood, saliva, gastric contents, etc.
  - –respiratory disease including upper airway infection.
  - –**smoking**.

If persistent, coughing may cause inadequate ventilation, and excessive intrathoracic pressures may reduce cardiac output (causing 'cough syncope' in non-anaesthetized patients). Deepening of anaesthesia, increased F_1O_2 and neuromuscular blockade may be required.

- The reflex is protective, helping to prevent sputum retention and **atelectasis**. Postoperatively, it may be reduced by:
  - –impaired mechanical movement, e.g. due to pain, muscle weakness, neuromuscular blockade or disease, central and peripheral nervous disorders.
  - –depressed cough reflex, e.g. depressant drugs, central lesions.

Opioid analgesic drugs, e.g. **codeine**, are sometimes used to suppress cough e.g. in malignant disease.

Cough-CPR. Maintenance of cerebral perfusion and consciousness during severe **arrhythmias**, e.g. **VF**, by repeated coughing. Each **cough** increases intrathoracic pressure and expels arterial blood from the thorax; each gasp draws in venous blood. Has been successful for up to 1–2 minutes pending availability of a defibrillator.
See also, Cardiopulmonary resuscitation

Coulomb. Unit of **charge**. One coulomb is the amount of charge passing any point in a circuit in 1 second when a current of 1 **ampere** is flowing.
[Charles Coulomb (1738–1806), French physicist]

CPAP, *see Continuous positive airway pressure*

CPD/CPD-A, Citrate–phosphate–dextrose/Citrate–phosphate–dextrose–adenine, *see Blood storage*

CPR, *see Cardiopulmonary resuscitation*

Cranial nerves. Comprised of 12 pairs, passing from the **brain** via foramina at the base of the **skull**. Convey motor and sensory fibres involved in somatic, parasympathetic (visceral) and special visceral (e.g. muscles of face and taste sensation) pathways:

- –I: olfactory nerves (convey smell sensation from the nasal mucosa); pass through the cribriform plate of the ethmoid bone to the olfactory bulb.
- –II: optic nerve (conveys visual sensation from the retina); passes through the optic canal and via the optic chiasma, tract and radiation to the visual cortex in the occipital lobe of the brain (*see Pupillary reflex*).
- –III: oculomotor nerve (somatic motor fibres supply

the extraocular muscles except superior oblique and lateral rectus; parasympathetic fibres supply the pupillary sphincter and ciliary muscles after synapsing in the ciliary ganglion). In the posterior fossa, the nerve passes from the upper midbrain between the cerebral peduncles and lies near the edge of the tentorium cerebelli (hence the early ipsilateral pupillary dilatation that occurs in acute rises of **ICP**, when the nerve is compressed against the edge of the tentorium (Hutchinson's pupil)). In the middle cranial fossa, it passes forwards on the lateral wall of the cavernous sinus as far as the supraorbital fissure. Before entering the fissure it divides into superior and inferior branches.
- –IV: trochlear nerve (motor supply to the superior oblique muscle). Passes from the dorsum of the lower midbrain, then forwards in the lateral wall of the cavernous sinus to enter the supraorbital fissure.
- –V: trigeminal nerve (sensory fibres supply the anterior dura, scalp and face, nasopharynx, nasal and oral cavities and air sinuses; motor fibres supply the muscles of mastication). The sensory nuclei are in the medulla, midbrain and pons. The nerve passes from the pons to the trigeminal ganglion lateral to the cavernous sinus, where it divides into ophthalmic, maxillary and mandibular divisions. The motor nucleus is in the pons; the root bypasses the ganglion to join the mandibular division.
  - –ophthalmic division (V^1): branches (lacrimal, frontal and nasociliary nerves) pass via the superior orbital fissure. Associated with the ciliary ganglion.
  - –maxillary division (V^2): passes via the foramen rotundum. Associated with the pterygopalatine ganglion. Branches (nasal, nasopalatine, palatine, pharyngeal, zygomatic, posterior superior alveolar and infraorbital nerves) are involved with lacrimation and sensory and sympathetic supply to the nose, nasopharynx, palate and orbit.
  - –mandibular division (V^3): passes via the foramen ovale. Associated with the otic (parotid gland) and submandibular (submandibular and sublingual glands) ganglia. Sensory branches are the meningeal, buccal, auriculotemporal, inferior alveolar and lingual nerves.

  (*See Gasserian ganglion block; Mandibular nerve blocks; Maxillary nerve blocks; Ophthalmic nerve blocks*).
- –VI: abducent nerve (motor supply to the lateral rectus). Passes from the lower pons through the cavernous sinus and supraorbital fissure. Often involved in injury to the skull.
- –VII: facial nerve (mixed sensory and motor nerve): passes laterally from the lower pons through the internal acoustic meatus to the geniculate ganglion. Passes through the temporal bone to emerge through the stylomastoid foramen. Runs forward to the parotid gland. Branches:
  - –motor supply to the muscles of facial expression: divides within the parotid gland into temporal, zygomatic, buccal, mandibular and cervical branches from above down. Branches also pass to the digastric, stylohyoid, auricular and occipital muscles.
  - –greater petrosal nerve: passes from the geniculate ganglion to the pterygopalatine ganglion and fossa, to supply the lacrimal gland.

–chorda tympani: leaves the facial nerve before it enters the stylomastoid foramen; conveys taste sensation from the anterior ⅔ of the **tongue** and parasympathetic fibres to the submandibular gland.

–VIII: vestibulocochlear nerve (special somatic sensory nerve): cochlear and vestibular components are involved in hearing and balance respectively. The nerve is formed in the internal acoustic meatus and passes to nuclei in the floor of the 4th ventricle. Connects centrally with cranial nerves III, IV, VI, XI and descending pathways to the upper cervical cord.

–IX: glossopharyngeal nerve (conveys sensation from the pharynx, back of the tongue and tonsil, middle ear, **carotid sinus** and **carotid body**, taste from the posterior ⅓ of the tongue, and parasympathetic fibres to the parotid gland; provides motor supply to stylopharyngeus). Passes from the medulla through the jugular foramen, and then passes between the internal and external **carotid arteries** to the pharynx.

–X: **vagus nerve** (provides parasympathetic afferent and efferent supply to the heart, lungs, and GIT as far as the splenic flexure, motor supply to the larynx, pharynx and palate, and conveys taste sensation from the valleculae and epiglottis, and sensation from the external ear canal and eardrum). Passes from the medulla via the jugular foramen.

–XI: accessory nerve (motor supply to the sternomastoid and trapezius muscles). Arises from the upper five cervical segments of the spinal cord, passing upwards through the foramen magnum to join the smaller cranial root. Leaves the skull through the jugular foramen; the cranial root joins the vagus (to the pharynx and larynx) and the spinal root passes to the sternomastoid.

–XII: hypoglossal nerve (motor supply to all muscles of the tongue except palatoglossus). Passes from the medulla, then through the hypoglossal canal behind the carotid sheath to the tongue.

• Cranial nerves may be assessed by testing:

–I: ability to smell substances, e.g. peppermint, cloves, etc. Irritant substances are avoided, since they may act via the Vth nerve.

–II:
  –visual acuity using distant objects/charts.
  –visual fields, e.g. ability to discern peripheral movement whilst looking straight ahead. Size of blind spot.
  –appearence of optic discs.
  –pupillary reflex to light and accommodation.

–III, IV, VI: full eye movements without diplopia. Results of specific lower **motor neurone** lesions:
  –III: eye displaced downwards and outwards, pupil dilated, ptosis.
  –IV: downward gaze impaired; eyeball rotated inwards by inferior rectus when attempted.
  –VI: lateral gaze impaired.
  Upper motor neurone lesions may cause impaired conjugate movements.

–V:
  –skin sensation in each division, e.g.:
    –ophthalmic: forehead, corneal reflex (afferent arc V, efferent pathway VII).
    –maxillary: cheek next to nose.
    –mandibular: side of jaw.
  –ability to open/close jaw against resistance.

–VII:
  –facial expression: ability to smile, show teeth, whistle, raise eyebrows, screw up eyes against resistance, blow out cheeks. Movement in the upper part of the face is preserved in upper motor neurone lesions, and lost in lower motor neurone lesions.
  –taste sensation of the anterior tongue, e.g. to salt, sugar, citric acid.

–VIII:
  –ability to hear, e.g. fingers rubbing next to the ear.
  –using a tuning fork: air conduction is lost in middle ear disease, with preservation of bone conduction (Rinne's test). Both are impaired in nerve damage. If the tuning fork is placed on the forehead, the sound is heard best on the affected side in middle ear disease, on the unaffected side in nerve disease (Weber's test).

–IX, X:
  –taste sensation of the posterior tongue.
  –soft palate elevation is equal on both sides.
  –**gag reflex**.
  –voice and phonation.

–XI: ability to raise shoulders, and rotate head to the side, against resistance.

–XII: protrusion of tongue in the midline (to the affected side if abnormal). Absence of wasting and ability to move from side to side.

[Sir Jonathan Hutchinson (1828–1913), English surgeon; Friedrich Rinne (1819–1868) and Friedrich Weber (1832–1891), German otologists]

'Crash induction', *see Induction, rapid sequence*

Creatinine. Basic compound formed mainly in skeletal **muscle** from phosphorylcreatine. The latter is formed from **ATP** and creatine, and is a source of ATP during exercise. Creatinine production remains fairly constant, hence the value of plasma creatinine measurement as a reflection of renal function (cf. **urea**, whose production varies with the amount of protein breakdown occurring). Normal value: 60–130 μmol/l; serial values are more useful indicators of renal function than single measurements. As **GFR** decreases, creatinine levels rise slowly up to about 200 μmol/l (GFR below 40 ml/min), rising greatly thereafter for small decreases of GFR. Thus measurement is less useful at high values, and values above 200 μmol/l represent severe renal impairment.

See also, Creatinine clearance

Creatinine clearance. Clearance of **creatinine**, used as an approximation for **GFR**. Although some creatinine is secreted by renal tubules, this source of error tends to be cancelled out by the overmeasurement of plasma creatinine at low levels. Commonly estimated, since creatinine is easily measured. Usually averaged over 24 hours to reduce error from inaccurate urine volume measurement. Normal value: 90–130 ml/min.

Cremophor EL. Polyoxyethylated castor oil, formed from ethylene oxide and castor oil. Used as an emulsifying agent in preparations of certain drugs. Implicated as causing **adverse drug reactions**, sometimes severe, after iv injection. Has led to the withdrawal of iv induction agents, e.g. **Althesin**, **propanidid** and the original formulation of

propofol, although injectable preparations of other drugs may still contain it (e.g. cyclosporin, miconazole and vitamin K).

Cricoid pressure (Sellick's manoeuvre). Digital pressure against the cricoid cartilage of the **larynx**, pushing it backwards. The oesophagus is thus compressed between the posterior aspect of the cricoid and the **vertebrae** behind. The cricoid cartilage is used since it forms the only complete ring of the larynx and trachea. Cricoid pressure prevents passive regurgitation of gastric and oesophageal contents, e.g. during **induction of anaesthesia**.

The cricoid cartilage is identified level with C6, and the index finger is placed against the cartilage in the midline, with the thumb and middle finger on either side. Moderate pressure may be applied before loss of consciousness, and firmer pressure maintained until the **cuff** of the tracheal tube is inflated.

The force required has been estimated to be 40 N. It must be released during active vomiting, to reduce risk of oesophageal rupture.

Also used in difficult tracheal intubation, to aid visualization of the larynx.

[Brian A Sellick, London anaesthetist]

Sellick BA (1961) Lancet; ii: 404–6

See also, Induction, rapid sequence

Cricothyrotomy. Puncture or incision of the cricothyroid membrane (passes between the thyroid cartilage above and the cricoid cartilage below) of the **larynx**. Performed to allow ventilation in **airway obstruction**, e.g. as a last resort following failed intubation.

With the neck extended, the cricoid cartilage is identified level with C6, and a cricothyrotomy device inserted in the midline above the cartilage. Most devices consist of a needle with or without a cannula, connected to a standard 15 mm fitting or needle hub. Aspiration of air confirms correct placement. Special tubes, introducers and guidewires are also available.

In emergencies, a wide bore needle or cannula may be used, connected to a means of ventilation in a number of different ways:

–via a 3.5 mm tracheal tube connector.

–via a 2 ml syringe with its plunger removed and an 8 mm tracheal tube connector inserted in its open end.

–via a syringe with plunger removed, inserted into the end of a rubber catheter mount.

–via an injector device, e.g. as used for **bronchoscopy**; connects directly to the needle hub.

• Ventilation may be achieved by:

–closing the expiratory valve of the anaesthetic breathing system, allowing the reservoir bag to distend as 6–8 l/min O_2 is delivered. Intermittent closure of the patient's mouth and nose results in ventilation. Spontaneous ventilation will also achieve oxygenation.

–IPPV using the injector device.

Exhaled gases must be free to escape, or **barotrauma** may result. In upper airway obstruction, further punctures may be required to allow exhalation. Incorrect cannula placement may cause severe subcutaneous emphysema. Haemorrhage may occur. The cannula should be firmly fixed in place.

Cricothyroid puncture is also performed for transtracheal injection of **lignocaine**, during awake intubation. The **minitracheotomy** device may also be used for sputum aspiration.

Crile, George Washington (1864–1943). Eminent US surgeon, a major contributor to regional anaesthesia. Described the combination of opioids, regional block and general anaesthesia in order to block separate facets of anaesthesia, calling the concept anociassociation (led to the concept of **balanced anaesthesia**). Also investigated the pathogenesis and treatment of **shock**, and described a pneumatic garment for its treatment in 1903.

Critical damping, *see Damping*

Critical flicker–fusion test, *see Recovery testing*

Critical pressure. Pressure required to liquify a **vapour** at its **critical temperature**. Examples:

–O_2: 50 bar.

–N_2O: 72 bar.

–CO_2: 73 bar.

–cyclopropane: 54 bar.

Critical temperature. Temperature above which a **vapour** cannot be liquified by any amount of pressure. Above this temperature, the substance is a gas; below it, the substance is a vapour. Examples:

–O_2: 118°C.

–N_2O: 36.5°C.

–CO_2: 31°C.

–cyclopropane: 125°C.

See also, Isotherms; Pseudocritical temperature

Critical velocity. Velocity above which laminar **flow** in a tube becomes turbulent.
Proportional to

$$\frac{\textbf{viscosity of fluid}}{\text{density of fluid} \times \text{radius of tube}};$$

thus refers to a specific fluid within a tube of specific radius.

At critical velocity, **Reynold's number** is greater than 2000.

Cromoglycate (Sodium cromoglycate). Drug used in the prophylaxis of **asthma**. Thought to stabilize **mast cells** by preventing **calcium** ion entry, thus preventing IgE-mediated release of inflammatory substances from granules. Particularly useful in allergic and exercise-induced asthma, especially in children. Should be taken regularly; will not terminate an acute attack. Administered as a powder, aerosol or nebulized solutions, usually 2–20 mg 4–6 times daily.

See also, Bronchodilator drugs

Cross-matching, *see Blood cross-matching*

Croup (Laryngotracheobronchitis). Upper respiratory obstruction and **stridor** in children due to viral infection affecting the larynx, trachea and bronchi; most commonly due to parainfluenza (especially type I), respiratory syncytial and influenza viruses. The typical barking 'croupy' cough, the child's age, (usually 6 months–2 years) and the gradual onset help distinguish it from **epiglottitis**, which is usually of more acute onset, affects children of 2–5 years, and is associated with greater systemic upset. Lateral neck X-ray helps exclude epiglottitis.

Treatment is supportive and includes humidified O_2 administration, adequate hydration, and careful observation and monitoring, with tracheal intubation if severe (managed as for epiglottitis).

Nebulized **adrenaline** has been used in an attempt to avoid intubation: racemic solution (equal amounts of D- and L-isomers) is widely used in the USA: 0.5 ml of 2.25% solution is diluted to 4 ml in saline. 5 ml of generally available nonracemic adrenaline 1:1000 (containing more active L-isomer) has been used in the UK.
Diaz JM (1985) Anesth Analg; 64: 621–3

Crush syndrome. Acute oliguric **renal failure** following **trauma** usually involving impaired circulation of a limb. May occur in direct trauma and in comatose patients who lie on a limb for prolonged periods. Muscle swelling and necrosis leads to release of myoglobin with resultant **myoglobinuria**. Renal impairment is compounded by any associated **hypotension** and **dehydration**. Potassium is also released from the damaged muscle; severe **hyperkalaemia** may be fatal unless **dialysis** is instituted.
Hyperphosphataemia and **hypocalcaemia** also occur.

Cryoanalgesia. Use of extreme cold to damage peripheral nerves and provide pain relief lasting up to several months. Causes axonal degeneration without epineurial or perineurial damage, allowing slow regeneration of the axon without neuritis or neuroma formation. Used in chronic **pain management**, and peroperatively to provide prolonged **postoperative analgesia**, e.g. applied to intercostal nerves in **thoracic surgery**.
See also, Cryoprobe; Refrigeration anaesthesia

Cryoprecipitate, *see Blood products*

Cryoprobe. Instrument used to freeze tissues. Compressed gas (e.g. CO_2 or N_2O) is passed through a narrow tube and allowed to expand suddenly at its tip. Work done by the gas as it expands results in a temperature drop (**Joule–Thomson effect**; an example of an **adiabatic change**) to as low as –70°C in the metal sheath of the probe. Used to destroy superficial lesions, e.g. in gynaecology and dermatology; also used in ophthalmology and to provide **cryoanalgesia**.

Crystalloid. Substance which, in solution, may pass through a semipermeable membrane (cf. **colloid**). **Saline solutions, dextrose solutions** and **Hartmann's solution** are commonly used clinically as **iv fluids**.

CSF, *see Cerebrospinal fluid*

CSM, *see Committee on Safety of Medicines*

CT scanning, *see Computed axial tomography*

CTZ, *see Chemoreceptor trigger zone*

Cuffs, of tracheal tubes. Required to seal the trachea to avoid gas leakage and contamination with liquids from above, e.g. blood, gastric contents, etc. Popularized by **Waters** and **Guedel** in the 1920s. Commonly inflated with

air following tracheal intubation, until the audible gas leak is just eliminated. The degree of distension of a pilot balloon, or measurement of cuff pressure, indicates the extent of cuff inflation.

- Main problems are related to pressure exerted by the cuff on the tracheal walls causing mucosal ischaemia:
  - may occur if capillary arteriolar pressure is exceeded (i.e. greater than about 25 mmHg). Intracuff pressures of up to 30 mmHg have been measured with high-volume low-pressure cuffs, and up to 200 mmHg with low-volume high-pressure cuffs (*see Laplace's law*). The former are therefore preferable, especially for prolonged intubation, e.g. in ICU. Hand-held cuff inflators may incorporate pressure gauges to indicate intracuff pressure during inflation.
  - intracuff pressure may increase during anaesthesia due to increased temperature or diffusion of N_2O into the cuff. Saline or N_2O mixtures have been used for cuff inflation, to avoid the latter problem. Monitoring of intracuff pressure, or intermittent deflation and inflation, have been suggested during long operations and in ICU.
  - the anterior tracheal wall is affected more than the posterior wall, since the former is less distensible due to the cartilage rings.
  - mucosal inflammation may lead to ulcer formation over cartilagenous rings; infection, tracheal dilatation and erosion of tracheal walls may follow. Tracheal stenosis may occur after extubation.
  - damage is worst after prolonged use, although some degree of ciliary damage may occur within a few hours of inflation.
  - damage is worse if wrinkles are formed by the cuff.
  Similar problems may occur with **tracheostomy** tubes. Recurrent **laryngeal nerve** injury may be caused by a cuff inflated just below the vocal cords. Cuff placement should be 1.5–2 cm below the cords. Trauma may be caused if tracheal extubation is performed without prior deflation of the cuff. Uncuffed tracheal tubes should be used for **paediatric anaesthesia**.

  Similar considerations apply to bronchial cuffs of **endobronchial tubes**; bronchial rupture may follow overvigorous inflation.
See also, Tracheal tubes

Cuirass ventilator, *see Intermittent negative pressure ventilation*

Curare. Dried plant extract used by South American Indians as arrow poison, containing **tubocurarine** (isolated in 1935) and other alkaloids. Described in Raleigh's writings in 1596. Used experimentally by **Waterton** and **Bernard**, amongst others, from the early/mid-1800s onwards. Used to treat **tetanus** and in psychiatric convulsive therapy. First used in anaesthesia by **Lawen** in 1912, but remained in short supply for many years. Its use became more widespread after **Griffith**'s famous description in 1942; his supply was brought back from Ecuador by Gill.
[Sir Walter Raleigh (1552–1618), English explorer; Richard C. Gill (1902–1958), US explorer]

Curling ulcers. Peptic ulcers occurring after severe **burns**. Most common in children.
[Thomas Curling (1811–1888), English surgeon]

Current. Flow of electrical **charge**. Direct current describes flow of charge continuously in one direction, e.g. from a battery. Direction of flow in an alternating current changes back and forth, e.g. mains power supply. SI **unit** is the **ampere**.

Current density. Current per unit area; important in **electrocution and electrical burns**. A low current density, e.g. when electrical contact is over a wide area, results in little heat production; a large current density, when the area of contact is small, causes greater heat production. Thus there is no tissue damage at the site of a **diathermy** plate, but intense heat at the site of the probe or forceps, where area of contact is very small. Similarly, a small current delivered directly to the heart over a very small area may produce the same current density as a much larger current delivered to the whole body, and may therefore be as dangerous (microshock).

Current-operated earth-leakage circuit breaker (COELCB). Device containing equally-sized coils of live and neutral wires, used in electrical circuits to prevent **electrocution**. The current in each wire induces magnetic flux equal and opposite to that induced by the other, so long as each wire carries the same current. Imbalance between the two currents, e.g. due to leakage of current to earth, results in unequal magnetic fluxes which do not cancel each other out. Resultant magnetic flux induces current in a third coil, causing rapid (within 5 ms) breakage of the circuit via a solenoid.

Cushing, Harvey Williams (1869–1939). US neurosurgeon, Professor of Surgery at Harvard. A pioneer in neurosurgery, he developed many techniques, including the use of **diathermy**, and clips for cerebral vessels. Advocated **record-keeping** and **monitoring** during anaesthesia, and investigated many aspects of neurophysiology and neuropathology, several of which bear his name. Won the Pulitzer Prize for his biography of Osler, and published many books and articles.
[Joseph Pulitzer (1847–1911), Hungarian-born US journalist; Sir William Osler (1849–1919), Canadian-born US and English physician]
Hirsch NP, Smith GB (1986) Anesth Analg; 65: 288–93

Cushing's disease. Cushing's syndrome caused by pituitary-dependent adrenal hyperplasia.
● Treatment:
  –formerly bilateral adrenalectomy.
  –pituitary surgery.
  –irradiation of the **pituitary gland** (either external irradiation or radioactive implantation.
  –medical treatment: metyrapone inhibits 11β-hydroxylase and reduces cortisol production. May be used before surgery, to improve the patient's condition, or after irradiation.

Cushing's reflex. Hypertension with compensatory bradycardia occurring with acutely raised **ICP**. Due to the effect of local **hypoxia** and **hypercapnia** on the **vasomotor centre** as **cerebral perfusion pressure** falls.
See also, Cushing

Cushing's syndrome. Clinical syndrome resulting from excessive endogenous or exogenous steroid levels.

● Features:
  –obesity, classically central rather than peripheral, i.e. limbs are spared ('lemon and toothpick' appearance). 'Buffalo hump' of fat behind the neck.
  –'moon face', greasy skin, acne, hirsutism.
  –skin atrophy and poor wound healing, with increased susceptibility to infection.
  –abdominal striae.
  –osteoporosis.
  –proximal muscle weakness.
  –psychiatric disturbances.
  –**hypertension**.
  –**hypernatraemia** and **hypokalaemia**.
  –**diabetes mellitus**.
● Caused by:
  –**Cushing's disease** (the most common non-iatrogenic cause).
  –adrenal tumours.
  –other hormone-secreting tumours, e.g. **bronchial carcinoma** secreting **ACTH**.
  –**steroid therapy**.
● Investigation:
  –raised urinary cortisol and 17–oxogenic steroids (cortisol precursors).
  –raised plasma cortisol levels; normally low at midnight, and low the morning after dexamethasone administration.
  –ACTH levels are raised in Cushing's disease and ACTH-secreting tumours. Metyrapone decreases adrenal cortisol production, causing ACTH to increase: this does not occur with adrenal tumours or ACTH-secreting tumours, but does occur in Cushing's disease. The ACTH increase is measured directly, or cortisol precursors (17–oxogenic steroids) are measured in the urine.
Hypertension and **cardiac failure**, hypernatraemia, hypokalaemia and diabetes, although not always present, may cause problems during anaesthesia. Steroid cover is required as for steroid therapy. Fragile skin and veins may be easily damaged. Postoperative fluid and electrolyte balance are particularly important.
See also, Cushing

Cushing's ulcers. Peptic ulcers occurring after **head injury**, associated with increased gastric acid secretion.
See also, Cushing

Cutoff effect. Reduced anaesthetic potency of larger molecules in a homologous series, despite increasing lipid solubility. Possibly due to membranes' inability to accomodate molecules above a certain size.
See also, Anaesthesia, mechanism of

CVA, see Cerebrovascular accident

Cyanide poisoning. May result from industrial accidents, self-administration, **smoke inhalation**, and prolonged use of **sodium nitroprusside**. Absorption may occur via stomach, skin, lungs, etc. (the latter may be rapidly fatal). Causes inhibition of the **cytochrome oxidase system** and other **enzymes**, interrupting cellular respiration. Tissues are thus unable to utilize delivered O_2 (histotoxic **hypoxia**). Cyanide is slowly converted to thiocyanate in the liver by the enzyme rhodanase; a small amount binds to methaemoglobin and a small amount to hydroxocobalamin.

- Features:
  - –non-specific: dizziness, headache, confusion, etc. Apnoea may follow initial tachypnoea.
  - –reduced **arteriovenous O$_2$ difference**, due to reduced uptake of O$_2$ by tissues. Metabolic **acidosis** with increased **lactate** results from tissue hypoxia.
  - –**convulsions** and cardiorespiratory collapse may occur.
  - –chronic poisoning causes **peripheral neuropathy**, ataxia and optic atrophy.

Measurement of plasma levels is technically difficult and may be unreliable unless performed rapidly.

- Treatment:
  - –general measures as for **poisoning and overdoses. O$_2$ therapy** is particularly important. Staff must avoid self-contamination.
  - –**gastric lavage** may be helpful.
  - –dicobalt edetate 300–600 mg iv over 1 minute; 300 mg repeated if necessary. Combines with cyanide to form inert compounds. May itself cause vomiting, hypertension and tachycardia; reservation for severe cases has been suggested.
  - –sodium thiosulphate 50%, 25 ml iv over 10 minutes. Converts cyanide to thiocyanate. Used together with:
    - –sodium nitrite 3%, 10 ml iv over 10–20 minutes. Converts haemoglobin to methaemoglobin, which binds cyanide. More efficacious than inhaled amyl nitrite. Methaemoglobin together with carboxyhaemoglobin if present should not exceed 40% total haemoglobin.
    - –hydroxocobalamin 40%, 10 ml iv over 20 minutes. Forms cyanocobalamin with cyanide. Has been used in cyanide poisoning and to reduce nitroprusside toxicity, but not widely used in the UK.

Cyanosis. Blue discoloration of tissues due to increased amounts of reduced **haemoglobin** in the blood. Clinically detectable at less than 5 g/100 ml reduced haemoglobin, although this value is often quoted as the minimum. Peripheral cyanosis, e.g. of fingernails, may result from reduced peripheral circulation. Central cyanosis, typically affecting the tongue, may result from heart or lung disease, including right-to-left shunts. **Methaemoglobinaemia** and **sulphaemoglobinaemia** may also cause bluish discoloration. Cyanosis may be further mimicked by grey or blue discolorization of skin, e.g. caused by heavy metals (e.g. iron, gold and lead) or drugs (e.g. amiodarone and phenothiazines).

Cyclazocine. Opioid analgesic drug, similar to **pentazocine**. Produces unacceptable psychomimetic effects, but was used in **morphine** overdose and dependence before the availability of newer drugs.

Cyclic AMP, *see Adenosine monophosphate, cyclic*

Cycling of ventilators, *see Ventilators*

Cyclizine hydrochloride/tartrate/lactate. Antiemetic drug, with antihistamine and anticholinergic actions. Available alone or combined with **opioid analgesic drugs** and ergotamine.
- Dosage: 50 mg 8 hourly, orally/im/iv.
- Side effects include drowsiness and blurred vision.

Cyclopropane. (CH$_2$)$_3$. **Inhalational anaesthetic agent**, first used in the early 1930s. Available in the UK but not in many other countries.
- Properties:
  - –sweet smelling colourless gas, 1.4 times denser than air.
  - –mw 42.
  - –boiling point –33°C.
  - –**critical temperature** 125°C.
  - –**partition coefficients**:
    - –blood/gas 0.45.
    - –oil/gas 11.4.
  - –**MAC** 9.2.
  - –explosive in O$_2$ between 2.5 and 60%; in air between 2.5 and 10%.
  - –diffuses through rubber.
  - –supplied in orange cylinders at a pressure of 5 bar.
- Effects:
  - –CNS: fast onset of and recovery from anaesthesia.
  - –RS: marked respiratory depression; **hypercapnia** is common with spontaneous respiration.
  - –CVS:
    - –myocardial depression but with sympathetic and parasympathetic discharge; usually, cardiac output and BP are maintained, but they may fall after opioid premedication. Vasoconstriction is common.
    - –withdrawal of cyclopropane may cause hypotension, due to decreasd vasoconstriction and catecholamine levels ('cyclopropane shock').
    - –ventricular **arrhythmias** are common with hypercapnia, **hypoxaemia**, and **atropine** or **adrenaline** administration.
    - –vagally mediated bradycardia is common after opioid premedication.
    - –reduced renal and hepatic blood flow.
  - –other:
    - –reduced uterine tone at high concentrations only.
    - –nausea and vomiting are common.

Excreted largely unchanged via the lungs. Its use is diminishing, mainly due to its high cost and explosion risk. Main use is for paediatric induction, using 50% in O$_2$; e.g. 1 l/min of each.

Cylinders. Made of molybdenum or chromium steel. Provide medical gases either directly to an output, e.g. attached to an **anaesthetic machine**, or from a bank of cylinders (manifold) via pipelines.
- The valve block screws into the open end of the cylinder and has the following features:
  - –marked with:
    - –serial number.
    - –tare (weight of the empty cylinder and valve block; used for calculation of contents by weight).
    - –pressure of the last hydraulic test.
    - –symbol of the contained gas.
  - –the valve is opened by turning a longitudinal spindle, set within a gland (stuffing box) screwed tightly into the valve block. Compression of a nylon ring around the spindle prevents leakage of gas along the spindle shaft.
  - –bears the **pin-index system** on the same face as the gas outlet.
  - –a safety outlet is fitted to the valve block (USA) or between the block and cylinder neck (UK); it melts

Table 13. Colour-coding of cylinders

Gas	UK		USA	Recommended international system
	Shoulder	Body		
O_2	White	Black	Green	White
N_2O	Blue	Blue	Blue	Blue
CO_2	Grey	Grey	Grey	Grey
Cyclopropane	Orange	Orange	Orange	Orange
Entonox	White/blue quarters	Blue		
Helium	Brown	Brown	Brown	Brown
O_2 21% helium	White/brown quarters	Black	Brown/yellow	Brown/white
Air	Black/white quarters	Grey	Yellow	Black/white

at low temperatures, allowing escape of gas in case of fire.

–a testing collar is attached (see below).

Colour-coding (UK): shoulder colour(s) represent the predominant gas(es) in the cylinder (Table 13a). USA colour-coding is different. An international colouring system has been recommended, taking one of the colours from the UK system (Table 13).

- Bodies are labelled with:
  –name and symbol of the gas.
  –volume and pressure of contained gas.
  –information and warnings about explosions and flammability where appropriate. When the gas supply is turned on suddenly, compression of the gas within the valves and pipes causes a rise in temperature. Oil or grease in the system may ignite, hence the warning against these lubricants.
- Testing:
  –every hundredth cylinder is cut into strips and tested at manufacture .
  –each cylinder is tested 5-yearly to withstand high hydraulic pressures (about 200–250 bar). Cylinders are filled with water under pressure, within a water jacket. Expansion and elastic recoil of the metal are then measured.
  –internal inspection with an endoscope.
  –a plastic disc is placed around the valve block neck; its colour and shape are coded for the date of the last test. The year in which testing is due is stamped on the disc, and a hole punched to indicate the quarter of the year.
- Cylinder pressures:
  –**O_2**: 137 bar.
  –**N_2O**: 40 bar.
  –**CO_2**: 50 bar.
  –**cyclopropane**: 5 bar.
  –**air**:
  –**O_2/helium**: } 137 bar.
  –**O_2/N_2O**:
    (maximal values at 15°C, as marked on the cylinders)
  Modern pressure gauges are marked in kPa $\times$ 100 (1 bar = 100 kPa).

N_2O, cyclopropane and CO_2 cylinders contain liquid; as such a cylinder empties, pressure is maintained by evaporation of liquid (although a slight drop in pressure does occur as temperature falls) until the liquid is depleted. Pressure then falls rapidly with further emptying. Gas-filled cylinders, e.g. containing O_2, provide gas whose pressure is proportional to cylinder contents.

Large **Entonox** cylinders contain connecting tubes from the valve block to the lower part of the cylinder, to reduce risk of hypoxic gas delivery should separation of gases occur below the **pseudocritical temperature**.
- Sizes of cylinders are denoted by capital letters. Usual sizes on anaesthetic machines:
  –O_2: E (contains 680 litres).
  –N_2O: E (contains 1800 litres).
  –CO_2: C (contains 450 litres).
  –cyclopropane: B (contains 180 litres).

See also, Filling ratio; Piped gas supply

Cystic fibrosis. Autosomal recessive genetic disease; the commonest lethal inherited illness in Caucasians, affecting 1 in 1500 live births. Affects exocrine gland function resulting in abnormally viscous secretions.
- Features:
  –repeated respiratory infection, usually by Staphylococcus and Pseudomonas, leading to **bronchiectasis**, **pulmonary fibrosis** and eventually **pulmonary hypertension** and **cor pulmonale**. Nasal polyps are common. **Pneumothorax** may occur. $\dot{V}/\dot{Q}$ mismatch, restrictive and obstructive defects and increased residual capacity often result in **hypoxaemia**. Arterial $P\text{CO}_2$ is usually reduced unless lung disease is severe. **Laryngospasm** and coughing are common during anaesthesia.
  –pancreatic insufficiency with malabsorption and intestinal obstruction (e.g. meconium ileus in the newborn). **Diabetes mellitus** is more common than in normal patients. Obstructive **jaundice** may occur.
  –renal impairment and amyloidosis may occur.

Survival into the 2nd and 3rd decade is now common with intensive **physiotherapy**, antibiotic therapy and pancreatic supplementation.
- Anaesthetic management:
  –careful **preoperative assessment** and continuation of physiotherapy, etc. **Coagulation** may be impaired. Opioid premedication is usually avoided. **Anticholinergic drugs** may increase secretion viscosity but are commonly used to reduce the incidence of bradycardia; they may be given on induction.
  –regional techniques where appropriate.
  –inhalational induction is prolonged because of $\dot{V}/\dot{Q}$ mismatch. **Ketamine** increases bronchial secretions.
  –usual technique: tracheal intubation and IPPV, with tracheobronchial suction as required. Extubation is performed awake. **Humidification** of gases is important.
  –careful fluid balance to avoid dehydration.

–postoperative observation, physiotherapy, analgesia and humidified O_2 administration are important.
Lamberty JM, Rubin BK (1985) Anaesthesia; 40: 448–59

Cystic hygroma. Congenital multiloculated cystic mass arising from the jugular lymph sac, the embryonic precursor of part of the thoracic duct. Contains lymph; characteristically transilluminates very well. Usually presents soon after birth. Sometimes sclerosant treatment is used; surgery is difficult because of widespread cystic tissue throughout neck. The tongue and pharynx may be involved. Main anaesthetic problems are related to **airway obstruction** and difficult intubation. Manual IPPV via a facepiece may be impossible; therefore spontaneous ventilation is usually maintained until intubation is achieved.
See also, Intubation, difficult

Cytochrome oxidase system. Series of iron-containing **enzymes** within mitochondrial inner membranes. Electron transport from oxidized nicotinamide adenine dinucleotide (NADH) or succinate proceeds via sequential cytochromes, the iron component becoming alternatively reduced and oxidized as the electron is passed to the next in line. Their structure and arrangement within the membrane is thought to be crucial to their function. Electron flow is coupled to **ATP** formation; 3 molecules of ATP are formed per 1 of NADH and 2 ATP per 1 of succinate. Cytochrome oxidase itself is the cytochrome binding to molecular O_2 to form water, and is inhibited in **cyanide poisoning** and **carbon monoxide poisoning**.

Similar enzymes exist in other membranes, e.g. cytochrome P_{450} in smooth endoplasmic reticulum (microsomal portion of centrifuged cellular material), responsible for metabolism of many drugs.

Cytokines. Extremely potent substances released by cells in miniscule amounts; include certain interleukins, interferons, and **tumour necrosis factor**, considered the most important one. Involved in the cellular response to infection, and tend to have positive feedback action on further production.
Bellomo R (1992) Anaesth Intensive Care; 20: 288–302

D

δ wave, *see Wolff–Parkinson–White syndrome*

DA examination (Diploma in Anaesthetics). First specialist examination in anaesthetics; first held in 1935 in London. Originally intended for anaesthetists with at least 2 years' experience of 2000 anaesthetics, later reduced to 1 year's residence in an approved hospital. A two-part examination was introduced in 1947, in order to ensure anaesthetists' equal footing with other specialists prior to establishment of the NHS. This examination became the **FFARCS examination** in 1953; the single-part DA remained separate until 1984, when the DA (UK) became the first part of the new three-part FFARCS.

Dalteparin sodium, *see Heparin*

Dalton's law. The pressure exerted by a fixed amount of a gas in a mixture equals the pressure it would exert if alone; thus the pressure exerted by a mixture of gases equals the sum of the partial pressures exerted by each gas.
[John Dalton (1766–1844), English chemist]

Damping. Progressive diminution of amplitude of oscillations in a resonant system, caused by dissipation of stored energy. Important in recording systems, e.g. direct **arterial BP measurement**. In the latter, damping mainly arises from viscous drag of fluid in the cannula and connecting tubing, compression of entrapped air bubbles, blood clots within the system and kinking. Excess damping causes a flattened trace which may be distorted (**phase shift**). The degree of damping is described by the damping factor (D); if a sudden change is imposed on a system, $D = 1$ if no overshoot of the trace occurs (critical damping; Fig. 42a). A marked overshoot followed by many oscillations occurs if $D \ll 1$ (Fig. 42b), and an excessively delayed response occurs if $D \gg 1$ (Fig. 42c). Optimal damping is 0.6–0.7 of critical damping, and produces the fastest response without excessive oscillations. D depends on the properties of the liquid within the system and the dimensions of the cannula and tubing.

Dandy–Walker syndrome, *see Hydrocephalus*

Dantrolene sodium. Skeletal **muscle** relaxant which acts by interfering with **calcium** ion release from sarcoplasmic reticulum. Used to treat spastic muscle spasm and **MH**.
- Dosage:
  - 25–400 mg orally daily for muscle spasm.
  - 5 mg/kg orally the day before surgery, as prophylaxis in MH susceptible patients (rarely used now that the iv form is available).
  - 1 mg/kg iv for treatment of MH, repeated up to 10 mg/kg. The solution is irritant with pH 9–10, and is best infused into a large vein. Presented in bottles of 20 mg orange powder with 3 g mannitol and sodium hydroxide, each requiring mixing with 60 ml water. Thus preparation is lengthy. Once prepared, the solution lasts 6 hours at 15–30°C. Dry powder has a shelf-life of 9 months.
- Side effects: hepatotoxicity has occurred after prolonged oral use; muscle weakness and sedation may follow iv injection. The high pH of the iv solution (9–10) may cause venous thrombosis following prolonged infusion, and tissue necrosis following extravasation.

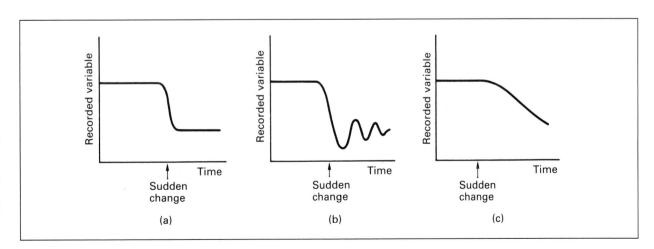

Figure 42 *Damping. (a) D=1; (b) D<<1; (c) D>>1*

Darrow's solution. Solution designed for **iv fluid** replacement in children suffering from gastroenteritis. Composed of sodium 122 mmol/l, chloride 104 mmol/l, lactate 53 mmol/l and potassium 35 mmol/l.
[Daniel Darrow (1895–1965), US paediatrician]

Data. In **statistics**, a series of observations or measurements.

- Data may be:
  - continuous; e.g. length in metres. The difference between 2 m and 3 m is the same as that between 35 m and 36 m, and 10 m is twice as long as 5 m.
    - interval data, i.e. cannot include zero value, e.g. patients' weight.
    - ratio data, i.e. includes zero value, e.g. plasma drug levels.

  If normally distributed, continuous data are described by the **mean** and **standard deviation** as indicators of central tendency and scatter respectively (described as for ordinal data if not normally distributed).
  - categorical:
    - ordinal data, e.g. pain scores. The difference between pain denoted by scores of 2 and 3 does not equal that between scores of 4 and 5, and a score of 4 is not 'twice as painful' as a score of 2. Ordinal data are described by the **median** and **percentiles** (or range).
    - nominal data, e.g. diagnosis, hair colour. May be dichotomous, e.g. male/female; alive/dead. Nominal data are described by the **mode** and a list of possible categories.

Different kinds of data require different **statistical tests** for correct analyses and comparisons: parametric tests for normally-distributed data (most continuous data), and non-parametric tests for non-normally distributed data (categorical and some continuous data). The latter may often be 'normalized' by mathematical transformation, allowing application of the more sensitive parametric tests.

See also, Clinical trials; Statistical frequency distributions

Davenport diagram. Graph of plasma **bicarbonate** concentration against **pH**, useful in interpreting and explaining disturbances of **acid–base balance**. Different lines may be drawn for different arterial P_{CO_2} values, but for each line, bicarbonate falls as pH falls, and increases as pH increases (Fig. 43).

- Can be used to demonstrate what happens in various acid–base disorders:
  - line BAD represents part of the titration curve for blood.
  - point A represents normal plasma.
  - point B represents respiratory **acidosis**; i.e. a rise in arterial P_{CO_2}, reducing pH and increasing bicarbonate. In order to return pH towards normal, compensatory mechanisms increase bicarbonate; i.e. move towards point C.
  - point D represents respiratory **alkalosis**; compensation results in a move towards point E.
  - point F represents metabolic acidosis; respiratory compensation (hyperventilation with a fall in arterial P_{CO_2}) causes a move towards point E.
  - point G represents metabolic alkalosis; compensatory hypoventilation causes a move towards point C.

The same relationship may be displayed in different ways,

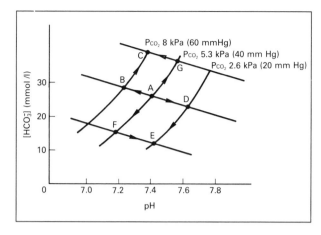

Figure 43 *Davenport diagram (see text)*

e.g. the **Siggaard-Andersen nomogram**, which contains more information and is more useful clinically.
[Horace W Davenport, US physiologist]

Davy, Sir Humphrey (1778–1892). Cornish-born scientist, inventor of the miner's safety lamp. Discovered sodium, potassium, calcium and barium. Suggested the use of **N₂O** (which he named 'laughing gas') for analgesia in 1799, whilst director of the Medical Pneumatic Institution in Bristol. Later became President of the Royal Society.

Day-case surgery. Surgery in which the patient presents to hospital and returns home on the day of operation. Increasingly performed, as it has many advantages over traditional inpatient surgery:
  - minimal psychological upheaval for the patient, especially children.
  - reduced requirement for nursing and medical supervision and hospital services, thus cheaper.
  - allows large number of patients to be treated.
  - reduced risk of hospital-acquired infection.

Standards of anaesthetic and surgical care and equipment (including preoperative preparation, **monitoring** and **recovery** facilities) should be as for inpatient surgery. Consultant surgical and anaesthetic supervision is considered mandatory.

- Patients may be managed within:
  - separate dedicated day-case units within hospitals: provide geographical, staffing, and some political independence from the main hospital, but require access to hospital facilities if required, e.g. X-ray, laboratories, wards, ICU, etc.
  - traditional inpatient lists.
  - completely separate units, without a nearby hospital.
- Patient selection:
  - age limits are controversial. Children under 1 year are usually excluded, but younger babies have been included without problems if fit and not premature (the latter have increased risk of apnoea postoperatively). Upper limits of 65–70 years are often applied, but other factors may be more important, e.g. fitness, home situation, etc.
  - usually restricted to **ASA physical status** I or II. Mild systemic disease, e.g. well-controlled **diabetes melli-**

tus, **hypertension**, etc. are not considered contraindicative by many authorities. **Obesity** is associated with higher complication rates and obese patients are therefore often excluded.

–patients are excluded unless escorted home by a responsible adult who can stay with them overnight. Other considerations include housing conditions, and availability of a telephone.

–operations expected to last less than 60 minutes are preferable. Surgery should be minor, with low rates of complications which if they occur should be mild. Expected pain should be mild.

Less stringent requirements are usually applied if the surgery is very minor and performed under local infiltration.

Patients are informed of the requirements for fasting, home arrangements, etc.

● Anaesthetic technique:
–patients are fully assessed preoperatively (often using a questionnaire). Anaesthetic outpatient clinics have been used. Time of last oral intake is checked.
–**premedication** is usually omitted, although short-acting drugs e.g. **temazepam** are sometimes used.
–general principles are as for any anaesthetic, but rapid recovery is particularly desirable. Thus short-acting drugs are usually used, e.g. **propofol**, **methohexitone**, **fentanyl**, **alfentanil**. Use of the more expensive drugs is controversial, since recovery testing some hours postoperatively may not reveal much difference between them and the cheaper drugs. Propofol is widely used, however, as immediate wakening is far superior than with other induction agents. There is little difference between the volatile agents. Tracheal intubation is acceptable but is usually avoided if possible. **Suxamethonium** is often avoided since muscle pains are more likely in ambulant patients.
–regional techniques may be suitable (often combined with general anaesthesia to provide postoperative analgesia). **Extradural** and **spinal anaesthesia** have been successfully performed, although uncommonly in the UK.
–oral analgesics and antiemetics are prescribed postoperatively.
–facilities for admission to an inpatient ward must be available in case of excessive bleeding or other complications (required in under 5% of cases).
● Postoperative assessment must be performed before discharge; the following are usually required:
–full orientation and responsiveness.
–ability to walk, dress and drink.
–adequately controlled pain.
–controlled bleeding and swelling.
–stable vital signs.

Written and verbal instructions are given to the patient, not to take depressant drugs or alcohol, or indulge in potentially dangerous activities (e.g. operating machinery, driving, frying food, etc.) for 24 hours usually; 48 hours has been suggested. These instructions may not always be followed.

Smith I, White PF (1992) Curr Anaesth Crit Care; 3: 77–83

Dead space. Volume of inspired air that takes no part in gas exchange. Divided into:
–anatomical dead space: mouth, nose, pharynx and large airways not lined with respiratory epithelium.

Measured by **Fowler's method**.
–alveolar dead space: ventilated lung normally contributing to gas exchange, but not doing so because of impaired perfusion. Thus represents one extreme of $\dot{V}/\dot{Q}$ **mismatch**.

Physiological dead space equals anatomical plus alveolar dead space. It is measured using the **Bohr equation**. Assessment may be useful in monitoring $\dot{V}/\dot{Q}$ mismatch in patients with extensive respiratory disease, especially when combined with estimation of **shunt** fraction. Normally equals 2–3 ml/kg; i.e. 30% of normal tidal volume. In rapid shallow breathing, **alveolar ventilation** is reduced despite a normal minute ventilation, beacause a greater proportion of tidal volume is dead space.

● Increased by:
–increased lung volumes.
–bronchodilatation.
–extension of neck.
–**PE/air embolism**.
–old age.
–hypotension.
–haemorrhage.
–pulmonary disease.
–general anaesthesia and **IPPV**.
–**atropine** and **hyoscine**.
–apparatus (see below).
● Decreased by:
–tracheal intubation and **tracheostomy**.
–supine position.

Apparatus dead space represents 'wasted' fresh gas within anaesthetic tubing, etc. Minimal lengths of tubing should lie between the fresh gas inlet of a T-piece and the patient, especially in children, whose tidal volumes are small. **Facepieces** and their connections may considerably increase dead space.

Fletcher R (1985) Br J Anaesth; 57: 245–9

Debrisoquine sulphate. Antihypertensive drug, acting by preventing **noradrenaline** release from postganglionic adrenergic neurones. Similar in effects to **guanethidine**, but does not deplete noradrenaline stores.

Decamethonium dibromide/diiodide. Depolarizing **neuromuscular blocking drug**, introduced in 1948. Blockade lasts 15–20 minutes. May cause muscle fasciculation and pains, ganglion blockade and bradycardia; repeated doses may cause **dual block**. No longer in use in the UK.

Decerebrate posture. Abnormal posture resulting experimentally from transection of the upper **brainstem**. Composed of internal rotation and hyperextension of all limbs, with hyperextension of neck and spine, and absent righting reflexes. Similar posturing may be seen in severe structural brain damage or **coning**.
See also, Decorticate posture

Declamping syndrome, *see Aortic aneurysm, abdominal*

Decompression sickness. Syndrome following rapid passage from a high atmospheric pressure environment to one of lower atmospheric pressure, e.g. surfacing after underwater diving, especially if followed by air transport at high altitude. Caused by formation of **nitrogen** bubbles as the gas comes out of solution, which it does readily because of its low solubility. Bubbles may embolize to or form in various tissues, giving rise to widespread symptoms: the joints ('the bends'); the CNS ('the staggers'); the skin ('the creeps'); the lungs ('the chokes'). Treated by immediate recompression.

Decontamination of anaesthetic equipment, *see Contamination of anaesthetic equipment*

Decorticate posture. Abnormal posture resulting from lesions of the cerebral cortex, with preservation of basal ganglia and brainstem function. Composed of leg extension, internal rotation and plantar flexion, with moderate arm flexion. Passive rotation of the head to one side causes extension of the ipsilateral arm, with full flexion of the contralateral arm, due to intact tonic neck reflexes. The contralateral leg may flex. Occurs in severe structural brain damage.
See also, Decerebrate posture

Deep vein thrombosis (DVT). Thrombus formation in the deep veins, usually of the leg and pelvis. A common postoperative complication, especially following prostatectomy, hip surgery and splenectomy. The true incidence is unknown but may exceed 50% in high-risk patients. Carries high risk of **PE**. May rarely cause systemic embolization via a patent foramen ovale (present in 30% of the population at autopsy).
- Triad of predisposing factors described by Virchow in 1856:
  - venous stasis, e.g. low cardiac output (e.g. **cardiac failure**, **MI**, **dehydration**), pelvic venous obstruction, prolonged immobility.
  - vessel wall damage, e.g. direct trauma, inflammation, varicosities, infiltration.
  - increased blood coagulability, e.g. trauma, **malignancy**, puerperium, oestrogen or antifibrinolytic administration, hereditary hypercoagulability, possibly **smoking**.

More common in old age, sepsis and **obesity**. Increased risk after surgery is thought to be related to increased **platelet** adhesiveness and activation of the **coagulation** cascade caused by tissue trauma, exacerbated by possible venous damage and postoperative immobility.

Clinical diagnosis is unreliable but suggested by tenderness, swelling and increased temperature of the calf, and pain on passive dorsiflexion of the foot (Homans' sign). The upper leg may also be involved. Accompanying superficial thrombophlebitis may be absent. Investigations include **Doppler** ultrasound, impedance plethysmography, thermography, uptake of radiolabelled fibrinogen or platelets, and venography. The latter is the most reliable.

Treated by systemic anticoagulation with **heparin** 500–1500 units/h iv titrated to a partial thromboplastin time of 2–4 × control. **Warfarin** is administered orally, and heparin discontinued when a prothrombin time of 2–3 × normal is achieved. Long-term interruption of leg blood flow may not be prevented, and prevention of PE has never been proven. Initial bed rest, leg elevation and analgesia are also prescribed. Surgical removal of thrombus has been performed, but reaccumulation usually occurs, possibly due to vessel wall damage. Use of **fibrinolytic drugs** is controversial.
- Prophylaxis should be considered for all but minor surgery, and in patients immobile in ICUs. Methods used:

- reduction of stasis:
  - heel cushion to prevent pressure on calf veins.
  - elevation of legs.
  - intermittent pneumatic compression of the legs.
  - graduated compression stockings.
  - electrical stimulation of leg muscles.
  - encouragement of postoperative leg exercises and early mobility.
- reduction of intravascular coagulation
  - fibrinolytic and **antiplatelet drugs**: not shown to prevent DVT, except for **dextrans** (shown to reduce fatal PEs). Reduction in blood **viscosity** may be important.
  - heparin and warfarin anticoagulation: effective but with risk of haemorrhage. Low dose heparin is widely used (5000 units sc 2 hours preoperatively then 8–12 hourly) and has been shown to be effective in reducing DVT and fatal PE. Low mw heparin reduces DVT without haemorrhagic side effects (*for doses, see Heparin*). Dihydroergotamine has been used together with heparin, and is thought to reduce the incidence further, possibly via venous vasoconstriction.
  - discontinuation of oral **contraceptives** 1–3 months preoperatively.
  - **extradural/spinal anaesthesia** is thought to be associated with increased **fibrinolysis** and reduced risk of DVT.

Low-dose heparin and compression stockings are most commonly used.
[Rudolph LW Virchow (1821–1902), German pathologist; John Homans (1877–1954), US surgeon]
Lowe GDO, Greer IA, Cooke TG et al (1992) Br Med J; 305: 567–74
See also, Coagulation studies

Defibrillation. Application of an electric current across the heart, to convert (ventricular) fibrillation to sinus rhythm. Use of electricity was described in the late 1700s/early 1800s, but modern use arose from experiments in the 1930s-1950s, largely by Kouwenhoven. Direct current is more effective and less damaging than alternating current.

Modern defibrillators contain a capacitor, with potential difference between its plates of up to 8000 V. Stored charge is released during discharge; the energy released is proportional to the potential difference. Up to 400 J is used for external defibrillation, and 20–50 J for internal defibrillation. The current pulse (up to 30 A) causes synchronous contraction of the heart muscle, hopefully allowing sinus rhythm to occur following a refractory period.

For external use, 200 J may be tried first. Firm application of large paddles over the sternum and heart apex, using conductive jelly or pads, increases efficiency. The paddles may also be placed on the front and back of the chest. Thoracic **impedance** is reduced by the first shock, so a second discharge at the same setting will deliver greater energy to the heart. If still unsuccessful, the energy level may be increased. For children, 2–5 J/kg is used. Lower energy levels are used in **cardioversion**. Repeated shocks may result in myocardial damage. **Electrocution** of members of the resuscitation team has occurred; all personnel should stand clear during discharge.

Automatic defibrillators identify life-threatening arrhythmias and deliver shocks, completely automatically or with the operator's approval. Their impact on resuscitation by non-medical staff has yet to be evaluated. Implantable defibrillators for patients with recurrent arrhythmias have also been described.

[William Kouwenhoven (1886–1975), US engineer]

See also, individual arrhythmias; Cardiopulmonary resuscitation

Deflation reflex. Stimulation of inspiration by lung deflation, initiated by **pulmonary stretch receptors**. Of uncertain significance in humans.

See also, Hering–Breuer reflex

Degrees of freedom. In **statistics**, the number of observations in a sample that can vary independently of other observations. For n observations, each observation may be compared with $n–1$ others; i.e. degress of freedom = $n–1$. For chi-squared analysis, it equals the product of (number of rows – 1) and (number of columns – 1).

Dehydration. Reflects loss of water from **ECF**, alone or with **intracellular fluid** (ICF) depletion. Sodium is usually lost concurrently, giving rise to **hypernatraemia** or **hyponatraemia**, depending on the relative degress of loss. If ECF **osmolality** rises, water passes from ICF into ECF by **osmosis**. A predominant water loss is shared by both ICF and ECF; water and sodium loss is borne mainly by ECF if osmolality is not greatly affected. Thus fever, lack of intake, **diabetes inspidus**, osmotic diuresis, etc. (mainly water loss) may be tolerated for longer periods than severe vomiting, diarrhoea, intestinal obstruction, diuretic therapy, etc. (water and sodium loss), although reduced water intake often accompanies the latter conditions.

The physiological response to dehydration includes increased thirst, **vasopressin** secretion and **renin/angiotensin system** activation, and CVS compensation for **hypovolaemia** via **osmoreceptor** and **baroreceptor** mechanisms.

Children are particularly prone to dehydration, as they exchange a greater proportion of body water each day.

- Clinical features are related to the extent of water loss:
  –5% of body weight: thirst, dry mouth.
  –5–10% of body weight: decreased intraocular pressure, peripheral perfusion and skin turgor, oliguria, orthostatic hypotension. **JVP/CVP** are reduced.
  –10–15%: shock, coma.

Blood **urea** and **haematocrit** are increased, and urine has high osmolality (over 300 msomol/kg) and low sodium content (under 10 mmol/l).

Treatment includes **iv fluid** administration: dextrose solutions are favoured for combinations of ICF and ECF losses and electrolyte solutions for ECF losses alone. Dehydration should be corrected preoperatively.

See also, Fluid balance; Fluids, body; Hypovolaemia

Delerium tremens. Condition seen following **alcohol** withdrawal in chronic heavy drinkers. Characterized by:
  –tremor, agitation.
  –confusion, disorientation, hallucinations (usually visual).
  –sweating, tachycardia, hypertension.
  –**dehydration**.

Usually occurs 2–3 days after withdrawal of alcohol, lasting 3–4 days. May thus occur perioperatively.

Treated by sedation, e.g. with **diazepam** or **chlormethiazole** (orally if possible, since iv therapy may be hazardous if liver function is impaired).

- Prevention: chlormethiazole capsules, up to 12/day over the first few days after withdrawal.

Demand valves. Valves which allow self-administration of **inhalational anaesthetic agents**; they may form part of **intermittent flow anaesthetic machines**, or be used to administer **Entonox**. The standard Entonox valve was developed from underwater breathing apparatus, and contains a two-stage **pressure regulator** within one unit which fits directly to the **cylinder**. The first stage regulator is similar to those on anaesthetic machines. At the second stage, gas flow is prevented by a rod which seals the valve. The patient's inspiratory effort moves a sensing diaphragm and tilts the rod, opening the valve. Very small negative pressures are required to produce gas flow of up to 300 l/min. An expiratory valve is attached to the mask/mouthpiece elbow piece. A safety (overpressure) valve is also incorporated. Other demand valves for use with Entonox have the second stage (demand) regulator attached to the patient's mask.

Demyelinating diseases. Non-specific group of disorders, with abnormality of the axonal **myelin** sheath as the predominant feature. Defective myelin may be present at birth (dysmyelinating) or may arise in areas of previously normal myelin (demyelinating). Multiple (disseminated) sclerosis (MS) is the commonest of the latter and is considered below; others include postimmunization or parainfectious encephalomyelitis.

Aetiology of MS is unknown but is probably multifactorial, involving climatic, geographical, genetic, viral and immune factors. Plaques of demyelination occur throughout the CNS, with preservation of axon continuity. Optic nerve, brainstem and spinal cord are particularly affected, with sparing of peripheral nerves. Neurological lesions are separated temporally and spatially, producing a variable clinical picture. Common presentations include limb weakness, spasticity, hyperreflexia, visual disturbances, parasthesiae and incoordination. Progression is variable with relapses associated with trauma, infection, stress and rise in body temperature.

Diagnosed clinically, supported by CSF lymphocytosis and altered CSF protein distribution. **Evoked potential** testing, CAT scanning and magnetic resonance imaging have been used, but are not diagnostic.

Treatment is supportive, but may include **steroid therapy**. Hyperbaric O_2 therapy has been advocated but is of unproven value.

Anaesthetic implications are unclear, since effects of stress, surgery and anaesthesia cannot be separated from the spontaneity of new lesion formation. Thus case reports are often conflicting in their conclusions. Increases in body temperature should be avoided; avoidance of **anticholinergic drugs** has been suggested. An abnormal response to **neuromuscular blocking drugs**, including **hyperkalaemia** following **suxamethonium**, has been suggested but without direct evidence. Prolonged muscle spasms may occur, but epilepsy is rare. Increased tendency to **DVT** has been suggested. Impairment of respiratory and autonomic control has been reported. Although not contraindicated, **extradural** or **spinal anaesthesia** is often avoided for medicolegal reasons.

Jones RM, Healy TEJ (1980) Anaesthesia; 35: 879–84

Denervation hypersensitivity. Increased sensitivity of denervated skeletal **muscle** to **acetylcholine**. Develops approximately 4–5 days after denervation, and is due to proliferation of extrajunctional **acetylcholine receptors** over the entire muscle membrane, instead of their being restricted to the **neuromuscular junction**. Thought to be the mechanism underlying the exaggerated hyperkalaemic response to **suxamethonium** seen after peripheral nerve injuries. Its cause is unclear. Also occurs in smooth muscle.

Density. For a substance, defined as its mass per unit volume. Relative density (**specific gravity**) is the mass of any volume of substance divided by the mass of the same volume of water.

Dental nerve blocks, *see Mandibular nerve blocks; Maxillary nerve blocks*

Dental surgery. Anaesthesia may be required for tooth extraction, conservative dental surgery or **faciomaxillary surgery**.
- For outpatient ambulatory surgery, the following may be used:
  - –**mandibular** and **maxillary nerve blocks**.
  - –**relative analgesia**.
  - –iv **sedation**, e.g. **Jorgensen technique** and variants.
  - –**inhalational anaesthetic agents**, including **N₂O** and/or volatile agents. Traditionally administered from **intermittent flow anaesthetic machines**, using **nasal inhalers**, although continuous flow machines are increasingly used. **Quantiflex apparatus** is also used. Occupational exposure to N₂O is a hazard, especially in small dental surgeries.
  - –iv **anaesthetic agents**.

The use of general anaesthesia for dental surgery is declining, with local anaesthetic techniques becoming more common, especially for conservative dentistry. General anaesthesia is usually indicated for patients who are mentally retarded or extremely nervous, children, those undergoing multiple extractions, and those with local infection (infiltration is less effective, and may spread infection). Most general anaesthetics are now performed by anaesthetists within hospitals. Adequate **monitoring** should be used, and full resuscitative equipment and suction must be available. Single operator/anaesthetist practice has been condemned.
- General anaesthetic principles are as for **day-case surgery**; main problems:
  - –high proportion of children, usually anxious and unpremedicated. **Preoperative assessment**, including checking for adequate starvation, should be performed.
  - –shared airway as for **ENT surgery**. **Airway obstruction**, mouth breathing during nasally-administered anaesthesia, airway soiling and breath holding may occur.
  - –**arrhythmias** are common, especially when **halothane** is used.
- Controversy exists over the best position of the patient:
  - –supine: the most familiar position for anaesthetists, and hypotension and reduced cerebral blood flow are less likely.
  - –sitting: the most familiar position for dentists, with less risk of airway contamination with blood, teeth,

etc., and possibly less risk of regurgitation and aspiration.

Fears over 'fainting' during anaesthesia are opposed by lack of increased mortality when the sitting position is used. The reclining position, with the foot of the chair/table raised, has been suggested as a compromise. Mouth packs are usually employed to prevent mouth breathing, soak up blood, and prevent airway soiling. They should be placed under the tongue, pushing the tongue back to seal the mouth from the airway. **Mouth gags** or props are often used to hold the mouth open; the former are often held by the anaesthetist from behind the patient's head.

Dental surgery is performed on an inpatient surgery basis if airway obstruction, cardiac or respiratory disease, **coagulation disorders** or extreme **obesity** are present. Nasotracheal intubation is usually performed, and a throat pack placed. Arrhythmias may occur, although the incidence is reduced with the use of IPPV. Use of concentrated **adrenaline** solutions by dentists is still common, e.g. 1:80 000, despite anaesthetists' opposition.

Depolarizing neuromuscular blockade (Phase I block). Follows depolarization of the **neuromuscular junction** postsynaptic membrane via activation of its **acetylcholine receptors**, but without repolarization. Effect of depolarization of presynaptic receptors is unclear. **Suxamethonium** is the most commonly used and widely available drug; previously used drugs include **decamethonium** and **suxethonium**.
- Features:
  - –may be preceded by **fasciculation**.
  - –does not exhibit **fade** or **post-tetanic potentiation**.
  - –increased by **acetylcholinesterase inhibitors**.
  - –potentiated by respiratory **alkalosis**, **hypothermia**, **hyperkalaemia** and **hypermagnesaemia**.
  - –antagonized by non-depolarizing neuromuscular blocking drugs.
  - –development of **dual block** with excessive dosage of drug.

See also, Neuromuscular blockade monitoring; Non-depolarizing neuromuscular blockade

Dermatomes. Lateral walls of somites (segmental units appearing longitudinally early in embryonic development), which form the skin and subcutaneous tissues. Cutaneous sensation retains the somatic distribution, corresponding to segmental spinal levels. Thus areas of skin are supplied by particular **spinal nerves**; useful in determining the extent of regional anaesthetic blocks and localizing neurological lesions (Fig. 44).
See also, Myotomes

Dermatomyositis, *see Polymyositis*

Desensitization block, *see Dual block*

Desflurane. CF₃CFHOCF₂H, 1–fluoro-2,2,2–trifluoro-ethyl difluoromethyl ether. **Inhalational anaesthetic agent**, synthesized in the 1960s but only recently studied clinically. Chemical structure is the same as **isoflurane**, but with the chlorine atom replaced by fluorine. Has similar clinical effects to isoflurane, but with **SVP** over 2.5 times as high, and blood/gas **partition coefficient** three times lower. Thus uptake and recovery are extremely rapid.

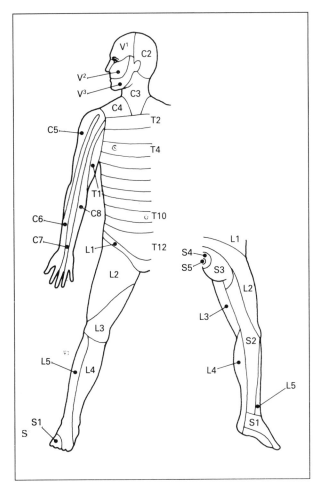

Figure 44 *Dermatomal nerve supply*

Less pungent than isoflurane. Chemically stable, with **MAC** 5–10%.
Supplement (1992) Anesth Analg; 75: S1–54

Desmopressin (1–deamino-8–D-arginine-vasopressin; DDAVP). Analogue of **vasopressin**, with a longer lasting antidiuretic effect but minimal vasoconstrictor actions. May be given intranasally or by injection. Used to diagnose and treat non-nephrogenic **diabetes insipidus**. May also be used to increase factor VIII and von Willebrand factor levels by 2–4 times in mild **haemophilia** or **von Willebrand's disease**. Has also been used to reduce blood loss in **cardiac surgery**.
- Dosage:
  –diabetes insipidus: 10–20 µg intranasally once-twice daily, or 1–4 µg/day iv.
  –to increase factor VIII levels: 0.4 µg/kg in 50 ml saline iv 1 hour preoperatively, repeated at 4 and 24 hours.
May cause pallor, abdominal cramps, and angina in susceptible patients.

Dew point. Temperature at which ambient air is saturated with water vapour. As air of a certain water content cools, e.g. when it is in contact with a cold surface, condensation occurs when dew point is reached (e.g.

misting on the surface of spectacles on entering a warm room from the cold). This process may be used to measure **humidity**.

Dexamethasone, *see Steroid therapy*

Dexmedetomidine. Selective α_2–adrenergic receptor agonist, currently being investigated for perioperative use. Reduces the **MAC** of **inhalational anaesthetic agents**, attenuates the hypertensive response to tracheal intubation, and reduces the requirements for postoperative **opioid analgesic drugs**.
Peden CJ, Prys-Roberts C (1992) Br J Anaesth; 68: 123–5

Dextrans. Group of branched polysaccharides of 200 000 glucose units, derived from the action of bacteria (*Leuconostoc mesenteroides*) on sucrose. Partial hydrolysis produces molecules of average mw 40 000, 70 000 and 110 000 (dextrans 40, 70 and 110 respectively). Dextran 40 is used to promote peripheral blood flow, e.g. in arterial insufficiency and in prophylaxis of **DVT**. Dextrans 70 and 110 are used mainly for plasma expansion; the latter is now rarely used. Dextrans increase peripheral blood flow by reducing **viscosity**, and may coat both endothelium and cellular elements of blood, reducing their interaction. They impair **platelet** adhesiveness, and possibly impair factor VIII activity.

Size of dextran molecules determines degree of plasma expansion produced and the molecules' circulation time. **Half-life** ranges from 15 minutes for small molecules, to several days for larger ones. Major route of excretion is via the kidneys.

Supplied in 5% dextrose or 0.9% saline, as 6% (dextrans 70 and 110) or 10% (dextran 40) solutions.
- Side effects:
  –**renal failure** caused by tubular obstruction by dextran casts; mainly occurs with dextran 40 when used in **hypovolaemia**; concurrent water and electrolyte administration should be provided.
  –**anaphylactic reactions**: thought to result from previous cross-immunization against bacterial antigens. Its incidence is reduced from 1:4500 to 1:84 000 by pretreatment with 3 g dextran 1 (mw 1000), to occupy and block antigen binding sites of circulating antibodies to dextran.
  –interference with **blood cross-matching**.
  –bleeding tendency. Initial administration should be limited to 500–1000 ml, and the total amount administered restricted to 10 (dextran 40) and 20 (dextran 70) ml/kg/day.
  –osmotic diuresis.
Dextrans have also been used locally to prolong the action of **local anaesthetic agents**, possibly by trapping the latter molecules within large macromolecules in the tissues. Inconsistent results have been reported.
Ramsay G (1989) BMJ; 296: 1422–3
See also, Colloids

Dextromoramide tartrate. Opioid analgesic drug, related to **methadone**. Introduced in 1956. Less sedating, and shorter acting (duration 2–3 hours) than **morphine**, but with similar effects.
- Dosage:
  –5–15 mg orally, sc or im.
  –10 mg rectally.

Dextropropoxyphene hydrochloride/napsylate. Opioid **analgesic drug**, related to **methadone**. Prepared in 1953. Has weak properties alone, but powerful when combined with **paracetamol** (as co-proxamol). Overdose of this combination is particularly dangerous; initial respiratory depression and coma (due to dextroproxyphene) may be treated correctly but later liver failure (due to paracetamol) may occur if prophylaxis with *N*-acetylcysteine or methionine is not undertaken.

- Dosage:
  - 65 mg 6 hourly, orally.
  - 32.5 mg with 325 mg paracetamol; 1–2 tablets 4 hourly, up to 8 tablets/24 h.

Dextrose solutions. **IV fluids** available as 5, 10, 20, 25 and 50% solutions in water (50, 100, 200, 250 and 500 g/l respectively). Once administered, the glucose is metabolized by red blood cells, and the water distributed to all body fluid compartments. Thus used in **hypoglycaemia**, and to replace water losses. Also used with **insulin** to treat acute **hyperkalaemia**.

Excess administration, e.g. perioperatively, may result in **hyponatraemia**. Solutions of higher concentrations are increasingly hypertonic, acidic and viscous; they may cause thrombophlebitis if infused peripherally. Osmolality of 5% dextrose solution is 278 mosmol/kg; of 10% solution 523 mosmol/kg. pH of 5% solution is approximately 4.0.

See also, Fluids, body; Intravenous fluid administration

Dezocine. Synthetic **opioid analgesic drug**, available in the USA but not in the UK. Comparable in potency, onset and duration of action to **morphine**. Has some **opioid receptor antagonist** activity, less than that of **nalorphine** but greater than that of **pentazocine**. Administered im or iv in doses of 2.5–20 mg.

Diabetes insipidus. Polyuria and polydipsia associated with reduced **vasopressin** activity, either because secretion by the **pituitary** is reduced (cranial) or the kidneys are unresponsive (nephrogenic):
- cranial: occurs in **head injury**, **neurosurgery**, intracranial tumours, etc. Rarely familial.
- nephrogenic: caused by drugs, e.g. **lithium**, demeclocycline and gentamicin; a rare X-linked recessive form may also occur.

Characterized by inappropriate passage of large volumes of dilute urine, with raised plasma **osmolality**. Patients cannot concentrate their urine in response to water deprivation. The two types are distinguished by their response to administered vasopressin.
- Treatment:
  - cranial: **desmopressin** (synthetic vasopressin analogue) 1–4 μg/day iv or 10–20 μg 12 hourly by nasal inhalation.
  - nephrogenic: **thiazide diuretics**.

Anaesthetic considerations are related to impaired **fluid balance** with **hypovolaemia**, **dehydration**, **hypernatraemia** and other electrolyte imbalance. Careful attention to **fluid balance**, with regular monitoring of urine and plasma osmolality and electrolytes, is required.

Blevins LS, Wand GS (1992) Crit Care Med; 20: 69–79

Diabetes mellitus. Disorder of **glucose** metabolism characterized by relative or total lack of **insulin**. This results in lipolysis, gluconeogenesis and glycogenolysis, with hepatic conversion of fatty acids to **ketone bodies**, and **hyperglycaemia**. The resultant glycosuria causes an osmotic diuresis, with polyuria, polydipsia and excessive sodium and potassium loss.

Affects 1–2% of the population; over 80% are over 80 years old and 50% are likely to require surgery.
- May be:
  - primary: thought to be related to genetic, infective and immunological factors, but the aetiology is unclear.
  - secondary:
    - pancreatic disease, e.g. **pancreatitis**, malignancy.
    - insulin antagonism, e.g. **steroid therapy**, **Cushing's syndrome**, **acromegaly**, **phaeochromocytoma**.
    - drugs, e.g. **thiazide diuretics**.

Classically divided into type I (insulin-dependent; IDDM) presenting in children, and type II (non-insulin-dependent; NIDDM), presenting in adults who are usually obese. The former is treated with insulin, the latter with diet, weight control and oral hypoglycaemic drugs. Resistance to insulin has been shown in type II. Further subdivision has been suggested. Although the criteria for diagnosis are controversial, a random plasma glucose above 11 mmol/l, or a fasting glucose above 8 mmol/l, have been suggested.
- Complications:
  - renal impairment, caused by glomerulosclerosis, vascular insufficiency, infection and papillary necrosis.
  - arteriosclerosis causing **ischaemic heart disease**, peripheral vascular insufficiency, and cerebrovascular disease with increased risk of **CVA**. Microvascular involvement may cause **cardiac failure** and impaired ventricular function. **Hypertension** is more common than in non-diabetic subjects.
  - **autonomic** and **peripheral neuropathy**, the latter sensory or motor. Single nerves may also be affected, including **cranial nerves**.
  - retinopathy and cataract formation.
  - skin: collagen thickening, blisters, necrobiosis lipoidica.
  - increased susceptibility to infection and delayed wound healing.
  - **diabetic coma**.
- Anaesthetic management is related to the above complications and to the perioperative control of blood sugar. Mortality and morbidity is increased when compared with non-diabetic patients.

Ideally, patients are admitted 1–2 days preoperatively, fully assessed for fitness and diabetic control, and scheduled for surgery at the beginning of the operating list. The aim is to avoid hyperglycaemia, **ketoacidosis** and **hypoglycaemia**:
  - NIDDM patients: for minor surgery, careful monitoring of blood sugar levels is usually all that is required. Chlorpropramide is withheld for 48 hours before surgery; shorter-acting **sulphonylureas** and **biguanides** are withheld on the morning of surgery. Glucose levels under 12 mmol/l are thought to be acceptable. Patients are treated as for IDDM when undergoing major surgery. Oral medication is restarted when eating postoperatively.
  - IDDM: patients are starved preoperatively, with morning insulin omitted. They should receive insulin

and dextrose iv throughout the perioperative period, to avoid hyper- and hypoglycaemia and maintain plasma glucose between 6 and 10 mmol/l. Dextrose and insulin infusions should be through the same iv cannula, to reduce risk of accidental overdose of one infusion should the other infusion cease running. Several regimens have been successfully used:

- Alberti regimen: 100 ml 10% dextrose + 10 U soluble insulin + 10 mmol potassium infused at 100 ml/h. The infusion is changed to contain more or less insulin according to regular testing with **glucose reagent sticks**. The preoperative insulin regimen is restarted when the patient is drinking and eating normally.
- the total daily insulin requirement is divided by four, adding the result to 500 ml 5% dextrose + 5–10 mmol potassium. The bag is infused at 100 ml/h, with regular checking of blood glucose levels.
- 5% dextrose + 5–10 mmol potassium is infused at 100 ml/h, with insulin infused via a syringe pump, adjusted according to a sliding scale.

Preoperative conversion to soluble insulin therapy has been used.

Since the symptoms of hypoglycaemia are masked by general anaesthesia, regular peroperative monitoring of plasma glucose is required. Administration of lactate-containing solutions is usually avoided for fear of increasing plasma glucose levels.

Modern anaesthetic agents have minimal effects on diabetic control (cf. **diethyl ether**), but regional techniques are often preferred because they interfere less with oral intake. Insulin requirements may be increased after major surgery as part of the **stress response to surgery**.

Emergency surgery is particularly hazardous, especially if diabetes is poorly controlled. Adequate resuscitation must be performed, with treatment of ketoacidosis if present. Hyperglycaemia may present with abdominal pain, and abdominal surgery may reveal no abnormality.

Pregnancy may precipitate or worsen diabetes, and close medical supervision is required. During labour, regimens usually involve iv infusions of 5% dextrose, e.g. 500 ml/8 h, with iv insulin rate adjusted according to regular stick testing. **Extradural anaesthesia** is usually suggested, since it reduces acidosis in labour and allows **Caesarean section** if indicated.

[Kurt GMM Alberti, Newcastle physician]

Milaskiewicz RM, Hall GM (1992) Br J Anaesth; 68: 198–206

Diabetic coma. Coma in **diabetes mellitus** may be caused by:

- **hypoglycaemia**: caused by excessive antidiabetic therapy, excessive exertion or decreased food intake. Treatment includes iv glucose; iv/im **glucagon** may occasionally be useful.
- **ketoacidosis**: more common in insulin-dependent diabetics. Mortality is about 10%, highest in old age. Often precipitated by other illness, e.g. infection and **MI**, since **insulin** requirements are increased. May develop insidiously.
  Features:
  - of **dehydration**, e.g. hypotension, tachycardia, etc.
  - of **acidosis**, e.g. hyperventilation.
  - vomiting, diarrhoea, abdominal pain; the latter may simulate an acute surgical emergency, requiring careful review of the diagnosis.
  - smell of acetone on the breath.
  Management:
  - measurement of urea and electrolytes, glucose, arterial blood gases, full blood count. Ketone stick tests are available. Chest X-ray and blood cultures, etc.
  - general management: O_2, nasogastric tube (gastric dilatation is common), urinary catheter, **CVP** measurement, ECG and clinical monitoring, etc. Antibiotics are administered if infection is suspected. Prophylactic **heparin** is usually suggested for high risk patients.
  - fluid therapy: guided by CVP measurement; up to 6–8 litre may be required. Suitable starting regimen: 1 litre of 0.9% saline over 30 minutes, then hourly for 2 hours, then 2 hourly, then 2–4 hourly. This is changed to 5% dextrose when blood glucose is 10–15 mmol/l (180–270 mg/dl). Hypotonic saline is used in hyperosmolar coma as below.
  - potassium supplementation is required despite any initial **hyperkalaemia**, since the body potassium deficit will be revealed once tissue uptake is stimulated by insulin. Suitable starting regimen: 10–20 mmol in the first litre of fluid; 10–40 mmol thereafter depending on the plasma potassium after 1 hour (repeated every few hours).
  - insulin is preferably given iv, e.g. 6 units as a bolus, then 6 units/h (0.1 units/kg/h in children) until plasma glucose is 10–15 mmol/l; 2–4 units/h thereafter. Glucose is monitored hourly; a reduction of 3–5 mmol/l/h (55–90 mg/dl) is aimed for. Insulin may also be given im: 20 units initially followed by 6 units hourly; then 2 hourly when glucose is 10–15 mmol/l. Insulin is given sc when food is taken orally.
  - **bicarbonate** therapy is given if pH is under 7.0–7.1. Administration is guided by **base excess**.
  - **hypophosphataemia** may require replacement, e.g. with potassium phosphate. 5–20 mmol/h has been suggested.
- hyperosmolar non-ketotic coma: usually occurs in elderly patients. Typically of slow onset with polyuria and progressive dehydration. Blood glucose levels and osmolality are very high, with little or no ketonuria. Treatment includes small doses of insulin and 0.45% saline administered slowly iv. **Cerebral oedema** and **convulsions** may occur if rehydration is too rapid.
- **lactic acidosis**: usually occurs in elderly patients taking **biguanides**. Blood glucose may be normal, with little or no ketonuria.

Table 14. Features of different types of diabetic coma

Type	Blood glucose (mmol/l)	Dehydration	Ketones
Hypoglycaemia	<2	0	0
Ketoacidosis	>14	+++	++
Hyperosmolar non-ketotic	>14	+++	0
Lactic acidosis	Variable	+	0 to +

Clinical distinction between different types of diabetic coma is unreliable. Features aiding the diagnosis are shown in Table 14.

Dialysis. Removal of solutes and water from blood by their passage across a semipermeable membrane into dialysis fluid (dialysate). Indications include **renal failure**, fluid overload and **pulmonary oedema**, electrolyte disturbances, severe **acidosis** and some cases of drug **overdose and poisoning**.

- Two main forms are commonly used:
  - haemodialysis (HD):
    - principles: vascular access, passage of blood via an extracorporeal circuit to a semipermeable cellophane membrane or hollow fibre system, and return of blood to the patient. Dialysate may be passed on the other side of the membrane, usually in a counter-current fashion. Modern machines may incorporate alarms and monitors for air bubbles.
    - vascular access is usually via:
      - double-lumen central venous catheter (or two single ones).
      - silastic arteriovenous shunt connecting adjacent vessels e.g. radial artery/cephalic vein (Scribner shunt).
      - permanent arteriovenous fistula.
      Infiltration, regional or general anaesthesia may be used for arteriovenous shunt insertion/formation. Blood flow is usually 150–300 ml/min.
    - anticoagulation of the extracorporeal circuit is required, e.g. with **heparin** 500–1000 units/h infused into the line upstream to the dialysis machine. Control of coagulation with infusion of **protamine** to the downstream line has been used but may be difficult. **Prostacyclin** has also been used.
    - solutes pass by **diffusion** from blood to dialysate, depending on the concentration gradient, size of solute, membrane porosity and duration of dialysis. Thus fluids of different composition may be used to remove different amounts of solute as required. Most dialysis fluids contain sodium, chloride, calcium, magnesium, acetate or bicarbonate (as an alkali source), and variable amounts of glucose and potassium.
    - water is removed by applying a hydrostatic pressure across the membrane (ultrafiltration). The amount of water extracted depends on the magnitude of the pressure gradient; positive pressure may be applied to the blood side of the membrane, or negative pressure to the dialysate side. Solute is also removed in this way (convective transport).
    - performed intermittently, e.g. for 4–6 hours daily/weekly as required.
    - complications:
      - related to vascular access and bleeding.
      - hypotension: may be related to hypovolaemia, dysequilibrium syndrome or acetate in dialysate.
      - dysequilibrium syndrome: nausea, vomiting, headache, hypotension, convulsions; thought to be caused by an acute decrease in plasma **osmolality**, with **cerebral oedema**.
      - hypoxaemia: mechanism is unclear.
      - electrolyte and acid-base disturbances.
    - modifications of the standard HD principle have

been developed, including:
  - intermittent isolated ultrafiltration (IIUF): similar to HD but without dialysate. Since solute and water are removed together, plasma osmolality is unchanged. Up to 1.5 l/h may be removed for 2–6 hour periods.
  - slow continuous ultrafiltration (SCUF): as above, but performed continuously, using the patient's arterial pressure to drive the system instead of a pump. Blood flows of 100–150 ml/h may be adequate. Negative pressure may be applied by placing the ultrafiltrate compartment below the level of the membrane. Tolerated better than HD.
    Sudden upsets in BP are avoided by the continuous process. Risk of **air embolism** is reduced by avoiding a pump.
  - continuous arteriovenous haemofiltration (CAVH): similar to SCUF; fluid is removed by ultrafiltration but at over 500 ml/h. Replacement fluid containing electrolytes is infused iv downstream of the filter, thereby maintaining circulatory volume.
  - continuous venovenous haemofiltration (CVVH): similar to CAVH but avoiding arterial cannulation and using a pump. Haemodynamic stability is usual.
  - continuous arteriovenous or venovenous haemodialysis (CAVHD or CVVHD): also called haemodiafiltration. Similar to CAVH and CVVH but involves the passage of dialysate on the filtrate side of the filter. Particularly useful when solute clearance is insufficient during CAVH/CVVH.
  - newer polymer membranes appear to be associated with less damage to platelets and white cells.
  - HD increases the rate of removal of many drugs including salicylates, phenobarbitone, methanol, ethylene glycol, disopyramide, methyldopa, lithium, theophylline, and many antibacterial drugs.
  - peritoneal dialysis (PD):
    - uses the peritoneum as the dialysing membrane.
    - prewarmed dialysate is admitted and drained via plastic PD catheters placed through the lower anterior abdominal wall.
    - solute clearance depends on the peritoneal permeability and blood flow, and dialysate composition and rate of exchange. Allowing the dialysate to remain in the abdomen for a 'dwell' period reduces overall solute removal.
    - removal of water depends on dialysate osmolality and dwell time. 2 litres dialysate is usually exchanged over 1 hour.
    - PD dialysate contains sodium, chloride, calcium, magnesium, lactate and a variable amount of glucose and potassium. Osmolality is 346–485 mosmol/kg, depending on glucose content, which varies from 1.3–4.5%. Potassium-free solutions are also available.
    - complications include pain, bleeding, visceral perforation, peritonitis, hyperglycaemia, hypoproteinaemia, hypokalaemia, overhydration or dehydration, and respiratory embarrassment. Contraindications include abdominal surgery,

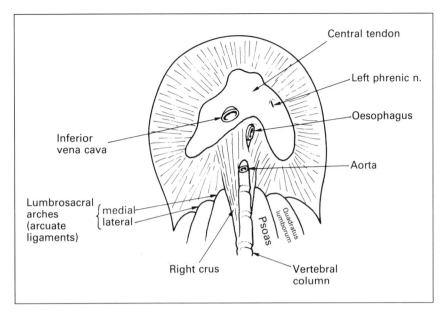

Figure 45 *Inferior aspect of diaphragm*

drains, ileus, adhesions, etc. Simpler to perform than HD but less reliable.

Monitoring includes cardiovasular monitoring, electrolyte measurement, careful measurement of **fluid balance** and daily weighing.

Drugs are removed from plasma during both types of dialysis and alterations in dosage may be required.

[Belding H Scribner, Seattle nephrologist]

Dickson DM, Hillman KM (1990) Anaesth Intensive Care; 18: 76–92

See also, Haemoperfusion

Diamorphine hydrochloride (Diacetylmorphine; Heroin). **Opioid analgesic drug**, introduced in 1898; causes less constipation, nausea and hypotension than **morphine**, but is more likely to cause addiction. Also suppresses coughing to a greater extent. More soluble than morphine, thus smaller volumes of injectate are required. Duration of action is half that of morphine.

• Dosage: 5 mg is equivalent to 10 mg morphine. It may be given im, iv, sc, orally or epidurally.

Metabolized to morphine and excreted renally.

Diaphragm. Fibromuscular sheet separating the thorax from the abdomen. The main **respiratory muscle**, it flattens and descends vertically during inspiration, expanding the thoracic cavity. During expiration, it relaxes; in forced expiration, contraction of the anterior abdominal muscles pushes the diaphragm upwards.

• Consists of (Fig. 45):
  –central tendon, attached to the pericardium above.
  –peripheral muscular part. Attachments:
    –posteriorly via the medial and lateral lumbrosacral arches (arcuate ligaments), to fascia covering psoas and quadratus lumborum muscles respectively. The right and left crura attach to vertebrae L1–3 and L1–2 respectively; between them lies the median lumbrosacral arch (median arcuate ligament).

–to the lower six ribs and costal cartilages anteriorly, and xiphisternum medially.

• Has three main openings which transmit the following structures:
  –inferior vena cava and right phrenic nerve at the level of T8.
  –oesophagus, vagus and gastric nerves and branches of the left gastric vessels at the level of T10.
  –aorta, thoracic duct and azygos vein at the level of T12.

The diaphragm is also pierced by the left phrenic nerve and splanchnic nerves.

The sympathetic chain passes behind the medial lumbrosacral arch.

• Nerve supply: from C3–5 via the **phrenic nerves**, with some sensory supply to the periphery via the lower intercostal nerves.

• Development:
  –originally in the neck; descends during development, retaining its cervical nerve supply.
  –formed from :
    –oesophageal mesentery dorsally.
    –right and left pleuroperitoneal membranes laterally.
    –septum transversum anteriorly (forming the central tendon).
    –small peripheral contribution from body wall.

Defects in development may produce **diaphragmatic herniae**.

See also, Hiatus hernia

Diaphragmatic herniae. Herniation of abdominal viscera through the **diaphragm** into the thorax.

Congenital herniae occur in approximately 1 in 4000 of live births (1 in 2500 of all births), and are caused by failure of fusion of the various components of the diaphragm, e.g.:
  –foramen of Bochdalek: through a defective pleuroperitoneal membrane, usually left-sided. The most common form (80%).

–foramen of Morgagni: between xiphoid and costal origins; more common on the right side.

–through the central tendon or oesophageal hiatus.

Other congenital defects may be present.

Causes respiratory distress, cyanosis, scaphoid abdomen and bowel sounds audible in the thorax. Diagnosed clinically and by X-ray. The lung on the affected side is often hypoplastic, with decreased **compliance** and increased **pulmonary vascular resistance** (PVR). Arterial **hypoxaemia** reflects immature lung tissue and reduced ventilation caused by presence of thoracic bowel, and persistent **fetal circulation** caused by the raised PVR. PVR is further increased by **hypoxic pulmonary vasoconstriction**.

Immediate management includes gastric decompression, improving oxygenation and decreasing PVR. IPPV by facepiece may increase gastric distension and should be avoided. IPPV is best performed using a tracheal tube, avoiding excessive inflation pressures since **pneumothorax** may easily occur. PVR may be reduced by avoiding **hypocapnia** and **hypothermia**, treating **acidosis**, and infusing **vasodilator drugs** centrally, e.g. **tolazoline** 1 mg/kg/h, or **sodium nitroprusside** 1–2 µg/kg/min. **Prostacyclin** 5–10 ng/kg/min has also been used.

Anaesthesia for surgical correction is as for **paediatric anaesthesia**. N_2O is avoided because of distension of thoracic bowel. Excessive inflation of the hypoplastic lung at the end of the procedure should be avoided, since pneumothorax may occur. Abdominal closure may be difficult once the bowel is returned to the abdomen; postoperative IPPV may be required. The hypoplastic lung slowly re-expands, usually within a few days/weeks.

Surgery is usually delayed in severe cases, until respiratory stability is achieved. **High frequency ventilation** and **extracorporeal membrane oxygenation** have been used. Mortality is high if pneumothorax occurs and lung compliance is low.

Acquired acute herniae may follow blunt or penetrating **trauma** or surgery. They may impair ventilation, or only cause symptoms if strangulation or obstruction occur. **Hiatus hernia** is gradual in onset.

[Giovanni B Morgagni (1682–1771), Italian anatomist; Victor A Bochdalek (1801–1883), Czech anatomist]

See also, Cardiopulmonary resuscitation, neonatal

Diastole, *see Cardiac cycle; Diastolic interval*

Diastolic blood pressure. Lowest **arterial BP** during diastole. Represents the pressure head for **coronary blood flow**, but otherwise generally thought to be less important than systolic blood pressure and **MAP**, although it contributes to the latter.

Diastolic BP has been used to guide therapy in **hypertension**, treatment usually being advocated if it exceeds 90 mmHg, but this is controversial.

Diastolic interval. Duration of diastole. Shortened when **heart rate** is increased; e.g. equals about 0.62 seconds at 65 beats/min, but only 0.14 seconds at 200 beats/min. Short diastolic intervals reduce **coronary blood flow** and ventricular filling.

Diastolic pressure time index (DPTI). Area between tracings of left ventricular pressure and aortic root pressure during diastole (*see Fig. 52; Endocardial viability ratio*). Represents the pressure head and time available

for **coronary blood flow**; used to calculate endocardial viability ratio.

See also, Cardiac cycle

Diathermy (Bovie machine). Device used to coagulate blood vessels, and cut and destroy tissues during surgery, by the heating effect of an electric current passed through them. Alternating current with a frequency of 0.5–1 MHz is used; a sine wave pattern is employed for cutting and a damped or pulsed sine wave pattern for coagulation. Effects on skeletal and cardiac muscle are negligible at these high frequencies. The **current density** is kept high at the site of intended damage by using small electrodes at this site, e.g. forceps tips.

- Diathermy may be:
  - unipolar:
    - forceps, etc. act as one electrode;
    - large plate strapped to the patient's leg acts as the other electrode, often at earth potential. Current density at this site is low because of the large area of tissue through which current passes; thus little heating occurs.
  - bipolar: current is passed across tissue held between the two tips of one pair of forceps. The power used is small and the current dispersal through other tissues is negligible; thus used for more delicate surgery, e.g. eye surgery and neurosurgery. No plate electrode is required.
- Hazards:
  - interference with **monitoring** equipment, especially when the old spark gap diathermy machines are used; interference is less likely with modern solid state machines.
  - incorrect attachment of the plate may cause burns, e.g. if contact is only made over a small surface area.
  - burns may occur if the surgeon activates the diathermy accidentally, or if the forceps are touching the patient or lying on saline or blood-soaked drapes. When not used, the forceps should be kept in a protective non-conducting holder. An audible buzzer warns that the device is operating.
  - if the plate electrode is earthed, and connections are faulty, current may take other routes to reach earth. Thus current may flow through any earthed metal conductor the patient touches, e.g. drip stands, ECG leads, etc., causing burns at the site of contact. In addition, the mains (50 Hz) current may flow through the system. A capacitor within the circuit will prevent the latter, whilst allowing the diathermy current to flow. Risks from flow of current to earth are reduced if the circuit is completely isolated from earth ('floating'), since current will no longer take these other routes.
  - may act as an ignition source of flammable substances, e.g. anaesthetic agents, bowel gases.
  - may interfere with pacemaker function.

[William T Bovie (1882–1958), US biophysicist]

See also, Cardiac pacing; Electrocution and electrical burns; Explosions and fires

Diazepam. Benzodiazepine, widely used for **sedation**, anxiolysis and as an **anticonvulsant drug**. Has been used as **premedication**, and to supplement or induce anaesthesia. Insoluble in water; original preparations caused pain on injection and thrombophlebitis. These are rare with

Diazemuls, an emulsion of diazepam in soya bean oil. Effects on the nervous system are via the **limbic system** and polysynaptic spinal pathways. Propagation of epileptiform waves is suppressed.

Injection iv may cause respiratory depression, especially in the elderly. Reduced cardiac output and vasodilatation may occur with large doses. Drowsiness and confusion, especially in the elderly, may persist for several hours after large iv doses. Absorption after im injection is unreliable and the injection is painful.

Half-life is 20–70 hours, with formation of active metabolites (e.g. nordiazepam, whose half-life is up to 120 hours). Thus repeated doses, e.g. in ICU, may lead to delayed recovery.

- Dosage:
  - –10–30 mg orally for premedication (0.5 mg/kg in children, up to 10 mg).
  - –5–10 mg iv for sedation or anticonvulsant effect, repeated as necessary. Rectal adminstration is also effective.

Diazoxide. Vasodilator drug, used for emergency treatment of severe **hypertension**. Acts directly on blood vessel walls. Increases blood **glucose** level by increasing **catecholamine** levels and by reducing **insulin** release; may be used orally to treat chronic **hypoglycaemia** (previously used iv to treat acute hypoglycaemia).

- Dosage: 1–3 mg/kg (up to 150 mg) iv in **hypertensive crises**, repeated after 5–15 minutes if required. **MI** and **CVA** have followed larger doses. Quickly bound to plasma proteins, therefore must be given rapidly.
- Side effects: tachycardia, **hyperglycaemia**, fluid retention.

Dibucaine, *see Cinchocaine*

Dibucaine number. Degree of inhibition of plasma **cholinesterase** by dibucaine (**cinchocaine**). Sample plasma is added to a benzoylcholine solution, and breakdown of the latter is observed using measurement of light absorption. This is repeated using plasma pretreated with 10^{-5} molar solution dibucaine; the percentage inhibition of benzoylcholine breakdown by the enzyme is the dibucaine number. Abnormal variants of cholinesterase are inhibited to lesser degrees, with dibucaine numbers less than the normal 75–85%. Thus useful in the analysis and typing of different abnormal variants, which may give rise to prolonged paralysis following **suxamethonium** administration.

Similar testing may be performed using inhibition by fluoride, chloride, suxamethonium itself and other compounds.

DIC, *see Disseminated intravascular coagulation*

Dichlorphenamide. Carbonic anhydrase inhibitor, used to treat **glaucoma** but also to stimulate respiration, possibly via lowering CSF pH. Actions are similar to those of **acetazolamide**, but longer lasting. Has been used to assist **weaning** in ICU. 100–200 mg are given orally, followed by 100 mg 12 hourly.

Diclofenac sodium. NSAID, available for parenteral use. Has been used for **postoperative analgesia**, thus reducing requirements for opioids. Also used for renal colic and other painful conditions. May also be given enterally.

- Dosage:
  - –1 mg/kg im up to 75 mg, as a single dose or once-twice daily for up to 2 days. Should be given by deep intragluteal injection.
  - –75–150 mg orally/day in divided doses (1–3 mg/kg in children). 100 mg and 12.5 mg suppositories are available.
- Side effects: as for NSAIDs. Should be used with caution in renal impairment. Muscle damage after im injection has been indicated by increased plasma creatine kinase levels. Sterile abscesses have occured after superficial injection.

Dicrotic notch, *see Arterial waveform*

Diethyl ether. $C_2H_5OC_2H_5$. **Inhalational anaesthetic agent**, first prepared in 1540. **Paracelsus** described its effects on animals in the same year. Produced by heating concentrated sulphuric acid with ethanol. First used for anaesthesia in 1842 by **Clarke** and **Long**, who did not publish their work until later. Introduced publicly by **Morton** in the USA in 1846; used in London by **Boott** and in **Dumfries** in the same year. Classically given by **open-drop techniques**, and more recently using a **draw-over technique** (e.g. using the EMO **vaporizer**), or by standard plenum vaporizer. Inspired concentrations of up to 20% may be required during induction of anaesthesia.

No longer generally available in the UK, although widely considered one of the safest inhalational agents, largely because respiratory depression is late and precedes cardiovascular depression. Still used worldwide, because of its safety and low cost.

Its many disadvantages include flammability, high blood/gas **partition coefficient** resulting in slow uptake and recovery, respiratory irritation causing coughing and laryngospasm, stimulation of salivary secretions, high incidence of nausea and vomiting, and occurrence of convulsions postoperatively, typically associated with pyrexia and **atropine** administration. Sympathetic stimulation maintains BP with low incidence of arrhythmias, but **hyperglycaemia** may occur.

Has been used in severe **asthma** because of its bronchodilator properties.

10–15% metabolized, to alcohol, acetaldehyde and acetic acid.

Difficult intubation, *see Intubation, difficult*

Diffusing capacity (Transfer factor). Volume of a substance (usually carbon monoxide (CO)) transferred across the alveoli per minute per unit alveolar partial pressure. CO is used because it is rapidly taken up by **haemoglobin** in the blood; thus its transfer from alveoli to blood is limited mainly by diffusion across the alveolar membrane.

- Measurement:
  - –a single breath of gas containing 0.3% CO and 10% helium is held for 10–20 seconds. Initial alveolar partial pressure of CO is derived by measuring the dilution of helium that has occurred. Expired partial pressure of CO is measured.
  - –continuous breathing of gas containing 0.3% CO, for up to a minute. Rate of uptake of CO is measured when steady state is reached.

• Normal value: 17–25 ml/min/mmHg.

Reduction in pulmonary diseases, e.g. **pulmonary fibrosis**, has been traditionally attributed to increased alveolar membrane thickness. However, $\dot{V}/\dot{Q}$ **mismatch** may be more important than alveolar thickening in these conditions. Also reduced when alveolar membrane area is reduced, e.g. after pneumonectomy (corrected by calculation of diffusing coefficient: diffusing capacity per litre of available lung volume).

The term 'transfer factor' is sometimes used because the measurement refers to overall measurement of gas transfer, which may be affected by ventilation, perfusion and diffusion defects distributed unevenly throughout the lung. Correlation with clinical examination is not always reliable for these reasons.

Diffusion. Movement of a substance from an area of high concentration to one of low concentration, resulting from spontaneous random movement of its constituent particles. May occur across **membranes**, e.g. from alveoli to bloodstream.

• Rate of diffusion across a membrane is proportional to:
  –available area of membrane.
  –concentration gradient across the membrane (**Fick's law**).
  –$\dfrac{1}{\sqrt{mw}\text{ of the substance}}$ (**Graham's law**).

For diffusion of a gas across a membrane into a liquid, e.g. across the alveolar membrane, concentration gradient is proportional to the pressure gradient, and is maintained if the gas is soluble in the liquid; i.e. rate of diffusion is proportional to **solubility**.

Diffusion hypoxia, *see Fink effect*

Digital nerve block. Each digit is supplied by two palmar and two dorsal digital nerves. A fine needle is introduced from the dorsal side of the base of the digit, and 2–3 ml **local anaesthetic agent** (without **adrenaline**) injected on each side, between bone and skin.

Digoxin. Most widely used **cardiac glycoside**, used to treat supraventricular **arrhythmias**, e.g. **AF**, **atrial flutter** and **SVT**. Described and investigated by Withering in 1785 in his *Account of the Foxglove*. Slows atrioventricular conduction and increases **myocardial contractility**. Its prolonged use in **cardiac failure** is controversial. Volume of distribution is large (700 litres) and **half-life** long (36 hours); elimination is therefore lengthy after termination of treatment. Dosage must be reduced in renal impairment and in the elderly. Therapeutic plasma levels: 1–2 ng/ml (blood is taken 1 hour after an iv dose, 8 hours after an oral dose).

Contraindicated in **Wolff–Parkinson–White syndrome**, since atrioventricular block may encourage conduction through accessory pathways with resultant arrhythmia.

• Dosage:
  –loading dose for rapid digitalization:
    –0.75–1.5 mg orally, followed by 0.25 mg 6 hourly until effects are seen, or:
    –0.5–1.0 mg iv by slow infusion, as 1–3 divided doses. Effects are usually seen within 10 minutes, and are maximal in 2 hours. Fast injection may cause vasoconstriction and coronary ischaemia. IM injection is painful and unreliable.

  –children: 10–20 µg/kg given 6 hourly until effects are seen.
  –maintenance: 0.125–0.25 mg daily (10–20 µg/kg daily in children).

• Side effects and toxicity:
  –more common in **hypokalaemia**, **hypercalcaemia** or **hypomagnesaemia**.
  –nausea, vomiting, diarrhoea.
  –headache, malaise, confusion. Impaired colour vision (typically for yellow) is an early symptom.
  –any cardiac arrhythmia may occur; bradycardia, heart block, and ventricular ectopics including bi- and trigemini are commonest.
  –ECG findings:
    –prolonged **P–R interval** and **heart block**.
    –**T wave** inversion.
    –**S–T segment** depression (the 'reverse tick').
  –arrhythmias should be treated as appropriate, if severe. Potassium replacement may be required. **Cardioversion** may result in severe arrhythmias, and should be avoided. **Phenytoin** is particularly useful in ventricular arrhythmias. Digoxin-specific antibody fragments are available for use in severe toxicity.

[William Withering (1741–99), English physician]

Dihydrocodeine tartrate. Opioid analgesic drug, of similar potency to **codeine**. Prepared in 1911. Causes fewer side effects than **morphine** or **pethidine** at equivalent analgesic doses. Also has a marked antitussive effect.

• Dosage: 30 mg orally or 50 mg im, 4–6 hourly; 0.5–1 mg/kg in children.

Dilution techniques. Used for measuring body compartment volumes. A known quantity of tracer substance is introduced into the space to be measured, and its concentration measured after complete mixing:

$$C_1 \times V_1 = C_2 \times (V_1 + V_2)$$

where C_1 = initial concentration of indicator
C_2 = final concentration of indicator
V_1 = volume of indicator
V_2 = volume to be measured.

The technique may be used to measure volume of blood, plasma, ECF, etc. Tracer substances include dyes and **radioisotopes**; the latter may be injected as radioactive ions or attached to proteins, red blood cells, etc. Gaseous markers may be used to study **lung volumes**, e.g. helium to measure **FRC**.

The principle may be extended for **cardiac output measurement**, where radioisotope, dye or ice-cold crystalloid solution is injected as a bolus proximal to the right ventricle, and its concentration measured distally, e.g. radial or pulmonary artery. A concentration-time curve is plotted to enable calculation of cardiac output.

Dimethyl tubocurarine chloride/bromide. Non-depolarizing **neuromuscular blocking drug**, derived from **tubocurarine**; introduced in 1948. More potent and longer-lasting (up to 2 hours) than tubocurarine, and with less ganglion blockade and **histamine** release; i.e. more cardiostable. No longer used in the UK, although recently popular in the USA as metocurine. Excreted almost exclusively via the urine.

• Intubating dose: 0.2–0.4 mg/kg; acts within 3–5 minutes.

Dinoprost/dinoprostone, *see Prostaglandins*

2,3–Diphosphoglycerate (2,3–DPG). Substance formed within red blood cells from phosphoglyceraldehyde, produced during **glycolysis**. Binds strongly to the β chains of deoxygenated **haemoglobin**, reducing O_2 binding and shifting the **oxyhaemoglobin dissociation curve** to the right; i.e. favours O_2 liberation to the tissues. Binds poorly to the γ chains of **fetal haemoglobin**.
- Levels are increased by:
  –**anaemia**.
  –**alkalosis**.
  –chronic **hypoxaemia**, e.g. in cyanotic heart disease.
  –high **altitude**.
  –exercise.
  –**pregnancy**.
  –**hyperthyroidism**.
  –hyperphosphataemia.
  –certain red cell enzyme abnormalities.
- Levels are decreased by:
  –**acidosis**, e.g. in stored blood; requires 12–24 hours for levels to be restored.
  –**hypophosphataemia**.
  –**hypothyroidism**.
  –**hypopituitarism**.

Diphtheria. Infection caused by *Corynebacterium diphtheriae*, a Gram-positive rod. Now rare in the Western world, due to immunization, but formerly a major cause of death, particularly in children.
- Features:
  –symptoms of upper respiratory infection.
  –increasing malaise and fever. Diphtheria toxin may affect CNS, heart and other organs. **Cranial nerve** palsies, visual disturbances, and **cardiac failure** with conduction defects and **arrhythmias** may occur.
  –a thick exudative membrane may form across the posterior pharynx/larynx, causing complete obstruction.
- Treatment:
  –as for **airway obstruction**.
  –antitoxin administration.
  –iv penicillin.

Dipipanone hydrochloride. Opioid analgesic drug, similar to **methadone** and **dextromoramide**. Prepared in 1950. Available in the UK for oral use as tablets of 10 mg combined with **cyclizine** 30 mg.
- Dosage: up to 3 tablets 6 hourly. Anticholinergic effects of cyclizine may limit its use.

Dipyrimadole. Antiplatelet drug, used to prevent arterial thrombus formation, e.g. on prosthetic heart valves. Modifies **platelet** aggregation, adhesion and survival. Also given iv for stress testing during diagnostic cardiac imaging; causes marked vasodilatation. May cause **coronary steal**.
- Dosage: 100–150 mg orally, 6–8 hourly.
- Side effects: may be hazardous in severe coronary and aortic stenosis due to its vasodilating effects. Nausea, vomiting and headache may also occur.

Disinfection of anaesthetic equipment, *see Contamination of anaesthetic equipment*

Disopyramide phosphate. Class Ia **antiarrhythmic drug,** used to treat ventricular and supraventricular arrhythmias. **Half-life** is 7 hours.
- Dosage:
  –2 mg/kg up to 150 mg iv over at least 5 minutes, followed by 0.4 mg/kg/h infusion.
  –300–800 mg/day orally in divided doses.
- Side effects: myocardial depression, hypotension, anticholinergic effects, e.g. urinary retention, atrioventricular block.

Disseminated intravascular coagulation (DIC). Pathological activation of **coagulation** by a disease process, leading to fibrin clot formation, consumption of **platelets** and coagulation factors (I, II and XIII), and secondary **fibrinolysis**. May be precipitated by **shock, septicaemia, haemolysis, malignancy, trauma, burns,** major surgery, **PE, extracorporeal circulation,** and obstetric conditions, e.g. **pre-eclampsia, amniotic fluid embolism,** intrauterine death and placental abruption.
- Effects:
  –may occur chronically, with little clinical abnormality.
  –bruising, bleeding from wounds, venepuncture sites, GIT, lung, urinary tract and uteroplacental bed.
  –capillary microthrombosis may cause multiple organ failure.
  –shock, **acidosis** and **hypoxaemia** may occur.
  Haematological investigation may reveal low titres of fibrinogen, coagulation factors and antithrombin III, **thrombocytopenia,** high titres of **fibrin degradation products** and prolonged prothrombin, partial thromboplastin and thrombin times.
- Treatment:
  –directed at underlying causes.
  –supportive.
  –administration of fresh frozen plasma, platelets, and possibly cryoprecipitate.
  –the role of **heparin** is still unclear, but it should be considered if initial therapy does not improve the patient's condition. Heparin has been used mainly in the treatment of chronic DIC without major coagulopathy.

Risberg B, Andreasson S, Eriksson E (1991) Acta Anaesthesiol Scand; 95: Suppl 60–71
See also, Blood products; Coagulation disorders; Coagulation studies

Disseminated sclerosis, *see Demyelinating diseases*

Dissociation curves, *see Carbon dioxide dissociation curve; Oxyhaemoglobin dissociation curve*

Dissociative anaesthesia, *see Ketamine*

Distigmine bromide. Acetylcholinesterase inhibitor, used in the treatment of **myasthenia gravis**. Duration of action is up to 24 hours. Risk of accumulation and **cholinergic crisis** is greater than with shorter acting drugs, and thus it is usually reserved for supplementation of other drugs. Also used in the treatment of urinary retention and intestinal atony.
- Dosage: 5–20 mg daily, orally.

Distribution curves, statistical, *see Statistical frequency distributions*

Diuresis, forced, *see Forced diuresis*

Diuretics. Drugs increasing the rate of urine production by the kidney.
- Divided into:
  - **thiazide diuretics**: act at the proximal part of the distal convoluted tubule of the **nephron**, and also at the proximal tubule. Have low ceilings of action; i.e. maximal effects are produced by small doses. May cause **hypokalaemia**, **hypomagnesaemia**, hyperuricaemia, **hyperglycaemia** and hypercholesterolaemia.
  - osmotic diuretics, e.g. **mannitol**: increase **renal blood flow** by plasma expansion, then draw water into the renal tubules by an osmotic effect. Other small molecules which are filtered but not reabsorbed may have similar osmotic diuretic actions, e.g. glucose, urea and sucrose.
  - potassium sparing diuretics, e.g. triamterene, amiloride, **spironolactone**: act at the distal convoluted tubule, where most potassium is normally lost; spironolactone acts by **aldosterone** inhibition. May cause **hyperkalaemia** and **hyponatraemia.**
  - loop diuretics, e.g. **frusemide**, **bumetanide**, ethacrynic acid: act at the ascending loop of Henle. More potent, with high ceilings of action. Immediate benefit in fluid overload/cardiac failure is thought to be due to vasodilatation. May cause hypokalaemia, hyperuricaemia, hypomagnesaemia and hyperglycaemia. Damage to 8th cranial nerve may occur, especially following rapid iv injection and with concurrent aminoglycoside therapy.
  - other substances causing diuresis:
    - mercurials: no longer used. Reduce sodium and chloride reabsorption at several sites. Hypochloraemic acidosis is common.
    - **carbonic anhydrase** inhibitors, e.g. **acetazolamide**.
    - **xanthines**, e.g. **aminophylline**: reduces sodium excretion and increases **GFR**.
    - **dopamine**: increases renal blood flow and GFR; also reduces sodium absorption.
    - water and ethanol inhibit **vasopressin** secretion.
    - acidifying salts, e.g. ammonium chloride: increases hydrogen ion and sodium excretion.
    - demeclocycline: blocks the action of vasopressin on the distal tubule and collecting duct; used in the **syndrome of inappropriate antidiuretic hormone**.

Anaesthesia for patients taking diuretics: **hypovolaemia** and electrolyte disturbances are possible, especially in the elderly. Hypokalaemia may represent severe body potassium depletion; conversely potassium supplements and potassium sparing diuretics may cause hyperkalaemia. Severe hyponatraemia may follow treatment with potassium sparing diuretics. Combinations of different types of diuretics tend to be synergistic.
[Friedrich GJ Henle (1809–1885), German anatomist]

Diving reflex. Decreased respiration, vagal bradycardia and splanchnic and muscle bed vasoconstriction following immersion of the face in water. Cerebral and cardiac circulations are preserved. Occurs in mammals, birds and reptiles; it has been suggested that it may aid survival in man, e.g. in boating and skiing accidents.

Divinyl ether. Inhalational anaesthetic agent, introduced in 1933 and no longer used. Similar in potency and explo-siveness to **diethyl ether**, but less irritant. Liver damage resulted from prolonged use. Combined 1:4 with ether as Vinesthene Anaesthetic Mixture.

$\dot{D}O_2$, *see Oxygen delivery*

Dobutamine hydrochloride. Synthetic **catecholamine**, used as an **inotropic drug** e.g. after **cardiac surgery**, and in **septic** or **cardiogenic shock**. Stimulates β_1–**adrenergic receptors**, with weak stimulation of β_2 and α receptors. Does not affect **dopamine receptors**. Increases myocardial contractility, with less increase in myocardial O_2 consumption than other catecholamines. Causes less tachycardia than dopamine or **isoprenaline**, probably because of a reduced effect on the sinoatrial node, and less activation of the **baroreceptor reflex**. Reduces **left ventricular end-diastolic pressure** if raised.

Plasma **half-life** is about 2 minutes. Excreted via the urine. Supplied as a solution for dilution with saline or 5% dextrose prior to use.
- Usual dosage: 2.5–10 µg/kg/min by infusion; higher rates may be required.
- Side effects: tachycardia and ventricular arrhythmias at high doses.

Doll's eye movements (Oculocephalic reflex). Reflex elicited in unconscious patients by quickly turning the patient's head to one side and holding it there. The eyes move to the right when the head is turned to the left, and vice versa; i.e. they continue to point in the original position in relation to the body, as if fixed on a distant object. They then move to the midposition. The reflex involves bilateral vesibular apparatus and nerves, brain-stem, and oculomotor nerves; it is therefore absent in **brainstem death**. Normally absent because of cerebral activity influencing eye movement; i.e. becomes apparent if cerebral activity is supressed or interrupted.

Domperidone maleate. Antiemetic drug related to **metoclopramide**, and with similar actions. Crosses the **blood–brain barrier** only slowly, thus less likely to cause sedation and **dystonic reactions** than other antiemetic drugs. No longer available for iv use, because of associated ventricular arrhythmias.
- Dosage:
  - 10–20 mg 4–8 hourly, orally.
  - 30–60 mg 4–8 hourly, rectally.

Donnan effect (Gibbs–Donnan effect). Effect of charged particles on one side of a **membrane** on the distribution of other charged particles, when the former cannot diffuse through the membrane but the latter can. For example, intracellular proteins (negatively charged) are confined within the cell. The distribution of potassium ions (positively charged) and chloride ions (negatively charged) on either side of the membrane is therefore affected by the electrical gradient produced by the proteins, as well as their own concentration gradients. There is a fixed ratio between the concentration of diffusible ions on one side of the membrane, and the concentration of those on the other. This ratio is the same for all the ions distributed about a particular membrane under the same conditions.
[Frederick Donnan (1870–1956), English chemist; Josiah Gibbs (1839–1903), US physicist]

Dopamine. Naturally-occurring **catecholamine** and **neurotransmitter**, found in postganglionic sympathetic nerve endings and the adrenal medulla. A precursor of **adrenaline** and **noradrenaline**. Used as an **inotropic drug**, e.g. in **cardiogenic** or **septic shock**. Also used to maintain splanchnic blood flow (e.g. to maintain urine output when renal function is compromised).

Supplied as the hydrochloride in a concentrated solution for dilution in saline or 5% dextrose, or as a ready-made iv solution in dextrose. Inactivated by alkali.
- Effects depend on the dose used:
  –up to 5 μg/kg/min: stimulates **dopamine receptors**, causing renal and mesenteric vasodilatation. **Renal blood flow**, **GFR**, urine output and sodium excretion are increased. These effects are inhibited by **phenothiazines**, **butyrophenones** and **metoclopramide**. Tubular sodium reabsorption may also be reduced independently of the increased renal blood flow.
  –5–15 μg/kg/min: stimulates β_1-**adrenergic receptors**; myocardial contractility, cardiac output, BP, and O_2 consumption are increased. **Pulmonary capillary wedge pressure** may paradoxically increase, possibly because of increased venous return secondary to venoconstriction. Some α_2-stimulation also occurs.
  –over 15 μg/kg/min: stimulates α_1-receptors, causing peripheral vasoconstriction.

Rapidly taken up by tissues and metabolized by dopamine β-hydroxylase and **monoamine oxidase** pathways, with renal excretion of metabolites. Plasma **half-life** is about 1 minute. Dosage must be reduced if the patient is taking **monoamine oxidase inhibitors**.
- Side effects: tachycardia and ventricular arrhythmias are common at higher doses. Severe tissue necrosis may follow peripheral extravasation; it should thus be administered into a large vein (preferably central).

Dopamine receptors. Found peripherally and in the CNS. Subdivided into:
  –central:
    –D_1 receptors: function is uncertain. Thought to be activated via **cAMP**.
    –D_2 receptors: found in pathways involving the basal ganglia and hypothalamus, concerned with coordination of movement, behaviour and inhibition of prolactin release. Also present in the **chemoreceptor trigger zone** where stimulation results in vomiting, and in the spinal cord. **Butyrophenones** are the classical antagonists; others include **phenothiazines** and **metoclopramide**. Bromocriptine is an agonist.
  –peripheral:
    –DA_1 receptors: postsynaptic; thought to be analogous to central D_1 receptors. Stimulation causes vasodilatation in renal and mesenteric vascular beds.
    –DA_2 receptors: presynaptic; stimulation inhibits **noradrenaline** release via negative feedback. Inhibition of cAMP formation may be involved. May also be present at cholinergic nerve endings. Inhibited by butyrophenones; i.e. thought to be analogous to central D_2 receptors.
Further subclasses of **dopamine** receptors may also exist.

Dopexamine hydrochloride. Analogue of **dopamine**, used as an **inotropic drug** in **cardiac failure** e.g. after cardiac surgery. Stimulates peripheral **dopamine receptors** and β_2-**adrenergic receptors**, with indirect stimulation of β_1-adrenergic receptors via inhibition of neuronal reuptake of **catecholamines**. Causes peripheral (including renal) vasodilatation with reduced BP and increased cardiac output. 40% bound to red blood cells.
- Dosage: 0.5–6.0 μg/kg/min.
- Side effects include tachycardia (usually mild) and arrhythmias, nausea, vomiting, and tremor.

Doppler effect. Increase in observed frequency of a signal when the signal source approaches the observer, and decrease when the source moves away. For example, the wavefronts in front of a moving car horn will be closer together than when the horn is stationary, because when each wavefront is emitted, the horn moves forward before emitting another. Similarly, the wavefronts behind the horn are further apart. To the observer, the tone of the horn changes from higher-pitched to lower-pitched as the horn approaches and passes, although the actual frequency emitted has not changed.

The principle is used clinically to determine velocities and flow rates of moving substances, e.g. in **cardiac output measurement**. An **ultrasound** beam may be directed along the path of flow; the sound waves reflect from the surfaces of the blood cells as they approach or move away. Analysis of the reflected frequencies allows determination of velocity of flow. Doppler probes contain both emitter and detector in the probe tip.

May also be used to detect arterial wall movement in **arterial BP measurement**; onset of movement occurs at systolic pressure, and cessation at diastolic pressure, as the cuff is deflated from high pressure. The ultrasonic beam is directed across the artery.
[Christian Doppler (1803–1853), Austrian physicist]
Allan PL (1992) Hosp Update; 18: 182–6 and 254–62

Dorsal column stimulation. Technique used in intractable **pain management**. Has been performed percutaneously using a wire electrode connected to an external power source, but an implantable system is usually employed. Electrodes may be placed at open laminectomy, or inserted into the extradural space through a needle. The electrodes are placed above the highest level of the pain, and connected to a subcutaneous inductance coil, usually on the abdominal wall, by insulated wires. The patient applies an external power source over the coil for pain relief. Implantable power sources may be used.

Dose–response curves. Curves describing the relationship between dose of a drug or other physiological agent and the resultant response. A logarithmic scale is usually used for the abscissa. The classic curve is sigmoid-shaped, with increasing response as dose is increased until a plateau is reached (Fig. 46).
- Different curves are characterized by their:
  –position on the abscissa (related to **potency**).
  –maximal height (**efficacy**).
  –slope (influenced by the number of receptors that must be activated before a drug has an effect).
Drugs A and B are both **agonists**, but A is more potent. Drug C is less efficacious and is therefore a partial agonist. Addition of a competitive **antagonist**, D, to A shifts the curve to the right (i.e. reduced potency) but without altering its height (i.e. same efficacy). A non-

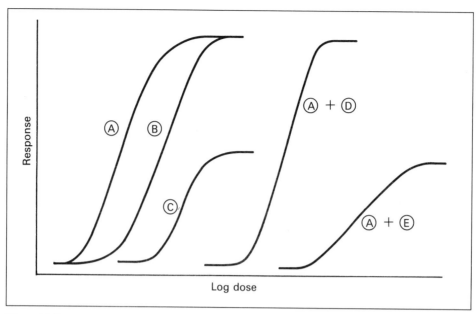

Figure 46 *Dose–response curves (see text)*

competitive antagonist, E, shifts the curve to the right, reduces its height and alters its slope.

The curves are affected by individual variability in response, related to differences in **pharmacokinetics** and **pharmacodynamics**. The dose of drug required to produce a certain response in a given percentage of the population ($n\%$) is described as the effective dose, ED_n.

See also, Receptor theory

Double-blind studies, *see Clinical trials*

Double-lumen tubes, *see Endobronchial tubes*

Down's syndrome. Syndrome resulting from presence of an extra chromosome 21 (hence the term trisomy 21). Usually due to non-dysjunction of chromosomes during germ cell formation, and rarely due to translocation in parental cells.
- Features:
  - round head and face, slanting eyes with prominent and wide epicanthic folds. Ears are low set; the mouth is small with a large tongue.
  - broad short hands, with a single transverse palmar crease; the gap between first and second toes is large.
  - congenital heart disease is common, especially **ASD** and **VSD**, **Fallot's tetralogy** and patent **ductus arteriosus**.
  - duodenal atresia and other congenital abnormalities are common.
  - leukaemia is common.
  - hypotonicity.
  - mental retardation.
- Anaesthetic problems:
  - cardiac abnormalities.
  - airway difficulties, including difficult tracheal intubation. Excessive secretions are common.
  - hypotonia.
  - atlantoaxial subluxation and instability.

[John Down (1828–1896), English physician]

Doxacurium chloride. Non-depolarizing **neuromuscular blocking drug**, introduced into the USA in 1991. Has similar features to **pancuronium**, but without cardiovascular effects. Dosage range: 25–80 μg/kg; intubation may be performed 4–6 minutes after the initial dose. Effects last 1–3 hours, depending on dosage. Excreted unchanged via the kidneys and liver. Causes **histamine** release only at much higher doses than required clinically. Has been suggested for prolonged surgery where cardiovascular stability is required, e.g. neurosurgery or cardiac surgery.

Maddineni VR, Cooper R, Stanley JC, et al (1992) Anaesthesia; 47: 554–7

Doxapram hydrochloride. **Analeptic drug,** used for its respiratory stimulant properties. Acts on peripheral **chemoreceptors**, increasing tidal volume more than respiratory rate. May be administered by infusion in ventilatory failure in patients with **COAD**, in an attempt to avoid the need for IPPV. Also used in postoperative respiratory depression, without reversing opioid-induced analgesia. Has been used routinely to reduce postoperative pulmonary complications, especially in at-risk patients. **Half-life** is 2–4 hours.
- Dosage:
  - 1–1.5 mg/kg iv over 30 seconds; repeated hourly.
  - 1.5–4 mg/min by infusion, according to response. Steady-state plasma levels are produced by:
    - 4 mg/min for 15 minutes,
    - 3 mg/min for 15 minutes,
    - 2 mg/min for 30 minutes,
    - 1.5 mg/min thereafter.
- Side effects: hypertension, tachycardia (resulting from vasomotor stimulation), restlessness. Convulsions may occur with high doses.

Contraindicated in coronary artery disease, severe hypertension, thyrotoxicosis, asthma and epilepsy. Effects are said to be potentiated by **monoamine oxidase inhibitors**.

2,3–DPG, *see 2,3–Diphosphoglycerate*

Draw-over techniques. Anaesthesia in which the patient's inspiratory effort draws room air (with or without added O_2) over a volatile agent with each breath. More sophisticated, but similar to, **open-drop techniques**. There should be minimal resistance in the breathing system and **vaporizer**. Incorporation of **bellows** or a **self-inflating bag** into the breathing system allows IPPV, and provides a reservoir if continuous flow of O_2 is added. **Non-rebreathing valves** prevent exhalation back into the vaporizer; a unidirectional valve is necessary upstream of the bellows or bag, if used, to allow IPPV (Fig. 47).
- Uses:
    - shortage of compressed gas supplies, e.g. battlefields, accident sites, Third World countries.
    - inhalational analgesia in obstetrics (no longer used).

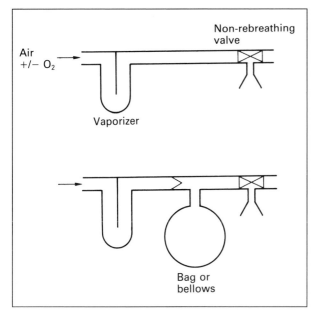

Figure 47 *Draw-over systems*

Dreaming, *see Awareness*

Droperidol. **Butyrophenone**, used as an antipsychotic drug in psychiatry, as an **antiemetic drug**, for **premedication** and for **neuroleptanaesthesia**. Has also been used to reduce the incidence of **emergence phenomena** after **ketamine**. Thought to interfere with **GABA receptors**. A powerful dopamine antagonist, related to haloperidol but of shorter duration of action (6–12 hours; cf. haloperidol 24–48 hours). May cause apparent outward sedation but internal distress, especially when concurrently administered opioids have short duration of action.
- Dosage:
    - premedication: up to 10 mg orally/im, 1 hour preoperatively.
    - neuroleptanaesthesia: 5–15 mg iv (children: 0.02–0.075 mg/kg).
    - antiemetic effect: as above. 0.5–2.0 mg iv has been shown to have effective antiemetic actions without noticable central effects.

– psychiatry: up to 20 mg by the above routes.
Side effects are unlikely after anaesthetic use; as for butyrophenones after chronic use. May lower BP slightly; said to be via α-adrenergic blockade although this has been disputed.

Drowning, *see Near-drowning*

Drug absorption, distribution, metabolism and excretion, *see Pharmacokinetics*

Drug addiction (Drug dependence). State of psychological and/or physical dependence on a drug, associated with **tolerance** and withdrawal symptoms. Usually associated with substance abuse.
- Potential anaesthetic problems:
    - **alcohol** abuse and **malnutrition** are common. **Solvent abuse** is more common in young patients.
    - effects of iv use, often with non-sterile needles (e.g. **opioid analgesic drugs**, **barbiturates**):
        - high risk of sepsis, thrombophlebitis, cellulitis, bacterial **endocarditis** and septic systemic and pulmonary embolism.
        - veins are often difficult to find and cannulate.
        - high risk group for **hepatitis** and **HIV infection**.
    - chronic effects of the substance, e.g. hepatic impairment/**enzyme induction** (e.g. opioids, barbiturates); **cardiomyopathy** (**cocaine**). **Thrombocytopenia** may occur in cocaine and opioid abuse.
    - acute effects:
        - depressant, e.g. opioids, barbiturates: respiratory depression, hypotension.
        - excitatory, e.g. **amphetamines**, cocaine, lysergic acid diethylamide (LSD): tachycardia, hypertension, arrhythmias, pyrexia. Hallucinations may occur postoperatively. **Anticholinergic drugs**, drugs which sensitize the myocardium to **catecholamines**, and indirectly acting **sympathomimetic drugs** should be avoided. LSD may impair plasma **cholinesterase**.
    - effects of withdrawal:
        - opioids: tachycardia, tremor, acute anxiety, GIT symptoms, piloerection and sweating ('cold turkey'). Unpleasant but rarely life-threatening.
        - barbiturates: anxiety, tremor, hallucinations and convulsions. May be life-threatening.
- Conduct of anaesthesia:
    - patients may be resistant to iv anaesthetic agents, with rapid recovery.
    - surgical cut-down, central venous cannulation or inhalational induction may be required if peripheral venous cannulation is impossible.
    - estimation of appropriate doses of opioids may be difficult, especially in opioid addicts. Inhalational and regional techniques are often preferred. **Opioid antagonists** may provoke acute withdrawal and should be avoided.
    - withdrawal states may occur postoperatively.
See also, Abuse of anaesthetic agents; Barbiturate poisoning; Misuse of Drugs Act; Opioid poisoning

Drug development. New drugs or indications for old drugs may arise from:
    - incidental observation, e.g. antiplatelet action of aspirin.

–modification of the structure of known natural substances, e.g. H₂ receptor antagonists.
–modification of existing drugs, e.g. opioid analgesics.
–screening of new compounds.
● Stages of development:
–identification of the substance.
–*in vitro* studies.
–animal studies:
  –effects, interactions, **pharmacokinetics**, etc.
  –toxicology: acute/chronic (usually up to 2 years) effects, **therapeutic index**; use of different animals, routes, doses etc. Include histological/biochemical effects on organs, bacterial mutagenicity, teratogenicity, carcinogenicity, and effects on fertility.
    Doubts have been expressed over the humanity of animal experiments and problems caused by possible species differences (e.g. thalidomide was free of teratogenicity in mice and rats but had devastating effects in humans).
–chemical details, e.g. formulation, manufacture, quality, storage, etc.
–human studies:
  –phase I (clinical pharmacology): 20–50 subjects, usually healthy volunteers. Pharmacokinetic and pharmacodynamic effects, safety, etc.
  –phase II (clinical investigation): 50–300 patients. Further information as above, plus effective dose ranges and regimens.
  –phase III (formal **clinical trials**): 250–1000+ patients. Comparison with other treatments. Frequent side effects are noted.
  –phase IV (postmarketing surveillance): 2000–10 000+ patients. Rare side effects are noted, e.g. oculomucocutaneous syndrome following oral practolol therapy. Techniques used:
    –cohort studies: large numbers are observed over long periods, noting side effects when they occur. May detect rare effects (less than 1:500), but costly and difficult to organize. May examine specific groups, e.g. the elderly, previously excluded.
    –case control studies: records of patients with a suspected side effect are analysed for previous drug exposure. Easier and cheaper than cohort studies, but less precise and more susceptible to bias. May detect side effects with frequency up to 1:500. Prove association, not causation; give relative risk.
    –voluntary reporting (yellow card system in UK). Specific anaesthetic cards are available.
    –general statistics, e.g. recording sudden changes in disease incidence, etc.
Statutory regulatory bodies are concerned with drug development from the animal study stage onwards: the **Committee on Safety of Medicines** in the UK, the **Food and Drug Administration** in the USA. A product licence is granted after phase III trials, and reviewed every 5 years in the UK. Financial costs of new drug development are considerable and often prohibitive.

Drug interactions. Common cause of morbidity and mortality, especially in hospital, although some interactions are beneficial.
● May be:
–**pharmacokinetic:**
  –outside the body, e.g. precipitation of **thiopentone/atracurium** mixture.
  –at site of absorption, e.g. effect of opioids and **metoclopramide** on **gastric emptying**, use of vasoconstrictors to delay local anaesthetic drug absorption, **second gas effect**.
  –affecting distribution, e.g. displacement of **warfarin** from protein bindings sites by **salicylates**.
  –affecting metabolism, e.g. peripheral conversion of levodopa to **dopamine** inhibition by concurrently administered carbidopa, **enzyme induction/inhibition** e.g by **cimetidine** (inhibition) or **barbiturates** (induction).
  –affecting elimination, e.g. decreased penicillin excretion caused by probenecid.
–**pharmacodynamic:**
  –additive:
    –summation: net effect equals the sum of individual drug effects.
    –synergism: net effect exceeds the sum of individual effects.
    –potentiation: one drug increases the effect of another.
  Examples: decreased requirement for anaesthetic agents when opioids and other sedatives are used, and the increase in **non-depolarizing neuromuscular blockade** caused by aminoglycosides and phenytoin.
  –**antagonism**: may be competitive, physiological, etc.
  –indirect effects, e.g. **hypokalaemia** induced by **diuretics** increases **digoxin** toxicity; **pethidine** interaction with **monoamine oxidase inhibitors**; sensitization of the myocardium to catecholamines by **halothane**.

Dual block (Phase II block). Phenomenon seen when large amounts of **suxamethonium** or related drugs are administered, in which features of **non-depolarizing neuromuscular blockade** gradually replace those of **depolarizing neuromuscular blockade**.
 Typically, tachyphylaxis to suxamethonium develops after administration of 400–500 mg by infusion or repeated doses, although individual variation is wide. This is followed by non-depolarizing neuromuscular blockade which may be reversed by **neostigmine**, although reversal is inconsistent. In doubtful cases, **edrophonium** 10 mg has been suggested as a test; the block worsens if depolarizing, reverses if non-depolarizing. Use of nerve stimulators has largely superseded this test.
 Has also been termed desensitization block, and sometimes subdivided into different phases. The mechanism is unclear; depolarization is thought not to persist despite continued presence of the drug. Pre- or postjunctional receptor modulation may be involved.
See also, Neuromuscular blockade monitoring

Ductus arteriosus, patent (Arterial duct). Accounts for 10–15% of **congenital heart disease**. The duct normally closes within a few days of birth; bradykinin, **prostaglandins** and a rise in PO_2 are thought to be involved, although the precise mechanism is unclear. If it remains open, significant left to right **shunt** may occur.
● Features:
–neonates/infants: **cardiac failure**, **respiratory failure**.

–older patients:
  –may be symptomless; cardiac failure or bacterial **endocarditis** may occur.
  –signs: continuous murmur heard at the left sternal edge, louder on expiration; may be systolic only, if the shunt is large. A pulmonary regurgitant murmur may be present.
  –pulmonary plethora and cardiomegaly on chest X-ray.
  –**pulmonary hypertension** may develop when older.
- Treatment:
  –medical (neonates): indomethacin 200 µg/kg iv, then two doses of 100 µg/kg (up to 8 hours old), 200 µg/kg (2–7 days old) or 250 µg/kg (over 7 days old) at 12–24 hour intervals.
  –surgical: ligation/division of duct; left thoracotomy is usually performed. Haemorrhage, recurrent laryngeal nerve or thoracic duct damage may occur. Postoperative IPPV may be required, especially in babies.
- Anaesthesia: as for congenital heart disease.
Prostaglandin E_1 may be used to prevent ductal closure in babies with congenital heart disease awaiting surgery, e.g. permitting right to left shunting to allow perfusion of the legs in severe aortic coarctation, or left to right shunting to allow pulmonary perfusion in severe **Fallot's tetralogy**.
See also, Fetal circulation

Dumfries, Scotland. Site of the first use of **diethyl ether** for surgery in the UK by Scott, on December 19th 1846, although **Liston's** use 2 days later is more famous. News of **Morton's** demonstration in Boston had travelled to Dumfries with Fraser, ship's surgeon aboard the Royal Mail steamship Acadia, which had reached Liverpool from America 3 days previously.
[William Scott (1820–1887) and William Fraser (1819–1863), Scottish surgeons]

Dumping valve. Device preventing application of excessive negative pressure to patients' airways, used in **scavenging** systems and some breathing attachments. Usually opens at –0.5 cmH$_2$O, allowing air to be drawn in.

Dural tap, *see Extradural anaesthesia*

Durrans' sign. Increased rate and depth of breathing following rapid injection of solution into the extradural space. More common in unconscious patients.
[Sidney F Durrans, Dorset anaesthetist]
See also, Extradural anaesthesia

DVT, *see Deep vein thrombosis*

Dye dilution techniques, *see Dilution techniques*

Dyne. Unit of **force** in the **cgs system of units**. 1 dyne is the force required to accelerate a mass of 1 gram by 1 centimetre per second per second. 1 newton = 100 000 dyne.

Dynorphins. Endogenous opioid peptides; dynorphin 1–8 (8 amino acids) is found in the CNS, especially hypothalamus and posterior pituitary; dynorphin 1–17 (17 amino acids) is found in the duodenum. Thought to be involved as **neurotransmitters**, possibly in **pain pathways**; more active at κ than at µ and δ **opioid receptors**.

Dysaesthesia. Abnormal unpleasant sensation, whether spontaneous or evoked; e.g. **hyperalgesia**, **allodynia**.

Dysequilibrium syndrome, *see Dialysis*

Dyspnoea. Feeling of breathlessness. Mechanism is unclear, but thought to be associated with the medullary interaction between abnormal respiratory drive and the motor output to respiratory muscles.
- May occur in:
  –increased respiratory drive, e.g. due to **hypoxaemia**, **hypercapnia**, **acidosis**, pulmonary receptor acitivity.
  –increased work of breathing.
  –impaired neuromuscular function of respiratory muscles.
Dyspnoea related to exercise tolerance is useful as a means of assessing respiratory/cardiovascular function, e.g. during **preoperative assessment**. Certain patterns are characteristically associated with certain disease processes, e.g. orthopnoea (left ventricular failure, also severe restrictive lung disease) or paroxysmal nocturnal dyspnoea (left ventricular failure).
See also, Breathing, control of

Dyspnoeic index. Difference between **maximal voluntary ventilation** and maximum minute ventilation reached during exercise, as a percentage of maximal voluntary ventilation. Has been used to try to relate the subjective feeling of breathlessness to an objective measure of cardiorespiratory function.

Dysrhythmias, *see Arrhythmias*

Dystonic reaction. Acute side effect of dopamine antagonist drugs, e.g. many **antiemetic drugs**. May follow oral therapy, but particularly common after parenteral administration. More common after **phenothiazine** administration, e.g. **prochlorperazine** and **perphenazine**, than after **metoclopramide**, but the latter is especially likely to cause it in children and young women.
Consists of involuntary muscle contraction, especially involving the face. Oculogyric crisis (involuntary conjugate deviation of the eyes, usually upwards) may also occur.
- Treatment: diazepam 5–10 mg iv; benztropine 1–2 mg iv/im; procyclidine 5–10 mg iv/im.

Dystrophia myotonica. Inherited disease (autosomal dominant) of muscle and other tissues.
- Features:
  –**cardiomyopathy**.
  –mental retardation.
  –frontal balding, sternomastoid and temporal muscle wasting, ptosis, cataracts.
  –weakness of forearm and calf muscles.
  –testicular atrophy.
  –impaired pulmonary ventilation.
  –thyroid dysfunction, adrenal impairment.
  –inability of muscle to relax after contraction (myotonia). Exacerbated by cold.
- Anaesthetic problems:
  –**suxamethonium** and **neostigmine** cause prolonged muscle contraction.
  –relaxation may be unpredictable following non-depolarizing **neuromuscular blocking drugs**.

E

Ear, nose and throat surgery (ENT surgery). Anaesthetic considerations:
- preoperatively:
  - most patients are young; many are children. Older patients with known or suspected tumours are more likely to have airway problems, and to be smokers/drinkers.
  - **airway obstruction** may be present. Potential difficulty with intubation should be considered. Teeth, caps etc. are particularly at risk if rigid endoscopy is planned. **Tracheostomy** may be performed under local anaesthesia preoperatively.
  - specific problems include bleeding **tonsil**, inhaled **foreign body**, **epiglottitis**, and peritonsillar abscess.
  - **premedication** is according to preference; specifically it may act as an adjunct to the subsequent anaesthetic technique, e.g. **hypotensive anaesthesia**. Reduction of secretions is helpful for procedures involving the mouth, nose and throat.
- peroperatively:
  - induction as for children/difficult airway/etc. Smooth induction is particularly desirable, to reduce bleeding.
  - shared airway: a **tracheal tube** is required for most procedures, with a throat pack if bleeding or debris is anticipated. Preformed tubes are useful. Special **connectors** are available. Oral intubation is suitable for most procedures including laryngectomy and tonsillectomy. A small diameter (5 mm) tube, passed orally or nasally, is usually suitable for microlaryngoscopy. Nasal intubation is usually performed for major surgery involving the face and mouth. The nasal cavity may be prepared with local anaesthetic solutions. **Cocaine** paste or spray or Moffett's solution reduces nasal bleeding (*see Nose*). **Laryngoscopy** or **bronchoscopy** may be performed using **injector techniques**. **Lignocaine** spray to the vocal cords is usually omitted if postoperative aspiration of blood is possible.
  - minor ear operations may be performed without intubation, e.g. myringotomy/grommets.
  - access to the airway is restricted, therefore **monitoring** is particularly important. **Coaxial anaesthetic breathing systems** are convenient and light. Obstruction of the tracheal tube is possible, especially during tonsillectomy if a mouth gag is used.
  - advantages and disadvantages of spontaneous ventilation versus **IPPV** are controversial. Neuromuscular blockade is often avoided in parotid surgery, to allow direct stimulation and identification of facial nerve branches during dissection. Spontaneous ventilation, or IPPV using opioids, volatile agent and induced hypocapnia may be employed in this case.
  - N_2O is sometimes avoided in middle ear surgery, because of expansion of gas-filled cavities.
  - hypotensive anaesthesia is sometimes used, especially for major reconstructive surgery, laryngectomy, mastoidectomy and middle ear surgery.
  - thoracotomy is occasionally required, e.g. mobilization of the stomach for anastomosis.
  - **laser surgery** is sometimes used.
  - blood loss should be monitored carefully especially in children, e.g. during tonsillectomy.
  - **adrenaline** solutions are often used by the surgeon.
  - if used, the throat pack must be removed before the patient wakes. The pharynx may be inspected to ensure an absence of bleeding.
  - tracheal **extubation** is performed with the patient deeply anaesthetized or awake (but not in between, because of the risk of **laryngospasm**) and in the head down, lateral position to reduce airway soiling.
- postoperatively: as for any surgery. Major procedures may require ICU/IPPV postoperatively.

See also, Mandibular nerve blocks; Maxillary nerve blocks

Earth-leakage circuit-breaker, *see Current-operated earth-leakage circuit-breaker*

East–Freeman automatic vent, *see Ventilators*

Eaton–Lambert syndrome, *see Myasthenic syndrome*

Ebstein's anomaly. Congenital heart defect characterized by:
- abnormal origin of tricuspid valve cusps, which arise from the right ventricle below the atrioventricular ring.
- abnormally thin right ventricle.
- **ASD** is usually present.

May lead to **arrhythmias**, conduction defects, right ventricular failure and cyanosis. Surgery may be indicated in severe cases.

[Wilhelm Ebstein (1836–1912), German physician]

See also, Congenital heart disease; Tricuspid valve lesions

ECF, *see Extracellular fluid*

ECG, *see Electrocardiography*

Echocardiography. Cardiac imaging using reflection of **ultrasound** pulses from interfaces between tissue planes. A single beam may be studied as it passes through the heart, displaying movement of tissue planes over time, usually recorded on moving paper (M mode). Alternatively, beams are directed in different directions from the same point, covering a sector of tissue; a moving cross-section may then be displayed on a screen. Analysis of the frequencies of reflected pulses may provide information about the velocity of moving structures and blood flow (**Doppler effect**); flow characteristics may be colour-coded and superimposed on sector images. The passage of injected saline may be studied as it travels through the heart, probably due to entrainment of small air bubbles.

Useful in diagnosing and quantifying **valvular heart disease**, **congenital heart disease**, myocardial and pericardial disease, and in assessing myocardial function. Techniques for the latter involve measurement of left ventricular dimensions and provide information about the:
- –fractional systolic shortening of internal ventricular diameter, and rate of shortening.
- –change in ventricular cavity area and wall thickness.

Has been used to estimate **ejection fraction** and **cardiac output**. Abnormalities of ventricular wall movement occur in the early stages of **myocardial ischaemia**, before ECG changes occur.

Transoesophageal echocardiography gives a good view of much of the heart, and has been used peroperatively to monitor left ventricular function.

Cahalan MK, Litt L, Botvinick EH, Schiller NB (1987) Anesthesiology; 66: 356–72

Eclampsia. Convulsions caused by hypertensive disease of pregnancy (**pre-eclampsia**).
- Carries risk of:
  - –complications of pre-eclampsia, especially coagulopathy.
  - –**cerebral oedema**/haemorrhage, coma, death.
  - –**aspiration of gastric contents**, **cardiac failure**, **pulmonary oedema**.
  - –fetal death.

Occurs antepartum in 50%, intrapartum in 30% and postpartum (up to several days) in 20% of patients. Premonitory signs of headache, photophobia, hyperreflexia, etc., may not precede convulsions, which may recur if untreated. Mortality is up to 5%, usually from CVA.
- Treatment:
  - –O$_2$ administration. Tracheal intubation and IPPV may be required; the former may be difficult because of oedema.
  - –**anticonvulsant drugs**; **diazepam** (Diazemuls) is commonly used in the UK. **Thiopentone** is suitable if the trachea is intubated or about to be. **Magnesium sulphate** is widely used in the USA, Australia, etc.
  - –left lateral position, head down, if the trachea is unprotected.
  - –lowering of BP as for pre-eclampsia.
  - –delivery of the fetus.

Ecothiopate iodide. Organophosphorus compound, used as eye drops to treat severe **glaucoma**. Plasma **cholinesterase** levels may be reduced for 3–4 weeks following its use, prolonging the action of **suxamethonium**.

ECT, *see Electroconvulsive therapy*

Ectopic beats, *see Atrial ectopic beats; Junctional arrhythmias; Ventricular ectopic beats*

ED$_{50}$, *see Therapeutic index/ratio*

Edema, *see Oedema*

EDRF, *see Endothelium-derived relaxing factor*

Edrophonium chloride. Acetylcholinesterase inhibitor, used to reverse **non-depolarizing neuromuscular blockade**, and in the diagnosis of **myasthenia gravis** (MG) and **dual block**. Has also been used to treat **SVT**. Binds reversibly to **acetylcholinesterase**, with duration of action about 10 minutes after a single dose. Of faster onset than **neostigmine**, and with fewer muscarinic side effects.
- Dosage:
  - –reversal of neuromuscular blockade: 1 mg/kg iv with **atropine**.
  - –diagnosis of MG: 2 mg, followed by 8 mg if no adverse reaction has occurred. Improvement in muscle strength occurs in MG.
  - –differentiation between myasthenic and **cholinergic crises**: 2 mg, 1 hour after the last dose of cholinergic drug. Increased muscle strength occurs in myasthenic crisis; worsening of weakness in cholinergic crisis.
  - –diagnosis of dual block: 10 mg; causes transient improvement in muscle power.
  - –treatment of SVT: 5–20 mg.
- Side effects: bradycardia, hypotension, nausea, vomiting, diarrhoea, abdominal cramps, increased salivation, muscle fasciculation. Convulsions and bronchospasm may also occur. The **ECG** should always be monitored when edrophonium is administered, and atropine must always be available.

EEG, *see Electroencephalography*

Efficacy. Maximal effect attainable by a drug; e.g. **morphine** is more efficacious than **codeine**.
See also, Dose–response curves; Potency

EGTA, Esophageal gastric tube airway, *see Oesophageal obturators and airways*

Eisenmenger's syndrome. Right-to-left cardiac **shunt** developing after long-standing left-to-right shunt, because of increased **pulmonary vascular resistance** and **pulmonary hypertension** secondary to the increased pulmonary blood flow. Once it occurs, prognosis is poor, since pulmonary hypertension is not affected by surgical correction of the shunt. May follow any left-to-right shunt, although the original description referred to **VSD**. May occur late in **ASD** and patent **ductus arteriosus**.
- Features:
  - –dyspnoea, effort syncope, angina, haemoptysis.
  - –supraventricular **arrhythmias**, right ventricular failure, features of pulmonary hypertension.

Anaesthesia is tolerated badly; any drop in peripheral resistance increases the shunt with worsening hypoxaemia, which in turn further increases pulmonary vascular resistance. Factors which decrease pulmonary blood flow also exacerbate the right-to-left shunt, e.g. **IPPV**. Risk of systemic **air embolism** following iv injection of bubbles is high.

Pregnancy is also tolerated badly; maternal mortality exceeds 25%. Very cautious **extradural anesthesia** has been suggested if pregnancy progresses to term.

Heart–lung transplantation is the only definitive treatment once established.

[Victor Eisenmenger (1864–1932), German physician]

Ejection fraction. Left ventricular **stroke volume** as a fraction of end-diastolic volume.

Equals: $\dfrac{\text{end-diastolic volume} - \text{end systolic volume}}{\text{end-diastolic volume}}$

Useful as an indication of the heart's ability to eject stroke volume. Measured using **nuclear cardiology**, **echocardiography** or contrast angiography. Normally greater than 60%. May also be determined for the right ventricle.

Vincent JL (1988) Br J Anaesth; 60: 113S-15S

Ejector flowmeter. Device used for **scavenging** from **anaesthetic breathing systems**. O_2 or air passing through the ejector causes entrainment of waste gases by the **Venturi principle**. The rate of removal is adjusted using a **flowmeter** until it equals the rate of fresh gas supply. Several litres of driving gas may be required per minute, at a pressure of at least 1 bar.

EKG, *see Electrocardiography*

Elastance. Reciprocal of **compliance**. Total elastance for lungs + chest wall is approximately 10 cmH₂O/l.

Elbow, nerve blocks. Used for minor surgery to the hand and lateral side of the arm.

- The following nerves are blocked (Fig. 48):
  - **median** (C5–T1): lies immediately medial to the brachial artery in the **antecubital fossa**. A needle is inserted with the elbow extended, level with the epicondyles, to approximately 5 mm, and 5 ml **local anaesthetic agent** injected. Subcutaneous infiltration blocks cutaneous branches.
  - **radial** (C5–T1): lies in the antecubital fossa in the groove between biceps tendon medially and brachio-

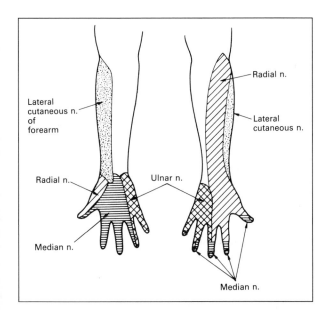

Figure 48 *Cutaneous distribution of nerves blocked at the elbow. (a) Anterior; (b) posterior*

radialis muscle laterally. A needle is inserted level with the epicondyles with the elbow extended, and directed proximally and laterally to contact the lateral epicondyle. 2–4 ml solution is injected, and a further 5 ml during withdrawal to skin. This is repeated with the needle directed more proximally.
  - lateral cutaneous nerve of the forearm (C5–7): lies alongside the radial nerve. It is a continuation of the musculoskeletal nerve of the **brachial plexus**. May be blocked by subcutaneous infiltration between biceps and brachioradialis, using the same puncture site as for the radial nerve.
  - **ulnar** (C6–T1): passes through the ulnar groove behind the medial humeral epicondyle. With the elbow flexed to 90°, a fine needle is inserted 1–2 cm proximal to the groove, pointing distally. At 1–2 cm depth, 2–5 ml solution is injected. Neuritis may follow injection into the nerve, or block within the ulnar groove.

See also, Brachial plexus block; Wrist, nerve blocks

Elderly, anaesthesia for. Becoming increasingly common as the population ages. Mortality and morbidity are higher in older patients.

- Anaesthetic considerations, compared with younger patients:
  - CVS:
    - **ischaemic heart disease** is likely, with reduced ventricular compliance and contractility, and cardiac output.
    - decreased blood flow to vital organs, e.g. kidneys, liver, etc.
    - cerebrovascular insufficiency is common.
    - widespread **atherosclerosis** with a more rigid arterial system. Hypertension is common.
    - veins are more tortuous and thickened, but more prone to damage; venepuncture is more difficult.
    - **DVT** is more common.
  - RS:
    - increased **closing capacity**, therefore more airway collapse with resultant increase in **alveolar–arterial O_2 difference**. Normal alveolar P_{O_2} is approximately:

$$13.3 - \frac{\text{age}}{30} \text{ kPa} \left(100 - \frac{\text{age}}{4} \text{ mmHg}\right).$$

  - decreased response to **hypercapnia** and **hypoxaemia**.
  - greater incidence of **atelectasis**, **PE** and **chest infection** postoperatively.
  - pharmacology:
    - increased sensitivity to many drugs, especially CNS depressants.
    - drug distribution, metabolism and elimination are altered. A greater proportion of body weight is fat, due to a decrease in total body water. Plasma proteins are reduced with altered drug binding.
    - **half-lives** of many drugs are increased.
  - metabolic:
    - metabolic rate is lower.
    - impaired renal function, thought to be due to decreased renal blood flow; suggested decrease in GFR is 1% per year over 20.
    - **fluid balance** is more critical. **Dehydration** is common following trauma and illness.

–**diabetes mellitus** and **malnutrition** are more common.
–nervous system:
  –cerebrovascular disease is common.
  –**confusion** is more likely, and may be caused by hypoxia, drugs, hospitalization, any illness, and possibly peroperative **hyperventilation**.
  –impaired hearing and memory are common.
–other considerations:
  –**heat loss during anaesthesia** is more likely due to impairment of both central control and compensatory mechanisms.
  –**hiatus hernia** is more common, with risk of regurgitation and aspiration.
  –systemic diseases and multiple drug therapy are more common.
  –cervical spondylosis is common, with reduced neck movement. Pain from arthritis may cause great discomfort, e.g. during local anaesthetic techniques. Ligaments are often calcified and tough.

In general, patients are more frail, with greater likelihood of per- and postoperative complications and slower healing. Attention to detail, e.g. fluid balance, is more important than with younger patients, since physiological reserves are less. Smaller doses of most agents are required, and **arm–brain circulation time** is prolonged.

Warming blankets, adequate **humidification**, and appropriate monitoring, e.g. of urine output, should be provided. Postoperative O_2 therapy should be instituted immediately and possibly continued overnight, since hypoxia may readily occur.

The appearance and activity of the patient are thought to be more relevant than the actual age: e.g. fit 90-year-olds may present less risk than frail 70-year-olds.
Jones RM (1989) Anaesthesia; 44: 377–8

Electrical anaesthesia. Induction of unconsciousness by passing high frequency alternating current across the head. Has been used in experimental animals and in human studies. Current has also been passed across the spinal cord to produce more local effects.

Electroacupuncture, *see Acupuncture*

Electrocardiography (ECG). Recording and display of cardiac electrical activity. First performed through the intact chest in 1887. Used for investigation of cardiac disease, particularly **ischaemic heart disease** and **arrhythmias**, also for **monitoring** cardiac rhythm.
• Standard modern ECG recordings are obtained from different combinations of chest and limb leads, each set recording from a different direction, and providing information about a different part of the heart:
  –standard leads:
    –I: between right arm and left arm.
    –II: between left leg and right arm.
    –III: between left leg and left arm.
  –augmented unipolar leads (reference electrode is obtained by connecting all three):
    –aVR: right arm.
    –aVL: left arm.
    –aVF: left leg.
  –unipolar chest leads (reference electrode is formed by the combined aV leads):

  –V_1: 4th intercostal space, right sternal edge.
  –V_2: 4th intercostal space, left sternal edge.
  –V_3: midway between V_2 and V_4.
  –V_4: 5th intercostal space, left midclavicular line.
  –V_5: 5th intercostal space, left anterior axillary line.
  –V_6: 5th intercostal space, left midaxillary line.

The display is recorded on to an **oscilloscope** or moving paper. Frequency range is 0.5–80 Hz. Magnitude of deflection is proportional to the amount of heart muscle, but reduced by passage through the chest. High skin resistance is reduced by cleaning with alcohol and skin abrasion. Electrodes are usually silver/silver chloride with chloride conducting gel, to reduce generation of potentials in the electrode by the recorded potential, and reduce **impedance** variability. Electrodes of differing compounds may generate potential by a battery-like effect. Interference may result from muscle activity, radiofrequency waves from **diathermy** and other equipment, and **inductance** by electrical equipment. 24–hour recordings have been used to detect infrequent arrhythmias, **myocardial ischaemia**, etc.

The leads may be represented on the chest and heart as in Fig. 49a. Thus abnormalities of the inferior portion of the heart will be demonstrated in the inferior leads (i.e. aVF, II and III); abnormalities of the anterolateral heart in aVL, I, II, etc. V_{1-2} demonstrate electrical activity from the right side of the heart, V_{3-4} from the septum and front, and V_{5-6} from the left side. Atrial activity may be investigated using an oesophageal lead.

Depolarization towards a lead (or repolarization away) results in a positive deflection; depolarization away (or repolarization towards) causes negative deflection. Thus in the normal ECG recording, polarity of deflection varies in the different leads.
• Plan for the interpretation of standard ECG, with normal values (Fig. 49b):
  –patient's name, date, etc.
  –usual speed of recording is 25 mm/s; usual calibration is 1 mV/cm.
  –rate: **heart rate** in beats/min is calculated by dividing the number of 5 mm squares between successive **QRS complexes** into 300.
  –rhythm:
    –regular or irregular. An irregular rhythm may be regularly (e.g. missing every third QRS) or irregularly (completely random in **AF**) irregular.
    –presence/absence of **P waves**, flutter waves in **atrial flutter**, **ventricular ectopic beats**, pacing spikes, etc.
  –axis: summation of electrical potentials from the standard and aV leads, plotted as vectors. The normal axis lies between –30° and +90° (Fig. 49c).
    Simple method of determination: since leads I and aVF are at right angles to each other, they can be used alone; e.g. if the QRS deflection is positive in both, the axis lies between 0 and 90°. If I is positive and aVF negative, the axis lies between 0 and –90°, etc.
  Left axis deviation (<30°) may occur in:
    –normal subjects (especially if pregnant), ascites, etc.
    –left **bundle branch block**, left anterior hemiblock.
    –left ventricular hypertrophy.
  Right axis deviation (>90°) may occur in:
    –normal subjects.
    –right ventricular hypertrophy.

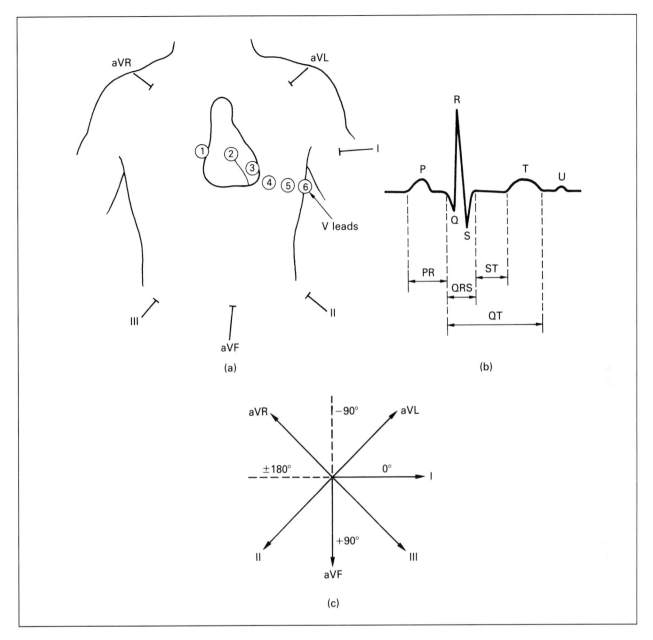

Figure 49 *The ECG: (a) arrangement of leads; (b) normal ECG; (c) electrical axis*

–right bundle branch block, left posterior hemiblock.
–P wave (atrial depolarization):
  –positive in I, II, and V$_{4–6}$; negative in aVR, since depolarization moves downwards and to the left.
  –height <2.5 mm.
  –width <3 mm.
  –shape.
–P–R interval: normally 0.12–0.2 seconds (3–5 mm squares).
–QRS complex (ventricular depolarization):
  –usually positive in I, II and V$_{4–6}$; negative in aVR and V$_{1–2}$, since depolarization moves downwards and to the left. Progresses smoothly across the chest leads, e.g. stepwise increase in height from V$_1$ to V$_4$; either increases or decreases in V$_{5–6}$.

  –duration is 0.04–0.12 seconds (1–3 mm squares).
  –amplitude in I+II+III >5 mm. Left ventricular hypertrophy exists if the **R wave** in V$_6$ + **S wave** in V$_1$ >35 mm. In right ventricular hypertrophy the R:S ratio >1 in V$_{1–2}$.
  –shape; presence of **Q waves**.
  –extra waves, e.g. J and δ waves in **hypothermia** and **Wolff–Parkinson–White syndrome** respectively.
–**S–T segment**:
  –level within 1 mm of baseline.
  –shape.
–**T wave** (ventricular repolarization):
  –orientation as for QRS complexes.
  –height < 5 mm.
  –shape.

–**Q–T interval**: corrected Q–T

$$\left(= \frac{\text{measured Q–T}}{\sqrt{\text{cycle length}}} \right) < 4.2 \text{ s.}$$

–**U wave**.

During anaesthesia/intensive care, lead II is often selected for continuous monitoring. Many simple ECG monitors only use three leads, as rate and rhythm are usually sufficient information. Myocardial ischaemia usually affects the left ventricle, and may be detected by various versions of V_5, e.g. CM_5 lead configuration (central manubrium V_5), which looks at the left ventricle:

–right arm electrode in suprasternal notch.
–left arm electrode over apex of heart (V_5 position).
–left leg electrode on left shoulder or leg serves as ground.

Other lead configurations are also used, e.g. CH_5, CC_5 and CS_5, with right arm electrode on the patient's head, right side of chest and subscapular regions respectively. The CB_5 configuration with electrode over the right scapula is better for demonstrating arrhythmias.

See also, Cardiac cycle; Heart block: His bundle electrography; Myocardial infarction

Electroconvulsive therapy

Electroconvulsive therapy (ECT). Passage of electric current, usually alternating, across the skull to produce convulsions; used to treat severe depressive psychosis. 30–45 J is usually given over 0.5–1.5 seconds; it may also be given as repeated ultrashort bursts. Usually given in courses over a few weeks. First used in the late 1930s.

Brief general anaesthesia is required; partial muscle relaxation is usually provided, to allow assessment of resultant convulsions whilst reducing the risk of vertebral fractures and other trauma.

- Anaesthetic considerations:
  –preoperatively:
  –patients should be prepared, starved and investigated as for any anaesthetic procedure. Particular care is required if cardiovascular disease or intracranial pathology coexists.
  –concurrent drug therapy may include **antidepressant drugs** including **monoamine oxidase inhibitors**, **lithium**, etc.
  –premedication is usually omitted.
  –peroperatively:
  –**monitoring** is required as for any procedure.
  –a single 'minimal sleep dose' of iv agent is usually given. **Methohexitone** is often considered the drug of choice because of its short action and convulsant properties; **propofol** is also used but its effect on convulsions is controversial. Other agents may be used.
  –**suxamethonium** 0.5 mg/kg is commonly given, although smaller doses have been used.
  –a soft mouth guard is inserted to protect the teeth and gums.
  –the lungs are ventilated with O_2 by facepiece before and after convulsions. The need for preoxygenation and ventilation during convulsions is controversial (often performed on the basis that it cannot do harm).
  –intense parasympathetic discharge may follow passage of current, and may be followed by increased sympathetic activity. **Atropine** should always be available; routine administration has been suggested.

–**recovery** facilities: as normal. Confusion may follow.

Marks RJ (1984) Can Anaesth Soc J; 31: 541–8

Electrocution and electrical burns. Hazard of using electrical equipment; during anaesthesia, malfunction or improper use of **diathermy**, **monitoring** equipment, infusion devices, etc. may cause sudden **cardiac arrest** or unnoticed burns.

Current flows between opposite poles for direct current, or from live wire to earth for alternating current, e.g. mains power. Mains voltage is 240 V at 50 Hz in the UK and 110 V at 60 Hz in the USA. Current flows via the path of least resistance; if this path includes a person, e.g. patient or doctor via earthed equipment, ECG lead, floor, etc., electrocution occurs.

- Effects:
  –heat production due to high resistance of tissues. Amount of heat is related to **current density**. May produce burns at sites of current entry/departure.
  –nerve and muscle stimulation; e.g. effect of current across chest (approximate values):
    –1 mA: tingling felt.
    –5 mA: pain.
    –15 mA: tonic muscle contraction, i.e. 'can't let go' threshold.
    –50 mA: respiratory arrest.
    –100 mA: VF.
    –>5 A: tonic contraction of the myocardium (utilized in **defibrillation**).

Magnitude of current depends on the resistance to flow, which is reduced if contacts are wet or have large surface area. Current density at the myocardium is important; thus 100 μA is sufficient to cause VF if delivered directly to the heart (microshock). Other important factors include:
  –frequency of alternating current: 50–60 Hz is particularly dangerous but cheap to provide.
  –timing of shock (e.g. **R on T phenomenon**).

- Methods of protection:
  –regular checking and maintenance of electrical equipment.
  –use of batteries only (impractical).
  –connection of equipment casing to earth (defined as class I equipment). Accidental contact between the live wire and casing then causes a large current to flow to earth, with melting of protective fuses and breakage of the circuit. Fuses are made of thin wire which melts at certain current loads; they serve to protect equipment in case of faults, but do not melt quickly enough to prevent dangerous currents flowing. Fuses are usually placed in live and neutral wires and mains plug.
  –double-insulation of all conducting wires within equipment (class II).
  –use of isolated circuits, e.g. in diathermy, ECG, etc.: patients are not connected directly to earth via plates and electrodes, but via transformers within each piece of apparatus. Current thus cannot reach earth through the patient if contact with a live supply occurs. Class III equipment uses internal transformers to reduce voltage, e.g. to under 24 V. Internal transformers are cheaper and more practical than large external transformers, e.g. one for an operating suite.

–reduction of stray leakage currents, e.g. due to drops in potential along the length of conductors, caused by **capacitance** between casing and innards or **inductance**. Leakage currents may be sufficient to produce microshock. Earth conductors are connected to each other to reduce differences between them. **Current-operated earth-leakage circuit breakers** may be used. Standards for leakage currents are defined, e.g. 10 μA maximum from the casing or delivered to the patient for intracardiac equipment; 100–500 μA for other equipment, depending on usage.

–reduction of the risk of microshock by avoiding conducting solutions, e.g. saline in intracardiac lines such as CVP manometers. Needle electrodes are also avoided, since their resistance is low.

–electrical equipment, plugs, etc. should not be placed on the floor where solutions may fall on them.

Buczko GB, McKay WPS (1987) Can J Anaesth; 34: 315–22

Electroencephalography (EEG). Recording of electrical activity of the brain. Signals from different combinations of 20–22 scalp electrodes are presented as 16 continuous traces on paper sheets. Shape, distribution, incidence and symmetry of waves are analysed to give information about underlying brain activity, in conjunction with clinical details. Concealed abnormalities may be revealed during hyperventilation.

• Different rhythms:
  –alpha: normal 8–10 Hz waves. Prominent at the parieto-occipital area at rest with the eyes shut.
  –beta: normal 13–30 Hz waves. Prominent over the frontal area.
  –delta: abnormal 4 Hz waves; may be normal in children and during **sleep**.
  –theta: 4–8 Hz waves; sometimes abnormal.

As age increases, infantile beta activity is slowly replaced by adult alpha activity. Characteristic patterns occur in normal sleep. During anaesthesia, alpha rhythms become depressed, and are replaced by high frequency rhythms. Slow rhythms may re-appear at deeper levels of anaesthesia, followed by periods of little or no activity separated by bursts of activity (burst supression). The pattern differs with different agents used. Large amounts of paper are produced, making its peroperative use awkward. There may be electrical interference, and interpretation is difficult. Modified forms of EEG have therefore been developed, e.g. **cerebral function monitor**, **cerebral function analysing monitor**, **power spectrum analysis**. Used to investigate intracranial activity in e.g. **head injury**, **epilepsy**, cerebrovascular disease, coma, encephalopathies, surgery, etc. Similar principles are involved in measuring **evoked potentials**.
See also, Anaesthesia, depth of

Electrolyte. Compound which dissociates in solution to produce ions, allowing conduction of electricity; also refers to the ions themselves. **Sodium, potassium, calcium, magnesium** and **hydrogen ions** are the most important cations in the body, chloride and **bicarbonate** ions the most important anions.
See also, Fluids, body; Intravenous fluids

Electrolyte imbalance, *see individual disorders*

Electrolyte solutions, *see Intravenous Fluids*

Electromagnetic flow measurement. Relies on the principle that a moving conductor within a magnetic field induces current which is proportional to the rate of movement (Faraday's law). Relationship of movement, field and current is described by Fleming's right-hand rule, with thumb, forefinger and middle finger of the right hand extended at mutual right angles (e.g. forefinger pointing forward, thumb upward and middle finger medially). If the forefinger points in the direction of the field, and thumb in the direction of movement, the middle finger will point in the direction of the induced current.

Electromagnets within a semicircular probe are placed around an artery, and the moving blood is the conductor. The potential difference between the walls of the vessel is measured, and average velocity of blood flow determined. Alternating current is used for magnetic field generation, to avoid the effect of induction of current in the detector electrode circuit.
[Michael Faraday (1791–1867), English chemist; Sir John Fleming (1849–1945), English electrical engineer]

Electromechanical dissociation. Absence of adequate cardiac output despite apparently adequate cardiac electrical activity. It does not respond to **inotropic drugs**. At **cardiac arrest**, it may represent irreversible cessation of myocardial contractility or massive **PE**, and prognosis is poor. Treatable mechanical causes, e.g. tension **pneumothorax**, profound **hypovolaemia** or **cardiac tamponade**, must be excluded.

Electromyography (EMG). Method of investigating neuromuscular function. Involves recording of spontaneous or evoked electrical activity from skeletal muscle; velocity of nerve conduction may be measured following stimulation at different sites along a nerve pathway. Thus useful in distinguishing between disorders of muscle, isolated or generalized nerve disease or lesions, and disorders affecting the neuromuscular junction.

In anaesthesia, it has been used to determine frontalis muscle tone to monitor depth of anaesthesia. Also used in **neuromuscular blockade monitoring**; nerve stimulation and muscle action potential recording are achieved using surface skin electrodes, although needle electrodes have been used. Less convenient than devices measuring mechanical muscle response, it may detect electrical activity when mechanical contraction is undetectable. Has also been used to investigate neuromuscular function of the eye, bladder, GIT, etc.
See also, Anaesthesia, depth of

Electron capture detector. Device used in the analysis of gas mixtures that have been separated by, for example, **gas chromatography**; particularly useful in detecting halogenated compounds. Electrons within an ionization chamber pass from cathode to anode, but are 'captured' by the halogenated substance blown though the chamber. The current passing across the chamber is therefore reduced, depending on how many electrons are captured. Used to quantify the amount of known substances, not to identify unknown ones.
See also, Gas analysis

Embryo, see *Environmental safety of anaesthetists; Fetus, effect of anaesthetic agents on*

EMD, see *Electromechanical dissociation*

Emergence phenomena. Usually consist of agitation and **confusion**, with laryngospasm, breath-holding, etc.; may be equivalent to the second stage of anaesthesia seen on induction, or be due to other causes of confusion, including the **central anticholinergic syndrome** and **dystonic reactions**. Hallucinations and frightening dreams are common after **ketamine**.

Emergency surgery. Usually refers to surgery occurring within 24 hours of admission or diagnosis; i.e. includes those cases where surgery follows resuscitation, and those where surgery and resuscitation proceed simultaneously (e.g. ruptured aortic aneurysm).
- Problems may be related to:
    - –inadequate preparation of patients for surgery:
        - –not starved, i.e. risk of **aspiration of gastric contents**.
        - –untreated pre-existing disease, electrolyte imbalance, etc.
        - –appropriate investigations and cross-matching of blood not performed or not ready.
    - –the presenting complaint:
        - –**haemorrhage** and **hypovolaemia**.
        - –intestinal obstruction/intra-abdominal pathology: **dehydration** and hypovolaemia, electrolyte imbalance, etc. Further risk of aspiration due to delayed gastric emptying and vomiting/haematemesis.
        - –**trauma**: haemorrhage, **head injury**, **chest trauma**, etc.
        - –**airway obstruction**/inhaled **foreign body**.
        - –related to specialist surgery, e.g. **cardiac surgery**, **neurosurgery**.

The balance between the need for preoperative treatment and urgency of surgery is sometimes difficult, but inadequate preoperative correction of fluid and electrolyte disturbance is consistently associated with increased perioperative mortality. Treatment of **cardiac failure** is also important whenever possible. Careful **preoperative assessment** and discussion with the surgeon is vital. Anaesthetic management is as for routine surgery but with the above considerations. Thus smaller doses of drugs than usual are given initially. Rapid sequence induction is usually employed. Measures against **heat loss** are important. Invasive monitoring and postoperative HDU/ICU and IPPV should be considered.

Regional techniques are particularly useful for limb surgery, but **extradural/spinal anaesthesia** is hazardous if hypovolaemia is present.
See also, specific procedures; Anaesthetic morbidity and mortality

Emesis, see *Vomiting*

Emetic drugs. Given to empty the stomach, e.g. following **poisoning**, or preoperatively to reduce risk of **aspiration pneumonitis**. Less widely used now, because of the risk of causing aspiration, they are particularly dangerous if corrosive or petroleum derivatives have been ingested, or in unconscious patients. Also extremely unpleasant, and not always effective.
- Drugs used include:
    - –**apomorphine**.

- –ipecacuanha 30 ml (adult); 10–15 ml (child), followed by a cup of water and repeated after 20 minutes as necessary. Irritates the stomach and stimulates the vomiting centre.
- –copper sulphate and sodium chloride: no longer used because of reported deaths following their use.

EMG, see *Electromyography*

EMLA cream (Eutectic mixture of local anaesthetics). Mixture of **prilocaine** base 2.5% and **lignocaine** base 2.5% as an oil–water emulsion. The melting point of each local anaesthetic agent is lowered by the presence of the other; the resultant mixture is effective in providing analgesia of the skin 60–90 minutes after topical application and covering with an occlusive dressing. May continue to be released from skin depots even after removal of surface cream. Particularly useful in children. May produce blanching of the skin; increases in methaemoglobin have been reported several hours after application.

EMMV, Extended mandatory minute ventilation, see *Mandatory minute ventilation*

EMO inhaler, see *Vaporizers*

Emphysema, see *Chronic obstructive airways disease*

Emphysema, subcutaneous. Presence of gas in subcutaneous tissues.
May be caused by:
- –trauma, including surgery (hence the term 'surgical emphysema'); gas arises from the atmosphere, viscera or air sinuses.
- –**pneumothorax** or rupture of a viscus, e.g. oesophagus.
- –**barotrauma**.
- –infection with gas-producing organisms (**gas–gangrene**).

Often palpable under the skin, and may be visible on X-ray. Rarely dangerous in itself although often alarming if severe. The gas is slowly absorbed once the cause is treated. Multiple skin puncture has been performed to allow escape of gas, and high F_IO_2 suggested to increase absorption (O_2 being more soluble than nitrogen), but the value of these measures is unknown.

Enalapril maleate. Angiotensin converting enzyme inhibitor, used to treat **hypertension** and **cardiac failure**. Longer acting than **captopril**, with onset of action within 2 hours; **half-life** is up to 35 hours via active metabolites.
- Dosage: 2.5–40 mg daily, orally.
- Side effects: hypotension following the first dose or following induction of anaesthesia, cough, dizziness, weakness, nausea, diarrhoea, rash, renal impairment.

Endobronchial blockers (Bronchial blockers). Used in **thoracic surgery** to isolate a portion of lung, e.g. to avoid air leaks during IPPV or prevent contamination of normal lung with secretions, pus, blood, etc. Less often used now, except for paediatric surgery, **endobronchial tubes** being more popular and versatile. Usually inserted under direct vision via a bronchoscope before tracheal intubation, although they may be passed blindly through a tracheal tube.

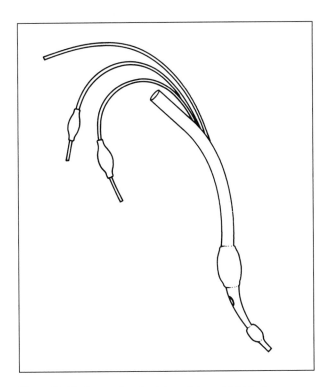

Figure 50 *Macintosh–Leatherdale endobronchial blocker*

• Examples:
 –**Magill** (1943): long red rubber catheter with a distal inflatable balloon, inserted using a wire stilette.
 –Vernon Thompson (1943): similar to Magill's, with separate channels for suction and cuff inflation (with water); inserted using a stilette. A nylon mesh covers the balloon to aid grip and reduce risk of damage during surgery.
 –Fogarty catheter: available in different sizes: 5–14 mm balloon diameter. Originally described for percutaneous arterial embolectomy.
 –combined with a tracheal tube:
  –**Macintosh**–Leatherdale (1955; Fig. 50): tracheal and blocker components, each with a separate cuff. The blocker component passes into the left main bronchus, with a narrow suction port opening at the tip. Resembles an endobronchial tube at first glance. Designed for surgery on the left lung.
  –plastic tracheal tubes incorporating an advanceable blocker are also available.
 –combined with an endobronchial tube: Vellacott (1954) and Green (1958): both are designed to be passed into the right main bronchus, blocking the right upper lobe bronchus with left lung ventilation via an opening between tracheal and bronchial cuffs. The former tube has one bronchial cuff; the latter has two (one on either side of the right upper lobe bronchus) with a suction catheter opening between them and a carinal hook. Placed using a bronchoscope.
[Vernon C Thompson, London surgeon; Thomas J Fogarty, US surgeon; Robert AL Leatherdale, Dorset anaesthetist; William N Vellacott, Worcester anaesthetist; Ronald A Green, London anaesthetist]

Endobronchial tubes. Used in **thoracic surgery** to allow sleeve resection of the bronchus, or to isolate infected lung or potential air leak, e.g. in **bronchopleural fistula** or emphysematous lung cysts. Other pulmonary surgery, e.g. pneumonectomy/lobectomy, pleural, aortic, oesophageal and mediastinal surgery, is possible with conventional tracheal tubes, although surgery may be made easier by collapsing one lung. Risks of **one-lung anaesthesia** should be considered before choosing their use.
• Examples:
 –single-lumen (Fig. 51a); usually mounted over a bronchoscope for insertion:
  –**Magill** (1936) and others: for left or right bronchial placement.
  –Gordon–Green (1955): passed into the right main bronchus. Has tracheal and bronchial cuffs, the latter with a slit to allow ventilation of the right upper bronchus. Has a carinal hook. Designed for surgery on the left lung.
  –**Macintosh**–Leatherdale (1955): passed blindly into the left main bronchus. Bears tracheal and bronchial cuffs, with a suction port opening between them. Designed for surgery on the right lung.
  –Brompton–Pallister (1959): passed into the left main bronchus, with tracheal cuff and two bronchial cuffs in case one is damaged. The second bronchial cuff has no pilot balloon. Designed for sleeve resection of the right upper bronchus.
 –double-lumen (Fig. 51b): all have cuffed endobronchial portions, and tracheal cuffs. The endobronchial portions are curved to the left or right as appropriate; the oropharyngeal parts are concave anteriorly. They are passed blindly. Most are made of red rubber. The main problem of right-sided tubes is related to the short length of the right main bronchus before giving off the upper lobe bronchus.
  –Carlens (1950): passed into the left main bronchus. One lumen runs anterior to the other. A carinal hook aids correct placement but may hinder passage through the glottis. Designed for differential bronchospirometry. Available in sizes 35–41 FG.
  –Bryce-Smith (1959): similar to Carlens', but with longer bronchial portion and fenestrated tracheal opening. Has no carinal hook.
  –Bryce-Smith–Salt (1960): right-sided version of the Bryce-Smith tube. The bronchial portion and cuff are slotted to allow ventilation of the right upper bronchus.
  –White (1960): right-sided version of the Carlens tube. Has a small slit in the bronchial portion and bronchial cuff.
  –Robertshaw (1962): the lumina are side by side and wider than in the others, with reduced resistance. Left- and right-sided versions are available, the latter with a slotted bronchial cuff. Available in large, medium and small sizes.
  –plastic disposable tubes, with thinner walls and low-pressure cuffs. Left- and right-sided tubes are available; the latter's cuff is deflected around a slot for the right upper bronchus.
Left-sided tubes are usually preferred, even for right-sided surgery, because of the risk of inadequate ventilation of the right upper lobe if incorrectly positioned.

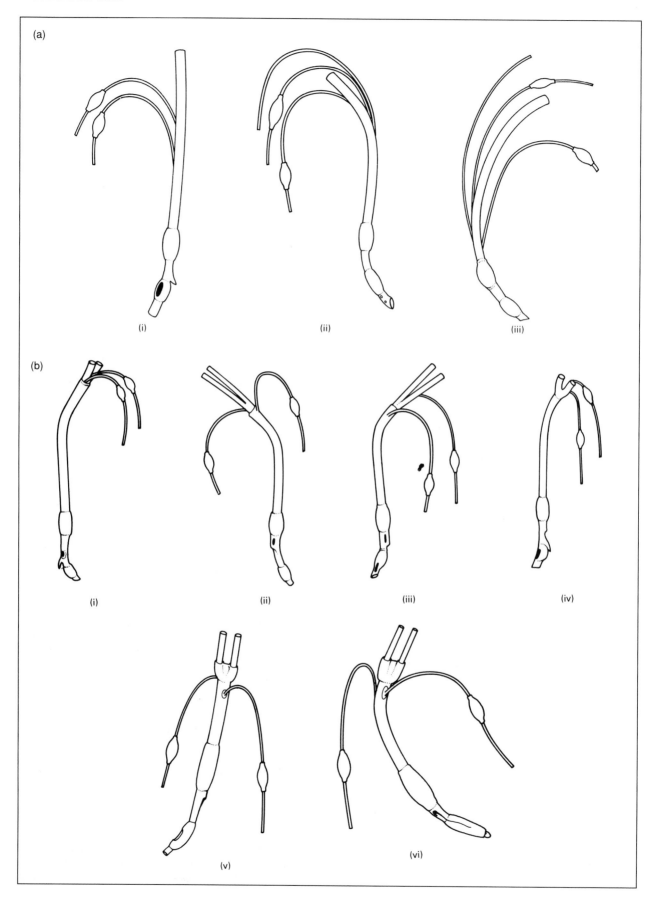

Figure 51 *Endobronchial tubes: (a) single lumen: (i) Gordon–Green; (ii) Macintosh–Leatherdale; (iii) Brompton–Pallister; (b) double lumen: (i) Carlens; (ii) Bryce-Smith; (iii) Bryce-Smith–Salt; (iv) White; (v) Robertshaw (right-sided); (vi) Robertshaw (left-sided)*

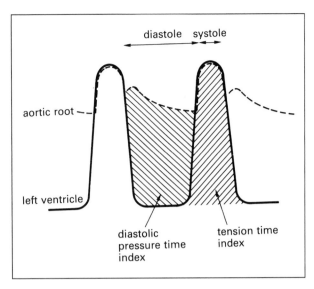

Figure 52 *Left ventricular and aortic root pressure tracings*

Right-sided tubes are often preferred if the left main bronchus is compressed by aortic aneurysm, to prevent traumatic haemorrhage.

- Insertion:
  - –as for tracheal tubes initially, with the bronchial curve concave anteriorly to aid passage through the pharynx.
  - –rotated 90° when the tip is through the larynx, to direct the endobronchial part to the appropriate side. The Carlens tube must be rotated 180°, so that the hook passes through the anterior part of the glottis, before further rotation by 90°.
  - –connected to the breathing system via a double catheter mount, each lumen connected via a capped connector and rubber tubing. Cuff inflation:
    - –the tracheal cuff is inflated until the air leak stops; both sides of the chest are checked for ventilation.
    - –the catheter mount to the tracheal lumen is clamped, and the tracheal lumen opened to air.
    - –the lung is inflated via the bronchial lumen only, inflating the bronchial cuff until no air leak is heard from the tracheal lumen. Only the selected side of the chest should now move.
    - –the tracheal lumen is reconnected and both sides of the chest are checked as before.
    - –both lungs should now be able to be ventilated separately, by inflating via one lumen only and opening the other to air.

Fibreoptic endoscopy is the best way of checking correct positioning, since clinical assessment may not be reliable; it is especially useful with right-sided tubes. It may also be used to check for cuff herniation causing tube or bronchial obstruction.

Complications are as for tracheal intubation (*see Intubation, complications of*). Bronchial rupture may occur if excessive volumes are used for cuff inflation. Incorrect positioning, or movement during positioning of the patient, may result in uneven ventilation and impaired gas exchange.

[Eric Carlens, Swedish otolaryngologist; Wally Gordon, English surgeon; Ronald A Green and William K Pallister, London anaesthetists; Robert AL Leatherdale, Dorset anaesthetist; Roger Bryce-Smith, Oxford anaesthetist; George MJ White, Middlesborough anaesthetist; Frank L Robertshaw (1918–1991), Manchester anaesthetist; Richard Salt, Oxford anaesthetic technician]

See also, Tracheobronchial tree

Endocardial viability ratio (EVR). Ratio of **diastolic pressure time index** to **tension time index**, obtained by recording left ventricular and aortic root pressure tracings (Fig. 52). May indicate myocardial O_2 supply/demand ratio and likelihood of **myocardial ischaemia** (thought to be likely when the ratio is under 0.7).

Endocarditis, infective. Infective inflammation of the endocardial lining of the heart and valves, most commonly the aortic valve (previously the mitral valve). Often associated with abnormal valves, e.g. rheumatic or prosthetic valves, or **congenital heart disease**. Results in tissue destruction and vegetations of platelets, macrophages and organisms, with systemic embolization. Systemic immune complex deposition may also occur.

- Traditionally divided into acute and subacute, although definitions are imprecise:
  - –acute:
    - –usually due to virulent organisms, e.g. *Streptococcus pneumoniae, Staphylococcus aureus.*
    - –presents early with rapid progression to death unless early aggressive treatment is instituted.
  - –subacute:
    - –usually due to viridans streptococcus.
    - –underlying structural heart disease is usual.
    - –chronic malaise and slow course of disease is typical.

Infection with atypical organisms, e.g. fungi, and Staphylococci is more common in iv drug abusers.

- Features:
  - –fever, malaise, etc.
  - –**heart murmurs, cardiac failure,** valve lesions.
  - –peripheral embolization, e.g. fingertips (Osler's nodes, splinter haemorrhages), kidneys (causing haematuria), CNS (causing **CVA**), etc. Splenomegaly and clubbing may occur.

Blood culture and serology, **ECG** and **echocardiography** are used in diagnosis. Treatment is supportive with antimicrobial therapy depending on the infecting organism. Cardiac valve replacement may be necessary. Prophylaxis in structural disease is as for congenital heart disease.

[Sir William Osler (1849–1919), Canadian-born US and English physician]

Endocrine disorders, *see individual diseases*

Endorphins. Endogenous opioid peptides found in the CNS, especially the pituitary and hypothalamus. β-Endorphin (31 amino acids) is the most potent endogenous opioid, active mainly at μ and δ **opioid receptors**. Derived from pro-opiomelanocortin (99 amino acids), from which ACTH is derived. Thought to be involved in central **pain pathways**, emotion, etc. May also be involved in **shock**, especially septic; thought to reduce SVR, cardiac output and BP, whilst decreasing GIT motility and sympathetic activity and enhancing parasympathetic activity. This may explain why **naloxone** sometimes improves cardiovascular parameters in shock.

Endothelium-derived relaxing factor (EDRF). Substance (thought to be nitric oxide or a related compound, e.g. nitrosothiol) released from vascular endothelium, which causes vascular smooth muscle relaxation and thus vasodilatation. Acts via formation of guanosine monophosphate from guanosine triphosphate. Release is increased by raised intracellular levels of **calcium** ions, e.g. caused by **ATP**, bradykinin and **histamine**. Thought to be important in intercellular communication and regulation of cell function; it also inhibits **platelet** aggregation, is involved in the immune system and may be a central **neurotransmitter**. It is thought to mediate the action of certain vasodilator drugs, e.g. **glyceryl trinitrate** and **sodium nitroprusside**.
Searle NR, Sahab P (1992) Can J Anaesth; 39: 838–57

Endotoxins. Lipopolysaccharides present on the surface of Gram-negative bacteria. Specific to each strain, with common chemical features. Released when the bacteria die, and extremely toxic, probably via release and activation of many inflammatory substances including **tumour necrosis factor**. Endotoxaemia is thought to be involved in the aetiology of **septic shock**; GIT organisms are most often implicated. A leaking gut wall is thought to allow increased passage of endotoxin into the circulation in critical illness. Attempts have been made to prevent endotoxaemia by killing gut organisms, and to treat established endotoxaemia with **antiendotoxin antibodies**.
Brock-Utne JG, Gaffin SL (1989) Anaesth Intensive Care; 17: 49–55

Endotracheal tubes, *see Tracheal tubes*

End-plate potentials. Depolarization potentials produced at the postsynaptic motor end-plate of the **neuromuscular junction** by binding of **acetylcholine** (ACh) to receptors. Their size and duration depends on the amount of ACh released, the number of ACh receptors free and the activity of **acetylcholinesterase**. Minature end-plate potentials (under 1 mV) are thought to be produced by random release of ACh from single vesicles (**quantal theory**), and are too small to initiate **muscle contraction**. Simultaneous release of ACh from many vesicles follows arrival of a nerve impulse at the **synapse**; the resultant large end-plate potential causes depolarization of adjacent muscle membrane, and muscle contraction.
See also, Neuromuscular transmission

End-tidal gas sampling. Gives the approximate composition of alveolar gas, unless major $\dot{V}/\dot{Q}$ mismatch exists or tidal volume is very small. Useful for estimating alveolar and hence arterial $P\text{CO}_2$, for monitoring adequacy of ventilation, etc. Alveolar concentrations of inhalational anaesthetic agents may also be monitored. May also indicate extent and rate of uptake of inhalational agents, if expired and inspired concentrations are compared, and the state of O_2 supply/demand. On-line multiple gas monitors are now available, providing breath-by-breath measurements.
See also, Carbon dioxide, end-tidal; Gas analysis

Energy. Capacity to perform **work**, whether mechanical, chemical, electrical, etc. Kinetic energy is the energy of a body due to its motion; potential energy is the energy of a body due to its state or position. Thus a body on a table has potential energy due to the effect of gravity; when it falls, this is converted to kinetic energy. Similarly, the potential energy of a stretched spring is converted to kinetic energy as it recoils. The law of conservation of energy states that energy cannot be destroyed or created, but only converted to other forms of energy, e.g. heat, light, sound, etc. Molecules within a body have potential energy due to their chemical composition and forces between them, and kinetic energy due to their movement. SI unit is the **joule**, although the **Calorie** is widely used for dietary energy estimations.

Energy is liberated in the body by breakdown of chemical bonds within foodstuffs, e.g. approximately 4 Cal/g **carbohydrate** and **protein**, 9 Cal/g **fat**, 7 Cal/g **alcohol**. It may be stored in high phosphate bonds, e.g. in **ATP**, and in other compounds, e.g. **glycogen**. Energy balance refers to the ratio between energy intake and energy loss, e.g. as heat and work done. If demand exceeds supply (negative balance), stores are broken down with resultant weight loss. Particularly important when **nutrition** is provided for critically ill patients, e.g. in TPN.
See also, Basal metabolic rate; Metabolism

Enflurane. 2–Chloro-1,1,2–trifluoroethyl difluoromethyl ether (Fig. 53). **Inhalational anaesthetic agent**, introduced in 1966.

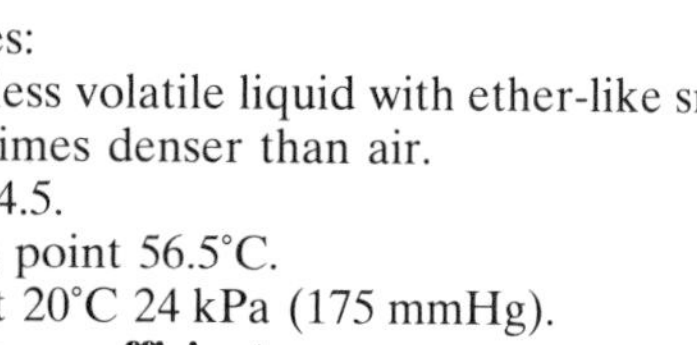

Figure 53 *Structure of enflurane*

- Properties:
  - colourless volatile liquid with ether-like smell; vapour is 7.5 times denser than air.
  - mw 184.5.
  - boiling point 56.5°C.
  - **SVP** at 20°C 24 kPa (175 mmHg).
  - **partition coefficients**:
    - blood/gas 1.9.
    - oil/gas 98.
  - **MAC** 1.68.
  - non-flammable and non-corrosive. Stable without additives and unaffected by light.
- Effects:
  - CNS:
    - smooth and rapid induction and recovery.
    - epileptiform EEG activity may occur especially at high doses, particularly with coexisting **hypocapnia**. **Convulsions** may occur postoperatively.

–increased **cerebral blood flow** but reduced **intraocular pressure**.

–has weak analgesic properties.

–RS:

–depresses airway reflexes less than **halothane** and therefore tracheal intubation is more difficult when the patient is breathing spontaneously.

–causes greater respiratory depression than halothane or **isoflurane**; an increased respiratory rate is common, with decreased tidal volume.

–bronchodilatation.

–CVS:

–causes greater myocardial depression than halothane. SVR is reduced, with compensatory tachycardia. Hypotension is common.

–causes fewer arrhythmias than halothane, and less sensitization of the myocardium to catecholamines.

–other:

–dose dependent uterine relaxation.

–nausea and vomiting are uncommon.

–muscular relaxation and potentiation of non-depolarizing neuromuscular blocking drugs is greater than that seen with halothane or isoflurane.

–may precipitate **MH**.

About 2% metabolized, the rest excreted via the lungs. Although **fluoride ions** may be produced by metabolism, toxic levels are usually not reached, although they have been reported in obese patients after prolonged anaesthesia. Patients with pre-existing renal impairment or receiving other nephrotoxic drugs or enzyme-inducing drugs, e.g. isoniazid, are also thought to be at risk.

Hepatitis has been reported following enflurane; cross-sensitivity with halothane has been suggested but this is disputed.

Inspired concentrations of 1–3% are usually adequate for anaesthesia, with higher concentrations for induction.

Enkephalins. Endogenous opioid peptides, found in the CNS, especially:

–periaqueductal grey matter.

–periventricular grey matter

–limbic system.

–medullary raphe nucleus.

–spinal cord, especially laminae I and II of the dorsal horn.

Methionine enkephalin and leucine enkephalin (each 5 amino acids) are derived from proenkephalin; they are thought to be involved as **neurotransmitters** in **pain pathways**, e.g. **gate control**. Active mainly at δ **opioid receptors**.

See also, Endorphins

Enoxaparin, *see Heparin*

Enoximone. **Phosphodiesterase inhibitor** unrelated to **catecholamines** or **cardiac glycosides**. Used as an **inotropic drug.** Increases cardiac contractility and stroke volume without much tachycardia, and without increasing myocardial O_2 demand. Also causes vasodilatation, reducing both **preload** and **afterload**, and decreases left and right ventricular filling pressures. BP may fall.

Acts directly on cardiac muscle. Adrenergic and other receptors are thought to be uninvolved.

Has been used in cardiogenic or other types of **shock**, after **cardiac surgery**, and in patients awaiting heart trans-

plants. Parenteral preparation contains alcohol, propylene glycol and sodium hydroxide (pH 12). Crystal formation may occur with glass syringes, etc. and if mixed with other drugs and dextrose solutions.

Undergoes hepatic metabolism to partially active metabolites, excreted renally.

- Dosage: 0.5–1 mg/kg over 10 minutes iv, repeated 1/2 hourly up to 3.0 mg/kg, then 5–20 µg/kg/min, up to 24 mg/kg/day.
- Side effects: hypotension, nausea and vomiting, insomnia, headache.

ENT surgery, *see Ear, nose and throat surgery*

Enteral nutrition, *see Nutrition, enteral*

Entonox. Trade name for gaseous N_2O/O_2 50:50 mixture, supplied in **cylinders** at a pressure of 137 bar. Cylinders are coloured blue with blue/white quartered shoulders. May also be supplied by pipeline. Formed by bubbling O_2 through liquid N_2O (**Poynting effect**).

Cylinders must be kept above 7°C (**pseudocritical temperature**) to prevent liquefacation of the N_2O. If this occurs and gas is drawn from the top of the cylinder, O_2 will be delivered first, followed by almost pure N_2O. In the large cylinders used for connection to a pipeline system via a manifold, gas is therefore drawn first from the bottom of the cylinder by a tube; should liquefacation of N_2O now occur, N_2O containing about 20% O_2 is delivered first. Warming and repeated inversion of the cylinders will reconstitute the gaseous mixture.

Widely used for inhalational analgesia for trauma, labour and minor procedures, e.g. physiotherapy or change of dressings; most commonly used with a **demand valve** for self-administration. Onset of analgesia is rapid, with minimal cardiovascular, respiratory or neurological side effects. Should unconsciousness occur, the patient drops the mask and recovery rapidly occurs.

Continuous use, e.g. in ICU, has declined because of interaction of N_2O with the **methionine** synthase system.

Environmental safety of anaesthetists. Hazards faced may be due to:

–inhalational agents: fears were expressed especially in the 1960s because of reported high incidence of lymphoid tumours in anaesthetists. Chronic exposure to low concentrations of volatile agent was thought to be responsible, hence attempts to remove excesses from the immediate atmosphere by adsorption or **scavenging**. Such an association is not supported by subsequent studies, and effects of breathing small amounts of volatile agents are thought to be minimal, if any. Effects of N_2O are now considered potentially more harmful; increased incidence of spontaneous abortion and possibly congenital malformation in theatre workers or their spouses is suspected but has never been conclusively proven. This may be via **methionine** synthase inhibition.

Effect on performance is controversial; there is no conclusive evidence that the low atmospheric concentrations measured are deleterious.

Any risks are reduced by testing apparatus for leaks, scavenging, avoiding spillage and monitoring contamination levels. Maximal allowed levels of 2 ppm halothane and 25–30 ppm N_2O are usually quoted, although levels may vary at different sites within operating theatres, and at different times. Levels may be higher in small unscavenged rooms, classically small dental surgeries.

–infection, e.g. with **hepatitis** or **HIV** infection. Risks are reduced by immunization against hepatitis, wearing of gloves and goggles, avoidance of needles wherever possible, and careful disposal of any contaminated equipment. Needles should never be resheathed. In case of accidental needlestick injuries:

–wash with soap and water.

–encourage bleeding.

–send patient and victim serum for testing for hepatitis, with immunoglobulin therapy if appropriate. Testing for HIV infection requires informed patient consent and counselling. Zidovudine therapy following needlestick injury is controversial.

Risk of infection after accidental exposure of health care workers is thought to be under 1% for HIV infection and 7–30% for hepatitis B.

–risk of **electrocution and burns**, **explosions and fires**, **radiation** exposure, back injury, stress and fatigue, etc. Access to addictive drugs makes **abuse of anaesthetic agents** easier. **Alcohol** abuse is common among doctors. Increased risk of suicide is suspected but not proven.

Redfern N (1990) Br J Hosp Med; 43: 377–81

See also, Contamination of anaesthetic equipment; COSHH regulations

Enzyme. Protein accelerating the chemical reaction of a substance (the substrate) but remaining unchanged itself, i.e. a catalyst. May be highly specific for a substrate. Sensitive to pH and temperature.

● Classified according to the reaction catalysed:

–oxidoreductases: oxidation/reduction, e.g. metabolism of many drugs.

–transferases: transfer of groups between molecules, e.g. transaminases.

–hydrolases: hydrolytic cleavage or reverse, e.g. **acetylcholinesterase**.

–lysases: cleavage of C–C, C–N, etc. without oxidation, reduction or hydrolysis, e.g. decarboxylases.

–isomerases: intramolecular rearrangements, e.g. mutases.

–ligases: reactions involving high energy bonds, e.g. **ATP**, and formation of C–C, C–N, etc.

Reactions involve formation of intermediate structures, with formation of reaction products and re-formation of enzyme.

See also, Enzyme induction/inhibition; Michaelis–Menten kinetics

Enzyme induction/inhibition. Certain drugs may alter the activity of **enzymes** involved in their metabolism, most importantly in the liver. Induction involves an increase in the amount of enzyme, caused by increased synthesis or decreased breakdown. It is usually related to the duration and extent of drug exposure. The cytochrome P_{450} system is often involved. Inhibition involves a reduction in the amount of enzyme or impairment of its activity.

● May affect metabolism of the original drug and other drugs, leading to **drug interactions**, e.g.:

–enzyme induction:

barbiturates increase metabolism of **warfarin**, **phenytoin** and **chlorpromazine**.

–phenytoin increases metabolism of digitoxin, thyroxine and **tricyclic antidepressants**.

–**alcohol** increases metabolism of warfarin, barbiturates and phenytoin.

–**smoking** increases metabolism of **aminophylline**, chlorpromazine and phenobarbitone.

–enzyme inhibition:

ecothiopate reduces metabolism of **suxamethonium**.

–metronidazole reduces metabolism of acetaldehyde produced by alcohol metabolism.

cimetidine reduces metabolism of **lignocaine**, **labetalol**, **propranolol** and **nifedipine**.

EOA, Esophageal obturator airway, *see Oesophageal obturators and airways*

Ephedrine hydrochloride. Sympathomimetic and **vasopressor drug**, mainly used to treat hypotension (especially in **spinal** and **extradural anaesthesia**). Sometimes used in the treatment of **bronchospasm**.

● Actions:

–directly stimulates α- and β-**adrenergic receptors**.

–releases **noradrenaline** from nerve endings.

–inhibits **monoamine oxidase**.

● Effects:

–increased cardiac rate, force of contraction and BP.

–vasoconstriction.

–bronchodilatation.

–central arousal and pupillary dilatation.

–increased sphincter tone.

–placental and uterine blood flow are maintained; thus it is the agent of choice in obstetric regional anaesthesia.

● Dosage:

–iv in increments (usually 3–10 mg), up to 50 mg.

–may be given orally (15–60 mg) or im.

–tachyphylaxis occurs with repeated administration.

May cause restlessness and palpatations in overdose.

Epidural..., *see Extradural...*

Epiglottis, *see Larynx*

Epiglottitis. Infection often caused by *Haemophilus influenzae* type B, causing enlargement of the epiglottis with upper **airway obstruction**. Most common in children aged 2–5 years. Classically follows an acute course, with fever, marked systemic upset, **stridor** and adoption of the sitting position with open drooling mouth. These features, plus absence of cough, help distinguish it from **croup**. Epiglottitis may progress to complete airway obstruction, which may be provoked by pharyngeal examination, iv cannulation, etc. Although lateral X-rays of the neck may reveal epiglottic enlargement, they may also provoke obstruction, and clinical assessment is sufficient in severe cases. **Pulmonary oedema** may occur if obstruction is severe.

● Management:

–assessment:

–general state: exhaustion, toxaemia, etc.

–respiratory distress: stridor, use of accessory **respiratory muscles** including flaring of the nostrils, intercostal and suprasternal recession, tachypnoea, cyanosis.

–experienced anaesthetic, paediatric and ENT help should be sought.

–humidified O_2 administration.

–**iv fluids** and **antibacterial drugs** are required, although iv cannulation should not be attempted before relief of the airway obstruction. Chloramphenicol or ampicillin are traditionally used.

–anaesthesia is as for airway obstruction, classically using **halothane** in O_2 with the patient sitting until tracheal intubation is possible. Induction is usually slow. Apparatus for difficult intubation plus facilities for urgent tracheostomy must be available. **Atropine** may be given once an iv cannula is sited. An oral tracheal tube is passed initially, and is changed for a nasal tube to allow better fixation and comfort.

–intubation is usually required for under 24 hours. Spontaneous ventilation is usually acceptable. **Humidification** is essential. **Sedation** may not be required, but the arms should be restrained to prevent accidental self-extubation.

–extubation is performed when the clinical condition has improved, and a leak is present around the tube. Extubation may be performed under inhalational anaesthesia but this may not be necessary.

Diaz JM (1985) Anesth Analg; 64: 621–3
See also, Paediatric anaesthesia

Epilepsy. Tendency to epileptic seizures, associated with paroxysmal discharge of cerebral neurones.

● Traditionally classified into:
  –generalized:
    –grand mal (tonic–clonic; **convulsions**): tonic (sustained muscle contraction) followed by clonic (jerking) phases lasting about 30 seconds each with loss of consciousness. May be preceded by prodromal symptoms hours or days before, and an aura minutes before.
    –petit mal (absence seizures): characterized by 3 Hz synchronized spikes on the EEG. Rarely associated with loss of consciousness and clonic movements.
  –partial (focal):
    –may occur with or without loss of consciousness.
    –classic presentations:
      –temporal: associated with auditory, visual or olfactory hallucinations and emotional or mood changes.
      –Jacksonian: clonic movements spreading from an extremity, e.g. single digit, to involve the whole body.

Definition of disease is difficult because certain stimuli will induce convulsions in normal subjects, e.g. hypoxia. Usually idiopathic, especially in childhood; intracranial lesions must be excluded in adults presenting with a single seizure. Pyrexia is a common cause in children; other causes are as for convulsions.

Treatment is with **anticonvulsant drugs**, and is directed at any underlying cause.

● Anaesthetic considerations:
  –**preoperative assessment**: frequency of seizures, date of last seizure, drug therapy, etc. Identification of cause if known.
  –therapy is maintained up to surgery; **benzodiazepines** are often used for premedication because of their anticonvulsant activity.
  –anaesthetic drugs associated with convulsions are

avoided, e.g. **methohexitone**, **enflurane** and possibly **propofol**. **Ketamine** is usually avoided. **Thiopentone**, **halothane** and **isoflurane** are known to have anticonvulsant properties and are therefore the drugs of choice. **Doxapram** is avoided. **Hypocapnia** reduces the threshold to epileptiform activity.

  –regional techniques are not contraindicated, but are often avoided for fear of reduced convulsive threshold to **local anaesthetic agents**, and risk of convulsions during the procedure.
  –anticonvulsant therapy is restarted as soon as possible postoperatively.

[John H Jackson (1835–1911), English neurologist]
See also, Status epilepticus

Epinephrine, *see Adrenaline*

Epistaxis. Nasal bleeding. May occur from:
  –veins of the nasal septum (younger patients).
  –arterial anastomoses of the lower part of the nasal septum (older patients). May be associated with **hypertension**.

Usually follows trauma, but predisposing conditions include bleeding disorders, hereditary telangiectasia and raised venous pressure. Bleeding may be caused by nasal intubation or passage of a nasal airway, especially if a vasoconstrictor, e.g. **cocaine**, is not used first.

Usually managed by nasal packing but may require ligation of the maxillary or anterior ethmoidal arteries, the former via the neck or oral route; the latter from the front of the **nose**.

Anaesthetic management is similar to that of the bleeding tonsil (*see Tonsil, bleeding*).

Epoprostenol, *see Prostacyclin*

EPSP, Excitatory postsynaptic potential, *see Synaptic transmission*

Equivalence. Amount of a substance divided by its **valence**. Equivalent weight (gram equivalent) is the weight of substance combining with or chemically equivalent to 8 g O_2, or 1 g hydrogen.

Electrical equivalence is the number of moles of ionized substance divided by valence.

Erg. cgs system unit of work. 1 erg = work done by a force of 1 dyne acting through a distance of 1 centimetre.

Ergometrine maleate. Uterine muscle stimulant, used to reduce postpartum or postabortion uterine bleeding. Uterine contraction occurs 5 minutes after im injection and 1 minute after iv injection; it lasts up to an hour. Slowly being replaced by synthetic **oxytocin** because of its adverse effects (nausea, vomiting, and vasoconstriction causing a marked rise in BP and CVP; the latter is exacerbated by autotransfusion of blood from the uterus, and lasts up to several hours). Hazardous therefore in patients with cardiovascular disease, particularly **pre-eclampsia**. Despite this, it is often given routinely combined with oxytocin at the end of the second stage of labour. An aggravating role of ergometrine-induced vasoconstriction has been suggested in **aspiration pneumonitis**. Has been used as a vasopressor, e.g. in **spinal anaesthesia**.

● Dosage: 0.1–0.5 mg im/iv; 0.5–1.0 mg orally.

See also, Uterus

Errors

Errors. In **statistics**, may lead to incorrect conclusions because of inadequate test design and analysis, too small a sample size or inaccurate data collection. May be:
- –type I (α; false positive): acceptance of a result as significant when it is not. Represented by the *P* value (**probability**); a value of 0.05 is usually accepted as the maximum acceptable.
- –type II (β; false negative): rejection of a result as not significant when it is. A value of 0.2 is usually considered the maximum acceptable.

It is thus easier to demonstrate a non-significant result than a significant one. As the required *P* value is made smaller, the risk of rejecting a real result (i.e. type II error) increases. Errors may limit the usefulness of an investigation, e.g. blood test, described by its **sensitivity**, **specificity** and **predictive value**.

Erythrocytes (Red blood cells). Biconcave discs, about 2 μm thick and 8 μm in diameter. Produced by red bone marrow. Contain **haemoglobin**, maintained in an appropriate state for **O_2 transport** (i.e. containing iron in the reduced state, and with generation of **2,3–DPG**). Maintenance of structural integrity and osmotic stability is via membrane pumps; the main energy source is aerobic **glycolysis**.

Circulating lifespan is about 120 days; they are removed by the reticuloendothelial system and broken down, with salvage and reuse of iron and amino acids from haemoglobin.
- Normal laboratory findings (adult):
  - –red cell count (RBC): 4.5–6.0 × 10^{12}/l blood (male). 4.0–5.2 × 10^{12}/l blood (female).
  - –reticulocyte count: under 2% of red cells. Increased in red cell loss from **haemolysis** or **haemorrhage**, signifying a normal bone marrow response. Also increased in treatment of deficiency **anaemias**.
  - –mean corpuscle volume (MCV): 80–100 fl. Decreased in iron deficiency or defective haemoglobin synthesis. Increased when reticulocyte count is increased, or due to megaloblastic cell formation (e.g. vitamin B_{12}/folate deficiency). Also increased in alcoholism.
  - –mean corpuscle haemoglobin (MCH): 26–34 pg.
  - –mean corpuscle haemoglobin concentration (MCHC): 32–36 g/dl. Decreased in iron deficiency or defective haemoglobin synthesis.
  - –erythrocyte sedimentation rate (ESR): <10 mm/h. Measure of the rate at which red cells settle when a column of blood is left for 1 hour. High values indicate reduced settling. Increased in many inflammatory and infective diseases, malignancy, old age and pregnancy.

Examination of the peripheral blood film gives information about haematological disease, e.g. abnormally shaped erythrocytes (**sickle cell anaemia**, hereditary spherocytosis, target cells in impaired haemoglobin production or liver disease, etc.).
See also, Erythropoiesis

Erythropoiesis. Formation of **erythrocytes**, usually resticted to the vertebrae, sternum, ribs, upper long bones and iliac crests in adults. Requires iron, vitamin B_{12} and folate, and possibly other vitamins and minerals. Stepwise differentiation from stem cells includes **haemoglobin** synthesis and nuclear extrusion to form reticulocytes, taking about 7 days. Stimulated by **erythropoietin**.

Erythropoietin. Glycoprotein hormone secreted mainly by the kidneys, but also by the liver. Secretion is increased by **haemorrhage** and **hypoxia** (possibly via **prostaglandin** synthesis), and inhibited by increased numbers of circulating **erythrocytes**. Causes increased **erythropoiesis**. Infusion of erythropoietin produced by recombinant genetic engineering has been used to treat anaemia in renal failure, but treatment is very expensive. It has also been used to increase the yield of blood collected for autologous **blood transfusion**.

Escape beats. On the **ECG**, complexes arising from sites other than the sinoatrial node, when the latter does not discharge (i.e. sinus arrest or severe bradycardia). Distinct from ectopic beats, which arise prematurely in the cardiac cycle.

Esmolol hydrochloride. Cardioselective **β-adrenergic receptor antagonist**, with no **intrinsic sympathomimetic activity**. Hydrolysed by red blood and other esterases, with a **half-life** of 9 minutes. Used to treat **AF**, atrial flutter and **SVT**, and during anaesthesia to prevent/treat tachycardia, e.g. associated with tracheal intubation. Has been used in **hypotensive anaesthesia**.
- Dosage:
  - – SVT etc.: 500 μg/kg/min loading dose iv for 1 minute, then 50 μg/kg/min maintenance for 4 minutes. If the response is inadequate, the loading dose may be repeated and the maintenance dose increased to 100 μg/kg/min, and so on until a maintenance dose of 200 μg/kg/min is reached.
  - –perioperative use: 0.5–1.0 mg/kg iv over 15–30 seconds, followed by 50–300 μg/kg/min infusion.
- Side effects: bradycardia, hypotension, sweating, nausea, confusion, thrombophlebitis. Bronchospasm may occur in susceptible patients.

Esophagus, *see Oesophagus*

ESR, Erythrocyte sedimentation rate, *see Erythrocytes*

Ethanol, *see Alcohol*

Ether, *see Diethyl ether*

Ethmoidal nerve block, anterior, *see Ophthalmic nerve blocks*

Ethoheptazine citrate. Analgesic drug, used for mild/moderate pain. Combined with meprobromate, a sedative muscular antispasmodic, and **aspirin**.
- Dosage: 75–150 mg 8 hourly, orally.
- Side effects: are largely related to meprobromate and include drowsiness and hypersensitivity.

Ethyl alcohol, *see Alcohol*

Ethyl chloride. Inhalational anaesthetic agent, first described in 1848; popular in the 1920s particularly for induction of anaesthesia because of its rapid action. Extremely volatile (boiling point 13°C) and difficult to control; also inflammable. Now used solely for its cooling action when sprayed on to skin, to cause anaesthesia or to test the extent of regional blockade.

166

Ethylene. Inhalational anaesthesic agent, used clinically in 1923. A gas of similar blood /gas solubility to **N₂O**, but more potent. Also extremely explosive and unpleasant to breathe. Cylinder body and shoulder are coloured violet.

Ethylene oxide, *see Contamination of anaesthetic equipment*

Etidocaine hydrochloride. Local anaesthetic agent introduced in 1972, derived from **lignocaine**. Onset is rapid, and duration of action is similar to that of **bupivacaine**. Produces motor blockade which may exceed sensory blockade. Used in 1–1.5% solutions. Maximal safe dose is 2 mg/kg. Not available in the UK.

Etomidate. IV anaesthetic agent, introduced in 1973. A carboxylated imidazole (five-membered ring containing three carbon atoms and two nitrogen atoms) compound (Fig. 54), presented in 35% propylene glycol; pH is 8.1. 75% bound to plasma proteins after injection.

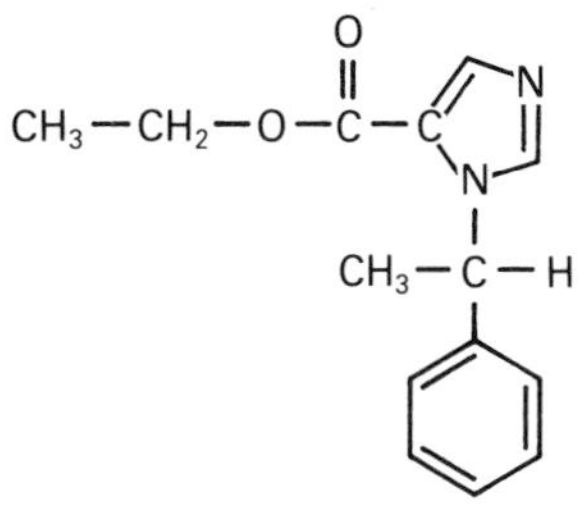

Figure 54 *Structure of etomidate*

- Effects:
  - induction:
    - rapid onset of sleep, lasting up to 8 minutes after a single dose.
    - muscle movements are common; reduced by use of opioids.
    - pain is common when injected into small veins; reduced by mixing with 2 ml 1% lignocaine. Thrombosis is rare.
  - CVS/RS:
    - causes less hypotension than **thiopentone**; thus often used in shocked patients, the elderly and those with cardiovascular disease.
    - respiratory depression is less than with thiopentone.
  - CNS:
    - not analgesic.
    - not associated with epileptiform discharges.
    - reduces **cerebral blood flow** and **intraocular pressure**.
  - other:
    - increases the incidence of postoperative nausea and vomiting.
    - does not cause **histamine** release.
- Metabolism:
  - rapidly metabolized by the liver; elimination **half-life** is about 70 minutes. Largely excreted via the urine. Not cumulative.
  - interferes with adrenal steroid synthesis by inhibiting

11-β-hydroxylase and 17-α-hydroxylase. IV infusion for sedation on ICU has been implicated as increasing mortality; it is now contraindicated for this purpose. Following a single induction dose, the rise in plasma cortisol normally seen after surgery is delayed for up to 6 hours. The significance of this is disputed.
- Dose: 0.2–0.3 mg/kg.

Etorphine hydrochloride. Analogue of thebaine, a naturally-occurring **opioid**. 400 times as potent as **morphine**. Used to immobilize large animals.

Evoked potentials (EPs). Electrical activity recorded from the CNS or peripherally following repetitive peripheral or central stimulation. Used to investigate demyelinating disease, neuropathies and brain tumours, and in monitoring of head injury and coma. Also used to monitor and investigate depth of anaesthesia or CNS integrity during surgery.

Requires complex equipment to increase recording sensitivity and reduce interference. Recorded potentials are small (usually 1–2 μV) compared with background electrical activity (over 100 μV); the signal is amplified and (random) background activity averaged out using computer averaging. Filters reduce noise. Displayed as a plot of voltage against time; a stimulation spike occurs within 1 ms, followed by a composite pattern representing potentials from near and distant structures along the conduction pathway, depending on the sites of stimulation and recording. Upward peaks represent negative potentials by convention. Latency is the time between the stimulation spike and the first major peak; amplitude is the height from this peak to the following trough.
- Different types:
  - sensory EPs:
    - somatosensory (SEPs):
      - stimulation of the posterior tibial or median nerves, using supramaximal stimulation. Direct spinal cord stimulation may be performed to monitor cord integrity during spinal surgery.
      - recording from:
        - scalp EEG electrodes, e.g. one over the sensory area appropriate to the site of stimulus plus a reference electrode elsewhere. May also examine transmission between different sites along the conduction pathway, e.g. central conduction time (CCT) between activity at the level of C5 to cortical activity.

          In general, most anaesthetic agents increase latency and decrease amplitude (**etomidate** consistently increases amplitude) in a dose-related manner. Amplitude increases following tracheal intubation or skin incision, suggesting SEPs represent level of arousal rather than anaesthetic depth itself. The technique has also been used to monitor function during craniotomy, e.g. measuring CCT: impaired conduction may represent physical damage, hypoxia or ischaemia.
        - extradural space in spinal surgery; e.g. bipolar electrodes placed via an extradural needle at the lower cervical level. Electrodes may also be placed in the subdural space if the dura is opened. Skin/vertebral recording is less reliable.

Anaesthetic agents have small effect, thus technique is useful for investigating spinal conduction at any anaesthetic depth. Each side is tested individually; amplitude reduction greater than 50% during surgery is likely to indicate postoperative neurological deficit. Used for surgery for **kyphoscoliosis**, tumours, vascular lesions, etc., also for surgery of the brachial plexus, aortic arch, etc.

–auditory (AEPs):
  –stimulation of the 8th cranial nerves bilaterally using headphones emitting clicks, usually at 6–10 Hz.
  –recording from scalp electrodes, e.g. vertex, mastoid and reference on the forehead.
  –recorded pattern represents brainstem, and early and late cortical responses. Brainstem EPs are little affected by anaesthetics; early cortical EPs are most consistently affected as for SEPs.
–visual (VEPs):
  –stimulation of optic nerves using swimming goggles incorporating light-emitting diodes; 2 Hz is usually employed.
  –recording from the occiput.
  –thought to be less reliable than SEPs or AEPs, but have been used to monitor function during surgery for lesions involving the optic nerve and chiasma, pituitary gland, etc.
–motor EPs:
  –stimulation of the scalp using large voltages, or the motor cortex directly. Induction of potential using magnetic fields has been used.
  –recording from the median or posterior tibial nerve, or EMG of limb muscles. Very sensitive to anaesthetic agents, thus not suitable for monitoring anaesthetic depth. Recording from the extradural space is thought to be less affected by anaesthetics, and has been used for spinal surgery.

See also, Anaesthesia, depth of

Exercise testing. Most commonly, involves **ECG** recording whilst performing exercise, e.g. using a treadmill or bicycle, with workload increased in steps.

Exercise increases cardiac output, mainly via increased heart rate, with a small increase in stroke volume. Arterial BP rises, despite a fall in SVR. Increased myocardial O_2 demand is normally met by increased coronary blood flow.

Testing is used to help diagnose obscure chest pain, and to indicate prognosis in **ischaemic heart disease**, especially following **MI**. ST depression is the most significant sign during exercise, but other changes, e.g. S–T elevation, Q waves, etc., may occur. Chest pain, hypotension and arrhythmias may also be provoked. Testing may be combined with other measurements, e.g. arterial BP, respiratory rate, tidal volume, O_2 consumption, CO_2 output, arterial blood gases and cardiac output. Useful in distinguishing respiratory from cardiovascular components of breathlessness. Rarely formally performed preoperatively, but the patient's own exercise tolerance, e.g. distance able to be walked or stairs climbed, remains a useful indicator of cardiorespiratory function.

Exomphalos, *see Gastroschisis and exomphalos*

Expiratory flow rate, *see Forced expiratory flow rate*

Expiratory pause, *see Inspiratory:expiratory ratio*

Expiratory reserve volume (ERV). **FRC** minus **residual volume**. Normally 1–1.2 l. Reduced ERV is usually the cause of reduced FRC.
See also, Lung volumes

Expiratory valve, *see Adjustable pressure-limiting valve*

Expired air ventilation. Forms part of **CPR**. Said to be referred to in the bible (2 Kings 4: 34–5). Reported in the 1700s and 1800s, but only became medically accepted practice in the 1950s, following demonstration that it was effective in apnoea during anaesthesia. Adequate oxygenation may be maintained with expired air of O_2 concentration 15–16%. Oxygenation is improved by the operator's inspiring O_2 between ventilations.

Having cleared the airway of food, dentures, etc., and with the patient supine, the neck is extended and the jaw held forward. In adults, the nose is pinched closed and the operator's mouth placed firmly over that of the patient (mouth-to-mouth respiration). Slow deep exhalations are made whilst observing the patient's chest for expansion. Passive exhalation is allowed. May also be performed through the patient's nose (mouth-to-nose respiration). In children, the operator's mouth is placed over the patient's nose and mouth.

Regurgitation of gastric contents may occur during expired air ventilation; this may be reduced by application of **cricoid pressure** if another person is available.

Various devices, some with valves, are available for avoidance of direct mouth-to-mouth contact, to improve aesthetic acceptability and reduce risk of cross-contamination; most hinder efficient ventilation. The Brook airway has a flange to cover the victim's mouth, a one-way valve and pharyngeal airway incorporated, but is now less widely used. An anaesthetic facepiece is suitable; specially designed facepieces which incorporate a one-way valve are available. Expired air ventilation may be perfomed through a correctly placed tracheal tube.
[Joseph and Morris Brook (described 1964), Canadian life-support instructors]

Explosions and fires. Occur when a substance combines with O_2 or another oxidizing agent, with release of **energy**. **Activation energy** is required to start the process, with utilization of energy produced to maintain combustion. If the reaction proceeds very fast, large amounts of heat, light and sound are given out, i.e. an explosion occurs. Speed of reaction is greatest for **stoichiometric mixtures**.

• The following are required for explosions to occur:
  –combustible substance:
    –anaesthetic agents, e.g. **cyclopropane**, **diethyl ether**. C–C bonds are susceptible to breakdown; C–F bonds are resistant, hence the non-**flammability** of **halothane**, **enflurane** and **isoflurane**.
    –alcohol used to clean skin.
    –gases, e.g. methane and hydrogen in the patient's GIT.
    –grease/oil in anaesthetic pressure gauges (*see Adiabatic change*).
  –gas to support combustion: O_2 is standard in most anaesthetic techniques. N_2O breaks down to O_2 and nitrogen with heat, and producing further energy;

thus reactions may be more vigorous with N_2O than with O_2 alone.

  –energy source: About $1\,\mu J$ is required for most reactions with O_2; about $100\,\mu J$ with air. Sources include:
  –sparks from:
    –build-up of static electricity.
    –electrical equipment e.g. **diathermy**, monitors, switches, etc.
  –naked flames, cigarettes, hot wires, diathermy, light sources etc.
  –equipment for **laser surgery**.

May result in **burns**, direct **trauma**, **smoke inhalation**, etc. Although uncommon now with modern agents and techniques, explosions and fires continue to be reported.

● Precautions during anaesthesia include:
  –avoidance of flammable agents: complete avoidance has been suggested, especially as precautions are expensive (particularly antistatic flooring). Following use of flammable agents, e.g. cyclopropane for induction, 5 minutes' use with non-flammable gas mixtures is thought to be sufficient to prevent subsequent explosion. If used, a **zone of risk** has been defined.
  –**antistatic precautions**, e.g. conductive rubber, floor, etc.
  –checking and maintenance of all electrical equipment. Use of spark-free switches.
  –use of air instead of N_2O.
  –use of **circle systems**.
  –air conditioning and **scavenging**, to reduce levels of anaesthetic agents. Sparks are reduced by maintaining relative humidity above 50%, and temperature above 20°C.

Fire-fighting equipment should be present in every operating department.

Non-combustion explosions may occur if **cylinders** are faulty or internal pressure excessively high.

See also, Ignition temperature

Exponential process. One in which the rate of change of a variable at any one time depends on the value of the variable at that time.

● Different types:
  –exponential decay (negative exponential), e.g. lung deflation after a breath, radioactive decay, **washout curves** (Fig. 55a). Similar curves are obtained in **pharmacokinetics**, in which several curves may be superimposed.

For exponential decay:

$$y = ab^{-cx}$$

where c = a constant,
  a = y at time zero,
  x = time,
  b = a particular base, usually e (2.718) because mathmatical manipulations are easier. The equation now becomes:

$$y = ae^{-x/\tau}$$

where τ = **time constant** (time taken for completion of the process at the initial rate of change). At time τ:

$$y = ae^{-1}$$

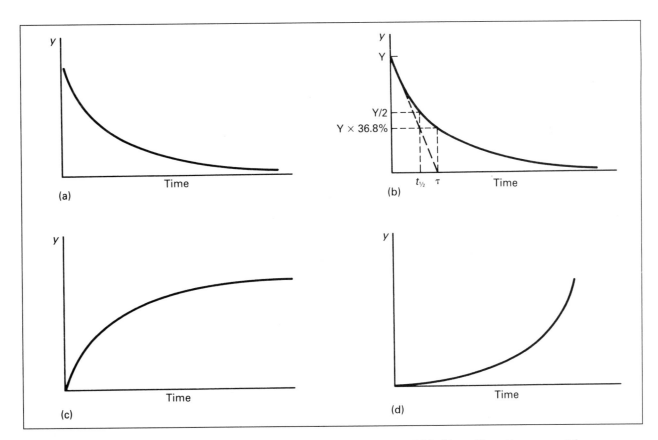

Figure 55 *Types of exponential processes: (a) and (b) exponential decay; (c) exponential build-up; (d) positive exponential*

Thus y at time $\tau = 1/e$ of its original value, $= 36.8\%$. The duration of the process is also indicated by **half-life** (time taken for original value to fall by half; (Fig. 55b).

–build-up exponential (wash-in curve), e.g. lung inflation with a constant-pressure generator ventilator, or uptake of inhalational anaesthetic agents (Fig. 55c).

–positive exponential (breakaway function), e.g. growth of bacteria (Fig. 55d).

Plotted on semi-logarithmic paper, exponential processes assume straight lines, e.g. used in the analysis of washout curves.

Extended mandatory minute ventilation, *see Mandatory minute ventilation*

Extracellular fluid. Body fluid compartment; volume is about 14 litres (20% of body weight). Consists of **interstitial fluid** and **plasma**. Transcellular fluid (approximately 1 litre, comprised of **CSF**, synovial fluid, etc.) and fluid within dense connective tissue, bone, etc., are usually excluded from the definition since these fluids are not readily exchangeable.

Measurement by **dilution techniques** is difficult because of eventual exchange with the above compartments, and because the substance used must remain extracellular. Substances used include inulin labelled with carbon-14, mannitol, sucrose, chloride-36 ions, bromide-82 ions, sulphate and thiosulphate. Slightly different values are obtained for each.

Compositions of plasma and interstitial fluid are different (*see Fluids, body*).

See also, Dehydration; Fluid balance

Extracorporeal carbon dioxide removal (ECCO$_2$R). Method of ventilatory support for extremely hypoxaemic patients. CO$_2$ is removed via a venovenous extracorporeal circuit and oxygenation is maintained by either **apnoeic oxygenation** or IPPV at very slow rates (1–4 breaths/min). The extracorporeal circuit runs at only 1 l/min; thus lung ischaemia is less likely than with **extracorporeal membrane oxygenation**. Initial human studies showed improved survival rates compared with conventional IPPV.

Practical considerations and complications are as for **cardiopulmonary bypass**.

Mudaliar MY, Hunter DN, Morgan C, Evans TW (1991) Hosp Update 17; 410–5

Extracorporeal circulation, *see Cardiopulmonary bypass; Dialysis; Extracorporeal carbon dioxide removal; Extracorporeal membrane oxygenation; Haemoperfusion; Plasmapheresis*

Extracorporeal membrane oxygenation (ECMO). Method of ventilatory support for extremely hypoxaemic patients. An arteriovenous extracorporeal circuit provides oxygenation and removal of CO$_2$ from anticoagulated blood. Very successful in neonates, e.g. with **respiratory distress syndrome**, but results are less clear in adults, in whom it is used mainly for temporary support prior to lung transplantation. Removal of a large proportion of the cardiac output by the arteriovenous circuit may exacerbate lung ischaemia.

Practical considerations and complications are as for **cardiopulmonary bypass**.

Mudaliar MY, Hunter DN, Morgan C, Evans TW (1991) Hosp Update 17; 410–5

Extracorporeal shock wave lithotripsy. Introduced in the early 1980s for fragmentation of renal calculi. Has been used more recently for gallstones. Shock waves generated by the underwater discharge of a spark plug (18–24 000 V) are focused on the calculus by a computer-controlled reflector, with the patient suspended in a waterbath on a hydraulic supportive cradle. At the interface between tissue fluid and calculus, energy released from the shock wave fragments the stone. Approximately 1000–2000 shocks are required to disintegrate an average stone, taking about 30–60 minutes. Shocks are triggered by the ECG R wave to avoid arrhythmias. Contraindications include cardiac pacemakers unless reprogrammed (timing may be modified), aortic calcification, pregnancy and presence of orthopaedic prostheses.

Energy may be released at any interface and cause pain, e.g. at water/skin interfaces; therefore anaesthesia is required. General and regional techniques have been used. **High frequency ventilation** has been used, since diaphragmatic movement is reduced. Air bubbles following loss of resistance techniques using air in **extradural anaesthesia** have been suggested as causing neurological damage. Other anaesthetic considerations are related to positioning, temperature control, inaccessibility of the patient and monitoring, effects of immersion (increased CVP and pulmonary artery pressure), and requests for pharmacological intervention to increase heart rate and thus rate of discharge.

Renal bleeding may occur if coagulation is impaired.

Extraction ratio (ER). Measure of the amount of removal of drug by an organ, e.g. liver:

$$ER = \frac{C_i - C_o}{C_i}$$

where C_i = drug concentration in blood entering the organ,

C_o = drug concentration in blood leaving the organ.

Drugs with high ER (approaching unity), e.g. **lignocaine** and **propranolol**, undergo significant **first-pass metabolism** in the liver after oral administration. The rate of elimination is thus dependent on hepatic blood flow as well as hepatic function, and is sensitive to **enzyme induction/inhibition**.

Drugs with low ER include **diazepam**, **digoxin** and **phenytoin**.

Extradural anaesthesia. Can be divided anatomically into cervical, thoracic, lumbar and caudal types. Involves the placement of **local anaesthetic agent** into the **extradural space**. **Caudal analgesia** was first performed in 1901; lumbar blockade was performed by Pages in 1921 and popularized by Dogliotti in the 1920s–1930s, although it was probably produced by **Corning** following his initial experiments. Continuous catheter techniques were introduced in the late 1940s.

Following injection, local anaesthetic may act at extradural, paravertebral or subarachnoid nerve roots, or directly at the **spinal cord**.

Indications are as for **spinal anaesthesia**; main advantages are avoidance of **postspinal headache**, and those related to catheter technique, i.e. allows control over onset, extent and duration of blockade. Thus used for per- and **postoperative analgesia**, analgesia following **chest trauma**, **obstetric analgesia and anaesthesia**, and treatment of intractable **pain**. However, blockade is less intense than spinal anaesthesia, with greater chance of missed segments, and the dose of drug injected is potentially dangerous if incorrectly placed.

Opioid analgesic drugs may be injected into the extradural space to provide analgesia.

(*For anatomy, path taken by needle, etc., see Extradural space.*)

- Technique (lumbar block):
  - performed with the patient sitting or lying. Preparation of patient, avoidance of spillage of cleansing solution, etc., is as for spinal anaesthesia. Full aseptic technique including sterile gown is usual in the UK, especially when a catheter is inserted.
  - median/paramedian approaches are used as for spinal anaesthesia. Easier catheter insertion, with less risk of dural or vascular puncture, is claimed for the latter approach. It may also be easier in the elderly, particularly if back flexion is difficult or the ligaments are calcified.
  - after deep and superficial infiltration with local anaesthetic, the skin is punctured with a lancet, to avoid pushing a skin plug into the tissues.
  - 16–19 G Tuohy **needles** are usually employed, especially for catheter insertion. The curved blunt tip reduces the risk of dural puncture and facilitates catheter direction (Fig. 56). The needle is usually marked at 1 cm intervals (Lee markings), and may be winged. The Crawford needle (straight-tipped with an oblique bevel) is sometimes used. The stilette is removed when the needle tip is gripped by the interspinous ligament (*see Vertebral ligaments*). Less damage to the longitudinal ligamentous fibres has been claimed if the needle is inserted with the bevel facing laterally; the needle may then be rotated 90° once the space is entered. However, insertion with the bevel facing cranially has also been advocated, since this avoids the possible risk of dural puncture during rotation of the needle.
  - the extradural space is identified by using tests of the negative pressure that is usually present therein, e.g. **hanging drop technique**, bubble indicator placed at

needle hub, collapsing balloons (e.g. **Macintosh**'s) etc., or by the 'loss of resistance' technique:
  - a low-resistance syringe, e.g. glass, is attached to the needle (after checking first to ensure a smooth action). It may be filled with:
    - saline: minimal 'give' when compressed, thus easier to judge resistance to injection. May be confused with **CSF** if dural puncture occurs (differentiated by detection of glucose in CSF but not in saline, using glucose reagent strips).
    - air: avoids confusion with CSF but compressible in the syringe, i.e. 'bounces'; judgement of loss of resistance is therefore harder. Neck ache is common; it is thought to be caused by small air emboli (may be detected by sensitive **Doppler** ultrasound).
    - local anaesthetic: may be less painful during insertion, but risks iv or subarachnoid injection.
  - continuous pressure is applied to the plunger as the needle is advanced, until a sudden 'give' is felt. Alternatively, pressure is applied intermittently after each (small) advance of the needle. The former technique is thought to be more likely to push the dura away from the needle when the extradural space is entered. In either case, the operator's other hand controls advancement, e.g. by placing the back of the hand against the patient's back and gripping the needle firmly between thumb and fingers.
  - high resistance to injection is encountered whilst the needle tip is in the ligamentum flavum; sudden loss of resistance with easy injection occurs when the extradural space is entered.
- injection of a **test dose** through the needle is controversial and rarely performed, especially if a catheter is to be inserted.
- injection through the needle may be 'single shot' or fractionated; faster onset and higher block are claimed for the former but better control and safety claimed for the latter.
- catheter technique:
  - a 16–18 G catheter is inserted through the needle and directed usually upwards within the extradural space. Incidence of bloody tap is thought to be reduced if saline is injected before the catheter is inserted. If insertion is difficult, injection of 5–10 ml saline or slight straightening of the legs may help. The catheter should never be pulled back through the needle, as its tip may be sheared off. 23 G needles are available for children.
  - the needle is removed over the catheter. 2–5 cm of the latter is usually left in the space; too little may increase risk of its falling out; too much may increase risk of inadequate block, e.g. by passing through an intervertebral foramen. After observation for CSF or blood drainage, the catheter is fixed to the patient's back, usually with plastic spray, swabs and waterproof plaster.
  - catheter types:
    - single end-hole: thought to be more likely to obstruct, and to produce incomplete blockade, e.g. if the tip is near an intervertebral foramen.
    - closed end with (usually three) side-holes: may account for development of extensive blockade, e.g. if the distal hole is located in the subarach-

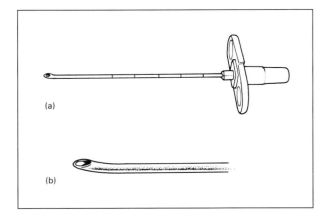

Figure 56 *(a) Winged Tuohy needle. (b) Detail of tip*

noid space and the proximal hole is in the extradural space. Solution injected slowly is thought to leave via the proximal hole with extradural block as expected; rapid injection may produce subarachnoid injection. Similar events may occur with iv placement of the tip.

–a 0.2 μm filter is attached to the proximal end of the catheter to reduce bacterial contamination and injection of glass fragments from ampoules.

–test doses of 2–3 ml local anaesthetic are commonly used to detect accidental subarachnoid or intravascular placement of the catheter, although the use of test doses is controversial.

–single or fractionated injections are controversial as above.

–assessment and management of blockade: as for spinal anaesthesia.

• Thoracic block:
–especially useful for postoperative analgesia and pain relief following trauma. Allows selective blockade of required thoracic segments with sparing of lower segments.

–general principles are as above. The paramedian approach is usually employed, since thoracic spinous processes are angled more steeply caudally, making the median approach difficult. The negative pressure is of greatest magnitude in the thoracic region; this may aid identification of the extradural space.

–the needle is inserted lateral to the interspace below that to be blocked, and directed slightly medially to encounter the lamina. It is then walked off cranially to enter the ligamentum flavum.

–a catheter technique is almost always used.

• Cervical block: has been performed for pain therapy, and for carotid artery, thyroid and arm surgery. General principles are as above.

• Solutions used:
–**bupivacaine** 0.25–0.75% and **lignocaine** 1–2% are most commonly used in the UK. Onset with bupivacaine is about 15–30 minutes; effects last about 1.5–2.5 hours. Onset with lignocaine is about 5–15 minutes; effects last about 1–1.5 hours if 1: 200 000 adrenaline is added. Other agents include **prilocaine**, **mepivacaine**, **etidocaine** and **chloroprocaine**, the latter three not available in the UK. The more concentrated solutions are used if muscle relaxation is required. Carbonated and pH-adjusted solutions are thought to produce faster onset of denser blockade.

–lumbar blockade: 10–30 ml is usually adequate. Rough guide: 1.5 ml/segment to be blocked, including sacral segments; 1.0 ml/segment if over 50 years or in **pregnancy**; 0.75 ml/segment if over 80 years.

Reduction of requirement with age is thought to be due to decreased leakage e.g. through intervertebral foramina. The above scheme does not take into account body size or site of injection/catheter insertion.

Effect of gravity: the dependent side tends to experience faster and denser block, but not consistenly in clinical trials.

–thoracic block: 3–5 ml is used to block 2–4 segments at the required level.

–cervical block: 6–8 ml is usually used.

–infusions are used in obstetrics, postoperatively and in pain therapy, e.g. 10–15 ml/h of 0.1–0.2% bupivacaine. Opioids are also commonly used (*see Spinal opioids*).

–tachyphylaxis is common; it may be related to local pH changes but the precise mechanism is unclear.

• Effects: similar to spinal anaesthesia, but block (and hypotension) are slower in onset. Density of block and muscle relaxation are less, with greater incidence of incomplete block.

• Contraindications: as for spinal anaesthesia.

• Complications:
–related to insertion of needle/catheter:
–trauma:
–local bruising/pain.
–neurological damage is rare, although restriction of the technique to awake patients has been suggested, especially for thoracic or cervical block. This suggestion is controversial.

–bloody tap: if bleeding occurs through the needle, it should be withdrawn and a different space used. If blood is obtained through the catheter (vigorous aspiration is avoided as it may collapse the veins), withdrawal of the catheter 1 cm following saline flushing may be performed. If blood is still obtained when flushed, and when the open end is held below the level of the patient, a different space should be used. If no further flow of blood occurs, the catheter may be fixed as above. Subsequent injection of local anaesthetic is performed with care in case the catheter still lies (at least partially) within a vein.

–extradural haematoma: as for spinal anaesthesia. Extradural catheters may be placed safely in patients undergoing subsequent anticoagulant therapy, provided the catheter is in place before anticoagulation is commenced.

–dural tap: usually obvious if caused by the extradural needle, as CSF flows back. Puncture by the extradural catheter may be harder to detect; flow of CSF may not be obvious, especially if saline was used to identify the extradural space. Management:

–leave the needle/catheter *in situ*.
–consider conversion of the block into spinal anaesthesia, especially in non-obstetric patients. Consider abandoning the procedure.
–resite the catheter in an adjacent interspace. Withdraw the original needle/catheter.
–cautious administration of test dose and subsequent doses (fractionated injection is safer, as partial subarachnoid injection may occur).
–administer 1 litre saline over 24 hours through the catheter to reduce the incidence of postspinal headache. Maintain good hydration. Use of laxatives has been suggested as a means of reducing straining. Abdominal binders have also been suggested as reducing the incidence of headache.
–administer simple analgesics as required. Consider **blood patch** if headache persists.
–in obstetrics, outlet forceps delivery has been suggested to avoid straining during the second stage of labour, but this may not be necessary. The suggestion is often avoided in practice because of fear of litigation, should difficult or

traumatic forceps delivery occur; the causative role of dural tap in altering the course of labour cannot then be disputed.

Postspinal headache may rarely occur without suspected dural puncture.

–shearing of the catheter tip: should be documented and the patient informed. Thought not to have adverse effects.

–knotting of the catheter is possible if excessive lengths are inserted.

–following injection of drug:

–hypotension as for spinal anaesthesia. A further contribution may be made by systemic absorption of local anaesthetic agent.

–iv injection of local anaesthetic.

–extensive blockade:

–accidental spinal blockade (subarachnoid): onset is usually within a few minutes. May lead to total spinal block if a large amount of drug is injected, with rapidly ascending motor and sensory blockade, respiratory paralysis and central apnoea, **cranial nerve** involvement with fixed dilated pupils, and loss of consciousness. Management includes oxygenation with tracheal intubation and IPPV, and cardiovascular support. Recovery without adverse effects is usual if hypoxaemia and hypotension are avoided.

–subdural blockade: piercing by the catheter of the dura but not arachnoid. Onset is typically within 20–30 minutes; blockade may be unilateral and include cranial nerve lesions.

–unexplained, with correct extradural placement of the catheter. Partial subarachnoid or subdural catheter placement are thought to be responsible for the many patchy blocks encountered in practice. Catheter migration may occur during prolonged blockade, e.g. in obstetrics.

–isolated cranial nerve palsies, e.g. 5th and 6th, and **Horner's syndrome**, have been reported.

Extensive blocks may develop after top-up injections during apparently normal extradural blocks.

–incomplete blockade: missed segments/unilateral block. Management: as for obstetric analgesia and anaesthesia.

–nerve damage due to injection of incorrect drugs/solutions. In addition, preservatives in certain preparations of local anaesthetics are suspected as causing damage, as are skin cleansing solutions.

–**shivering**.

–prolonged blockade: uncommon; has lasted up to 8–12 hours after the last injection.

–**anterior spinal artery syndrome**: thought to be related to severe hypotension, not to the technique itself.

–**adverse drug reactions** to agents used: rare.

–late:

–**arachnoiditis**.

–abscess formation/meningitis: thought to be rare if aseptic techniques are used.

[Fidel Pages (1886–1924), Spanish surgeon; Achilles Dogliotti (1897–1966), Italian surgeon; Edward B Tuohy (1908–1959), US anaesthetist; John Alfred Lee (1906–1989), Southend anaesthetist; Jeffrey S Crawford (1922–1989), Birmingham anaesthetist]

Extradural haemorrhage. Haemorrhage between the periosteum and dura.

● May be:

–intracranial: may occur from meningeal vessels (classically the middle meningeal artery), dural sinuses, or fractured bone. Features are as for **head injury**; typically progressive signs follow a lucid period of a few hours after recovery from relatively minor trauma. Management: as for head injury, with urgent evacuation of the clot.

–spinal: may occur spontaneously in patients with impaired coagulation, or following lumbar puncture, and **spinal** or **extradural anaesthesia**. Marked haemorrhage with haematoma formation may cause **spinal cord**/nerve compression, which may be masked by regional blockade.

Extradural opioids, *see Spinal opioids*

Extradural space. Continuous space within the vertebral column, extending from the foramen magnum to the sacrococcygeal membrane of the **sacral canal**. The **vertebral canal** becomes triangular in cross-section in the lumbar region, its base anterior; the extradural space is that part external to the spinal dura. It is very narrow anteriorly, and up to 5 mm wide posteriorly.

● Boundaries:

–internal: dura mater of the **spinal cord** (at the foramen magnum, reflected back as the periosteal lining of the vertebral canal).

–external:

–posteriorly: ligamenta flava, and periosteum lining the vertebral laminae.

–anteriorly: posterior longitudinal ligament.

–laterally: intervertebral foramina, and periosteum lining the vertebral pedicles. The space may extend through the intervertebral foramina into the paravertebral spaces.

Contains extradural fat, extradural veins (**Batson's plexus**), lymphatics and spinal nerve roots. Connective tissue layers have been demonstrated by radiology and endoscopy within the extradural space, in some cases dividing it into right and left portions.

● Pressure in the extradural space is found to be negative in most cases, occasionally positive. Postulated explanations include:

–artefactual or transient negative pressure:

–anterior dimpling of the dura by the needle.

–anterior indentation of the ligamentum flavum by the needle, followed by its sudden posterior recoil when punctured.

–back flexion causing stretching of the dural sac, and/or squeezing out **CSF**.

–true negative pressure:

–transmitted negative intrapleural pressure via thoracic paravertebral spaces.

–relative overgrowth of the vertebral canal compared with the dural sac.

–true positive pressure: bulging of dura due to pressure of CSF.

● Passage taken by an extradural needle when entering the extradural space (median approach):

–1: skin.

–2: subcutaneous tissues.

–3: supraspinous ligament (along the tips of spinous processes from C7 to sacrum).

–4: interspinous ligament (between spinous processes of adjacent vertebrae).

–5: ligamentum flavum (between laminae of adjacent vertebrae).

–6: extradural space.

The normal distance between the skin and the extradural space varies between 2 and 9 cm.

For the lateral approach: 1,2,5,6.

Hogan QH (1991) Anesthesiology; 75: 767–75

See also, Extradural anaesthesia; Vertebrae; Vertebral ligaments

Extubation, tracheal. Problems that may occur include the following:

- –cardiovascular response: similar to that on tracheal intubation but usually of reduced magnitude.
- –coughing and **laryngospasm**: the latter is especially likely to occur at light planes of anaesthesia and in children.
- –regurgitation and **aspiration of gastric contents**.
- –**airway obstruction**.
- –laryngeal trauma caused by the **cuff** if still inflated.

At the end of anaesthesia, tracheal extubation is traditionally performed with the patient either deeply anaesthetized or awake. Whilst the former avoids complications such as coughing, hypertension, etc., the latter option allows return of the patient's respiratory and laryngeal reflexes and is safer in those at risk of aspiration (in whom extubation should be performed in the lateral position) or airway obstruction. Extubation should be preceded by suction to the pharynx and larynx, preferably under direct vision, to remove secretions, etc. which might otherwise be inhaled. Secretions are particularly marked in unpremedicated patients and following **neostigmine**. Inflation of the lungs with O_2 immediately before and during extubation provides an O_2 reserve in case of laryngospasm and helps expel sputum, etc. from the larynx. Facilities for reintubation should be available.

Similar considerations apply to patients in ICU after successful **weaning from ventilators**.

Eye, penetrating injury. Anaesthetic considerations:

- –as for any intraocular **ophthalmic surgery**.
- –risk of expulsion of intraocular contents should **intraocular pressure** (IOP) rise.
- –may present as an acute emergency following **trauma**, for eye or other surgery; i.e. with risk of **aspiration of gastric contents**.

● Management:

- –preoperatively:
  - –general assessment, particularly of airway and risk of difficult intubation.
  - –delaying surgery should be considered if possible, to allow **gastric emptying**. Risk of **aspiration pneumonitis** may be reduced by **metoclopramide**, **H_2 receptor antagonists**, etc.
- –peroperatively: choice to be made, if surgery cannot wait:
  - –to risk the rise in IOP caused by **suxamethonium** whilst performing rapid sequence induction. Risks may be reduced by:
    - –pressure bandage to the eye.
    - –methods used to reduce the rise in IOP, although not always reliable:
      - –'generous' dose of induction agent, or a supplementary dose before intubation, especially using **propofol**.
      - –iv **β-adrenergic receptor antagonists**, **lignocaine**, opioids, **acetazolamide**, and nondepolarizing neuromuscular blocking drug pretreatment have been studied, with mixed results.

    Some centres have reported that use of suxamethonium need not result in loss of intraocular contents.
  - –to use alternative means of achieving tracheal intubation (although laryngoscopy and intubation themselves raise IOP):
    - –modified rapid sequence induction, using **vecuronium** or **atracurium**. Requires injection of the neuromuscular blocking drug before injection of the induction agent; intubating conditions may be suboptimal and with increased risk if intubation fails. The **priming principle** has been used.
    - –inhalational induction/awake intubation: however, coughing and straining increases IOP.
    - –the above may be combined with measures to reduce risk from aspiration.

The decision is controversial; i.e. 'to save the eye or the lungs'. The individual patient's medical condition and severity of injury, and the skill of the anaesthetist, should be carefully considered before deciding on the most appropriate technique. Ultimately, safe tracheal intubation must take precedence over protection of the eye. Other drugs known to increase IOP, e.g. **ketamine**, should be avoided.

Libonati MM, Leahy JJ, Ellison N (1985) Anesthesiology; 62: 637–40

F

F wave, *see Atrial flutter.*

Facepieces. Most commonly made of black antistatic rubber, with soft edges or inflatable rims. Some have transparent plastic central portions, allowing condensation of breath or vomitus to be seen. Ideally, they should have minimal **dead space** and make an airtight seal with the patient's face. Some are malleable to improve fit. Damage may be caused to eyes, nose and face if excessive pressure is used. Dead space may be measured using water, and may be up to 200 ml if the elbow attachment is included. Paediatric facepieces may be small versions of adult ones, or may be specially designed to minimize dead space, e.g. Rendell-Baker's (anatomically moulded to fit the face).
[Leslie Rendell-Baker, Californian anaesthetist]
See also, Open-drop techniques

Facetal injection. Injection of the posterior facets of the intervertebral joints, performed in patients with mechanical low back pain not associated with leg symptoms or signs of root irritation/compression. The posterior primary ramus of each **spinal nerve** divides into lateral and medial branches; the latter supplies the lower portion of the facet joint capsule at that spinal level and the upper portion of the capsule below. Thus two posterior primary rami must be blocked to anaesthetize one facet joint.

With the patient prone, the joint is located using image intensification radiography, and a needle inserted under local anaesthesia. It is walked medially and superiorly off the transverse process of the vertebra to reach the angle where the lateral edge of the facet joint meets the superomedial aspect of the transverse process. **Local anaesthetic agent** may be injected, or longer-lasting relief obtained by destroying the facet joint nerve using radiofrequency rhizolysis.

Facial deformities, congenital. Patients may present for radiological assessment and corrective cosmetic surgery.
- Anaesthetic considerations are usually related to:
  - airway difficulties including difficult intubation.
  - other congenital abnormalities, e.g. CVS, renal, CNS, etc.
  - general problems of **paediatric anaesthesia** and **plastic surgery**, e.g. fluid balance, heat and blood loss during prolonged procedures. Topical vasoconstrictors may be used to reduce bleeding.
  - repeat anaesthetics.
- Common conditions:
  - cleft lip and palate: incidence is about 1 in 600; it may involve the lip only (right, left or bilateral), palate only, or combinations thereof. Other abnormalities are present in up to 15% of cases. Swallowing abnormalities may be present, with risk of **aspiration**

pneumonitis. Surgery for cleft lip is usually performed at 3–6 months, for cleft palate at 6–12 months.

Induction of anaesthesia is as for standard paediatric anaesthesia, but tracheal intubation may be difficult if the **laryngoscope blade** slips into the cleft. To prevent this the cleft may be packed with gauze or the Oxford blade used. Preformed or rigid **tracheal tubes** are usually employed, with a throat pack. Further surgery may be required in later years.
- mandibular hypoplasia: e.g. in Pierre Robin syndrome (macroglossia, cleft palate and cardiac defects) and Treacher Collins syndrome (**choanal atresia**, downwards sloping eyes, deafness, low-set ears and cardiac defects). The small mandible leaves little room for the tongue, the larynx appearing anterior. Intubation may be extremely difficult; deep inhalational anaesthesia, awake or blind nasal intubation, **cricothyrotomy** and **tracheostomy** have been employed.
- hypertelorism (increased distance between the eyes): associated with many other abnormalities or syndromes, including airway abnormalities. Corrective surgery may include mandibular or maxillary osteotomies, craniotomy and multiple rib grafts, and is often prolonged with much haemorrhage.
- other deformities which may produce airway problems include macroglossia, **cystic hygroma** and branchial cyst. Raised **ICP** may occur with **hydrocephalus** and craniosynostosis (premature closure of the cranial sutures).
[Edward Treacher Collins (1862–1919), English ophthalmologist; Pierre Robin (1867–1950), French paediatrician]
See also, Intubation, difficult

Facial nerve block. Performed to prevent blepharospasm during ophthalmic surgery, e.g. with **retrobulbar block**.
- Methods:
  - local anaesthetic infiltration between muscle and bone along the lateral and inferior margins of the orbit.
  - injection of 5 ml solution over the condyloid process of the mandible, just anterior to the ear and below the zygoma.

Facilitation, post-tetanic, *see Post-tetanic potentiation*

Faciomaxillary surgery. Anaesthesia may be required for elective surgery (e.g. for **facial deformities**) or because of **trauma**, the latter commonly due to assault or road accidents. Main considerations are as for the fractured **jaw**; in particular, risk of **airway obstruction**, **aspiration of gastric contents**, intraoral haemorrhage, and associated other injuries, e.g. **head**, **chest**, neck and **spinal cord injuries**.

- Classification of facial injuries:
  –maxillary fractures: often more serious, and associated with significant head injury. Classified by Le Fort after dropping heavy objects on to the faces of cadavers:
    –I: transverse fractures of mid–lower maxilla.
    –II: triangular fracture from top of the nose to base of the maxilla.
    –III: severe fractures, with disruption of facial bones from the skull. Cribriform plate disruption and CSF leak are common.
  –zygomatic fractures: may hinder mouth opening.
  –nasal fractures: may require reduction under anaesthesia; tracheal intubation and insertion of a throat pack should always be performed in case of epistaxis, even though reduction is usually quick.

Similar considerations exist for elective procedures. Surgery may be long and bloody as for **plastic surgery**. Bradycardia may occur during procedures around the face (*see Oculocardiac reflex*).
[René Le Fort (1829–93), French surgeon]
See also, Dental surgery

Faculty of Anaesthetists, Royal College of Surgeons of England.

Founded in 1948 at the request of the **Association of Anaesthetists**, in order to manage the academic side of anaesthesia whilst the latter body concentrated on general and political aspects. Organized and regulated the **FFARCS examination**, training of junior anaesthetists, anaesthetic research, etc., until it became the **College of Anaesthetists** in 1988. The corresponding Faculty in Ireland was founded in 1959.

Fade.

Gradual decrease in strength of **muscle contraction** during tetanic stimulation, exaggerated in **non-depolarizing neuromuscular blockade**. Thought to be caused partly by inadequate mobilization of **acetylcholine** in presynaptic nerve endings at the **neuromuscular junction** compared with the rate of release. Block of prejunctional **acetylcholine receptors**, which normally increase mobilization by a positive feedback mechanism, is thought to be involved during neuromuscular blockade. Thus patterns of fade are different with different blocking drugs, reflecting their different affinities for prejunctional receptors (e.g. greater with **tubocurarine** than with **pancuronium**).

Failed intubation, *see Intubation, failed*

Fallot's tetralogy.

Accounts for 5–10% of **congenital heart disease**, and is the commonest cause of cyanotic heart disease (65%).

- Consists of:
  –**VSD**.
  –pulmonary stenosis (ranges from subvalvular stenosis to pulmonary atresia.
  –overriding aorta.
  –right ventricular hypertrophy.

Blood flow from right ventricle to pulmonary artery is reduced, with shunting through the VSD and aortopulmonary collaterals.

- Features:
  –**hypoxaemia** and cyanosis, usually from birth, with secondary **polycythaemia**. Dyspnoea occurs on effort.
  –acute exacerbations of shunt are traditionally blamed

on infundibular spasm; increased **pulmonary vascular resistance** secondary to hypoxia has also been suggested. Features include worsening cyanosis, syncope and metabolic acidosis. Squatting is classically described in children; thought to increase SVR and encourage pulmonary blood flow.
  –supraventricular arrhythmias; right heart failure in adults.
  –a loud pulmonary murmur suggests mild stenosis. A large VSD may be unaccompanied by a murmur.

Corrective surgery is usually performed within the first year of life. The VSD and right ventricular outflow are repaired with patches; right ventricular pressure measurement indicates whether there has been adequate relief of obstruction. Shunt procedures are performed for palliation if marked polycythaemia or pulmonary arterial hypoplasia are present.

- Anaesthetic management:
  –as for congenital heart disease, VSD, **cardiac surgery**, **paediatric anaesthesia**.
  –infundibular spasm is provoked by fear, anxiety, etc. and may be treated with **β-adrenergic receptor antagonists**. Sedative **premedication** is often given.
  –avoidance of air bubbles in iv injectate, because of the risk of systemic embolization.
  –peripheral vasodilatation worsens shunt and cyanosis. **Vasopressor drugs**, e.g. **phenylephrine** may be used to increase SVR and pulmonary blood flow.

[Etienne-Louis Fallot (1850–1911), French physician]

False negative/false positive, *see Errors*

Familial periodic paralysis.

Rare group of hereditary (autosomal dominant) muscular diseases involving episodes of muscle weakness. May cause **aspiration of gastric contents**, **respiratory failure** or postoperative weakness.

- Three variants are described:
  –hypokalaemic: attacks are provoked by carbohydrate meals, cold, infection or stress, and last several hours. Commonest in young adults.
  –normokalaemic: attacks may last for weeks.
  –hyperkalaemic: attacks last less than an hour, occurring at a younger age and also during rest.

Careful use of **neuromuscular blocking drugs** is required, with close monitoring of perioperative potassium levels. **Arrhythmias** may accompany potassium changes. **Acetazolamide** has been used to prevent attacks in all three variants.

Fascicular block, *see Bundle branch block*

Fasciculation.

Visible contraction of skeletal muscle fibre fasciculi, seen following use of **suxamethonium** and other depolarizing **neuromuscular blocking drugs**. Possible damage to fibres is suggested by increased serum myoglobin and creatine kinase following suxamethonium; it may also be partly responsible for the raised potassium that occurs. Possibly related to post-suxamethonium myalgia, since measures to reduce the latter often reduce visible fasciculation.

Also occurs in **motor neurone disease**, spinal **motor neurone** lesions, and rarely in myopathies. Muscle fibre fibrillation, e.g. occurring after denervation injury, is invisible.

Fat, brown, *see Brown fat*

Fat embolism. Dispersion of fat droplets into the circulation, usually following major **trauma**. Post-mortem evidence of fat embolism is found in 90% of fatal trauma cases. Fat is thought to be liberated from fractured bone or blood lipids. Fat embolism may possibly occur during adverse reactions to orthopaedic **methylmethacrylate cement**, although other possible mechanisms have also been suggested. Incidence after trauma is thought to be reduced by early fixation of fractures.

- The fat embolism syndrome occurs in under 10%, typically occurring 1–3 days after long bone fractures. Features may be due to blood vessel obstruction or toxic effect of fats on tissues:
    - confusion, restlessness, **coma**, **convulsions**.
    - dyspnoea, cough, haemoptysis. **Hypoxaemia** is almost inevitable. **Pulmonary hypertension** and **pulmonary oedema** may occur. Typically, gives a 'snowstorm' appearance on the chest X-ray, but radiography may be normal. May contribute to development of **ARDS**.
    - petechial rash, typically affecting the trunk, pharynx, axillae and conjunctivae.
    - tachycardia, hypotension, pyrexia.
    - **platelets** are reduced in 50%; **hypocalcaemia** is also common.
    - fat droplets may be found in urine and sputum.
    Systemic embolism is thought to occur via pulmonary arteriovenous shunts or a patent foramen ovale.
- Management:
    - O_2 therapy; IPPV may be required.
    - supportive therapy. Fluid restriction has been advocated for reducing lung water.
    - **heparin**, **aprotinin**, **steroid therapy**, **aspirin**, clofibrate, **prostacyclin**, **dextran** and alcohol infusion have all been tried, without conclusive benefit.
    Prognosis is unpredictable and unrelated to severity.
    Van Besouw JP, Hinds CJ (1989) Br J Hosp Med; 42: 304–11

Fats (Lipids). Four main classes are present in plasma and cells:
- triglycerides:
    - composed of glycerol and fatty acids. Formed in the GIT, liver and adipose tissue.
    - the main source of dietary fat; digested in the small bowel. Initially emulsified by bile salts and broken down to monoglycerides, free fatty acids (FFAs) and glycerol by lipases within the GIT. Undigested triglycerides are only minimally absorbed but glycerol and FFAs are taken up readily. Short-chain fatty acids pass directly into the portal vein and circulate as FFAs; long-chain FFAs (over 10–12 carbon atoms) are reconstituted with glycerol to reform triglycerides prior to incorporation into chylomicrons.
    - endogenous triglycerides are synthesized in the liver and secreted as very low-density lipoproteins (VLDLs). These are hydrolysed in the blood by lipoprotein lipase; the FFAs released are taken up by tissues for resynthesis of triglycerides or remain free in the plasma. During starvation, intracellular hormone-sensitive lipase breaks down adipose triglycerides to FFAs and glycerol (increased by β-adrenergic stimulation; decreased by **insulin**).
- sterols:
    - include steroids, bile salts and cholesterol (from which the former two are derived).
    - plasma cholesterol is esterified with fatty acids, or circulates within low-density, high-density and intermediate-density lipoproteins (LDLs, HDLs and IDLs respectively) and VLDLs, especially the first. Unesterified cholesterol forms a major component of cell **membranes**.
    - cholesterol is either synthesized, mainly in the liver, or absorbed from the GIT and delivered to the liver in chylomicrons.
- phospholipids:
    - mainly synthesized in the liver or small intestine mucosa.
    - circulate in the plasma in lipoproteins and constitute important cellular components, but not part of the depot fats. Present in **myelin** and cell membranes.
- fatty acids:
    - may be saturated (no double bonds between carbon atoms) or unsaturated (variable number of double bonds). Deficiency of certain polyunsaturated fatty acids may impair capillary, hepatic, immune and GIT function, hence they are termed essential.
    - esterified with triglycerides, cholesterol or phospholipids, or bound to circulating albumin as FFAs.
    - FFAs are used as an energy source by most tissues.
    Lipoproteins are classified according to their size: chylomicrons 80–500 nm; VLDLs 30–80 nm; IDLs 25–40 nm; LDLs 20 nm; HDLs 7.5–10 nm. LDLs and IDLs are formed from VLDLs; HDLs are formed in the liver. High levels of cholesterol, LDLs and VLDLs are associated with **ischaemic heart disease**, although the role of each is controversial. HDLs may be protective.

Fazadinium bromide. Non-depolarizing **neuromuscular blocking drug**, first used in 1972. Onset of action is within 1 minute, hence its initial suggestion as an alternative to **suxamethonium**. Lasts for 40–60 minutes. Causes marked vagal blockade. Excreted renally, therefore contraindicated in renal failure. Unavailable for use in the UK or USA.

FCAnaes. examination (Fellowship of the **College of Anaesthetists**). Replaced the **FFARCS examination** in 1989.

FDA, *see Food and Drug Administration*

FDP, *see Fibrin degradation products*

Felypressin. Analogue of **vasopressin**, used as a locally-acting vasoconstrictor. Has minimal effects on the myocardium, therefore safer than **adrenaline** when used during inhalational anaesthesia. Available in combination with **prilocaine** for local infiltration.

Femoral nerve block. Useful as an adjunct to general anaesthesia for operations involving the anterior thigh and medial lower leg. May be combined with **sciatic nerve block** and/or **obturator nerve block** for more extensive surgery, but dangerously large amounts of solution may

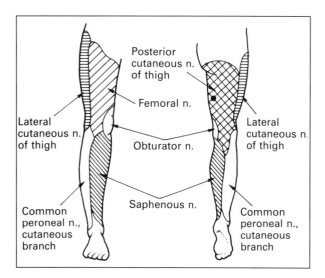

Figure 57 *Nerve supply of leg (*for nerve supply of ankle and foot, see Fig. 7, ankle, nerve blocks*)*

be required. Has been used for analgesia in leg and thigh fractures.

● Anatomy:
–the femoral nerve (L2–4) arises from the **lumbar plexus**, passing under the inguinal ligament lateral to the femoral artery. Divides into terminal branches within 3–6 cm.
–supplies muscles of the anterior thigh, hip and knee joints. Also supplies skin of the anterior thigh and knee, and medial lower leg and foot via the saphenous branch (Fig. 57).

● Block:
–the femoral artery is palpated below the midpoint of the inguinal ligament (i.e. halfway between the superior anterior iliac spine and pubic tubercle); the femoral vein lies medially and the nerve laterally.
–a needle is introduced through a wheal 1–2 cm lateral to the pulsation, and directed slightly cranially, to a depth of 3–4 cm.
–after aspiration to exclude arterial puncture, 10–15 ml **local anaesthetic agent** is injected. A further 5–10 ml is injected in a fan laterally as the needle is withdrawn, in case cutaneous branches arise higher than normal.
–injection of 30–40 ml solution at the initial site, with distal compression, will force solution cranially to the lumbar plexus, lying between psoas and quadratus lumborum muscles (three-in-one block). The femoral and obturator nerves, and lateral cutaneous nerve of the thigh are blocked, providing analgesia of the whole of the anterior thigh.

Fentanyl citrate. Synthetic **opioid analgesic drug**, derived from **pethidine**. Developed in 1960. 100 times as potent as **morphine**. Mainly used during anaesthesia; has also been used for induction in high doses, for premedication, and **sedation**, e.g. in ICU. Onset of action is within 1–2 minutes after iv injection; peak effect is within 4–5 minutes. Duration of action is about 20 minutes, limited by redistribution initially as plasma **clearance** is less than for morphine. Postoperative respiratory depression is

possible if large doses are used, especially if opioid premedication and other depressant drugs are used. Causes minimal **histamine** release or cardiovascular changes, although bradycardia has been reported.

● Dosage:
–for premedication: 50–100 µg im (rarely used).
–to obtund the pressor response to laryngoscopy: 7–10 µg/kg.
–during anaesthesia: 1–3 µg/kg with spontaneous ventilation; 5–10 µg/kg with IPPV. Up to 100 µg/kg has been used for **cardiac surgery**. Muscular rigidity and hypotension are more common after high dosage. Has been used in **neuroleptanaesthesia**.
–by infusion: 1–5 µg/kg/h, e.g. for sedation.

Fetal circulation. Oxygenated blood from the **placenta** passes through the single umbilical vein, and enters the inferior vena cava, about 50% bypassing the liver via the ductus venosus. Most of it is diverted through the foramen ovale into the left atrium, passing to the brain via the carotid arteries (Fig. 58). Deoxygenated blood from the brain enters the right atrium via the superior vena cava, and passes through the tricuspid valve to the right ventricle. Because the resistance of the pulmonary vessels within the collapsed lungs is high, the blood passes from the pulmonary artery trunk through the ductus arteriosus to enter the aortic arch downstream from the origin of the carotid arteries. Thus relatively O_2–rich blood is conserved for the brain, and the rest of the body is perfused with the less oxygenated blood. Deoxygenated blood reaches the placenta via the two umbilical arteries, arising from the internal iliac arteries; they receive about 60% of cardiac output.

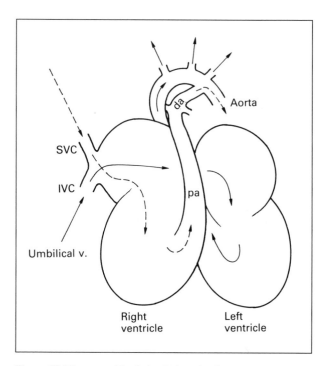

Figure 58 *Diagram of fetal circulation. da, ductus arteriosus; pa, pulmonary artery; IVC, inferior vena cava; SVC, superior vena cava; →, flow of oxygenated blood; – – →, flow of deoxygenated blood*

- Approximate values:
  - umbilical vein:
    - P_{O_2} 4 kPa (30 mmHg).
    - P_{CO_2} 6 kPa (45 mmHg).
    - pH 7.2
  - umbilical artery:
    - P_{O_2} 2 kPa (15 mmHg).
    - P_{CO_2} 7 kPa (53 mmHg).

At birth, placental blood flow ceases, and peripheral resistance increases. Lung expansion lowers **pulmonary vascular resistance**, both directly and via reduction of **hypoxic pulmonary vasoconstriction**. Thus pulmonary and right heart pressures fall, and aortic and left heart pressures rise. Pulmonary blood flow increases, and flow through the ductus arteriosus and foramen ovale ceases. Pulmonary artery pressure, pulmonary vascular resistance and pulmonary blood flow approach adult values by 4–6 weeks.

Neonates may resort to persistent fetal circulation, with decreased pulmonary blood flow and right to left **shunt** through the ductus arteriosus, foramen ovale or both. This may occur if pulmonary vascular resistance is increased, e.g. by **hypoxia**, **hypothermia**, **hypercapnia**, **acidosis**, polycythaemia, etc. It may occur during surgery if anaesthesia is too light or if the patient 'bucks' on the tracheal tube. Right to left shunt increases with worsening hypoxia and further reflex vasoconstriction. Ductal shunting may be demonstrated clinically by measuring O_2 saturation (e.g. by pulse **oximetry**) in the arm and leg simultaneously; a large difference (higher saturation in the arm) represents significant ductal blood flow (i.e. pulmonary artery pressure exceeds aortic pressure). If the right ventricle fails, right atrial pressure exceeds left atrial pressure, increasing shunt through the foramen ovale.

Treatment of persistent fetal circulation includes O_2 therapy, correction of acidosis, hypercapnia and hypothermia, and inotropes and fluid administration. Drugs which lower pulmonary vascular resistance, e.g. **tolazoline**, **isoprenaline**, etc. may be given. **Extracorporeal membrane oxygenation** has been used.

See also, Ductus arteriosus, patent

Fetal haemoglobin. Consists of two α chains and two γ chains, the latter differing from β chains by 37 amino acids. Binds **2,3–DPG** less avidly than **haemoglobin** A (adult), thus shifting the **oxyhaemoglobin dissociation curve** to the left (P_{50} is 2.4 kPa [18 mmHg]) and favouring O_2 transfer from mother to fetus. At the low fetal P_{O_2}, it gives up more O_2 to the tissues than adult haemoglobin would, because its dissociation curve is steeper in this part. Forms 80% of circulating haemoglobin at birth; replaced by haemoglobin A normally within 3–5 months. May persist in the **haemoglobinopathies**.

Embryonic haemoglobin is present up to 2–3 months of gestation.

Fetal wellbeing, during labour. Assessed by:
- presence of meconium in amniotic fluid: usually represents fetal distress, and presents risk of meconium aspiration on delivery.
- heart rate, especially related to uterine contractions. Now usually performed with electronic equipment (cardiotocograph), measuring heart rate by external ultrasonography or fetal scalp electrode, and contractions by external transducer or intrauterine probe:
  - normal heart rate is 120–160/min, with beat to beat variability of 10–25/min, related to autonomic activity. Increased baseline and reduced variability may be related to distress, although they may also be caused by administration of depressant drugs to the mother, maternal pyrexia, etc.
  - accelerations are usually related to reactivity and wellbeing.
  - decelerations: usual significance:
    - early (type I), i.e. with contractions: vagally mediated, due to head compression.
    - late (type II), i.e. after contractions: represent hypoxia, although not always with acidosis.
    - variable: usually due to cord compression; they may indicate distress if severe.
    Prolonged decelerations are more sinister, and may represent severe fetal distress.

  Signs of fetal distress may be related to treatable conditions, e.g. uterine hypertonicity associated with excessive oxytocin administration, maternal hypotension, etc. **Aortocaval compression** should always be considered, especially if extradural blockade has been provided. Predictive value of cardiotocography is poor in low-risk patients, hence some controversy surrounds its routine use.
  - fetal blood sample: pH under 7.2 represents severe acidosis. May be measured serially to observe trends.
  - fetal scalp oximetry, EEG, ECG and continuous pH measurement have been investigated but are not routinely available.

Post delivery, cord blood gas analysis (pH represents degree of acidosis at time of delivery), **Apgar scoring**, **time to sustained respiration** and **neurobehavioural testing of neonates** may be assessed; these may be useful prognostically.

Guay J (1991) Can J Anaesth; 38: R83–8

Fetus, effects of anaesthetic drugs on. The fetus is usually defined as such from the fourth month of gestation, or when the embryo becomes recognizably human. Most major organ structures develop earlier than this.
- Main anaesthetic considerations:
  - effect of anaesthetic drugs on fetal development and spontaneous abortion:
    - animal studies suggest increased fetal loss and abnormalities following prolonged exposure to high concentrations of volatile agents and **N_2O**.
    - human studies have produced conflicting results. It is generally accepted that general anaesthesia should be avoided where possible during pregnancy, particularly during the first trimester.
    - N_2O has been implicated (but not proven) as increasing the incidence of spontaneous abortion in health workers chronically exposed; current opinion holds that its use is not contraindicated in pregnant patients.
    - new drugs should be avoided during early pregnancy, until more information becomes available.
  - effect of anaesthetic drugs given during labour on the **neonate**:
    - indirect effects:
      - reduced uteroplacental blood flow, e.g. due to oxytocin, etc., or hypotension following regional blockade or general anaesthesia.

–maternal hypoxia, e.g. due to drug-induced respiratory depression, total spinal block, convulsions, etc.

–increased maternal catecholamine levels during general anaesthesia with **awareness**; uteroplacental vasoconstriction and fetal acidosis may result. Levels are reduced in labour following extradural block; this is thought to reduce fetal acidosis.

–direct effects:
  –related to fetal plasma levels, affected by:
    –uteroplacental blood flow.
    –placental, maternal and fetal protein concentrations and drug binding. May be the most important factor.
    –peak maternal plasma drug levels and their duration.
    –**diffusion** of drug across the **placenta**, depending on membrane thickness, molecular size and shape, degree of ionization and lipid solubility.
    –reduced fetal hepatic and renal function. Most drugs bypasses the fetal liver via the ductus venosus.
    –umbilical vein drug levels: reduced by dilution with blood from the rest of the body. Thus umbilical vein levels may not reflect fetal levels.
    –fetal hypoxia and acidosis: cause trapping of basic drugs, e.g. opioids and **local anaesthetic agents**, and increase blood flow to vital centres e.g. brain. Thus brain levels may be increased.

–specific drugs:
  –**opioid analgesic drugs**:
    –fetal respiratory and neurobehavioural depression are well recognized.
    –fetal opioid levels are increased by acidosis. Peak levels occur 2–5 hours after im **pethidine**, 6 minutes after iv injection.
    –**half-life** in the fetus is prolonged; e.g. pethidine: up to 20 hours; that of norpethidine is longer.
    –**naloxone** crosses the placenta easily, but its administration is usually reserved for the fetus.
  –**iv anaesthetic agents**:
    –all cross the placenta rapidly, but have usually redistributed by the time of delivery. **Thiopentone** selectively accumulates in fetal liver.
    –neurobehavioural depression has been shown following their use, although the effect is small.
  –**inhalational anaesthetic agents**:
    –at low inspired concentrations, any effect is small.
    –benefits of their use include uteroplacental vasodilatation and prevention of maternal awareness.
  –**neuromuscular blocking drugs**:
    –very little transfer follows normal use.
    –**gallamine** and **alcuronium** cross the placenta to a slightly greater extent than the others.
  –local anaesthetic agents:
    –transfer varies according to dose, site of injection (e.g. high fetal levels following **paracervical block**), use of vasoconstrictors and different plasma protein binding characteristics of the fetus and mother for certain drugs; e.g. umbilical vein/maternal blood levels:

–**prilocaine**: >1.
–**lignocaine**: 0.5.
–**bupivacaine**: 0.3.
–**etidocaine**: 0.2.
–subtle neurobehavioural effects have been shown; initial fears about adverse effects of lignocaine compared with bupivacaine are now thought to be unfounded.
–fetal **methaemoglobinaemia** may follow excessive doses of prilocaine.
–**procaine** and **2–chloroprocaine** are metabolized by esterases in maternal and fetal plasma.
–others, e.g. **benzodiazepines**, **phenothiazines**, etc.:
  –all cross the placenta to some extent.
  –**diazepam** is more strongly bound to fetal than to maternal protein, and has been associated with neonatal hypotonia and hypothermia. Umbilical vein/maternal blood ratio is 2.0.
  –all drugs that may cause central effects, and therefore cross the blood–brain barrier, may cross the placenta to similar extents, e.g. atropine, propranolol, etc.

See also, Environmental safety of anaesthetists; Fetal wellbeing, during labour; Neurobehavioural testing of neonates

FEV$_1$, *see Forced expiratory volume*

FFARCS examination (Fellowship of the **Faculty of Anaesthetists at the Royal College of Surgeons of England**). First held in 1953; became the **FCAnaes. examination** in 1989 following the founding of the **College of Anaesthetists**. Since 1985 it has consisted of three parts: I, relating to the fundamentals of clinical anaesthesia; II, relating to the basic sciences; III, relating to the practice of anaesthesia as a whole. Pass rates are in the order of 40–50%, 30–40% and 20–40%, respectively. The Irish equivalent exam (FFARCSI) was first held in 1961.

FFP, Fresh frozen plasma, *see Blood products*

Fibreoptic instruments. First use of a fibreoptic instrument (choledocoscope) for tracheal intubation was in 1967. Fibreoptic bronchoscopes were introduced in 1968. Flexible fibreoptic intubating bronchoscopes of down to 3–4 mm diameter are now available.

• Features:
  –rely on internal reflection of light within bundles of glass fibres, about 20 μm diameter.
  –each fibre is encased in glass of different refractive index, the interface acting as the reflective surface.
  –fibres are lubricated and flexible; the instrument's tip can be flexed using controls at the proximal end.
  –each instrument contains bundles for passage of light for illumination, and bundles for passage of the image back to the proximal end. The arrangement of the image-bearing bundles is identical at each end of the instrument, allowing accurate spatial representation of the object.
  –a lens at each end allows focusing.
  –may contain channels for suction, passage of gas, liquid, forceps, etc.
  –very delicate instruments; easily damaged e.g. by teeth, etc. Careful cleaning is required; passage of disinfectant into the scope may disrupt lubrication between fibres.

• Apart from diagnostic and therapeutic use (e.g. removal of secretions and foreign bodies, etc.), they have been used in anaesthesia for:

–tracheal intubation, with the patient awake or anaesthetized. Especially useful in cases of known difficult intubation. The endoscope may be passed through a tracheal tube, and then guided via the mouth or nose into the larynx. Lignocaine may be sprayed through a side-port. The tube is passed over the scope into the trachea. Alternatively, the scope and tube are passed together, the former protruding a short distance from the latter. Has been used with endobronchial tubes.

–checking the position of tracheal or endobronchial tubes, etc., once placed. Particularly useful for endobronchial tubes. May be passed through special connectors with rubber ports, thus allowing undisturbed delivery of anaesthetic gases.

–assessing the tracheobronchial tree before, during and after thoracic surgery.

Widely used in the USA but less so in the UK, partly related to the cost of equipment. Considerable practice is required to achieve adequate skill in their use, which has been suggested as being desirable during all anaesthetists' training.

Fibreoptic sensors have also been used for clinical measurement of e.g. pressure, flow and chemical concentrations.

See also, Intubation, awake; Intubation, difficult; Intubation, endobronchial; Intubation, tracheal

Fibrin degradation products (FDPs). Products of fibrin breakdown by plasmin; thus blood levels reflect the rate of **fibrinolysis**. **Half-life** is about 9 hours. May inhibit clot formation by competing for fibrin polymerization sites. Also interfere with **platelet** function and thrombin; thus excess fibrinolysis may impair further **coagulation**. May possibly damage vascular endothelium.

Non-specific testing for FDPs has been replaced in many centres by testing for the D-dimer portion of fibrin, which is released only during fibrinolysis and is not present on fibrinogen nor released during the latter's breakdown.

Normal levels: <10 mg/l (FDPs); <500 ng/ml (D-dimer).

See also, Coagulation studies

Fibrinogen, *see Coagulation*

Fibrinolysis. Dissolution of fibrin; occurs following clot formation allowing blood vessel remodelling, and also after wound healing. Fibrinolytic and **coagulation** pathways are in equilibrium normally, each composed of a series of plasma precursor molecules.

Plasminogen, a globulin, is activated to form plasmin, a fibrinolytic enzyme. Activation involves clotting factors XII and XI, **kallikrein** and **kinins**, and leucocyte products. Activation of tissue plasminogen is caused by products released by endothelial cells. Plasminogen activators and plasminogen itself bind to fibrin, with plasmin formation thus localized to the site of fibrin formation. Fibrin is degraded to **fibrin degradation products**, with **complement** and **platelet** activation. Fibrinolysis may be decreased by stress, including surgery; effects are greatest 2–3 days postoperatively. It may be increased by **fibrinolytic drugs**, and following **DIC** as a response to the large amount of fibrin formed. Also increased by venous occlusion, **catecholamines**, and possibly **extradural** and **spinal anaesthesia**. Primary fibrinolysis may occur in certain malignancies.

Fibrinolytic drugs. Drugs causing **fibrinolysis** by activating plasminogen. Used iv and intra-arterially to prevent thrombosis, and to break up established thrombi, e.g. **PE**. Have been shown to reduce mortality in acute **MI** when given iv within 24 hours, especially within 6 hours. Main side effects are related to bleeding. Allergic reactions may occur, especially following repeated administration of **streptokinase**. Allergic reactions are less common with urokinase, used mainly for thrombolysis in the eye and arteriovenous shunts. Recombinant tissue plasminogen activator has recently been introduced; it is activated by fibrin and therefore has less effect on circulating clotting factors.

Fibrocystic disease, *see Cystic fibrosis*

Fick principle. Blood flow to an organ in unit time =

$$\frac{\text{amount of a marker substance taken up by the organ in that time}}{\text{concentration difference of the substance in the vessels supplying and draining the organ}}$$

The amount of a substance given up by an organ can also be used, e.g. CO_2 (see below).

May be used to determine blood flow to individual organs, e.g. **cerebral blood flow (Kety–Schmidt technique)** or **renal blood flow**.

May also be used to determine **cardiac output**, using O_2 or CO_2 as the substance measured, and the heart as the organ concerned:

cardiac output (l/min)

$$= \frac{O_2 \text{ consumption (ml/min)}}{\text{arterial} - \text{mixed venous } O_2 \text{ concentration (ml/l)}}$$

substituting normal values:

$$= \frac{250 \text{ ml/min}}{200-150 \text{ ml/l}}$$

$$= 5 \text{ l/min}$$

using CO_2:

cardiac output

$$= \frac{CO_2 \text{ ouput (ml/min)}}{\text{mixed venous} - \text{arterial } CO_2 \text{ concentration (ml/l)}}$$

substituting normal values:

$$= \frac{200}{540-500 \text{ ml/l}}$$

$$= 5 \text{ l/min}$$

[Adolf Fick (1829–1901), German physiologist]

Fick's law of diffusion. Rate of **diffusion** across a **membrane** is proportional to the concentration gradient across that membrane.

See also, Fick principle

Filling ratio. Extent to which **cylinders** are underfilled with liquid substances. The presence of gas above the liquid reduces the pressure increase caused by any temperature rise, reducing the risk of pressure build-up and rupture. Defined as the weight of substance contained in the cylinder, divided by the weight of water it could contain.

- Applicable to substances at temperatures below their **critical temperatures**, e.g.:
  N_2O:
  –0.75 (temperate climate).
  –0.67 (tropical climate).
  CO_2: as for N_2O.
  cyclopropane:
  –0.51 (temperate climate).
  –0.48 (tropical climate).

Filtration fraction. Ratio of **GFR** to renal plasma flow (RPF). As RPF falls, GFR remains fairly constant because of efferent arteriolar constriction, causing filtration fraction to rise. Normally 0.16–0.2.

Fink effect. Reduced alveolar concentration of a gas, and thus reduced uptake, resulting from its dilution by another gas leaving the bloodstream and entering the alveoli. Analogous but opposite to the **second gas effect**. At the end of anaesthesia, it may cause **diffusion hypoxia** as N_2O leaving the bloodstream dilutes alveolar O_2.
[Bernard Raymond Fink, Seattle anaesthetist]

F_1O_2. Fractional inspired concentration of O_2. By convention, expressed as a decimalized fraction, e.g. 0.21, 0.5, etc., although previously expressed as a percentage.

First-pass metabolism. Metabolism of a substance once absorbed, reducing the amount of substance before it reaches systemic circulation. Active metabolites may be formed. Most commonly refers to metabolism by the liver following oral administration of drugs, e.g. **propranolol, morphine, lignocaine** and **glyceryl trinitrate** (i.e. drugs with a high **extraction ratio**). Drugs may be given by alternative routes to bypass the liver, e.g. parenterally, sublingually or rectally. May also occur in the intestinal mucosa following oral administration of e.g. **methyldopa, chlorpromazine** and **isoprenaline**, and in the bronchial mucosa following inhalation of isoprenaline.

Flail chest. Disruption of chest wall integrity, where a portion of the thoracic cage becomes detached from the bony structure of the rest. The flail segment no longer moves outwards on inspiration, but is free to be drawn inwards by negative intrathoracic pressure; it is pushed out during expiration whilst the rest of the thorax contracts. Occurs in severe **chest trauma** with multiple fractures involving several **ribs** with or without the sternum. May result from trauma or surgery.
- Features:
  - **hypoventilation**, with reduced tidal volume and vital capacity. **Pendulluft** is now thought not to occur; mediastinal shift results in air entry to both lungs, although overall hypoventilation may be severe. Hypoventilation is further exacerbated by pain. Ability to cough is reduced due to mechanical impairment and pain.
  - underlying lung contusion/**atelectasis/pneumothorax** with resultant **shunt** and **$\dot{V}/\dot{Q}$ mismatch**; thought to be more important than hypoventilation.
  - associated injuries, e.g. to mediastinum, head, abdomen, etc.
  - mediastinal shift may affect cardiac output.
- Management is as for chest trauma, i.e.:
  - O_2 administration,
  - analgesia (e.g. systemic opioids/**intercostal nerve block/extradural analgesia**).
  - treatment of hypovolaemia and associated injuries.
  - **chest drainage** if required.
  - **physiotherapy**.
  - nasogastric drainage helps prevent gastric dilatation.
  - if arterial blood gases are acceptable, no further treatment may be required. Improved oxygenation and chest wall splinting may be achieved by **CPAP**.
  - tracheal intubation and IPPV. May be continued until the underlying lung improves or surgical fixation of the flail segment (i.e. up to several weeks). **IMV** has been used.
  - surgical fixation of rib fractures is preferred by some surgeons.

Flame ionization detector. Device used in analysis of gas mixtures, separated e.g. by **gas chromatography**. A potential difference is applied across a flame of hydrogen gas burning in air. Addition of organic vapour to the gas stream causes a change in current flow across the flame, the amount of change proportional to the amount of substance present. Used only to quantify the amount of a known substance, not to identify unknown ones.
See also, Gas analysis

Flammability. Ability to support combustion. Dependant on molecular structure; e.g. C–C bonds readily break down with heat and O_2 to form carbon monoxide/dioxide, whereas C–F bonds are resistant. Flammability limits refer to concentrations of a substance which will support combustion; e.g.:
  –cyclopropane:
    –2.5–60% in O_2.
    –2.5–10% in air.
    –1.5–30% in N_2O.
  –diethyl ether:
    –2–82% in O_2.
    –2–35% in air.
    –1.5–24% in N_2O.
Ranges for explosive mixtures occur within these limits, especially with high O_2 concentration. The **stoichiometric mixture** lies within the explosive range. Flammability is greater in N_2O than in O_2, because the former decomposes to produce O_2 with release of energy. Addition of water vapour reduces flammability.

'Non-flammable' agents, e.g. halothane, enflurane, isoflurane, will ignite only at higher concentrations than occur during anaesthesia, and require much greater amounts of energy to initiate ignition (**activation energy**).
See also, Explosions and fires

Flash-point. Lowest temperature at which a saturated vapour of a liquid ignites when exposed to a flame, in the presence of one or more other gas(es).

Flecainide acetate. Class Ic **antiarrhythmic drug**. Slows impulse conduction, without affecting action potential duration. Used for severe VT and extrasystoles, and SVT, especially those involving accessory pathways (e.g. **Wolff–Parkinson–White syndrome**).

- Dosage:
  - –2 mg/kg up to 150 mg, over 10–30 minutes iv.
  - –by infusion: 1.5 mg/kg/h for 1 hour; 0.1–0.25 mg/kg/h thereafter.
  - –100–400 mg orally.
- Side effects:
  - –giddiness, visual disturbances, corneal deposits.
  - –myocardial depression (minor), **proarrhythmias**.
  - –resistance to endocardial pacing.
  - –increased plasma levels in hepatic/renal failure (levels should be monitored).
  - –has been associated with increased risk of cardiac arrest after MI, therefore reserved for life-threatening arrhythmias.

Flow. Amount of **fluid** moving per unit time. Flow through a tube may be:
- –laminar: flow is smooth and without eddies. Molecules at the tube's edges move more slowly; those at the centre more rapidly (Fig. 59)

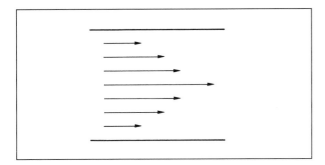

Figure 59 *Laminar flow profile*

laminar flow =

$$\frac{\text{pressure gradient along tube} \times \text{radius}^4 \times \pi}{\text{tube length} \times \textbf{viscosity of fluid} \times 8}$$

(Hagen-Poiseuille equation).
- –turbulent: caused when the tube is unevenly shaped, or when the fluid flows through an orifice, around sharp edges, etc. Also occurs from laminar flow when flow velocity is too fast, exceeding the **critical velocity**. **Reynold's number** describes the relationship between tube and fluid characteristics and velocity at which turbulent flow occurs. Turbulent flow is proportional to:
  - –radius^2.
  - –√pressure gradient.
  - –1/length.
  - –1/density of fluid.

Flow in the airways and blood vessels is a mixture of laminar and turbulent, but behaves approximately according to the above principles.
- Measurement:
  - –gas: **flowmeters**.
  - –liquid: **dilution techniques**, **electromagnetic flow measurement**, **Fick principle**. Similar flowmeters to those used for gases may also be used.
  - –measurement of volume over a certain time.

Flow-directed balloon-tipped pulmonary artery catheters, *see Pulmonary artery catheterization*

Flow generators, *see Ventilators*

Flowmasta, *see Ventilators*

Flowmeters. Devices for measuring **flow**. Usually refer to measurement of gas flow, e.g. from cylinders and anaesthetic machines, or in breathing systems.
- May be:
  - –constant orifice, variable pressure. Since flow through an orifice is proportional to the pressure difference across it, flow may be deduced by measuring the pressure difference across a fixed orifice. In the first two examples, only the downstream pressure is measured, since the pressure upstream of the orifice is constant:
    - –simple pressure gauge downstream from the outlet of an O_2 cylinder. The gauge may be calibrated directly for flow, e.g. litres/min.
    - –water depression flowmeter. The pressure is measured with a simple water manometer.
    - –**pneumotachograph**. Pressure is measured electronically using transducers.
  - –constant pressure, variable orifice. If the pressure across a variable orifice remains constant, the size of the orifice depends on the gas flow. Examples:
    - –**Rotameter**, simple ball flowmeter and dry bobbin flowmeter. The size of the orifice is determined by the height of the bobbin in its tube: the greater the height, the larger the orifice. In the rotameter and ball flowmeter, the tube is of tapered bore, being wider at the top than at the bottom. The dry bobbin flowmeter tube is of uniform diameter, with small holes arranged longitudinally. The variability of the effective orifice size is provided by the number of holes below the bobbin, i.e. the bobbin's height.
    - –Heidbrink flowmeter. The 'bobbin' is extended vertically to form a rod; its bottom end sits in a tapered tube whilst its top end lies opposite a linear scale above the tapered part. It functions in a similar way to the rotameter, but without rotating.
    - –**peakflow meters**.
  - –variable pressure, variable orifice. In the watersight flowmeter, gas passes through a tube with holes along its length, immersed into water. At low gas flows, gas bubbles from the upper holes only; at higher flow rates, from the lower holes as well. The holes are marked with according flow rates. Orifice variability results from the different number of holes through which gas may pass; pressure variability arises because pressure is higher at greater depth of water.
  - –constant pressure, constant orifice. Bubble flowmeters may be used for calibration at low flow rates. Gas passes along a uniform tube, carrying a thin soap film with it. Flow is deduced by measuring the velocity of the film along the tube using a timer.
- Other flowmeters include:
  - –thermistor flowmeter: the cooling effect of a gas stream on a thermistor varies with flow rate.
  - –ultrasonic flowmeter: turbulent eddies are formed around a rod in the gas path. The frequency of oscillation of the eddies, measured by **Doppler** probe, is proportional to flow rate.

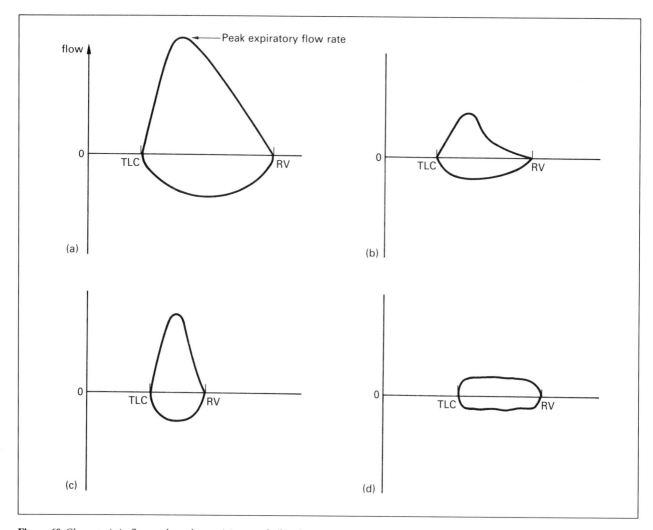

Figure 60 *Characteristic flow–volume loops: (a) normal; (b) obstructive lung disease; (c) restrictive lung disease; (d) tracheal/largyngeal obstruction. TLC, total lung capacity; RV, residual volume*

Flow can also be determined by measuring the volume of gas per unit time, e.g. using a **respirometer**.
[Jay A Heidbrink (1875–1957), US anaesthetist]

Flow–volume loops. Curves resulting from simultaneous measurement and plotting of air flow and lung volume during a maximal forced expiration. If **residual volume** is known, lung volume may be determined by measuring expired volume. Characteristic loops are obtained in certain conditions, although the loops obtained in practice are rarely as easily distinguishable (Fig. 60).

Much of the information from studying **forced expiration** may be obtained from flow–volume loops, e.g. **forced expiratory flow rate**, **forced expiratory volume**, and **peak expiratory flow rate**.
See also, Lung function tests

Fluid. Form of matter whose shape is continuously changed when subjected to a shearing force, i.e. gas or liquid. Continuous shearing force results in **flow**; resistance to flow is proportional to **viscosity**. For a Newtonian fluid, viscosity is constant for different shear rates and

over time; for a non-Newtonian fluid (e.g. blood), it varies with shear rates or over time.
[Sir Isaac Newton (1642–1727), English scientist]
See also, Fluidics

Fluid balance. Normal approximate fluid intake of a 70 kg adult:

      1500 ml liquid
       750 ml in food
       250 ml from **metabolism** within the body.
total: 2500 ml
Normal output:
      1500 ml urine
       100 ml in faeces
       900 ml **insensible water loss**.
total: 2500 ml
Loss in sweat is normally negligible but may exceed several litres in hot environments. Insensible losses are also increased in high temperatures. About 5% of body water is exchanged per day in adults, 15% in infants; hence the increased risk of **dehydration** in the latter.

Balance is normally regulated to maintain **ECF** volume and **osmolality**; changes are detected by **baroreceptors** and **osmoreceptors**, with resultant compensatory mechanisms:

  –water intake is regulated by thirst; increased by **hypovolaemia** and **hyperosmolality**.
  –cardiovascular compensation for hypovolaemia.
  –urinary output is regulated by **vasopressin**, **atrial natriuretic peptide** and **renin/angiotensin system**.

• Fluid balance may be disturbed in patients presenting for anaesthesia, perioperatively and in ICU:

  –reduced intake, e.g. coma, dysphagia, nausea, nil by mouth instructions.
  –increased intake, e.g. excessive iv administration.
  –redistribution, e.g. to **third space**.
  –reduced output, e.g. **syndrome of inappropriate anti-diuretic hormone**.
  –increased output, e.g sweating, polyuria, vomiting, diarrhoea.

Routine administration of **iv fluids** peroperatively is controversial; excessive dextrose administration may lead to **hyperglycaemia** and **hyponatraemia**, whilst excessive salt solution administration may cause peripheral and pulmonary **oedema**. Improved recovery has been claimed following fluid administration (especially containing dextrose) during minor surgery compared with no fluids. The **colloid/crystalloid controversy** adds to the confused picture.

• **IV fluid administration** should be guided by the following:

  –maintenance requirements: 40 ml/kg/day
   (1.6 ml/kg/h). Requirements are greater in **paediatric** anaesthesia.
  –replacement of **blood loss** (*see Haemorrhage*).
  –third space losses: with peroperative evaporative losses, approximately 10–15 ml/kg/h during major abdominal surgery.
  –other losses, e.g. nasogastric aspirate.

Careful attention to fluid balance is required in all perioperative and critically ill patients to prevent complications, e.g. **hypernatraemia**, hyponatraemia, **dehydration**, **renal failure**, etc. Therapy is guided by **CVP**, urine output, BP, pulse and electrolyte balance. Body weight is a useful supplement to fluid intake/output charts.

See also, Fluids, body

Fluid therapy, *see Intravenous fluids*

Fluidics. Technology of operating control systems by utilizing flow characteristics of gases or liquids. Has been used in control mechanisms of ventilators, e.g. employing the **Coanda effect**. The direction of a jet of gas in a valve may be switched by 'signal' jets of driving gas across the main jet. Combinations of signal jets allow complex manipulation of the valve output, without moving parts.

Pneumatic spool valves may contain moving shuttles, driven by gas from either end. The valve chamber is divided into segments by seals through which the shuttle passes; the valve output depends on the lining up of ports and channels in the shuttle and valve wall. The output may be used to drive cylinders which may be driven from either end.

Fluids, body. Approximately 60% of male body weight is water; 50–55% in females (greater proportion of fat). Total body water may be measured using a **dilution technique** with deuterium oxide (heavy water). Its main constituent compartments are **intracellular fluid** (ICF), **ECF**, **plasma** and **interstitial fluid** (Fig. 61). Approximately 1 litre is contained within the GIT, CSF, etc. (transcellular fluid).

In **neonates**, ECF exceeds 30% (but plasma is still 5%), and ICF is less than 40%. These differences are greatest in premature babies, when ECF exceeds ICF. During childhood, the adult situation slowly develops.

Composition of fluid compartments are shown in Table 15.

• Main methods of movement of ions and molecules between compartments:

  –**diffusion**.
  –facilitated diffusion: carrier molecules transport substances from high to low concentrations, requiring no energy.
  –**active transport**.
  –filtration.

Movement of substances are also affected by other substances, e.g. **Donnan effect**.

Water moves across **membranes** from solutions of low concentrations to those of high concentrations (**osmosis**). Depending on their constitution, different **iv fluids** will fill certain compartments more than others.

See also, Blood volume; Fluid balance

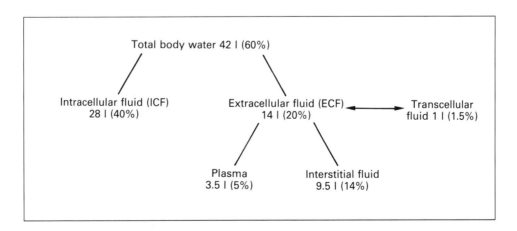

Figure 61 *Composition of body fluids, with volumes for an average 70 kg man (% body weight)*

Table 15. Approximate composition of body fluid compartments (mmol/l)

Compartment	Na^+	K^+	HCO_3^-	Cl^-	Ca^{2+}	Mg^{2+}	SO_4^{2-}	$HPO_4^{2-} + PO_4^{3-}$
Intracellular fluid	10	150	10	3	3	30	20	100
Interstitial fluid	140	5	30	110	5	3	1	2
Plasma	140	5	28	110	5	3	1	2

Flumazenil. Benzodiazepine agonist, introduced in 1987. Acts specifically at central benzodiazepine receptors. Has been used to reverse excessive sedation due to benzodiazepines, e.g. following attempted suicide, prolonged sedation with benzodiazepines in ICU, and iatrogenic overdose. Benzodiazepine metabolism is unaffected.
- Dosage: 0.2 mg iv, repeated slowly as necessary up to 1–2 mg. May also be given by infusion (0.1–0.4 mg/h).
- Has caused excessive excitement and convulsions, especially in patients maintained on long-term benzodiazepines, e.g. for epilepsy. Because of its short **half-life** (less than 1 hour), its effects may wear off with recurrence of sedation.

Fluoride ions. Nephrotoxic ions implicated in the high output renal failure seen following **methoxyflurane** administration. Evidence for their role:
   –degree of renal impairment is proportional to plasma concentration:
      –subclinical evidence of renal impairment occurs above 50 μmol/l.
      –polyuria, decreased urinary osmolality and increased plasma sodium and osmolality occur above 80–100 μmol/l.
   –infusion of fluoride ions into rats produces similar renal effects.
Mechanism of renal damage is unclear but may involve impairment of both renal Na/K/ATPase systems and **vasopressin** action.
- Levels are highest after methoxyflurane, but may be raised after other halogenated volatile agents:
   –methoxyflurane: 50–60 μmol/l after 2.5 MAC hours; 90–120 μmol/l after 5 MAC hours.
   –**enflurane**: up to 30 μmol/l after prolonged use (over 9 hours). Plasma levels are highest in obese patients. **Enzyme induction** with isoniazid is thought to increase levels.
   –**isoflurane**: under 5 μmol/l even after prolonged surgery. Levels of up to 90 μmol/l have been reported after several days' use for sedation in ICU.
   –**halothane**: minimal production of fluoride ions.

Fluotec vaporizer, *see Vaporizers*

Fluroxene (Trifluoroethyl vinyl ether). **Inhalational anaesthetic agent**, introduced in 1954. The first fluorine-containing volatile agent, now unavailable. Explosive, possibly mutagenic, and toxic to experimental animals due to biotransformation to trifluoroethanol.

Flurpitine maleate. Non-opioid centrally acting **analgesic drug**, recently investigated. Thought to act via central adrenergic pathway stimulation, although the precise mechanism is unclear.

Flying squad, obstetric. Mobile team including anaesthetist, obstetrician and midwife; first suggested in 1929, and organized in Glasgow in 1933. The usual problems of **obstetric anaesthesia** and neonatal resuscitation are compounded by the abnormal location, limitation of facilities, requiring portable equipment, and lack of patient preparation. Commonest emergency is postpartum haemorrhage caused by retained placenta. Use of a flying squad has declined as the number of home deliveries has decreased. The above problems have led many units to withdraw anaesthetic cover from such squads, with emphasis on rapid transfer of the patient to hospital.
Davies CK (1969) Br J Anaesth; 41: 545–50

Foetal, *see Fetal*

Food and Drug Administration (FDA). US body, involved in testing new drugs and reviewing test results. Also controls imports, and regulates foods and cosmetics. Companies must apply to the FDA before initiating **clinical trials**. Evolved after World War II from the 1938 Food, Drug and Cosmetics Act, restricting labelling and advertising of drugs; amended in 1968 to require that drugs be shown to be efficacious as well as safe. Thus enforces laws enacted by the US Congress. Previously, the Pure Food and Drugs Act of 1906 and subsequent amendments attempted to prevent improper labelling and fraudulent claims by manufacturers.
See also, Committee on Safety of Medicines

Foot, nerve blocks, *see Ankle, nerve blocks; Digital nerve block*

Force. That which changes a body's state of rest or motion. SI **unit** of force is the **newton**.

Forced diuresis. Method of increasing renal excretion of certain drugs, sometimes used in **poisoning and overdoses**. By manipulating urinary pH, excretion may be increased by 'trapping' the ionized fraction of a drug in urine, preventing its diffusion back into the bloodstream, since charged molecules diffuse poorly across biological membranes.
- Forced alkaline diuresis:
   –used in poisoning with acid drugs, e.g. **salicylates** and **barbiturates**.
   –500 ml/h of the following fluids are administered in rotation:
      –500 ml 1.26% sodium bicarbonate.
      –500 ml 5% dextrose.
      –500 ml 0.9% saline.
   –CVP, urine output and pH, blood gas measurement and plasma electrolytes (especially potassium) must be closely monitored. Infusion rate is reduced in the elderly.

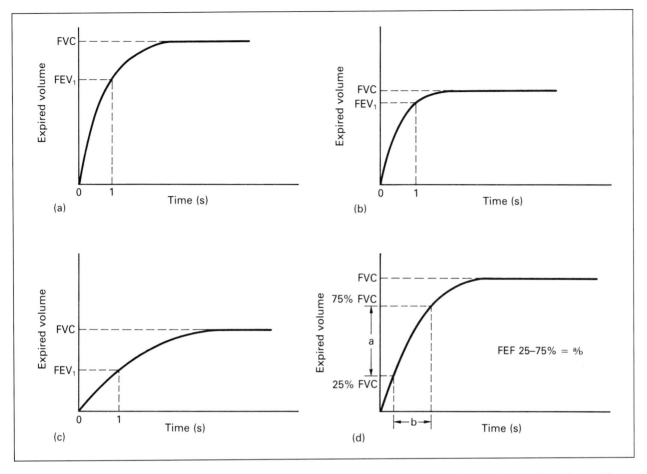

Figure 62 *Typical forced expiratory patterns: (a) normal; (b) showing calculation of FEF (25–75%); (c) obstructive lung disease; (d) restrictive lung disease*

- Forced acid diuresis:
  - –used in poisoning with alkaline drugs, e.g. phency-clidines.
  - –1000 ml/h of the following fluids are administered in rotation:
    - –500 ml 5% dextrose + 1.5 g ammonium chloride.
    - –500 ml 5% dextrose.
    - –500 ml 0.9% saline.
  - –monitoring as above.

Severe metabolic upset and circulatory overload may occur.

Forced expiration. Means of investigating lung function, from which may be measured: **forced expiratory flow rate** ($FEF_{25-75\%}$), **FEV**, **FVC** and **peak expiratory flow rate**. Other suggested measurements exclude the first 200 ml of expiration, or analyse the flow rate at 50% of vital capacity.

    Flow–volume loops and data from **spirometers** (e.g. the Vitalograph) may be analysed (Fig. 62). Repetition following bronchodilator therapy may indicate the extent of reversible airway obstruction.

    At lung volumes of up to 60% of vital capacity, maximal expiratory flow rate is independent of effort; increasing effort raises intrathoracic pressure, increasing the pressure difference across the airways, and leading to airway collapse.

See also, Lung function tests

Forced expiratory flow rate ($FEF_{25-75\%}$). Average flow rate measured at between 25% and 75% of forced maximal expired volume (Fig. 62). Usually changes with **forced expiratory volume**, but has wider spread of normal values.

See also, Forced expiration; Lung function tests; Peak expiratory flow rate

Forced expiratory volume (FEV). Volume of gas forcibly exhaled from full inspiration, in a set period of time (normally 1 second; the volume is then called FEV_1). Normally 80% of **FVC**, which may be measured at the same time using a **spirometer**. Reduced in obstructive lung disease, as is the FEV_1/FVC ratio. In restrictive disease, FEV_1 may be normal, but FVC isreduced.

    Easier and more comfortable to measure than **maximal voluntary ventilation**.

See also, Forced expiration; Lung function tests

Forced vital capacity (FVC). **Vital capacity** measured when expiration is forced. Closure of some airways may

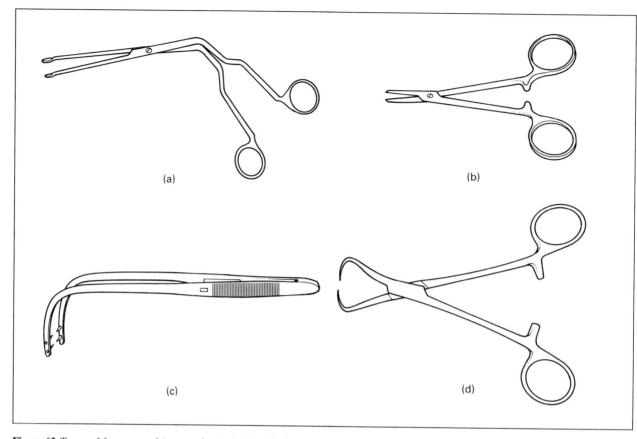

Figure 63 *Types of forceps used in anaesthesia: (a) Magill; (b) Spencer Wells; (c) Krause; (d) Moynihan tongue forceps*

occur when intrathoracic pressure is high, causing air-trapping. FVC thus may be less than 'true' vital capacity. Reduced in restrictive disease, the supine position, the elderly, muscle weakness, abdominal swelling, pain, and when premature airway closing occurs during forced expiration, e.g. emphysema.

See also, Forced expiration; Lung function tests; Lung volumes

Forceps. Many varieties may be used by anaesthetists, e.g. (Fig. 63):
- **Magill**'s forceps: introduced originally in 1920 to assist placement of gum-elastic bougies for insufflation anaesthesia. Used to guide tracheal tubes into the larynx, or nasogastric tubes into the oesophagus, under direct vision. May damage the tracheal tube cuff if grasped. Also used to place pharyngeal packs or to remove foreign bodies. The operator's hand is held out of the line of vision by the angled handles. Adult and paediatric sizes are available. Many modifications have been described.
- Spencer Wells artery forceps: used mainly to clamp the pilot tube of the tracheal cuff to prevent deflation. Also used for fixing tubing, etc.
- Krause's forceps: used to hold local anaesthetic-soaked pledgets in the piriform fossae for blocking the superior laryngeal nerves for awake intubation. They bear a spring catch and spiked jaws.
- several tongue forceps exist; formerly used to pull the tongue forward to relieve airway obstruction, but now more likely to be used for fixing tubing, etc.

[Thomas Spencer Wells (1818–1897), English surgeon; Herman Krause (1848–1921), German laryngologist; Berkley GA Moynihan (1865–1936), English surgeon]
See also, Mouth gags

Foreign body, inhaled. Most common in children. May obstruct upper or lower airways. Should be considered in any child with **stridor** or persistent cough and chest infections. Most small objects lodge in the right main bronchus, because of its more vertical angle of origin and greater width. Organic matter, e.g. peanuts, may cause intense bronchial inflammatory reactions within a few hours, with oedema and possibly bronchial obstruction. Other features may include:
- distal **atelectasis**.
- distal air-trapping if the object acts as a ball-valve. Chest X-ray in expiration may reveal unilateral overinflation.
- features of **airway obstruction**.
- infection.
- Removal is via rigid **bronchoscopy**. Anaesthetic management:
  - preoperatively:
    - assessment for severity of airway obstruction.
    - **premedication** with **atropine**. Sedative drugs are suggested by some as being helpful; by others as being a hindrance.
  - peroperatively:
    - an experienced anaesthetist's presence is mandatory.

–classically, an inhalational induction is performed, using **halothane** in O_2. **N_2O** is avoided in case of distal air-trapping, and to raise F_1O_2. Induction may be slow.

–iv induction is preferred by some.

–**lignocaine** spray to the vocal cords may reduce risk of per- and postoperative **laryngospasm**.

–classically, spontaneous ventilation is employed using ether, with bronchoscopy performed as anaesthesia lightens. Halothane is most commonly used now. Avoidance of IPPV is usually advocated, to reduce risk of blowing the object further distally. In practice, adequate depth of anaesthesia and oxygenation may be difficult to maintain with spontaneous ventilation, without excessive hypercapnia.

–postoperatively:

–close monitoring is required in case of bronchospasm or laryngospasm.

–humidified O_2 administration by mask.

Forward failure, *see Cardiac failure*

Fourier analysis. Mathematical breakdown of **waveforms** into simple sine wave constituents. Any complex waveform consists of sine waves of different frequencies: the slowest (fundamental) frequency and **harmonics** thereof. Used in analysis and reconstruction of waveforms, e.g. transmission of electrical signals. The higher the frequencies analysed, the more accurate the reproduction.

[Baron Jean-Baptiste Fourier (1768–1830), French mathematician]

Fowler's method (Single breath nitrogen washout). Method of investigation of **lung volumes**. The subject breathes air normally, and takes a maximal breath of O_2 (i.e. to **vital capacity**) from the the end of normal expiration (i.e. **FRC**). Exhaled nitrogen concentration is measured during maximal slow expiration (i.e. to **residual volume**), and plotted against volume of expired gas.

● Four phases are described (Fig. 64):

–phase 1: O_2 from the conducting airways (anatomical **dead space**), containing no nitrogen.

–phase 2: mixture of dead space gas and alveolar gas.

–phase 3: alveolar gas, containing the nitrogen present in the alveoli before the O_2 breath started. There is a slight upward slope normally, increased in lung disease.

–phase 4: at **closing capacity**, lower alveoli and airways collapse, thus the exhaled gas comes from upper airways only. At the onset of the O_2 inspiration, the upper airways were already considerably expanded (with nitrogen-containing air) compared with lower ones, since most ventilation is of upper lung regions at normal tidal volume. Most of the inspired O_2 therefore entered the lower alveoli, since they started off smaller. When they collapse, nitrogen-rich gas from the upper alveoli is exhaled, giving rise to phase 4.

Anatomical dead space is measured to the mid-point of phase 2.

CO_2 measurement may be used in a similar way, using **capnography**.

[Ward S Fowler, US physiologist]

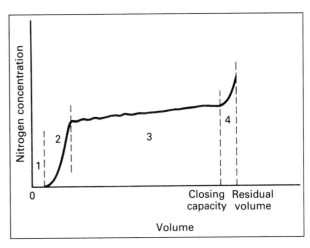

Figure 64 *Fowler's method of estimating anatomical dead space and closing capacity (see text)*

Frankenhauser's plexus block, *see Paracervical block*

FRC, *see Functional residual capacity*

Free radicals. Atoms or molecules with unpaired electrons, i.e. only one within an orbital. Produced as intermediaries during stages of certain biological reactions, e.g. involving reduction of molecular O_2 to oxide ions, with production of oxygen-derived free radicals (OFRs) including superoxide (O_2^-), hydroxyl ($OH^·$) and hydroperoxy ($HO_2^·$) radicals, the latter two particularly reactive. Hydrogen peroxide is involved in formation of many OFRs. Thought to be involved in normal phagocyte function and host defence; released into phagosomes to destroy bacteria, etc. May also be produced by radiation and certain chemicals, and increased production has been implicated in many disease processes including pulmonary **O_2 toxicity, halothane hepatitis, ARDS, paracetamol poisoning, burns,** carcinogenesis and ischaemic colitis. Defence mechanisms against normal free radical formation may be overwhelmed, resulting in oxidation of tissues, especially cell membrane lipids, proteins, nucleic acids and extracellular matrix. Reactions with free radicals may liberate further free radicals, with further injury, etc.

Defence mechanisms include the enzymes superoxide dismutase (SOD) and catalase, and antioxidants (free radical scavengers) e.g. glutathione and vitamin E. Increasing these substances indirectly, or administering them directly, may reduce tissue injury in some experimental models, especially involving O_2 toxicity, but extrapolation to clinical use is unclear.

Royston D (1988) Anaesthesia; 43: 315–20

Free water clearance, *see Clearance, free water*

Freud, Sigmund (1856–1939). Austrian neurologist and psychiatrist, the inventor of psychoanalysis. Postulated that **cocaine** might be a treatment for morphine addiction, and a stimulant for psychoneurotic patients. Investigated the drug with his friend **Koller**, who introduced it as the first local anaesthetic drug. Fled from Vienna to London in 1938 to escape the Nazis.

Friedreich's ataxia. Hereditary (autosomal recessive) condition consisting of progressive degeneration of spinocerebellar and pyramidal tracts and dorsal root ganglia, mainly affecting the legs. Onset is in childhood or teens.

- Features:
  - upper **motor neurone** weakness, with upgoing plantar reflexes (if present).
  - ataxia, dysarthria and nystagmus.
  - impaired joint position, vibration and touch sense. Reflexes may be absent.
  - **kyphoscoliosis** and pes cavus.
  - **cardiomyopathy** in over 50% of patients, with risk of **cardiac failure** and **arrhythmias**.
- Anaesthesic precautions:
  - **preoperative assessment** of neurological, cardiovascular and respiratory systems.
  - cautious use of **neuromuscular blocking drugs**.
  - risk of respiratory insufficiency postoperatively; physiotherapy, O_2 therapy and adequate analgesia are required.

  Other rarer, hereditary ataxias also exist.

[Nikolaus Friedreich (1825–1882), German neurologist]

Frontal nerve block, *see Ophthalmic nerve blocks*

Frusemide. Loop **diuretic**, derived from sulphonamides. Decreases renal sodium and water reabsorption, with potassium loss. IV injection causes vasodilatation, with diuresis within 30 minutes.

- Dosage:
  - depends on renal function and response: 5–10 mg may cause considerable diuresis given orally or iv (less than 4 mg/min) to healthy patients. Up to 500 mg may be given in severe renal impairment.
  - suitable starting dose in fluid retention or cardiac failure: 0.5–1.0 mg/kg.
- Side effects:
  - ototoxicity, especially after rapid iv injection.
  - **hypokalaemia**.
  - raised creatinine, urea and uric acid may occur.
  - rash, thrombocytopenia and leucopenia rarely.

Fuel cell, *see Oxygen measurement*

Functional residual capacity (FRC). **Lung volume**, the sum of **residual volume** and **expiratory reserve volume**. Normally 2.5–3.0 litres for an average male.

- Measurement:
  - helium dilution: breathing of air with a known concentration of helium from a **spirometer**, starting from the end of normal expiration. CO_2 is absorbed using soda lime, and O_2 replaced as it is used. The helium distributes between spirometer, tubing and the subject's lungs, with minimal uptake by the bloodstream. After equilibrium is reached, the new concentration of helium is measured:

    total amount of helium in the system

    = initial concentration × volume of apparatus

    = new concentration × volume of (apparatus + lungs)

  - **nitrogen washout**. The subject breathes 100% O_2 from end of normal expiration, and total volume of expired gas over several minutes is analysed for nitrogen content. This amount of nitrogen was originally contained in the FRC to give a concentration of 79%; thus FRC may be calculated.
  - **body plethysmograph**.

  The helium dilution and nitrogen washout techniques do not include collapsed portions of lung, or those with poor air entry (if not enough time is allowed for equilibration). Measurements using the body plethysmograph include these areas, which may not participate in gas exchange. Comparison of the tests may indicate the degree of airway collapse/hypoventilation.

- FRC is important because **hypoxaemia** may result if it is reduced:
  - if **closing capacity** (CC) exceeds FRC, airway closure occurs with quiet breathing, with $\dot{V}/\dot{Q}$ mismatch. Hypoxaemia of old age is thought to result from this, since CC rises with age.
  - FRC serves as an O_2 reserve; thus a reduced FRC holds less O_2 e.g. should airway obstruction occur. The FRC O_2 store helps prevent large swings in arterial Po_2 during respiration.

  Reduced FRC may also reduce lung **compliance** and increase **pulmonary vascular resistance**.

- Reduced by:
  - supine position.
  - **obesity**.
  - **pregnancy**.
  - anaesthesia, even with IPPV (mechanism is unknown, but thought to involve decreased muscle tone and shift of thoracic and peripheral blood to the abdomen).
  - restrictive lung disease, e.g. **pulmonary fibrosis**; it may also be reduced in **pulmonary oedema**, infection, **atelectasis**, **ARDS**, etc.
- Increased by:
  - **PEEP** and **CPAP**.
  - increased airway resistance, e.g. **asthma**.

Furosemide, *see Frusemide*

FVC, *see Forced vital capacity*

G

G6PD deficiency, *see Glucose 6–phosphate dehydroge-nase deficiency*

GABA, *see γ-Aminobutyric acid*

Gag reflex. Elevation and constriction of the pharynx following stimulation of the posterior pharyngeal wall. The afferent pathway is via the glossopharyngeal nerve; the efferent is via the vagus. Elevation of the soft palate when it is touched relies on afferent fibres in the maxillary division of the trigeminal nerve; often the two reflexes are elicited together. The gag reflex is abolished following local anaesthesia and lesions of the pharynx, lesions involving the vagal nuclei in the medulla, and deep anaesthesia or coma. Absence of the gag reflex may indicate that the airway is at risk, e.g. from aspiration of vomitus.

Gain, electrical. Ratio of output signal amplitude to input signal amplitude. Thus a measure of amplification of signal, e.g. in **monitoring** equipment. May be specified as voltage, current or power gain; expressed as a simple ratio, or for power gain, also expressed as logarithm (base 10) of the ratio (in bels or decibels).
[Alexander Bell (1847–1922), Scottish-born US inventor]

Gallamine triethiodide. Non-depolarizing **neuromuscular blocking drug**, first used in 1948. Initial dose is 1–2 mg/kg, acting within 1–2 minutes and providing relaxation for about 20–30 minutes. Supplementary dose: 0.5 mg/kg. Causes marked tachycardia due to an anticholinergic action. Crosses the **placenta** more readily than other neuromuscular blocking drugs, thus not used in obstetrics. Anaphylaxis is rare. Mostly excreted via the kidneys, therefore avoided in renal failure.

Galvanic skin response (Skin conductance response; Sympathogalvanic response). Test of sympathetic afferent, efferent and spinal interconnecting pathways, used to assess the effects of **sympathetic nerve blocks**. Has also been used to assess other regional blocks in which sympathetic blockade occurs, e.g. **extradural anaesthesia**, **brachial plexus block**. Skin electrodes are placed on dorsal and ventral surfaces of the hand/foot, with a reference electrode elsewhere. Opposite sides of the body are normally compared. The output is displayed on an **oscilloscope** (e.g. ECG machine); a steady line results. With intact sympathetic pathways, pinching the skin causes altered skin conductance via changes in sweat gland secretion, displayed as a deflection lasting under 5 seconds. Deflection is abolished by successful blockade. The response may be diminished by use of **atropine**, repeated testing and in the elderly.

Preblockade size of deflection has also been used to assess suitability for subsequent sympathetic block.
Changes in skin potential may also be measured.

Ganglion blocking drugs. Nicotinic **acetylcholine receptor** antagonists acting at autonomic ganglia. The first drugs used to treat **hypertension**, now rarely used because of widespread side effects caused by sympathetic blockade (postural and exertional hypotension, decreased sweating) and parasympathetic blockade (constipation, urinary retention, impotence, dry mouth, blurring of vision). May first stimulate then block receptors (e.g. nicotine) or exhibit competetive antagonism (e.g. **hexamethonium, pentolinium, trimetaphan**). Hexamethonium and pentamethonium are no longer used, but pentolinium and trimetaphan are used in **hypotensive anaesthesia**.

Because of the similarity between neuromuscular and ganglionic nicotinic receptors, ganglion blockers (e.g. hexamethonium) may cause neuromuscular blockade, and **neuromuscular blocking drugs** (e.g. **tubocurarine**) may cause ganglionic blockade.
See also, Antihypertensive drugs

Gas. Form of matter whose constituent molecules or atoms are constantly moving, and whose mean positions are far apart. Tends to expand in all directions, and diffuse and mix with other gases. Governed by the gas laws under ideal circumstances. Formed by a **liquid** above its **critical temperature**. The constituent particles are sufficiently far apart for the forces (e.g. **Van der Waals forces**) between them to be almost negligible, unless the gas is compressed. Pressure exerted by a gas is proportional to the number of collisions of atoms/molecules against the container's walls.
See also, Boyle's law; Charles' law; Ideal gas law

Gas analysis. Possible methods:
–chemical: the gas reacts chemically with other substances to form non-gaseous compounds, with reduction of overall volume (e.g. **Haldane apparatus**) or pressure (e.g. **van Slyke apparatus**).
–physical:
  –spectroscopy:
    –infrared absorption, e.g. by CO_2, N_2O and halothane/enflurane/isoflurane (the volatile agents cannot be distinguished by this method). The amount of light absorbed is measured indirectly by comparison with reference gas, or by detection of sound emitted by the excited molecules (photoacoustic spectroscopy). Used in **capnography**.
    –halothane meter (ultraviolet absorption). Requires lengthy warming-up and frequent calibration; now rarely used routinely.

–Raman spectroscopy: light is scattered by passage through the sample gas, with some alteration of frequency. The pattern of scattered light is used to identify and quantify specific gas and vapour components. Multiple gas analysers are available using laser light.

–gas discharge meter: used to measure nitrogen concentration. 1500 V potential is passed across the gas sample in a tube. Intensity of purple light at a specific wavelength is measured.

–adsorption of vapours on to surfaces:

–rubber strips, e.g. in the Dräger Narkotest. Tension of the strips is reduced by volatile agents; the extent is proportional to their concentration. Temperature compensated with a bimetallic strip. Adjustable for use with different agents and in the presence of N_2O, to which it is also sensitive. Has a slow response; now rarely used.

–silicone polymer coating a vibrating quartz crystal, e.g. in the Engström Emma. Change in frequency of vibration (caused by passing current through the crystal) is proportional to the concentration of volatile agent, which may be specified.

–interferometer: a light beam is split and passed through two chambers, one for reference and the other for samples. The beams are delayed to different extents; thus the emergent beams are out of phase. The resultant interference pattern is visualized through a telescope, and is displaced when gas is drawn into the sample chamber. Degree of change is related to the sample concentration. Used for calibration, e.g. of vaporizers, not for peroperative monitoring.

–**mass spectrometer**.

–**gas chromatography** and detectors, e.g. **katharometer**, **flame ionization detector**, **electron capture detector**.

–fuel cell, and paramagnetic and polarographic analysers, used for **O_2 measurement**.

–other methods, e.g. depending on different viscosities of gases, or velocity of sound through gases, are rarely used now.

–fibreoptic sensors have been used to measure P_{CO_2} and P_{O_2} in arterial blood, by detecting changes in intensity or wavelength of light reflecting off a reagent on the fibre tip.

[Chandrasekhara V Raman (1888–1970), Indian physicist; Heinrich Dräger (1847–1917), German engineer; Carl-Gunnar Engström, Swedish physician]
See also, Carbon dioxide measurement

Gas chromatography. Technique used for **gas analysis**. The sample mixture is injected into a stream of inert carrier gas, e.g. nitrogen, helium or argon (mobile phase), which passes through a column of silica–alumina particles coated in oil or wax (stationary phase). Separation of the sample component gases occurs along the column's length, depending on their relative solubilities in the two phases. Temperature of the column is carefully controlled, e.g. in an oven. Liquids may also be analysed. Suitable detectors, e.g. **katharometer**, **flame ionization detector** or **electron capture detector**, are required.

Gas flow. Principles of **flow** are as for any **fluid**. Clinical applications:

–flow is turbulent in the upper airway, trachea and bronchi, especially during forceful breathing; i.e. gas **viscosity** is more important than density. Thus in upper **airway obstruction**, flow is increased if low density gas is used, e.g. **helium**.

–flow is laminar in small bronchioles; i.e. **viscosity** is important; although tube radius is very small, velocity is also very low. Helium is of no use in improving laminar flow, e.g. in **asthma**.

–flow may be mostly laminar during quiet breathing, with turbulence at branches in the trachea and bronchi. Turbulence is more likely at midinspiration/expiration, when flow rate is highest (e.g. up to 50 l/min).

Turbulence usually occurs in **anaesthetic breathing systems** during peak flow, especially if sharp-angled bends are present, e.g. at connections between components. Turbulence is more likely with narrow tubing and tubes.

–other applications include the **Venturi principle**, **fluidics**, **flow–volume loops** and **flowmeters**.
See also, Airway resistance

Gas gangrene. Infection due to clostridium species, usually *Cl. perfringens* (formerly *welchii*), a spore-forming Gram-positive anaerobic bacillus found in soil and faeces. Classically associated with deep war wounds, especially those contaminated with dirt or foreign bodies, but may follow any **trauma**, e.g. surgery. The incubation period is under 4 days, usually under 1 day.

The organism produces gas within tissues, often detectable clinically as subcutaneous emphysema. **Endotoxin** production causes generalized debilitation and toxaemia; local spread is rapid, with oedema, pain and tissue necrosis.

Prevented by cleansing of wounds and excision of dead tissue. Penicillin is effective prophylaxis. In established infection, penicillin therapy and surgical excision of all affected tissue are required. Hyperbaric O_2 therapy has been used to increase local tissue O_2 content; antitoxin therapy is more controversial.
See also, Oxygen, hyperbaric

Gas laws, *see Avogadro's hypothesis; Boyle's law; Charles' law; Dalton's law; Henry's law; Ideal gas law*

Gas transport, *see Carbon dioxide transport; Oxygen transport*

Gasp reflex. Production of a deep slow breath following a large positive pressure inflation of the lungs. Originally described in cats and dogs, but may be seen in newborn babies; during neonatal resuscitation, it may occur within primary **apnoea**. A similar response may also be seen after opioid administration in anaesthetized patients.

Head's paradoxical reflex, although similar, is produced under different experimental circumstances.
See also, Cardiopulmonary resuscitation, neonatal

Gasserian ganglion block. Block of the trigeminal ganglion which lies medially in the middle cranial fossa within a dural reflection (Meckel's cave), lateral to the internal carotid artery and cavernous sinus. Results in anaesthesia of the face, forehead, and anterior scalp (Fig. 65). Used mainly for treatment of **trigeminal neuralgia**, but also for surgery to the face.

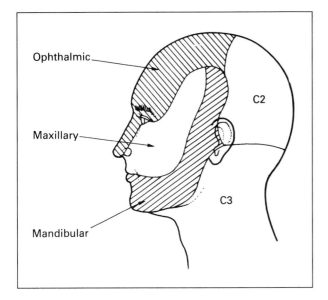

Figure 65 *Innervation of the face*

- Technique:
  - with the patient supine and looking straight ahead, a 22 G 10 cm needle is introduced 3 cm lateral to the angle of the mouth, level with the second upper molar. Aiming at the pupil from the front, and the midpoint of the zygoma from the side, it is inserted until it contacts bone (greater wing of sphenoid, anterior to the foramen ovale). It is redirected posteriorly 1–1.5 cm deeper, passing through the foramen (paraesthesiae radiating to the distribution of the appropriate branch). Electrical stimulation of the needle and X-ray imaging may be used to confirm correct positioning.
  - after careful aspiration, 1–2 ml solution, e.g. 1% **lignocaine**, is injected. Alcohol injection or thermocoagulation may follow if ablative therapy is required. Accidental subarachnoid injection may occur.

May be painful; general anaesthesia or sedation may be employed, with waking up or reversal to confirm paraesthesiae, followed by resedation for ablation. **Propofol** or a **midazolam/flumazenil** combination have been used.

[Johann Gasser (1723–1765), Austrian anatomist; Johann Meckel (1714–1774), German anatomist]

See also, Mandibular nerve block; Maxillary nerve block; Ophthalmic nerve block

Gastric contents. Anaesthetic importance:
  - absorption of orally administered drugs; e.g. related to **gastric emptying**, pH, and **drug interactions** within the stomach.
  - **aspiration of gastric contents**; severity of **aspiration pneumonitis** is related to the pH and volume of aspirate, although particulate nature of the aspirate is also important.
- Gastric secretion is increased by:
  - presence of food in the mouth (vagal reflex).
  - anger, stress.
  - presence of food in the stomach (local reflex).
  - protein meal, via duodenal gastrin secretion.

  - **hypoglycaemia**.
  - **alcohol, caffeine**.
- Gastric secretion and acidity are decreased by:
  - **H₂ receptor antagonists**.
  - **omeprazole**.
  - drinking water.

Gastric acidity is decreased by **antacids**.

Gastric volume is related to gastric emptying and intake. Volume is reduced by H₂ antagonists and omeprazole, but increased by antacids.

Gastric emptying. Normally results from peristaltic waves of contraction passing through the cardia, antrum, pylorus and duodenum, occurring up to three times/minute after a meal. Small amounts of liquid traverse the pylorus, which closes as the contraction wave reaches it, redirecting most of the propelled (solid) material back into the proximal stomach for further mixing. Thus liquids leave faster than solids. Carbohydrates leave faster than proteins and fats are slowest, via inhibitory feedback mechanisms involving duodenal hormone secretion.
- Slowed by:
  - lying down.
  - anxiety, fear, pain, etc.
  - mechanical obstruction and duodenal distension.
  - **pregnancy**.
  - drugs, e.g. **opioid analgesic drugs, anticholinergic drugs, alcohol**, dopamine.
- Increased by:
  - gastric distension.
  - drugs, e.g. **metoclopramide, domperidone** (opioid-induced gastric stasis is not reversed; cf. **cisapride**).

Rate of emptying is important because of the risks of nausea, vomiting, regurgitation and **aspiration of gastric contents**. Emptying also affects absorption of orally administered drugs. Traditionally, 4–6 hours' starvation is usually required preoperatively in all but life-threatening emergencies, depending on the nature of the food/drink; gastric emptying is assumed to be complete in this time. However, **gastric contents** may be considerable, particularly after solid food. Small amounts of water (150 ml) given 2–3 hours preoperatively have been shown to reduce the volume and acidity of gastric contents.
- Measurement:
  - measurement of plasma levels of orally administered substance, e.g. paracetamol (absorbed from the small intestine, not from the stomach).
  - serial nasogastric aspiration, with measurement of orally administered marker substance.
  - measurement of **impedance** across the lower chest/upper abdomen; alters as composition of tissues, i.e. gastric contents, changes.
  - oral administration of radioisotope, with measurement of radioactivity over the stomach.
  - ultrasound imaging.
  - X-ray imaging following oral contrast medium.

Emptying can be aided by naso- or orogastric aspiration. The latter is more efficient, using a wide bore tube with multiple holes and lumina, but is unpleasant and rarely used now. **Emetic drugs** are also rarely used.

Gastric intramucosal pH. Measured indirectly by measuring gastric luminal $P\text{CO}_2$ (which approximates to intramucosal $P\text{CO}_2$) and arterial **bicarbonate** concentration (which approximates to mucosal bicarbonate concentration). A tonometer incorporating a saline-filled balloon is placed via the oesophagus into the stomach, and luminal P_{CO_2} determined by measuring P_{CO_2} in the saline. **H₂ receptor antagonist** administration is required to eliminate the effect of gastric acid combining with pancreatic bicarbonate to release CO_2. Direct measurement is also possible but involves trauma to the mucosa and is less reliable.

Used as an indicator of gastric (and therefore GIT) mucosal **O₂ delivery** and consumption, intramucosal acidosis indicating impaired O_2 delivery or impaired utilization. Measurement has been suggested as a guide to resuscitation in critical illness (e.g. to increase intramucosal pH above 7.35) and as a guide to mortality on **ICU**. Fiddian-Green RG (1988) Ann R Coll Surg Engl; 70: 128–34

Gastric lavage. Performed for removal of drugs, poisons, etc. following **poisoning and overdose**; usually recommended up to 4 hours after ingestion (longer if gastric emptying is delayed, e.g. by anticholinergic drugs, aspirin), or at any time if the patient is unconscious. Involves passage of a wide bore orogastric tube, with aspiration to ensure the trachea has not been entered inadvertently. 300–600 ml warm water is introduced and allowed to drain under gravity; this is repeated until the aspirate is clear. Pulmonary aspiration may occur; the patient should be placed in the head-down lateral position with suction available. Tracheal intubation is required if laryngeal reflexes are absent. Lavage should not be performed if petroleum derivatives have been ingested, since pulmonary aspiration is particularly hazardous. Oesophageal/gastric perforation is also likely if caustic substances have been ingested.

Gastro-oesophageal reflux. Normally prevented by the **lower oesophageal sphincter** and anatomical arrangement of the oesophagus and stomach. Common in, but not exclusive to, **hiatus hernia** and **obesity**. May cause burning retrosternal pain, especially on stooping/lying. Regurgitation of bitter fluid into the mouth may also occur. Associated oesophagitis may cause pain after meals, especially if spicy. Medical treatment is as for **peptic ulcer disease/** hiatus hernia; it includes losing weight and avoidance of provocative postures. Anaesthetic management is as for hiatus hernia.

Gastro-oesophageal sphincter, *see Lower oesophageal sphincter*

Gastroschisis and exomphalos. Congenital malformations of the abdominal wall, associated with protrusion of abdominal contents:
  –gastroschisis: abdominal wall defect, not associated with the midline or umbilicus. Incidence is 1:30 000.
  –exomphalos: midline defect, related to the umbilicus. Incidence is 1:5–10 000.
- Associated with:
  –prematurity.
  –other congenital abnormalities, e.g. cardiac defects (especially VSD), other GIT malformations and genitourinary abnormalities.
- Initial problems:
  –damage to exposed organs.
  –fluid and electrolyte balance.

  –heat loss.
  –infection.
- Treatment:
  –the bowel is covered with a dry towel/plastic bag.
  –primary surgical closure is preferable to delayed closure if possible.
- Anaesthetic considerations: as for **paediatric anaesthesia** plus the above considerations. In addition:
  –**N₂O** diffuses into the bowel, increasing its size, and is avoided.
  –abdominal closure may be difficult, with increased intra-abdominal pressure. Postoperative IPPV may be necessary. Staged closure may be performed using a Silastic pouch, if adverse effects of primary closure are excessive.
  –postoperative nutrition and prevention/treatment of infection are important.

Gate control theory of pain. Proposed in 1965 by Melzack and Wall to account for the influence of psychological and physiological variables on **pain** transmission. Suggests that impulses flow from periphery to brain through a 'gate' at spinal level, the opening or closure of which is influenced by other neural pathways. Pain is felt when impulse flow exceeds a certain critical level. The gate is closed by descending and large ascending (Aβ) fibres and opened by small ascending (C) fibres. It is thought to be located in the substantia gelatinosa (SG), lamina II of the dorsal horn; interneurones project to target cells which then project cranially. The theory has been modified since conception to account for expanding experimental and clinical evidence of neurotransmitter and receptor involvement (Fig. 66):
  –C fibres from deep receptors (e.g. chemical damage) project to SG cells, probably via **substance P** ('pushes' gate open). Cranial projection is via spinoreticular fibres.

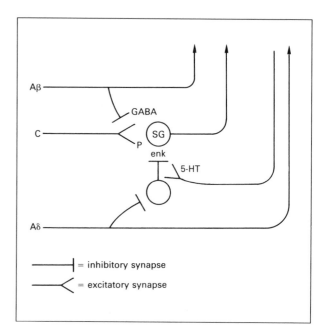

Figure 66 *Gate control theory of pain. enk, encephalin; P, substance P; SG, substantia gelatinosa cell*

Table 16. Components of gelatin solutions

Solution	Gelatin (g/l)	Sodium (mmol/l)	Chloride (mmol/l)	Calcium (mmol/l)	Potassium (mmol/l)
Haemaccel	35 urea-linked	145	145	6.26	5.1
Gelofusine	40 succinylated	154	125	0.4	0.4

–Aβ fibres (activated by e.g. high frequency low amplitude **TENS**) inhibit the above synapse presynaptically; **GABA** is thought to be the neurotransmitter (closes gate). The Aβ fibres also project cranially.

–Aδ fibres from superficial receptors (e.g. temperature, pinprick, **acupuncture**, low frequency TENS) project cranially, via spinothalamic fibres. Cause **5HT**-mediated descending pathways to close the gate via **enkephalin**-secreting interneurones acting on target cells.

Descending fibres are also affected by mood, emotion, etc.

Aδ fibres also project directly on to interneurones inhibiting enkephalin secretion (i.e. opens gate).

[Patrick D Wall, London anatomist; Ronald Melzack, Montreal psychologist]

Gay-Lussac's law, *see Charles' law*

Gelatin solutions. Colloid solutions derived from animal gelatin, a derivative of collagen. Commonly used forms contain urea-linked (Haemaccel) or succinylated (Gelofusine) gelatin components (Table 16); average mw is about 35 000. Used clinically as plasma substitutes, e.g. in **haemorrhage** and **shock**. Cheaper than albumin solutions and **hydroxyethyl starch**, but with shorter **half-life** (about 4 hours). Allergic (**anaphylactoid**) **reactions** have followed rapid infusion, especially of Haemaccel (said to be reduced in its new form); usually mild but occasionally severe. The incidence is of reactions is less than 0.15%.

Renal function, blood cross-matching and haemostasis are unaffected, although the calcium in Haemaccel may coagulate stored blood if infused through the same giving set without first flushing with crystalloid.

Saddler JM, Horsey PJ (1987) Anaesthesia; 42: 998–1004

Gelofusine, *see Gelatin solutions*

Genitofemoral nerve block, *see Inguinal hernia field block*

Geriatric patient, *see Elderly, anaesthesia for*

GFR, *see Glomerular filtration rate*

GHBA, *see γ-Hydroxybutyric acid*

Gland/gland nut, *see Cylinders*

Glasgow coma scale. Scoring system originally suggested for assessment of patients with **head injury**; now widely applied to other causes of **coma**. A maximum of 15 points may be scored, according to the following criteria:

–Best motor response:
  –movement in response to command: 6 points
  –localizes pain: 5 points
  –withdraws from pain: 4 points
  –flexes in response to pain: 3 points
  –extends in response to pain: 2 points
  –no response: 1 point
–Best verbal response:
  –fully orientated: 5 points
  –confused: 4 points
  –inappropriate words: 3 points
  –incomprehensible sounds: 2 points
  –no response: 1 point
–Best eye response:
  –eyes spontaneously open: 4 points
  –eyes open to command: 3 points
  –eyes open in response to pain: 2 points
  –eyes remain closed: 1 point

Scores may be expressed as totals, or separated into the three categories. Changes in scores over time are more useful than single values.

Teasdale G, Jennett B (1974) Lancet ii: 81–3

See also, Coma scales; Trauma scales

Glaucoma. Damage to the eye associated with raised **intraocular pressure** (IOP).
• Anaesthetic considerations:
  –related to IOP:
    –avoidance of drugs which raise IOP, e.g. **ketamine**. Systemic **atropine** is safe; topical use may cause mydriasis and obstruction of drainage of aqueous humour.
    –avoidance of trauma to the eye, steep head-down position, coughing, straining, etc., which may increase IOP.
    –IOP may be reduced by specific measures, e.g. iv **mannitol, acetazolamide**, etc.
  –related to concurrent drug therapy:
    –timolol drops and related drugs: systemic absorption and β-blockade may occur.
    –**ecothiopate** drops: may prolong **suxamethonium**'s action.
    –pilocarpine and **physostigmine** drops: systemic absorption and bradycardia may occur.
    –acetazolamide: electrolyte imbalance may occur.

Glomerular filtration rate (GFR). Volume (ml) of plasma filtered by the **kidneys** per minute. Normally 120 ml/min.
• Depends on:
  –effective glomerular surface area: reduced by contraction of mesangial cells within the glomerulus, e.g. in response to angiotensin II, **vasopressin**,

noradrenaline, leukotrienes, histamine and certain prostaglandins. Dopamine and atrial natriuretic peptide cause relaxation.

–permeability of the capillary wall, basement membrane and glomerular epithelium. Dependent on size (molecules under 4–8 nm pass through relatively easily), protein-binding and charge (filtration of cations is favoured over that of anions because of the negative charge of the glomerular wall). Increased in certain diseases.

–hydrostatic gradient across the capillary walls. Affected by:

   –renal blood flow and capillary vascular tone (e.g. noradrenaline constricts the afferent arterioles predominantly, whilst angiotensin II constricts the efferent arterioles). Autoregulation is thought to involve afferent arteriolar vascular tone.

   –ureteric obstruction/renal oedema.

–osmotic gradient: rarely clinically important.

Measured by iv infusion of a substance which is freely filtered and neither reabsorbed nor secreted by the renal tubules. It must also be non-toxic, not metabolized and have no effect on GFR. At steady state, the clearance of the substance is calculated. The volume of plasma cleared per minute then equals the volume filtered per minute i.e.:

$$\text{GFR} = \frac{\text{urine concentration} \times \text{urinary volume/min}}{\text{plasma concentration}}$$

Inulin, a carbohydrate derived from plant tubers, is usually used. Radioactive chromium-labelled EDTA may also be used.

Provides an indication of renal function, but is difficult to measure routinely. Creatinine clearance approximates to GFR, and is commonly measured instead. Creatinine is actually secreted by the renal tubules to a small degree, but measurement of plasma levels overestimates by a small amount, tending to cancel any error.

See also, Nephron; Renin/angiotensin system

Glomerulonephritis. Renal disease of usually unknown aetiology, but often involving renal immune complex deposition or antibodies against glomerular basement membrane. Histological classification is unrelated to clinical presentation, which may include:

–oliguria, salt and water retention, hypervolaemia and hypertension due to impaired glomerular filtration (nephritic syndrome). Classically follows streptococcal infection.

–proteinuria, causing hypoproteinaemia and marked oedema if severe (nephrotic syndrome).

–others: hypertension, haematuria, loin pain, renal failure (acute and chronic).

● Anaesthetic considerations:

–impaired renal function.

–oedema and hypoproteinaemia.

–hypertension.

–drug therapy: may include antihypertensive drugs and steroid therapy.

Glomus tumours. Rare tumours arising from glomus bodies (arteriovenous anastomoses adjacent to blood vessels, richly innervated and thought to be involved with regulating local blood flow). More common in the limbs, but may arise from the glomus jugulare (tympanic body) in the upper jugular bulb. The latter may extend into the cerebellum and brainstem, middle ear, internal jugular vein or laterally into the neck. Thus associated with neurological lesions, including of lower cranial nerves. May rarely secrete catecholamines. Anaesthesic concerns include excessive length of surgery and blood loss, and those of neurosurgery.

Glossopharyngeal nerve block. Used to supplement topical anaesthesia and/or superior laryngeal nerve block; also used for tonsillectomy and glossopharyngeal neuralgia.

Having applied topical anaesthesia to the tongue, it is depressed and an angled needle inserted behind the middle of the posterior tonsillar pillar, to 1 cm depth. After aspiration, 3 ml local anaesthetic agent is injected. Produces anaesthesia of the posterior third of the tongue, oropharynx and tonsils, with block of the gag reflex.

May also be blocked by injecting 5–6 ml solution just behind and deep to the styloid process, found 2–4 cm deep, midway between the tip of the mastoid process and angle of the jaw. Internal carotid and jugular vessels lie very close.

Glossopharyngeal neuralgia. Recurrent, sudden stabbing pain in the distribution of the glossopharyngeal nerve. May result from nerve compression by vertebral or posterior inferior cerebellar arteries, local musculoskeletal anomalies, or trauma. May be relieved by topical local anaesthetic to oropharyngeal trigger areas. Treatment includes glossopharyngeal nerve block using local anaesthetic at weekly intervals; alcohol injection or surgical resection of the glossopharyngeal rootlets may be required.

Glottis, *see Larynx*

Glucagon. Hormone secreted by the A cells of pancreatic islets. Causes hepatic adenylate cyclase stimulation, leading to glycogen breakdown and release of glucose. Also increases hepatic glucose formation from amino acids, and breakdown of fats to form ketone bodies. Stimulates secretion of growth hormone, insulin and somatostatin. Has inotropic and chronotropic actions on the heart, unrelated to adrenergic receptors. Thought to increase calcium transport into myocardial cells, possibly via adenylate cyclase activation; it has been used in the treatment of overdose of β-adrenergic antagonists. Half-life is less than 10 minutes.

Secretion is increased by β-adrenergic stimulation, stress, exercise, amino acids, gastrin and starvation. It is decreased by hyperglycaemia, somatostatin, ketone bodies, fatty acids, insulin and α-adrenergic stimulation.

Glucocorticoids. Hormones secreted by the adrenal cortex; consist mainly of cortisol and corticosterone. Thought to act via interaction with cellular nuclear proteins, with alteration of enzyme synthesis and cell function. Secretion is increased by ACTH.

● Actions:

–increased glycogen and protein breakdown, and glucose synthesis, with increased blood glucose levels.

–required for efficient functioning of catecholamines on metabolism, bronchi and CVS, also for correct movement of fluid across the vascular endothelium and fluid balance. This may explain the hypotension seen in adrenocortical insufficiency.

–required for efficient muscle contraction and nerve conduction; also involved in inflammatory/immunological responses.

–mild **aldosterone**-like activity.

Large doses of glucocorticoids suppress inflammation, and are used in many inflammatory and immunological diseases.

See also, Steroid therapy

Glucose. Carbohydrate, of central importance as an **energy** source within the body.

- Main metabolic pathways:
  - production:
    - from breakdown of carbohydrate foodstuffs.
    - from **glycogen** stores, or other endogenous molecules (e.g. **protein**, **fats**) via intermediate steps in glucose metabolism; occurs in the liver during starvation, exercise, etc. Produces glucose 6–phosphate, which is converted by hepatic glucose 6–phosphatase to glucose which enters the bloodstream. Other tissues, e.g. muscle, lack this enzyme, and glucose 6–phosphate is catabolized directly via the glycolytic pathway.
  - uptake:
    - from the GIT via carrier-assisted transport, i.e. as part of an **active transport** mechanism for sodium ions. Thus indirectly utilizes energy.
    - from the bloodstream into cells by the action of **insulin**.
  - utilization for energy production: via conversion into glucose 6–phosphate and subsequent breakdown (**glycolysis**).
  - conversion to glycogen via glucose 6–phosphate and glucose 1–phosphate.
  - hexose/pentose monophosphate shunt: alternate energy producing pathway from glucose 6–phosphate, with reduction of nicotinamide adenine dinucleotide phosphate (NADP).
  - conversion to fats and proteins.

Fasting plasma levels are maintained at 4–6 mmol/l (72–108 mg/dl) by the action of various hormones mainly on the liver; e.g. insulin decreases blood glucose, whilst **glucagon**, **catecholamines**, **growth hormone**, **glucocorticoids** and thyroid hormones increase it.

Filtered and reabsorbed in the kidneys; renal capacity for reabsorption is exceeded above plasma levels of about 10 mmol/l (180 mg/dl). Congenital inability to reabsorb glucose results in renal glycosuria at normal plasma levels. The renal threshold may also be reduced in **pregnancy** and tubular damage.

See also, Catabolism; Diabetes mellitus; Metabolism; Nutrition

Glucose–insulin–potassium infusion. Infusion regimen used in an attempt to reduce the size of **MI**, increase cardiac output and reduce arrhythmias; its efficacy is yet to be proven. Thought to reduce plasma free fatty acid levels, reducing myocardial energy and O_2 requirements; it possibly augments anaerobic metabolism by increasing **ATP** supply. 50 units insulin and 50 mmol potassium are added to 500 ml of 50% glucose, infused iv at 100 ml/h. Glucose/insulin infusion has also been used in **hyponatraemia** due to the 'sick cell syndrome'; it supposedly restores ionic balance.

Glucose 6–phosphate dehydrogenase deficiency (G6PD deficiency). Sex-linked inherited disorder of red blood cell metabolism, common in Mediterranean, African, Middle Eastern and South East Asian populations. Impairs the hexose monophosphate shunt of **glucose** metabolism, required for cell protection against products of oxidation. Results in **haemolysis**, which may be chronic or associated with infection and drugs, e.g. antimalarials, sulphonamides, aspirin and related drugs, and methylene blue. Reduction of **methaemoglobin** is impaired, thus avoidance of **prilocaine** has been suggested.

Chronic haemolysis is also associated with other **inborn errors of metabolism**, e.g. pyruvate kinase deficiency.

Glucose reagent sticks. Plastic strips bearing reagents, used to measure **glucose** concentration, e.g. in blood or urine. Glucose is converted by glucose oxidase to gluconic acid and hydrogen peroxide, the latter oxidizing a dye to produce a colour change. Accuracy is increased by using reflectance colorimeters to quantify the colour change, and may be reduced by use of alcohol swabs for cleaning the skin. They are less accurate at lower (hypoglycaemic) glucose levels. Useful as a bedside test, and for home monitoring of glucose levels.

Glucose tolerance test. Investigation used in the diagnosis of **diabetes mellitus**. Involves administration of glucose either orally or iv, usually the former. 1.75 g/kg is given orally up to 75 g, in at least 250 ml water. Blood glucose normally rises from fasting levels to a peak at 10–60 minutes, declining thereafter. Fasting and 2 hour levels used for diagnosis:
  - venous plasma glucose under 7.8 mmol/l (140 mg/dl) fasting and at 2 hours: normal.
  - venous plasma glucose over 11.1 mmol/l (200 mg/dl) at 2 hours: diabetic.
  - intermediate values: 'impaired glucose tolerance'.

Diabetes is usually diagnosed on random and fasting blood sugar estimations alone. The tolerance test is mainly used to investigate diabetes in pregnancy.

Glutamate. Amino acid, thought to be active as an excitatory **neurotransmitter** throughout the CNS, especially brain. Increases **membrane** sodium conductance, causing postsynaptic depolarization. Aspartate is thought to have similar properties. Thought to build up in **cerebral ischaemia**; resultant receptor-specific **calcium** ion entry into cells increases electrical activity and exacerbates cell damage. Specific antagonists may possibly be beneficial in **cerebral protection/resuscitation**, e.g. at the *N*-methyl-D-aspartate receptor.

Glyceryl trinitrate (GTN; Nitroglycerin). **Vasodilator drug**, used to treat **myocardial ischaemia** and **cardiac failure**, and to lower BP, e.g. in **hypertensive crisis** and **hypotensive anaesthesia**. Acts directly on vascular smooth muscle (mainly venous), lowering **preload** and reducing **SVR** and **pulmonary vascular resistance**. Also increases **coronary blood flow**. A cutaneous slow-release patch may be applied preoperatively in patients with **ischaemic heart disease**, and these have also been applied to sites of **iv fluid administration**, reducing infusion failure by up to 60%.

- Dosage:
  - sublingually 0.3–1.0 mg, repeated as required. Lasts about 20–30 minutes. Available as 0.3 mg or 0.5 mg tablets; also as 0.2 mg or 0.4 mg/dose spray.
  - orally as slow-release tablets: 2.6–6.4 mg, 8–12 hourly.

–cutaneously: 5–10 mg/day applied to the chest; 5 mg 3–4 hourly to infusion sites.

–iv: 0.2–5 µg/kg/min. Effects occur within 2–5 minutes and last 5–10 minutes after stopping the infusion. Some preparations contain 30–50% propylene glycol and alcohol. GTN is adsorbed on to PVC; polyethylene and rigid plastic/glass infusion sets are acceptable.

● Side effects: headache, flushing, hypotension, tachycardia. Tachyphylaxis is common.

Glycine. Amino acid, thought to be active as an inhibitory **neurotransmitter** at spinal interneurones. Increases membrane chloride conductance, causing postsynaptic hyperpolarization. May also be involved in inhibitory pathways within the **ascending reticular activating system**. Used as an irrigating solution for **TURP**. Systemic absorption is thought possibly to be associated with CNS symptoms, e.g. transient blindness, either via central inhibitory pathways or conversion to ammonia.

Glycogen. Storage form of **glucose**; consists of glucose molecules linked together into a branched polymer. Found mainly in liver and skeletal muscle, and formed from glucose 1–phosphate, derived from glucose 6–phosphate. Glycogenolysis provides glucose for **glycolysis**, and is increased by **adrenaline** via liver β-receptors (via **cAMP**) and α-receptors (via intracellular **calcium**). Defects in the various storage and breakdown pathways result in the **glycogen storage disorders**.

Glycogen storage disorders. Inborn errors of metabolism affecting **glycogen** and **glucose** metabolism. All are rare, and almost all are autosomal recessive. Classified according to the deficient enzyme and the site of abnormal glycogen storage; 12 types have been described. Common to most are **hypoglycaemia** and **acidosis** with hepatomegaly; cardiac, mental and renal impairment may also occur.

● The following are of particular concern:
 –type I: von Gierke's disease: glucose 6–phosphatase deficiency; i.e. cannot convert glucose to glycogen. Hypoglycaemia, acidosis, mental and growth retardation, hepatomegaly, platelet dysfunction and renal impairment may occur, with death within early childhood.
 –type II: Pompe's disease: glycogen is deposited in skeletal, cardiac and smooth muscle. **Cardiac failure** and generalized muscle weakness are common. The tongue may be enlarged.
 –type V: McArdle's disease: skeletal muscle phosphorylase deficiency, impairing glycogenolysis. Muscle weakness and **myoglobinuria** may occur, the latter e.g. following **suxamethonium**. Muscle atrophy may follow use of tourniquets for surgery. Hypoglycaemia and acidosis are common.

[Edgar von Gierke (1877–1945), German pathologist; JC Pompe (1901–1945), Dutch pathologist; Brian McArdle, English physician]

Glycolysis. Breakdown of **glucose** (6 carbon atoms) to pyruvic acid or **lactate** (3 carbon atoms). Each step in the pathway (Fig. 67) is catalysed by a specific enzyme. **Energy** released during the process is utilized by production of **ATP**. The reactions occur anaerobically, with net gain of

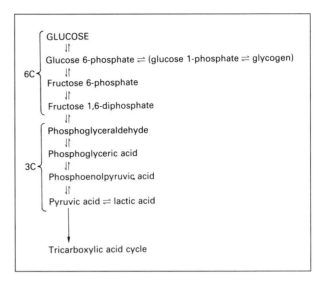

Figure 67 *Glycolytic pathway*

2 moles ATP per mole of glucose. Under aerobic conditions, pyruvic acid enters the **tricarboxylic acid cycle** with net gain of 36 more moles ATP. Anaerobic energy production is less efficient; formation of lactate from pyruvate limits ATP production to 2 moles per mole glucose. This may occur in exercising muscle and red blood cells.

Passage of glucose into muscle and fat cells is increased by **insulin**, with increased glycolysis; most other cell membranes are relatively permeable to glucose. In the liver, glucose 6–phosphatase levels control the rate of glycolysis; insulin causes increased levels and starvation decreased levels.

Other pathways may branch from the glycolytic pathway, e.g. the hexose monophosphate shunt from glucose 6–phosphate in red blood cells. Protein and fat derivatives may enter the glycolytic chain and **glycogen** may be broken down to glucose 6–phosphate via glucose 1–phosphate.

Glycopyrronium bromide (Glycopyrrolate). **Anticholinergic drug,** used as **premedication** and pre- and peroperatively to prevent bradycardia. Also used to prevent muscarinic effects of **acetylcholinesterase inhibitors** used to reverse neuromuscular blockade. A quaternary ammonium compound; therefore has minimal central effects, as opposed to **atropine** and **hyoscine**. Also less likely to cause tachycardia, mydriasis and blurred vision, but markedly reduces sweat and salivary gland activity. Its action persists for longer than that of atropine, reducing postoperative bradycardia. Dry mouth may persist postoperatively. About twice as expensive as atropine, thus often reserved for elderly patients, or those with cardiovascular disease or tachycardia.

● Dosage:
 –4–5 µg/kg im/iv.
 –with acetylcholinesterase inhibitors: 10–15 µg/kg.

Goldman cardiac risk index, *see Cardiac risk index*

Goldman constant-field equation. Describes the relationship between sodium, potassium and chloride ions, and **membrane** permeability to each:

$$V = \frac{RT}{F} \ln \frac{(P_{K^+}[K_o^+] + P_{Na^+}[Na_o^+] + P_{Cl^-}[Cl_i^-])}{(P_{K^+}[K_i^+] + P_{Na^+}[Na_i^+] + P_{Cl^-}[Cl_o^-])}$$

where V = **membrane potential**.

R = gas constant.

F = faraday constant.

P_{K^+}, P_{Na^+}, P_{Cl^-} = permeability to potassium, sodium and chloride respectively.

$[K_o^+]$, $[Na_o^+]$, $[Cl_o^-]$ = outside concentration of ions.

$[K_i^+]$, $[Na_i^+]$, $[Cl_i^-]$ = inside concentration of ions.

[David E Goldman, US physiologist; Michael Faraday (1791–1867), English chemist]

Graham's law. Rate of **diffusion** of a gas is inversely proportional to the square root of its mw.

[Thomas Graham (1805–1869), Scottish chemist]

Gravity suit, *see Antigravity suit*

Greener, Hannah (1832–1848). Fifteen-year-old girl, generally accepted as being the first recorded death under anaesthesia in January 1848, although other (dubious) reports had been made the year before. She was having a toenail removed under open **chloroform** anaesthesia, when she suddenly collapsed and died, despite attempted revival with brandy.

Griffith, Harold Randall (1894–1985). Canadian anaesthetist in Montreal; famous for the use of **curare** in anaesthesia in 1942. None of the patients described required respiratory assistance. Active in many other areas of anaesthetic research, including the properties of **cyclopropane**. Of world renown, he received many honours and medals.

Seldon TH (1986) Anesth Analg; 65: 1051–3

Growth hormone. Polypeptide hormone released from the anterior **pituitary gland**. Release is increased by:

–**hypoglycaemia** and exercise.

–stress; i.e. produced as part of the **stress response to surgery**.

–protein meal and **glucagon.**

–**dopamine receptor** agonists.

Growth hormone-releasing and -inhibiting hormones (the latter is **somatostatin**) are released by the hypothalamus; growth hormone release is inhibited by growth hormone itself.

- Effects:

–increased skeletal growth and cell division.

–increased protein synthesis, lipolysis and gluconeogenesis (anti-insulin effect).

Oversecretion causes gigantism before puberty, **acromegaly** thereafter.

G-suit, *see Antigravity suit*

GTN, *see Glyceryl trinitrate*

GTT, *see Glucose tolerance test*

Guanethidine monosulphate. Antihypertensive drug, depleting adrenergic neurones of **noradrenaline** and preventing its release. Rarely used for hypertension now, but sometimes useful in **causalgia** and **reflex sympathetic**

dystrophy; e.g. 10–25 mg in 20 ml saline injected iv into the exsanguinated arm (30–40 mg in 40 ml for leg), and the tourniquet kept inflated for 10–20 minutes. Close cardiovascular observation is required afterwards; hypotension may be delayed. A small amount of lignocaine is sometimes added. The procedure may be repeated, e.g. on alternate days for a number of weeks, often with long-lasting results.

May causes diarrhoea and postural hypotension.

Guedel, Arthur Ernest (1883–1956). US anaesthetist, practising in Indiana, then California. Considered a pioneer of modern anaesthesia; published extensively on many subjects, including tracheal tube **cuffs**, **divinyl ether**, **cyclopropane**, his pharyngeal airway, and a classic description of the stages of anaesthesia. Received many honours and medals.

Guillain–Barré syndrome (Acute inflammatory/post-infection polyneuropathy). Neuropathy described in 1916, although previously reported in 1859. Incidence is 1–2 per 100 000, affecting all ages. 50–60% of cases follow viral illness within the preceding month; up to 10% follow vaccination or surgery. A diarrhoeal illness involving Campylobacter is a common association.

The mechanism of the disease is unclear, but it involves lymphocytic infiltration and demyelination of spinal and cranial nerves and nerve roots, with axonal damage if severe. Autonomic nerves are sometimes affected. Pyramidal or cerebellar impairment is rare. Immune involvement is suggested by animal experimental models, detection of antineurone antibodies, and the response to **plasmapheresis**.

- Features:

–weakness, usually bilateral and symmetrical; typically ascending from the legs but it may affect any region first. Bulbar involvement may occur. May develop over 1–2 days to 2–3 weeks; 90% of patients are maximally affected within 3–4 weeks. Areflexia occurs. 30% require respiratory support. Recovery takes from several weeks to months, and up to years if severe. 10–15% are left with residual disability; 5% relapse.

–sensory disturbance: paraesthesiae occur in 50%, usually with glove and stocking distribution. Reduced touch, sensation and joint position sense may also occur. Pain may occur, e.g. in the calves and back.

–features of autonomic disturbance include hypotension or hypertension, tachycardia, arrhythmias, ileus and incontinence.

Diagnosed by history/clinical features. CSF protein is raised in over 90% of patients after a few days. Nerve conduction studies may suggest demyelination or axonal damage.

The differential diagnosis is extensive and includes **diabetes mellitus**, **poliomyelitis**, **porphyria**, lead and solvent poisoning, **botulism**, and other causes of **peripheral neuropathy**.

- Management:

–supportive:

–careful turning/nursing care/physiotherapy.

–**heparin** prophylaxis against **DVT**.

–adequate **nutrition**.

–prompt treatment of infection, e.g. urinary, respiratory, etc.

–treatment of cardiovascular abnormalities as appropriate.

–respiratory: close monitoring, usually of **vital capacity**; 15 ml/kg is usually taken as the minimum before IPPV is instituted, together with other features of **respiratory failure**. **Sedation** is rarely required. Tracheal intubation is also required if laryngeal reflexes are impaired. **Tracheostomy** is often performed as prolonged respiratory support may be required.

–**plasmapheresis**: most beneficial if performed within the first 2 weeks, and before ventilatory support is required. It is usually performed daily for 4–5 days.

–high dose immunoglobulin therapy has recently been used.

–steroids have been used but their benefit is disputed.

[Georges Guillain (1876–1961) and Jean A Barré (1880–1967), French neurologists]

Ropper AH (1992) New Engl J Med; 326: 1130–6

H

H₂ receptor antagonists. Used to reduce **histamine**-mediated gastric acid secretion, e.g. in **peptic ulcer disease**, **gastro-oesophageal reflux**, to reduce risk from **aspiration of gastric contents**, and to reduce gastric/duodenal bleeding in patients in ICU. Have also been used with **antihistamine drugs** to reduce the severity of **adverse drug reactions** and other allergic responses involving histamine.

- Drugs include:
  - **cimetidine**: introduced first. Cheapest, but with more side effects. Inhibits hepatic microsomal enzymes.
  - **ranitidine**: fewer side effects. Longer duration of action.
  - famotidine: fewer side effects. Duration of action is 10 hours.
  - nizatidine: similar to ranitidine.

Haemaccel, *see Gelatin solutions*

Haematocrit (Hct). Total red cell volume as a proportion of **blood volume**; expressed as a fraction of unity (formerly expressed as a percentage). Slightly higher in venous blood than in arterial blood, because of entry of chloride ions (**chloride shift**) into red cells with accompanying water entry by **osmosis**. An easily measured index of O_2 carrying ability of the blood, assuming normal red cell **haemoglobin** concentration. Normal values: 0.4–0.54 (male); 0.37–0.47 (female). Reduced hct of 0.3–0.35 (**haemodilution**) is thought to be beneficial for tissue O_2 delivery, e.g. in severely ill patients, because of reduced blood **viscosity** and increased **flow**; a value below this level is thought to be undesirable because of reduced O_2-carrying capacity despite increased **blood flow**.

- Useful as a guide to adequate fluid replacement therapy, e.g.:
  - **blood loss**: indicates relative need for red cells/colloid.
  - plasma loss, e.g. **burns**: plasma deficit may be determined:

  fall in plasma volume (%) =

$$100 \times \left[1 - \left(\frac{1 - \text{new Hct}}{\text{new Hct}} \times \frac{\text{original Hct}}{1 - \text{original Hct}} \right) \right]$$

See also, Investigations, preoperative

Haemoconcentration. Increase in **haematocrit** and **haemoglobin** concentration following **dehydration** or plasma loss. Degree of haemoconcentration may indicate the extent of fluid deficiency. Does not occur initially after **haemorrhage**, since red cells and plasma are lost together; compensatory mechanisms restoring blood volume cause subsequent **haemodilution**. In prolonged severe 'irreversible' **shock**, however, fluid leaves the capillaries with resulting haemoconcentration.

Haemodialysis, *see Dialysis*

Haemodilution. Lowering of **haematocrit** and **haemoglobin** concentration due to fluid shift, retention or administration. May follow compensatory restoration of blood volume after **haemorrhage**, or iv fluid therapy with only partial replacement of red cell losses. Also occurs as a physiological process in **pregnancy**. Reduction of haematocrit lowers blood **viscosity** and increases **blood flow**, although O_2 content falls. Optimal haematocrit following acute blood loss is thought to be about 0.3; in addition to improved tissue blood flow, hazards of **blood transfusion** and risk of **DVT** are reduced.
Crosby ET (1992) Can J Anaesth; 39: 695–707

Haemofiltration, *see Dialysis*

Haemoglobin (Hb). Red-coloured pigment in **erythrocytes**, composed of:
  - globin: four polypeptide subunits, in two pairs. Different types of haemoglobin contain different types of polypeptide:
    - Hb A (adult): two α chains, two β chains.
    - Hb A₂ (usually 2–3%): two α chains, two δ chains.
    - Hb F (fetal): two α chains, two γ chains.
  There are 141 amino acid residues in α chains; 146 in β, δ and γ chains.

  Fetal Hb is normally replaced by Hb A within 6 months of birth, unless polypeptide chain production is abnormal, e.g.:
    - **thalassaemia**: reduced synthesis of normal chains.
    - **haemoglobinopathies**, e.g. **sickle cell anaemia**: abnormal β chains are synthesized.
  - haem: porphyrin derivative containing iron in the ferrous (Fe^{2+}) state. One haem moiety, containing one iron atom, is conjugated to each polypeptide. Oxidation of the iron to the ferric (Fe^{3+}) state forms methaemoglobin.

- Reactions of Hb:
  - the iron atom in each haem moiety, remaining in the ferrous state but sharing one of its electrons, can reversibly bind one O_2 molecule, forming oxyhaemoglobin. Thus each Hb molecule can bind four O_2 molecules. Binding of one O_2 molecule increases the affinity for further binding, resulting in the sigmoid shaped **oxyhaemoglobin dissociation curve**. Affinity is reduced by increasing PCO_2 (**Bohr effect**), acidity, temperature and amount of **2,3–DPG** present. Fetal Hb has greater affinity for O_2 than has adult Hb.
  - CO_2 may bind reversibly to amino groups of the polypeptide chains, forming carbamino compounds ($RNH_2 + CO_2 \rightarrow RNHCO_2H$). Deoxygenated Hb reacts in this way more than oxygenated (**Haldane effect**).

–imidazole groups of histidine residues act as **buffers** in the blood. A large buffering capacity results from the many histidine residues contained in Hb, and the large amount of Hb in the blood. Deoxygenated Hb is a weaker acid and better buffer than oxygenated.
–others:
  –with carbon monoxide, forming carboxyhaemoglobin.
  –formation of methaemoglobin.
  –causing **sulphaemoglobinaemia**.
  –prolonged exposure to raised glucose levels in **diabetes mellitus**, forming glycosylated Hb.
Normal blood Hb concentration is 13–17 g/dl (men), 12–16 g/dl (women).

Hb is split into globin and haem portions when erythrocytes are destroyed. The iron is extracted and reused, the porphyrin ring opened to form biliverdin. The latter is converted to bilirubin and excreted via bile.
See also, Anaemia; Carbon dioxide transport; Carbon monoxide poisoning; Methaemoglobinaemia; Myoglobin; Oxygen transport

Haemoglobinopathies. Disorders of abnormal **haemoglobin** production (cf. **thalassaemias**: impaired production of normal haemoglobin). Over 300 variants have been described, mostly due to single amino acid substitutions. Originally named after letters of the alphabet, then after the place of origin of the first patient described. Most are clinically insignificant, but some may lead to acute or chronic **haemolysis**, and some are associated with impaired O_2 binding and secondary **polycythaemia**. **Sickle cell anaemia** is the most important; it may be combined with other abnormalities, e.g. haemoglobin C. The latter on its own may cause mild haemolytic **anaemia** and splenomegaly.

Haemolysis. Abnormal destruction of **erythrocytes**. Normal red cell survival is about 120 days; bone marrow compensation may restore red cell volume if the lifespan is shortened. **Anaemia** may result if haemolysis is excessive, bone marrow abnormal, or iron, etc. deficient.
● Caused by:
  –genetic red cell abnormalities:
    –membrane abnormalities, e.g. hereditary spherocytosis, elliptocytosis.
    –**haemoglobinopathies, thalassaemia**.
    –enzyme deficiencies, e.g. **glucose 6–phosphate dehydrogenase deficiency**.
  –acquired disorders:
    –immune:
      –autoimmune:
        –primary.
        –secondary to:
          –**connective tissue diseases**.
          –**malignancy**.
          –infection, e.g. viral, mycoplasma.
          –drugs, e.g. penicillins, methyldopa, rifampicin, sulphonamides.
      –incompatible **blood transfusion** (including **rhesus blood group** incompatibility).
    Antibodies bound to red blood cells may be detected by the direct Coombs' test; those circulating in the blood may be detected by the indirect Coombs' test.
    –non-immune:
      –infection, e.g. **malaria, septicaemia**.

–drugs, e.g. sulphonamides, phenacetin.
–**renal** and **hepatic failure**.
–hypersplenism.
–trauma, e.g. prosthetic heart valves, extracorporeal circuits. Also associated with red cell damage following contact with vasculitic endothelium (e.g. haemolytic-uraemic syndromes: endothelial damage causes renal impairment and complement/coagulation activation, with red cell damage and consumptive coagulopathy. This may occur in **pre-eclampsia/ eclampsia**, postpartum renal failure, and childhood haemolytic-uraemic syndrome).
–**paroxysmal nocturnal haemoglobinuria**.
● Haemolysis may be:
  –extravascular: most common type; involves sequestration of red cells from the circulation.
  –intravascular, e.g. haemolytic-uraemic syndromes, paroxysmal nocturnal haemoglobinuria, incompatible blood transfusion. In the latter, renal damage results from immune complex and red cell stroma deposition. Haemoglobin is released into the plasma and binds to haptoglobulin; the resultant complex is rapidly removed by the liver. Thus the amount of plasma haptoglobulin is inversely related to the degree of haemolysis. If haemolysis is severe, free haemoglobin may appear in glomerular filtrate; if proximal tubular reabsorption is exceeded, haemoglobinuria and haemosiderinuria may result.
[Robin RA Coombs, Cambridge immunologist]

Haemoperfusion. Removal of toxic substances from plasma by adsorption on to special filters, e.g. amberlite resin, **activated charcoal** granules coated in acrylic gel or cellulose. Performed in **poisoning and overdose**, and **hepatic failure**. Modern devices are extremely efficient; complete removal of toxin from the body is limited by tissue binding. Thus haemoperfusion is most effective for poisons with small **volumes of distribution**, e.g. **barbiturates, disopyramide, theophylline**, meprobamate and methaqualone; these are rarely taken in overdose. **Tricyclic antidepressants** are not removed. Requires vascular cannulation (e.g. femoral vein), pump and heparinization. Blood flow of 100–200 ml/min is employed, continued for several hours according to the clinical condition or plasma toxin levels.
● Complications: as for **dialysis**. Thrombocytopenia was common with earlier adsorption columns.

Haemophilia. The most common hereditary **coagulation disorder**, inherited as a sex-linked recessive defect. Thus affects males, although female carriers may exhibit mild disease. Female homozygotes virtually always die *in utero*. Results in deficiency of factor VIII (haemophilia A) or IX (haemophilia B; Christmas disease; one tenth as common), leading to increased bleeding into muscles, joints and internal organs. The intrinsic **coagulation** pathway is slowed, with activated partial thromboplastin time prolonged and bleeding time normal. Specific factor VIII/IX assay reveals reduced activity, and von Willebrand factor assay is normal.
● Anaesthetic considerations
  –risk of haemorrhage:
    –spontaneous bleeding may occur at factor VIII levels below 5%; prolonged bleeding may follow

surgery or trauma at 5–15%. At 15–35%, bleeding is likely only if surgery or trauma is major; it is unlikely if levels exceed 35%, but over 50% is suggested for surgery where possible.

–factor VIII is given as a concentrate (preferred), as cryoprecipitate, or as fresh frozen plasma, with haematological advice and monitoring of blood levels. Some patients have cirulating antibodies to factor VIII. **Half-life** is 8–12 hours; adequate levels are required for at least a week postoperatively.

  Desmopressin 0.4 µg/kg iv may increase levels of factor VIII transiently in mild cases, and tranexamic acid 1 g orally may also be given.

  –im injections are avoided.

  –NSAIDs and antiplatelet drugs should be avoided.

–high risk of HIV infection in haemophiliacs given pooled factor VIII before recombinant factor VIII became available in the mid/late 1980s. The risk is still present for factor IX.

[Christmas; name of patient in whom the disease was first described]

See also, Coagulation studies; von Willebrand's disease

Haemorrhage. Physiological effects of acute haemorrhage:

  –**blood volume** is reduced, leading to reduced **venous return** and **cardiac output**.

  –arterial BP falls, with activation of the **baroreceptor reflex**, reduced parasympathetic activity and increased sympathetic activity.

  –tachycardia, peripheral arterial vasoconstriction (to skin, viscera and kidneys) and venous constriction restore BP (unless volume loss is severe). Healthy adults can tolerate about 500 ml blood loss over a few minutes with little effect. Tachycardia and postural hypotension are likely with about 1000 ml loss, **shock** with 1500–2000 ml loss. Bradycardia and hypotension may occur with over 20% of blood volume; it is thought to be vagally-mediated, due to cardiac afferent C-fibre discharge caused by ventricular distortion and underfilling.

  –increased **vasopressin** secretion and **renin/angiotensin system** activity causes vasoconstriction, sodium and water retention and thirst.

  –**catecholamine** and steroid secretion increase as part of the **stress response**.

  –increased movement of interstitial fluid to the intravascular compartment and **third space**.

● Long-term effects:

  –increased **2,3–DPG** production, increasing tissue O_2 delivery.

  –increased plasma protein synthesis.

  –increased **erythopoietin** secretion and **erythropoiesis**.

Volume restoration takes 1–3 days after moderate haemorrhage, with reduction of **haematocrit** and plasma protein concentration.

● Features: as for **hypovolaemia**.

● Management:

  –local pressure and haemostasis, supine position, raising the feet, O_2 therapy, etc.

  –iv fluids:

    –cross-matched blood is best (but some benefit in cardiac output and tissue flow is derived from **haemodilution**).

    –O Rhesus-negative blood is used in life-threatening

haemorrhage, but ABO compatible blood should be used if available.

    –**colloid** maintains intravascular expansion for longer than **crystalloid**.

    –crystalloid: saline is more effective than dextrose.

  –**CVP** and **urine** output measurement are useful for monitoring volume replacement.

See also, Blood loss, peroperative; Blood transfusion; Colloid/crystalloid controversy

Haemostasis, *see Coagulation*

HAFOE, High air-flow oxygen enrichment, *see Oxygen therapy*

Hagen–Poiseuille equation. For laminar **flow** of a **fluid** of **viscosity** η through a tube of length L and radius r, with pressure gradient P across the length of the tube:

$$\text{Flow} = \frac{P\, r^4\, \pi}{8\, \eta\, L}$$

Originally derived by observing flow of liquid through rigid cylinders of different dimensions, with different driving pressures. Applied to **blood flow** through blood vessels, and **gas flow** through breathing systems and airways, although these tubes are neither rigid nor perfect cylinders.

[Jean Poiseuille (1797–1869), French physiologist; Gotthilf HL Hagen (1797–1884), German engineer]

Haldane apparatus. Burette for measuring gas volumes before and after removal of CO_2 by reaction with potassium hydroxide. The volume percentage of CO_2 in the original gas mixture may thus be determined. Similar determination of O_2 concentration may be performed, using pyrogallol as the absorbant.

[John Haldane (1860–1936), Scottish-born English physiologist]

See also, Carbon dioxide measurement; Gas analysis

Haldane effect. Increased capacity of deoxygenated blood for CO_2 **transport** compared with oxygenated blood.

● Results from:

  –increased buffering ability of reduced **haemoglobin**, allowing more CO_2 to be transported as bicarbonate.

  –increased binding of reduced haemoglobin to CO_2, forming carbamino groups.

See also, Haldane apparatus

Half-life ($t_{1/2}$). In an **exponential process**, the time taken for the variable to reach half its original value. Remains constant, whatever its starting point; thus indicates the rate of such a process, usually a decay.

● Examples:

  –radioactive half-life (time taken for half the original number of atoms to disintegrate).

  –drug half-life (time taken for drug concentration to fall by half, whether resulting from redistribution, elimination, etc.).

See also, Pharmacokinetics; Time constant

Hall, Richard, *see Halsted, William Stewart*

Halothane. 2–Bromo-2–chloro-1,1,1–trifluoroethane (Fig. 68). **Inhalational anaesthetic agent**, introduced in 1956. Its

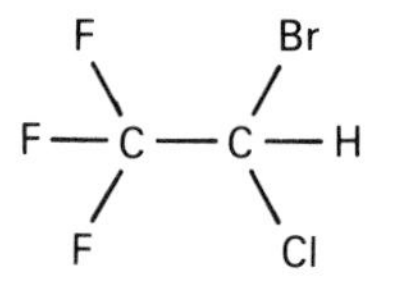

Figure 68 *Structure of halothana*

use rapidly spread because of its greater potency, ease of use, non-irritability and non-inflammability compared with **diethyl ether** and **cyclopropane**. Fears over liver damage on repeated administration (**halothane hepatitis**) have led to a decline in its use; its place in current anaesthetic practice is controversial because of this, although its superiority over alternative agents for upper **airway obstruction** is generally accepted.

• Properties:
  –colourless liquid; vapour has characteristic pleasant smell and is 6.8 times denser than air.
  –mw 197.
  –boiling point 50°C.
  –SVP at 20°C 32 kPa (243 mmHg).
  –**partition coefficients**:
    –blood/gas 2.5.
    –oil/gas 225.
  –**MAC** 0.76.
  –non-flammable.
  –adsorbed on to rubber.
  –may corrode aluminium, tin and certain alloys when moist.
  –supplied in liquid form with **thymol** 0.01%; decomposes slightly in light.
• Effects:
  –CNS:
    –smooth rapid induction, with rapid recovery.
    –anticonvulsant action.
    –increases **cerebral blood flow** but reduces **intraocular pressure**.
    –poor analgesic properties.
  –RS:
    –non-irritant. Pharyngeal, laryngeal and cough reflexes are abolished early, hence its value in difficult airways.
    –respiratory depressant, with increased respiratory rate and reduced tidal volume.
    –bronchodilatation and inhibition of secretions.
  –CVS:
    –myocardial depression possibly via reduction of intracellular calcium mobilization, and bradycardia via increased vagal tone. Has ganglion blocking and central vasomotor depressant actions. Hypotension is common.
    –myocardial O_2 demand decreases.
    –slight vasodilatation only.
    –**arrhythmias** are common, e.g. bradycardia, nodal rhythm, ventricular ectopics/bigemini.
    –sensitizes the myocardium to catecholamines, e.g. endogenous or injected **adrenaline**.
  –other:
    –dose-dependent uterine relaxation.
    –nausea/vomiting is uncommon. GIT motility is decreased.

–skeletal muscle relaxation; non-depolarizing neuromuscular blocking drugs may be potentiated. **Shivering** is common during recovery.
–may precipitate **MH**.

Up to 20% is metabolized in the liver, usually via oxidative pathways. Reduction is thought to be more likely under hypoxic conditions, and may be important in the development of hepatitis. Metabolites include bromine, chlorine and trifluoroacetic acid; negligible amounts of **fluoride ions** are produced. Repeated administration after recent use may result in hepatitis.

0.5–2.0% is usually adequate for maintenance of anaesthesia, with higher concentrations for induction. Tracheal intubation may be performed easily with spontaneous respiration, under halothane anaesthesia.
See also, Vaporizers

Halothane hepatitis. **Hepatitis** following **halothane** exposure; first reported in 1958. Incidence and characteristics are controversial and difficult to study, because of its rarity and other causes of hepatic impairment after surgery. In the USA, the National Halothane Study (1969) reported 850 000 hepatitis cases occurring within 6 weeks of anaesthesia, 250 000 of whom had received halothane. Only nine cases were unexplained by other causes; seven of these had received halothane. Studies since then do support the existence of the condition. Its incidence is 1:6000 to 1:30 000, although mild hepatic dysfunction as indicated by deranged liver function tests may occur in up to 20% of patients receiving halothane. Hepatitis is more common following repeated use, especially in rapid succession, although the safe time interval is not known. It may be more common in middle-aged women and in obese patients. There may be a genetic predisposition. Incidence is unrelated to pre-existing liver disease. Previously considered not to affect children, it has recently been shown to occur although less commonly than in adults.

Most patients are thought to be unharmed by repeated administration; some show mild impairment of liver function and a few progress to **hepatic failure**, with poor prognosis.

• Main theories of mechanism:
  –a toxic metabolite of halothane causes direct liver damage. Supported by the need in certain animal models for increased halothane metabolism via **enzyme induction** (e.g. with barbiturate pretreatment) before hepatitis occurs. Hypoxia is also required, suggesting involvement of reductive metabolism (normally oxidative metabolism occurs). However, the theory is not supported by similar hepatotoxicity following **enflurane** and **isoflurane** under similar circumstances, despite their low metabolism. Also, reductive metabolites themselves are not hepatotoxic, and other factors may increase toxicity without increasing metabolism, e.g. fasting, or high doses for short periods.
  –immune reaction to halothane or hepatocytes altered by halothane. Suggested by finding increased autoimmune antibodies in affected patients' sera. Antibodies reacting with rabbit halothane-altered hepatocyte membrane determinants are found in 75% of affected patients, and may be used as a diagnostic test. Immune reaction to a metabolite may be involved; trifluoroacetyl halide has been implicated.

–hepatic O_2 supply reduced by cardiovascular effects of halothane, causing ischaemic necrosis. Enzyme induction caused by barbiturates increases O_2 demand, exacerbating supply/demand imbalance. Although hypoxia is thought to contribute to hepatitis, this theory is not considered the most important.

Much experimental work has been performed in animals, with interspecies variation; extrapolation to humans is difficult.

- The **Committee on Safety of Medicines** in 1986 recommended avoidance of halothane following:
  –history of previous exposure and adverse reactions.
  –previous exposure within 3 months unless the indications are felt clinically overriding.
  –history of unexplained jaundice/pyrexia after previous exposure to halothane.

This recommendation led to much controversy amongst UK anaesthetists, some supporting the routine use of alternative agents and some defending halothane as the best drug for most anaesthetics, and worried that it might eventually be withdrawn. Hepatitis has followed exposure to enflurane and isoflurane, but their repeated use is generally felt to be safe.

Elliott RH, Strunin L (1993) Br J Anaesth; 70: 339–48

'Halothane shakes', *see Shivering, postoperative*

Halsted, William Stewart (1852–1922). US surgeon, considered the founder of local anaesthetic nerve blocks with Hall and others in New York from 1884, using **cocaine**. He and Hall described blocks of most of the nerves of the face, head and limbs, experimenting on each other and becoming cocaine addicts in the process. Highly regarded for his surgical skills, becoming Professor at Baltimore. Also introduced rubber gloves into surgery.
[Richard J Hall (1856–97), Irish-born US surgeon]

Hamburger shift, *see Chloride shift*

Hanging drop technique. Method of identifying the **extradural space**, e.g. during **extradural** or **spinal anaesthesia**. A drop of saline is placed at the hub of a needle which is advanced towards the extradural space; when the space has been entered the drop is drawn into the needle by the negative pressure within the space. Not always reliable, since negative pressure is not always present.

Haptoglobin, *see Haemolysis*

Harmonics. Related sine waveforms; the frequency of each is a multiple of the fundamental frequency of the first harmonic, the slowest component of the series. Complex **waveforms** may be produced by adding higher harmonics to the first (fundamental) harmonic (**Fourier analysis**). **Monitoring** equipment must be able to reproduce harmonics of high enough frequency for the signal recorded; e.g. up to the 10th harmonic for many recorders. More harmonics are required for more complex wavefroms with higher frequncies, increasing the required frequency response of the monitor concerned, e.g. **ECG** 0.5–80 Hz, **EEG** 1–60 Hz, **EMG** 2–1200 Hz.

Harnesses. Used to secure breathing attachments or facepieces to the patient. May damage soft tissues around the face, and **airway obstruction** may still occur.

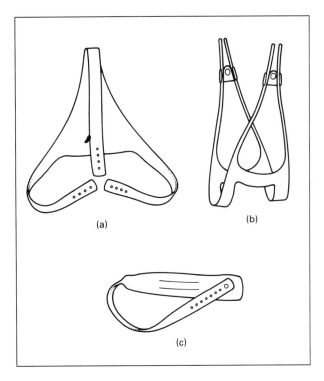

Figure 69 *Examples of harnesses: (a) Clausen; (b) Connell; (c) Hudson*

- Examples (Fig. 69):
  –Clausen harness: triangular, with straps at each corner for attachment to hooks around the facepiece.
  –Connell harness: square back, with attachments at each end for the sides of the facepiece.
  –Hudson harness (for dental surgery): long strap for fixation of the catheter mount from the nasotracheal tube; binds around the patient's forehead.
[RJ Clausen (1890–1966), English anaesthetist; Karl Connell (1873–1941), US surgeon; Maurice WP Hudson, London anaesthetist]

Hartmann's solution (Ringer's lactate; Compound sodium lactate). **IV fluid** containing sodium 131 mmol/l, potassium 5 mmol/l, calcium 2 mmol/l, chloride 111 mmol/l and lactate 29 mmol/l. pH is 5–7. Originally formulated from **Ringer's solution** to allow fluid replacement and treatment of metabolic acidosis in sick children, using an isotonic solution containing more sodium than chloride. Lactate is metabolized to **bicarbonate** within a few hours, and the hazards of bicarbonate administration avoided. Now widely used as the crystalloid of choice for **ECF** replacement, since it closely resembles this fluid in make-up; however, its advantage over saline solutions for routine use has been questioned.

Often avoided in patients with renal failure because of the risk of **hyperkalaemia**, in sick patients or those with hepatic failure because of the risk of **lactic acidosis**, and in diabetics because of the risk of lactate metabolism to glucose.
[Alexis Hartmann (1898–1964), US paediatrician]

Hb, *see Haemoglobin*

HBE, *see His bundle electrography*

Hct, *see Haematocrit*

HDU, *see High dependency unit*

Head injury. Common cause of morbidity and mortality in **trauma**, especially in young males; it should be suspected in all trauma cases. Once admitted to hospital, further damage is thought to be mostly preventable. Brain dysfunction may follow:

   –direct trauma on the side of injury or opposite (contrecoup). Damage may be gross or microscopic, the latter often diffuse.
   –compression due to **cerebral oedema** or intracerebral, intraventricular, **extradural** or **subdural haemorrhage**; the first two are usually associated with direct brain injury.
   –impaired CNS oxygenation, e.g. due to **hypoxaemia** or **hypotension** associated with other injuries, **hypoventilation** or **airway obstruction** due to depressed consciousness, etc.

- Features:
   –external signs of head injury, e.g. bruising, lacerations, etc. Neck fractures should be assumed until proven otherwise. **Chest trauma** is common. Other injuries may be present.
   –impaired consciousness and **amnesia**. Often associated with **alcohol** or other cause of **coma**. **Brainstem death** may occur.
   –**pupils**: the 3rd **cranial nerve** on the side of an expanding cerebral lesion is stretched over the edge of the tentorium cerebelli, causing ipsilateral dilatation and absence of light reflex with consensual light reflex preserved. Eventually, the contralateral pupil is affected too.
   –bradycardia and hypertension may occur (**Cushing's reflex**), and irregular respiration as compression continues.
   –hemiparesis/hemiplegia, upward plantar reflexes, and **convulsions** may occur. Cranial nerve involvement may reflect the site of injury; e.g. 1–6 in anterior fossa, 7–8 in middle fossa and 9–10 in posterior fossa injuries. Other CNS signs are often variable.
   –other complications:
      –infection.
      –**Cushing's ulcers.**
      –convulsions.
      –disturbance of **CSF** dynamics, causing CSF leak or **hydrocephalus**.
      –respiratory, e.g. **aspiration pneumonitis**, infection, **PE**, **pulmonary oedema**, **ARDS**, etc.
      –**diabetes insipidus** or **syndrome of inappropriate antidiuretic hormone secretion.**
      –**DIC.**
- Management:
   –as for coma and trauma, i.e. **CPR**: O_2 administration, airway, breathing, circulation, etc. **Glasgow coma scale** is widely used for assessment. Continuing assessment is important.
   –**opioid analgesic drugs** are avoided in spontaneously breathing patients, because of the risk of central and respiratory depression and their effects on the pupils; **codeine** is traditionally used, as these effects are held to be less, but this may represent codeine's lesser potency.

   –skull and neck X-rays to identify fractures, and CAT scanning to identify haemorrhage, oedema, etc. Ultrasound has been used to identify midline shift, before subsequent CAT scanning.
   Criteria for skull X-ray:
      –unconsciousness or amnesia at any time.
      –neurological signs.
      –CSF/blood from nose or ear.
      –serious scalp injury.
      –difficulty in assessment, e.g. confusion, alcohol, etc.
   Criteria for CAT scan:
      –deterioration in conscious level, pupillary signs or other observations.
      –focal neurological signs.
      –fractured skull and confusion.
      –continuing unconsciousness.
   Transfer for CAT scan requires tracheal intubation if conscious level is depressed.
   –if injury is severe, tracheal intubation and IPPV are performed to reduce **ICP** and cerebral oedema, with other measures, e.g. **mannitol**, etc. IPPV is usually continued for 24–48 hours. Indications vary but include:
      –hypoxaemia.
      –respiratory irregularity, hypo- or hyperventilation.
      –uncontrolled convulsions, raised ICP or hyperthermia.
      –extensor or flexor posturing.
   Patients are likely to be at risk of regurgitating gastric contents. A nasogastric tube is required to prevent gastric dilatation. **ICP monitoring** is instituted in some centres. **EEG** and related monitoring, and **evoked potentials** have been used to monitor progress.
   –**cerebral protection/resuscitation**; not yet generally proven nor accepted.
   –drug therapy:
      –to reduce ICP: diuretics for acute increases in ICP associated with a mass lesion, i.e. haematoma. A beneficial effect of steroids has yet to be shown.
      –for **sedation**/paralysis/analgesia.
      –usually a sulphonamide, e.g. sulphadimidine 0.5–1 g 4 hourly if CSF leak is suspected, since sulphonamides easily penetrate the blood–brain barrier.
      –**H₂ receptor antagonists**.
      –**anticonvulsant drugs**, e.g. **phenytoin**, if required. They may be given prophylactically, e.g. if craniotomy is required.
   Surgery may be required for associated injuries, elevation of depressed fractures or evacuation of intracranial haemorrhage; the latter may require burr holes or craniotomy.
- Anaesthesia for patients with head injuries: as for **neurosurgery** and **emergency surgery**. In particular:
   –other injuries may be present.
   –regional techniques are often difficult, especially if the patient is confused. Sedation is dangerous. Burr holes may be drilled under local anaesthesia.
   –spontaneous ventilation must be avoided, even for minor procedures, since a small increase in **cerebral blood flow** and intracranial volume may cause a catastrophic rise in ICP. All patients should be managed as if ICP is raised.

Borel C, Hanley D, Diringer MN, Rogers MC (1990)
Chest; 98: 180–9
See also, Cerebral metabolic rate for oxygen; Cerebral perfusion pressure; Coning; Faciomaxillary surgery

Head's paradoxical reflex. Sustained diaphragmatic contraction, followed by shallow respiration, following a small passive lung inflation. Seen only in rabbits, and following cooling and partial rewarming of the vagi. Significance is unknown.
[Sir Henry Head (1861–1940), English neurologist]
See also, Gasp reflex

Heart. Develops from a single tube which doubles up forming primitive atrium and ventricle; divided by septa into left and right sides (*see Atrial septal defect; Ventricular septal defect*). The primitive arterial outlet (truncus arteriosus) splits spirally to form the aorta and pulmonary trunk; the venous inlet (truncus venosus) absorbs into the smooth-walled part of the right atrium.
- Surface anatomy:
  - right border: from 3rd to 6th right costal cartilages, 1–1.5 cm from the left sternal edge.
  - left border: from 2nd left costal cartilage, 1–1.5 cm from the left sternal edge, to the apex beat (usually at the 5th left intercostal space in the midclavicular line).
  - upper limit: level with the angle of Louis (T4–5).
  - base: level with the xiphisternum (T8–9).

The left border is composed mainly of left ventricle, the right border mainly of right atrium, and the base mainly of right ventricle as on the **chest X-ray**. Weighs about 300 g. Encased within **pericardium**.
- Chambers:
  - right atrium:
    - bears the auricular appendage (remnant of the original atrium).
    - receives superior and inferior venae cavae, and coronary sinus.
  - right ventricle:
    - crescent-shaped in cross-section, due to bulging of the left ventricle.
    - tendinous cords from the interventricular septum and papillary muscles attach to the tricuspid valve.
    - pulmonary valve: comprised of three cusps.
  - left atrium: receives four non-valved pulmonary veins.
  - left ventricle:
    - thick walled.
    - the two-cusped mitral valve is anchored with tendinous cords as for the tricuspid valve. The anterior cusp is bigger than the posterior.
    - aortic valve: comprised of three semilunar cusps, one anterior and two posterior.
- Blood supply: *see Coronary circulation*
- Nerve supply: from **vagus** and **sympathetic nervous system** from upper thoracic and cervical ganglia; mainly T1–4. The cardiac plexus receives branches from both components of the autonomic nervous system.
[Antoine Louis (1723–1792), French surgeon]
See also, Action potential; Atrial...; Cardiac...; Coronary...; Heart, conducting system; Left Ventricular...; Myocardial...; Ventricular...

Heart, artificial. Device used to replace or assist the heart in end-stage disease when **heart transplantation** is

unavailable, or following **cardiac surgery**. Permanent replacement is not feasible at present, but temporary support is increasingly used as a short-term measure.
- Types:
  - ventricular assist devices:
    - assist either or both ventricles.
    - roller or centrifugal pumps provide non-pulsatile flow; pneumatic pumps provide pulsatile flow.
  - permanent devices: pneumatically or electrically powered, with an external power source.

Main problems are related to infection, thromboembolism, and reliability and flexibility of the devices.
Graham TR, Chalmers JAC (1989) Br J Hosp Med; 41: 420–5 and 520–4

Heart block. Usually refers to atrioventricular (AV) block, i.e. interruption of impulse propagation between atria and ventricles. **Bundle branch block** refers to interruption distal to the atrioventricular node.
- Classification:
  - 1st degree (Fig. 70a): delay at the AV node; block is never complete:
    - **P–R interval** > 0.2 seconds at normal heart rate.
    - usually clinically insignificant.
    - caused by:
      - ageing.
      - **ischaemic heart disease**.
      - increased vagal tone.

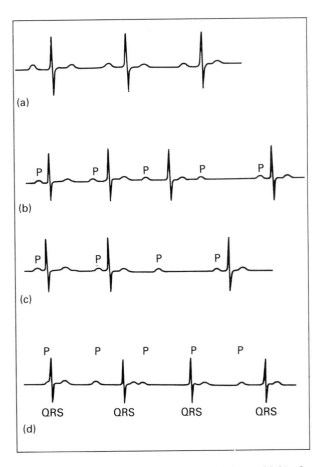

Figure 70 *Heart block: (a) 1st degree; (b) 2nd degree, Mobitz I; (c) 2nd degree, Mobitz II; (d) 3rd degree*

–drugs, e.g. **halothane**, **digoxin**.
–**cardiomyopathy**, myocarditis, etc.
–2nd degree: occasional complete block. May be:
  –Mobitz type I (Wenckebach phenomenon) (Fig. 70b):
    –AV delay; P–R interval lengthens with successive **P waves** until complete AV block occurs, and no **QRS complex** follows the P wave. The cycle then repeats.
    –usually due to AV conduction delay.
    –rarely proceeds to complete heart block.
  –Mobitz type II (Fig. 70c):
    –sudden block below the AV node; i.e. P–R interval may be normal. May occur regularly, e.g. every third complex.
    –at risk of developing complete heart block, particularly if it occurs regularly.
  –3rd degree (Fig. 70d): complete heart block, at the AV node or below (the latter is trifascicular block. If incomplete, it may appear as bifascicular block with P–R prolongation):
    –**ECG** demonstrates independent atrial and ventricular activity, the latter arising from an ectopic site. The ventricular rate is usually slow, especially if the ectopic site is far from the AV node (wide QRS complexes; rate <45/min).
    –clinical findings:
      –hypotension is common.
      –wide pulse pressure (large stroke volume).
      –cannon waves in the **JVP**.
      –escape ventricular arrhythmias may occur.
    –caused by:
      –old age.
      –**ischaemic heart disease**.
      –myocarditis/**cardiomyopathy**.
      –**cardiac surgery**.
      –increased vagal tone.
      –**β-adrenergic antagonists**, digoxin.
      –**hyperkalaemia**.
      –congenital abnormality.
Complete heart block and predisposing conditions should be treated by insertion of pacing wires preoperatively. Drugs decreasing AV conduction, e.g. β-receptor antagonists and halothane, should be avoided. **Isoprenaline** 0.02–0.2 µg/kg/min may be used to increase ventricular rate in complete heart block, and should be available, as should a back-up pacing box. Cardiac output should be maintained where possible. **Antiarrhythmic drugs** supressing ventricular activity should be avoided.
[Karl Wenckebach (1848–1904), Dutch physician; Woldemar Mobitz (1889–?), German cardiologist]
For management of patients with pacemakers, see Cardiac pacing

Heart, conducting system. Composed of:
–sinoatrial node: at the junction of the superior vena cava and right atrium. Normally discharges more rapidly than the rest of the heart, thus setting the rate of contraction, although all cardiac muscle is capable of originating electrical impulses spontaneously.
–atrioventricular node (AV node): lies in the atrial septum, above the coronary sinus opening. Normally the only means of conduction between atria and ventricles.
–bundle of His (or Kent): divides into left and right bundle branches above the interventricular septum, passing down on either side subendocardially:

–the left bundle branch divides into anterior and posterior fascicles.
–Purkinje fibres spread from the ends of bundle branches/fascicles to the rest of the ventricles.
Impulses pass from node to node through normal atrial muscle, then via specialized cardiac muscle cells, insulated from the rest of the myocardium by connective tissue sheaths. Conduction through each of the following takes about 0.1 seconds:
–atria.
–AV node.
–bundle of His/Purkinje system.
Vagal and sympathetic innervation is directed to both nodes; conduction through the AV node is slowed by the former and speeded by the latter.
  Ventricular depolarization begins at the heart's apex and spreads outwards and upwards, encouraging upward expulsion of blood from the ventricles.
  Interruption of impulse conduction may result in **bundle branch block** and **heart block**.
[Wilhelm His (1863–1934), German anatomist; Albert Kent (1863–1958), English physiologist and radiologist; Johannes von Purkinje (1787–1869), Czech physiologist]

Heart failure, *see Cardiac failure*

Heart–lung transplantation. First performed in 1968 but with poor results; since 1980 over 150 have been performed, mainly in the Universities of Pittsburgh and Stanford (USA), and in Harefield (UK). Isolated lung transplantation has produced poor results but interest has increased recently.
• Indications: usually **pulmonary hypertension** or **Eisenmenger's syndrome**. Has been performed for **pulmonary fibrosis**, **cystic fibrosis**, emphysema, etc.
• Donor:
  –as for **heart transplantation**, with normal chest X-ray, minimal sputum and no history of aspiration or pulmonary oedema. Arterial P_{O_2} should exceed 13.3 kPa (100 mmHg) with $F_{I}O_2$ 0.4.
  –the heart and lungs are placed into a bag and immersed in cold electrolyte solution, with IPPV at low rates and perfusion of the coronary arteries with donor blood. Whole body transfer using cardiopulmonary bypass has also been used.
• Recipient:
  –immunosuppression and general management as for heart transplantation.
  –the trachea is divided above the carina. Damage to vagi, phrenic and recurrent laryngeal nerves is possible.
  –**PEEP** and inotropes are usually required; **isoprenaline** is particularly useful because of its ablity to reduce **pulmonary vascular resistance**. Pulmonary oedema and sputum retention are common. The cough reflex is destroyed and **ciliary activity** impaired.
  –**weaning** from IPPV is as for cardiac surgery.
  –lung rejection may occur without heart rejection, and may be difficult to detect.
Freeman JW, Lilley JP (1990) Curr Opin Anaesth; 3: 71–6

Heart murmurs. General principles:
–caused by turbulent flow of blood, including abnormal flow through a normal valve or normal flow though an abnormal valve or orifice.

–systolic murmurs may be physiological; diastolic murmurs are always pathological.

–stenotic murmurs are harsh and usually immediate; regurgitant murmurs are soft and usually follow a pause.

–low murmurs are heard best with the stethoscope bell, high pitched ones with the diaphragm.

–left-sided murmurs are heard best in expiration; right-sided ones best in inspiration.

–murmurs radiate usually in the direction of turbulent flow.

–when auscultating the heart, murmurs are best described by:

–time of occurrence.

–site and radiation.

–character including relation to respiration. Loudness is usually expressed as score of 1–5: 1 = only just audible; 5 = audible without a stethoscope.

–associated **heart sounds**.

- Classification:

–systolic:

–pansystolic:

–**VSD**.

–**mitral regurgitation**.

–tricuspid regurgitation.

–ejection:

–**aortic stenosis**.

–pulmonary stenosis.

–**ASD**.

–diastolic:

–**mitral stenosis**.

–**aortic regurgitation**.

–continuous:

–patent **ductus arteriosus**.

(NB. Venous hum: due to kinking of major neck veins, especially in children. Abolished by pressure on the neck).

See also, Cardiac cycle; Preoperative assessment; Pulmonary valve lesions; Tricuspid valve lesions

Heart rate. Normal range in adults is usually defined as 60–100 beats/min, but it may be less than 50/min in fit young subjects, and increase up to 200/min on exercise. Rate is about 100/min in the heart denervated of sympathetic and parasympathetic innervation.

- Rate is increased by:

–sympathetic activity, e.g. secondary to **hypotension**, **hypoxaemia**, **hypercapnia**, pain, fear, anger, exercise, inspiration.

–hormones, e.g. **catecholamines**, thyroxine.

–infection and fever.

–**Bainbridge reflex**.

–drugs, e.g. **salbutamol**.

- Rate is decreased by:

–parasympathetic activity via the **vagus nerve**, e.g. secondary to the **baroreceptor reflex**, fear, pain, raised **ICP**, expiration.

–**hypoxaemia**.

–drugs, e.g. **neostigmine**.

See also, Arrhythmias; Pacemaker cells; Sinus arrhythmia; Sinus bradycardia; Sinus rhythm; Sinus tachycardia

Heart sounds. The first sound is due to closure of the tricuspid and mitral valves; it lasts 0.15 seconds with frequency 25–45 Hz. The second is due to closure of the aortic and pulmonary valves; it lasts 0.12 seconds with frequency 50 Hz. Valve opening is normally silent.

- Intensity:

–quiet in obese or well-built subjects.

–2nd sound is quiet in **aortic stenosis**, since valve mobility is reduced.

–1st sound is quiet in **mitral regurgitation**, since valve closure is incomplete.

–1st sound is increased in **mitral stenosis**, since the valve is kept open right up to systole by increased left atrial pressure, instead of gradual closure at end of diastole.

- Splitting of the second sound:

–heard at the left sternal edge.

–the aortic component normally precedes the pulmonary component, since left ventricular contraction is faster than that of the right.

–increased in inspiration, when right ventricular contraction is delayed by increased preload. Fixed in **ASD**; reversed in left **bundle branch block** and severe aortic stenosis, when left ventricular contraction is markedly delayed.

- Extra sounds:

–3rd heart sound (thought to be due to ventricular filling). Occurs shortly after the 2nd sound. May occur in normal subjects, also in reduced ventricular compliance/increased volume, e.g. in **cardiac failure**, mitral regurgitation, **VSD**.

–4th heart sound (thought to be due to atrial contraction under pressure with forceful ventricular distension). Occurs shortly before the 1st sound. May occur in aortic stenosis, pulmonary stenosis, **hypertension**.

–gallop rhythm: all four sounds, e.g. cardiac failure.

–others, e.g. the late ejection click of aortic stenosis, the late systolic click of **mitral valve prolapse**, and the early diastolic opening snap of mitral stenosis.

–**heart murmurs**.

See also, Cardiac cycle; Preoperative assessment

Heart transplantation. First performed in humans in 1967 by Barnard. Initial problems were infection and rejection. Interest resurged in the late 1970s with the introduction of cyclosporin, leading to establishment of centres worldwide.

- Indications: mostly end-stage **ischaemic heart disease** and **cardiomyopathy**; also **congenital heart disease**, valvular disease and others.

- Contraindications include age over 50 years, insulin-dependent **diabetes mellitus**, active infection, and recent **PE/MI**; these contraindications have been relaxed as expertise increases and chances of survival improve.

- Donor:

–normal past medical history/examination and ECG. A short period of cardiac arrest, and minimal requirements for inotropic support are acceptable. Age should be under 40. ABO compatibility with the recipient is required.

–initial management including **heparin** and **cardioplegia** is as for **cardiac surgery**. The heart is placed in cold crystalloid solution and both the atria opened; it is transported in ice.

- Recipient:

–most patients are prepared for the possibility of emergency transplantation. By definition, they are in poor general health, i.e. high risk.

209

–**immunodepressant drugs** include cyclosporin, steroids, azathioprine and anti-thymocyte immuno-globulin.

–all iv lines, tracheal tube, laryngoscope, tubing, etc., are sterile to reduce infection, with gown and gloves worn.

–general management is as for cardiac surgery. After **cardiopulmonary bypass** and aortic cross-clamping, the ventricles are removed, leaving most of the atria. The atria and aortas are anastomosed. The donor heart may also be piggy-backed next to the original heart, anastomosing left atria, aortas, pulmonary arteries and venae cavae.

–inotropes are usually required for over 24 hours. The denervated heart rate is usually faster than that of the innervated heart, with no response to indirectly-acting drugs, e.g. **atropine**. Directly-acting drugs, e.g. **isoprenaline**, are used. The rate responds slowly to circulating catecholamines.

Postoperative care is as routine, but barrier nursing is required.

–regular endocardial biopsy via the right internal jugular vein is performed to detect rejection, e.g. weekly, then monthly for 3 months, then 6 monthly.

For anaesthesia in a heart recipient, aseptic techniques are used, and directly-acting cardiovascular drugs as above. Otherwise, management is as for any high risk cardiac case.

[Christian Barnard, South African surgeon]

White DA, Latimer RD (1991) Curr Opin Anaesth; 4: 83–9.

See also, Heart–lung transplantation

Heat. Form of **energy** associated with movement of molecules, atoms and smaller structural units; it moves from one site to another owing to a **temperature** difference between them.

- Heat is transferred by:
  –radiation: especially from bright shiny bodies to dark matt bodies.
  –convection: as air next to a warm body is warmed, it expands and becomes less dense, rising and being replaced by colder air.
  –evaporation: heat is transferred to liquid molecules, providing the energy required to break the bonds between them in forming a vapour.
  –conduction: especially via good conductors of heat, e.g. metals.

All these routes may be important in **heat loss during anaesthesia**.

See also, Temperature regulation

Heat capacity. Quantity of **heat** required to raise the **temperature** of a mass by 1 K (J/K). Specific heat capacity (C) is the quantity of heat required to raise the temperature of unit mass of substance by 1 K (J/kg/K). The total heat capacity of an object may be calculated from knowledge of the mass and values for C of its constituent parts.

- Examples of C:
  –human tissues, including blood: 3.5 kJ/kg/K.
  –water: 4.18 kJ/kg/K (1 Cal/kg/°C).

For a gas, C_p is specific heat capacity at constant pressure, and C_v is specific heat capacity at constant volume. $C_p - C_v$ equals the work done in expansion of the gas. For an ideal gas, $C_p - C_v = R$ (**universal gas constant**).

Since gases are much less dense than liquids, the energy required to heat unit volume is much less. Thus little energy is expended in heating inspired air (although significant energy is expended humidifying it).

See also, Latent heat

Heat loss, during anaesthesia. Prevention is important because of the adverse effects of **hypothermia** and the increased postoperative O_2 consumption (up to 10 times) caused by **shivering**. In addition, the duration of action of neuromuscular blocking drugs is prolonged and drug excretion delayed. Particularly important in **neonates** and children, and in the **elderly**, because of reduced reserves.

- Temperature may fall by several °C during prolonged surgery, via:
  –increased loss of **heat**:
    –radiation: increased if the patient is uncovered and surrounded by cold objects. Also increased by vasodilatation.
    –convection : increased if the patient is uncovered.
    –evaporation: increased if a body cavity is opened, e.g. abdomen, especially if environmental humidity is low. Heat loss via evaporation in the trachea and airways may be considerable if inspired gases are unhumidified.
    –conduction: usually a less important route; increased by use of cold irrigating solutions, etc.
  –reduced heat production and impaired **temperature regulation**. The latter may be peripheral (e.g. vasodilatation, shivering and impaired piloerection) or central (central effects of drugs).
- Prevention:
  –identification of high risk patients:
    –elderly.
    –children.
    –severely ill patients with malnutrition.
    –prolonged surgery.
    –major blood loss.
    –open body cavity.
    –**sickle cell anaemia**.
  –**temperature measurement** during anaesthesia.
  –covering during transfer to the operating suite.
  –maintenance of ambient temperature at 22–24°C and humidity about 50% (compromise between patient temperature and staff comfort).
  –covering with drapes, reflective garments and head coverings (especially children).
  –warming of all skin cleansing solutions and iv fluids.
  –**humidification** of inspired gases.
  –warming blankets, e.g. using heated water or air.
  –warming of the bed, etc. postoperatively.

Imrie MM, Hall GM (1990) Br J Anaesth; 64: 346–54

Heat–moisture exchanger, *see Humidification*

Heat of vaporization, *see Latent heat*

Heatstroke, *see Hyperthermia*

Hedonal. Obsolete anaesthetic agent, one of the first to be used iv (1905); also used rectally and orally. Poorly water soluble, requiring large volumes of injectate. Of very slow onset and prolonged duration of action.

Heidbrink valve, *see Adjustable pressure-limiting valve*

Heimlich manoeuvre. Method of relieving upper **airway obstruction** caused by a foreign body using rapid compression of the upper abdomen. The resultant rise in intrathoracic pressure expels the object from the upper airway. The operator stands behind the subject with hands clenched over the subject's epigastrium, the operator's arms passing under the subject's. A sharp thrust is delivered inwards and upwards. A similar manoeuvre may be performed with the subject lying. Compression of the lower chest has been found to be as effective. Clearance of one's own airway by falling forwards on to the back of a chair has been reported.
[Henry J Heimlich, US surgeon]

Helium. Inert gas, present in natural gas and to a lesser extent in **air**. Less dense than nitrogen. Thus, if **flow** is turbulent, greater flow of a helium/O_2 mixture will occur than of a nitrogen/O_2 mixture, as turbulent flow depends on fluid density. Used therefore to increase alveolar O_2 supply in upper **airway obstruction**. Of no use in lower airway obstruction, e.g. **asthma**, because flow is laminar and therefore depends on viscosity, which is greater for helium/O_2 mixtures than for nitrogen/O_2.

Supplied in **cylinders** with brown shoulders and body, at 137 bar. Also available with 21% O_2, in brown-bodied cylinders with brown and white quartered shoulders, at the same pressure.

Has also been used to investigate small airway resistance to flow, by comparing **flow-volume loops** breathing air and helium/O_2. The two curves are more similar in small airway obstruction than in normal lungs.

Because of its very low solubility, helium is also used in measurement of **lung volumes**.

Hemicholinium. Synthetic compound which blocks choline transport into cholinergic nerve endings. Thus reduces **acetylcholine** synthesis and storage. Used in experimental pharmacology.

Hemo..., *see Haemo*...

Henderson–Hasselbalch equation. Originally derived to describe **pH** changes resulting from addition of **base** or **acid** to any **buffer** system; now often specifically applied to the **bicarbonate** buffer system.

For the reaction of CO_2 with water to form carbonic acid, which dissociates to form bicarbonate and **hydrogen ions**:

$$CO_2 + H_2O \rightleftharpoons H_2CO_3 \rightleftharpoons H^+ + HCO_3^-$$

The dissociation constant K_a for the dissociation of H_2CO_3 then equals

$$\frac{[H^+]\,[HCO_3^-]}{[H_2CO_3]}$$

Taking logarithms of both sides:

$$\log K_a = \log [H^+] + \log \frac{[HCO_3^-]}{[H_2CO_3]}$$

therefore $-\log pH = -\log K_a + \log \dfrac{[HCO_3^-]}{[H_2CO_3]}$

or, $pH = pK_a + \log \dfrac{[HCO_3^-]}{[H_2CO_3]}$

Since $[H_2CO_3]$ is related to $[CO_2]$ by the original reaction, and $[CO_2]$ is related to $P\text{CO}_2$ and a solubility factor (0.03 mmol/l/mmHg, or 0.23 mmol/l/kPa),

$$pH = pK_a + \log \frac{[HCO_3^-]}{P\text{CO}_2 \times 0.03}$$

with $P\text{CO}_2$ measured in mmHg

or $pKa + \log \dfrac{[HCO_3^-]}{P\text{CO}_2 \times 0.23}$

with $P\text{CO}_2$ measured in kPa.

Describes what happens to pH, $P\text{CO}_2$ and $[HCO_3^-]$ in various acid–base disturbances.

Maximal efficiency of a buffering system occurs at pH values close to its pKa. pKa for carbonic acid/bicarbonate is 6.1 at body temperature; its importance arises from the ability to excrete CO_2 via the lungs.
[Lawrence Henderson (1878–1942), US biochemist; Karl Hasselbalch (1874–1962), Danish physiologist]
See also, Acid–base balance

Henry's law. Amount of gas dissolved in a solvent is proportional to its partial pressure above the solvent, at constant temperature.
[William Henry (1744–1836), English chemist]

Heparin sodium/calcium. **Anticoagulant drug**, used to prevent and treat thromboembolism. Has also been used in **DIC**. Discovered in 1916. Mucopolysaccharide, derived from animal lung and intestine. Strongly acidic and electronegative, binding strongly to proteins and amines.
- Actions:
    –accelerates the action of antithrombin III, a naturally occurring inhibitor of activated **coagulation** factors XII, XI, IX, X and thrombin.
    –inhibits **platelet** aggregation by fibrin.
    –activates lipoprotein lipase, involved in fat transport.
    –thought to be involved in immunological/inflammatory reactions, possibly via binding to **histamine** and **5–HT**. Contained within **mast cells**.

Short acting, with **half-life** of about 90 minutes; therefore most effectively given by iv infusion (heparin sodium). Effects persist for 4–6 hours. Effects are monitored by measuring the activated partial thromboplastin time (APTT), although thrombin and clotting times are also prolonged.

Given sc (heparin sodium or calcium) to prevent **DVT**, e.g. perioperatively, but possibly with wide individual variation in effect. Low mw heparin sodium is thought to cause minimal systemic anticoagulant effects, by inhibiting factor X only. It also has less effect on platelet function and a longer half-life.

'Units' are defined according to the anticoagulant effect on sheep's blood under standard conditions; 1 mg is approximately equivalent to 100–110 units.

Metabolized by hepatic heparinase to products excreted via urine.
- Dosage:
    –for treatment of thrombosis, 5000 units iv, then 1000–2000 units/h (14–28 units/kg/h) by infusion, or 5000–10 000 units iv 4 hourly by bolus. APPT is kept at 1.5–2.5 times normal.
    –for prophylaxis of DVT, 5000 units sc 2 hours preoperatively, then 8–12 hourly until the patient is

walking. 10 000 units sc 12 hourly is used in pregnancy. For low mw heparin:
- –dalteparin sodium: 2500 units sc 1–2 hours preoperatively (repeated after 12 hours in high risk patients), followed by 2500 units once daily (5000 units if high risk) for 5 days.
- –enoxaparin: 2000 units sc 1–2 hours preoperatively (4000 units 12 hours preoperatively in high risk patients), followed by 2000 units once daily (4000 units if high risk) for 7–10 days.
- –during arterial surgery, 100 units/kg iv; for **cardiac surgery**, 300 units/kg.
- Side effects: bleeding, thrombocytopenia, hypersensitivity, osteoporosis. Cessation of infusion is usually adequate if bleeding occurs; **protamine**, a specific antidote, may be given.

Hirsh J (1991) New Engl J Med; 324: 1565–74
See also, Coagulation studies

Hepatic failure. May follow:
- –chronic disease and cirrhosis:
  - –chronic autoimmune **hepatitis**.
  - –chronic viral hepatitis.
  - –drugs, e.g. **methyldopa, alcohol**.
  - –metabolic disease, e.g. haemochromatosis, Wilson's disease, α_1–antitrypsin deficiency, other **inborn errors of metabolism**.
  - –biliary disease, e.g. primary biliary cirrhosis.
  - –vascular lesions, e.g. venous occlusion, chronic **cardiac failure**.
- –acute disease (fulminant hepatic failure):
  - –acute viral hepatitis.
  - –drugs, e.g. **paracetamol, halothane, chloroform, chlorpromazine, monoamine oxidase inhibitors, phenytoin**, isoniazid.
  - –others: less common, including:
    - –poisons, e.g. carbon tetrachloride.
    - –portal vein thrombosis.
    - –pregnancy.
    - –**shock.**
    - –**Reye' s syndrome**.
- Features:
  - –chronic liver disease:
    - –malaise, GIT symptoms.
    - –**jaundice**.
    - –skin: spider naevi, palmar erythema, leukonychia, finger clubbing, Dupuytren's contracture, bruising, pigmentation.
    - –hepatic fetor.
    - –gynaecomastia and testicular atrophy, caused by decreased metabolism of circulating oestrogens.
    - –neurological impairment: thought to be caused by reduced metabolism of toxic waste products, e.g. ammonia, methionine and fatty acids. May be provoked by stress, including surgery, trauma and infection. Classified thus:
      - –stage 1: impaired personality or thinking. EEG is usually normal.
      - –stage 2: confusion, abnormal sleep and drowsiness. Asterixis and increased reflexes, with plantar response up or down. EEG is abnormal.
      - –stage 3: marked confusion, with inability to perform fine movement. Responds to painful stimuli.
      - –stage 4: comatose with depressed reflexes.

Treatment includes reduction of nitrogen intake, and oral administration of lactulose (20–50 ml/day) and/or neomycin (1 g 4–6 hourly) to reduce ammonia-producing GIT bacteria and encourage nitrogen-utilizing bacteria.
- –portal hypertension is caused by vascular occlusion, possibly due to fibrotic changes in cirrhosis. It may cause splenomegaly and enlargement of portal–systemic vascular anastomoses, e.g. oesophagogastric junction, retroperitoneal and umbilical vessels. Oesophageal varices may cause severe haemorrhage; treatment may include injection of varices with sclerosant, iv infusion of **vasopressin** or analogues, administration of **somatostatin**, use of a **Sengstaken–Blakemore tube**, or rarely surgery.
- –GIT haemorrhage: apart from oesophageal varices, may also be caused by gastric erosions or **peptic ulcer disease. Coagulation** factors and **platelets** may be reduced. **Anaemia** is common.
- –**hypoproteinaemia**, with reduced plasma **oncotic pressure**, drug binding, **immunoglobulins, cholinesterase** and coagulation factors.
- –fluid retention: may cause ascites, **pleural effusion**, peripheral **oedema** and hyperdynamic circulation. Treatment includes **spironolactone**, sodium restriction and drainage of ascites/pleural effusion.
- –hypoxaemia is common, caused by $\dot{V}/\dot{Q}$ **mismatch, atelectasis**, diaphragmatic splinting or pleural effusion.
- –infection is common, especially bacterial.
- –renal impairment may occur.
- –metabolic and respiratory **alkalosis** may occur.
- –acute fulminant hepatic failure: defined as hepatic failure occurring within 8 weeks of illness, in a previously normal liver. It presents with rapidly progressing encephalopathy, coma and **cerebral oedema**, with **hypoglycaemia, hyponatraemia, hypokalaemia**, alkalosis, **hypothermia, respiratory failure**, haemorrhage, and **renal failure**. Renal failure may be due to **hepatorenal syndrome** or acute tubular necrosis. Jaundice is uncommon initially. **DIC** and infection may occur. Treatment is supportive, including nutritional support with dextrose. **Haemoperfusion** has been used.
- Anaesthetic management of patients with hepatic failure or chronic liver disease:
  - –directed towards the above complications, particularly **preoperative assessment** for, and improvement of:
    - –encephalopathy, and haematological and coagulation abnormalities.
    - –pulmonary and renal function.
    - –fluid, acid–base and electrolyte disturbance.
  - **Vitamin K** may be administered if coagulation is abnormal, plasma if surgery is urgent.
  - –anaesthetic technique: increased doses of iv agents and neuromuscular blocking drugs may be required in cirrhosis, due to increased **volume of distribution**, but elimination may be prolonged. Opioids should be used cautiously. All sedative drugs require careful use if encephalopathy is present. Drug metabolism is reduced; **isoflurane** and **atracurium** are often preferred as reliance on metabolism is less than with other agents. Halothane is often avoided because of

Table 17. Scoring system for anaesthesia in hepatic failure

| | Points scored | | |
	1	2	3
Bilirubin (μmol/l)	<25	25–40	>40
Albumin (g/l)	>35	28–35	<28
Prothrombin time prolongation (s)	<4	4–6	>6
Encephalopathy stage	0	1–2	3–4

halothane hepatitis, although its incidence is not increased in hepatic impairment. Halothane may reduce hepatic blood flow more than isoflurane or **enflurane**; **cyclopropane** is especially detrimental. **Hypocapnia** exacerbates the reduction in hepatic blood flow during general anaesthesia.
–screening for infectious hepatitis should be performed.
–maintenance of good per- and postoperative renal function is important (*see Jaundice*).
A scoring system has been devised for assessment of risk, depending on preoperative blood tests and clinical assessment (Table 17). Good operative risk is suggested by < 6 points, moderate by 7–9 points, and poor risk by > 10 points.
[Baron Guillaume Dupuytren (1777–1835), French surgeon; Samuel AK Wilson (1878–1937), US-born English neurologist]
O'Grady J, Williams R (1987) Hosp Update; 13: 481–94

Hepatitis. Acute hepatitis may be:
–viral:
  –hepatitis A:
    –RNA enterovirus, spread via the orofaecal route. Incubation period is 3–5 weeks.
    –causes fever, headache, GIT symptoms, impaired **liver function tests**, **jaundice** and hepatomegaly.
    –recovery is usually within 6 weeks, although malaise may persist longer.
    –passive immunization with immunoglobulin is available.
  –hepatitis B:
    –DNA virus, spread mainly via blood/blood products and body secretions, including homosexual contact, tattooing, iv drug abuse and childbirth. Incubation period is 2–6 months.
    –features are as for hepatitis A but more severe. May lead to recovery, death or a chronic infective state. The latter includes asymptomatic carriage or chronic hepatitis which may lead to hepatocellular carcinoma or **hepatic failure**.
    –serological markers include surface (Australia) antigen (HBsAg), e antigen (HBeAg), corresponding antibodies (anti-HBs, anti-HBe) and antibody to core antigen (anti-HBc). Pattern:
      –HBsAg: increases 1 month after exposure, peaks at 2–3 months, and falls at 4–5 months.
      –HBeAg: increases at 1 month, peaks at 2 months, and falls at 3 months.
      –anti-HBc: increases at 2 months, peaks at 4 months, and falls slowly thereafter.

      –anti-HBe: increases at 2–3 months, remaining elevated.
      –anti-HBs: increases at 1–2 months, remaining elevated.
    –asymptomatic carrier state is associated with HBsAg, HBeAg and anti-HBc expression. Its incidence is under 0.1% in the West, and up to 20% in South East Asia.
    –prevention:
      –active immunization (against HBsAg) of medical workers and high risk groups, e.g. homosexuals, drug abusers, multiple blood transfusion recipients, renal dialysis patients, babies of infected mothers, and inmates of mental institutions.
      –passive immunization using immunoglobulin; preferably performed within 24 hours of exposure and certainly within 7 days.
      –screening of blood for transfusion, use of disposable needles, etc.; operating theatre precautions as for **HIV infection**.
  –hepatitis C (causes most cases of what was previously called non-A non-B hepatitis):
    –RNA virus; a serological marker was recently discovered. Previously diagnosed by exclusion.
    –thought to be responsible for over 90% of post-transfusion hepatitis in the Western world. Also common in patients receiving renal dialysis.
    –causes a similar spectrum of disease to hepatitis A and B, but with incubation period up to 60 days. High rates of chronic infection and cirrhosis occur.
  –hepatitis D (delta): RNA virus, dependent on coexistent hepatitis B infection.
  –hepatitis E (enteral non-A non-B infection): RNA virus, recently characterized.
  –other viral infections include cytomegalovirus and glandular fever.
–due to other infections, e.g. toxoplasmosis, leptospirosis.
–chemical:
  –idiosyncratic, e.g. **phenothiazines**, **monoamine oxidase inhibitors**, **tricyclic antidepressants**, **halothane**, **chloroform**, **methyldopa**, **indomethacin**, erythromycin, rifampicin, chlorpropamide.
  –dose-related, e.g. **paracetamol**, carbon tetrachloride, **alcohol**.
–metabolic, e.g. Wilson's disease, or associated with pregnancy.
–associated with circulatory abnormalities, e.g. right ventricular failure, severe hypotension.
The cause of postoperative hepatitis is difficult to determine because many factors may be involved. 1 in 700 fit patients may have incidental impaired liver function tests preoperatively. Chronic hepatitis is one cause of chronic liver disease and cirrhosis leading to hepatic failure.
[Samuel AK Wilson (1878–1937), US-born English neurologist]
See also, Environmental safety of anaesthetists

Hepatorenal syndrome. Renal impairment secondary to hepatic dysfunction. Thought to be caused by renal vasoconstriction, possibly due to excess **endotoxin** reaching the kidneys caused by bile salt deficiency. Excess bilirubin within renal tubules may also contribute. May occur perioperatively in patients with **hepatic failure** and **jaundice**, especially if dehydration exists.

Causes oliguria, with concentrated urine containing little sodium and few granular casts; i.e. resembles prerenal **renal failure**, but does not improve with fluid replacement. Blood urea may be low because of impaired production by the liver.

Prognosis is poor unless hepatic function improves. Acute tubular necrosis may also occur perioperatively (high urinary sodium concentration and isosmotic urine) and has a better prognosis.

Maintenance of adequate **urine** output, e.g. using **mannitol**, reduces the incidence of renal failure in hepatic disease. Both forms of renal impairment are more likely in sepsis.

Wilkinson SP (1987) Intensive Care Med; 13: 145–7

Hereditary angioneurotic oedema. Congenital deficiency of C1 esterase inhibitor, or inhibition of its action, leading to **complement** activation with inflammatory swelling affecting the face, mouth, skin and intestine. Of autosomal recessive inheritance. May occur spontaneously or following trauma, possibly via activation of **kinins**, plasmins or other proteases. A similar form may occur in lymphomas. May cause upper **airway obstruction**. Management of an acute episode is as for airway obstruction; iv adrenaline, steroids, antihistamines, aprotinin, antifibrinolytic drugs and danazol have been tried, with varying results. Fresh frozen plasma (which contains C1 esterase inhibitor) is a specific treatment; 2–4 units may be given. 10 days' preoperative treatment with danazol has been suggested, and avoidance of upper airway instrumentation if possible.

Hering–Breuer reflex (Inflation reflex). Inhibition of respiratory muscles following lung inflation, leading to curtailment of inspiration. Afferent pathway is thought to be from **pulmonary stretch receptors** via the vagus. Of minor importance in man, but active in many other mammals; bilateral vagotomy produces slow deep breathing in the latter but not the former.
[Karl Hering (1834–1918), German physiologist; Josef Breuer (1852–1925), Austrian psychiatrist]

Heroin, *see Diamorphine*

Hertz. SI **unit** of frequency. 1 Hz = 1 cycle per second.
[Heinrich Hertz (1857–1894), German physicist]

Hespan, *see Hetastarch*

Hetastarch. Synthetic **colloid**. Of similar structure to **glycogen**, consisting of chains of glucose molecules, 70% of which are linked with hydroxyethyl groups. Mean mw is 450 000 and median mw 70 000; i.e. most molecules are small, but some are very large. The smallest molecules (mw < 50 000) are excreted rapidly in the urine; the larger ones are broken down slowly, although the glucose-hydroxyethyl bonds remain unbroken.

Used as an **iv fluid**; it causes sustained increase in plasma volume, by just over the volume infused, for over 24 hours. Elimination **half-life** is approximately 17 days; some remnants have been found in the reticuloendothelial system several years after administration, although the significance of this is unknown.

Slightly prolonged coagulation may occur after large infused volumes. Allergic reactions are very rare and mild. Does not interfere with blood cross-matching after up to 20% of blood volume.

Presented as 6% hetastarch in 0.9% saline; pH is about 5.5.

A lower mw analogue, **pentastarch**, has been developed.

Hewer, Christopher Langton (1896–1986). English anaesthetist, of major importance in the establishment and evolution of anaesthesia in the UK. Popularized the use of **trichloroethylene** in 1941. Edited *Anaesthesia* for its first 20 years, also *Recent Advances in Anaesthesia and Analgesia* for 50 years. Received many honours and medals.

Hewitt, Frederick (1857–1916). English anaesthetist, practised at St George's Hospital. Renowned for many contributions to anaesthesia, including the first fixed-proportion N_2O/O_2 machine, also inhalers, airways and other equipment. A strong advocate of teaching and high standards in anaesthesia. Knighted in 1911.

Hexaflourenium. Drug formerly used to prolong the action of **suxamethonium** by up to 10 times, by inhibiting plasma **cholinesterase**. Injected before suxamethonium; it may reduce muscle fasciculation due to a mild non-depolarizing action. Arrhythmias and bronchospasm have occurred.

Hexamethonium. Ganglion blocking drug, formerly used iv for **hypotensive anaesthesia**.

HFJV, HFPPV, HFO, HFV, *see High frequency ventilation*

Hiatus hernia. Protrusion of stomach through the diaphragmatic crura into the thorax. May be sliding (type I), when the oesophagocardiac junction and upper stomach move into the thorax, or rolling (type II), when this junction remains intra-abdominal but part of the fundus herniates. The former is more common and more likely to cause gastro-oesophageal valve incompetence; the latter is more likely to strangulate.
More common in the elderly and in **obesity**.
- Symptoms:
  –epigastric pain, belching, indigestion.
  –regurgitation; may lead to stricture formation.
  –GIT bleeding may occur.
- Anaesthetic problems:
  –**aspiration of gastric contents**:
    –chronic pulmonary damage due to repeated aspiration.
    –risk of acute aspiration perioperatively.
  –chronic **anaemia**.
- Management:
  –medical: weight loss, **antacids**, **H$_2$ receptor antagonists**.
  –surgical: repair of the diaphragmatic defect and fundoplasty: the oesphagogastric junction is invaginated into a sleeve of fundus (Nissen's plication). Requires laparotomy and possibly thoracotomy, and may be lengthy.
[Rudolph Nissen, Swiss surgeon]
See also, Diaphragmatic herniae; Gastro-oesophageal reflux; Lower oesophageal sphincter

Hiccups. Spasmodic diaphragmatic contractions, causing sudden inspiration and glottic closure. May involve phrenic or vagal afferents. During anaestheia, may be provoked by surgical stimulation, especially around the diaphragm, and particularly in the presence of inadequate paralysis and/or light anaesthesia. May follow use of **methohexitone** and **etomidate**, and may occur during **spinal/extradural anaesthesia**.

- Rarely troublesome, but the following have been suggested as treatment:
  - –deepening anaesthesia.
  - –increasing analgesia and muscle relaxation.
  - –hyperventilation.
  - –nasal/pharyngeal stimulation.
  - –**metoclopramide** 10 mg or **chlorpromazine** 25 mg iv.

May also occur in **hepatic failure**, **uraemia**, and lesions and infections affecting the medulla.

Hickman, Henry Hill (1800–1830). English surgeon, practising in Ludlow and Shifnall, Shropshire. First described the production of insensibility in animals by exposure to a gas (CO_2) and suggested its use for painless surgery, in 1824. His efforts to publicise his experiments were unsuccessful, both in the UK and abroad.

Hickman line, *see Central venous cannulation, long-term*

High dependency unit (HDU). Area for patients who require more intensive monitoring or treatment than is available on a general ward, but who do not require IPPV or intensive care. Used for care of patients with medical or surgical conditions, postoperative care of high-risk patients including those undergoing major surgery, monitoring of respiration in patients receiving **spinal opioids**, care of patients discharged from **ICU** but not yet ready for general ward care, etc. Costs and nursing requirements are midway between those of general wards and ICUs.

High frequency ventilation (HFV). Mechanism of respiratory support developed in the 1970s. Small breaths are delivered at high frequencies, maintaining gas exchange without **barotrauma** or other deleterious effects of **IPPV**. May be superimposed on spontaneous ventilation.

- Three modes are used:
  - –high frequency positive-pressure ventilation (HFPPV): 60–150 cycles/min, delivered via an intratracheal insufflation catheter, bronchoscope or **tracheal tube**. Tidal volumes of 100–400 ml are used. Fluidic valves are often used, without moving parts. Possible using some conventional **ventilators**, especially paediatric ones.
  - –high frequency jet ventilation (HFJV). 60–600 cycles/min, delivered via a cannula inserted through the cricothyroid membrane, placed within a bronchoscope, etc., or incorporated near the tip of a tracheal tube. Expiration is continuous through the open system. Principles of gas entrainment are as for **injector techniques**. Tidal volume is up to 150 ml. Produces positive airway pressure of about 5 cmH2O. Most ventilators employ electrical solenoid valves.
  - –high frequency oscillation (HFO). 500–3000 cycles/min; the gas column is oscillated with an O_2 input via a side arm. CO_2 exits via another side arm.

The mechanism of gas exchange is unclear but is thought to involve continuous mixing of gases. HFJV is most commonly used, especially in paediatrics, thoracic procedures and ENT endoscopy. HFO is also used in children, and in combination with low frequency ventilation.

Initial enthusiasm has waned because of costly, complicated and noisy equipment. Difficulties of using inhalational anaesthetic agents and monitoring also limit its use. However, it has been advocated for **ENT surgery**, sleeve resection of bronchi, tracheal surgery and **bronchopleural fistula**, where increased airway pressure and excessive movement may be detrimental. Tracheal suction is possible without interruption of ventilation. HFV has also been used in **weaning from ventilators** and in **ARDS**. HFJV via crycothyrotomy has been suggested as an alternative to tracheal intubation and IPPV in **respiratory failure**.
Smith BE (1990) Br J Anaesth; 65: 130–8

His bundle electrography. Technique for investigating cardiac conduction defects and tachycardias, using transvenous intracardiac bipolar electrodes at various sites. Concurrent recording of a formal **ECG** is usually undertaken. Information may be obtained about conduction through different parts of the **heart conducting system**, and the site of delayed conduction identified. May also be used to distinguish supraventricular from ventricular arrhythmias; ventricular complexes in the former are preceded by His bundle activity. The effects of pacing stimuli at different sites may also be observed, e.g. in assessment of refractory tachycardias.
[Wilhelm His (1863–1934), German anatomist]

Histamine and histamine receptors. Histamine is present in **mast cells**, basophils, gastric mucosa and the CNS. It is involved in the inflammatory response and gastric acid secretion, and is thought to be a **neurotransmitter**, although its role as the latter is unclear. Synthesized by decarboxylation of L-histidine, and broken down by deamination and/or methylation.

- Histamine receptor subsets have been identified:
  - –H1:
    - –cause smooth muscle contraction in the GIT and uterus, and bronchoconstriction via cholinergic pathways following stimulation of irritant pulmonary receptors.
    - –cause vascular smooth muscle relaxation and dilatation, with increased vascular permeability.
    - –cause stimulation and irritation of cutaneous nerve endings.
  - –H2:
    - –cause some vasodilatation (but less then H1 receptors).
    - –have direct inotropic and chronotropic effects on isolated hearts, but hypotension usually results from vasodilatation.
    - –increase acid, pepsin and intrinsic factor secretion from gastric mucosa.
  - –H3: presynaptic; thought to inhibit histamine release.

H2 actions are thought to be mediated via **cAMP**, and H1 via cyclic guanosine monophosphate.
Specific receptor antagonists have been developed; they are called **antihistamine drugs** (H1) and **H2 receptor antagonists** largely for historical reasons (the latter were discovered many years after the former).

Histamine is released from mast cells following iv injection of certain drugs, e.g. **tubocurarine** and **morphine**. The amount released depends partially on the rate of injection. Skin wheals, hypotension and bronchospasm may occur.
See also, Anaphylactoid reactions; Carcinoid syndrome

Histamine receptor antagonists, *see Antihistamine drugs; H₂ receptor antagonists*

HIV, *see Human immunodeficiency viral infection*

Hofmann degradation. Spontaneous degradation of amides (RCONH₂) to amines (RNH₂), and quaternary ammonium salts to tertiary ones, under certain physical conditions. **Atracurium** (a quaternary ammonium compound) spontaneously degrades to **laudanosine** at body temperature and plasma pH.
[August von Hofmann (1818–1892), German chemist]

Holmes, Oliver Wendell (1809–1894). US physician, poet and author; Professor of Anatomy at Harvard, Boston. Famous for his treatise on puerperal fever and its prevention, and for his non-medical writing. Suggested **anaesthesia** as a suitable term for ether narcosis.

Homeostasis. Maintenance of physiological variables within normal limits, allowing optimal functioning of tissues and cells. Includes maintenance of **acid–base balance**, **fluid balance**, **temperature regulation**, **arterial BP**, hormone secretion, etc. Most mechanisms involve negative feedback; i.e. an increase of a substance or parameter causes direct inhibition of mechanisms which increase it, bringing about its restoration to normal; deficiency results in stimulation of these mechanisms.

Horner's syndrome. Clinical picture resulting from interruption of sympathetic innervation to the head. Originally described with cervical lesions, it may be due to lesions anywhere along the sympathetic pathway. Consists of partial ptosis, meiosis, apparent enophthalmos, lack of sweating and nasal stuffiness on the affected side.
[Johann Horner (1831–1886), Swiss ophthalmologist]

5–HT, *see 5–Hydroxytryptamine*

Hüfner constant. The volume of O₂ carried by 1 g **haemoglobin**; e.g. used in the calculation of **O₂ delivery** and **O₂ flux**. Figures vary, according to whether it is measured *in vitro* or *in vivo*; 1.39 and 1.34 ml are most commonly quoted, respectively. The latter value is most relevant clinically.
[Carl von Hüfner (1840–1908), German physician]

Human immunodeficiency viral infection (HIV infection). First recognized in 1981 in the US as the acquired immunodeficiency syndrome (AIDS) in otherwise healthy homosexual males. The retrovirus, human immunodeficiency virus (HIV-I), was previously called human T-cell lymphotrophic virus type III (HTLV-III), or lymphadenopathy associated virus (LAV). HIV-II has been identified, mainly in West Africa, where the disease is thought to have originated.
Infection has been estimated to be present in up to 1 000 000 people in the USA and 50 000to 150 000 in the UK.
• Transmitted mainly via semen and blood, i.e. via:

–homosexual, and heterosexual (especially male to female) contact.
–transfusion of **blood products**.
–infected needles, e.g. used by drug addicts.
–transplacentally or at delivery.
–spillage of infected blood on to broken skin, or into the eye.
The virus may be isolated from other body fluids, e.g. vaginal secretions, saliva, tears, etc.. Transmission by mouth to mouth contact, e.g. during **CPR**, is not thought to occur.
High risk groups include promiscuous homo- and heterosexuals and their partners, iv drug abusers, haemophiliacs, Haitians and Central/West Africans.
Causes impaired helper T lymphocyte function, with increased susceptibilty to infection and malignancy; it may also affect the CNS. Mortality is unknown, but is thought to approach 100% for AIDS.
• Features:
–most infected people are thought to be asymptomatic.
–an acute flu-like illness may occur 1–3 weeks after infection. The incubation period may be as long as several years.
–weight loss, diarrhoea, fever and thrush (AIDS-related complex) commonly progress to AIDS itself. Persistent generalized lymphadenopathy is thought to progress less often. Thrombocytopenic purpura and anaemia, dementia, encephalitis and psychosis may occur, related to HIV infection itself or secondary infection by other organisms.
–AIDS: opportunistic infection (especially *Pneumocystis carinii* chest infection), Kaposi's sarcoma, lymphoma.
A more recent re-definition has been suggested:
–acute infection.
–asymptomatic infection.
–persistent generalized lymphadenopathy.
–others, including generalized malaise, secondary infection/malignancy, neurological and other disease.
Diagnosed clinically and by serum antibody detection. Time between infection and seroconversion is thought to be approximately 3 months. HIV infection reduces the helper T4 population (defined by the CD4 surface antigen, thought to be the major receptor for the virus on target cells). The CD4 count may fall gradually or suddenly; a count below 200/mm³ may indicate increased risk of opportunistic infection. Early in HIV infection, the suppressor/cytotoxic T cell population (defined by the CD8 antigen) may increase, subsequently becoming normal or reduced. The CD4:CD8 ratio has been used to monitor progress of the infection.
• Treatment:
–supportive, e.g. nutrition, treatment of infection, etc. Co-trimoxazole and pentamidine are usually used for Pneumocystis infection; the latter may be given iv, im, or by nebulizer to reduce side effects (and as prophylaxis). Side effects include hypotension, hypoglycaemia, renal and hepatic impairment, blood dyscrasias and arrhythmias.
–disease suppression, either of AIDS or related states: zidovudine (AZT) interferes with viral DNA replication and is increasingly used. Anaemia and leucopenia are common; nausea and peripheral neuropathy may occur.
• Anaesthetic considerations:
–features of illness and drug therapy as above.

–patients are at risk from infection as for **immunodeficiency**.

–measures to protect staff and other patients from HIV infection:
  –simple hygiene.
  –avoidance of use of needles/parenteral medication.
  –wearing of gowns, goggles, gloves and overshoes.
  –careful disposal of sharps and other equipment. Needles should not be resheathed after use. Hospitals should have policies for management of accidental needlestick injuries (*see Environmental safety of anaesthetists*).
  –use of disposable equipment where possible.
  –minimal equipment in operating theatre.
  –induction of anaesthesia and recovery in theatre.
  –filters on breathing tubing if not disposable.
  –all non-disposable equipment is soaked in hypochlorite or gluteraldehyde solution after use; theatre equipment, walls, floors, etc. are washed down.
  –general considerations:
    –blood and its products are used increasingly sparingly; although donor blood is screened for anti-HIV antibodies, virus infection without seroconversion cannot be excluded.
    –iv equipment should not be used for more than one patient.
  –selection of cases requiring high risk procedures:
    (i) performed on every patient as routine.
    (ii) performed only for high risk groups as above.
    (iii) performed only if seropositive.
    The first option is increasingly employed, especially in the USA, although costly and time consuming. Routine testing is controversial, because of the implications of a positive test result on employment, social standing, life assurance, etc. Testing in the USA is more common than in the UK, and requires full consent and appropriate pretest counselling.
  –ICU treatment is along similar lines, but protective wear is required less for routine care. Admission of HIV infected patients is controversial; in general, they are admitted only for treatment of acute, curable episodes, e.g. chest infections.

[Moricz K Kaposi (1837–1902), Austrian dermatologist]
Cantineau JP (1989) Curr Opin Anaesth; 2: 349–52

Humidification. Inspired air is normally maximally humidified in the naso-/oropharynx, becoming saturated by the time it reaches the trachea. Absolute **humidity** in the upper trachea is 34 g/m³ (i.e. fully saturated at 34°C); in alveoli it is 43 g/m³ (i.e. fully saturated at 37°C). Delivery of dry gases to the trachea, e.g. via a tracheal tube or tracheostomy, may cause drying of the respiratory mucosa with reduced **ciliary activity**, keratinization and ulceration, and increased tenacity of mucus with plugging of airways, atelectasis and reduced gas exchange. Humidification of inspired gases prevents this and reduces heat loss, partly by warming the gases (under 2% of total basal heat loss) but more importantly by avoiding the requirement for **latent heat** of vaporization (10–15% of total basal heat loss) within the trachea.

Humidification is thus required during ventilation on ICUs. It is also particularly important during prolonged anaesthesia, and in the elderly, children, severely ill patients and those with respiratory disease. It has been suggested as being mandatory during all anaesthetics.

• Humidification of the patient's environment may be achieved, e.g. with an O_2 tent, but it is usually restricted to inspired gases only. Methods:
  –passive:
    –tracheal water/saline instillation; inefficient and potentially dangerous.
    –bubbling inspired gas through cold water; simple but relatively inefficient (up to 10 g/m³ produced). Vaporization cools the water, increasing inefficiency.
    –heat–moisture exchanger (Swedish nose; hygroscopic condenser); fits on the end of tracheal/tracheostomy tubes. Contains material (e.g. sponges or metal gauze) which can absorb large amounts of water. As expired gas passes through, water vapour condenses on the sponge which is also heated. The water and heat are given up when dry cool inspiratory gas passes through. May be disposable or refillable. Light and cheap; with up to 90% efficiency for modern devices. However, they increase dead space and may act as an infection source with prolonged use. They may also increases resistance to spontaneous ventilation.
  –active, i.e. energy source required; commonly used in ICU because efficiency is high:
    –hot water bath: up to 60°C is employed in some, to reduce bacterial contamination. Inspired gas is passed over or through the water. Efficiency is increased by passing gas through a perforated screen to form tiny bubbles (cascade humidifier), or using absorbent wicks to increase surface area. Humidified gas is unsaturated at the working temperature, but becomes near-saturated as the temperature falls along the tubing to the patient. Condensation of water within the tubing may be reduced by heating wires within the tubing, giving closer control of the temperature drop between machine and patient. Risk of delivering excessively hot gases is reduced by monitoring the temperature within the humidifier and at the patient end of the tubing (usually kept at about 35°C), using thermostat controls and alarms.
    –other heated humidifiers, e.g. dropping water on to a heated element.
  –**nebulizers**.

Infection risks (typically with Pseudomonas) are reduced by addition of antiseptic to the water, maintenance at high temperature where appropriate, and changing tubing and water regularly (e.g. every 24 hours). Condensation within tubing may provide foci for infection, obstruct ventilation, or drain water into the patient's airways. The level of the water source should be kept below that of the patient. Overheating and **electrocution** may also occur.

Shelly MP, Lloyd GM, Park GR (1988) Intensive Care Med; 14: 1–9

Humidity. Absolute humidity is the amount of water vapour per unit volume of gas at given temperature and pressure, in g/m³ or mg/l.

Relative humidity (%) is the absolute humidity divided by the amount present when the gas is fully saturated at the same temperature and pressure.

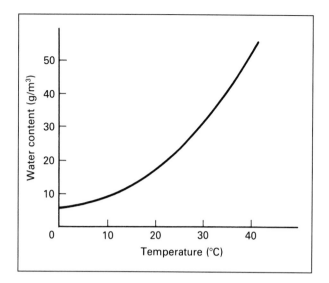

Figure 71 *Water content of saturated air at different temperatures*

Maximal possible water content varies with temperature (Fig. 71). Thus heating a gas does not affect its absolute humidity, since the amount of water contained remains constant, but relative humidity is reduced, because warmer gas can contain more water vapour.
- Normal values of absolute humidity in:
    –upper trachea: 34 g/m³ (fully saturated at 34°C)
    –alveoli: 43 g/m³ (fully saturated at 37°C)
Usual value of relative humidity in operating theatres: 50–60%. Higher values are too uncomfortable; lower values increase risk of sparks. Measured using a **hygrometer**.
See also, Humidification

Hunter's disease, *see Inborn errors of metabolism*

Huntington's chorea. Rare autosomal dominant inherited disorder, resulting in neurological degeneration in middle life. Ataxia, dementia and choreiform movements occur, with emaciation and death usually within 15 years. Increased sensitivity to **barbiturates** and prolonged action of **suxamethonium** have been reported.
[George Huntington (1850–1916), US physician]

Hurler's disease, *see Inborn errors of metabolism*

Hyaline membrane disease, *see Respiratory distress syndrome*

Hyaluronidase. Enzyme which reversibly depolymerizes hyaluronic acid, a polysaccharide present in connective tissue. Aids dispersal and absorption of drugs, fluids, etc., given sc or im, by intention or accident. Has also been mixed with **local anaesthetic agents** to aid spread. Administration: 1500 international units (one ampoule) in 1–2 ml water is injected into the absorption site, before, after or together with the drug. May be injected through a sc cannula prior to administration of fluid (hypodermoclysis), allowing up to 1000 ml to be given into the thigh, calf, chest, abdomen or back regions.

Hydralazine hydrochloride. Vasodilator drug, acting mainly on arterioles. Used to lower BP, e.g. in **hypertension**, **hypotensive anaesthesia** and **pre-eclampsia**. **Half-life** is 2–3 hours; up to 16 hours in renal failure. Certain patients acetylate the drug quickly, reducing half-life to under 1 hour. Its onset of action may be up to 15 minutes after iv bolus, with effects lasting up to 90 minutes.
- Dosage:
    –25–50 mg orally 12 hourly.
    –5–20 mg iv.
    –200–300 µg/min by infusion initially, then 50–150 µg/min.
- Side effects:
    –hypotension, tachycardia, fluid retention, nausea.
    –systemic lupus erythematosus syndrome, especially in slow acetylators and following prolonged oral therapy at a dose greater than 100 mg/day.

Hydrocephalus. Increased **CSF** volume. May be caused by increased production or decreased drainage, usually the latter:
    –non-communicating: blockage between the lateral ventricles and 4th ventricular outlets.
    –communicating: blockage distal to the 4th ventricular outlets, e.g. at the basal cisterns.
- Causes:
    –congenital, e.g. narrowed aqueduct, obstruction of 4th ventricle outlet by a membrane (Dandy–Walker syndrome), herniation of the cerebellar tonsils through the foramen magnum (Arnold–Chiari syndrome), etc.
    –acquired: **meningitis** with adhesions, surgery, **head injury**, tumour, etc..
Usually accompanied by increased **ICP**; it may be acute, requiring urgent drainage. Pressure may be normal in some chronic forms, with slow ventricular enlargement. Head size is increased in children, with bulging of fontanelles. Cerebral or cerebellar atrophy may be present.
- Treatment:
    –surgery to the obstructive lesion.
    –shunt insertion:
        –bypassing the obstructed portion only.
        –from lateral ventricle to peritoneum or right atrium.
- Anaesthesic considerations:
    –as for **neonates/paediatric anaesthesia**.
    –as for **neurosurgery**.
    –head enlargement may hinder tracheal intubation.
[Walter E Dandy (1886–1946) and Alvin E Walker, US neurosurgeons; Julius Arnold (1835–1915), German pathologist; Hans von Chiari (1851–1916), Austrian pathologist]

Hydrocodone bitartrate. Opioid analgesic drug, available in the USA together with other ingredients in oral preparations for cough and pain.

Hydrocortisone, *see Steroid therapy*

Hydrogen ions (H⁺). About 12 500–13 000 mmol are produced in the body per day, mainly from the reaction of CO_2 (produced during respiration) with water. Also produced during metabolism of foodstuffs, etc. **Acid–base balance** requires buffering and excretion to maintain extracellular hydrogen ion concentration at 34–46 nmol/l,

equivalent to **pH** of 7.34–7.46. Hydrogen ion homeostasis is required to maintain proper functioning of proteins (especially **enzymes**), etc.
See also, Acidosis; Alkalosis; Buffers

Hydromorphone hydrochloride. Opioid analgesic drug, widely used in the USA but not available in the UK. 1.5 mg is equivalent to 10 mg **morphine**, from which it is derived. Action lasts 3–5 hours. Available for rectal, oral and parenteral administration.

Hydrostatic pressure, *see Starling forces*

γ-Hydroxybutyric acid. Drug related to **GABA** and used as an **iv anaesthetic agent** in the 1960s and 1970s. Present as a **neurotransmitter**, especially in the hypothalamus and basal ganglia. Causes slow onset of anaesthesia, lasting up to 90 minutes. Has been used for paediatric anaesthesia (especially cardiac catheterization) because of its relative lack of cardiorespiratory depression, although bradycardia may occur. No longer available.

Hydroxydione. Obsolete **iv anaesthetic agent**, introduced in 1955. A steroid derivative, it produced slow induction of anaesthesia and delayed recovery, with a high incidence of thrombophlebitis.

Hydroxyethyl starch, *see Hetastarch*

5-Hydroxytryptamine (5-HT, Serotonin). Substance found in GIT enterochromaffin cells (90%) and other tissues, e.g. **platelets**, **mast cells** and CNS.
● Involved in:
  –inflammatory mechanisms: increases vascular permeability and platelet aggregation, causes bronchoconstriction, and causes vasodilatation and constriction at different vascular beds.
  –GIT function: increases motility, water and electrolyte secretion.
  –arousal, muscle tone, hypothalamic/parasympathetic regulatory mechanisms, mood, memory and spinal modulation of **pain** sensation. Functions as an inhibitory **neurotransmitter** in the brainstem, descending spinal pathways, hypothalamic, cortical, limbic and extrapyramidal systems.
Formed by hydroxylation and decarboxylation of tryptophan. Taken up from synaptic clefts via the presynaptic membrane and metabolized by **monoamine oxidase** to form 5–hydroxyindoleacetic acid; urinary levels of the latter reflect rate of metabolism.
● Acts via receptors, divided into three types:
  –5-HT$_1$: cause vascular and gut smooth muscle relaxation, hypotension and tachycardia. Thought to be subdivided into 4 subtypes.
  –5-HT$_2$: cause vascular, gut and bronchial smooth muscle contraction, and hypertension. Involved in platelet aggregation.
  –5-HT$_3$: cause bradycardia and vomiting. Involved in pain transmission.
Ondansetron, a 5-HT$_3$ receptor antagonist, is used orally or iv to reduce vomiting caused by chemotherapy or radiotherapy. Granisetron, a similar drug, has recently been made available for iv use. Other drugs are being developed for possible use in psychiatry and treatment of migraine (e.g. sumatriptan, a 5-HT$_1$ receptor agonist).

Agents which block uptake of 5-HT have been developed for use in depression.
See also, Carcinoid syndrome

Hygrometer. Device for measuring atmospheric **humidity**.
● Examples:
  –hair hygrometer: pointer attached to a hair whose length changes with differing humidity. Human hair, animal tissue or paper have been used. Inaccurate but simple.
  –Regnault's hygrometer: silver tube containing ether; cooled by blowing air through it with a rubber bulb. When condensation appears on the outside, the air is saturated with water at that temperature (**dew point**). From a graph of water content of saturated air against temperature, water content at dew point and that at room temperature may be found. Relative humidity is the latter divided by the former.
  –wet and dry bulb hygrometer: consists of two thermometer bulbs: one dry, the other wrapped in a wet wick. The wet thermometer bulb loses heat due to water evaporation, depending on atmospheric humidity. Humidity is read from tables, according to the temperatures measured by the two thermometers. Accuracy depends on adequate air movement.
  –humidity **transducers**: electrical properties of certain compounds, e.g. lithium chloride, alter as they absorb water. Electrical resistance or capacitance is usually measured.
  –**mass spectrometer**.
  –ultraviolet light absorption: depends on water content of air.
[Henri Regnault (1810–1878), French physicist]

Hygroscopic condensers, *see Humidification*

Hyoscine hydrobromide. Anticholinergic drug, used mainly for **premedication**. Tertiary ammonium compound, an ester of tropic acid and scopine; found naturally in the henbane plant. Has greater sedative, antiemetic and antisialogogue action than **atropine**, but with less action on the heart and bronchial muscle. Also used to prevent travel sickness, and (as the quaternary ammonium compound, hyoscine butylbromide) to prevent or reduce gut spasm.
● Effects:
  –sedation, **amnesia**, mydriasis, antiemetic action via the vomiting centre; may cause the **central anticholinergic syndrome**.
  –reduced bronchial and GIT secretions; reduced gut motility.
  –tachycardia (bradycardia is possible following a small dose).
● Dosage:
  –4 μg/kg for im premedication. Confusion is more likely in the elderly.
  –0.3 mg, repeated twice 6 hourly for travel sickness. Slow-release cutaneous patches are available, and have been used to reduce postoperative nausea and vomiting.
  –20 mg butylbromide orally/iv/im for GIT spasm.

Hyperaesthesia. Increased sensitivity to a sensory stimulus, excluding the special senses. Includes **allodynia** and **hyperalgesia**.

Hyperaldosteronism. Excessive **aldosterone** secretion. May be:

–primary (Conn's Syndrome):
  –causes include adrenal adenoma (most common), hyperplasia and carcinoma. Twice as common in women.
  –causes **hypertension**, **hypervolaemia**, **hypokalaemia** and metabolic **alkalosis**.
  –**spironolactone** (aldosterone inhibitor) is used to treat hyperplasia. Some forms are corrected by dexamethasone. Adenomas are treated by surgery.
  –anaesthetic considerations are related to appropriate preoperative correction of electrolyte, fluid and acid-base imbalances. Spironolactone is useful preoperatively. Cardiovascular instability may occur per- and postoperatively. Postoperative mineralocorticoid deficiency may be treated with fludrocortisone 100–300 µg/day orally.
–secondary: may occur in cardiac and hepatic failure, malignant hypertension and renal artery stenosis.
[Jerome Conn, US physician]
Weatherill D, Spence AA (1984) Br J Anaesth; 56: 741–9

Hyperalgesia. Increased **pain** from a normally painful stimulus. The term usually refers to a feature of chronic pain, but is similar to the **antanalgesia** seen with certain centrally depressant drugs.

Hyperalimentation, *see Nutrition, total parenteral*

Hypercalcaemia. Effects are due to raised ionized calcium levels; symptoms are usually present when total calcium exceeds 3.5 mmol/l.
- Caused by:
  –**hyperparathyroidism**.
  –malignancy, both primary and bony metastases.
  –less commonly:
    –increased intake , e.g. milk-alkali syndrome.
    –others: **hyperthyroidism**, **sarcoidosis**, **adrenocortical insufficiency**, immobilization, thiazide diuretics.
- Features:
  –psychiatric disturbances.
  –**dehydration**, polyuria/polydipsia.
  –nausea/vomiting, constipation.
  –muscle weakness.
  –drowsiness, **coma**.
  –shortened **Q–T interval**; prolonged **P–R interval** on the **ECG**.
  –may lead to renal calculi/nephrocalcinosis and **renal failure**.
- Treatment:
  –of underlying cause.
  –rehydration followed by induced diuresis to increase renal calcium loss, e.g. with **frusemide** and saline administration. Careful fluid balance and CVP monitoring are required.
  –in severe hypercalcaemia, especially associated with malignancy:
    –bi- (previously di-) phosphonates, e.g. disodium pamidronate 15–60 mg iv over 4 hours, with fluids. Reduces bone resorption.
    –corticosteroids, e.g. prednisolone up to 120 mg/day. Reduces bone resorption and increases renal calcium loss.
    –plicamycin (mithramycin): cytotoxic agent; may impair coagulation and bone marrow function. Hepatic and renal impairment are also reported. 25 µg/kg is given iv over 4–6 hours, repeated 1–3 times weekly. Reduces bone resorption.
    –calcitonin 4 units/kg im/sc 8–24 hourly. Reduces bone resorption.
    –trisodium edetate up to 70 mg/kg/day iv over 3 hours; rapidly acting but may cause renal failure. Chelates circulating calcium.
    –oral/iv phosphate may precipitate calcium phosphate into tissues, e.g. kidneys, especially if phosphate levels are already high. Also reduces bone resorption and GIT calcium absorption.
    –**dialysis** has been used.

Hypercapnia. Arterial P_{CO_2} over 6 kPa (45 mmHg).
- Caused by:
  –increased production, e.g. **MH**, TPN using high carbohydrate content. Average normal production is approximately 200 ml/min.
  –reduced **alveolar ventilation**.
  –$\dot{V}/\dot{Q}$ **mismatch**, e.g. severe COAD.
  –increased inspired CO_2.
- Effects:
  –respiratory:
    –arterial O_2 saturation falls below about 90% at an alveolar P_{CO_2} over about 8 kPa (60 mmHg), breathing air.
    –increased respiratory drive via central/peripheral chemoreceptors. Tidal volume and respiratory rate increase; the extent varies with other factors (*see Carbon dioxide response curve*). Respiration may become depressed at very high levels.
    –response to **hypoxaemia** is increased.
    –**oxyhaemoglobin dissociation curve** shifts to the right.
  –cardiovascular:
    –increased sympathetic activity (causing increases in circulating catecholamine levels, heart rate and arterial BP), overriding CO_2's direct myocardial depressant effect. **Arrhythmias** may occur.
    –increased **cerebral blood flow**, **ICP** and **intraocular pressure**.
  –other:
    –dilated pupils, with sluggish response.
    –respiratory **acidosis** and **hyperkalaemia**. Initial **bicarbonate** increase is about 0.76 mmol/l per kPa rise above 5.3 if hypercapnia is acute (1 mmol/l per 10 mmHg above 40). Renal compensation includes bicarbonate retention and excreting hydrogen ions; bicarbonate increase in chronic hypercapnia is about 3 mmol/l per kPa (4 mmol/l per 10 mmHg).
    –confusion, headache and coma may result (**CO₂ narcosis**).
The CNS may adjust to higher CO_2 levels than normal in chronic hypercapnia.
Treated according to cause. If P_{CO_2} is reduced too rapidly, **alkalosis** and potassium shift may occur, causing convulsions, hypotension and arrhythmias.
See also, Breathing, control of

Hyperglycaemia. Plasma **glucose** over 6.0 mmol/l (108 mg/dl).
- Caused by:

–pancreatic failure, e.g. **diabetes mellitus, pancreatitis,** sepsis, pancreatectomy.
–stress response, due to actions of **catecholamines, growth hormone, glucocorticoids, glucagon.** May occur following trauma, surgery, burns, etc. (*see Stress response to surgery*).
–administration of glucose, e.g. TPN.
–drugs, e.g. **diethyl ether, thiazide diuretics.**
● Effects:
–osmotic diuresis, causing **dehydration**, sodium and potassium loss.
–**diabetic coma**, e.g. **ketoacidosis.**
–increased blood **osmolality** and **viscosity.**
–may impair **platelet** function, increase susceptibility to infection and exacerbate effects of **cerebral ischaemia.**
–chronic effects of diabetes.
● Treatment:
–of primary cause.
–oral hypoglycaemic drugs (**biguanides** and **sulphonyl-ureas**).
–**insulin.**

Hyperkalaemia. Plasma **potassium** over 5.0 mmol/l.
● Caused by:
–increased intake, e.g. iv administration, rapid **blood transfusion.**
–decreased renal output:
 –**renal failure**:
  –acute: related to intake.
  –chronic: occurs only when **GFR** falls below 15 ml/h.
 –**adrenocortical insufficiency.**
 –drugs: cyclosporin, **angiotensin converting enzyme inhibitors**, potassium-sparing **diuretics,** e.g. amiloride, **spironolactone.**
–movement of potassium out of cells:
 –**trauma, crush syndrome**, rhabdomyolysis, **MH.**
 –action of **suxamethonium**; exaggerated in **burns,** nerve injury, etc.
 –**acidosis.**
 –**familial periodic paralysis**, etc.
–artefactual, e.g. haemolysed blood sample, very high white cell counts.
● Effects:
–nausea, vomiting, diarrhoea, muscle weakness.
–myocardial depression, **ECG** changes (peaked **T waves**, absent **P waves**, widened **QRS complexes**, and slurring of **S–T segments** into T waves). Ventricular **arrhythmias** including **VF** are common at above 7 mmol/l. **Cardiac arrest** may occur in diastole.
● Treatment:
–oral/rectal ion exchange resin, e.g. calcium resonium 15 g/30–50 g respectively, 8 hourly.
–**insulin** 20 units in 100 ml of 20% dextrose iv over 30–60 minutes (drives potassium into cells).
–**bicarbonate** 50 mmol iv may be given (exchanges potassium ions for hydrogen ions across cell membranes).
–**calcium** 5–10 mmol iv if severe (acts as a physiological antagonist of potassium).
–**dialysis.**
Hyperkalaemia should be corrected before anaesthesia and surgery, although the ratio of intracellular: extracellular potassium is more important than isolated plasma levels.
Vitez T (1987) Can J Anaesth; 34: S30–1

Hypermagnesaemia. Plasma **magnesium** over 1.05 mmol/l.
● Caused by:
–**renal failure**.
–magnesium administration.
–laxative/antacid abuse .
–**adrenocortical insufficiency**, myxoedema.
● Effects:
–vasodilatation, hypotension, cardiac conduction defects.
–sedation, coma, weakness, respiratory depression. Potentiation of **non-depolarizing neuromuscular blockade.**
● Treatment:
–encourage diuresis.
–iv **calcium**.

Hypernatraemia. Plasma **sodium** over 145 mmol/l.
● Caused by:
–sodium excess (urine sodium >20 mmol/l):
 –**hyperaldosteronism.**
 –**Cushing's syndrome.**
 –iatrogenic, e.g. sodium **bicarbonate**, hypertonic saline administration.
–water depletion (urine sodium variable):
 –renal loss, e.g. **diabetes insipidus.**
 –other:
  –**insensible water loss.**
  –insufficient water intake.
–sodium deficiency, with greater water deficiency:
 –renal loss (urine sodium >20 mmol/l), e.g. osmotic diuresis caused by **mannitol**, glucose, urea, etc.
 –other (urine sodium <10 mmol/l):
  –vomiting, diarrhoea.
  –sweating, weeping wounds.
  –**adrenocortical insufficiency.**
● Effects:
–features of **dehydration** if present.
–thirst, drowsiness, confusion, coma. Cerebral dehydration, with ruptured vessels and intracranial haemorrhage, may occur.
● Treatment:
–of underlying cause.
–oral water is given when possible, and/or diuretics in sodium excess. Normal saline may be given iv, hypotonic saline in severe water and sodium deficiency. Rapid infusion may lead to cerebral oedema and convulsions. Optimal rate of correction is controversial but full correction should take at least 48 hours.
Oh MS, Carroll HJ (1992) Crit Care Med; 20: 94–103

Hyperosmolality. Plasma **osmolality** over 305 mosmol/kg. Features are as for **hypernatraemia**, which usually accompanies it. May also occur in **hyperglycaemia**, e.g. due to **diabetic coma**, TPN, and ingestion/administration of osmotically active substances, e.g. hypertonic **mannitol** solutions or **alcohol**. Detected by hypothalamic **osmoreceptors**, causing compensatory changes in water ingestion/secretion.

Hyperparathyroidism. Increased parathyroid hormone production:
–primary: usually from a single adenoma; multiple adenomata and carcinoma may also be responsible.

May be associated with **multiple endocrine adenomatosis**.

–secondary: hyperplasia arising from prolonged **hypocalcaemia**, e.g. in **renal failure**.

–tertiary: secondary hyperparathyroidism where autonomous secretion develops, e.g. after renal transplantation.

Hormone secretion may occur in certain tumours, e.g. **bronchial carcinoma** (pseudohyperparathyroidism). May be asymptomatic.

• Features:
  –those of **hypercalcaemia**. Renal stones are common.
  –bony erosion and cystic changes may occur.

• Treatment:
  –as for hypercalcaemia.
  –surgery; primary adenomata may be difficult to find.

• Anaesthetic considerations:
  –preoperative hypercalcaemia, **dehydration** and renal impairment should be corrected before surgery.
  –decalcified bone is easily fractured, e.g. during positioning.
  –practical management of anaesthesia is as for **hyperthyroidism**.

Hyperpathia. Increased sensation from a sensory stimulus, but with raised threshold of sensation. **Pain** may increase during stimulation, and linger afterwards.

Hyperpyrexia, malignant, *see Malignant hyperthermia*

Hypersensitivity, *see Adverse drug reactions; Atopy*

Hypertension. Raised **arterial BP**; definition is difficult because of observer and subject variation, and arbitrariness of cutoff values. Upper normal limit is often taken as 140/90 mmHg for the general population. The relative importance of systolic or diastolic pressure is also controversial. BP increases with age in normal subjects.

• In 5% of cases, hypertension is secondary to:
  –adrenal disorders, e.g. **hyperaldosteronism, Cushing's syndrome, phaeochromocytoma**.
  –unilateral or bilateral renal disease, e.g. renal artery stenosis, infection, reflux, **glomerulonephritis**, congenital abnormalities, **diabetes mellitus, connective tissue diseases**, obstruction, tumour, etc.
  –others: **coarctation of the aorta, pre-eclampsia**, drugs, e.g. **steroid therapy**, oral **contraceptives**.

In the remaining 95% of cases, hypertension is termed 'essential', i.e. has no apparent cause. Associated with family history and obesity, possibly alcohol and salt intake, diet and stress. Caffeine and smoking increase BP.

• Pathophysiological effects:
  –arteriolar wall thickening, with greater reduction in vessel radius for a given vasoconstrictive stimulus.
  –degenerative changes (e.g. fibrinoid necrosis and atheroma formation) lead to reduced blood flow and propensity to aneurysm formation and rupture.
  –**baroreceptor** sensitivity is reduced.
  –increased myocardial workload, with left ventricular hypertrophy. Increased end-diastolic pressure and coronary atheromatous plaques reduce **coronary blood flow** despite increased O_2 demand. Angina and/or **cardiac failure** may result.

• Features:

  –of **ischaemic heart disease**.
  –of cardiac failure.
  –**CVA**, encephalopathy.
  –due to renal impairment.
  –**hypertensive crisis** may occur.
  –hypertensive retinopathy: arteriovenous nipping, increased light reflex, increased tortuosity, cotton wool exudates, haemorrhages and papilloedema.
  –**ECG** features include those of ischaemia and left ventricular hypertrophy. **Chest X-ray** features may include left ventricular dilatation and those of left ventricular failure.

• Treatment:
  –weight loss, cessation of smoking, physical exercise.
  –thiazide **diuretics, β-adrenergic receptor antagonists** and **vasodilator drugs** are commonly used first, singly and in combination (*see Antihypertensive drugs*).
  –benefits of treating severe hypertension are undoubted; those of treating milder forms are controversial. The incidence of CVA is thought to be reduced if diastolic pressures above 90 mmHg are treated. Screening is widely practised.

• Anaesthesia for patients with hypertension:
  –preoperatively:
    –assessment for ischaemic heart disease, cardiac failure, cerebrovascular disease and renal impairment.
    –if not on treatment, surgery should be cancelled unless it is an emergency. Patients with diastolic pressure above 110 mmHg should be investigated and hypertension treated before anaesthesia and surgery, since morbidity and mortality are greater if untreated. Antihypertensive drugs are continued up to the morning of surgery.
    –sedative **premedication** is usually advocated to reduce endogenous catecholamine levels.
  –peroperatively:
    –induction and maintenance as for ischaemic heart disease. Large swings in BP are more likely because of arteriolar hypertrophy; e.g. hypotension due on induction and hypertension on intubation (*see Intubation, complications of*), etc.
    –marked cardiovascular instability may accompany **spinal/extradural anaesthesia**, especially if hypertension is uncontrolled.
  –postoperatively:
    –adequate analgesia is particularly important.
    –treatment of persistent hypertension may be required.

• Hypertension during (or persisting after) anaesthesia may be due to:
  –inadequate anaesthesia/analgesia.
  –tracheal intubation/extubation.
  –inadequate paralysis.
  –underlying hypertensive disease.
  –aortic clamping.
  –**hypercapnia, hypoxaemia**.
  –**cerebral ischaemia**, CVA, etc.; raised **ICP**.
  –drugs, e.g. **ketamine, adrenaline**.
  –rarely, **MH**, phaeochromocytoma, **thyroid crisis, carcinoid syndrome**.

In the elderly, **atherosclerosis** is suggested by normal or low diastolic pressure. Altered baroreceptor activity is common. Postoperatively urinary retention, pain and anxiety may cause hypertension.

Management is directed towards the underlying cause. **Labetalol, hydralazine, nifedipine, sodium nitroprusside** and **glyceryl trinitrate** are commonly used to control BP, as for hypertensive crisis; the first three drugs are usually most convenient. Vasodilator therapy is less likely to be successful in atherosclerosis, since the arterial tree is relatively rigid; labetalol or other β-adrenergic antagonists may be more effective.

Mangano DT (1990) Anesthesiology; 72: 153–84

Hypertensive crisis. May occur as a feature of hypertensive disease (malignant **hypertension**), postoperatively after cardiac/vascular surgery, or other conditions including **pre-eclampsia** and **phaeochromocytoma**.

- Features:
  - –severe progressive hypertension.
  - –renal impairment.
  - –encephalopathy: confusion, headache, visual disturbances, convulsions, coma.
  - –retinal haemorrhage and papilloedema.
  - –**cardiac failure** and **CVA** may occur.
- Treatment: if associated with hypertensive disease, oral therapy as for hypertension is usually preferred, to avoid precipitous falls in BP. For rapid control, the following are commonly used:
  - –**diazoxide** up to 150 mg iv, repeated after 10 minutes.
  - –**nifedipine** 10 mg sublingually.
  - –**hydralazine** 5–10 mg iv, repeated after 10 minutes.
  - –**sodium nitroprusside** 0.5–8 µg/kg/min, or **glyceryl trinitrate** 0.2–5 µg/kg/min, iv.
  - –**labetalol** up to 50 mg iv.

Other drugs include **phentolamine, trimetaphan**.

Calhoun DA, Oparil S (1990) New Engl J Med; 323: 1177–83

Hyperthermia. Raised body temperature, sometimes defined as greater than 41.6°C (107°F). Pyrexia tends to refer to body temperature above 37.2°C (99°F) caused by illness, drugs, etc. Heatstroke is the clinical syndrome caused by increased temperature itself. May follow several hours' exposure to excessive environmental temperature, especially if unaccustomed, and if **temperature regulation** is impaired. May also be caused by increased metabolic rate and heat production, and 'resetting' of the central thermostat.

- Causes of raised temperature:
  - –drugs:
    - –**adverse drug reactions**, e.g. **MH, neuroleptic malignant syndrome**.
    - –centrally acting drugs, **phenothiaziones, barbiturates, anticholinergic drugs**.
    - –drugs interfering with sweating/vasodilatation, e.g. anticholinergic drugs.
  - –systemic disease, e.g. **malignancy, hyperthyroidism, phaeochromocytoma**, sepsis.
  - –**autonomic neuropathy, e.g.** due to diabetes.
  - –central lesions, e.g. due to tumour, surgery, **CVA**.
  - –excessive warming during anaesthesia.

Features of heatstroke include dry hot skin, confusion, headache, coma and raised temperature. Hyperventilation may be followed by metabolic acidosis, convulsions, and cardiovascular and multisystem failure.

- Treatment:
  - –specific, e.g. MH.
  - –cooling with tepid water; cold water may induce

peripheral vasoconstriction with impairment of further heat exchange. Cold iv fluids and irrigation of body cavities may be used.
  - –drugs, e.g. **aspirin, paracetamol**.

Hyperthermia, malignant, *see Malignant hyperthermia*

Hyperthyroidism (Thyrotoxicosis). In 99% of cases, hyperthyroidism is caused by primary thyroid overactivity produced by thyroid-stimulating autoantibodies (Graves' disease) or hyperactive nodules. It is rarely due to carcinoma, thyroid stimulating hormone secretion, or administration of thyroid hormones. 7–10 times more common in women.

- Features:
  - –malaise, anxiety, sweating, heat intolerance, tremor, psychological changes, myopathy (usually proximal).
  - –weight loss, increased appetite, diarrhoea.
  - –palpatations, tachycardia, **AF, cardiac failure**.
  - –goitre, oligomenorrhoea, gynaecomastia.
  - –eye features: usually lid retraction and mild proptosis; occasionally severe with visual disturbances. May be associated with pretibial myxoedema (pink/brown subcutaneous infiltration on the lower leg), pseudo-clubbing.
  - –**thyroid crisis** may occur, triggered by surgery, infection, etc..
- Investigation: measurement of plasma thyroxine and triiodothyronine (either or both of which may be raised), thyroid stimulating hormone, and rarely thyrotrophin releasing hormone. Radioisotope and ultrasound scanning may be performed.
- Treatment:
  - –antithyroid drugs:
    - –carbimazole (UK) or methimazole (USA); propyluracil: prevent formation of thyroid hormones. Pruritus and rash are common; agranulocytosis may occur. Increase vascularity of the gland, therefore sometimes stopped 2 weeks preoperatively. Usually given for a course of 1–1.5 years. Act within at least 1–2 weeks.
    - –iodine: temporarily inhibits hormone release; sometimes given for 2 weeks preoperatively to reduce glandular vascularity.
    - –radioactive iodine: increasingly used as fears of subsequent sterility and tumours diminish.
  - –**β-adrenergic receptor antagonists**: reduce the peripheral effects of hyperthyroidism directly and by reducing conversion of thyroxine to triiodothyronine. Act within 12–24 hours.
  - –surgery: requires adequate control of the disease preoperatively, in order to prevent thyroid crisis.
- Anaesthetic management:
  - –preoperatively:
    - –assessment of thyroid state, especially cardiovascular and neurological aspects. Emergency treatment is as for thyroid crisis. Other **autoimmune disease** may be present, e.g. **myasthenia gravis**.
    - –assessment for possible upper **airway obstruction**. **Chest X-ray** including **thoracic inlet** views are useful. Elective **tracheostomy** is sometimes performed if the goitre is very large. Indirect laryngoscopy is performed to assess vocal cord function in case of pre-existing or peroperative damage to the **laryngeal nerves**.

–peroperatively:
  –tracheal intubation may be difficult. IPPV is usually used; spontaneous ventilation is preferred by some. Reinforced tracheal tubes are sometimes preferred.
  –the eyes should be protected from pressure.
  –operative bleeding may be reduced by infiltration with adrenaline solutions, head-up position, and **hypotensive anaesthesia**.
  –**arrhythmias** may result from poor thyroid control or manipulation of the **carotid sinus**. Risk of **air embolism** exists in the steep head-up position.
  –**pneumothorax** and tracheal trauma may occur.
  –regional anaesthesia may also be used in poor risk patients, using 0.5% **prilocaine** or **lignocaine** with adrenaline:
    –from the midpoint of the sternomastoid muscle on both sides, 10 ml is injected into the muscle body, 10 ml anteriorly, and 10 ml infiltrated caudally and cranially.
    –20 ml is injected sc to each side from the midline, below the thyroid gland.
–postoperatively:
  –activity of the vocal cords is assessed by the anaesthetist using direct laryngoscopy on extubation.
  –airway obstruction may be caused by:
    –haemorrhage into the tissues of the neck. Skin sutures or clips must be easily removable.
    –floppy collapsible trachea (tracheomalacia) if the goitre is large. Reintubation or tracheostomy may be required.
    –laryngeal nerve damage.
    –**hypoparathyroidism** causing **hypocalcaemia** and **tetany** may occur from several hours to several days later.
  –thyroid crisis or subsequent **hypothyroidism** may also occur.
[Robert Graves (1796–1853), Irish physician]
See also, Neck, cross-sectional anatomy; Thyroid gland

Hypertonic intravenous solutions. Have been used in small volumes (under 500 ml) for initial resuscitation in, e.g. **haemorrhage** in animals and humans. Thought to draw fluid into the vasculature, possibly to cause vasodilatation and increase myocardial contractility causing increased tissue and organ flow, and possibly to affect central cardiovascular control mechanisms. Solutions used include 7.5% **saline**, **dextrans**, and others.
Vincent JL (1991) Br J Anaesth; 67: 185–93

Hyperventilation. Commonly performed during **IPPV**, intentionally or unintentionally. Its main effects are related to resultant **hypocapnia**, or the adverse cardiovascular effects of IPPV. It may occur in both awake and anaesthetized spontaneously breathing patients, e.g. due to pain, **hypoxaemia**, **hypercapnia**, **acidosis** and **pregnancy**. Sometimes occurs in midbrain/pontine lesions. Increases the work of breathing, although it aids excretion of the increased CO_2 it produces. Hypocapnia in spontaneously breathing patients may result in **tetany**.

Hypnosis. Sleep-like state, with persistence of certain behavioural responses. The subject is susceptible to, and may respond to, the hypnotist's suggestions concerning aspects of behaviour, environment, memory, etc., despite possible contradiction by actual stimuli and character. The effects may persist after return to normal consciousness, but possibly without recall of the hypnotic state.
● Has been used:
  –to help the giving up of smoking, etc.
  –to aid recall of subconscious thoughts, e.g. psychiatric/psychological research and therapy, investigation of **awareness** under anaesthesia.
  –to modify pain perception, e.g. in obstetrics, perioperatively, and in chronic pain.
  –for entertainment.
Originally expounded as **mesmerism** in the mid/late 1700s, although evidence of similar techniques date back thousands of years. The term was coined in the 1840s.
  Whether hypnosis represents a separate physiological state, or an interpersonal social interaction (i.e. obeyer/commander) is controversial. Certainly suggestion is widely used, e.g. by doctors and dentists to reduce fear, anxiety, use of drugs, etc.
[Hypnos, Greek god of sleep]

Hypoaesthesia. Reduced sensitivity to a sensory stimulus, excluding special senses.

Hypoalgesia. Reduced **pain** from a normally painful stimulus.

Hypocalcaemia. Effects are usually present when total plasma **calcium** is under 2.0 mmol/l, and are due to decreased plasma ionized calcium. Although total calcium is reduced in **hypoproteinaemia**, the ionized portion is normal and clinical features are absent.
● Caused by:
  –**hypoparathyroidism**, e.g. postoperative.
  –disorders of vitamin D metabolism, e.g. chronic **renal failure**, intestinal malabsorption, inadequate diet.
  –**pancreatitis**, rapid **blood transfusion**, severe illness.
  –**alkalosis**, e.g. due to **hyperventilation**.
● Features (exacerbated by **hypomagnesaemia**):
  –paraesthesiae.
  –muscle cramps/spasm/**tetany**. **Stridor** may occur. Chvostek's sign is facial spasm following tapping over the facial nerve. Trousseau's sign is carpopedal spasm following inflation of a tourniquet around the arm.
  –mental excitability, **convulsions**.
  –prolonged **Q–T interval** on the **ECG**; decreased cardiac output.
● Treatment:
  –of predisposing cause.
  –supportive (airway, etc.).
  –iv calcium if severe, e.g. chloride 5–10 ml or gluconate 10–20 ml slowly, followed by infusion if required.
  –magnesium if deficient.
[Frantisek Chvostek (1835–1884), Austrian physician; Armand Trousseau (1801–1867), French physician]

Hypocapnia. Arterial P_{CO_2} under 4.7 kPa (35 mmHg).
● Caused by:
  –**hyperventilation**.
  –reduced CO_2 production.
● Effects:
  –vasoconstriction; reduced **cerebral blood flow** may cause dizziness, light-headedness and confusion. Risk of **convulsions** if predisposed, e.g. if **enflurane** is used.

Placental blood flow is reduced. If **IPPV** is employed, cardiovascular effects are increased.

–**alkalosis**; **hypokalaemia** and **hypocalcaemia** may occur.

–reduced respiratory drive; apnoea may occur postoperatively.

–reduced requirement for anaesthetic agents has been shown in some studies, but not in others.

Corrected by reducing **alveolar ventilation**, e.g. by increasing **dead space** and rebreathing, or reducing minute volume.

Hypoglycaemia. Low plasma **glucose** level; symptoms are uncommon until level falls to 2–3 mmol/l (40–50 mg/dl); the threshold is lower in chronic hypoglycaemia and higher in chronic hyperglycaemia.

- Types:
  - –fasting, i.e. only after several hours without food:
    - –reduced glucose output from liver:
      - –starvation (especially children).
      - –**alcohol** ingestion.
      - –**hepatic failure**.
      - –**adrenocortical insufficiency**.
      - –**renal failure**, **growth hormone** deficiency, **pregnancy**.
    - –increased **insulin** activity:
      - –insulin/**sulphonylurea** administration.
      - –insulinoma. Over 90% are benign.
      - –sarcoma, hepatoma, adrenocortical and other tumours. Thought to be caused by secretion of an insulin-like factor.
      - –**septicaemia**, **malaria**.
  - –reactive, i.e. 2–5 hours postprandially:
    - –idiopathic.
    - –gastric surgery; causes rapid glucose absorption and excessive insulin release (cf. dumping syndrome, due to sudden osmotic load and/or other gut hormone release).
    - –may occur in **diabetes mellitus**.
    - –**inborn errors of metabolism**.
  - –rebound hypoglycaemia may follow sudden cessation of TPN, due to high levels of circulating insulin.
- Features:
  - –secretion of hyperglycaemic hormones, e.g. **adrenaline**, **glucagon**, **growth hormone** and cortisol; the former causes tachycardia, sweating and pallor.
  - –confusion, restlessness, dysarthria, diplopia, convulsions, coma. Permanent brain damage may occur with coma of increasing duration, but is rare if under 4 hours. May be exacerbated by hypoxaemia and hypotension. **Cerebral oedema** may contribute.
  - –may be masked during anaesthesia, presenting only during recovery.
- Treatment:
  - –25–50 ml 50% glucose iv if unconscious, repeated as necessary. Risk of venous thrombosis is reduced by flushing the cannula with saline after injection. Oral glucose is given if able to drink.
  - –glucagon 1 mg has been used im, but is ineffective in hepatic dysfunction and alcohol ingestion, and may exacerbate insulinoma-induced hypoglycaemia.
  - –**mannitol** and dexamethasone have been used if cerebral oedema is suspected and coma persists.

Hypoglycaemic drugs, *see Biguanides; Insulin; Sulphonylureas*

Hypokalaemia. Plasma **potassium** under 3.5 mmol/l. Symptoms usually occur below 2.5 mmol/l. Total deficit may be up to 500 mmol.

- Caused by:
  - –reduced intake, e.g. iv fluid therapy without potassium supplementation.
  - –excessive losses:
    - –renal:
      - –solute diuresis, e.g. saline, glucose, **mannitol**, urea.
      - –**diuretic** therapy.
      - –**hyperaldosteronism** and disorders of the **renin/angiotensin system**.
      - –**Cushing's syndrome**.
      - –diuretic phase of acute **renal failure**.
    - –GIT, e. g. diarrhoea, vomiting, fistulae, etc.
  - –movement of potassium into cells:
    - –**alkalosis**.
    - –drugs, e.g. **insulin**, **catecholamines**.
- Effects:
  - –muscle weakness, ileus.
  - –**arrhythmias**, ECG changes (S–T segment depression, Q–T and P–R prolongation, **T wave** inversion, **U wave**). **Cardiac arrest** may occur.
  - –impaired renal concentrating ability.
  - –increased sensitivity to non-depolarizing **neuromuscular blocking drugs**.
  - –increased adverse effects of **digoxin**.
  - –may cause metabolic alkalosis.
- Treatment:
  - –oral supplementation: up to 200 mmol (15 g)/day.
  - –iv potassium chloride: up to 40 mmol (3 g)/l fluid usually, infused at up to 40 mmol/h. Excessively concentrated solutions may cause vascular necrosis, and too rapid administration may cause **VF**; in severe cases, the above limits may be exceeded with ECG monitoring.

Hypokalaemia should be corrected before anaesthesia and surgery, although the ratio of intracellular: extracellular potassium is more important than isolated plasma levels.

Vitez T (1987) Can J Anaesth; 34: S30–1

Hypomagnesaemia. Plasma **magnesium** under 0.75 mmol/l. Because only 1% of magnesium is present in ECF, plasma levels may not correlate with clinical features.

- Caused by :
  - –reduced magnesium intake, e.g. **TPN**, alcoholism.
  - –malabsorption.
  - –increased loss, e.g. GIT, renal.
- Features:
  - –**arrhythmias**.
  - –neurological: confusion, irritability, tremor, convulsions.
  - –exacerbation of the effects of **hypocalcaemia**.
- Treatment: magnesium replacement, up to 50 mmol/day.

Hyponatraemia. Plasma **sodium** under 135 mmol/l. Usually results in hypo-osmolar plasma (not always, e.g. **hyperglycaemia** or hypertonic **mannitol** infusion causing hyperosmolar plasma).

- Caused by:
  - –water excess:

–excessive intake (urine sodium <10 mmol/l):
  –iv administration of sodium-deficient fluids.
  –TURP syndrome.
  –excessive drinking.
–reduced excretion (urine sodium >20 mmol/l):
  –syndrome of inappropriate antidiuretic hormone secretion (SIADH).
  –drugs, e.g. chlorpropramide, oxytocin (have antidiuretic effect).
–water excess with smaller sodium excess (urine sodium <10 mmol/l):
  –cardiac and hepatic failure.
  –nephrotic syndrome.
–water deficiency with greater sodium deficiency:
  –renal loss (urine sodium >20 mmol/l):
    –diuretic therapy.
    –hypoadrenalism.
    –salt-losing nephritis.
    –renal tubular acidosis.
    –post-relief of urinary obstruction.
  –other loss (urine sodium < 10 mmol/l):
    –diarrhoea and vomiting.
    –pancreatitis.
–redistribution of sodium/water:
  –sick cell syndrome in terminally ill patients: thought to be caused by impaired cell membrane sodium/potassium transport, resulting in sodium redistribution to the intracellular compartment.
  –water shift from intracellular to extracellular compartments, e.g. due to hyperglycaemia. Corrected plasma sodium concentration in hyperglycaemia: $[Na^+]$ + $([glucose]/4)$.
–pseudohyponatraemia, e.g. in hyperlipidaemia: the sodium-poor lipid portion is analysed together with the aqueous portion. Modern equipment analyses only the aqueous portion.
- Features:
  –of **dehydration** and **hypovolaemia** in sodium deficiency.
  –symptoms are unlikely above 120 mmol/l in water excess; they include headache, nausea, confusion, coma and convulsions, with possibly permanent neurological defects (especially in women). Thought to be caused by water entering cells by **osmosis**.
- Treatment:
  –of underlying cause.
  –as for SIADH: water restriction, demeclocycline.
  –iv hypertonic saline (1.8%, 4.5% or 5%) has been used in severe cases of sodium and water deficiency (sodium under 115 mmol/l). The optimal rate of plasma sodium increase is controversial, but correction should be slow, since subdural haemorrhage, pontine lesions and cardiac failure may occur if too rapid. 5–10 mmol/l/day has been suggested as the maximal safe rate; up to 2 mmol/l/h until a plasma sodium of 120 mmol/l is reached. Total sodium deficit (mmol) assuming distribution throughout total body water = (125 - measured sodium) × 60% of body weight (kg). Normal saline with frusemide has been used in less severe cases.

Oh MS, Carroll HJ (1992) Crit Care Med; 20: 94–103

Hypo-osmolality. Plasma **osmolality** under 280 mosmol/kg. Features are as for **hyponatraemia**. Detected by hypothalamic **osmoreceptors**, causing compensatory changes in water ingestion and secretion.

Hypoparathyroidism. Most commonly occurs postoperatively, e.g. following parathyroid/thyroid/laryngeal surgery; may be acute or occur several years later. May also be idiopathic, sometimes familial.

Pseudohypoparathyroidism: same features, due to peripheral lack of response to parathyroid hormone; may be associated with **hypothyroidism**.

Pseudopseudohypoparathyroidism: features of pseudohypoparathyroidism but with normal **calcium** and **phosphate** levels.
- Features:
  –hypocalcaemia.
  –hyperphosphataemia.
- Treatment: calcium and vitamin D supplements.
Anaesthetic considerations are related to hypocalcaemia.
See also, Thyroid gland

Hypophosphataemia. Plasma **phosphate** under 0.8 mmol/l.
- Caused by:
  –mild: **hyperparathyroidism**, osteomalacia, increased carbohydrate metabolism, **hypomagnesaemia**, haemodialysis, acute **alkalosis**.
  –severe: **ketoacidosis**, TPN and refeeding after starvation, chronic alcoholism/withdrawal.
- Effects:
  –muscle weakness, myocardial depression.
  –irritability, dysarthria, encephalopathy, peripheral neuropathy, convulsions, coma.
  –rhabdomyolysis, haemolysis, platelet and leucocyte dysfunction.
- Treatment: sodium or potassium phosphate: 10–20 mmol orally or 5–20 mmol/h iv. Overtreatment and resultant hyperphosphataemia may cause **hypocalcaemia** and hypomagnesaemia.
Berkelhammer C, Bear RA (1984) Can Med Assoc J; 130: 17–23

Hypopituitarism. Reduced secretion of the anterior **pituitary gland** (hyposecretion of posterior portion causes **diabetes insipidus**). Most commonly caused by pituitary tumour; may also follow surgery/radiotherapy, granulomatous disease, cysts, and classically ischaemic necrosis after haemorrhage during labour (Sheehan's syndrome).
- Features:
  –absent axillary/pubic hair, breast and genital atrophy, pale skin, muscle wasting.
  –of **hypothyroidism** and **adrenocortical insufficiency**.
Main anaesthetic considerations are related to the latter two features, and any oversecretion due to tumour, e.g. **Cushing's syndrome**, **acromegaly**.
[Harold Sheehan, English pathologist]

Hypoproteinaemia. Plasma proteins under 60 g/l. Most commonly due to low **albumin** levels (under 35 g/l). May occur in **hepatic/renal failure**, protein-losing nephropathy or enteropathy, and in severely ill catabolic patients, e.g. on ICU.
- Anaesthetic significance:
  –for drugs which are largely protein-bound, reduced available binding sites increase the proportion of unbound drug after iv injection, increasing the clinical effect; e.g. **opioid analgesic drugs**, **thiopentone**. Effects are increased further if available binding sites are already occupied by other protein-bound drugs.

Albumin is usually involved in **protein-binding,** but others are also involved, e.g. gammaglobulin and acid α_1-glycoprotein.

–decreased plasma **oncotic pressure** may lead to tissue **oedema**.

–specific protein deficiencies, e.g. **coagulation disorders**, plasma **cholinesterase** deficiency.

Hypotension. Since **MAP** = **cardiac output** (CO) × **SVR**, hypotension may result from reduction of:

- –CO:
  - –reduced **heart rate**:
    - –vagal reflexes.
    - –drugs, e.g. **halothane, β-adrenergic receptor antagonists, neostigmine.**
    - –arrhythmias.
  - –reduced **stroke volume**:
    - –reduced **venous return.**, e.g. **hypovolaemia**, head-up posture, **aortocaval compression, IPPV**, tension **pneumothorax, cardiac tamponade.**
    - –arrhythmias.
    - –increased **afterload**, e.g. **aortic stenosis, PE** (including **air** and **amniotic fluid embolism**), pneumothorax, tamponade.
    - –reduced **myocardial contractility**, e.g. drugs, **hypoxia, hypercapnia, ischaemic heart disease, MI, cardiomyopathy**, myocarditis, etc.; **cardiac failure, acidosis, hypothermia.**
- –SVR:
  - – drugs, e.g. **vasodilator drugs**, volatile and iv anaesthetic agents.
  - –**adverse drug reactions**.
  - –**spinal/extradural/caudal anaesthesia**.
  - –**septicaemia**.

Reduction in blood flow to vital organs may result, with risk of permanent ischaemic damage, e.g. **CVA, MI, renal failure. Autoregulation** maintains **cerebral, coronary** and **renal blood flows** at systolic BP of approximately 70–80 mmHg.

Treatment consists of O_2 administration, raising the feet and specific treatment directed towards the cause.

Hypotensive anaesthesia. Usually defined as deliberate lowering of BP during anaesthesia by more than 30% of resting value. Techniques usually involve reduction of systolic BP to about 80 mmHg (**MAP** 50–60 mmHg), although levels of 60–70 mmHg (MAP 40 mmHg) have been employed. Performed in circumstances where surgery may be hindered by bleeding and to reduce **blood loss**, e.g. middle ear surgery, **neurosurgery, plastic surgery**, and extensive major surgery, e.g. cystectomy, pelvic clearance. Its use is controversial, since hypotension may cause organ ischaemia, dysfunction and infarction, particularly heart, liver, kidneys, brain and spinal cord. Considered by some to be too dangerous for non life-saving surgery, but by others to be routinely acceptable. Risks are lowest in fit young patients, but consequences of major infarction are more dramatic and tragic in this group.

- Contraindications are also controversial, but include:
  - –impaired organ blood flow or function, e.g. **ischaemic heart disease**, renal disease, cerebrovascular disease, age (implies the foregoing).
  - –**hypertension**.
  - –**diabetes mellitus**: there may be increased sensitivity to hypotensive agents as autonomic function may be

impaired already. Increased sensitivity to insulin has followed ganglion blockade.

  - –severe respiratory disease. **Bronchospasm** may follow use of **ganglion-blocking drugs** or **β-adrenergic receptor antagonists** in asthmatics.
  - –**pregnancy, anaemia, hypovolaemia.**
  - –anaesthetist and surgeon unfamiliar with the technique.
- Originally achieved in the 1940s by deliberate hypovolaemia and/or high **spinal anaesthesia**. Now achieved by using:
  - –anaesthetic drugs/techniques which lower BP:
    - –reduced **cardiac output**, e.g. **IPPV**, head-up **positioning** of the patient, **halothane.**
    - –reduced **SVR**, e.g. **tubocurarine, isoflurane**, spinal/ **extradural anaesthesia.**
  - –specific hypotensive drugs, e.g.:
    - –β-receptor antagonists including **labetalol.**
    - –**vasodilator drugs**, e.g. **sodium nitroprusside, glyceryl trinitrate, hydralazine.**
    - –ganglion-blocking drugs, e.g. **trimetaphan, pentolinium.**
- Management:
  - –**preoperative assessment** with regard to contraindications.
  - –**premedication** is usually given, to improve smoothness of induction. **Atropine** is avoided.
  - –smooth induction of anaesthesia, with minimal coughing, straining, etc. Attempts may be made to reduce the hypertensive response to intubation (*see Intubation, complications of*). Drugs increasing heart rate or BP are avoided, e.g. atropine, **ketamine, pancuronium.**
  - –tracheal intubation is usually performed. Spontaneous ventilation is preferred by some, since it may indicate adequacy of brainstem blood flow. IPPV is often employed to avoid **hypercapnia** and vasodilatation associated with spontaneous respiration; it also reduces venous return. **PEEP** has been used to augment the latter but may increase venous bleeding. **Dead space** and $\dot{V}/\dot{Q}$ **mismatch** are increased at low blood pressures, therefore F_1O_2 is usually increased to 0.5.
  - –intra-arterial BP measurement is usually employed if profound hypotension or infusions of powerful hypotensive agents are used; otherwise indirect methods of measurement are usually adequate. Pulse **oximetry** and **capnography** are particularly useful. **CVP** measurement is useful in major surgery. A large-bore iv cannula is required. **EEG** and its derivatives have been used to monitor cerebral activity.
  - –careful positioning of patient, with the site of surgery raised above the heart, and avoidance of venous kinking and obstruction. Head-up tilt is introduced gradually to avoid sudden severe hypotension. 20–30° tilt is usually sufficient; BP at the head is about 15–20 mmHg less than that at the heart.
  - –a typical anaesthetic sequence consists of **thiopentone**, tubocurarine, IPPV using halothane or isoflurane, with increments of labetalol or hydralazine. Infusions of nitroprusside, glyceryl trinitrate, or others including trimetaphan may be used. Choice of agent is largely personal. Relative importance of BP over **blood flow** is controversial, e.g. whether use of vasodilators is better than reduction of cardiac output.

–careful postoperative observation is important, since cardiovascular instability may persist.
Simpson P (1992) Br J Anaesth; 69: 498–507

Hypothalamus. Part of the **brain** forming the floor of the 3rd ventricle. Lies posterior to the optic chiasma and infundibular stalk attached to the posterior lobe of the **pituitary gland**. Important controlling area for **autonomic nervous system** activity; sympathetic mainly restricted to the posteromedial part, parasympathetic to the anterolateral part. Involved in **temperature regulation** and regulation of hormone secretion by the pituitary, also of thirst, hunger, sexual activity, etc.

Hypothermia. Core temperature below 36°C. May result from exposure or immersion (**near-drowning**), e.g. complicating **trauma** and **coma** from any cause, especially involving depressant drug overdose, **hypothyroidism** and **phenothiazine** therapy. May also result from excessive **heat loss during anaesthesia**. Induced for surgery, e.g. **cardiac surgery**; techniques include surface cooling by sponging or immersion, central cooling with heat exchangers, and irrigation of body cavities with cold solutions.
- Effects:
  –cardiovascular:
    –reduced cardiac output (a 30% reduction at 30°C).
    –J waves (positive deflections at the end of **QRS complexes**) may appear on the **ECG** at 30°C (Fig. 72). They are clinically insignificant.

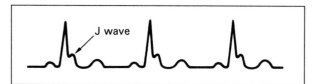

Figure 72 *ECG showing J waves*

–ventricular **arrhythmias** at 30°C, **VF** at 28°C.
–vasoconstriction. Vasodilatation occurs below 20°C.
–increased blood **viscosity**.
–increased **haematocrit** below 30°C. **Thrombocytopenia** may be caused by sequestration, mainly hepatic but also splenic.
–respiratory:
  –apnoea at 24°C.
  –reduced tissue O_2 delivery because of reduced cardiac output, vasoconstriction, increased viscosity and shift of the **oxyhaemoglobin dissociation curve** to the left, despite increased dissolved volume of O_2 in blood.
  –reduced O_2 demand and CO_2 production.
  –arterial blood gas tensions are measured at 37°C; values are traditionally corrected to body temperature but correction is now considered unnecessary.
–neurological:
  –confusion below 35°C.
  –unconsciousness at 30°C.
  –reduced requirement for volatile agents.
  –cessation of all cerebral electrical activity below 18°C.
–other:
  –diuresis due to inability to reabsorb sodium and water. GFR is reduced by 50% at 30°C.

–respiratory and metabolic acidosis. Increased blood glucose and potassium.
–metabolic rate increases initially, then decreases. **Hyperglycaemia** and increased fat mobilization may occur.
- Management:
  –investigation: both routine and as for coma, in particular those causes mentioned above.
  –routine ICU monitoring.
  –treatment of hypoxia/hypoventilation/acidosis as required. Antiarrhythmic treatment may be ineffective at low temperatures.
  –rewarming methods include:
    –heating-blankets and baths.
    –irrigation of body cavities (e.g. bladder, abdomen and stomach) with warm solution.
    –**humidification** and warming of inspired gases.
    –**extracorporeal circulation** using heat exchangers.
  External warming may cause peripheral vasodilatation and hypotension, or subsequent rebound hypothermia if the core is relatively unwarmed. Rapid rewarming is thought to be best in hypothermia of rapid onset; gradual rewarming if of gradual onset (i.e. up to 1°C/h).
  –treatment of the underlying cause.
Stoneham MD, Squires SJ (1992) Anaesthesia; 47: 784–8
See also, Temperature regulation

Hypothesis testing, *see Null hypothesis*

Hypothyroidism. Usually follows thyroid disease (e.g. autoimmune) or treatment for **hyperthyroidism** (including surgery and radiotherapy). May also follow treatment with other drugs, e.g. **amiodarone** and **lithium**. Rarely due to pituitary disease. Approximately ten times more common in women; the incidence increases with age.
- Features:
  –lethargy, slowed reactions, delayed relaxation of tendon reflexes (classically plantar reflex).
  –coarse skin and hair. Loss of the outer part of the eyebrows is classically described but is uncommon. Pretibial myxoedema is non-pitting oedema caused by subcutaneous mucopolysaccharide deposition.
  –weight gain, reduced appetite, constipation.
  –hoarse voice, lowered temperature.
  –**anaemia**: from menorrhagia or associated pernicious anaemia.
  –bradycardia, cardiomegaly and pericardial effusion may occur. Typical **ECG** findings include low voltage complexes, bradycardia and T wave flattening/inversion.
  –nerve entrapment, myopathy, confusion. **Coma** may occur (see below).
- Investigations: thyroxine (T_4) and triiodothyronine (T_3) are low. Thyroid stimulating hormone is high in primary thyroid failure, and low in pituitary failure.
- Treatment: thryoxine replacement (50–200 µg/day). Initial dosage is reduced in the elderly and those with heart disease, to reduce the risk of **myocardial ischaemia**.
- Hypothyroid coma (myxoedema coma):
  –particularly common during winter when **hypothermia** is common, especially in the elderly. May be precipitated by infection, CVA, anaesthesia, etc.
  –mortality may exceed 50%.

–treatment:

–T_3 (liothyronine) 5–20 µg slowly iv, repeated 4–12 hourly depending on severity and response. Alternatively, 50 µg iv may be followed by 25 µg 8 hourly, reducing to 25 µg 12 hourly. ECG monitoring is required.

–hydrocortisone is often given but its place is uncertain if **adrenocortical insufficiency** is not present.

–treatment of **hypoventilation**, hypothermia, hypotension, bradycardia, **acidosis, hyponatraemia, hypoglycaemia** and **convulsions** as required. Fluid restriction is usually advocated for treatment of hyponatraemia and prevention of cardiac failure.

● Anaesthetic considerations in hypothyroidism:

–other **autoimmune diseases** may be present, e.g. **myasthenia gravis**.

–patients show increased sensitivity to depressant drugs, especially opioids.

–CO_2 and heat production, and drug metabolism/ excretion are reduced.

–hypoventilation and coma may occur.

Hypoventilation. Reduced **alveolar ventilation**; it may result from reduction of respiratory rate and/or tidal volume.

● Caused by:

–reduced central respiratory drive:

–drugs, e.g. **opioid analgesic drugs, barbiturates, inhalational anaesthetic agents**.

–**hypocapnia**, e.g. following IPPV. Also may occur in extreme **hypercapnia**.

–metabolic disturbances, e.g. severe **acidosis, hyperglycaemia**, etc.

–administration of high F_IO_2 to patients with **COAD**.

–intracranial pathology, e.g. **CVA**, tumour, infection, **head injury**, raised **ICP**, etc.

–**hypothermia**.

–**alveolar hypoventilation** and **sleep apnoea** syndromes.

–impaired peripheral mechanism of breathing:

–**airway obstruction**.

–restriction due to pain, **obesity**, severe ascites, tight bandages, etc.

–chest disease, e.g. COAD, **pneumothorax, asthma, flail chest**, etc.

–muscular weakness, e.g. electrolyte disturbances, **muscular dystrophy, dystrophia myotonica**, etc.

–**neuromuscular junction** impairment, e.g. **nondepolarizing** and **depolarizing neuromuscular blockade, myasthenia gravis**.

–nerve lesions, e.g. **spinal cord injury, phrenic nerve** injury, **motor neurone disease, poliomyelitis, Guillain–Barré syndrome**, etc.

–increased **dead space**, e.g. embolism, anaesthetic apparatus.

Effects are those of hypercapnia, respiratory **acidosis** and **hypoxaemia**. Uptake of inhalational anaesthetic agents, or recovery from them, is slowed.

● Treatment:

–**O_2 therapy**. Restores alveolar PO_2 as indicated by the **alveolar air equation**. Assisted or controlled ventilation may be required.

–directed at the cause. **Neuromuscular blockade monitoring** helps distinguish central from peripheral causes.

–**doxapram** has been used perioperatively to reduce or treat hypoventilation, and in COAD. **Naloxone** is used in opioid overdose.

See also, Carbon dioxide response curve

Hypovolaemia. Reduced circulating blood volume. May be caused by deficiency of:

–blood; i.e. **haemorrhage**.

–plasma; e.g. **burns**.

–extracellular and/or intracellular fluid;, e.g. **dehydration**, diuretic therapy, haemodialysis, **third space** and evaporative losses during surgery.

'Relative hypovolaemia' refers to pooling of blood, e.g. in the legs following **spinal anaesthesia**, or drug-induced vasodilatation. Less blood is available for circulation despite an unchanged blood volume.

● Results in increased sympathetic activity, reduced parasympathetic activity and other compensatory mechanisms, as in acute haemorrhage. Important clinically because:

–many patients presenting for **emergency surgery** have a degree of hypovolaemia.

–BP and perfusion of vital organs (e.g. heart, brain) are maintained largely by sympathetically-mediated vasoconstriction and tachycardia. Drugs (e.g. anaesthetic agents) which cause vasodilatation or reduce cardiac output may thus cause severe hypotension, as may **spinal/extradural anaesthesia**.

–vital organs receive a greater proportion of cardiac output than normal, at the expense of other tissues, e.g. skin and GIT. Smaller doses of anaesthetic agents are therefore required to produce clinical effects, including side effects (e.g. myocardial depression).

–**renal failure** may occur.

Hypovolaemia should therefore be detected and corrected wherever possible before induction of anaesthesia, and treated promptly when it occurs per- and postoperatively.

● Features:

–pallor (peripheral vasoconstriction).

–tachycardia.

–hypotension with low **CVP**.

–oliguria, thirst.

–reduced O_2 delivery, e.g. :

–to tissues: **lactic acidosis**.

–to brain: confusion, restlessness.

–to carotid/aortic bodies: breathlessness.

–to heart: angina if susceptible.

–haematocrit and urea and electrolyte abnormalities depending on aetiology.

● Treatment:

–O_2 administration, supine position and raising the feet.

–fluid replacement.

Hypoxaemia. Arterial PO_2 under 12 kPa (90 mmHg).

● Caused by:

–**hypoventilation** (see Alveolar air equation).

–**diffusion** impairment, e.g. due to **pulmonary fibrosis, connective tissue diseases**; $\dot{V}/\dot{Q}$ **mismatch** is thought to be more significant.

–**shunt**.

–$\dot{V}/\dot{Q}$ mismatch.

–reduced F_IO_2, e.g. due to high **altitude** or inadvertent hypoxic gas delivery during anaesthesia.

During anaesthesia, hypoxaemia may occur because of respiratory depression, **airway obstruction**, **atelectasis** and $\dot{V}/\dot{Q}$ mismatch, including reduced **FRC**. It is especially common after upper abdominal surgery, due to the same factors plus hypoventilation caused by pain and depressant drugs and inability to cough. Impaired **ciliary activity** may also contribute. Hypoxaemia may persist for 2–3 days after upper abdominal surgery. Impaired sleep control may contribute to obstructive apnoea following anaesthesia.

- Effects:
  - direct effects:
    - **cyanosis**.
    - confusion, drowsiness, excitement, headache, nausea. Unconsciousness, convulsions and death follow unless corrected.
    - myocardial depression, arrhythmias, bradycardia, coronary and cerebral vasodilatation.
    - **hypoxic pulmonary vasoconstriction** and **pulmonary hypertension**.
    - renal impairment.
  - effects of **carotid** and **aortic body** stimulation:
    - tachycardia, hypertension.
    - hyperventilation.

Acute hypoxaemia with 85% **haemoglobin** saturation may cause mental impairment, becoming severe at 75% saturation. Unconsciousness usually occurs at 65% saturation. Chronic hypoxaemia, e.g. at altitude leads to adaptation.

- Treatment:
  - directed at the cause.
  - **O_2 therapy**: increases alveolar P_{O_2}, resulting in increased arterial P_{O_2}. The increase will be minimal in shunt.

See also, Breathing, control of; Hypoxia; Respiratory failure

Hypoxia. Reduced O_2 for tissue respiration.
- Classically divided into:
  - hypoxic hypoxia (**hypoxaemia**).
  - anaemic hypoxia: normal arterial P_{O_2} but reduced available **haemoglobin**, e.g. due to **anaemia**, **carbon monoxide poisoning**.
  - stagnant (ischaemic) hypoxia: normal arterial P_{O_2} and haemoglobin availability, but reduced tissue blood flow; may be due to reduced cardiac output or local interruption of blood flow.
  - histotoxic (cytotoxic) hypoxia: normal arterial P_{O_2},

haemoglobin availability and blood flow, but inability of tissues to utilize O_2, e.g. due to **cyanide poisoning**, carbon monoxide poisoning.
- Effects:
  - aerobic metabolism at the **cytochrome oxidase system** is replaced by anaerobic metabolism, with increasing **lactate** production. Membrane pumps cease functioning, with impairment of normal intra/extracellular ion balance; irreversible cell damage may follow. Brain and heart are most susceptible. Other tissues may continue for long periods under hypoxic conditions. The critical value for intracellular O_2 tension is not known, but is thought to be about 0.13 kPa (1 mmHg) at the mitochondrial level.
  - local stagnant hypoxia effects depending on the tissue involved.
  - general effects of hypoxia are as for hypoxaemia. Stimulation of the **carotid** and **aortic bodies** occurs when arterial P_{O_2} falls; i.e. it may not occur in anaemic and histotoxic hypoxia.

See also, Oxygen cascade

Hypoxic pulmonary vasoconstriction. Reflex vasoconstriction of pulmonary arterioles in response to low P_{O_2} (under 11–13 kPa; 80–100 mmHg) in nearby alveoli. Does not rely on innervation of vessel walls, and is less dependent on P_{O_2} in blood; thus it occurs in isolated lung perfused with blood of high O_2 content and ventilated with gas of low O_2 content. Results in flow of blood away from poorly ventilated areas of lung, helping to reduce $\dot{V}/\dot{Q}$ **mismatch**.

Before birth, decreased pulmonary blood flow is thought to be caused by pulmonary vasoconstriction, relieved at birth when O_2 enters the lungs at the first breath.

Important in cardiac defects; **hypoxaemia** may cause a generalized increase in **pulmonary vascular resistance**, with increased right ventricular work and increased right-to-left shunting, particularly if SVR is lowered.

- Reduced by:
  - **hypocapnia**.
  - increased distension of arterioles.
  - **vasodilator** drugs.
  - volatile anaesthetic agents in animal and laboratory experiments; the clinical relevance of this is controversial.

Eisenkraft JB (1990) Br J Anaesth; 65: 63–78

I

Iceberg theory, *see Clathrates*

ICP, *see Intracranial pressure*

ICU, *see Intensive care unit*

I–D interval. Time between induction of anaesthesia and delivery of the infant in **Caesarean section**. Infant **thiopentone** levels may be high if the interval is very short. If very long, **inhalational anaesthetic agents** may accumulate in the infant. An I–D interval of less than 30 minutes is not thought to influence fetal acidosis if **aortocaval compression** and **hypoxaemia** are avoided.

Ideal gas law. For a perfect **gas**;

$$\frac{\text{pressure } P \times \text{volume } V}{\text{temperature } T} = \text{constant}$$

rearranged as $PV = nRT$,
where n = number of moles of gas
$\quad\quad$ R = **universal gas constant**.
Thus a combination of **Boyle's law**, **Charles' law** and **Avogadro's hypothesis**.

Idioventricular rhythm, *see Atrioventricular dissociation*

I:E ratio, *see Inspiratory:expiratory ratio*

Ignition temperature. Lowest temperature at which combustible mixtures ignite (energy required = **activation energy**). Lowest for **stoichiometric mixtures**.
See also, Explosions and fires

IHD, *see Ischaemic heart disease*

Ileus, postoperative. Intestinal atony; occurs to some extent after most abdominal operations. Small bowel activity may continue despite gastric and colonic stasis.
• Aetiology is thought to include:
  –reflex response of the bowel to intraoperative manipulation.
  –sympathetic overactivity.
  –peritoneal irritation due to blood, etc.
  –electrolyte imbalance, especially **hypokalaemia**.
May cause fluid and electrolyte loss, and abdominal distension with possible impairment of ventilation. Presence of colicky pain and increased bowel sounds suggest development of mechanical obstruction, which may follow paralytic ileus.
Ileus usually resolves within 48 hours, although return of bowel sounds is not a reliable indicator. Routine early administration of oral clear fluids has been suggested in uncomplicated abdominal cases. **Metoclopramide** or **cisapride** have been used in certain cases.

Iliac crest block. Blocks the ilioinguinal, iliohypogastric and lower 2–3 intercostal nerves, providing anaesthesia of the lower ipsilateral abdomen. An 8 cm needle is introduced 2–3 cm inferior and medial to the superior anterior iliac spine, and directed cranially and laterally to reach the inner ilium. 10 ml **local anaesthetic agent** is injected whilst the needle is withdrawn. Injection is repeated, directed more deeply.
See also, Inguinal hernia field block

Iliohypogastric nerve block/Ilioinguinal nerve block, *see Iliac crest block; Inguinal hernia field block*

Immune system, anaesthesia and. Normal immune defences may be:
  –non-specific, e.g. epithelial surface barriers, secreted **immunoglobulins**, local inflammatory responses including phagocytes and macrophages, **complement** system.
  –specific:
    –humoral: B lymphocytes form plasma cells which secrete specific immunoglobulins.
    –cellular: T lymphocytes conditioned in the thymus have killer activity and regulatory effects via helper/suppressor subsets.
    –natural killer cells.
• Main areas of anaesthetic importance:
  –patients with **immunodeficiency**.
  –**adverse drug reactions**, **blood cross-matching**, etc.
  –effects of anaesthesia on immunocompetence, especially against infection and malignancy. Difficult to study clinically, because of other factors, e.g. surgery, drugs, pre-existing disease, **stress response to surgery**, etc., although phagocyte, monocyte and B lymphocyte activity is reduced during anaesthesia. **Ciliary activity** may be affected. *In vitro* testing has revealed depression of monocyte and phagocyte activity and migration, e.g. in response to mitogen or antigen provocation. Natural killer cell activity, lymphocyte proliferation and plasma cell formation are also reduced following anaesthesia with most inhalational agents. Lysosomal **free radical** formation may also be suppressed. Effects on spread and metastasis of malignancy are controversial, although spread in animals may be increased by anaesthesia, and **blood transfusion** may be detrimental in colonic cancer surgery.
Stevenson GW, Hall SC, Rudnick S et al (1990) Anesthesiology; 72: 542–52

Immunodeficiency. Results in increased susceptibility to infection and **malignancy**, the former a more common problem acutely. May result from deficient cell-mediated (T cell lymphocyte) or antibody-mediated (B cell lymphocyte) function, phagocytic activity or **complement** activity. Results in repeated and persistent infection, typically with unusual organisms.

- May be:
  - –primary, e.g. B cell or T cell deficiency, often inherited. Specific **immunoglobulin** types may be deficient. Neutrophil and complement disorders may also be inherited.
  - –secondary to:
    - –infection, e.g. viral (e.g. **HIV infection**), **septicaemia**.
    - –drugs, e.g. **immunosuppressant drugs**, gold, penicillamine.
    - –**connective tissue diseases**.
    - –severe illness, **trauma**, **burns**, etc.; i.e. it may occur in any severely ill patient on ICU.
    - –malignancy.
    - –splenectomy.
- Management:
  - –prevention of infection, e.g. meticulous aseptic technique, barrier nursing, prophylactic antibacterial therapy, etc.
  - –prompt diagnosis and treatment of infection.
  - –treatment of the underlying cause.
  - –immunoglobulin administration.
  - –immune stimulant therapy is not generally available, although some, e.g. interferons, have been used.

Immunoglobulins (Antibodies). Proteins secreted by plasma cells, involved in immunological defence systems. Each molecule consists of two heavy chains (which determine the class of immunoglobulin) and two light chains. The Y-shaped molecule presents two highly specific antigen-binding sites, each made up of portions of heavy and light chains, at one end (the Fab portion). The other end (the Fc portion) is made up of heavy chain only, and may bind to **complement**, or to the surface of mediator cells, e.g. **mast cells**, macrophages.

- Types of immunoglobulins:
  - –IgG: the most abundant in plasma. Involved in complement fixation.
  - –IgA: secreted from epithelial barriers, e.g. GIT.
  - –IgM: comprised of five joined molecules; involved in complement fixation.
  - –IgD: involved in antigen recognition by lymphocytes.
  - –IgE: on the surface of mast cells; involved in **histamine** release and **anaphylactic reactions**.

  Most **adverse drug reactions** to anaesthetic drugs via immunoglobulins involve IgG and IgM (complement activation) or IgE (anaphylaxis).
- Immunoglobulins may be administered to humans, and are obtained from:
  - –pooled human plasma:
    - –from blood donated for transfusion (normal immunoglobulin): given im for prophylaxis of certain infections, e.g. measles, **hepatitis**, rubella in pregnant women. Certain forms may be given iv as replacement therapy in **immunodeficiency**.
    - –from donors who are convalescing, or whose antibody production has been boosted (specific immunoglobulins): given im and available against hepatitis B, tetanus, rabies, Rhesus D antigen and herpes viruses.

    They are screened for hepatitis and **HIV infection**.
  - –monoclonal cell biology and recombinant genetic engineering: not yet widespread. Monoclonal IgM

directed against **endotoxin** has been used in sepsis, but has recently been withdrawn.

Hypersensitivity reactions are more likely with immunoglobulins from pooled plasma. **Digoxin**-specific antibody fragments (Fab) derived from sheep immunoglobulins are available for use in digoxin toxicity.

Immunosuppressive drugs. Used to treat inflammatory/**autoimmune diseases**, and to prevent rejection following **transplantation**.

- Different types of drug used:
  - –**antimitotic drugs**, e.g. azathioprine, cyclophosphamide, chlorambucil.
  - –**steroid therapy**.
  - –cyclosporin. Side effects include renal and hepatic impairment, GIT upset, tremor, hyperkalaemia, fluid retention and convulsions.

Impedance. Resistance to flow of an alternating **current** in an electrical circuit, dependent on the current's frequency. Represented by the letter Z, although measured in **ohms**. Different components within circuits, e.g. loudspeakers, monitor screens, etc., should be matched for impedance, to maximize efficiency. Amplifiers in **monitoring** equipment generally have high input impedance to minimize the effect of poor contact with the patient; any increased impedance because of the latter makes little difference to the overall input impedance.
See also, Impedance plethysmography

Impedance plethysmography. Method of determining changes in intrathoracic gas and fluid volumes by measuring transthoracic **impedance**, which varies according to the composition of thoracic contents.

- Used for:
  - –**monitoring** respiration, e.g. on ICU: a small high-frequency current is passed between ECG electrodes; the changes in impedance between them represents ventilatory movements.
  - –**cardiac output measurement**: two sets of circular wire electrodes are placed around the chest and neck. Current is passed between the outer two, with measurement of potential difference between the inner two. Maximal rate of change of impedance ocurs with peak aortic flow, although absolute values do not correlate well.
  - –others, e.g. lung water measurement.

  May also be applied to other parts of the body, e.g. leg veins to diagnose **DVT**.

IMV, *see Intermittent mandatory ventilation*

Inborn errors of metabolism. Group of disorders caused by inherited single **enzyme** defects. Over 200 are known; some are clinically insignificant and others fatal. Most are rare (1:20 000–500 000), are caused by autosomal recessive genes, and present in infancy/early childhood.

- Include disorders of:
  - –porphyrin metabolism (*see Porphyrias*).
  - –**carbohydrate** metabolism, e.g. **glycogen storage disorders**, galactosaemia and fructose metabolic disorders. Liver, brain, skeletal and cardiac muscle may be affected. **Hypoglycaemia** is common, also metabolic **acidosis** and electrolyte imbalance.
  - –**amino acid** metabolism, e.g. phenylketonuria, homo-

cystinuria, alcaptonuria. Mental handicap, neurological abnormalities and metabolic disturbances are common. Skeletal abnormalities may present difficulty with tracheal intubation in the latter two disorders. Hypoglycaemia may occur.

–lysosomal storage; results in accumulation of macromolecules within lysosomes. Most conditions cause severe mental retardation and neurological abnormalities, with death in childhood. Include:

–sphingolipidoses, e.g. Gaucher's disease; coagulation abnormalities and hepatosplenomegaly are common.

–mucopolysaccharidoses, e.g. Hurler's and Hunter's diseases (the latter is sex-linked recessive). CNS, skeleton and viscera are affected. Characteristic 'gargoyle' facies occur, with possible upper respiratory obstruction, and thoracic spinous deformities. Hurler's syndrome is more severe than Hunter's, with corneal clouding, valvular and **ischaemic heart disease**.

–purine metabolism: may lead to gout, with tissue deposition of urate crystals, especially in the joints. This group includes Lesch–Nyhan syndrome, with mental and neurological abnormalities.

–red blood cell metabolism, e.g. **glucose 6–phosphate dehydrogenase deficiency**. **Haemolysis** may also feature in other defects.

–copper metabolism (Wilson's disease): impaired hepatic and central nervous motor function.

–iron metabolism (haemochromatosis): hepatic and myocardial impairment are common; **diabetes mellitus** may occur.

[Philippe Gaucher (1854–1918), French physician; Gertrud Hurler, German paediatrician; Charles Hunter (1872–1955), US physician; Michael Lesch and William Nyhan, US paediatricians; Samuel Wilson (1878–1937), US-born English neurologist]

Incentive breathing. Encouragement of deep breathing to reduce **atelactasis** and improve respiratory muscle function, e.g. postoperatively.

● Apart from verbal encouragement and teaching of breathing exercises, the following techniques have been used:

–inspiration from bellows; when the preset tidal volume has been reached, a light illuminates.

–inspiration or expiration through flowmeters, e.g. glass cylinders containing coloured balls; the patient attempts to reach preset targets.

–inflation of a balloon on expiration.

–expiration through a blow-bottle: the patient breathes out through a tube passing into a sealed jar containing water, which is displaced through a second tube into a second jar.

Recent evidence suggests that the technique is useful in reducing breathlessness in COAD.

See also, Physiotherapy

Indomethacin. NSAID, available for oral and rectal use. The latter route has been used for **postoperative analgesia** and to replace oral therapy withdrawn perioperatively.

● Dosage:

–100 mg rectally once-twice daily.

–25–50 mg orally, 6–8 hourly.

● Side effects: as for NSAIDs; in addition dizziness and headache may occur.

Indoramin hydrochloride. α-Adrenergic receptor antagonist, selective for α_1–receptors; used orally as an **antihypertensive drug**. Reflex tachycardia and postural hypotension are rarely problems, although sedation is common.

Inductance. Capacity for an electromotive force to be induced in an electrical circuit by a changing **current** flowing in that circuit, or in a neighbouring one. Flow of current induces a magnetic field, which in turn induces the electromotive force, the magnitude of which depends on the rate of change of current. May give rise to interference in electrical equipment, or occur intentionally in transformers. Has been used as a basis for **monitoring** respiration, by using two coils placed on the chest, e.g. one anteriorly, one posteriorly.

Induction agents, *see Intravenous anaesthetic agents*

Induction of anaesthesia. Transition from the awake to the anaesthetized state, although the end-point is difficult to define.

● Represents a period of great physiological change during which the following may occur:

–cardiovascular changes, e.g. **hypotension**, **arrhythmias**.

–**hypoventilation/apnoea**. Particularly dangerous in patients with airway problems.

–**aspiration of gastric contents**.

–**laryngospasm**, **vomiting**, etc. during the stage of excitement, particularly if disturbed by movement, noise, etc.

–**adverse drug reactions**, especially following iv injections.

–others, e.g. involuntary movement/**convulsions**, MH/**masseter spasm**.

Inhalational and iv techniques are most commonly used, although other routes (e.g. im or rectal) of drug administration are possible.

● Inhalational induction:

–usually reserved for children, patients with **airway obstruction**, and in difficult intubation. By allowing continuous spontaneous ventilation, the anaesthetist avoids being unable to ventilate an apnoeic patient. May also be used in patients with poor veins.

–the anaesthetic agent is gradually introduced to the patient in increasing concentrations. The characteristics of induction depend on the **inhalational anaesthetic agent** used. More rapid induction has been achieved using maximal breaths of high percentage of volatile agent, e.g. 4–5% **halothane** ('single breath induction').

–the different stages of anaesthesia may be seen in turn, especially in unpremedicated patients.

–induction is slower than with iv agents. The stage of excitement may be prolonged.

● IV induction:

–much faster, allowing rapid passage through the stage of excitement. Usually more pleasant for adults than an inhalational technique.

–an estimated appropriate dose should be given slowly, and the patient observed for its effect before injecting more. Considerable time may be required if the **arm–brain circulation time** is prolonged, e.g. in the elderly and those with cardiovascular disease.

–the characteristics of induction depend on the **iv anaesthetic agent** used.

–carries risk of extravasation, intra-arterial or painful injection, thrombosis, chemical reaction with other drugs in the cannula, and adverse drug reactions.

–movement, hiccupping, etc., may occur.

–overdosage is more likely because induction is faster, especially if injection is rapid and without pausing to observe the effect.

Respiratory and cardiac depression may follow both methods of induction, but are more sudden after iv induction, especially after rapid injection. Use of other depressant drugs, e.g. for **premedication**, may reduce the amount of induction agent required and allow smoother induction. Respiratory depressants, e.g. opioids, may slow inhalational induction.

Emergency drugs and equipment, a tipping trolley and skilled assistance should always be present before inducing anaesthesia. Equipment should always be checked before use.

See also, Anaesthesia, stages of; Checking of anaesthetic equipment; Induction, rapid sequence

Induction, rapid sequence ('Crash induction'). **Induction of anaesthesia** in which risks of regurgitation and **aspiration of gastric contents** are minimized by:

–presence of emergency drugs and equipment, a tipping trolley and skilled assistance (should be present before inducing anaesthesia in any patient, but especially important in rapid sequence induction, as is **checking of anaesthetic equipment**).

–**suction apparatus**: should be turned on before induction and be within easy reach of the anaesthetist.

–aspiration of gastric tube if in place, prior to induction. Pre-induction passage of a stomach tube is controversial, as is whether to leave a nasogastric tube *in situ* during induction, or whether to remove it in case **cricoid pressure** is made inefficient.

–use of a rapidly-acting iv induction agent and **suxamethonium** to achieve rapid muscle relaxation. **Vecuronium** or **atracurium** have been suggested as alternatives when suxamethonium is contraindicated, but are slower in onset. Regurgitation and aspiration have been reported during use of the **priming principle**. Other analgesic or sedative drugs should not precede the iv agent.

–application of cricoid pressure.

–avoidance of manual inflation of the lungs by facepiece, to prevent inflation of the stomach and thus increase risk of regurgitation. **Preoxygenation** is therefore required to prevent **hypoxaemia** during **apnoea** until tracheal intubation is achieved.

–tracheal intubation and inflation of the cuff before cricoid pressure is released.

Spare laryngoscopes, tubes, etc. must be prepared in advance, as must a plan in case of unexpectedly difficult or impossible intubation.

Rapid sequence induction should be performed in all cases known to be at risk of regurgitation or aspiration, including all emergency abdominal operations, except in cases where intubation is expected to be particularly difficult.

See also, Intubation, difficult; Intubation, failed; Nasogastric intubation

Inert gas narcosis. Loss of consciousness caused by inhalation of high partial pressures of inert gases, e.g.

xenon, neon, argon and nitrogen (nitrogen narcosis). Nitrogen has no anaesthetic properties at sea level pressures, but impairs intellectual and manual functions at partial pressures above 4–5 atmospheres, e.g. diving to depths greater than 30–40 metres whilst breathing air. Use of **helium** in breathing apparatus allows deeper dives.

Infiltration anaesthesia. Commonly performed for minor surgery, suturing, etc. Subcutaneous and intradermal infiltration is performed around the lesion, with further injection as required. May also be used for manipulations and more extensive surgery, e.g. **Caesarean section**, etc., in which the deeper tissues are also infiltrated. The maximal safe dose of **local anaesthetic agent** should not be exceeded. Dilute solutions are usually adequate. Excessive volumes of injectate containing adrenaline may cause skin necrosis. Adequate time must be allowed before starting surgery.

Inflation pressure, *see Airway pressure*

Inflation reflex, *see Hering–Breuer reflex*

Informed consent, *see Consent*

Infraorbital nerve block, *see Maxillary nerve blocks*

Infratrochlear nerve block, *see Ophthalmic nerve blocks*

Inguinal hernia field block. May be used as the sole technique for surgery in poor risk patients, or as an adjunct to general anaesthesia to reduce the anaesthetic requirement and to provide **postoperative analgesia**.

● Anatomy:

–the inguinal canal represents the path taken by the descending testicle, and contains the spermatic cord in the male (round ligament in the female). It runs downwards and medially, above and parallel to the inguinal ligament, which passes from the superior anterior iliac spine to the pubic tubercle.

–anterior abdominal wall muscle layers, from within outwards: transversus abdominis, internal oblique, external oblique.

–the canal emerges through the deep ring of the tranversalis fascia and transversus abdominis above the midpoint of the inguinal ligament. The internal oblique lies in front laterally, but its conjoint tendon (formed with tranversus abdominis) arches over the canal superiorly to lie behind it medially. The external oblique lies anteriorly along its length. The superficial ring is the defect in the external oblique aponeurosis just lateral and above the pubic tubercle.

–nerve supply (branches from the **lumbar plexus**):

–iliohypogastric (L1): anterior cutaneous branch is given off at the iliac crest; it passes between transversus abdominis and the internal oblique, piercing the latter 2 cm medial to the anterior superior iliac spine. It then runs deep to the aponeurosis of the external oblique, piercing it above the superficial ring to supply the skin above the pubis.

–ilioinguinal (L1): passes just caudal to the iliohypogastric nerve, passing through the superficial ring to supply the skin of the groin and scrotum/labia majora.

–genitofemoral (L1,2): genital branch passes with the spermatic cord through the deep ring, supplying the skin of the scrotum/labia majora.
- Technique of block:
  –iliohypogastric and ilioinguinal nerves: with the patient supine, a short-bevelled needle is introduced vertically downwards, 2 cm medial and caudal to the anterior superior iliac spine. A click is felt as the external oblique aponeurosis is penetrated. 10–20 ml **local anaesthetic agent** is injected, repeated with the needle directed medially and laterally. Subcutaneous infiltration from the pubis, 10 cm cranially, blocks fibres from the other side.
  –subcutaneous infiltration along the incision site.
  –genitofemoral nerve: injection of 20 ml solution at the deep ring, 1–2 cm above the midpoint of the inguinal ligament, deep to the external oblique aponeurosis as before. This may be left to the surgeon to reduce risk of vascular or peritoneal puncture.
  –the neck of the hernia sac may also be infiltrated by the surgeon.

Prilocaine 0.5% with adrenaline is suitable, and allows use of a large volume of solution. The maximal safe dose allowable is calculated and divided between the above injections. For an adjunct to general anaesthesia and postoperative analgesia, smaller volumes of **bupivacaine** with adrenaline may provide several hours' analgesia. Leg weakness has been reported.

Inhalational anaesthesic agents. Since the discovery of anaesthesia, a variety of gases and volatile agents have been tried and discarded, including: **diethyl ether** (first used in 1842), **N₂O** (1844), **chloroform** (1847), **ethyl chloride** (1848), **ethylene** (1923), **cyclopropane** (1930), **divinyl ether** (1933), **trichloroethylene** (1935), **halothane** and **fluroxene** (1956), **methoxyflurane** (1960), **enflurane** (1966), **isoflurane** (1971). **Sevoflurane** (available in Japan) and **desflurane** are still being evaluated. Some properties of inhalational agents are shown in Table 18.

Inhalational agents are popular because alveolar levels (and thus blood levels) are easily controllable by adjusting inspired concentration. However, side effects and **pollution** fears have led to increased use of **iv anaesthetic agents**, e.g. **TIVA**.

Volatile anaesthetic agents are convenient to supply and store, but require special **vaporizers**. Many are ethers; **flammability** and risk of **explosion and fires** is reduced by addition of halogen atoms to the basic molecule.

Gases are supplied in **cylinders** or via pipelines. Cylinders are bulky to store. Administration of gases is controlled using **flowmeters** alongside the O_2 flowmeter of an **anaesthetic machine**.
- Features of the ideal inhalational anaesthetic agent:
  –physical/chemical properties:
    –chemically stable, e.g. in the presence of heat, light, **soda lime**; long shelf-life. No additive required, e.g. **thymol**, and non-flammable.
    –non-irritant, with pleasant smell.
    –no corrosion of metal or adsorption on to rubber.
    –**SVP** should be high enough to enable production of clinically useful concentrations (depends on potency; **MAC**).
    –low blood/gas **partition coefficient**.
    –cheap.
  –pharmacology:
    –smooth rapid induction with no breath holding, laryngospasm, coughing, increased secretions, etc.
    –sufficiently potent to allow concurrent high F_1O_2.
    –analgesic, antiemetic and anticonvulsant properties, with skeletal muscle relaxation. No increase in **cerebral blood flow** or **ICP**.
    –no respiratory depression. Bronchodilatory action.
    –no cardiovascular depression or sensitization of myocardium to **catecholamines**. No decrease in coronary, renal or hepatic blood flow.
    –minimal metabolism, with excretion via the lungs. No **fluoride ion** production.
    –no adverse renal, hepatic or haematological effects.
    –non-trigger for **MH**.

Table 18. Properties of inhalational anaesthetic agents

Agent	Structure	Molecular weight	Boiling point (°C)	SVP at 20°C (kPa (mmHg)	MAC (% vol.)	Partition coefficients at 37°C Blood/gas	Oil/gas
Chloroform	$CHCl_3$	119	61	21 (160)	0.5	10	260
Cyclopropane	$(CH_2)_3$	42	–33	—	9.2	0.45	11.5
Desflurane	$CF_3–CHF–O–CF_2H$	168	23	88 (673)	5–10	0.42	19
Diethyl ether	$CH_3–CH_2–O–CH_2–CH_3$	74	35	59 (425)	1.9	12	65
Divinyl ether	$CH_2=CH–O–CH=CH_2$	70	28	74 (553)	3	2.8	60
Enflurane	$CHFCl–CF_2–O–CF_2H$	184.5	56	24 (175)	1.68	1.9	98
Ethyl chloride	$CH_3–CH_2Cl$	64.5	13	131 (988)	2	3	—
Ethylene	$CH_2=CH_2$	28	–104	—	65	0.4	1.3
Fluoroxene	$CF_3–CH_2–O–CH=CH_2$	126	43	38 (286)	3.4	1.4	48
Halothane	$CF_3–CHClBr$	197.4	50	32 (243)	0.76	2.4	225
Isoflurane	$CF_3–CHCl–O–CF_2H$	184.5	49	33 (250)	1.15	1.4	97
Methoxyflurane	$CF_2–CHCl–O–CH_3$	165	105	3 (23)	0.2	13	970
Nitrous oxide	N_2O	44	–88	—	105	0.47	1.4
Sevoflurane	$(CF_3)_2CH–O–CH_2F$	200	58	21 (160)	1.7–2	0.6	53
Trichloroethylene	$CCl_2=CHCl$	131	87	8 (60)	0.17	9	960
Xenon	Xe	131	—	—	71	0.17	1.9

–no effects on the **uterus**.
–non-teratogenic/carcinogenic.

No currently available agent fulfils all the above. All of the three volatile agents most commonly used (halothane, isoflurane and enflurane) have undesirable effects; in addition to those listed in Table 19, they all depress respiration, reduce uterine tone, and may trigger MH. All increase cerebral blood flow, although isoflurane less so than the other two. N_2O is not potent enough for use as a sole agent and is losing popularity because of effects on **methionine** metabolism, cardiovascular and cerebral function, and because it expands gas-containing cavities (e.g. **pneumothorax**). Trichloroethylene is analgesic and extremely cheap but is no longer produced because of costs associated with renewal of its product licence. Diethyl ether is only available on a named-patient basis. Cyclopropane is used mainly for induction of anaesthesia, especially in children; it is expensive and flammable, and its use is declining. Sevoflurane and desflurane are the latest to be developed.

Table 19. Undesirable features compared for halothane, isoflurane and enflurane

Feature	Halothane	Isoflurane	Enflurane
Thymol required	+	–	–
Solubility in rubber	++	+	+
Decomposed by light	+	–	–
Approximate cost/100 ml (£)	4–5	30–40	15–20
Irritant to breathe	–	+	+/–
Cardiac output	↓↓	↓	↓↓↓
SVR	(↓)	↓↓	↓
Heart rate	↓	↑	↑↑
BP	↓	↓↓↓	↓↓
Sensitization to catecholamines	+++	+	++
Metabolized (%)	20	0.2	2
Others	Halothane hepatitis	Coronary steal	Epileptiform EEG

• The potency of anaesthetic agents depends on their **solubility** in the CNS, estimated by the oil/gas partition coefficient. Brain concentration is related to arterial concentration which approximates to alveolar concentration. Thus steady-state brain concentration requires steady state alveolar concentration. Drug is distributed from alveoli via bloodstream to:
    –vessel-rich tissues (e.g. brain, heart, kidney, liver; receive 70–80% of cardiac output) until equilibrium is reached, then:
    –vessel-intermediate tissues (muscle, skin; 18% of cardiac output).
    –fat (6% of cardiac output) and other vessel-poor tissues, e.g. bone, ligaments, etc.
In prolonged anaesthesia, the agent accumulates in fat, especially if it is very fat soluble (i.e. potent). Thus it takes 80 minutes for the partial pressure of N_2O in fat to equal half that in arterial blood; halothane requires 32 hours.

• Factors affecting uptake:
    –delivery to alveoli:
        –vaporization: SVP, gas flow, temperature, vaporizer design, **pumping effect**.
        –**anaesthetic breathing system**: gas flow, volume of system and dilution of agent, adsorption on to rubber etc.
        –**alveolar ventilation**: agent in each breath is diluted by alveolar gas; the effect is most marked at induction, when uptake of agent is greatest, especially when the blood/gas partition coefficient is high (i.e. blood solubility is high). Hyperventilation thus increases uptake.
        –**concentration effect** and **second gas effect**.
    –uptake from alveoli:
        –blood/gas partition coefficient (solubility): if high, uptake into blood is rapid, thus alveolar concentration falls rapidly until the next breath. Build-up of stable alveolar concentration and thus arterial concentration is therefore slow. If solubility is low, only a small proportion of agent passes into blood, leaving a large reserve in the lungs. Thus alveolar and arterial concentrations build up rapidly, with rapid clinical effects. Changes in vaporizer settings are more rapidly reflected in arterial concentrations with insoluble agents than with soluble ones.
        –cardiac output and pulmonary blood flow: uptake is more rapid if cardiac output is high, leading to slow build-up of alveolar concentration. If cardiac output is low, alveolar concentration builds up more quickly; in addition, a greater proportion of cadiac output goes to vital organs, e.g. brain and heart, increasing clinical effects. Thus overdose is more likely if cardiac output is low. The effect is more marked with soluble agents.
        –concentration of agent in the pulmonary artery (i.e. mixed venous). As it approaches pulmonary venous concentration, alveolar and arterial levels approach equilibrium. Occurs as body tissues become saturated, or in severe low output states when tissue perfusion is reduced.
        –$\dot{V}/\dot{Q}$ **mismatch**: rarely significant unless large, e.g. accidental endobronchial intubation. Effects are greater for insoluble agents.
        –impaired diffusion across alveolar wall is rarely significant.
Factors affecting recovery are similar to those above. If body tissues are unsaturated, recovery is more rapid because the agent moves from arterial blood to both tissues and alveoli. If tissues are saturated after prolonged anaesthesia, recovery is slower, but is hastened by hyperventilation. However, drug movement from tissues into blood may cause reaccumulation of anaesthetic alveolar concentrations after initial wakening.

Heijke S, Smith G (1990) Br J Anaesth; 64: 3–6

See also, Anaesthesia, mechanisms of; Coronary steal; Halothane hepatitis; Meyer–Overton rule

Injector techniques. Use of intermittent jets of driving gas, usually O_2, for IPPV by entraining room air. The jet is delivered to the proximal end of a bronchoscope, etc., by a metal cannula (Sanders injector), and entrains stationary gas within the scope by **jet mixing**. Room air is drawn in from the open end to replace the air delivered to the lungs. Expiration occurs by passive recoil of the lungs. A 14–16 G cannula is suitable for adults (delivers up to 30–50 cmH$_2$O pressure); 17–18 G for adolescents and small adults (up to 25 cmH$_2$O); 19 G for children (up to 15 cmH$_2$O). The Carden jetting device was described for attachment to a bronchoscope side-arm; higher inflation pressures and F_1O_2 are achieved with lower driving pressures.

The system usually consists of tubing and a connector for wall socket or gas cylinder, a pressure reducing valve and gauge, a hand-operated trigger and attachment for the cannula. It may also be attached to commercially available **cricothyrotomy** devices, or to iv cannulae used for emergency cricothyrotomy. Similar principles are also used in high frequency jet ventilation.

Commonly used for **bronchoscopy** and laryngoscopy because of its convenience.
- Disadvantages:
   –tidal volume and minute ventilation are difficult to assess.
   –trachea is unprotected during airway surgery.
   –possible interference with surgery from movement of vocal cords during ventilation.
   –**barotrauma** is possible if expiration is obstructed.
   –volatile anaesthetic agents cannot be delivered.
[RD Sanders (described 1967), US anaesthetist; E Carden (described 1973), Canadian anaesthetist]
See also, High frequency ventilation

Inosine. Metabolite of **adenosine**, with some similar actions. Causes vasodilatation via a direct action on vascular smooth muscle. Also has a positive inotropic effect, but not via β-**adrenergic receptors**. Thought to improve cell survival following ischaemia and reperfusion, e.g. in cardiac and renal surgery, possibly by increasing intracellular levels of energy-rich phosphates and reducing **ATP** depletion. Has been used in high vascular and renal surgery; e.g. 30 mg/kg iv before clamping. Hypotension may occur.

Inotropic drugs. Drugs which increase **myocardial contractility**, increasing **cardiac output**; used in low cardiac output states.
- Drugs available include:
   –**catecholamines**: increase intracellular **cAMP** levels via adenylate cyclase stimulation; cAMP increases intracellular **calcium** ion mobilization and force of contraction.
      –**adrenaline**: β-**adrenergic receptor** agonist mainly at low doses, α-receptor agonist mainly at higher doses. Causes peripheral and renal vasoconstriction, especially at higher doses. Tachycardia and arrhythmias may occur, increasing myocardial O$_2$ demand.
      –**noradrenaline**: α-receptor agonist mainly, with some β-receptor agonist properties. Causes peripheral and renal vasoconstriction, with raised BP and compensatory bradycardia. Myocardial O$_2$ demand is increased markedly.
      –**isoprenaline**: β-receptor agonist only. Increases cardiac output and rate, with peripheral and pulmonary vasodilatation. Arrhythmias are common, and myocardial O$_2$ demand is increased; ischaemia may occur due to lowered BP.
      –**dopamine**: causes **dopamine receptor**-mediated renal and mesenteric vasodilatation, with diuresis, at low doses; β$_1$–receptor agonist at higher doses, with increased cardiac output and BP. α-Receptor-

mediated vasoconstriction occurs at even higher doses. Myocardial O$_2$ demand is increased, but ischaemia is less likely as BP also increases. Tachycardia is less common.
      –**dobutamine**: mainly a β$_1$-receptor agonist, with weak β$_2$- and weaker α-receptor agonist properties. Causes less tachycardia than other catecholamines for a given inotropic effect, possibly due to a smaller effect on the sino-atrial node, and activation of the **baroreceptor reflex** by increased BP. Coronary perfusion may increase as left ventricular end-diastolic pressure falls.
      –**dopexamine**. Derived from dopamine; more active at β$_2$-receptors and less active at dopaminergic receptors. Causes peripheral and renal vasodilatation, with little tachycardia.
      –**pirbuterol**: mainly a β$_1$-receptor agonist. Causes some vasodilatation.
      –**salbutamol**: not a direct inotrope but sometimes used in circulatory failure. A β$_2$-receptor agonist, reducing SVR. Tachycardia is common.
   –**phosphodiesterase inhibitors**:
      –specific for cardiac phosphodiesterase: **amrinone, milrinone, enoximone**. Cause vasodilatation and increased cardiac output.
      –non-specific, e.g. **aminophylline**.
   –others:
      –calcium: effect lasts for about 5 minutes. Used as a temporary measure. Ventricular arrhythmias may occur.
      –**cardiac glycosides, e.g. digoxin**. Increase cardiac output and reduce heart rate; possibly also cause vasoconstriction. Thought to increase intracellular calcium ion activity via other ionic effects. Their use in circulatory failure is controversial.
      –**glucagon**: mechanism is unclear; adrenergic receptors are thought not to be involved. Thought to increase calcium flux into myocardial muscle by stimulating adenylate cyclase.

Choice of drug depends on clinical circumstances. Dopamine is often used in low dosage for its renal effect; dobutamine is commonly used for cardiac support. Adrenaline and noradrenaline are occasionally used, the latter, e.g. when vasodilatation is a particular problem, e.g. **septic shock**. Enoximone is increasingly used, e.g. after **cardiac surgery**, where tachycardia is particularly undesirable. Isoprenaline is indicated in bradycardia, and raised pulmonary vascular resistance.

Combinations are often used, e.g. with **vasodilator drugs**, to reduce filling pressures whilst providing inotropic support. Enoximone and dopexamine especially fulfil both functions.

INPB, Intermittent negative pressure breathing, *see Intermittent negative pressure ventilation*

INPV, *see Intermittent negative pressure ventilation*

INR, International normalized ratio, *see Coagulation studies*

Insensible water loss. Unmeasurable volume of pure water lost per day (i.e. without solutes as in sweat), mainly through skin and lungs. Normally up to 1200 ml at rest, increasing with body temperature (by up to 20% per °C above normal) and metabolic rate, and also in tachypnoea. Reduced as ambient humidity increases. During IPPV, exhaled losses may be reduced by **humidification** of inspired gases.

See also, Fluid balance

Inspiratory capacity. Maximal possible volume of air inspired from **FRC**. Composed of **tidal volume** and **inspiratory reserve volume**. Normally 4.0–5.0 litres.

See also, Lung volumes

Inspiratory:expiratory ratio (I:E ratio). Ratio of inspiratory time to expiratory time. Usually 1:2, allowing recovery from the cardiovascular effects of **IPPV** during expiration. Adjustable on most **ventilators** between 1:1 and 1:4. If expiration is too short, air trapping may occur, with increasing intrathoracic volume and pressure, increasing adverse effects of IPPV. However, a reversed I:E ratio of up to 4:1 (**inverse ratio ventilation**) has been used to improve oxygenation in respiratory failure, especially combined with **PEEP**.

If expiration is too long, **dead space** is thought to increase.

Inspiratory pressure support. Augmentation of spontaneous inspiration with supplementary gas flow. A more refined form of **assisted ventilation**, provided by sophisticated **ventilators**. Inspiratory flow rate is adjusted to produce a preset inspiratory airway pressure; when flow rate falls to a certain value, inspiration ends. Increases tidal volume, reducing work of breathing and respiratory rate during **weaning from ventilators**. However, negative pressure must be generated by the patient before augmentation. Tidal volume may vary according to the patient's inspiratory flow pattern. During weaning, the amount of support supplied may be reduced either by lowering the preset airway pressure, or by increasing the negative pressure required to trigger the support.

Inspiratory reserve volume. Inspiratory capacity minus **tidal volume**. Normally 3.5–4.0 litres.

See also, Lung volumes

Insufflation techniques. Passage of 4–6 l/min fresh gas through a fine bore catheter, passed through the larynx into the trachea; the tip usually lies near the carina (tracheal insufflation). With spontaneous ventilation, fresh gas and room air are inhaled into the lungs, with exhaled gas passing out around the catheter. May also be used to maintain oxygenation in apnoeic patients, although with build-up of CO_2 (**apnoeic oxygenation**).

First used in the early 1900s. **Magill** and **Rowbotham** later provided a separate tube for expired gases, both tubes subsequently replaced by a single wide bore tracheal tube. Still used by some anaesthetists for **bronchoscopy**, **laryngoscopy**, etc., especially in children. Fresh gas may also be delivered via the rigid endoscope.

Pharyngeal insufflation is also possible, using a pharyngeal catheter, or by attaching the fresh gas source to a gag or airway.

Barotrauma may occur if escape of gas is obstructed.

Insulin. Hormone secreted by B (β) cells of the pancreatic islets of Langerhans (A [α] cells secrete **glucagon**, and D [δ] cells **somatostatin**). Composed of two polypeptide chains specific to species, linked by disulphide bridges. Synthesized as a precursor molecule, subsequently split before secretion.

- Secretion is increased by:
  - **glucose**, mannose, fructose.
  - **amino acids**.
  - glucagon and other gut hormones.
  - β-**adrenergic receptor** stimulation.
  - vagal stimulation.
  - phosphodiesterase inhibition, e.g. due to drugs.
  - **sulphonylureas**.
  - stress.
- Secretion is decreased by:
  - **hypoglycaemia**.
  - somatostatin.
  - α-receptor stimulation.
  - insulin itself.
  - drugs:
    - **diazoxide**.
    - **thiazide diuretics**.
    - β-**adrenergic receptor antagonists**.
- Actions:
  - increases:
    - glucose uptake by muscle and fat.
    - **glycogen** synthesis.
    - **fat** synthesis and deposition.
    - **protein** synthesis.
    - potassium uptake by cells.
  - decreases:
    - glycogen breakdown and gluconeogenesis.
    - fat breakdown.
    - protein breakdown.
    - **ketone body** synthesis in the liver.

Thus lowers blood glucose levels and increases glucose utilization. Thought to act via cell surface receptors, via phosphorylation of intracellular **enzymes**.

Insulins for therapeutic administration, e.g. in **diabetes mellitus**, are derived from beef or pork pancreatic extract; human insulin is obtained using recombinant genetic engineering or enzymatic modification of pork insulin. Pork insulin is nearer in structure to human insulin than is beef. All types may cause antibody production in the recipient. Changing from one type to another, especially from beef to human, may result in hypoglycaemia.

Usually administered sc; may also be injected iv, im and intraperitoneally.

- Three types of insulin are available:
  - short acting: soluble insulin. Acts within 30–60 minutes of sc injection, with effects lasting up to 8 hours (**half-life** is 5 minutes after iv injection, with effects lasting 30 minutes). Used for emergency treatment of **hyperglycaemia** and perioperatively; also to lower plasma potassium in **hyperkalaemia**. When added to iv infusions, adequate mixing is essential to prevent uneven administration. May be adsorbed on to the infusion set plastic.
  - intermediate acting: isophane insulin (suspension with protamine) and amorphous insulin zinc suspension. Acts within 1–2 hours, lasting up to 20 hours.
  - long acting: crystalline insulin zinc suspension. Acts within 1–2 hours, lasting up to 36 hours.

The last two groups are mainly used for maintenance sc administration. Several insulin mixtures are also available. Available as 100 units/ml in the UK; dosage is adjusted for each patient.

[Paul Langerhans (1847–1888), German pathologist]
See also, Glycolysis

Intensive care unit (ICU). Modern techniques originate from respiratory care units in 1940–1950 along with developments in **IPPV** and **CPR**. **Coronary care units** were the first specialized units, set up in the 1960s.

An ICU usually provides 1–2% of total hospital beds, apart from specialized requirements, e.g. cardiac surgery, neurosurgery, etc. Units larger than ten beds should be subdivided into specialized units; a minimum of four beds is recommended. 85% of ICUs are run by anaesthetists in the UK.

- Design considerations:
  - size of unit/bed space (approximately 20 m² suggested per patient); number of cubicles.
  - proximity to theatres, casualty department, X-ray and laboratory facilities.
  - equipment: **ventilators**, **monitoring**, infusion pumps, etc. Adequate electrical points, gas pipelines, suction, etc.
  - lighting, basins, etc.
  - staff and their facilities (one nurse per patient required for 24 h/day).
- Patient selection criteria:
  - major organ failure requiring artificial support, e.g. respiratory or cardiovascular, often in combination with other organ system failure (e.g. commonly renal).
  - intensive monitoring and treatment in severe disease states, e.g. **septicaemia**, **head injury**, **poisoning and overdose**, **burns**, etc.
  - postoperative monitoring of respiratory, cardiovascular, neurological systems, etc.
  - other considerations:
    - reasons for admission: the disease state should be potentially reversible.
    - premorbid general health, age and **mortality prediction scores**.
    - availability of beds.
- Problems may be related to:
  - original condition.
  - multiple organ failure; may follow many disease processes (e.g. **renal failure** and **ARDS** are common in critical illness of any cause). Prognosis worsens as more organ systems are involved.
  - infection, e.g. septicaemia.
  - adequate **nutrition**, and fluid and electrolyte balance.
  - gastric ulceration (**stress ulcers**). Prophylaxis is as for **peptic ulcer disease**; **H₂ receptor antagonists** are most commonly used, **sucralfate** increasingly so.
  - immobility: **DVT** and bed sores may occur. Prophylactic sc **heparin** is usually administered, and careful skin care, regular turning and physiotherapy instituted.
  - **sedation**.

See also, Selective decontamination of the digestive tract

Intercostal nerve block. Used for per- and **postoperative analgesia**, and for analgesia in patients with fractured **ribs**.

- Technique:
  - may be performed with the patient sitting, with shoulders flexed to pull the scapulae forwards (e.g. with the forearms resting on pillows), or in the lateral position, with the side to be blocked uppermost.
  - identification of selected ribs: by counting down from the spinous process of T1 (the most prominent palpable at the base of the neck) or up from L4–5 (level with the iliac crests). The rib is palpated laterally to the angle, about 6–10 cm from the midline. Injection at the angle blocks the lateral cutaneous branch of the intercostal nerve, which is missed if injection is performed in the mid- or posterior axillary line.
  - a needle (mounted on a syringe to prevent air entry if pleura is pierced) is introduced at the lower edge of the rib, directed cranially. It contacts bone, and is 'walked' inferiorly until it slips off the rib's inferior surface. It is then advanced 2–3 mm. The patient is asked to breath-hold to reduce lung movement and risk of **pneumothorax**.
  - stretching of the overlying skin cranially before needle insertion has been suggested: release of stretch following insertion aids angling of the needle tip into the subcostal groove.
  - following aspiration for blood, 3–5 ml of **local anaesthetic agent** is injected whilst moving the needle inwards and outwards 1–2 mm. **Bupivacaine** 0.25–0.5% with **adrenaline** may provide analgesia lasting up to 12 hours; **lignocaine** 1% with adrenaline up to 2–4 hours. Catheters have been inserted for repeated injections.
  - studies with dyes have shown extensive overlap of injected solution to adjacent spaces (and even to the other side). Systemic absorption of solution is significant; maximal 'safe' doses should not be exceeded.
  - pneumothorax and puncture of intercostal blood vessels may occur. Intra- or extradural spread via a dural cuff surrounding the proximal nerve is also possible.

See also, Intercostal spaces; Interpleural analgesia

Intercostal spaces. Contain the intercostal nerves and blood vessels as they run around the width of the body (Fig. 73).

- Muscle layers between **ribs**:
  - external intercostal muscle, passing down and forwards.
  - internal intercostal muscle, passing down and backwards. Becomes the internal intercostal membrane posterior to the rib angles.
  - innermost intercostal muscle, attached to the ribs' inner surfaces.
- Intercostal nerves:
  - ventral rami of **spinal nerves** T1–11. Each spinal nerve has dorsal and ventral roots, which join and then divide into dorsal and ventral rami. The dorsal rami supply the extensor muscles and skin of the back.
  - lie below the blood vessels in the intercostal space.
  - each (except the 1st) gives off a lateral cutaneous branch anterior to the rib angles, and ends as the anterior cutaneous branch.
  - collateral branch arises at the angle, passing forward with main nerve.
- Intercostal arteries:
  - two anterior and one posterior supply each space except the lower two (posterior only).
  - anterior arteries arise from the internal thoracic artery or its terminal branch. They anastomose with the posterior artery and its collateral.

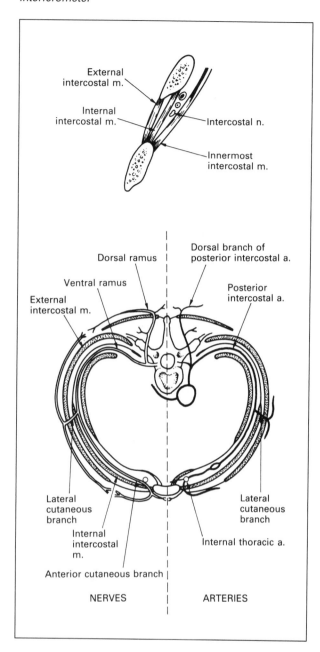

External intercostal m.

Internal intercostal m.

Intercostal n.

Innermost intercostal m.

Dorsal ramus

Dorsal branch of posterior intercostal a.

Ventral ramus

Posterior intercostal a.

External intercostal m.

Lateral cutaneous branch

Lateral cutaneous branch

Internal intercostal m.

Internal thoracic a.

Anterior cutaneous branch

NERVES

ARTERIES

Figure 73 *Anatomy of intercostal spaces*

–posterior arteries arise from the superior intercostal artery (1st and 2nd) or descending aorta. They each give off a collateral branch.
Venous drainage is via two anterior and one posterior intercostal veins, to internal thoracic and azygos veins.

Interferometer, *see Gas analysis*

Intermittent flow anaesthetic machines. To be distinguished from apparatus used for **draw-over techniques**, in which the patient's own inspiratory effort causes gas flow. Intermittent flow machines provide gas flow usually on demand, i.e. when triggered by the patient's inspiration, but are more sophisticated than simple **demand valves**.

Allow mixing of gases, usually O_2 and N_2O, and addition of volatile agents using conventional **vaporizers**. Minnitt's machine (described in 1933) using a N_2O cylinder with indrawn air was used for analgesia in labour. Inspiration reduces pressure within the apparatus, moving a valve and allowing gas flow. In the **McKesson** machine, the force opposing fresh gas flow may be adjusted, so that continuous low flow may be provided if required, between breaths. Further adjustment provides continuous high flow, as with conventional **anaesthetic machines**.

Some machines feature O_2 **warning devices**, O_2 flushes and valves to cut off N_2O in case of potentially hypoxic gas mixtures.

Traditionally used for **dental surgery**, but less commonly used now because of unfamiliarity, inaccuracy of flow rates and gas composition, and relative lack of safety features.
[Robert J Minnitt (1889–1974), Liverpool anaesthetist]

Intermittent mandatory ventilation (IMV). Ventilatory mode used to assist **weaning from ventilators**. A mandatory minute volume is preset and delivered by the ventilator, but the patient is allowed to breathe spontaneously from a reservoir between ventilator breaths. As the patient weans, the proportion of minute volume delivered by the ventilator may be reduced, usually by reducing the ventilator rate.

IMV reduces average intrathoracic pressures and risk of **barotrauma**. The patient's progress may be monitored by counting the spontaneous respiratory rate.

Some sophisticated ventilators will not deliver positive pressure breaths within a certain period of spontaneous breaths, to prevent over-distension of the patient's lungs and barotrauma (synchronized intermittent mandatory ventilation). Others simply incorporate a pressure-relief valve.

Although the weaning process is not shortened, IMV allows it to start earlier and be monitored more easily whilst requiring less **sedation**, and reducing risks of **IPPV**.
Cameron PD, Oh TE (1986) Anaesth Intensive Care; 14: 258–66

Intermittent negative pressure ventilation (INPV). Advocated in the 1800s as a means of controlled ventilation without the adverse effects of **IPPV**, although the latter were then overestimated. Tank **ventilators** were described first, then cuirass types; motor driven devices were used in the 1930s.

Avoids the risk of **barotrauma** and other dangers of IPPV, whilst allowing the respiratory muscles to rest. Does not require tracheal intubation, although the risks of regurgitation and aspiration are still present. Indrawing of the soft tissues of the neck may result in upper airway obstruction. **Sedation** is not required. Continuous end-expiratory negative extrathoracic pressure has similar beneficial effects to **PEEP**, but without its adverse effects.

Largely superseded by IPPV, but still used for chronic ventilation, e.g. domiciliary night-time ventilation for neuromuscular disease; it has been used to aid **weaning** from prolonged IPPV.
Shneerson JM (1989) Care Crit Ill; 5: 153–8

Intermittent positive pressure ventilation (IPPV). Form of controlled ventilation. Performed by Vesalius in

1543 (via a tracheotomy in a pig) and Hooke in 1667 (used bellows via a tracheotomy in a dog). Used initially for **CPR**; later employed in animal experiments with **curare** by **Waterton** in the 1820s. Used in the late 1800s/early 1900s during anaesthesia, but wider acceptance accompanied the introduction of **neuromuscular blocking drugs** in the 1940s. Use in **respiratory failure** developed largely following the 1952 Danish **poliomyelitis** epidemic.

Modified forms, e.g. **IMV, mandatory minute ventilation** etc., are mainly used in **ICU** during **weaning from ventilators**. **High frequency ventilation** was developed from the early 1970s. **Nasal positive pressure ventilation** has recently been introduced for patients with neuromuscular respiratory failure, and may be useful in COAD.

- Indications:
  - ICU:
    - respiratory failure.
    - **head injury**.
    - others, e.g. **coma**, post-CPR.
  - anaesthesia:
    - when neuromuscular blockade is required; often performed when tracheal intubation is indicated.
    - thoracic surgery.
    - when ventilation is inadequate.
    - to control arterial P_{CO_2}.
    - to reduce requirement for inhalational agents, e.g. in cardiovascular disease.
    - to ensure adequate air entry, e.g. in respiratory disease.
- Technique:
  - tracheal intubation is usually employed, but it may be performed via **laryngeal mask** or even **facepiece**.
  - manual ventilation was formerly used extensively; **ventilators** are now widespread. **Injector techniques** may also be used.
  - a tidal volume of 10–15 ml/kg, at a rate of 10–12 breaths/min, is commonly used, ideally adjusted to arterial (or end-tidal) P_{CO_2}. Intermittent 'sighs' of larger tidal volume were formerly used to reduce **atelectasis**, but are no longer considered effective. **Negative end-expiratory pressure** is no longer recommended.

    Mean intrathoracic pressure is lowest with accelerating gas flow, but ventilation is uneven. Ventilation is more uniform with decelerating flow, but mean pressure is highest. **Inspiratory : expiratory ratio** of 1:2 is usually employed but may be varied according to clinical requirements.
  - neuromuscular blockade is usually employed; deep anaesthesia using volatile agents may also be used, combined with **opioid analgesic drugs** and **hypocapnia** to suppress respiratory drive. Sedative/opioid infusions are commonly used in ICU (*see Sedation*).
  - **monitoring** is important to ensure adequate ventilation and gas exchange, and to detect disconnection.
- Physiological effects/hazards:
  - cardiovascular effects, due to increased intrathoracic pressure:
    - reduced **venous return** and **cardiac output**; may reduce BP, especially in **autonomic neuropathy** or **hypovolaemia**.
    - increased **pulmonary vascular resistance**, reducing right ventricular output.
    - reduced left ventricular **compliance** and filling, especially with **PEEP**. Bulging of the right ventricle

and direct effects of lung expansion are thought to be responsible.
  - measured **CVP** is raised, and venous drainage from head and neck is reduced. **ICP** may increase.
  - respiratory effects:
    - **intrapleural pressure** is about –5 cmH_2O during expiration and up to +5 cmH_2O during inspiration, in contrast to spontaneous ventilation.
    - lung compliance and **FRC** fall. Atelectasis occurs in dependent lung tissue, increasing **alveolar-arterial O_2 difference** and **dead space**. Adding PEEP and increasing tidal volume may reduce these effects.
  - others:
    - renal: reduced arterial BP and increased venous pressure lower renal perfusion. Glomerular filtration is reduced, and the **renin/angiotensin system** stimulated. **Atrial natriuretic peptide** secretion is lowered and **vasopressin** secretion may be increased. The overall effect is reduced urine output (by up to 40%) and sodium retention.
    - **ileus** is common with prolonged IPPV; the cause is unclear but may involve changes in GIT neural activity and pressures. It may also be related to concurrent illness or drug therapy.
    - risks of tracheal intubation.
    - **barotrauma**, undetected disconnection.

[Andreas Vesalius (1514–1564), German anatomist; Robert Hooke (1635–1703), Curator of the Royal Society, England]

Hillman DR (1986) Anaesth Intensive Care; 14: 226–35

See also, Intermittent negative pressure ventilation; Intubation, tracheal

Internal jugular venous cannulation. The internal **jugular vein** lies deep to the sternomastoid muscle, and follows a course from just anterior to the mastoid process to behind the sternoclavicular joint (Fig. 74). Cannulation may be performed at a number of sites; the most common are outlined below.

- Technique:
  - head-down position distends the vein and reduces the risk of **air embolism**. The head is turned to the contralateral side. Aseptic techniques are used.
  - the distended vein may be palpable (or even visible) in thin subjects, lateral to the carotid pulsation.
  - a right side approach is usually employed, since the right internal jugular vein, superior vena cava and right atrium are more directly aligned than on the left.
  - local anaesthetic is used if the patient is awake.
  - high approach:
    - the carotid pulsation is located level with the cricoid cartilage (C6). With the fingers of one hand guarding the artery, the needle is introduced just laterally, angled at 30° to the skin and directed towards the ipsilateral nipple. When blood is aspirated, the needle is lowered to align it more with the vein, and the cannula advanced or wire inserted (**Seldinger technique**). If no blood is aspirated, the needle may be redirected slightly medially. Some prefer to locate the vein with a small needle first before using the larger introducer needle. Ultrasound probes have also been used to aid location of the vein.

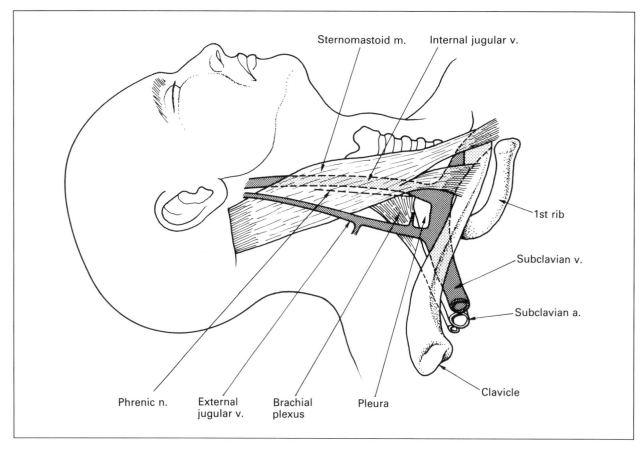

Figure 74 *Anatomy of right internal jugular vein*

–alternatively, a slightly lower approach involves needle insertion at the apex of the triangle formed by the two heads of sternomastoid, a more reliable landmark when the carotid pulsation is weak or absent (e.g. cardiac arrest).

–low approach: the needle is introduced just above the sternoclavicular joint and directed caudally. A higher incidence of **pneumothorax** may result from this approach.

For complications and comparisons with other techniques, see Central venous cannulation

International normalized ratio, *see Coagulation studies*

Interonium distance. Distance between quaternary ammonium groups in molecules of non-depolarizing **neuromuscular blocking drugs**. Thought to relate to drug activity in blocking **acetylcholine receptor** sites, thought originally to be placed 1.2–1.4 nm apart. Drugs with interonium distances of 0.6–0.7 nm are also active, suggesting cross-linkage between drugs or receptors.

Interpleural analgesia. Injection of **local anaesthetic agent** into the pleural cavity, performed for analgesia after thoracic and upper abdominal surgery and in **rib** fractures. Unilateral pain is the most suitable indication. An extradural catheter may be placed either under direct vision during thoracotomy, or via an extradural needle; the pleural space is identified using a loss of resistance syringe,

allowing the syringe plunger to be drawn in by the negative interpleural pressure. The patient's breath is held at end-inspiration if spontaneously breathing, or end-expiration if ventilated, to maintain maximal negative pressure during needle insertion. Alternatively, a catheter is pushed through the needle as the latter is advanced; unobstructed passage of the catheter occurs when the parietal pleura is punctured. Straw-coloured pleural fluid may be aspirated. The midaxillary line of the 4th–8th interspace is usually employed. 8–30 ml of 0.25–0.5% **bupivacaine** with **adrenaline** has been used, producing up to 24 hours' analgesia. 0.1–0.5 ml/kg/h infusion has also been used. Gravity and positioning may be used to extend the block if inadequate. Solution may also be instilled through a pleural drain. Mechanism of analgesia is unclear, but is thought to involve blockade of **intercostal nerves**.

Complications are uncommon, and include **pneumothorax**, local anaesthetic toxicity (maximal levels occur within 20 minutes of bolus injection), phrenic, recurrent laryngeal or sympathetic nerve blockade and haemorrhage.
Lewis GW (1989) Can J Anaesth; 36: 103–5

Interstitial fibrosis, *see Pulmonary fibrosis*

Interstitial fluid. Fluid compartment comprising most of the **ECF**. Volume is approximately 9.5 litres, about 14% of body weight of an average man; it is determined by subtracting **plasma** volume from ECF volume.
For composition etc., see Fluids, body

Intestinal obstruction, *see Emergency surgery*

Intra-aortic counter-pulsation balloon pump. Device used to support **cardiac output** by inflating a balloon within the descending aorta at the beginning of diastole, with deflation immediately before systole. Introduced percutaneously, e.g. via the femoral artery, and inflated with helium or CO_2. Triggered and timed according to the **ECG** and **arterial waveform**. Increases coronary and tissue blood flow, with reduced **afterload** and left ventricular work; i.e. increases myocardial O_2 supply whilst decreasing demand.

Used as a temporary measure, e.g. in left ventricular failure and **cardiogenic shock** pre/post **cardiac surgery** or after **MI**. Complications include trauma, haemorrhage, etc. during insertion, **aortic dissection** and rupture, distal thrombus, embolism and ischaemia, and trauma to platelets and red cells.

Maccioli GA, Lucas WJ, Norfleet EA (1988) J Cardiothorac Anesth; 2: 365–73

Intra-arterial regional anaesthesia. Injection of **local anaesthetic agent**, e.g. 10–20 ml 0.5% **lignocaine**, into the brachial artery, a tourniquet having been inflated proximally to above systolic BP. Produces anaesthesia of the arm using smaller amounts of drug than for **IVRA**, but now rarely performed. Described in 1908 by Goyanes.
[J Goyanes (1876–1964), Spanish surgeon]

Intracellular fluid. Similar in composition between different cells; thus considered a single fluid compartment comprising about 28 litres (40% of body weight) in an average man. Determined by subtracting **ECF** from total body water (measured using a **dilution technique** with deuterium oxide).
For composition etc., see Fluids, body

Intracranial haemorrhage, *see Cerebrovascular accident; Extradural haemorrhage; Head injury; Subarachnoid haemorrhage; Subdural haemorrhage*

Intracranial pressure (ICP). Normally 7–15 mmHg (1–2 kPa) supine; fluctuations may be revealed by **ICP monitoring**. Because the skull is a rigid box, and its contents incompressible, ICP depends on the volume of intracranial contents: normally 50–70 ml blood (5–7%), 50–120 ml **CSF** (5–12%), and 1.4 kg brain tissue (80–85%) (*see Monro–Kellie doctrine*).
- Effects of increased intracranial volume:
  - movement of CSF into the spinal canal, increased absorption of CSF into the venous circulation, and venous sinus compression. Thus ICP is maintained at near normal levels initially.
  - eventually, compensatory mechanisms are overwhelmed; small changes in volume are now accompanied by large increases in ICP (Fig. 75).
  - as ICP rises, **cerebral perfusion pressure** and **cerebral blood flow** are decreased. When venous blood vessels are obstructed, massive swelling occurs. Regional ischaemia, structural distortion and **coning** may follow. During surgery, raised ICP is prevented by the open skull, but the brain may bulge and hinder surgery or closure.
  - clinical features:

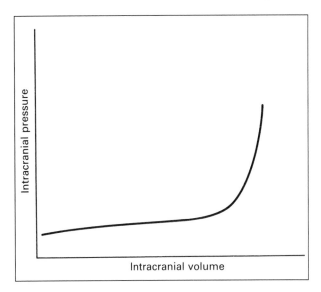

Figure 75 *Effects of increasing intracranial volume on intracranial pressure*

  - headache, nausea/vomiting, confusion. Headache is classically worse in the early morning and exacerbated by stooping or straining.
  - papilloedema, impaired consciousness, hypertension and bradycardia (**Cushing's reflex**) as ICP continues to rise.
  - hypotension, coma, irregular respiration or apnoea, fixed and dilated pupils.
- Raised ICP is caused by increased volume of the following compartments:
  - blood:
    - increased cerebral blood flow.
    - impaired venous drainage, e.g. coughing, straining, kinked jugular veins, head-down position.
  - brain:
    - tumour, abscess, haematoma.
    - **cerebral oedema**.
  - CSF: as for **hydrocephalus**.

Rarely, 'benign' intracranial hypertension is associated with none of the above, especially in young women. It may cause permanent visual impairment due to optic nerve damage. Its management includes repeated lumbar CSF drainage, steroids and shunt insertion.
- Treatment of raised ICP involves reduction in volume of:
  - blood:
    - IPPV with **hyperventilation** to arterial P_{CO_2} 3.5–4 kPa (27–30 mmHg), to produce cerebral vasoconstriction. Effectiveness may be limited to 24–48 hours.
    - encouragement of venous drainage: head up posture, adequate sedation/relaxation, avoiding jugular compression/kinking.
  - brain:
    - surgical decompression.
    - diuretics and steroids in certain circumstances (*see Cerebral oedema*).
    - fluid restriction to 1.5–2 l/day is often instituted.
  - CSF: drainage, e.g. via the lateral ventricle. Long-term shunts as for hydrocephalus.

- Effects of anaesthetic agents on ICP:
  - –iv agents: **barbiturates**, **etomidate**, **propofol**, **benzodiazepines**: reduce ICP. Opioids: no change or reduction, if normocapnia is maintained. **Ketamine** increases ICP.
  - –inhalational agents: **halothane**, **enflurane**, **isoflurane**: cause a dose-dependent increase in ICP via increasing cerebral blood flow. The effect is counteracted by hyperventilation and hypocapnia; this must be achieved before introduction of halothane or enflurane to prevent the rise in ICP but this is not necessary for isoflurane. **N$_2$O** may increase ICP via increased blood flow, or if air is contained in cavities within the skull, e.g. following surgery, head injury, etc.
  - –others: Non-depolarizing **neuromuscular blocking drugs** cause no change in ICP. **Suxamethonium** may cause a transient increase during fasciculation, due to an increase in intrathoracic pressure. ICP is increased by laryngoscopy and tracheal intubation.
  - –hypotensive drugs: ICP may increase following **sodium nitroprusside** and nitrates, probably via increased intracranial blood volume due to vasodilatation. No rise is associated with **trimetaphan**.

Anaesthesia for patients with raised ICP: as for **neurosurgery**.

See also, Cerebral protection/resuscitation

Intracranial pressure monitoring. Indications vary between units but may include any cause of **coma** and raised **ICP,** most commonly **head injury**, intracranial haemorrhage, postoperatively, encephalopathies, etc. Associated with significant risk of infection, especially with over 3 days' use.

- Types of monitoring:
  - –extradural fibreoptic probe, laid between the dura and skull via a burr hole. Easy to position, with low infection rates. CSF drainage is impossible, and accuracy is less reliable. Fully implantable devices have been described.
  - –subarachnoid screw, applied via a burr hole. Easy to position, but infection rate is higher. More accurate unless oedema is present. CSF drainage is sometimes possible. Subdural catheters have also been described.
  - –ventricular drain, placed during craniotomy. High accuracy but infection rate is highest. CSF drainage is easy. Fibreoptic devices may also be used, or a catheter attached to a subcutaneous device for percutaneous puncture, for chronic use.
  - –intracerebral transducer, placed within brain tissue itself.

Devices are flushed rarely using small volumes (under 0.2 ml). Continuous flow apparatus is not used. Output is best displayed as a continuous recording, ideally with simultaneous calculation of **cerebral perfusion pressure**, e.g. using a computer. Injecting small volumes into the ventricular system has been used to calculate ventricular compliance or pressure/volume index (volume required to raise CSF pressure by a factor of 10); these indices of distensibility are not routinely performed. The waveform obtained resembles the **arterial waveform**, corresponding to the pulsation of large vessels within the brain. The waveform also varies with respiration, reflecting changes in **CVP**. Mean ICP is calculated in a similar way to **MAP** and is normally 7–15 mmHg (1–2 kPa) in the supine position.

- Three variations in ICP have been described:
  - –A (plateau) waves: amplitude 50–100 mmHg, they last 5–20 minutes. Associated with cerebral vasodilatation. Most common in patients with intracranial tumours. Often associated with acute clinical deterioration and thus may be useful clinically.
  - –B waves: amplitude <50 mmHg; occur at about 1/min. Associated with changes in respiratory pattern. Less useful clinically.
  - –C waves: amplitude <20 mmHg; occur at 4–8/min. Related to systemic vasomotor tone and BP. Not useful clinically.

Active management is usually advocated at pressures exceeding 15–30 mmHg (2–3 kPa), depending on the underlying condition, speed of deterioration and clinical situation.

Doyle DJ, Mark PW (1992) J Clin Monit; 8: 81–90

Intractable pain, *see Pain; Pain management*

Intradural..., *see Spinal...*

Intramucosal pH, *see Gastric intramucosal pH*

Intraocular pressure (IOP). Normally 1.3–2 kPa (10–15 mmHg), increased in **glaucoma**. Important during open **ophthalmic surgery** because of the risk of expulsion of intraocular contents and haemorrhage, with subsequent distortion of anatomy, scarring and loss of vision.

- Related to:
  - –external pressure on the eye:
    - –from facepiece, leaning on the eye, etc.
    - –retrobulbar haematoma.
    - –extrinsic muscles.
    - –venous congestion of orbit.
  - –scleral rigidity: increased in severe myopia and in the elderly.
  - –intraocular contents:
    - –choroidal blood volume:
      - –increases with arterial PCO$_2$ and **hypoxaemia**, and vasodilatation.
      - –increases transiently with acute rises in systolic BP; falls at systolic pressure of under 80–90 mmHg.
      - –increases with **CVP**, e.g. due to straining, coughing, vomiting, head-down position, etc.
    - –aqueous humour:
      - –formed by the choroidal plexus of the posterior chamber, at about 0.08 ml/h. A small amount is formed in the anterior chamber.
      - –passes through the pupil to the anterior chamber; drains from the angle between the iris and cornea via the canal of Schlemm into the venous circulation.
      - –reduced by **acetazolamide**, although it also increases choroidal blood volume. Also reduced by oral glycerol and meiosis. Control is important in glaucoma, but less so during surgery.
    - –vitreous humour: may be reduced by administration of **mannitol** 0.5–1.5 g/kg iv, 45 minutes preoperatively. Urinary catheterization is usually required. Sucrose 50% 1 g/kg is shorter-acting.
    - –other structures, e.g . lens.

–sulphur hexafluoride (SF_6) is sometimes injected into the vitreous in retinal surgery to splint the retina; N_2O markedly expands the SF_6 volume and increases IOP by diffusing into the bubble faster than SF_6 diffuses out (blood/gas **solubility** of N_2O is over 100 times that of SF_6). When N_2O is stopped at the end of surgery, IOP may decrease markedly. N_2O is therefore usually discontinued before SF_6 injection, to reduce large swings in IOP. Atmospheric nitrogen diffuses into the bubble postoperatively, but its effect is smaller and slower because its blood/gas solubility is only 2–3 times that of SF_6.

- Effects of anaesthetic agents on IOP:
  –little effect, if any, of premedicant drugs.
  –no effect of **atropine**, unless administered topically to glaucomatous eyes (IOP may rise).
  –reduced by all iv induction agents except **ketamine**; **propofol** and **etomidate** cause a greater reduction than **thiopentone**.
  –reduced slightly by **benzodiazepines** and **neuroleptanaesthesia**.
  –reduced by all volatile agents; the mechanism is unclear. Unaffected by N_2O.
  –increased by **suxamethonium**, possibly via choroidal vasodilatation and extrinsic eye muscle contraction, although the increase in IOP still occurs when the muscles are cut. The increase lasts only a few minutes. The use of suxamethonium in the presence of penetrating eye injury is controversial (*see Eye, penetrating injury*).
  –non-depolarizing **neuromuscular blocking drugs** may lower IOP slightly.

Anaesthesia for open eye operations thus involves avoidance of factors increasing IOP, e.g. straining, vomiting, etc., and use of techniques and drugs which lower IOP, e.g. head-up tilt, hypocapnia, smooth anaesthesia, etc.

IOP is estimated by measuring corneal indentation by a weighted plunger, or by measuring the force required to flatten an area of cornea.

[Friedrich Schlemm (1795–1858), German anatomist]
Cunningham AJ, Barry P (1986) Can Anaesth Soc J; 33: 195–208

Intrapleural pressure. Pressure within the pleural cavity, perhaps better termed interpleural pressure. Measured indirectly using an oesophageal balloon catheter (i.e. within the thorax but outside the lungs). Normally negative, due to the thoracic cage's tendency to spring outwards, and the lungs' tendency to collapse inwards. In the erect posture at normal resting lung volume, intrapleural pressure equals approximately $-10\,cmH_2O$ at the lung apex, $-2.5\,cmH_2O$ at the base.

Increases in magnitude as lung volume (and thus elastic recoil) increases. During spontaneous ventilation, it thus becomes more negative during inspiration. Normally changes by 3–4 cmH_2O, more if **airway resistance** is increased or breathing forceful. During expiration, it returns to its original value unless expiration is forced or resistance increased; it may then exceed zero.

During IPPV, pressure increases from the resting value, depending on the inflating pressure (usually by 10–20 cmH_2O). Thus it usually exceeds zero during inspiration. Increased by **CPAP** and **PEEP** (i.e. towards or beyond zero).

Intrathecal..., *see Spinal*...

Intravenous anaesthetic agents. Development of drugs and iv techniques occurred later than for **inhalational anaesthetic agents**, but iv **induction of anaesthesia** is usually preferred now because it is faster with less risk of excitement, laryngospasm, etc. Popularized in the 1930s by **Weese**, **Lundy** and **Waters**, although **Oré** had used iv **chloral hydrate** in 1872. Subsequent agents include **hedonal** (1905), phenobarbitone (1912), **paraldehyde** (1913), **bromethol** (1927), hexobarbitone (1932; the first widely used iv **barbiturate**), thiopentone (1932), **hydroxydione** (1955), **methohexitone** (1957), **propranidid** (1956), γ-**hydroxybutyric acid** (1962), **ketamine** (1965), **Althesin** (1971), **etomidate** (1973), and **propofol** (1986). **Diethyl ether** has been injected iv.

Used for induction and maintenance of anaesthesia, including **TIVA**, and for **sedation**. Many iv agents have also been given im or rectally. **Benzodiazepines**, e.g. **midazolam** have been used for induction, as have high doses of **opioid analgesic drugs**.

- Have been classified thus:
  –rapid onset:
    –barbiturates: thiopentone, methohexitone.
    –imidazole compounds: etomidate.
    –alkyl phenol: propofol.
    –steroids: Althesin, **minaxolone**, hydroxydione.
    –eugenols: propranidid.
  –slow onset:
    –ketamine.
    –benzodiazepines.
    –opioids.
- Features of the ideal iv anaesethetic agent:
  –physical/chemical properties:
    –chemically stable; i.e. not requiring storage in a fridge or away from light. Long shelf-life.
    –water-soluble, not requiring reconstitution before use, nor any additives.
    –compatible with iv fluids, other drugs, etc.
  –pharmacology:
    –painless on injection, with low incidence of thrombophlebitis. Harmless on extravasation or intra-arterial injection.
    –low incidence of **adverse drug reactions**.
    –smooth onset of anaesthesia within one **arm–brain circulation time**, without unwanted movement, coughing, hiccup, etc.
    –anticonvulsant, antiemetic and analgesic properties. No increase in **cerebral blood flow**, **ICP** or **intraocular pressure**. Reduces **$CMRO_2$**.
    –no respiratory depression. Bronchodilator.
    –no cardiovascular depression or stimulation, or arrhythmias.
    –predictable recovery, related to the dose injected.
    –rapid metabolism to non-active metabolites; i.e. non-cumulative.
    –no impairment of renal or hepatic function or steroid synthesis.
    –no **emergence phenomena**.
    –no teratogenicity.

No currently available agent fulfils all of the above (Table 20).

Agents should be injected slowly, titrating against effect, especially if the patient has reduced cardiac output. Overdose is easily produced by rapid injection of a large dose.

Table 20. Properties of iv anaesthetic agents

Agent	Thiopentone	Methohexitone	Ketamine	Etomidate	Propofol	Midazolam
Additives	Sodium carbonate	Sodium carbonate	Benzethonium chloride	Propylene glycol	Soya-bean oil emulsion	–
Aqueous solution	+	+	+	–	–	+
Approximate cost/induction dose (£)	1	<1	2–3	1–2	<4	2–3
Painful injection	–	+	–	+	+	–
Rapid onset	+	+	–	+	+	–
Unwanted movement	–	+	±	+	–	–
Respiratory/cardiovascular depression	+	+	–	±	+	±
Analgesic	–	–	+	–	–	–
Vomiting	–	–	+	+	–	–
Steroid inhibition	–	–	–	+	–	–
Rapid recovery	+	+	–	+	+	–
Emergence phenomena	–	–	+	–	–	–
pK_a	7.6	7.9	7.5	4.2	11	6.2
Protein binding (%)	85	85	12	75	98	98
Volume of distribution (l/kg)	1.5–2.5	1–2	2–3	2–5	3–5	1–2
Distribution half-life (min)	2–6	5–6	10–15	1–4	1–2	7–15
Elimination half-life (h)	5–10	2–4	2–3	1–5	1–5	2–5
Clearance (ml/kg/min)	2–4	10–12	18–20	18–25	25–30	6–11

- Following iv injection, brain levels depend on the amount of drug crossing the **blood–brain barrier**, related to:
    - **protein binding**.
    - **ionization**:, e.g. at pH of 7.4, 61% of thiopentone, 75% of methohexitone and over 90% of propofol is unionized.
    - cerebral blood flow: increased as a proportion of cardiac output in **hypovolaemia**, etc.
    - fat solubility: high for most anaesthetic agents; propofol and ketamine are particularly fat soluble.
    - distribution, metabolism and excretion.

Recovery from, e.g., thiopentone occurs by redistribution from vessel-rich tissues (brain, heart, liver, kidney; 70–80% of cardiac output) to vessel-intermediate tissues (muscle, skin; 18% of cardiac output), thence to fat (6%) and vessel-poor tissues such as ligaments, etc. (Fig. 76). Thus significant amounts of thiopentone remain in the body after recovery, compared with more rapidly metabolized agents, e.g. propofol.

See also, Pharmacokinetics

Intravenous fluid administration. Described in the 1600s. **Saline solutions** were used sporadically in **dehydration** due to cholera, **diabetes mellitus** and diarrhoea in the 1800s. Infusions were widely used in World War I, including acacia as a **colloid**. Bacterial and chemical contamination and allergic reactions were common. Sterile fluids and administration sets became available in World War II; increasing investigation into **fluid balance** since then was prompted by subsequent wars, e.g. Korea, Vietnam. Balanced fluid therapy was developed in the 1950s–1960s.

- Practical considerations:
    - site of administration: usually forearm, since it is the least awkward for the patient. The arm or hand are preferred to the legs, since venous stasis is commoner in the latter. Placement near joints or known arteries is avoided when possible. **Central venous cannulation** is used for irritant or vasoactive drugs, if peripheral cannulation is unsuccessful or if long-term administration or CVP measurement is required.

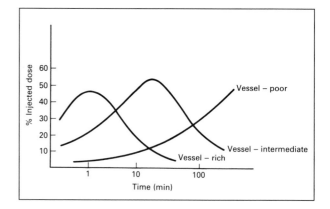

Figure 76 *Fate of thiopentone after iv injection*

- cannulation: venous filling is increased by gentle slapping, squeezing of the hand, or immersion of the limb in warm water for 10 minutes. Intradermal injection of local anaesthetic or use of **EMLA** reduces the pain of insertion of large cannulae. Attempts are made to cannulate distal veins first, moving proximally if unsuccessful. Rarely, cut-down may be required:
    - an anatomically constant venous site is chosen, e.g. long saphenous vein (above and anterior to the medial malleolus).
    - the vein is exposed and two ties placed around it; only the distal one is tightened.
    - the cannula is introduced and secured with the proximal tie.
    - cannulae: plastic cannulae were developed in the 1970s. Their general design is similar but flow characteristics differ widely between different makes. British Standard for determining flow rate: a constant pressure of 10 kPa is maintained using a constant-level tank of distilled water at 22°C. It is connected via 110 cm tubing (inside diameter 4 mm) to the

cannula, with the distal 4 cm and the cannula horizontal. The volume of water is collected over at least 30 seconds; an average of three readings is taken. Thus the flows are different from those achieved clinically, but the values are useful for comparison between differently-sized cannulae:

 –10 G : 550–600 ml/min.
 –12 G : 400–500 ml/min.
 –14 G : 250–360 ml/min.
 –16 G : 130–220 ml/min.
 –18 G : 75–120 ml/min.
 –20 G : 40–80 ml/min.

Gauge ('G') numbers are equivalent to those used for **needles**. Recently introduced colour-coding standard for iv cannulae:

 –14 G : orange
 –16 G : grey
 –18 G : green
 –20 G : pink
 –22 G : blue
 –24 G : yellow
 –26 G : black

–giving sets: internal diameter is 4 mm, but extra turbulence and resistance arises from extra length, drip chambers and filter (170 μm pore size). Non-blood giving sets have no filter or float, and are narrower and cheaper.
–syringe pumps, volumetric pumps, drip counters, etc.; high pressures may occur with the former two if obstruction to flow occurs. Some syringe pumps may empty rapidly if placed above the patient.
–microfiltration: not routinely used, but 0.2 μm filters are claimed to reduce phlebitis, especially when repeated drug injections are given. They may also retain **endotoxin** and prevent **air embolism**. The routine use of **blood filters** is controversial.
• Hazards:
–during cannulation: haemorrhage, haematoma, trauma.
–extravasation: especially harmful if the fluid is irritant, e.g. potassium or **bicarbonate** solutions, **thiopentone**, antimitotic drugs, etc. Flushing with saline, **hyaluronidase** or steroids has been suggested as treatment.
–thrombophlebitis: more common with small veins and highly concentrated or irritant infusates. Reduced if infusion sites are changed regularly, e.g. 24–48 hourly. May lead to thrombosis and/or infection. Infusion life may be prolonged with a **glyceryl trinitrate** patch applied topically. Addition of heparin or hydrocortisone to the fluid bag has also been used. Heparinoid cream is often applied to existing phlebitis.
–interactions between infused drugs or fluids, especially if multiple infusions are used through a single cannula.
–air embolism.
–related to the **iv fluid** infused, e.g. **hyponatraemia**, **pulmonary oedema**, etc.
–when one cannula is used for more than one infusion, temporary blockage of the cannula may lead to one infusion (e.g. of a drug) retrogradely filling the tubing of the second infusion (e.g. a saline infusion), especially if the former is driven by a pump. When the obstruction is relieved, a bolus of drug may be delivered instead of a saline flush.

Fluids may also be administered directly into bone (e.g. sternum), rectally, im or sc, the latter two aided by hyaluronidase.

Intravenous fluids. May be divided into **colloids** and **crystalloids** (Table 21).
• Simplistic effects of infused fluid on body fluid compartments:
–initial expansion of the vascular compartment. Extent and duration depends on whether it can freely cross the vascular endothelium; i.e. crystalloids do, colloids do so only slowly, e.g. **gelatine solutions** after a few hours. Colloids may draw water into the vascular

Table 21. Composition of commonly used iv fluids (in mmol/l unless otherwise stated)

Fluid	Na$^+$	K$^+$	Ca^{2+}	Cl$^-$	Other	pH
*Crystalloids**						
Saline 0.9% ('normal')	154	—	—	154	—	5.0
Dextrose 4% – saline 0.18%	30	—	—	30	Dextrose 40 g	4–5
Dextrose 5%	—	—	—	—	Dextrose 50 g	4.0
Hartmann's solution	131	5	2	111	Lactate 129	6.5
Bicarbonate						
8.4%	1000	—	—	—	HCO$_3^-$ 1000	8.0
1.26%	150	—	—	—	HCO$_3^-$ 150	7.0
Colloids†						
Haemaccel	145	5.1	6.25	145	Gelatin 35 g	7.4
Gelofusine	154	<0.4	<0.4	125	Gelatin 40 g Mg^{2+} <0.4	7.4
Hetastarch	154	—	—	154	Starch 60 g	5.5
Pentastarch	154	—	—	154	Starch 100 g	5.0
Albumin 4.5%	<160	<2	—	136	Albumin 40–50 g Citrate <15	7.4
Dextran In saline 0.9%: as above In dextrose 5%: as above } 60 g dextran 70 or 100 g dextran 40						4.5–5 5–6

*All have an osmolality of 280–300 mosmol/kg, except for bicarbonate 8.4% (2000 mosmol/kg)
†Osmolality ranges between approximately 280–320 mosmol/kg

space by **osmosis** in addition to the volume infused (hence '**plasma expanders**').

–expansion of the **interstitial fluid** compartment as fluids pass into it from the vascular compartment. Fluids distribute within the **ECF** thus: ¾ in interstitial fluid, ¼ in **plasma**.

–expansion of the intracellular space. Water moves across cell membranes by osmosis only if **osmolality** on one side of the membrane changes. Thus, if **saline** 0.9% is added to ECF, osmolality is unchanged, thus no movement of water occurs; i.e. saline is confined to ECF. With **dextrose solutions**, the dextrose is rapidly metabolized by erythrocytes, leaving water. The water enters the ECF causing dilution; thus water moves into the cells by osmosis.

● Thus:

–colloids cause greater expansion of the vascular compartment for the volume infused, and are ideally suited to replace plasma/blood losses.

–saline 0.9% and **Hartmann's solution** expand ECF (¾ interstitial, ¼ plasma), and are ideally suited to replace ECF losses.

–dextrose 5% expands total body water (⅓ ECF, ⅔ interstitial). Thus only ½ infused volume of dextrose 5% remains in the vascular compartment. The main use of dextrose is to replenish a water deficit; infusing pure water would cause haemolysis.

See also, Bicarbonate; Colloid/crystalloid controversy; Dextrans; Haemorrhage; Hypertonic intravenous solutions; Intravenous fluid administration; Pentastarch

Intravenous oxygenator (IVOX). Intravascular gas exchange device, consisting of a 30–40 cm long bundle of hollow gas-permeable polypropylene fibres (internal diameter 200 µm), which may be introduced into the superior and inferior venae cavae via the right internal jugular or femoral veins. O_2 is passed under low pressure through the lumina of the fibres, whilst blood returning to the heart via normal channels flows over the fibres' external surfaces. O_2 passes into the blood from the fibres, and CO_2 passes in the opposite direction. Currently being evaluated as an adjunct to conventional therapy in acute **respiratory failure**.
Kallis P, Al-Saady NM, Bennett ED, Treasure T (1992) Br J Hosp Med; 47: 824–8

Intravenous regional anaesthesia (IVRA; Bier block). First described in 1908 by **Bier**, who injected **procaine** iv into an exsanguinated portion of the arm between two inflated tourniquets, to provide distal analgesia.

● Modern technique (described in the 1960s):

–an iv cannula is placed in each hand.

–the limb is exsanguinated by raising it with the brachial artery compressed, or by using a rubber bandage.

–a **tourniquet** is inflated around the upper arm to a value higher than systolic BP (twice systolic BP is usually quoted).

–**local anaesthetic agent** is injected slowly.

–a more distal tourniquet may be inflated after 5–10 minutes and the original deflated, to reduce discomfort.

–motor and sensory block occurs within 5–10 minutes.

–for prolonged surgery, the cannula is left *in situ*. The

cuff may be deflated after 60–90 minutes for 5 minutes, the arm re-emptied of blood and the tourniquet reinflated. Half the initial dose is then injected. Thus safe tourniquet time is not exceeded.

● Solutions:

–**prilocaine** is safest but **lignocaine** may also used; 3 mg/kg (0.6 ml/kg) 0.5% solution is suitable, without adrenaline. Preservative-free solution is now available for IVRA, but for many years prior to its introduction, solution containing preservative was safely used.

–**bupivacaine** was previously used but is now contraindicated because of its toxicity.

● Mechanism of action is unclear, but may include:

–compression by the tourniquet.

–ischaemia.

–drug action on nerve trunks.

–drug action on nerve endings.

● IVRA is a potentially dangerous technique, involving direct iv injection of local anaesthetic; therefore the following must apply:

–all equipment is checked for leaks, etc.

–the patient is prepared and starved as for any local anaesthetic procedure, with resuscitative drugs and equipment available.

–full **monitoring** is applied throughout.

–rapid injection is avoided (may force solution past the tourniquet).

–injection near the antecubital fossa is avoided (solution may be forced into the systemic circulation).

–the technique is used with caution in patients with severe arteriosclerosis and **hypertension**, since the tourniquet may not completely compress their arteries. Similar caution has been suggested in **obesity**.

–avoidance has been suggested in prepubertal children, since intraosseous vessels may allow local anaesthetic to bypass the tourniquet.

–the tourniquet is deflated after at least 20 minutes. Intermittent deflation/reinflation has been suggested to reduce blood drug levels, e.g. deflation for 5–10 seconds, inflation for 1 second, etc.

–not to be used in patients with **sickle cell anaemia** or trait.

May be used for the leg, although larger volumes are required, e.g. 1.0 ml/kg. The block may be less effective than in the arm.

Has also been used for **sympathetic nerve block**, e.g. using **guanethidine** 10–25 mg in 20 ml saline for the arm (30–40 mg in 40 ml for the leg); lignocaine or prilocaine is often added. The tourniquet is deflated after 10–20 minutes. Hypotension may occur up to several hours later. It may be repeated for several weeks, e.g. on alternate days.
Goold JE (1985) Br J Hosp Med; 33: 335–40

Intrinsic activity. Ability of a substance, e.g. drug, to produce a response by interacting with a surface receptor. Refers to the amount of response produced, i.e. **efficacy**.
See also, Affinity

Intrinsic sympathomimetic activity (ISA). Ability of **β-adrenergic receptor antagonists** to stimulate **β-adrenergic receptors** as well as block them. Oxprenolol, **labetalol**, pindolol and acebutolol have ISA and are therefore partial **agonists**; they may cause less bradycardia than other β-receptor antagonists, although the importance of this is unclear.

Intubation aids. Used in difficult tracheal intubation.
● Designed for:
 –avoiding obstruction of the **laryngoscope** handle on the chest during insertion of the blade into the mouth:
  –laryngoscopes with adjustable handles or an increased angle between the blade and handle (e.g. polio **laryngoscope blade**).
  –adaptor to swing the handle to one side during insertion (Yentis adaptor).
  –short-handled laryngoscope.
 –improving the view of the glottis:
  –specialized laryngoscope blades.
  –**fibreoptic instruments**: may be flexible, rigid or malleable; extendable forceps, stylets, etc. may be attached.
  –optical devices and mirrors attached to or incorporated in the laryngoscope. The Huffman prism clips to a standard laryngoscope blade, allowing visualization of the larynx by refracting light 30° from its original path. It must be warmed before use to prevent misting.
 –enabling intubation despite poor view:
  –long flexible bougie (traditionally gum elastic); may be placed first and the **tracheal tube** passed over it, with gentle rotation if required. It may be placed blindly; correct placement is suggested by feeling the tracheal rings during insertion, and feeling the distal end reach the carina. Directional bougies, controllable from their proximal end, are also available.
  –malleable stylet, inserted through the tube before insertion. Plastic-coated ones are less traumatic than those of bare metal; trauma is reduced by avoiding protrusion of the stylet from the distal end of the tube.
  –**forceps** to guide the tube.
  –some tracheal tubes are able to be flexed by pulling a cord within their walls, aiding direction during placement.
  –laryngoscope blades have been described which incorporate forceps, allowing manipulation of the tracheal tube.
  –hooks introduced orally for pulling the tube anteriorly.
 –allowing intubation without laryngoscopy:
  –flexible lighted stylet (light wand): passed through the tube and introduced through the mouth, with observation of the anterior neck. The light may be followed down the anterior larynx into the trachea; it disappears if intraoesophageal.
  –retrograde extradural catheter technique: the catheter is introduced through the cricothyroid membrane via an extradural needle and passed upwards through the larynx and out of the mouth. The tracheal tube is advanced over it from the mouth into the trachea as the catheter is held from above. For nasal intubation, the catheter is tied with thread to a suction catheter passed through the nose and out through the mouth, then both are pulled out of the nose. Central venous cannulae, threads, etc., have also been used.
  –detecting oesophageal intubation.
Their use should be practised in easy cases.
[John P Huffman, US nurse-anaesthetist; SM Yentis, London anaesthetist]

Cobley M, Vaughan RS (1992) Br J Anaesth; 68: 90–7
See also, Intubation, difficult; Intubation; oesophageal; Intubation, tracheal

Intubation, awake. Indications:
 –known or suspected difficult airway or intubation, including an unstable cervical spine.
 –to isolate a leak and/or protect lung segments before applying IPPV, e.g. **bronchopleural fistula, tracheo-oesophageal fistula**.
 –in **neonates**: controversial, it is felt to be safer by many but with the possibility of causing undue stress, raised **ICP**, etc.
 –if the usual drugs given for intubation are withheld, e.g. because of the patient's poor condition.
● Requires anaesthesia of the **pharynx, larynx** and trachea, and **tongue** or nasal passages:
 –nose: cocaine spray 4–10% to provide anaesthesia and vasoconstriction (3 mg/kg maximum). Alternatively, xylometazoline 0.1% and **lignocaine** 1–4% may be used.
 –tongue and oropharynx: benzocaine lozenge 100 mg, sucked ½ hour beforehand.
 –pharynx and larynx above the vocal cords: lignocaine or **prilocaine** 1–4% via metered spray or swabs at increasing depths into the mouth, using a spatula or laryngoscope. Excessive dosage should not be administered. **Glossopharyngeal nerve block** has been used, but topical anaesthesia is easier to perform. Superior **laryngeal nerve** block provides anaesthesia of the epiglottis, base of tongue and mucosa down to the cords, and is performed thus:
  –holding a lignocaine-soaked pledget for 2–3 minutes in the piriform fossa on each side, e.g. using Krause's **forceps**. Alternatively, 2–3 ml 1% lignocaine may be injected from the front of the neck just below the greater cornu of the hyoid bone on each side, with the bone displaced towards the side to be blocked with the operator's other hand. A click may be felt as the thyrohyoid membrane is pierced.
 –trachea and larynx below the cords: rapid transtracheal injection of 3–5 ml 1% lignocaine through the cricothyroid membrane, following aspiration of air to confirm correct placement. The patient is asked to breathe out fully before injection; the resultant inspiration and coughing aids spread of solution within the upper **tracheobronchial tree**. The 21–23 G needle is withdrawn immediately following injection to reduce the risk of breakage during coughing. Use of an iv cannula has been suggested to reduce the risk of this and trauma; the needle is removed leaving the plastic cannula before injection.
 –nebulized 4% lignocaine may be used as the sole local anaesthetic.
Tracheal intubation then proceeds as usual, using laryngoscopy or a blind nasal technique.

The upper airways are rendered insensitive to aspirated material, and the patient should be kept nil by mouth for 4 hours. Patients already at risk of regurgitation and aspiration are placed further at risk.

A similar technique may be used for awake fibreoptic **bronchoscopy. Fibreoptic instruments** for bronchoscopy/intubation have injection ports through which local anaesthetic may be sprayed as the scope is advanced.

Benumof JL (1991) Anesthesiology; 75: 1087–110
See also, Intubation, blind nasal; Intubation, tracheal

Intubation, blind nasal. Technique of tracheal intubation without using laryngoscopes or other instruments; developed by **Magill** and **Rowbotham** as their first method of tracheal intubation (without use of neuromuscular blocking drugs). Of particular use in difficult intubation, since visualization of the larynx is not required. Also used in awake intubation.

Originally described in spontaneously breathing patients, with use of 5–10% inspired CO_2 to increase ventilation. May also be performed in paralysed patients, although induction of muscle paralysis may be hazardous in difficult intubation. Use of CO_2 is now generally considered dangerous.

- Technique:
  - the patient's head is positioned in the 'sniffing position'.
  - a lubricated tracheal tube is inserted into a nostril (usually the right, since most bevels face left). Uncuffed rubber tubes were originally used; cuffed tubes are also suitable. **Epistaxis** may occur; it is reduced if a soft tube, little force and **cocaine** paste or spray are used. Trauma to the nasopharynx may also occur, and the incidence of bacteraemia is higher than with oral intubation.
  - the tube is passed into the pharynx, keeping the head extended and mandible elevated. The head is rotated slightly towards the side of the nostril used.
  - in spontaneous ventilation, the opposite nostril is occluded. Audible breath sounds from the tube are used as a guide to the position of the tube's tip; i.e. if they disappear, the tube is withdrawn slightly and redirected.
  - the tube is gently inserted further; it may:
    - enter the trachea in approximately a third of cases.
    - enter the oesophagus; the tube is partially withdrawn and reinserted with the head extended further. Posterior external pressure on the larynx may help.
    - meet obstruction level with the larynx; the tube's tip may be:
      - lateral to the glottis, e.g. in a piriform fossa, or against a false cord or arytenoid cartilage. A bulge may be visible at one side of the larynx at the front of the neck. The tube is partially withdrawn, rotated and reinserted. Head rotation or lateral external pressure on the larynx may help.
      - against the anterior part of the cricoid or in the vallecula; tube rotation or head flexion may help.

  Practice is required to achieve proficiency. Differently curved tubes may be required.

See also, Intubation, awake; Intubation, difficult; Intubation, oesophageal; Intubation, tracheal

Intubation, complications of. Complications may occur at the time of tracheal intubation or afterwards.

- During intubation:
  - trauma:
    - caused by leaning on the eyes.
    - to the neck or jaw.
    - to the **teeth**, lips, nasal mucosa, mouth, **tongue**, **pharynx**, **larynx**, **laryngeal nerves** and trachea.

Infection, surgical emphysema and bleeding may result. Rigid introducers and bougies are particularly traumatic. Nasal polyps, etc. may be carried into the trachea during nasal intubation.

- hypertensive response:
  - associated with sympathetic activity and tachycardia.
  - may increase **ICP**.
  - particularly undesirable in patients with **hypertension**, **ischaemic heart disease**, etc.
  - caused by **laryngoscopy** alone; thus not obtunded by **lignocaine** spray.
  - methods to reduce the response:
    - **antihypertensive drugs**, e.g. **β-adrenergic receptor antagonists**, **hydralazine**, **nitroglycerine**, **sodium nitroprusside**. Some may be effective given orally, preoperatively, e.g. β-receptor antagonists, but bradycardia may occur.
    - **benzodiazepines**.
    - deep inhalational anaesthesia.
    - iv **lignocaine** 1–2 mg/kg.
    - **fentanyl** 6–8 µg/kg, **alfentanil** 30–50 µg/kg or **sufentanil** 0.5–1.0 µg/kg obtund the response if given 1–2 minutes before intubation.
- **arrhythmias**, particularly if **hypoxaemia** and **hypercapnia** are present.
- **laryngospasm**, **bronchospasm**, breath-holding, etc., if intubation is attempted too early.
- **aspiration of gastric contents**.
- misplaced tube, e.g. oesophageal or endobronchial. Auscultation over both lungs and axillae and the stomach should be performed following intubation and positioning.
- difficult/failed intubation: risk of misplacement of the tube. Hypoxaemia, hypercapnia, **awareness**, trauma and aspiration may occur during repeated attempts at intubation.
- bacteraemia has been reported but the clinical significance is unclear. More likely with nasal intubation.

- Once the trachea is intubated:
  - displacement of the tube:
    - **extubation**.
    - endobronchial intubation. Suggested by:
      - lightening anaesthesia.
      - increased **airway pressures**.
      - hypoxaemia.
      - unequal lung expansion.

      Usually occurs on the right side. It may cause collapse of the unventilated lung (± right upper lobe) and postoperative infection. On the **chest X-ray**, the tube's tip should be at T1–3 (carina lies at T4–5). The tube may move up to 2 cm with neck movement (caudad with flexion, cephalad with extension).
  - disconnection from the fresh gas supply.
  - **airway obstruction**:
    - blockage by sputum, blood, foreign object, etc.
    - compression by mouth gag, surgeon, kinking, etc.
  - related to the **cuff**.
  - tube ignition by **laser**.
  - complications of extubation.

- Late complications:
  - cord ulceration and granuloma: uncommon; typically occur at the junction of the posterior and middle thirds of the cord.

–damage to the recurrent/superior laryngeal nerves. Stretching and compression are thought to be the most likely causes. Slow recovery usually occurs.
–tracheal stenosis following prolonged intubation.
–nasal/oral ulceration.
–sinusitis may occur in prolonged nasotracheal intubation.

Tracheostomy is performed to avoid late complications after long-term intubation (traditionally at 2–3 weeks, although this is controversial).

See also, Anaesthetic morbidity and mortality; Intubation, difficult; Intubation, failed; Intubation, oesophageal; Intubation, tracheal

Intubation, difficult. Incidence is thought to be about 1% in the general population, although definitions vary.

• Widely accepted classification (of Cormack and Lehane) according to the best view possible at laryngoscopy (Fig. 77a):
  –grade I: complete glottis visible.
  –grade II: anterior glottis not seen.
  –grade III: epiglottis seen but not glottis.
  –grade IV: epiglottis not seen.
  Grades III and IV together are termed 'difficult'.
• Caused by:
  –difficulty inserting the laryngoscope into the mouth, e.g. because its handle is obstructed by the patient's chest or by the hand applying **cricoid pressure** (e.g. **obesity**, **Caesarean section**, barrel-chest). This may also occur with reduced mouth opening and neck mobility.
  –reduced neck mobility, e.g. caused by osteoarthrosis, **rheumatoid arthritis, ankylosing spondylitis**, surgical fixation/traction, etc.
  –reduced mouth opening, e.g. reduced **temporo-mandibular joint** (TMJ) mobility, **trismus**, scarring, fibrosis, local lesions/swelling.
  –lesions/swelling/fibrosis of **larynx, pharynx, tongue**, etc.
  –congenital conditions, often associated with the above, e.g. **facial deformities, achondroplasia, Marfan's syndrome, cystic hygroma**, etc.
  –anatomical variants of normal; they may be associated with the above but difficult intubation may occur in otherwise unremarkable patients.

Studies analysing cases of difficult intubation have described many features associated with difficulty; the large number of factors involved may make preoperative anticipation of problems difficult. Although many difficult cases may have common features, many patients with these features present no difficulty; i.e. the **specificity** of most tests is poor.

• Difficulty may be suggested by:
  –previous difficulty recorded in the medical notes.
  –obesity, with short neck and reduced movement at the **cervical spine**, especially the atlanto-occipito-axial complex. The latter is tested by asking for full neck flexion, then asking the patient to look up with the examiner's hand at the back of the neck, holding it flexed. Normal movement exceeds 15°.
  –reduced TMJ movement: anterior/posterior sliding of lower jaw (inability to protrude the lower teeth beyond the upper) or mouth opening (less than two fingers' width).
  –protruding teeth, small mouth, high, narrow arched palate, receding mandible.

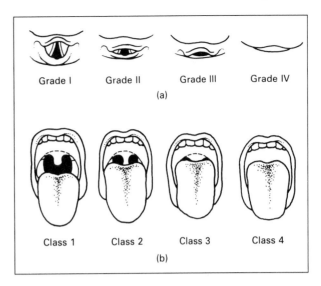

Figure 77 *(a) Cormack and Lehane classification of laryngoscopic views. (b) Modified Mallampati's classification of pharyngeal appearance.*

  –poor visualization of the fauces with open mouth and tongue protruded maximally, with the observer level with the seated patient. The modified Mallampati classification is commonly used (Fig. 77b): soft palate, uvula, fauces and pillars visible (class 1), soft palate, uvula and fauces visible (class 2), soft palate and base of uvula visible (class 3) and soft palate not visible (Class 4).
  –thyromental distance, with neck extended, of less than three fingers (<6.5 cm).
  –X-ray assessment: as above plus:

  $$\frac{\text{distance from TMJ to lower incisors}}{\text{distance between top of 3rd molar and ramus}}$$

  Difficulty is suggested if this ratio is under 3.6. Rarely performed.
  –neck in extension/flexion. Middle/upper vertebral movement is particularly important. There should be a gap between the occiput and posterior arch of the atlas. The gap should increase on neck flexion. An absent gap or little change on flexion suggests limited movement at the top of the spine.

  Rarely performed as routine, unless neck disease is suspected.

• Management:
  –known case:
    –consideration of alternatives to intubation:
      –**regional anaesthesia**.
      –**facepiece** +/- **airway**.
      –**laryngeal mask**.
      –**tracheostomy/cricothyrotomy**.
    –if oro/nasal intubation is deemed necessary, it may be performed with the patient awake or anaesthetized. In the latter case, inhalational induction is usually employed, with intubation whilst breathing spontaneously. **Halothane** is usually considered the agent of choice.

      IV induction should be avoided, since ability to maintain the airway or ventilate by facepiece is uncertain, should apnoea occur. If the patient is not at risk of regurgitation, small incremental doses of iv agent may be slowly given, maintaining spontaneous ventilation, and simultaneously deepening inhalational anaesthesia.

–techniques of intubation:
  –the position of the head should be optimized. **Cricoid pressure** may help if the larnyx is anteriorly placed.
  –blind nasal intubation.
  –use of **intubation aids**, e.g. bougies, **forceps, fibreoptic instruments**, specialized **laryngoscopes** and **tracheal tubes**, retrograde catheter technique, etc.

  Preoxygenation must precede all attempts at intubation. Muscle relaxation is avoided until the airway is secure, or ability to ventilate by facepiece has been confirmed. Experienced help and facilities for tracheostomy or cricothyrotomy should be available. Special considerations apply if **airway obstruction** is present.

  In patients at risk of regurgitation, risk of aspiration is increased if laryngeal protective reflexes are obtunded by local anaesthetic during awake intubation. If inhalational induction is chosen, the left lateral head-down position is considered safest, but intubation may be more awkward.

–unsuspected case:
  –maintenance of oxygenation.
  –consideration of alternative strategies:
    –allowing the patient to wake, with subsequent management as above.
    –continuing inhalational anaesthesia without intubation.
    –persisting in intubation attempts as above. Increases the risk of trauma, **awareness**, oesophageal intubation, etc.
    –a failed intubation drill should be instituted early, especially if at risk of regurgitation.
  –anaesthetic records and notes should be clearly marked to warn other anaesthetists. The patient should be visited postoperatively, to discuss the events and implications.

The use of a difficult intubation box, containing all the equipment required, and available for emergency use, has been suggested.

[Ronald S Cormack, London anaesthetist; John R Lehane, Oxford anaesthetist; S Rao Mallampati, Boston anaesthetist]

Cobley M, Vaughan RS (1992) Br J Anaesth; 68: 90–7

See also, Intubation, awake; Intubation, blind nasal; Intubation, complications of; Intubation, failed; Intubation, oesophageal; Intubation, tracheal

Intubation, endobronchial, *see Endobronchial blockers; Endobronchial tubes; Intubation, complications of; One-lung anaesthesia; Thoracic surgery*

Intubation, failed. Incidence is approximately 1:2500–3000 in general patients, and 1:300 in obstetrics. If it occurs, management is directed towards maintaining oxygenation and preventing **aspiration of gastric contents**.

• A failed intubation drill is widely practised for **Caesarean section**, but is applicable to all patients:
  –early recognition of failure is important; i.e. not persisting with attempts at intubation if the patient is becoming hypoxaemic.
  –help should be summoned.
  –**cricoid pressure** should be maintained and the patient positioned on the left side with head-down tilt (obtaining help from the surgeons if necessary). Suction should be used as required.
  –oxygenation should proceed via a facepiece, using 100% O_2. Oxygenation may be aided by:
    –an assistant squeezing the reservoir bag if both hands are needed to support the airway.
    –fully closing the expiratory valve, and turning on and locking the O_2 flush. By applying the facepiece intermittently, IPPV may be performed.
    –releasing cricoid pressure (if the patient is in the lateral, head-down position).
    –using an **oesophageal obturator/airway** if available. Deliberate oesophageal intubation using an ordinary tracheal tube may improve the airway. Oesophageal obturation has been suggested early if the patient cannot be turned into the lateral position.
    –use of a **laryngeal mask** has been suggested; however, this will not protect the airway from aspiration of gastric contents.
  –if surgery is not required as an emergency, e.g. elective Caesarean section, the patient should be kept oxygenated and allowed to wake up. Alternative techniques, e.g. regional techniques, awake intubation, etc., should be considered.
  –in emergency surgery, proceeding with inhalational anaesthesia may be considered, but only if the airway is clear. Cricoid pressure must remain applied if the airway is unprotected. The stomach should be emptied only in the head-down, left lateral position, using a wide bore tube. Local anaesthetic infiltration of the surgical field may reduce requirements for volatile agents.
  –if oxygenation is impossible by facemask, perform **cricothyrotomy**. Difficulty may be encountered, especially if the patient has a fat neck. A straight-through device, e.g. iv cannula, may be easier than performing separate puncture and insertion, when the original hole may be difficult to find. A 3 mm tracheal tube connector fits into the hub of an iv cannula; alternatively an 8 mm connector fits into the hub of a 2 ml syringe. Transtracheal ventilation may be performed by intermittent squeezing of the reservoir bag, use of the O_2 flush, or an injector system.

King TA, Adams AP (1990) Br J Anaesth; 65: 400–14

See also, Intubation, awake; Intubation, difficult

Intubation, oesophageal. A potential complication of attempted tracheal intubation. If undetected, it may lead to severe **hypoxaemia** resulting in death or brain injury. Particularly likely if intubation is difficult or the intubator unskilled. Detection is often difficult, since observation of chest movement and ausculation over the chest and stomach may wrongly suggest successful tracheal intubation. The belching noise on manual inflation that usually accompanies oesophageal intubation may be absent. The reservoir bag may move convincingly during spontaneous ventilation. Condensation of water vapour within the tube may occur in both oesophageal and tracheal intubation. **Preoxygenation** may delay subsequent hypoxaemia and cyanosis.

• Methods of detection:
  –tactile test for tracheal tube placement: the index finger is passed along the tube into the **pharynx**, and attempts made to palpate the interarytenoid groove at the back of the **larynx**, posterior to the tube. The larynx is moved cranially from the front of the neck, using the other hand.
  –sudden overdistension of the tracheal tube cuff has been suggested, with palpation over the front of the trachea at the sternal notch. Tracheal trauma may occur.
  –injection and withdrawal of air through the tube, using a large syringe or rubber bulb (oesophageal intubation detector device). Oesophageal intubation is suggested by a belch on inflation, followed by absent or obstructed withdrawal of air. Both components are silent and unobstructed if intubation is tracheal.
  –passage of an illuminated stylet down the tube; tracheal placement is suggested by visible light at the front of the neck.
  –**capnography**; although CO_2 may be present in the stomach, sustained levels in repeated expirations indicate tracheal intubation. Disposable indicators may be attached to the tube, giving breath-by-breath colour changes in response to exhaled CO_2.
  –fibreoptic endoscopy through the tube.

Removal of the tube has been advocated if there is any doubt as to its position. Alternatively, disconnecting the tube but leaving it in place may allow manual ventilation using a facepiece placed over it.

Birmingham PK, Cheney FW, Ward RJ (1986) Anesth Analg; 65: 886–91

Intubation, tracheal. Oro/nasal intubation was initially described for resuscitation, e.g. by **Kite** in 1788, and for laryngeal obstruction, although tracheal insufflation in animals had been described earlier. **Macewen** was the first to advocate tracheal intubation instead of **tracheostomy** for anaesthesia for head and neck surgery, in 1880. An intubating tube was described by **O'Dwyer** in 1885. **Laryngoscopy** was pioneered by **Kirstein**, **Killian** and **Jackson** between 1895 and 1915. Modern endotracheal anaesthesia and blind nasal intubation were developed by **Magill** and **Rowbotham** after World War I. **Tracheal tubes** and **laryngoscopes** are continually being developed and adapted.

• Indications for intubation:
  –anaesthetic:
    –restricted access to the patient, e.g. head and neck surgery, prone position.
    –to protect against tracheal soiling by gastric contents, blood, etc., e.g **dental**, **ENT** and **emergency surgery**.
    –to secure the airway, e.g. in **airway obstruction**.
    –when muscle relaxation is required, e.g. abdominal surgery.
    –when IPPV is required, e.g. respiratory disease, **thoracic** or **cardiac surgery**, **neurosurgery**, prolonged surgery.
  –non-anaesthetic:
    –**CPR**.
    –when IPPV is required, e.g. **respiratory failure**.
    –to secure/protect the airway, e.g. in airway obstruction, unconscious patients, impaired protective laryngeal reflexes, etc.
    –to allow aspiration of sputum/secretions.

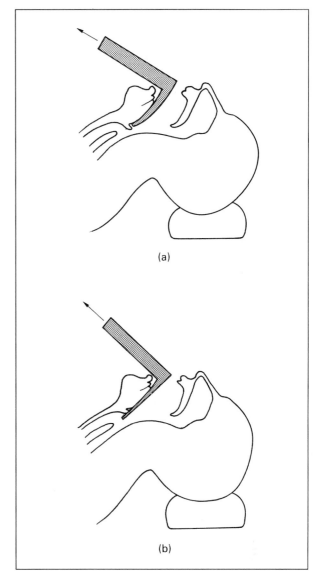

Figure 78 *Tracheal intubation using (a) curved, and (b) straight laryngoscope blades*

• Technique:
  –at least two laryngoscopes, a selection of tubes, syringe for **cuff** inflation, **suction apparatus**, **intubation aids**, emergency equipment and drugs should always be available and checked before use.
  –oral:
    –the patient is positioned with the neck flexed about 35° and head extended about 15° ('sniffing the morning air'). A pillow is required.
    –with the lungs oxygenated and the patient either paralysed or adequately anaesthetized if breathing spontaneously, the mouth is opened with the right hand and the laryngoscope introduced at the right side, using the left hand. The blade's tip is passed back along the upper surface of the tongue until the epiglottis is visible.
    –if a curved blade (e.g. **Macintosh's**) is used, the tip is placed between the epiglottis and the base of the

tongue, and the laryngoscope lifted in the direction of the handle, avoiding pivoting or pressure on the upper teeth. The glottis is visible under the epiglottis as the latter is lifted forward (Fig. 78a). This method is thought to be less stimulating than with a straight blade, because the dorsal surface of the epiglottis (innervated by the superior laryngeal branch of the vagus) is not touched.

–if a straight blade (e.g. Magill's) is used, the tip is placed posterior to the epiglottis and lifted as above. The glottis is visible beyond the tip (Fig. 78b). Alternatively, the tip is passed into the oesophagus and slowly withdrawn until the glottis appears. Epiglottic bruising is more likely with this technique.

–**lignocaine** spray 4% is sometimes applied to the larynx, to reduce stimulation by the tube once placed. Lignocaine gel is also available.

–size 9 mm tubes are usually used for men, 8 mm for women; average suitable length is 22–25 cm. The tube is inserted under direct vision if possible, from the right side of the mouth with conventional laryngoscopes. The view may be improved by backward pressure on the larynx from the front of the neck. If the view is incomplete or insertion difficult, intubation aids, e.g. stylet, bougie etc. may help. If the glottis is not seen, the bougie or tube may be placed blindly, by careful advancement posterior to the epiglottis or laryngoscope tip. Tracheal rings may be felt if placement is successful; oesophageal intubation must be excluded.

–the tube cuff is inflated slowly until the audible leak vanishes. Low-pressure inflators are available.

–observation of the chest and auscultation of both lungs, e.g. high in the axilla, are required to exclude accidental intubation of the right main bronchus. Auscultation over the stomach and in the suprasternal notch has also been suggested to help indicate gastric inflation and tracheal leak, respectively.

–the tube is tied or taped in position.

–other techniques include awake intubation, and use of **fibreoptic instruments**, **laryngeal mask**, retrograde catheters etc. Intubation may also be performed without instruments, by hooking the fingers or thumb of one hand over the back of the tongue, and guiding the tube by touch.

–nasal:

–**cocaine** paste/spray 10%, or xylometazoline 0.1% is used to reduce epistaxis, which may be severe.

–tubes of diameter 1 mm less than for oral intubation are usually employed; average suitable length is 25–28 cm. The lubricated tube is gently inserted directly backwards, twisting to ease its passage. Intubation is achieved blindly, or with laryngoscopy as above, using **forceps** to position the tube if required.

–checking/securing as above.

Special considerations apply for **paediatric anaesthesia**, or when risk of aspiration is present (*see Induction, rapid sequence*).

In ICU, nasal intubation is often preferred because of increased patient comfort, easier securing of tube and easier nursing care of the mouth. However, smaller longer tubes are required; thus suction is more difficult and

occlusion more likely. Tracheostomy is often performed after 2–3 weeks' intubation but this practice is controversial.

See also, Intubation, awake; Intubation, blind nasal; Intubation, complications of; Intubation, difficult; Intubation, oesophageal

Inverse ratio ventilation (IRV). Ventilatory mode used in neonatal **IPPV** and recently in **ARDS**. Consists of a prolonged inspiratory phase of up to four times the duration of the expiratory phase. Increases mean **airway pressure** and thought to improve alveolar inflation and splinting, with improved oxygenation. May require a few hours for alveolar recruitment to become apparent. Risk of **barotrauma** may be increased, and air trapping may occur if the expiratory phase is too short. Spontaneous ventilation is prevented by most ventilators during the long inspiratory phase; thus it is unsuitable for **weaning from ventilators**. Usually requires neuromuscular blockade and **sedation**.

Cameron PD, Oh TE (1986) Anaesth Intensive Care; 14: 258–66

Investigations, preoperative. Aid clinical **preoperative assessment** of patients' fitness for surgery, whether improvement is possible, and provide a baseline for subsequent testing. Indications and requirements vary and are sometimes controversial; history and examination are generally considered more useful in routine preoperative screening for disease. Unnecessary testing is expensive, time consuming and may be worrying for the patient; it may be performed because of ignorance, supposed medicolegal security, and to avoid postponement of surgery should a test result be required later. Conversely, anaesthetists are often pressed to proceed with anaesthesia despite inadequate investigation.

• Guidelines for investigation are related to:

–cost of testing.

–**sensitivity** and **specificity** of the test.

–incidence of abnormality in the population concerned.

–clinical significance of the result if abnormal.

• Typical guidelines:

–**chest X-ray**:

–cardiovascular/respiratory disease unless recent (under 6–12 months) films are available.

–new respiratory symptoms.

–possible metastases.

–recent immigrant from an area where **TB** is endemic, unless recents films are available.

–as a preoperative baseline in major surgery.

–age >60 years.

The first four indications are recommended by the Royal College of Radiologists.

–**ECG**: age over 40–50 years, earlier in smokers or in patients with cardiovascular disease.

–**haemoglobin**: age >50–60 years, evidence of anaemia, etc. Routine testing in all women and in all patients has been suggested.

–biochemistry: age >40–50, metabolic diseases, **dehydration**, etc., drug therapy known to alter biochemistry, e.g. **diuretics**, or whose actions are affected by abnormalities, e.g. **digoxin**. Creatinine has been suggested as a better routine test than **urea**. Urine testing for glucose has been suggested if blood is not tested.

–other investigations if suggested by history/examination include testing for **sickle cell anaemia**, **liver function tests**, **lung function tests**, **coagulation studies**, arterial **blood gas tensions**, **cervical spine** X-rays, etc.

Ionization of drugs. Important determinent of a drug's passage through **membranes**, since charged (ionized) particles are relatively lipid-insoluble and therefore do not cross easily. Once a drug has dissociated, passage across the membrane depends on the concentration of the unionized form. Weak **acids** dissociate in alkaline environments; thus passage across membranes is favoured by acid environments. The opposite applies for weak **bases**.

Degree of ionization is derived from the **Henderson–Hasselbalch equation**:

acidic drug: $pH - pK_a = \log \dfrac{[\text{ionized drug}]}{[\text{unionized drug}]}$

basic drug: $pH - pK_a = \log \dfrac{[\text{unionized drug}]}{[\text{ionized drug}]}$

At 50% ionization, $pH = pK_a$.
- Examples of acidic drugs:
  –**phenytoin**.
  –**barbiturates**, e.g. **thiopentone** (pK_a 7.6), **methohexitone** (pK_a 7.9).
  –**salicylates**.
  –penicillins.
- Examples of basic drugs:
  –**diazepam** (pK_a 3.3).
  –**local anaesthetic agents**, e.g. **lignocaine** (pK_a 7.9), **bupivacaine** (pK_a 8.1).
  –**opioid analgesic drugs**, e.g. **morphine** (pK_a 7.9), **pethidine** (pK_a 8.5).
  –non-depolarizing **neuromuscular blocking drugs**.
- Examples of anaesthetic relevance:
  –in **acidosis**, dissociation of thiopentone is decreased; thus the concentration of unionized portion increases. The amount of drug entering the brain therefore increases; thus the effect per mg increases.
  –**fentanyl** passes into the stomach from the circulation and is 'trapped' there by dissociation in acidic gastric fluid. This is now thought to be clinically insignificant.
  –'trapping' of drugs in the ionized form in urine, by manipulating urinary pH to aid excretion (**forced diuresis**).

See also, Pharmacokinetics

IPPV, *see Intermittent positive pressure ventilation*

Ipratropium bromide. Anticholinergic drug, used to treat **asthma** and chronic bronchitis. Has a quarternary amine structure. Of slower onset than **salbutamol** and similar drugs; there may be synergy between them.
- Dosage:
  –1–2 puffs aerosol (20–40 µg) 6–8 hourly.
  –0.1–0.5 mg nebulizer solution (0.4–2.0 ml 0.025% solution) 6–8 hourly. Paradoxical bronchospasm in earlier preparations is thought to have been caused by preservatives.
- Systemic anticholinergic effects are rare, although **glaucoma** has occurred in susceptible patients following delivery of nebulized ipratropium through poorly-fitting masks.

IPSP, Inhibitory postsynaptic potential, *see Synaptic transmission*

Iron lung, *see Intermittent negative pressure ventilation*

IRV, *see Inverse ratio ventilation*

ISA, *see Intrinsic sympathomimetic activity*

Ischaemic heart disease. Most common cause of death in the Western world (20–30%); its incidence is declining in the USA, Australia, Finland and Belgium but not the UK.
- Precise aetiology is uncertain but risk factors are as follows:
  –increasing age, maleness and family history.
  –**smoking**.
  –diet: associated with high cholesterol and saturated fatty acid intake, possibly sugar intake; their exact roles are controversial. Risk of mortality and morbidity may be lowered by treating hypercholesterolaemia if present.
  –**hypertension, diabetes mellitus**.
  –**obesity**, lack of exercise, poverty, stress, water softness and **alcohol** have been associated in some studies but the relationships are unclear.
- The main pathophysiological feature is reduction in coronary vessel lumen diameter by lipid atheromatous plaques, which may be exacerbated by coronary spasm. This may lead to:
  –**myocardial ischaemia** when O_2 demand exceeds supply (usually causing angina).
  –fissuring of plaques with thrombus formation; may lead to unstable angina, **MI** or sudden death.
- Clinical features:
  –chest pain. May be difficult to distinguish from oesophageal pain, even when related to exercise.
  –**dyspnoea** may occur, related to ischaemia, **cardiac failure** or associated chest disease caused by smoking.
  –palpatations, fainting attacks due to **arrhythmias** (including **heart block**).
  –hypertension, cardiomegaly, peripheral or **pulmonary oedema**.
  –fatty deposits due to hyperlipidaemia, e.g. around the eyes, arcus senilis in the cornea.
  –sudden death.
- Investigation:
  –**ECG**.
  –**exercise testing**.
  –**echocardiography**.
  –**nuclear cardiology** ± gated scanning.
  –**cardiac catheterization**.
  –**CAT scanning**.
  –**magnetic resonance imaging**.
  –digital subtraction angiography: computerized subtraction of background signals in order to enhance vessel images. Allows iv contrast injection instead of cardiac catheterization.
- Management:
  –first-line treatment is with nitrates (e.g. **glyceryl trinitrate, isosorbide**), **β-adrenergic receptor antagonists** and **calcium channel blocking drugs**. Oral/sublingual therapy is started first; iv nitrates and β-adrenergic antagonists are used in unstable angina.
  –drugs affecting coagulation, e.g. **warfarin**, **aspirin**, have been investigated. Reduced risk of death has been found using the latter.

–**percutaneous transluminal coronary angioplasty** is increasingly used to avoid surgery. Laser ablation of atheroma has also been used.
–**coronary artery bypass graft**.

- Anaesthetic management: the main aim is to prevent perioperative myocardial ischaemia and infarction (reinfarction rate is up to 6%, usually on the third day. Infarction rate if none previously is about 0.1–0.2%):
  –preoperatively:
    –**preoperative assessment** of risk factors and severity of disease. **Cardiac risk index** is sometimes used. Conditions are optimized before surgery if possible; e.g. treatment of cardiac failure, arrhythmias, etc.
    –continuation of antianginal therapy up to and including the morning of surgery.
    –addition of further therapy if required; e.g. glyceryl trinitrate skin patch.
    –sedative **premedication** is usually prescribed, to reduce anxiety and endogenous **catacholamine** secretion.
  –peroperatively:
    –full **monitoring** and iv lines are set up before **induction of anaesthesia**. Direct arterial BP monitoring is useful if disease is severe or surgery extensive. **Pulmonary artery catheterization** is controversial.
    –**preoxygenation**.
    –smooth induction, using a minimal dose of **iv anaesthetic agent** given slowly, as the **arm–brain circulation** time may be prolonged. **Etomidate** causes less myocardial depression than other drugs, but others are often used. **Ketamine** may increase cardiac work and is usually avoided.
    –maintenance of adequate oxygenation and avoidance of **hypercapnia** and excessive amounts of volatile agent are achieved by tracheal intubation and muscle relaxation for most procedures. Alternatively, light inhalational anaesthesia combined with local anaesthetic techniques avoids the cardiovascular effects of intubation. **Spinal** and **extradural anaesthesia** risk hypotension and worsening of myocardial ischaemia, although they may reduce **preload** and **afterload**.
    –hypertensive response to intubation increases myocardial O_2 demand with risk of myocardial ischaemia (*see Intubation, complications of*).
    –peroperative control of excessive changes in heart rate, BP, etc., is especially important. The combination of tachycardia and hypotension is particularly hazardous. In general, drugs with minimal cardiovascular effects are often chosen, e.g. **vecuronium**, **atracurium**, **fentanyl**, although bradycardia has been reported. **Pancuronium** is preferred by some because hypotension is less likely. Low concentrations of volatile agents are acceptable; large amounts cause myocardial depression. **Halothane** decreases heart rate and myocardial O_2 consumption, but **enflurane** and **isoflurane** cause tachycardia, which may be detrimental. Isoflurane has been implicated as causing **coronary steal**.
    –myocardial ischaemia may be demonstrated by ECG or also assessed by **rate–pressure product**, etc.
  –postoperatively:
    –admission to HDU/ICU if severe. Routine ICU admission with aggressive maintenance of cardiovascular stability is controversial.

–**postoperative analgesia** is particularly important, to reduce sympathetic overactivity.
Mangano DT (1990) Anesthesiology; 72: 153–84
See also, Arteriosclerosis

Isobestic point. Point at which two substances absorb a certain wavelength of light to the same extent. In **oximetry**, the different absorption profiles of oxyhaemoglobin and deoxyhaemoglobin are utilized to quantify the percentage saturation of **haemoglobin**. Isobestic points occur at 590 and 805 nm; these may be used as reference points where light absorption is independent of degree of saturation (*see Fig. 104; Oximetry*).

Isoflurane. 1–Chloro-2,2,2–trifluoroethyl difluoromethyl ether (Fig. 79). **Inhalational anaesthetic agent**, first synthesized in 1965 with its isomer **enflurane**, but not introduced until 1980 because of earlier (erroneous) reports of hepatic carcinogenicity in mice. Increasingly used despite being nine times as expensive as **halothane**.

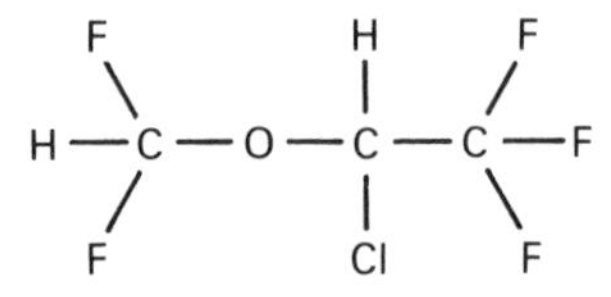

Figure 79 *Structure of isoflurane*

- Properties:
  –colourless liquid; pungent vapour, 7.5 times denser than air.
  –mw 184.5.
  –boiling point 49°C.
  –**SVP** at 20°C 33 kPa (250 mmHg).
  –**partition coefficients**:
    –blood/gas 1.4.
    –oil/gas 97.
  –**MAC** 1.15.
  –non-flammable, non-corrosive. Dissolves certain plastics, e.g. some makes of syringe, etc.
  –supplied in liquid form with no additive.
- Effects:
  –CNS:
    –smooth rapid induction, but speed of uptake is limited by respiratory irritation. Recovery is also rapid.
    –anticonvulsant properties, unlike enflurane. Causes more reduction of EEG activity than other agents.
    –increases **cerebral blood flow** and **ICP** (prevented by hyperventilation and hypocapnia even if achieved after introduction of isoflurane, unlike halothane).
    –decreases **intraocular pressure**.
    –has poor analgesic properties.
  –RS:
    –irritant; more likely to cause coughing, etc. than halothane and enflurane.
    –respiratory depressant, with increased rate and decreased tidal volume.
    –causes bronchodilatation.

–CVS:

–myocardial depression is less than with halothane and enflurane, but vasodilatation and hypotension commonly occur. Compensatory tachycardia is common, especially in young patients.

–myocardial O_2 demand decreases, but tachycardia and **coronary steal** may reduce myocardial O_2 supply, although this is controversial.

–arrhythmias are less common than with other agents. Little myocardial sensitization to **catecholamines**.

–other:

–dose-dependent uterine relaxation.

–nausea/vomiting is uncommon.

–skeletal muscle relaxation; **non-depolarizing neuro-muscular blockade** may be potentiated.

–may precipitate **MH**.

Less than 0.2% metabolized, the rest being excreted by the lungs. Thus considered the agent of choice in renal and hepatic impairment, and thought to be the least likely volatile agent to cause **hepatitis** after repeated use. Also widely used in **neurosurgery**, for the above properties. **Fluoride ion** production is minimal, even after prolonged surgery; higher levels have been reported after several days' use on ICU.

1–2.5% is usually adequate for maintenance of anaesthesia, with higher concentrations for induction. Tracheal intubation may be performed easily with spontaneous respiration, once the patient is adequately anaesthetized.
See also, Vaporizers

Isolated forearm technique. Method for detecting **awareness** during anaesthesia. A tourniquet is inflated on the upper arm to above systolic BP, before systemic injection of **neuromuscular blocking drug**. Arm movement, both spontaneous and in response to verbal command, can be observed during anaesthesia. Patients may respond to command without postoperative recall (wakefulness).
Tunstall ME (1977) BMJ; 1:1321

Isomerism. Existence of two or more ions or compounds that have the same atomic composition but different structural arrangement, often with different properties, e.g. **isoflurane** ($CF_3CHClOCHF_2$) and **enflurane** ($CHCLF-CF_2OCHF_2$). Optical isomers (enantiomers; chiral substances) are mirror images of each other, and rotate the plane of polarization of polarized light in opposite directions, e.g. the laevo- (*l*-) and dextro- (*d*-) rotatory forms of **catecholamines**. A racemic mixture is one containing equal amounts of the *l*- and *d*- forms. That such closely related isomers may have different effects is one piece of evidence supporting **receptor theory**.
Calvey TN (1992) Anaesthesia; 47: 93–4

Isoprenaline hydrochloride/sulphate. Catecholamine and **inotropic drug**. A non-selective β-adrenergic receptor agonist, used for its effects on heart rate, vasomotor tone and bronchial muscle.

• Actions:

–increased heart rate and force of myocardial contraction.

–peripheral and pulmonary vasodilatation.

–bronchodilatation.

–systolic BP may rise or fall; diastolic BP usually falls.

• Dosage:

–0.02–0.2 μg/kg/min iv for complete **heart block** or severe bradycardia. A bolus of 5–20 μg may also be given.

–may also be given orally, rectally or sublingually: 10–30 mg 8 hourly; absorption may be unreliable.

May cause tachycardia, tremor and ventricular arrhythmias. May worsen coronary perfusion in **ischaemic heart disease**.

Isosorbide di- and mononitrate. Vasodilator drugs, with similar actions to **glyceryl trinitrate** (GTN) but of longer duration (up to 12 hours with sustained release preparations). IV infusion of the dinitrate has been suggested in preference to infusion of GTN preparations because the latter contains additives (e.g. propylene glycol). The mononitrate is a metabolite of the dinitrate. Used in **ischaemic heart disease**, **cardiac failure**, and as an **antihypertensive drug** peroperatively.

• Dosage:

–dinitrate:

–5–10 mg sublingually.

–up to 240 mg/day orally; given 1–4 times daily.

–2–7 mg/h iv (0.5–2 μg/kg/min).

–mononitrate: 20–120 mg/day orally; given 1–4 times daily.

Isothermal change. Alteration in the state of a **gas** whilst **temperature** remains constant, e.g. by removal of **heat** produced during compression. Thus **Boyle's law** applies.
See also, Adiabatic change

Isotherms. Lines on a chart or graph denoting changes in volume or **pressure** with **temperature** remaining constant. The graph for an ideal gas would consist of rectangular hyperbolas according to the gas laws. In fact, for **N_2O** (Fig. 80), the isotherms approach those of an ideal gas at temperatures above its **critical temperature** (36.5°C). Compression of the N_2O below its critical temperature causes liquefaction, thus resisting an increase in pressure. Once all the N_2O is liquid, further compression causes a large increase in pressure, since liquids are less compressible than gases.

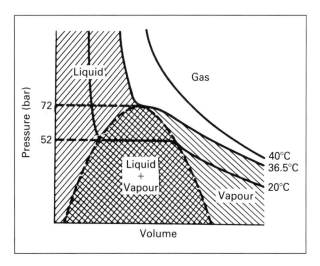

Figure 80 *Isotherms for N_2O*

ITU, Intensive therapy unit, *see Intensive care unit*

IVOX, *see Intravenous oxygenator*

IVRA, *see Intravenous regional anaesthesia*

J

J receptors, *see Juxtapulmonary capillary receptors*

J wave, *see Hypothermia*

Jackson, Charles T (1805–1880). US chemist, present at **Wells'** unsuccessful demonstration of **N₂O** in 1846; suggested **diethyl ether** to **Morton** for dental topical anaesthesia instead. Applied for the patent rights to ether jointly with Morton, the latter subsequently taking over 90% of Jackson's share. Jackson later claimed sole credit for the discovery of anaesthesia.

Jackson, Chevalier (1865–1958). Renowned US laryngologist. Perfected a direct vision **laryngoscope** in the early 1900s, and wrote extensively on laryngoscopy and tracheal insufflation.

Jaundice. Clinically detectable when plasma total bilirubin exceeds 50 μmol/l (normally under 17 μmol/l).
- Normal formation and metabolism of bilirubin:
  - **haemoglobin** is broken down to haem in the reticuloendothelial system. Lipid-soluble unconjugated bilirubin is transported to the **liver**.
  - unconjugated bilirubin is converted to conjugated bilirubin (water soluble) in the liver.
  - conjugated bilirubin is stored in the gallbladder with bile salts and acids, passing into the small bowel.
  - bilirubin is converted to urobilinogen and thence urobilin by gut bacteria. Reabsorbed from the gut, with some urobilinogen passing back to the liver to be re-excreted; a small amount is extracted by the kidneys.
- Causes of jaundice:
  - increased bilirubin production, e.g. **haemolysis**. Usually mild. Unconjugated and conjugated bilirubin levels are raised, with increased urinary urobilinogen.
  - impaired conjugation of bilirubin, e.g. **hepatitis**, cirrhosis, drug-induced (e.g. **α-methyldopa, paracetamol**), **hepatic failure**. Unconjugated bilirubin is raised; urinary urobilinogen may be raised because the liver is unable to re-excrete it.
  - congenital abnormalities of bilirubin transport are rare, except for Gilbert's syndrome (mild unconjugated bilirubinaemia with otherwise normal **liver function tests**, and no urinary bilirubin).
  - obstruction of bile drainage, e.g. gallstones, pancreatic carcinoma (extrahepatic), primary biliary cirrhosis, drug-induced, e.g. **contraceptives**. Conjugated bilirubin is raised, often markedly, spilling over into the urine which is dark (but with urobilinogen reduced). Faeces are pale. Itching is common.

The latter two types are frequently mixed and difficult to distinguish.

All jaundiced patients should be questioned for history of tattoos, drug-abuse, sexual contacts, contacts with jaundiced people, travel abroad, drugs, blood transfusions, alcohol, acupuncture, abdominal symptoms and recent anaesthetics.
- Anaesthetic management:
  - preoperative assessment as above, and for hepatic failure, depending on severity and cause.
  - risk of perioperative acute **renal failure** due to acute tubular necrosis or **hepatorenal syndrome**:
    - especially common with obstructive jaundice, since bilirubin levels are often highest.
    - more likely if dehydration or biliary sepsis are present.
    - plasma urea/creatinine is monitored preoperatively.
    - preoperative iv hydration is instituted to maintain urine flow above 1 ml/kg/h.
    - **mannitol** is usually infused if bilirubin is very high or urine output inadequate despite hydration. **Frusemide** has been used.
  - **antibacterial therapy**.
  - anaesthetic drugs and techniques as for hepatic failure.
- Postoperative jaundice may be due to:
  - Gilbert's syndrome.
  - underlying medical/surgical conditions.
  - drugs, including **halothane**.
  - haemolysis, e.g. due to **blood transfusion** reaction, or following extensive bruising and haematoma.
  - infection, e.g. transmitted via transfused blood, needles, etc., septicaemia, pre-existing subclinical hepatitis becoming apparent postoperatively, etc.
  - hepatic damage due to severe hypoxia/hypotension.
  - surgical iatrogenic biliary obstruction.

Jaundice is particularly hazardous in **neonates**; the immature blood–brain barrier allows penetration of bilirubin into the basal ganglia of the brain, causing kernicterus (convulsions may occur leading to brain damage).
[Nicolas Gilbert (1858–1927), French physician]
See also, Halothane hepatitis

Jaw, fractured. Anaesthetic considerations are related to the presence of other **trauma** (especially to head, chest and neck), **alcohol** ingestion, risk of **aspiration of gastric contents**, possible **airway obstruction** and difficult tracheal intubation, and postoperative management of the airway.
- Anaesthetic management:
  - preoperatively:
    - assessment for the above factors. Airway obstruction and major haemorrhage are more likely with bilateral fractures.

–**gastric contents** include food or drink (including alcohol), swallowed blood, etc. Fractures rarely require immediate surgery; thus a period of preoperative starvation is usually possible.

–the patient should be warned about postoperative inability to open the mouth if the jaw is wired.

–**premedication** is according to preference. Opioid premedication is usually restricted if inhalational **induction of anaesthesia** is planned or **head injury** suspected.

–peroperatively:

–rapid sequence induction may be necessary. Other techniques may be required if airway obstruction is present (e.g. awake fibreoptic tracheal intubation).

–nasal tracheal intubation is usually required. Oral intubation may be performed first to secure the airway.

–procedures often involve wiring of jaw segments together, and splinting of the mandible to the upper jaw. Silk threads are sometimes used. Plates may be applied, with wiring 1–2 days later.

–postoperatively:

–tracheal **extubation** (if appropriate) should be performed when the patient is awake and in the lateral position. If severe oedema is anticipated, the tracheal tube is left in place postoperatively until swelling has subsided. Oral suction may be impossible.

–the tracheal tube may be withdrawn into the pharynx to act as a nasal airway.

–postoperative care should be on HDU/ICU, since the airway must be closely watched for obstruction, bleeding, etc. Wire cutters should be next to the patient at all times.

See also, Dental surgery; Faciomaxillary surgery; Induction, rapid sequence

Jaw, nerve blocks, *see Gasserian ganglion block; Mandibular nerve blocks; Maxillary nerve blocks*

Jehovah's Witnesses. Religious group founded in the USA in the 1870s. Believe that they alone will survive the imminent destruction of the world, to rule over the resurrected. Also believe that to recieve blood products is against God's will, thus causing potential difficulties perioperatively. Special **consent** forms are usually employed. For paediatric surgery, a court order is required in order to overrule parents' wishes. Autologous **blood transfusion** is permitted only if contact of blood with the body is not broken.

Benson KT (1989) Anesth Analg; 69: 647–56

See also, Medicolegal aspects of anaesthesia

Jet mixing. Effect of a jet of **gas**, e.g. O_2, delivered from a nozzle into ambient gas, e.g. air. Energy is transferred from O_2 molecules to adjacent air molecules; the latter are entrained into the jet due to viscous shearing between the gas layers. Employed in **injector techniques** for IPPV, and in fixed performance O_2 masks. In the latter, air is entrained to a fixed degree depending on O_2 flow rate and the size of side ports in the entrainment device.

See also, Oxygen therapy; Venturi principle

Jet ventilators, *see High frequency ventilation; Injector techniques; Ventilators*

JG cells, *see Juxtaglomerular cells*

Jorgensen technique. **Sedation** using pentobarbitone (30–300 mg), **pethidine** (up to 25 mg) and **hyoscine** (0.3 mg) iv, to allow **dental surgery**. Although maintaining cardiovascular stability, nausea and delayed **recovery** may occur. Described in 1953.

[Niels B Jorgensen (1894–1974), Danish-born Californian dentist]

Joule. SI **unit** of **energy**. 1 joule = **work** done when the point of application of a **force** of 1 **newton** moves 1 metre in the direction of the force (1 J = 1 N × 1 m).

[James Joule (1818–89), English physicist]

Joule–Thomson effect (**Joule**–Kelvin effect). Lowering of temperature when a gas expands, e.g. passing from a **cylinder** under pressure to a large space. The principle is employed in the **cryoprobe**. Conversely, temperature rises if gas within a small space is compressed.

[William Thomson (Lord **Kelvin**) (1824–1907), Irish-born Scottish physicist]

See also, Adiabatic change

Jugular veins. Include the internal, external and anterior jugular veins (Fig. 81; *See also Fig. 97; Neck, cross-sectional anatomy*).

● Internal jugular vein:

–passes through the jugular foramen at the base of the **skull**, draining the intracranial structures via the sigmoid sinus.

–lies at first posterior, then lateral, to the internal **carotid artery**. Contained within the carotid sheath with the carotid artery and **vagus nerve**; the cervical sympathetic chain lies behind the sheath.

–receives tributaries from the pharynx, face, scalp, tongue and thyroid gland. Receives the thoracic duct on the left and right lymph duct on the right.

–has a dilatation at each end (jugular bulb), with valves above the lower bulb.

–terminates behind the sternoclavicular joint by joining with the subclavian vein to form the brachiocephalic vein.

● External jugular vein:

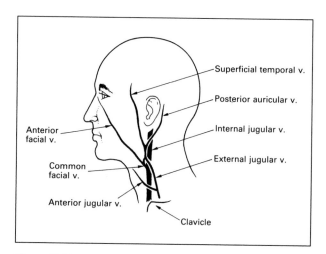

Figure 81 *Venous drainage of head and neck*

–drains the lateral parts of the head; passes over the sternomastoid muscle to join the subclavian vein behind the clavicle at its midpoint.

–receives the anterior jugular vein (passing down from in front of the hyoid bone) behind the clavicle.

See also, Cerebral circulation; Internal jugular cannulation

Jugular venous pressure (JVP). Assessed by observing the height (in cm) of visible pulsation in the **jugular veins** above the sternal angle, with the patient reclining at 45°. The normal value is zero; i.e. the venous pulsations are not normally visible. The JVP falls during inspiration, and rises during expiration and when pressure is applied to the abdomen (Q sign). Pulsations are usually non-palpable. The **venous waveform** may be apparent. JVP may be difficult to identify in obese patients.

Useful as a clinical guide to right atrial pressure; raised in right-sided **cardiac failure**, hypervolaemia, and mechanical obstruction, e.g. tricuspid stenosis or **superior vena caval obstruction**.

See also, Central venous pressure

Junctional arrhythmias (Nodal arrhythmias). **Arrhythmias** arising from the atrioventricular node. Common during anaesthesia, especially deep inhalational anaesthesia.

- May consist of:
  –ectopic beats.
  –bradycardia.
  –tachycardia.

On the **ECG**, inverted **P waves** may precede, follow, or be hidden by, the (normal) **QRS complexes**. Usually of little clinical significance, although cardiac output may be reduced. Cannon waves may be visible in the jugular **venous waveform**.

Atropine and **ephedrine** have been used to restore sinus rhythm in bradycardia; junctional tachycardias may respond to **lignocaine** and similar drugs.

See also, Heart, conducting system

Juxtaglomerular apparatus. System adjacent to renal glomeruli, composed of:

–juxtaglomerular cells; epithelioid cells within the media of afferent arterioles entering the glomeruli. Contain renin in granules.

–macula densa; specialized tubular epithelial cells, just before the start of the distal convoluted tubule. Thought to be involved in the control of renin secretion.

–granular cells within surrounding connective tissue; contain some renin granules.

Responds to reductions in renal perfusion pressure by secreting renin, although the exact mechanism is unclear. Possibly renal vasodilatation is involved, since **β-adrenergic receptor agonists**, **prostacyclin**, **bradykinin**, **dopamine**, **frusemide** and **vasodilator drugs** all increase renin secretion. Conversely, **α-adrenergic receptor agonists**, **vasopressin**, and angiotensin reduce renin secretion.

Richly innervated with adrenergic nerve fibres; β-adrenergic activity increases secretion, and antagonism reduces it, independantly of vasodilatation.

See also, Nephron; Renin/angiotensin system

Juxtapulmonary capillary receptors (J receptors). Receptors thought to be present in alveolar walls near the capillaries. Thought to be responsible for the tachypnoea seen in **pulmonary oedema** and interstitial lung disease, via vagal afferent fibres. Their role in normal lungs is unknown.

K

Kallikreins. Proteolytic **enzymes** in tissue and plasma, producing **kinins** from kininogens. May also catalyse formation of renin from prorenin. Plasma kallikrein is produced from prekallikrein by various activating substances, including part of activated **coagulation** factor XII. Plasmin, a fibrinolytic enzyme, catalyses the reaction, as does kallikrein itself. Inhibited by **aprotinin.**

Katharometer. Device used for **gas analysis**, following separation, e.g. by **gas chromatography**. A heated wire is placed in the gas flow; different gases have different thermal conductive properties and therefore produce different changes in electrical resistance of the wire. Particularly useful in detecting inorganic gases, e.g. helium, CO_2, N_2O, and O_2. Used to quantify the amount of a known gas, not to identify unknown ones.

KCT, Kaolin cephalin time, *see Coagulation studies*

Kelvin. SI **unit** of **temperature**. One kelvin (K) = 1/273.16 of the thermodynamic scale temperature of the triple point of water (point at which solid, liquid and gaseous water are at equilibrium). $nK = (n - 273.16)$ °C.
[William Thomson (1824–1907), Irish-born Scottish physicist; became Lord Kelvin in 1892]

Kerley's lines. Opaque markings seen on the **chest X-ray**:
  –type A: thin unbranched lines, radiating from the hila. Possibly represent interlobular septa.
  –type B: transverse lines, under 3 cm long, seen at the lung bases, especially costophrenic angles. Represent thickened interlobular septa, e.g. due to fluid (e.g. **pulmonary oedema**), fibrosis or tumour.
  –type C: spider's web appearance.
[Peter Kerley (1900–1978), Irish radiologist]

Ketamine hydrochloride. IV anaesthetic agent (Fig. 82), first used in 1965. Derivative of phencyclidine ('angel dust'), but less likely to cause hallucinations. Presented in 10, 50 and 100 mg/ml solutions, the latter two with

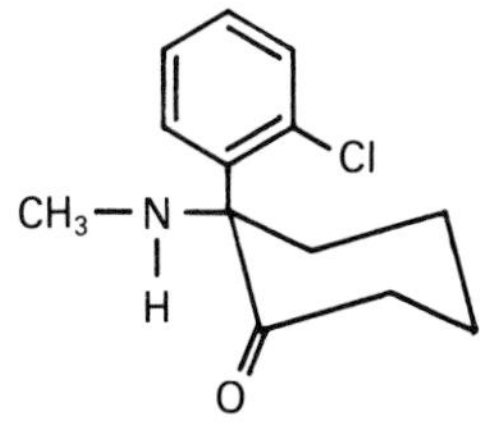

Figure 82 *Structure of ketamine*

benzethonium chloride 0.01% as a preservative. pH is 3.5–5.5; pK_a 7.5. 12% bound to plasma albumin. Elimination **half-life** is about 3 hours. Metabolized in the liver to weakly active metabolites, excreted in urine. Produces a state of 'dissociative anaesthesia': intense analgesia with light sleep. Increased thalamic and limbic activity occur, with dissociation from higher centres.

Used for **induction of anaesthesia**, traditionally in shocked patients. May also be used for maintenance as the sole agent, especially in **burns**, **trauma**, **radiotherapy**, radiological investigations, etc., because of its alleged preservation of upper airway reflexes. Has local anaesthetic properties, and has been used for **spinal** and **extradural anaesthesia**, in doses of up to 50 mg.
● Effects:
  –induction: smooth, but slower than **thiopentone** (about 30 seconds).
  –CVS/RS:
    –BP and heart rate usually increase; cardiac output is maintained. Changes are probably via direct myocardial and central sympathetic stimulation, and blockade of noradrenaline uptake by sympathetic nerve endings. Contraindicated in severe **ischaemic heart disease** and **hypertension**.
    –may cause respiratory depression after rapid injection, but less than with other agents.
    –traditionally held to preserve laryngeal and pharyngeal reflexes, with minimal upper airway obstruction. However, airway obstruction, laryngospasm and aspiration may still occur.
    –causes bronchodilatation via a direct action and sympathomimetic effects.
  –CNS:
    –causes analgesia, even at subanaesthetic doses.
    –may cause increased muscle tone, twitching, blinking and nystagmus.
    –increases **cerebral blood flow** and **ICP**; contraindicated in **pre-eclampsia** and severe intracranial pathology.
    –may cause anterograde amnesia.
    –may cause vivid dreams and **emergence phenomena**, e.g. hallucinations which are often frightening. Usually less distressing in patients below 15 years or above 65 years. Dreams are said to be reduced by **benzodiazepines**, and delirium by **butyrophenones**. **Physostigmine** has also been used. Preoperative counselling and opioid/hyoscine premedication may also reduce their incidence. In the past, patients have traditionally recovered in quiet darkened rooms.
  –other:
    –may cause nausea and vomiting. Salivation is increased.
    –may increase uterine tone.

Ketanserin

–increases **intraocular pressure**; contra-indicated in open eye operations, although it has been used for anaesthesia for measurement of intraocular pressures in children.
–does not cause **histamine** release.
- Dosage:
  –1–2 mg/kg iv for induction. Effects last for 5–10 minutes. Supplementary doses 0.5 mg/kg.
  –10 mg/kg im for induction; acts in 3–5 minutes, lasting 20–30 minutes.
  –may be used in smaller doses for **sedation**, e.g. prior to induction in agitated patients or whilst performing regional techniques, especially when moving painful limbs. Suitable doses: 2 mg/kg im, 10 mg increments iv, or 1–2 mg/kg/h infusion.
  –to treat severe **asthma**: 0.5–2.5 mg/kg/h infusion.

Ketanserin. 5-HT antagonist, and weak α_1–adrenergic **receptor antagonist**. Also has Class III antiarrhythmic properties. Has been used to prevent vasoconstriction and bronchospasm in **carcinoid syndrome**, and also to provide vasodilatation and hypotension in **cardiac surgery**.

Ketoacidosis. Metabolic **acidosis** due to accumulation of **ketone bodies** in plasma. May be associated with **hyperglycaemia**, especially in **diabetic coma**. May also occur in chronic **alcohol** abuse following a recent binge and starvation; hyperglycaemia is then not be a feature.
- Features:
  –of acidosis, including hyperventilation and **hyperkalaemia**.
  –characteristic sweet smell on the patient's breath due to ketosis (undetectable by a minority of clinicians).
  –nausea and vomiting, **dehydration**.
Treatment includes rehydration and correction of electrolyte imbalance. Diabetics require **insulin**; alcoholics require glucose.

Ketobemidone hydrochloride. Opioid analgesic drug, with similar potency and properties to **morphine**. Mainly used in Scandinavia.

Ketone bodies. Acetone, acetoacetic acid and hydroxybutyric acid; formed from hepatic metabolism of free fatty acids released from adipose tissue. Normally utilized by brain, heart and other tissues as an energy source, keeping blood levels low. Levels increase when **fat** metabolism increases, especially when intracellular **glucose** is deficient, e.g. in **diabetes mellitus**, starvation, and high fat/low **carbohydrate** diet. May occur in **alcohol** abuse, when glucose production is impaired. Increased levels may lead to **ketoacidosis**. Acetone may be detected on the breath.

Ketorolac trometamol/tromethamine. NSAID, available for im use. Has a marked analgesic effect with little anti-inflammatory effect; 30 mg is equivalent to 10 mg **morphine**. Has been used for **postoperative analgesia**, reducing opioid requirements. Maximal plasma levels occur within 60 minutes of im injection, with resultant analgesia lasting 4–6 hours. Highly protein-bound, with hepatic metabolism (reduced in the elderly). **Half-life** is 5–6 hours.
- Dosage: 10–30 mg im 4–6 hourly, up to 120 mg/day for up to 5 days. May also be given orally: 10 mg 4–6 hourly, up to 40 mg/day for up to 7 days.

- Side effects: as for NSAIDs. CNS effects including drowsiness, dizziness, psychological changes and convulsions have been reported.
Kenny GNC (1990) Br J Anaesth; 65: 445–7

Kety–Schmidt technique. Method of measuring **cerebral blood flow** using the **Fick principle**, using N_2O. 10% N_2O is inhaled for 10–15 minutes, and the jugular venous concentration is assumed to be equal to the brain concentration. Cerebral N_2O uptake is therefore calculated.
[Seymour S Kety, US neurophysiologist; Richard P Schmidt, US neurologist]

Key filling system. System for filling modern **vaporizers** with volatile anaesthetic agent, preventing filling with incorrect agent and supposedly reducing spillage and pollution by using closely fitting interlocking components.
- Composed of:
  –filler tube: a base at one end screws on to the bottle; the other end bears a plastic block which only fits into the correct vaporizer filling port.
  –collar round the neck of the bottle of volatile agent; protruding pegs slot into corresponding slots in the filler tube base. Position of pegs and slots are specific for each agent.
Collar, filler tube base and block are colour-coded for the particular agent (**halothane** - red; **enflurane** - orange; **isoflurane** - purple; **trichloroethylene** - blue; **methoxyflurane** - green). The name of the correct agent is written on the filler tube base.
See also, COSHH regulations; Environmental safety of anaesthetists

Kidney. Situated on the posterior abdominal wall, with the diaphragm and 11th and 12th ribs posteriorly. The renal hila are approximately level with the pylorus. Each kidney is about 10 cm long, 5 cm wide and 3 cm thick. Nerve supply is via the coeliac ganglion from T12 and L1. Blood supply is from the renal arteries which arise from the descending aorta, and venous drainage is via the renal veins into the inferior vena cava. **Renal blood flow** is 1200 ml/min (22% of cardiac output), about 400 ml/100 g/min. O_2 consumption is 20 ml/min, or 6 ml/100 g/min.

Composed of outer cortex and inner medulla forming pyramids. Functional unit is the **nephron**, with accompanying arterioles and capillaries.
- Functions:
  –filtration of plasma and excretion of waste products of **metabolism**, whilst maintaining water, **osmolality**, electrolyte and acid–base homeostasis.
  –secretion of renin.
  –secretion of **erythropoietin**.
  –formation of 1, 25–dihydroxycholecalciferol (important in **calcium** homeostasis).
  –metabolism and excretion of drugs.
- May be affected by anaesthesia/surgery:
  –drug effects, e.g. **methoxyflurane**, **diuretics**.
  –alteration of renal blood flow, e.g. **hypotension**, **aortic aneurysm** repair.
  –renal impairment following incompatible **blood transfusion**, severe **jaundice**, sepsis, obstetric emergencies, **crush syndrome**, etc.
See also, Acid–base balance; Fluid balance; Renal failure; Renal transplantation; Renin/angiotensin system

Killian, Gustav (1860–1921). German laryngologist; published extensively on the structure and function of the **larynx**. A former student of **Kirstein**, he helped popularize direct **laryngoscopy**. Also performed the first translaryngeal removal of a foreign body from the right main bronchus in 1897, using a rigid oesophagoscope and cocaine local anaesthesia, thus pioneering **bronchoscopy**.

Kilogram. SI **unit** of **mass**. The standard kilogram is the mass of a cylindrical piece of platinum–iridium alloy kept at Sèvres, France.

Kilogram weight. Weight of a **mass** of 1 **kilogram**. Also called kilogram force.
1 kg wt (or kgf) due to gravity = 1 kg × 9.81 m/s
$$= 9.81 \text{ newton.}$$

Kinins. Vasodilator peptides derived from precursor molecules (kininogens) by the action of **kallikreins**. Involved in many inflammatory and immune reactions, and possibly in **shock**. Also thought to be involved in the **carcinoid syndrome**. Bradykinin is the main plasma kinin, causing vasodilatation and increased vascular permeability. **Glucocorticoids** inhibit their release. Broken down by angiotensin converting enzyme, mainly in the lung. Elimination **half-life** is less than 15 seconds.

Kirstein, Alfred (1863–1922). German laryngologist; described the first direct **laryngoscopy** in 1895. His **laryngoscopes** could be placed anterior or posterior to the epiglottis. Stressed the importance of the 'sniffing position' for laryngoscopy. Also suggested translaryngeal removal of bronchial foreign bodies as being easier than via tracheostomy.
Hirsch NP, Smith GB, Hirsch PO (1986) Anaesthesia; 41: 42–5

Kite, Charles (1768–1811). English doctor, practising at Gravesend, Kent. Awarded the silver medal by the Humane Society (now Royal Humane Society) in 1787 for his *Essay on the Recovery of the Apparently Dead*, later published as a book. Described oro- and nasotracheal catheterization for lung inflation, and suggested laryngospasm as a cause for hypoxia in drowning.

Klippel–Feil syndrome. Congenitally fused cervical vertebrae, possibly with thoracic or lumbar fusion. Subdivided according to the extent of vertebral involvement. Most commonly restricted to C2–3 and C5–6. Scoliosis, other skeletal malformations, and cardiovascular and genitourinary abnormalities may also occur. Typically, the patient has a short neck with limited movement and a low posterior hair line. Both autosomal dominant and recessive inheritance has been suggested for different subtypes.
- Anaesthetic considerations:
  - cervical instability.
  - difficult intubation.
  - **extradural** and **spinal anaesthesia** may be technically difficult.
  - related to abnormalities of other systems.
[Maurice Klippel (1858–1942) and Andre Feil (1884–1955), French neurologists]
Naguib M, Farag H, Ibrahim AEW (1986) Can Anaesth Soc J; 33: 66–70

Knee, nerve blocks. Performed for surgery to the lower leg and foot.
- Nerves which may be blocked (*see Fig. 57; Femoral nerve block*):
  - tibial nerve (L4–S3): terminal branch of the sciatic nerve; supplies the anteromedial part of the sole of the foot via plantar branches. In the **popliteal fossa**, the nerve lies superficial and lateral to the popliteal vessels, with vein medially and artery most medial.

    With patient prone and knee extended, a needle is inserted in the midline of the popliteal fossa, level with the femoral condyles. 5–10 ml **local anaesthetic agent** is injected at a depth of 2–3 cm.
  - common peroneal (L4–S2): terminal branch of the sciatic nerve; supplies the dorsum of the foot via its superficial peroneal branch, and the area between the first and second toes via the deep peroneal branch. The region posterior to the head of the fibula is infiltrated with 5 ml solution. Some workers claim that neuritis is common, but this has been disputed.
  - sciatic (L4–S3): may be blocked before it divides into tibial and common peroneal nerves above the popliteal fossa, at a point 7 cm cranial to the skin crease behind the knee, and 1 cm lateral to the midline. 5–10 ml solution is injected at a depth of 3–5 cm.
  - saphenous (L4–5): a continuation of the femoral nerve; supplies the medial part of the lower leg, ankle and foot. May be blocked by infiltration from the medial border of the tibial tuberosity to the posterior edge of the tibia (taking care to avoid the saphenous vein).

Koller, Carl (1857–1944). Austrian ophthalmologist; first described the use of **local anaesthetic agent** (**cocaine**) for a surgical operation (for glaucoma) in Vienna in 1884, having previously investigated the drug with **Freud**. This was reported by a colleague at an ophthalmological congress in Heidelberg on the following day. Disappointed with his career's subsequent progress, he emigrated to New York in 1888.

Korotkoff sounds. Sounds heard during auscultation over the brachial artery, whilst a proximal cuff is slowly deflated from above systolic pressure. Thought to result from turbulent flow within the artery causing vessel wall vibration and resonance. Used in **arterial BP measurement**. Three phases were originally described by Korotkoff; these were subsequently increased to five:
  - phase I: intermittent tapping sound, corresponding to the heartbeat. Represents systolic pressure.
  - phase II: sounds quieten or even disappear (**auscultatory gap**).
  - phase III: sounds become louder again.
  - phase IV: sounds suddenly become muffled.
  - phase V: sounds disappear.
Argument over whether diastolic pressure is best recorded at phase IV or V continues; traditionally phase IV is used in the UK; phase V in the USA. Recording of both has been suggested, e.g. 120/80/75.
[Nicolai Korotkoff (1874–1920), Russian physician]

Krebs cycle, *see Tricarboxylic acid cycle*

Kuhn, Franz (1866–1929). German physician; wrote extensively on tracheal intubation for anaesthesia.

Described tracheal insufflation in 1900 and nasotracheal intubation in 1902.

Sweeney B (1985) Anaesthesia; 40: 1000–5

Kussmaul breathing (Air hunger). **Hyperventilation** originally described in diabetic hyperglycaemic **ketoacidosis**. Caused by stimulation of central chemoreceptors by hydrogen ions. Occurs in severe metabolic **acidosis** of any cause.

[Adolf Kussmaul (1822–1909), German physician]

Kussmaul's sign, *see Cardiac tamponade*

Kyphoscoliosis. Definitions:
   –kyphosis: posterior curvature of spine.
   –scoliosis: lateral curvature.
   There may also be rotational deformity.
May be associated with congenital skeletal, muscular or neurological abnormalities and diseases. Idiopathic scoliosis develops in childhood; vertebral rotation is common. Thoracic, rib and chest wall deformity may cause restriction of ventilation. Surgical fixation is usually performed before puberty. This may be performed using metal Harrington rods, allowing distraction of the vertebrae using a ratchet.
• Anaesthetic management:
   –preoperatively:
      –assessment for associated disease.
      –**MH** is commoner in this group.
      –assessment of RS: lung volumes and **compliance**

are reduced; the main defect is restrictive. $\dot{V}/\dot{Q}$ **mismatch** may be present. Repeated aspiration may occur in neuromuscular disease. **Chest X-ray** is mandatory; **lung function tests** and arterial blood gas analysis are useful.
   –chronic hypoxia may lead to **pulmonary hypertension** and **cor pulmonale.**
   –preoperative **physiotherapy**, antibiotics, etc. may be required.
–peroperatively :
   –tracheal intubation may be difficult, especially if the patient is unable to lie flat.
   –surgery may be prolonged, with risk of major blood loss, hypothermia, etc.
   –transthoracic surgery may involve anterior or posterior approaches.
   –**hypotensive anaesthesia** is advocated by some, to reduce blood loss and ease surgery. Others argue that possible ischaemia of the spinal cord precludes this. Careful positioning of patient is required to prevent pressure on the abdominal inferior vena cava.
   –risk of cord damage during distraction of **vertebrae** may be assessed by the **wake-up test** or monitoring of **evoked potentials.**
   –access to the patient may be restricted.
–postoperatively: ventilatory failure is possible; close monitoring is required. Chest X-ray is usual to exclude **pneumothorax.**

[Paul R Harrington, Texas surgeon]

L

Labat, Gaston (1877–1934). Anaesthetist, born in the Seychelles; worked in Paris and at the Mayo Clinic and New York University, USA. Pioneer of regional anaesthesia, writing a classic text on the subject in 1922. Founded the American Society of Regional Anaesthesia in 1923.

Labetalol hydrochloride. Combined β- and α-adrenergic receptor antagonist, with ratio of activities usually quoted between 2:1 and 5:1 respectively. Selective for α_1-receptors, but non-selective at β-receptors, with some **intrinsic sympathomimetic activity**. Used to treat severe **hypertension** and **pre-eclampsia**, and in **hypotensive anaesthesia**. 90% protein bound. **Half-life** is 4 hours. Metabolized in the liver and excreted in urine and faeces. Undergoes extensive **first-pass metabolism** when given orally.
- Dosage:
  - –5–50 mg iv by slow injection, up to 200 mg. Effects occur usually within 5 minutes, lasting 6 hours but possibly up to 18 hours.
  - –10–200 mg/h infusion.
  - –50–100 mg orally 12 hourly; increased up to a maximum 2.4 g/24 hours.
- Side effects:
  - –as for β-adrenergic receptor antagonists. Synergistic with halothane; marked hypotension may result.
  - –jaundice has occurred rarely.

Labour, active management of. Medical intervention depends on the plot of cervical dilatation and descent of the fetal head against time, usually starting from presentation in labour. The curve obtained is compared with curves derived from studies of normal labours, primiparous or multiparous as appropriate (partograms). The normal curve is comprised of latent (up to 3–4 cm cervical dilatation) and active (until 10 cm dilatation) phases. Delay in progress is represented by a lag of more than two hours to the right of the expected curve.
- Different patterns of delay may occur:
  - –prolonged latent phase: its existence is disputed by some obstetricians, since the definition of onset of labour is difficult and variable. Others claim up to 30% forceps rate and up to 15% Caesarean section (CS) rate. Commoner in primiparous women.
  - –primary delay: i.e. slow progress of the active phase, e.g. due to inefficient uterine contraction. Forceps rate is 7–8%, CS rate 4–5%. More common in primiparous women.
  - –secondary arrest: normal progress to 7–8 cm, then delay. Commonly due to malposition. Forceps rate is 2–3%, CS rate 1–2%.

Cephalopelvic disproportion may cause delay at any stage, but especially secondary delay. Most other causes are treated successfully with **oxytocic drugs**, monitoring **fetal wellbeing** and further progress.

Extradural blockade is often instituted to provide analgesia for augmented contractions, possibly to restore uterine coordinate activity, and in case of operative delivery.

Lack breathing system, *see Coaxial anaesthetic breathing systems*

Lactate. Byproduct of anaerobic **glycolysis**. **Hypoxia** prevents aerobic metabolism of pyruvate to CO_2 and water; instead lactate is formed, with consequent increases in plasma lactate/pyruvate ratio (normally 10) and plasma lactate (normally 0.6–1.8 mmol/l). Thus increased values may indicate failure of peripheral perfusion, e.g. in **shock**, and have been predictive of mortality in some studies. An initial increase in plasma lactate when perfusion improves may represent washout from previously underperfused tissues.

Lactate may also accumulate if gluconeogenesis is reduced, e.g. in type B **lactic acidosis**. Normal daily load is about 1.2 mol; 50% is eliminated by the liver.

Lactic acidosis. Metabolic **acidosis** accompanied by raised plasma **lactate** levels, usually defined as over 5–7 mmol/l.
- Causes are divided into:
  - –those with overt tissue hypoxia (type A):
    - –severe **hypoxaemia**.
    - –severe **anaemia**.
    - –**shock/haemorrhage/hypotension**.
    - –**cardiac failure**.
    - –severe exercise.
  - –those without apparent initial tissue hypoxia (type B):
    - –**diabetes mellitus**.
    - –**hepatic failure**.
    - –**renal failure**.
    - –severe infection, leukaemia, lymphoma.
    - –drug-induced, e.g. **biguanides**, **ethanol**/methanol, **salicylates**; xylitol, fructose and sorbitol in TPN (metabolized to lactate).
    - –**glycogen storage disorders, inborn errors of metabolism**.
- Treatment:
  - –directed at the underlying cause.
  - –cautious use of **bicarbonate** (increased lactate levels have followed its use).
  - –amine buffers, insulin and glucose infusions, and stimulation of pyruvate dehydrogenase with sodium dichloroacetate have also been tried.

Mizock BA, Falk JL (1992) Crit Care Med; 20: 80–93

Lambert–Beer law, *see Beer–Lambert law*

LAP, *see Left atrial pressure*

Laparoscopy. Common gynaecological procedure, requiring induced pneumoperitoneum, usually with CO_2. N_2O has also been used. Many other types of surgery, e.g. cholecystectomy, are increasingly being performed using laparoscopic techniques. Whilst postoperative pain and morbidity (and thus stay in hospital) are reduced compared with conventional surgery, patients may be exposed to the complications below. In addition, surgery may be prolonged whilst the technique is being learnt.

- Main problems are related to:
  - gas insufflation:
    - risk of trauma to intra-abdominal viscera (including stomach if previously distended with air during IPPV via facepiece) and great vessels when the trocar is introduced or gas insufflated.
    - risk of gas embolus if gas is inadvertently insufflated into blood vessels. CO_2 is rapidly absorbed from the blood, reducing the size of embolus, whereas N_2O is not.
    - subcutaneous/mediastinal emphysema and **pneumothorax** may occur.
    - caval compression reducing venous return if intra-peritoneal pressure exceeds 3–4 kPa. Higher pressures may compress the aorta.
    - gas may splint the diaphragm and reduce lung expansion.
    - raised intra-abdominal pressure may increase risk of regurgitation and **aspiration of gastric contents**.
    - CO_2 may be extensively absorbed across the peritoneum, requiring increased alveolar ventilation to maintain normocapnia. If N_2O is used, absorption provides some analgesia.
    - risk of explosion if laparoscopic diathermy is used with N_2O, but not with CO_2.
    - presence of peritoneal gas postoperatively may cause pain or discomfort, typically referred to the shoulder tip.
  - semilithotomy position:
    - reduced **FRC** and diaphragmatic splinting, with risk of **hypoxaemia** and **hypoventilation**.
    - risks of regurgitation are exacerbated.
    - venous return is increased when the legs are raised. Pooling of blood in the legs may occur when they are lowered afterwards, with resultant hypotension.
  - high incidence of severe **arrhythmias** and hypoventilation occurred in earlier studies involving deep halothane anaesthesia with spontaneous ventilation, thought to be related to the above. Bradycardia may occur even in ventilated patients.

Most patients are young fit women, but the above complications have made most anaesthetists choose tracheal intubation and IPPV as the technique of choice. Expired CO_2 monitoring is particularly useful.

- Recommended maximal safe limits for insufflation:
  - 4 l/min.
  - 3–5 litres total gas volume.
  - 3 kPa maximal intraperitoneal pressure.
  - 30–40 minutes total duration.

Laparoscopy may be performed using local anaesthesia, with infiltration of the abdominal puncture site. Discomfort may result from peritoneal stretching and pneumoperitoneum.

Laplace's law. For a hollow distensible structure:

$$P = \frac{T}{R_1} + \frac{T}{R_2}$$

where P = transmural pressure
T = tension in the wall
R_1 = radius of curvature in one direction
R_2 = radius of curvature in the other direction.

For a cylinder, one radius = infinity, therefore $P = \dfrac{T}{R}$

For a sphere, both radii are equal, therefore $P = \dfrac{2T}{R}$

- Physiological/clinical importance:
  - cylinders:
    - arteriolar smooth muscle response to fluctuating intraluminal pressure: wall tension varies in order to maintain constant radius and blood flow (one theory of the mechanism of **autoregulation**).
    - as intraluminal pressure in arterioles or airways falls, or external pressure rises, there is a critical closing pressure across the wall at which collapse may occur. In the lungs, this may occur during **forced expiration**, limiting expiratory air flow.
  - spheres:
    - ventricular cardiac muscle must generate greater tension when the heart is dilated than when of normal size, in order to produce the same intra-ventricular pressure. Thus an enlarged failing heart must contract more forcibly to sustain BP, hence the benefit of reducing **preload**.
    - in the lungs, alveoli would tend to collapse as they became smaller, were it not for **surfactant**, which reduces surface tension.
    - if the outlet of an **anaesthetic breathing system** is obstructed, the **reservoir bag** distends, thus limiting the dangerous build-up of pressure that would occur within a non-distensible bag.

[Pierre-Simon Laplace (1749–1827), French scientist]

Larrey, Baron Dominique Jean (1766–1842). French surgeon-in-chief to Napoleon. Employed **refrigeration anaesthesia** in 1807, and again in the Russian campaign to allow painless amputations in half-frozen soldiers. Also employed **triage**. Supported **Hickman** when the latter presented his experiments on 'suspended animation' to the French Academy in 1828.

[Napoleon Bonaparte (1769–1821), French Emperor]

Laryngeal mask (Brain airway). Device for supporting and maintaining the airway without tracheal intubation. Consists of an oval head attached to a connecting tube (Fig. 83). The head is inserted blindly into the pharynx to lie against the back of the larynx, and the circumferential cuff inflated to form a seal. Tolerated at lighter levels of anaesthesia than a tracheal tube. Has also been used for IPPV, using inflation pressures of up to 10–25 cmH_2O. Does not protect against **aspiration of gastric contents**.

- Originally supplied in four sizes; two more have been added:
  - 1: neonates/infants under 6.5 kg body weight.
  - 2: babies/children under 25 kg.
  - 2½: children 20–30 kg.
  - 3: ST children and small adults under 25 kg.

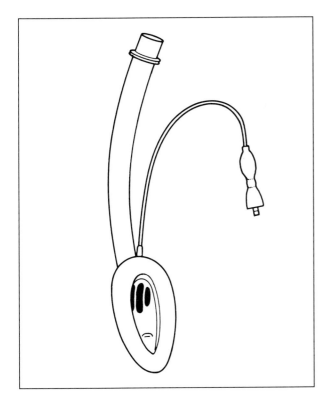

Figure 83 *Laryngeal mask*

–3: small adults.
–4: large adults.
Also available with reinforced tubes to prevent kinking.
• Its use has been suggested for:
 –routine inhalational anaesthesia.
 –inhalational anaesthesia where holding a facepiece may be difficult, e.g. due to the patient's positioning or site of surgery.
 –airway maintenance in difficult intubation, in both previously unsuspected and known cases.
 –emergency management of failed intubation.
 –**CPR**.
In difficult intubation, a bougie or fibreoptic instrument may be passed through it into the larynx, and a tracheal tube railroaded over it.
 Formerly placed with a metal introducer which is now considered unnecessary.
[Archibald IJ Brain, London anaesthetist]
Brimacombe J, Shorney N (1992) Br J Hosp Med; 47: 252–6

Laryngeal nerve blocks, *see Intubation, awake*

Laryngeal nerves. Derived from the **vagus nerves**:
 –superior laryngeal nerve:
  –arises at the base of the skull and passes deep to the carotid arteries.
  –divides into internal and external branches below and anterior to the greater cornua of the hyoid bone.
  –the internal laryngeal nerve pierces the thyrohyoid membrane with the superior laryngeal vessels, supplying the mucous membrane of the **larynx** down to the vocal cords.

 –the external laryngeal nerve passes deep to the superior thyroid artery, supplying cricothyroid muscle and the inferior constrictor muscle of the pharynx.
 –recurrent laryngeal nerve:
  –on the left, arises anterior to the ligamentum arteriosum, passes below and behind it and the aorta and ascends in the neck (*see Fig. 97; Neck, cross-sectional anatomy*).
  –on the right, given off at the right subclavian artery, passing below and behind it and ascending in the neck.
  –in the neck, ascends in the groove between the oesophagus posteriorly and trachea anteriorly.
  –enters the larynx posterior to the thyrocricoid joints, deep to the inferior constrictor. Supplies all the intrinsic laryngeal muscles except cricothyroid, and the mucous membrane of the larynx below the vocal cords.
 –afferent pathways also pass within the above nerves. Sympathetic branches pass with the arterial supply.
• Effects of nerve damage:
 –superior laryngeal: slack cord and weak voice.
 –recurrent laryngeal (partial): cord held in the midline because the abductors are affected more than the adductors (Semon's law). The voice is hoarse. If bilateral, severe airway obstruction may occur.
 –recurrent laryngeal (complete): cord held midway between the midline and abducted position. If bilateral, the cords may be snapped shut during inspiration, causing stridor. The voice is lost.
 –if one side only is affected, the contralateral cord may move across and restore the voice.
Branches may be damaged during surgery (e.g. thyroidectomy) and also by tracheal intubation, especially if undue force is used or the **cuff** is inflated within the larynx. The recurrent laryngeal nerve may be involved by lesions in the neck, or thorax or mediastinum (on the left).
 The superior laryngeal nerve may be blocked to allow awake tracheal intubation.
[Sir Felix Semon (1849–1921), German-born English laryngologist]
See also, Intubation, awake

Laryngeal reflex. Laryngospasm in response to touching of the laryngeal/hypopharyngeal mucosa. Afferent pathway is via the **laryngeal nerves**, **vagus** and **brainstem**.

Laryngoscope. Instrument used to perform **laryngoscopy**. The first direct-vision laryngoscope was invented by **Kirstein** and later developed by **Jackson**; the principle was later modified by **Magill**, **Macintosh** and others.
• Most consist of:
 –handle:
  –contains a battery power source (originally connected to mains electricity).
  –fibreoptic laryngoscopes have batteries and bulb in the handle, with transmission of light along a fibreoptic bundle set in the blade.
  –short or adjustable handles are available; smaller lighter handles are usually used for **paediatric anaesthesia**. The Anderson laryngoscope handle bears a hook for the left index finger, allowing laryngoscopy using only the thumb and index finger whilst the other fingers of the left hand are

free to apply pressure over the front of the infant's larynx. The hook and blade should be on the same side of the laryngoscope when correctly assembled.

–blade:
  –usually set at right angles to the handle.
  –many different **laryngoscope blades** have been described, most of them interchangeable when standard attachments are used.
  –older type of attachment: secured by screwing a pin through the handle and blade seatings (Longworth fitting). Newer forms employ a 'hook on' attachment at the base of the blade, locked on to the handle by a spring-loaded ball-bearing.

Flexible **fibreoptic instruments** are also available. The Bullard laryngoscope incorporates forceps, a smooth curved blade and a rigid fibreoptic channel with a proximal eye-piece within one instrument; the tracheal tube is advanced into the larynx using the forceps under visual control.

Surgical laryngoscopes resemble Jackson's more closely; they are comprised of a viewing tube with a right-angled handle, the two components together forming three sides of a rectangle. They are illuminated by an external light source attached to the proximal end of the tube.

[Sheila M Anderson (?–1986), London anaesthetist; Longworth Scientific Instrument Co. Ltd., original name for Penlon Ltd; Roger Bullard, Australian anaesthetist]

Laryngoscope blades. Parts of **laryngoscopes** inserted into the mouth.

• Consist of:

–base for attachment to handle.
–tongue: straight or curved; the former is designed for placement posterior to the epiglottis, the latter for anterior placement. The tip is usually blunt and thickened to reduce trauma.
–web: forms a shelf along one edge of the tongue, connecting the latter to the flange. Incorporates electric connections and bulb (or fibreoptic bundle). Connection channels are completely removable in older models, and fixed to the web in newer ones.
–flange: parallel to the tongue; usually only present for the proximal 1–2-thirds of the blade.

Most are designed for use with the laryngoscope handle held in the left hand; i.e. the tongue is pushed to the left side of the patient's mouth by the flange and web.

• Common varieties (Fig. 84a):
  –**Macintosh** (1943): tongue, web and flange form a reverse Z shape in cross-section. The most commonly used blade in the UK; also popular in the USA. Available in large adult, adult, child and baby sizes; the latter size was not designed by Macintosh and has been criticized by him as being anatomically incorrect. A 'left-handed' version is available, for use when anatomical features of the airway require insertion of the tracheal tube from the left side of the mouth instead of the right.
  –polio Macintosh (1950s): mounted at 135° to the handle, to allow intubation in patients confined to iron lung ventilators (e.g. in the Scandinavian polio

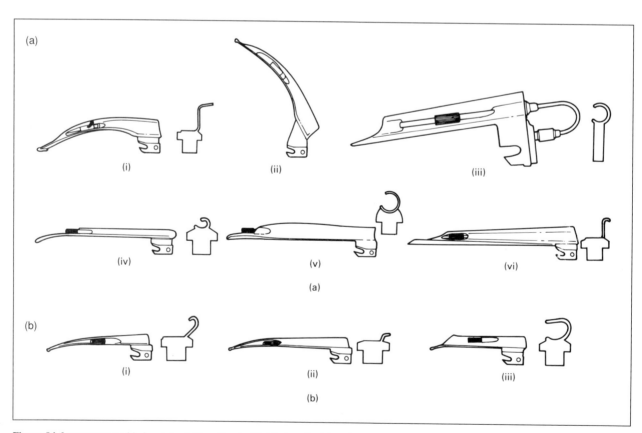

Figure 84 *Laryngoscope blades: (a) adult/paediatric: (i) Macintosh; (ii) polio Macintosh; (iii) Magill; (iv) Miller; (v) Wisconsin; (vi) Soper; (b) paediatric only: (i) Robertshaw; (ii) Seward; (iii) Oxford infant. (Not drawn to scale)*

epidemics of the 1950s). Useful when insertion of the blade into the mouth is hindered, e.g. by barrel chest, enlarged breasts, etc., especially in obstetrics.
- –**Magill** (1926): U-shaped in cross section. The most commonly used straight blade in the UK.
- –Miller (1941): similar to Magill's, but with a curved tip and flatter flange and web, requiring less mouth opening for insertion. Available in 4–5 sizes from premature baby to large adult. Popular in the USA.
- –Wisconsin (1941): bigger than Magill's, with the bulb nearer the tip. Available in similar sizes to Miller's blade. Popular in the USA.
- –Soper (1947): straight version of the Macintosh blade. The small transverse slot near the tip was designed to prevent the epiglottis slipping off the blade. Available in adult, child and baby sizes.
- • Specific paediatric blades (Fig. 84b):
  - –Robertshaw (1962): straight tongue with gently curving tip; the flange is folded inwards over the tongue. Available in infant and neonatal sizes.
  - –Seward (1957): similar to Robertshaw's but with the flange folded outwards. Available in child and baby sizes.
  - –Oxford infant (1952): straight tongue with slightly curved tip. Available in one size. Useful for intubation in children with cleft palate.
- • Others:
  - –**Guedel** and Flagg (1928): similar to Magill's, but with the bulb at the tip. Guedel's is set at an acute angle to the handle.
  - –Bowen–Jackson (1952): similar to Macintosh's but with a cleft tip, designed to straddle the glossoepiglottic fold.
  - –Siker (1956): angled blade incorporating a mirror at the angle.
  - –Bizzarri–Giuffrida (1958): similar to Macintosh's but with virtually no web and a very small flange; designed for patients with little mouth opening.
  - –Bellhouse (1988): angled blade comprised of two straight portions; used with an optical prism at the angle.

[Robert L Soper (1908–1973), RAF anaesthetist; Frank L Robertshaw (1918–1991), Manchester anaesthetist; Edgar H Seward, Oxford anaesthetist; Ronald A Bowen and Ian Jackson, London anaesthetists; Paluel Flagg (1886–1970), Robert A Miller (1906–1976), Ephraim S Siker, Dante V Bizzarri and Joseph G Giuffrida, US anaesthetists; Paul Bellhouse, Australian anaesthetist]
See also, Intubation aids; Intubation, tracheal

Laryngoscopy. Act of viewing the **larynx**. Indirect laryngoscopy was first described in 1855 in London by Garcia using a mirror. Direct laryngoscopy was pioneered by **Kirstein**, **Killian** and **Jackson** in the late 1800s/early 1900s, and is now the technique most commonly used for tracheal intubation. The view of the larynx during direct laryngoscopy is shown in Fig. 85.
Anaesthesia for diagnostic or therapeutic laryngoscopy must provide relaxation of the jaw and vocal cords, with rapid recovery of laryngeal reflexes without **laryngospasm**. Problems include sharing of the airway, the hypertensive response to laryngoscopy, contamination of the airway with blood, etc. Usually performed under general anaesthesia, with IPPV through a special 5–6 mm 'microlaryngoscopy' cuffed tracheal tube (resistance is too high for spontaneous

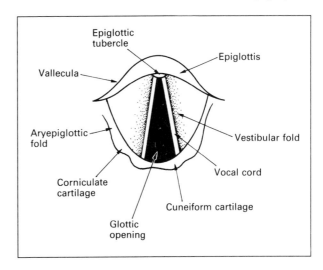

Figure 85 *View obtained during direct laryngoscopy*

ventilation). Other methods include **injector** and **insufflation techniques** as for **bronchoscopy**. Spraying the cords with **lignocaine** reduces postoperative laryngospasm but at the expense of diminshed laryngeal reflexes.
[Manuel Garcia (1805–1906), Spanish singing teacher]
See also, Intubation, complications of; Intubation, tracheal

Laryngospasm. Reflex closure of the glottis by adduction of the true and/or false cords. May persist after cessation of its stimulus. The precise mechanism is controversial; the lateral cricothyroid muscles are thought to be most important in adducting the cords whilst cricothyroid tenses them. The extrinsic muscles of the **larynx** may also have a role.
- • Caused by:
  - –local stimulation of the larnyx by saliva, blood, vomitus, foreign body (including laryngoscope, airway or tracheal tube), etc.
  - –response to other stimulation, e.g. surgery, movement, stimulation of anus, cervix, etc. (**Brewer–Luckhardt reflex**).

The reflex is abolished in planes 2–4 of anaesthesia; thus its occurrence may indicate insufficient depth of anaesthesia. Laryngeal reflexes are more sensitive in upper respiratory tract infections and in smokers.
May cause complete or partial **airway obstruction**, the latter often presenting as inspiratory stridor. Causes **hypoxaemia** and **hypoventilation**; **pulmonary oedema** has been reported.
- • Management:
  - –cessation of stimulus.
  - –administration of 100% O_2. Positive airway pressure may be applied by tightening the expiratory valve of the breathing system, thus increasing the intake of O_2 with each breath.
  - –when laryngospasm has subsided, depth of anaesthesia may be deepened.
  - –laryngeal muscle relaxation may be achieved with **suxamethonium**, followed by ventilation with O_2 and tracheal intubation if necessary.
- • Prevented by:
  - –achieving adequate depth of anaesthesia before attempting laryngoscopy, insertion of airway, surgery, etc.

–local anaesthetic spray to the larynx and **laryngeal nerve blocks**.

–use of neuromuscular blocking drugs and tracheal intubation.

Larynx.

* Functions:
  –protects the **tracheobronchial tree** and lungs, e.g. during swallowing.
  –allows coughing.
  –allows speech.
  –allows straining, e.g. during defaecation.

Extends from the root of the **tongue** to the cricoid cartilage, i.e. level with C3–6 (at higher level in children).

* Dimensions:
  –length: 45 mm (men); 35 mm (women).
  –anteroposterior: 35 mm (men); 25 mm (women).
  –transverse: 45 mm (men); 40 mm (women).

* Composed of hyoid bone, and epiglottic, thyroid, cricoid, arytenoid, corniculate and cuneiform cartilages, joined by several muscles and ligaments (Fig. 86):
  –hyoid bone:
    –level with C3.
    –U-shaped, with horizontal body and bilateral greater and lesser horns, which pass backwards and upwards respectively.
    –attached superiorly to the mandible and tongue (by hyoglossus, mylohyoid, geniohyoid and digastric muscles), and styloid process (by stylohyoid ligament and muscle).
    –attached inferiorly to the thyroid cartilage (by thyrohyoid membrane and muscle), sternum (by sternohyoid muscle) and clavicle (by omohyoid muscle).
    –attached posteriorly to the **pharynx** by the middle constrictor muscle.
  –epiglottis:
    –leaf-shaped, attached anteriorly to the base of the tongue, body of the hyoid and back of the thyroid cartilage above the vocal cords. The depression on either side of the midline glossoepiglottic fold is the vallecula, with the pharyngoepiglottic folds laterally.
    –attached to the arytenoid laterally by the aryepiglottic membrane.
  –thyroid cartilage:
    –formed from two quadrilateral halves, meeting anteriorly to form the thyroid notch level with C4. The posterior edge forms superior and inferior horns on each side, the latter articulating with the cricoid cartilage.
    –attached superiorly to the hyoid bone by the thyrohyoid membrane and muscle.
    –attached posteriorly to the pharynx (by inferior constrictor muscle, palatopharyngeus and salpingopharyngeus muscles) and styloid process (by stylothyroid muscle).
    –attached inferiorly to the cricoid (by cricothyroid membrane and muscle) and sternum (by sternothyroid muscle).
    –attached inferomedially to the arytenoids by thyroarytenoid muscle; part of it attaches to the free border of cricothyroid forming vocalis muscle and part attaches to the lateral epiglottis forming thyroepiglottic muscle.

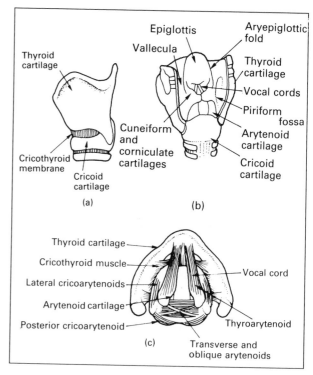

Figure 86 *Anatomy of the larynx: (a) lateral view; (b) posterior view; (c) superior view with intrinsic muscles*

–cricoid cartilage:
  –signet-ring shaped, broadest posteriorly. Level with C6. The lateral surface articulates with the inferior horn of the thyroid cartilage; its upper surface posteriorly articulates with the arytenoids.
  –attached via the superior surface to the thyroid cartilage by the cricothyroid membrane.
  –attached via the lateral surface to the thyroid cartilage (by cricothyroid muscle) and arytenoids (by lateral cricoarytenoid muscles).
  –attached via the posterior surface to the arytenoids by the posterior cricoarytenoid muscles.
  –attached inferiorly to the trachea by the cricotracheal membrane.
–arytenoid cartilages:
  –pyramid shaped, the bases articulating with the back of the cricoid.
  –also attached to the cricoid by posterior and lateral cricoarytenoid muscles.
  –the vocal cords pass from the vocal processes anteriorly to the back of the thyroid cartilage .
  –attached to the epiglottis superomedially via the aryepiglottic folds and muscles.
  –attached anterolaterally to the back of the thyroid cartilages by the thyroarytenoid muscles.
  –attached to each other by the transverse arytenoid muscle.
–corniculate cartilages: form tubercles in the posterior aryepiglottic folds, at the apex of the arytenoids.
–cuneiform cartilages: lie anterior to the corniculate cartilages, in the aryepiglottic folds.

* Membranes and areas of the larynx:
  –aryepiglottic membrane:

–passes from the anterior arytenoid to lateral epiglottis.

–forms the vestibular fold at the lower border. The area between vestibular folds is termed the rima vestibuli; that between the aryepiglottic fold and vestibular fold is the vestibule; the recess between the vocal and vestibular cords is the laryngeal sinus (saccule).

–cricothyroid membrane: free upper border forms the vocal cord (level with C5) between the back of the thyroid cartilage and vocal process of the arytenoid; it contains the vocal ligament beneath its mucosa. The area between vocal cords is the rima glottidis (glottis).

–thyrohyoid membrane: lateral borders are thickened to form the lateral thyrohyoid ligaments.

The entrance to the larynx slopes downwards and backwards, bounded anteriorly by the epiglottis, laterally by the aryepiglottic folds and posteriorly by the arytenoid cartilages. The piriform fossa is the recess on each side, between the aryepiglottic folds medially and thyroid cartilage and thyrohyoid membrane laterally.

The rima glottidis is the narrowest part of the airway in adults; the cricoid is the narrowest in children.

- Epithelium: squamous above the cords, columnar below. Mucosa of the cords is closely adherent.
- Muscle actions (Fig. 86c):
    –the cords are tensed by cricothyroid and relaxed by thyroarytenoid and vocalis muscles.
    –the cords are abducted by the posterior cricoarytenoids, causing outward rotation and movement of the arytenoids.
    –the cords are adducted by the lateral cricoarytenoids (causing inward rotation of the arytenoids) and transverse arytenoid muscle (causing the arytenoids to move together).
    –the inlet is opened by the thyroepiglottic muscle and closed by the aryepiglottic muscle.
    –the larynx is elevated by muscles from the pharynx and those above the hyoid, and depressed by sternothyroid.
- Nerve supply:
    –recurrent **laryngeal nerve**: all muscles except cricothyroid, and sensation below vocal cords.
    –superior laryngeal nerve: cricothyroid muscle, and sensation above vocal cords.
- Blood supply: branches of superior and inferior thyroid arteries and accompanying veins.
- Lymphatic drainage:
    –above cords: to upper deep cervical nodes.
    –below cords: to lower deep cervical nodes.

See also, Laryngoscopy

Laser surgery. Use of laser (Light Amplification by Stimulated Emission of Radiation) radiation to cause tissue destruction by producing intense local heat. Involves stimulation of atoms, ions or molecules within a tube using high voltage. Energy is absorbed and emitted by the particles; the emitted energy is amplified and allowed to escape as a parallel beam of coherent light, of precise wavelength and in phase.

- Effects of the laser beam on tissues depend on its wavelength:
    –CO_2 laser (wavelength 10 600 nm): used for precise surgical cutting and coagulation, e.g. in **ENT surgery**,

neurosurgery, general and gynaecological surgery and dermatology.

–neodymium yttrium–aluminium–garnet (NdYAG) laser (1060 nm): used for photocoagulation and debulking of tumours, e.g. bronchial carcinoma.

–argon or krypton (400–700 nm): used for photocoagulation in ophthalmology and dermatology.

- Risks to patient and operating staff:
    –ocular (corneal and retinal) damage: prevented by containment of the laser beam, and by wearing protective glasses. Most glasses will absorb energy from the CO_2 laser; specifically tinted goggles are required for the other types.
    –skin damage: prevented by appropriate towelling of the patient.
    –**explosions and fires**: particularly problematic during upper airway surgery, when the high energy beams may cause ignition of anaesthetic vapours, rubber, PVC or silicone tracheal tubes, drapes, etc. The following precautions have been suggested:
        –flexible metal tracheal tubes without cuffs.
        –metallic-coated tubes: expensive, and may still be susceptible to damage. Cuff inflation is with saline instead of air.
        –protection of the tube by wrapping in metallic tape: risks detachment of the tape within the airway, or damage to tissues by the tape's sharp edges.
        –avoidance of tracheal intubation:, e.g. use of **insufflation** or **injector techniques**, including **high frequency ventilation**.
        –use of non-explosive mixtures of gases, e.g. under 30% O_2 in nitrogen or helium. Intermittent flushing with 100% nitrogen or helium has been used.
        –limitation of laser power and duration of bursts.
    Vigilance should be high. If ignition occurs, the O_2 source should be disconnected and the operative site doused with water.
    –production of noxious/potentially infective fumes: adequate suction is required.

Rampil IJ (1992) Anesth Analg; 74: 424–35

Latent heat. Energy required solely to change the state of a substance, without changing its temperature, e.g.:
    –liquid to gas or vice versa (latent heat of vaporization).
    –solid to liquid or vice versa (latent heat of fusion).

Heat is required to change liquid to a gas, in order to overcome the attraction between molecules and expand the substance; heat is given out when the reverse occurs, e.g. when steam condenses.

Specific latent heat is the energy required to alter the state of unit mass of substance at specified temperature; e.g. specific latent heat of vaporization of water = 2.26 MJ/kg at 100°C. It is greater at lower temperatures, and falls at higher temperatures until it reaches zero at the **critical temperature**.

Lateral cutaneous nerve of the forearm, block, *see Elbow, nerve blocks*

Lateral cutaneous nerve of the thigh, block. Provides analgesia of the lateral thigh, e.g. following skin harvesting, and to reduce leg tourniquet pain.

The nerve (L2–3) arises from the **lumbar plexus** (may arise from the femoral nerve), passing under the inguinal ligament just medial to the anterior superior iliac spine to supply the skin of the lateral side of the thigh. A needle is inserted 2 cm medial and inferior to the iliac spine, at right angles to the skin. A click is felt as the fascia lata is pierced. 10–15 ml **local anaesthetic agent** is injected fanwise, mediolaterally.

May also be blocked via **femoral nerve block** (three-in-one block).

Laudanosine. Tertiary amine, a product of **atracurium** metabolism via **Hofmann degradation**. **Half-life** is about 2–3 hours, i.e. considerably longer than for atracurium; approximately doubled in renal failure. In anaesthetized dogs, causes epileptiform EEG changes at blood levels over 15 µg/ml. Blood levels in humans, even after several days' infusion in patients with renal and hepatic failure, rarely rise above 3–4 µg/ml, although fears have been expressed about central stimulation in patients at risk, e.g. those with an impaired blood–brain barrier.

Lavoisier, Antoine Laurent (1742–1794). French chemist. Disproved the **phlogiston** theory, showing that the gain in weight of sulphur or phosphorus on combustion was due to combination with air. Concluded that air consists of two elastic fluids: one necessary for combustion and respiration, and one that would support neither. Renamed the former (previously called dephlogisticated air) 'oxygene', estimating its concentration in air to be about 25%.

Lawen, Arthur (1876–1958). German surgeon, the first to perform **caudal analgesia** for abdominal surgery, using large volumes of **procaine**. Also described **paravertebral block**, and helped popularize regional anaesthesia. Described the use of **curare** to produce relaxation during surgery in 1912.

LBBB, Left bundle branch block, *see Bundle branch block*

LD$_{50}$, *see Therapeutic index/ratio*

Left atrial pressure (LAP). Mean pressure approximates to **left ventricular end-diastolic pressure**, unless the mitral valve is abnormal. Pressure wave and abnormalities are similar to the **venous waveform**, but with reference to mitral and aortic valves and systemic circulation, instead of tricuspid and pulmonary valves and pulmonary circulation.

May be measured via a catheter inserted directly into the left atrium, or indirectly via **pulmonary artery catheterization**, which measures **pulmonary capillary wedge pressure**. Usually measured from midaxilla or sternal angle. Normal value is 2–10 mmHg.

Left ventricular ejection time, *see Systolic time intervals*

Left ventricular end-diastolic pressure (LVEDP). Reflects the **preload** of the left ventricle. Provided ventricular compliance is constant, a constant relationship (exponential rather than linear) holds between LVEDP and **left ventricular end-diastolic volume**. Normal LVEDP does not ensure normal ventricular function, and abnormal LVEDP may not indicate degree of dysfunction. Elevations of LVEDP (normally under 12 mmHg) may reflect increased blood volume, reduced **myocardial contractility**, reduced ventricular compliance and increased **venous return**. May be measured directly via a ventricular cannula or arterial cannulation, or inferred via **pulmonary artery catheterization**.

Left ventricular end-diastolic volume. Nearest physiological variable to left ventricular **preload** as described by **Starling's law**. May be assessed using **echocardiography** or radiology, but indicators of **left ventricular end-diastolic pressure** are easier to measure. Normally 70–95 ml/m^2.

Left ventricular failure, *see Cardiac failure*

Left ventricular stroke work, *see Stroke work*

Legionnaire's disease, *see Chest infection*

LES, *see Lower oesophageal sphincter*

Letheon. Name given to **diethyl ether** by **Morton** when he patented his discovery. Despite this patent, ether was widely used without acknowledgement of Morton's claim. His attempts to enforce the patent and payments of royalties included approaching the governments of the USA and France, but were unsuccessful.

Leucocytes. White blood cells; total count in peripheral **blood** is 4–10 × 10^9/l.
- Exist as three morphologically different types:
  - granulocytes: derived from common bone marrow precursor stem cells:
    - neutrophils (60–70%; 2.5–7 × 10^9/l): phagocytic with high enzyme content.
    - eosinophils (1–4%; 0.01–0.4 × 10^9/l): contain **histamine** and are involved in cell-mediated allergic reactions.
    - basophils (0–1%; 0–0.2 × 10^9/l): contain histamine and **heparin**; non-phagocytic.
  - lymphocytes (23–35%: 1–3.5 × 10^9/l): derived from lymphoid stem cells throughout the body including bone marrow. Mainly concerned with immune mechanisms: B (bursa) cells with **immunoglobulin** production and T (thymus) cells with immune system regulation and killing of infected cells.
  - monocytes (4–8%; 0.2–0.8 × 10^9/l): formed in spleen, lymphoid tissue and marrow. Differentiate into phagocytic tissue macrophages.

See also, Erythrocytes; Platelets

Leukotrienes. Series of compounds derived from **arachidonic acid** by the action of lipoxygenases. Act as mediators of inflammation, and released from **mast cells**, **platelets** and some **leucocytes** following mechanical, thermal, chemical, infective and immunological stimuli. Most leukotrienes cause bronchoconstriction, vasoconstriction and increased vascular permeability; LTC$_4$ and LTD$_4$ probably account for the activity originally known as slow-reacting substance of anaphylaxis (SRS-A). LTB$_4$ is a potent chemotactic agent for other inflammatory cells. They have been implicated in the pathophysiology of **septicaemia** and **ARDS**.

Levallorphan tartrate. Opioid receptor **antagonist** with partial agonist properties, the *n*-allyl derivative of **levor-**

phanol. Synthesized in 1950. 1.25 mg levallorphan has been combined with 100 mg **pethidine** as Pethilorphan, but hopes of analgesia without respiratory depression were not realized. Its use has been superseded by **naloxone**.
- Dosage: 0.5–1.0 mg iv/im.

Levorphanol tartrate. Synthetic **opioid analgesic drug**, synthesized in 1949. Similar to **morphine** but less sedating. Onset of action is under 30 minutes, lasting for up to 8 hours.
- Dosage:
  - 1.5–4.5 mg orally, once–twice daily.
  - 0.05 mg/kg iv/im/sc.

Lidocaine, *see Lignocaine*

Life support, *see Cardiopulmonary resuscitation*

Lignocaine hydrochloride. Amide **local anaesthetic agent**, introduced in 1947 (revolutionizing regional anaesthesia because of its superior safety to previous agents). The standard drug against which other local anaesthetics are compared. pK_a is 7.9. 65% protein bound; 95% of an injected dose undergoes hepatic metabolism and is excreted renally. Onset is rapid by all routes; usual duration of action for 1% solution is about one hour, increased to 1.5–2 hours if **adrenaline** is added.
- Uses:
  - local anaesthesia. Often combined with adrenaline, since lignocaine tends to produce local vasodilatation; 1:200 000 and 1:80 000 solutions are commonly available, the latter is usually restricted to dental use.
  - iv administration:
    - depression of laryngeal and tracheal reflexes (e.g. during tracheal intubation/extubation). Commonly used to reduce the increase in **ICP** caused by laryngoscopy. Possibly reduces muscle pains and potassium increase after **suxamethonium**. It has been used to produce analgesia and general anaesthesia (although its **therapeutic ratio** is low).
    - class I **antiarrhythmic drug** in ventricular tachyarrhythmias.
- Many preparations are available, including:
  - 0.25–0.5% solutions for **infiltration anaesthesia** and **IVRA**.
  - 1–2% solutions for nerve blocks and **extradural anaesthesia**.
  - 4% solution (coloured pink) for **topical anaesthesia** of the mucous membranes of the mouth, pharynx and respiratory tract.
  - 10% spray for topical anaesthesia as above. Available in metered dose delivery systems (10 mg/spray).
  - also available in 1–2% gel for urethral instillation, and 5% ointment for skin, rectum and other mucous membranes. 5% hyperbaric solution has been used in **spinal anaesthesia**.
- Dosage:
  - depends on the block.
  - 1–2 mg/kg iv 2–5 minutes before intubation/extubation.
  - for ventricular arrhythmias: 1 mg/kg iv initially, then 4 mg/kg/min for 30 minutes, 2 mg/kg/min for 2 hours, and 1 mg/kg/min thereafter.

May be given via the tracheal tube in emergency at twice the iv dose.

Adverse effects are as for local anaesthetic agents. Maximal recommended dose: 3 mg/kg without adrenaline, 7 mg/kg with adrenaline. Toxic plasma levels: above about 10 µg/ml.

Limbic system. Part of the **brain**, formerly termed the rhinencephalon. Composed of left and right lobes, each consisting of:
  - rim of cortical tissue around the hilum of the cerebral hemisphere.
  - associated deep structures: hippocampus and gyrus, uncus, amygdala, cingulate gyrus, part of insula, septal area, isthmus, Broca's olfactory area and orbital surface of the frontal lobe.

Responsible for olfaction, feeding behaviour, motivation, sexual behaviour and generation of emotions. Damage to the amygdala is associated with rage reactions, hyperphagia and increased sexual activity; lesions in the uncus with olfactory and gustatory hallucinations.

Thought to be one site of action of **benzodiazepines** and possibly other anaesthetic drugs.
[Pierre P Broca (1824–1880), French surgeon]

Linear analogue scale (Visual analogue scale). Method of **pain evaluation**, e.g. for statistical analysis. A horizontal 10 cm line is drawn on plain paper, with 'no pain' written at the left-hand end, and 'worst possible pain' at the right-hand end. The patient marks his or her position on the line. Thought to be more reliable than assessments where patients choose the most appropriate number or word from a list, which may be influenced by personal preference for certain words or numbers and limited by the number of choices offered. Thought to be consistent for any individual; however, because patients may interpret the analogue scale differently, comparison between patients may be unreliable. May also be used for other symptoms or feelings, e.g. anxiety.

Lingual nerve block, *see Mandibular nerve blocks*

Lissive anaesthesia. Technique of anaesthesia, now considered unsafe, in which non-depolarizing neuromuscular blocking drugs (originally **tubocurarine**) were used to produce muscle relaxation without causing complete paralysis. Thus spontaneous respiration was allowed following small doses of tubocurarine, due to presumed 'diaphragmatic sparing'.

Liston, Robert (1794–1847). Scottish-born surgeon; moved to London after quarrelling with his colleagues. Performed the first operation under **diethyl ether** anaesthesia in England on 21st December 1846, at University College Hospital, London, having been told about ether by **Boott**. William Squire administered the anaesthetic from a glass inhaler made by his uncle Peter, whilst Frederick Churchill had an above-knee amputation. The operation allegedly lasted 25 seconds.
[William Squire (1825–1899), London medical student, later physician; Peter Squire (1798–1884), London chemist; Frederick Churchill (1810–?), English butler]

Lithium. Metal used to treat manic–depressive disease. Mimics **sodium** in the body, entering excitable cells during depolarization. Decreases release of central and peripheral neurotransmitters; may prolong **depolarizing neuro-**

muscular **blockade** and decrease requirements for anaesthetic agents. Termination 24 hours before anaesthesia has been suggested but this is disputed. Has low **therapeutic ratio**, with optimal plasma concentration of 0.4–1.0 mmol/l. Toxic effects include lethargy, **hypokalaemia**, **arrhythmias**, tremor, rigidity and **convulsions**. Toxicity is increased by **diuretics** and **dehydration**.

Litre. SI **unit** of volume. Originally defined as the volume of 1 kg pure water at 4°C, but redefined as equal to 1000 cm^3 in 1964, because of an error in the standard **kilogramme** constructed in 1889.

Liver. Largest body organ, weighing about 1200–1500 g, lying in the right upper abdominal quadrant. Two major lobes, right and left, are divided into lobules based on a central vein connected by a network of sinusoids to peripheral portal tracts. Central veins are tributaries of hepatic veins; portal tracts contain branches of the hepatic artery, portal vein, lymphatics and bile ducts. Blood from the hepatic arterial and portal venous systems is conveyed to the central veins via the sinusoids, lined with endothelial and phagocytic (Kupffer) cells and separated by hepatocytes. Bile canaliculi form networks between the hepatocytes, conveying bile towards terminal bile ducts.

Blood flow is about 20–30% of cardiac output (70% via the portal vein).

- Functions:
  - **carbohydrate** metabolism: **glycogen** storage and breakdown.
  - **protein** metabolism: synthesizes many, including **albumin**, globulins, **coagulation** factors, **complement** system components, transferrin, haptoglobulins, caeruloplasmin, plasma **cholinesterase** and α_1-antitrypsin. Important site of **amino acid** deamination prior to interconversion and oxidation. Ammonia produced by deamination is converted to **urea**.
  - **fat** metabolism: breakdown of dietary triglycerides and fatty acids, and synthesis of triglycerides, phospholipid and cholesterol, released into the bloodstream as lipoproteins. Cholesterol is also used to make bile acids.
  - bilirubin metabolism: unconjugated fat-soluble bilirubin is transported to the liver bound to albumin; it is conjugated with glucuronide to the water-soluble form.
  - formation of bile acids: cholic and chenodeoxycholic acids are produced from cholesterol and secreted in the bile. Reabsorbed via enterohepatic circulation.
  - vitamin storage: A, D, K, B$_{12}$ and folate.
  - hormone metabolism and inactivation: includes cortisol, oestrogens, **aldosterone**, **vasopressin** and thyroxine.
  - haematological role: site of haemopoiesis during fetal and early neonatal life. Also acts as a reservoir for blood which can be redistributed to the body by stimulation of the liver's autonomic innervation. Kupffer cells phagocytose antigens and bacteria absorbed from the GIT, and destroy old red cells.
  - drug metabolism: achieved by transforming lipid-soluble compounds into water-soluble ones via **enzymes** located in the hepatocyte microsomes. Several processes are involved, including oxidation, conjugation, reduction, hydrolysis, methylation and acetylation. Most drugs are metabolized by a combination of oxidation by the **cytochrome oxidase system**, and conjugation.
- Effects of anaesthetic agents:
  - both hepatic artery and portal vein blood flow is reduced by most agents, probably as a consequence of reduced cardiac output. The effect is opposed by hypercapnia and exacerbated by hypocapnia and IPPV, although this is thought to be rarely significant.
  - drug metabolism may be reduced in the presence of volatile agents, although whether due to alterations in hepatic blood flow or a direct inhibitory effect is unclear.
  - **enzyme induction** by volatile agents has been reported but is controversial.
  - toxic effects: e.g. **halothane hepatitis**.

[Karl W von Kupffer (1829–1902), German anatomist]

Liver failure, *see Hepatic failure*

Liver function tests. Most commonly measured:
- bilirubin (*see Jaundice*).
- liver enzymes:
  - aspartate aminotransferase (AST) and alanine aminotransferase (ALT): released by damaged hepatocytes. Highly raised values suggest **hepatitis**. Normally 5–40 iu/l.
  - alkaline phosphatase: highly raised in cholestasis, both intra- and extrahepatic. Isoenzyme analysis differentiates between hepatic and other sources, e.g. bone. Normally 40–110 iu/l.
  - γ-glutamyl transferase (γGT): non-specific, but often raised following drug ingestion, e.g. alcohol. Normally 10–50 iu/l.
- plasma proteins:
  - albumin: reduced in chronic liver disease after a few weeks. Normally 35–55 g/l.
  - globulins: increased to varying extents, depending on the underlying cause. Normally 25–35 g/l.
- **coagulation studies**.
- others, including:
  - bromsulphthalein excretion: rate of excretion depends on hepatic function.
  - α_1-fetoprotein, increased in hepatoma.
  - **cholinesterase**.
  - 5' nucleotidase, increased in biliary obstruction.

Liver transplantation. First performed in 1963. Indicated for end-stage **hepatic failure**, e.g. due to inherited disease, chronic **hepatitis**, acute toxic hepatitis, primary biliary cirrhosis and some cases of **liver** tumour. Surgery involves vascular and biliary isolation of the diseased organ with re-anastomosis of a donor cadaveric organ; partial donation by live donors has also been used. The recipient's liver is dissected to its vascular pedicle and venovenous bypass employed from the portal and femoral veins to the axillary vein (anhepatic phase) if the patient's weight exceeds 40 kg. The portal vein, hepatic artery and inferior vena cava above and below the liver are clamped, and the diseased organ removed. Donor liver viability is up to 8 hours from harvesting. It is flushed with crystalloid solution via the portal vein to remove the transport infusate and air bubbles. Anastomosis of the portal vein and hepatic artery is followed by release of vascular clamps, incorporating the donor liver into the recipient's circulation.

- Anaesthesia:
  - –as for hepatic failure. Opioid, volatile agent, neuromuscular blockade and IPPV are usual; N_2O is often avoided to reduce bowel distension and risk of **air embolism** during re-anastomosis. Aseptic techniques are used to reduce infection. Cyclosporin and steroids are given.
  - –monitoring and vascular lines include direct BP and CVP measurement, pulmonary artery catheterization, several large iv cannula (e.g. 8 G), temperature probes and urinary catheter.
  - –frequent estimation of plasma electrolytes, glucose, haemoglobin, platelets, arterial blood gases and **coagulation studies** is required. Thromboelastography is useful for coagulation studies.
  - –blood loss is usually 8–10 units but may be up to 200 units. Autologous **blood transfusion** is often used. Rapid transfusion devices are required to keep up with losses; they include a reservoir of several units of blood, driven by a pump. Venous return may also be reduced by surgical manipulation.
  - –SVR and cardiac rhythm may change frequently. Myocardial depression may be caused by **hypocalcaemia**, **hypothermia** and **acidosis**. Acidosis is common but treated cautiously, as postoperative metabolic **alkalosis** is also common, due to metabolism of lactate and citrate. **Inotropic drugs** are often required.
  - –**hypoglycaemia** and **hyperglycaemia** may occur, especially during the anhepatic phase.
  - –potassium levels fluctuate due to acid–base changes, flushing out of liver perfusate and uptake by the transplanted liver.
  - –surgery usually lasts 8–10 hours but may be up to 24 hours, with major biochemical, haematological and temperature disturbances which may persist postoperatively. IPPV is usually maintained for 24–48 hours. Postoperative problems include infection, atelectasis and **pleural effusion**, graft failure, hepatic artery thrombosis, biliary leaks or obstruction, neurological impairment, renal failure.

Borland LM, Roule M, Cook DR (1985) Anesth Analg; 64: 117–24

See also, Organ donation; Transplantation

Local anaesthesia, *see Infiltration anaesthesia; Local anaesthetic agents; Regional anaesthesia; Topical anaesthesia; specific blocks*

Local anaesthetic agents. Cocaine was introduced in 1884 by **Freud** and **Koller**; less toxic agents subsequently introduced include **procaine** and **stovaine** (1904), **cinchocaine** (1925), **amethocaine** (1931) and **lignocaine** (1947). Lignocaine was particularly non-toxic. Later drugs include **chloroprocaine** (1952), **mepivacaine** (1956), **prilocaine** (1959), **bupivacaine** (1963) and **etidocaine** (1972). **Ropivacaine** is currently being evaluated. Others are used only for **topical anaesthesia**, e.g. benzocaine.

- General properties (Table 22):
  - –poorly water soluble weak acids with $pK_a > 7.4$.
  - –comprised of hydrophilic and hydrophobic portions separated by an alkyl chain. The hydrophilic part is usually a tertiary amine; the lipophilic part (essential for local anaesthetic action) is usually an unsaturated aromatic ring, e.g. *para*-aminobenzoic acid.

Table 22. Properties of local anaesthetic agents.

Agent	pK_a	% Protein binding	Equivalent concentration (%)	Recommended maximal safe dose (mg/kg)
Esters				
Cocaine	8.7	—	1	3
Procaine	8.9	6	2	12
Amethocaine	8.5	76	0.25	1.5
Chloroprocaine	8.7	—	1	15
Amides				
Cinchocaine	7.9	—	0.25	2
Lignocaine	7.9	64	1	3–7
Mepivacaine	7.6	78	1	5
Prilocaine	7.9	55	1	5–8
Bupivacaine	8.1	96	0.25	2
Etidocaine	7.7	94	0.5	2

  - –modification of chemical structure (lengthening the alkyl chain or increasing the number of carbon atoms in the aromatic ring or tertiary amine) may alter lipid solubility, potency, rate of metabolism and duration of action.
  - –divided according to the nature of linkage between the amine and aromatic parts into ester or amide drugs:
    - –esters:
      - –allergic reactions are common.
      - –rapidly metabolized by plasma and liver **cholinesterase**. One metabolite, *para*-aminobenzoic acid, is thought to be responsible for allergic reactions. Metabolism may be prolonged when plasma cholinesterase level is low, e.g. liver disease, **pregnancy** or atypical enzymes.
    - –amides:
      - –allergic reactions are rare; they may be associated with the preservative vehicle.
      - –metabolized by liver microsomal enzymes, initially to aminocarboxylic acid and a cyclic aniline derivative, subsequently via N-dealkylation and hydroxylation respectively. Dependent on liver blood flow and function.
  - –presented in solution as acidic hydrochloride salts.
- Mechanism of action:
  - –produce reversible blockade of neural transmission in autonomic, sensory and motor nerve fibres, depending on the concentration of drug applied. Active peripherally and at the CNS.
  - –bind to **sodium** channels in the axon membrane from within, preventing sodium entry during depolarization. The threshold potential is thus not reached and the **action potential** of the nerve not propagated (membrane stabilizing effect).
  - –fate of injected drug:
    - –diffuses to axons; thus more effective the nearer the nerve it is deposited (*see Minimal blocking concentration*).
    - –crosses the membrane in the unionized form; thus activity depends on extracellular pH, since the degree of ionization and thus lipid solubility is increased by acidosis. The pH of infected tissue is lower than normal, hence the effects of local anaesthetics are reduced.

–dissociates within the axon to the unionized form; thus dependent on intracellular pH.

–binds to sodium channels.

–smallest **nerve fibres** are blocked first.

- Features of block are affected by:

–patient variables, e.g. age, fitness, pregnancy, etc.

–individual drug characteristics as below.

–concentration and dose used: e.g. higher concentrations and doses reduce onset time, and increase density and duration of block.

–site of injection, e.g. rapid onset of **spinal anaesthesia** but slow onset of **brachial plexus block**.

–additives:

–vasoconstrictors, e.g. **adrenaline, felypressin, phenylephrine**: reduce absorption and prolong the block. Intensity and onset may be improved. Effects are greatest with local anaesthetics that cause vasodilatation, e.g. lignocaine, and less with prilocaine and bupivacaine. Cocaine iteself causes vasoconstriction. **Noradrenaline** is less effective than adrenaline.

–CO_2 dissolved under pressure (carbonated solutions): passes into axons, lowering pH; intracellular dissociation is thus favoured, with faster block.

–sodium hydroxide: remains extracellular, raising pH and increasing the unionized fraction of drug; uptake into the axon is thus favoured.

–potassium: has been shown to increase duration of block.

–**dextrans**: used to prolong blocks, perhaps by combining with local anaesthetic and trapping it within the tissues. Results are inconsistent.

–**hyaluronidase**: formerly used to increase spread by breaking down tissue stroma. Benefits are doubtful; thus rarely used now.

–dextrose to increase baricity for spinal anaesthesia: affects spread.

- Toxicity:

–due to membrane stabilizing effects on other cells, especially heart and CNS. Features:

–tingling, typically around the mouth and tongue.

–lightheadedness, agitation and tremor.

–unconsciousness and/or convulsions.

–hypotension may be caused by hypoxaemia following central apnoea, direct myocardial depression or vasodilatation. Arrhythmias may occur; resistant ventricular arrhythmias are particularly likely with bupivacaine.

–may follow accidental iv injection, or systemic absorption, the latter affected by:

–total dose administered. Recommended maximal 'safe' doses are rough estimations only, since other factors are involved, but are useful as a guide (see above).

–site of injection:, e.g. absorption is large after topical anaesthesia and **intercostal block** and slow after **brachial plexus block** and **infiltration anaesthesia**. Affected by blood flow and tissue vascularity.

–vasoconstrictor additives.

–individual drug: e.g. lignocaine causes vasodilatation; bupivacaine binds extensively to tissues.

–effects are related to age and fitness of the patient, other drugs (e.g. anticonvulsants), etc. Uptake by the lungs reduces blood levels following iv injection,

shielding the heart and brain from higher levels.

–treatment: supportive, with oxygenation/cardiovascular support as for **CPR**. **Thiopentone** or **diazepam/midazolam** may be used for convulsions, although hypotension may be exacerbated. Recovery of consciousness is usually within a few minutes.

–other complications may be related to:

–vasoconstrictors, e.g. tachycardia, arrhythmias, pallor, agitation, etc. caused by adrenaline.

–regional technique, e.g. intraneural injection, hypotension following spinal anaesthesia, etc.

–preservatives, e.g. allergic reactions (e.g. to methylparaben), neurological damage and **arachnoiditis** (possibly due to sodium bisulphite).

See also, Regional anaesthesia; specific blocks

Lofentanil *cis*-oxalate. Opioid analgesic drug derived from **fentanyl**; developed in 1975. 20 times as potent as fentanyl and 6000 times as potent as **morphine** in animal studies. Of similar pK_a to fentanyl, highly lipophilic and with a particularly long duration of action due to persistent binding to **opioid receptors** (about 10 hours). Has been used via the extradural route to provide long-lasting analgesia, but not generally available.

Long, Crawford Williamson (1815–1878). US general practitioner; administered **diethyl ether** several times for minor surgery from 1842 in Georgia, but did not report it until after **Morton's** demonstration.

Lorazepam. Benzodiazepine, used for insomnia, **epilepsy, sedation** and **premedication. Half-life** is approximately 12 hours with prolonged duration of action. Said to produce more **amnesia** than other benzodiazepines. Similar rates of absorption follow im and oral administration. Metabolized to a non-active metabolite.

- Dosage:

–1–4 mg orally. If given the night before surgery, a further 1–2 mg may be given 1–2 hours preoperatively.

–1–4 mg iv (50 µg/kg).

LOS, *see Lower oesophageal sphincter*

Lower oesophageal sphincter. 2–5 cm portion of oesophagus of increased intraluminal pressure, extending above and below the diaphragm. Opens reflexly during swallowing, and helps to prevent retrograde passage of gastric contents into the oesophagus via:

–increased muscle tone: muscle of the sphincter zone, especially the inner circular layer, has higher resting tone than other oesophageal muscle, possibly via increased **calcium** ion uptake and utilization.

–neural input:

–vagal: muscle tone reflexly increases as intragastric pressure increases, thus maintaining barrier pressure (normally about 20 cmH_2O). The reflex is abolished by **atropine**.

–sympathetic: tone is increased by α-stimulation and β-blockade, and decreased by β-stimulation and α-blockade.

–mechanical factors:

–oesophageal compression by the diaphragm.

–acute angle of entry of the oesophagus into the stomach.

–mucosal flap or rosette at the oesophageal opening.

- Muscle tone is decreased by :
  - **anticholinergic** drugs given iv; possibly less with **glycopyrronium**. Atropine im does not affect sphincter pressure, but prevents the action of **metoclopramide**.
  - gut hormones, e.g. **vasoactive intestinal hormone, glucagon** and gastric inhibitory peptide. Gastrin may increase tone at very high levels.
  - progesterone.
  - **opioid analgesic drugs**, volatile anaesthetic agents and most iv anaesthetic agents.
  - **ganglion** blocking drugs.
- Tone is increased by:
  - metoclopramide, **domperidone, cisapride** and **prochlorperazine**.
  - **neostigmine**.
  - **antacids**, via increased pH.
  - **pancuronium**.

No change is found with **cimetidine/ranitidine**. Although **suxamethonium** may increase intragastric pressure, the corresponding increase in lower oesophageal sphincter tone maintains barrier pressure.

Sphincter incompetence may result in **gastrooesophageal reflux**. It becomes less competent in **hiatus hernia**, particularly if intra-abdominal pressure increases, e.g. by raising the legs.

Cotton BR, Smith G (1984) Br J Anaesth; 56: 37–46

Lown–Ganong–Levine syndrome. Tendency to **SVT** caused by an accessory conducting pathway bypassing the atrioventricular node. Impulses may pass directly from the atria to the distal **heart conducting system**, without the usual delay at the node.

Characterized by a normal **P wave**, short **P–R interval** and normal **QRS complex** on the **ECG**. Anaesthetic management is as for **Wolff–Parkinson–White syndrome**.

[Samuel A Levine (1891–1966) and Bernard Lown, US cardiologists; William F Ganong, US physiologist]

Ludwig's angina. Cellulitis of the floor of the mouth and submandibular region, with massive swelling. Often due to anaerobic infection. May progress to laryngeal obstruction and death unless treated with antibiotics initially, or by deep incision of the tissues under the mandible.

Anaesthetic management is as for **airway obstruction**; antibiotic therapy may reduce the swelling and improve obstruction preoperatively. Local anaesthesia may be preferable in extreme cases.

[Wilhelm von Ludwig (1790–1865), German surgeon]

Lumbar extradural anaesthesia, *see Extradural anaesthesia*

Lumbar plexus. Formed in front of the transverse processes of the lumbar vertebrae from the anterior primary rami of the first four lumbar nerves, occasionally with a contribution from T12 (Fig. 87).

May be blocked via **paravertebral, psoas compartment** and 'three-in-one' **femoral nerve blocks**. Individual nerves may also be blocked. Block is useful for surgery on the inner and outer aspects of the thigh and anterior gluteal region together with adjacent perineal and suprapubic areas.

See also, Inguinal hernia field block

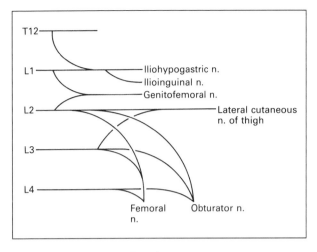

Figure 87 *Plan of the lumbar plexus*

Lumbar sympathetic block. Performed for peripheral vascular disease including incipient gangrene, and in chronic **pain management** (e.g. post-traumatic dystrophies).

The lumbar sympathetic chain lies on the anterolateral aspect of the lumbar vertebral bodies within a fascial compartment formed by the vertebral column, psoas sheath and posterior peritoneum.

With the patient in the lateral position and with a soft pillow between the iliac crest and costal margin to curve the spine laterally, skin wheals are raised 5–8 cm lateral to the upper borders of the spinous processes of L2–4. A 12–18 cm long needle is directed medially, to strike the transverse process at about 3–5 cm. The lateral aspect of the vertebral body is contacted usually 4–6 cm deeper, and the needle advanced a further 1–2 cm. Correct positioning is confirmed by negative aspiration for CSF or blood, and radiographic imaging: the needles should barely reach the anterior borders of the vertebral bodies in the lateral view, and should overlie their lateral edge in the anteroposterior view. Further confirmation of positioning is made by injecting contrast medium. 25–30 ml local anaesthetic solution, e.g. 0.5% **lignocaine** or **prilocaine**, is injected at L2, or 15 ml at L2 and L4. Catheters have been inserted for repeated injection. **Phenol** or absolute alcohol is used for chemical sympatholysis, 3 ml at each of L1, L2 and L3. The block may also be performed with patient prone.

Complications include hypotension, genitofemoral neuritis, bleeding into psoas, and extradural, subarachnoid or iv injection.

Similar blocks have been performed in the thoracic region but with risk of pneumothorax.

Lundy, John Silus (1894–1973). US anaesthetist; he became head of department at the Mayo Clinic in 1924. Co-founder of the **American Board of Anesthesiology**. An advocate and developer of regional techniques, **balanced anaesthesia, thiopentone** and post-anaesthetic **recovery rooms**.

Lung. Organ of respiration. Continues to develop after birth, with alveolar proliferation complete at about eight years.

- Anatomy:
  - cone-shaped, with bases applied to the **diaphragm**.
  - enveloped in **pleura**, attached to the **mediastinum** at the hila.
  - the right lung is larger than the left and divided into three lobes separated by the oblique and transverse fissures.
  - the left lung is divided into two lobes by the oblique fissure. The lingula is the anteroinferior portion of the upper lobe.
  - lobes are divided into segments (*see Tracheobronchial tree*).
  - surface anatomy:
    - as for pleura, except for the lower border, which lies two ribs cranial to the caudal pleural limit.
    - on the left side, the medial anterior border lies 2–3 cm lateral to the sternum at the 5th and 6th costal cartilages (cardiac notch).
    - the oblique fissure follows a line from the spine of T4 downwards and outwards to the 6th costal cartilage.
    - the transverse fissure follows a horizontal line from the 4th costal cartilage until it hits the previous line.
- Blood supply: via bronchial and pulmonary arteries (*see Pulmonary circulation*).
- Nerve supply: sympathetic and vagal plexuses; sensory pathways are mainly via the latter.
- Lymph drainage: via bronchopulmonary, tracheobronchial and paratracheal nodes to mediastinal lymph trunks and thence brachiocephalic veins.

- Functions:
  - gas exchange.
  - synthesis of associated phospholipids, e.g. **surfactant**, carbohydrates (e.g. **mucopolysaccharides**) and proteins (e.g. collagen).
  - metabolism and deactivation of certain compounds, e.g. angiotensin, bradykinin and **5–HT**. Takes up amide **local anaesthetic agents**.
  - synthesis and release of compounds, e.g. **prostaglandins** and **histamine**.
  - involvement in the immune system and possibly coagulation.
  - acts as a reservoir for blood; the pulmonary circulation contains 500–900 ml blood.

See also, Alveolus; Lung volumes; Pulmonary ....

Lung function tests. Used to determine the nature and extent of pulmonary disorders. Clinical assessment, e.g. ability to walk up stairs, breath-hold for > 30 seconds, or blow out a lighted match held six inches (15 cm) away, are imprecise and non-specific indicators.

- Include tests of:
  - ventilation mechanics:
    - measurement of static **lung volumes**: cumbersome apparatus is required. **Dead space** and **closing capacity** may be measured.
    - assessment of **forced expiration** and derived variables (e.g. **FEV₁**, **FVC**, **forced expiratory flow rate**, etc.), e.g. using a **spirometer**. The FEV_1/FVC ratio typically is reduced in obstructive lung

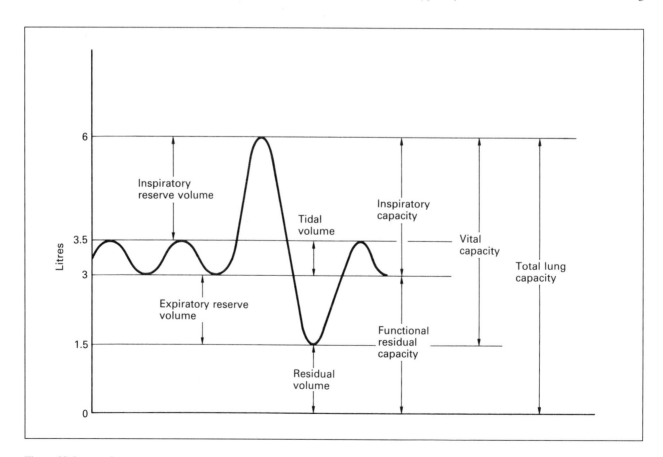

Figure 88 *Lung volumes*

disease, and is normal or high in restrictive disease. **Peak expiratory flow rate** is another simple bedside test for obstructive disease. Airway reactivity is assessed by challenging with histamine or methacholine whilst measuring FEV_1.
- **flow–volume loops** require more sophisticated apparatus, with instantaneous flow rate measurement.
- **airway resistance** itself may be measured, and lung **compliance**.
- **maximal voluntary ventilation** is non-specific and related to effort as well as pulmonary function.
- **respiratory muscle** function may be assessed, e.g. maximal mouth pressures when breathing against a closed valve. Work of breathing and O_2 consumption may also be measured.
- gas exchange:
  - analysis of **blood gas tensions** and pulse **oximetry**.
  - **diffusing capacity** for carbon monoxide (transfer factor); now thought to be related more to $\dot{V}/\dot{Q}$ **mismatch** than to diffusion impairment.
  - distribution of ventilation and perfusion as for $\dot{V}/\dot{Q}$ mismatch.
- pulmonary circulation: assessment is difficult. **Radioisotope** scanning may be used as for $\dot{V}/\dot{Q}$ mismatch.
- control of breathing: CO_2 **response curve** or response to hypoxia may be used.
- response to exercise, using the above tests.

Laszlo G (1991) Br J Hosp Med; 46: 311–22
See also, Body plethysmograph; Nitrogen washout

Lung volumes. Functional, not anatomical, volumes of the lungs, usually expressed as if both lungs comprise one unit. May be derived from a **spirometer** tracing of inhaled/exhaled volumes, with maximal inspiration and expiration following normal quiet tidal breathing (Fig. 88).
- Approximate normal values for a 70 kg man:
  - **tidal volume**: 0.5 litres
  - **inspiratory reserve volume**: 2.5 litres
  - **inspiratory capacity**: 3.0 litres
  - **vital capacity**: 4.5 litres
  - **expiratory reserve volume**: 1.5 litres
  - **residual volume**: 1.5 litres
  - **FRC**: 3.0 litres
  - **total lung capacity**: 6.0 litres

  Capacities are sums of volumes.

Tidal volume, inspiratory reserve volume, expiratory reserve volume, and capacities derived from them may be measured using a wet spirometer. Residual volume may be measured using helium dilution or the **body plethysmograph**.

Other lung volumes measured include **dead space** and **closing capacity**. Differential spirometry is used to examine function of single lungs.
See also, Lung function tests

LVEDP, *see Left ventricular end-diastolic pressure*

LVEDV, *see Left ventricular end-diastolic volume*

LVET, Left ventricular ejection time, *see Systolic time intervals*

LVF, Left ventricular failure, *see Cardiac failure*

LVH, Left ventricular hypertrophy, *see Cardiac failure*

Lytic cocktail. Mixture of **chlorpromazine**, **promethazine** and **pethidine** (e.g. 50–100 mg of each added to an iv infusion), described in the 1940s as a means of **sedation**, e.g. for unpleasant procedures, premedication and labour. Produced a state of drowsiness and apathy ('artificial hibernation') but effects were long-lasting and accompanied by hypotension. The technique is now refined as **neuroleptanaesthesia and analgesia**.

Sometimes used for premedication in children, e.g. a mixture containing chlorpromazine 7 mg, promethazine 7 mg and pethidine 28 mg per ml; 0.05 ml/kg im or 0.1 ml/kg rectally.

M

MAC, *see Minimal alveolar concentration*

Macewen, William (1847–1924). Eminent Scottish surgeon; Professor at Glasgow University, knighted in 1902. Advocated and practised tracheal intubation, usually oral, for laryngeal obstruction, e.g. due to **diphtheria**; he performed this by touch without anaesthetic. Was the first to advocate tracheal intubation instead of tracheotomy for head and neck surgery, in 1880. The tube was inserted prior to introduction of **chloroform**, and the patient allowed to breathe spontaneously. Packing around the tube achieved a seal.

Macintosh, Robert Reynolds (1897–1989). New Zealand-born anaesthetist, he became the first British Professor of Anaesthetics in Oxford in 1937. Lord Nuffield, a friend of Macintosh, had insisted that such a chair be set up as a precondition for endowing further chairs in Medicine, Surgery and Obstetrics and Gynaecology. Established Oxford as a centre for anaesthesia, and helped to establish anaesthesia as a medical specialty. Wrote books and articles about many aspects of local and general anaesthesia, and designed many pieces of equipment, including his **laryngoscope, spray, endobronchial tube, vaporizers** and devices for locating the extradural space. Also helped research the hazards of aviation and seafaring. Knighted in 1955, and recieved many other medals and awards.
[William Morris (1877–1963), English automobile industrialist and philanthropist; created Lord Nuffield in 1934]
Mushin WW (1989) Anaesthesia; 44: 951–2

McKesson, Elmer Isaac (1881–1935). US anaesthetist, practising in Toledo, Ohio. Founder and member of many US and international anaesthetic bodies. Also inventor and manufacturer of expiratory valves, **pressure regulators, flowmeters, suction apparatus, vaporizers** and **intermittent flow anaesthetic machines**. A major proponent of the use of **N₂O** in modern anaesthesia.

McMechan, Francis Hoeffer (1879–1939). US anaesthetist, practising in Cincinnati. A pioneer of the development of anaesthesia in the USA. Founded the American Association of Anesthetists in 1912, and instrumental in founding the National Anesthetic Research Society (subsequently the International Anaesthesia Research Society) whose publication (which became *Anesthesia and Analgesia*) he edited.

Magill breathing system, *see Anaesthetic breathing systems*

Magill, Ivan Whiteside (1888–1986). Irish-born anaesthetist, responsible for much of the innovation in, and development of, modern anaesthesia. With **Rowbotham** in Sidcup after World War I, he developed endotracheal anaesthesia as an alternative to **insufflation techniques**, originally for facial plastic surgery. Introduced his own **anaesthetic breathing system, forceps, laryngoscope,** and **connectors,** and developed blind nasal intubation. A pioneer of anaesthesia for thoracic surgery, he developed **one-lung anaesthesia, endobronchial tubes** and **bronchial blockers**. Also introduced bobbin **flowmeters,** portable anaesthetic apparatus and other equipment.

Helped found the **Association of Anaesthetists of Great Britain and Ireland**, and was involved in the setting up of the **DA Examination**, the **Faculty of Anaesthetists** and the **FFARCS Examination**. Worked at the Westminster and Brompton Hospitals, London. Knighted in 1960, and recieved many other medals and awards.
Edridge AW (1987) Anaesthesia; 42: 231–3

Magnesium. Largely intracellular ion, present mainly in bone (over 50%) and skeletal muscle (20%); the remainder is found in the heart, liver and other organs. 1% is in the **ECF**. Normal plasma levels: 0.75–1.05 mmol/l (although the value of measurement has been questioned, since most magnesium is intracellular). Required for protein and nucleic acid synthesis, regulation of intracellular **calcium** and **potassium**, and many enzymatic reactions including all those involving **ATP** synthesis/hydrolysis. Its actions are opposed by calcium.
See also, Hypermagnesaemia; Hypomagnesaemia.

Magnesium sulphate. Drug used mainly as an **anticonvulsant drug** in **pre-eclampsia**. Also causes vasodilatation, helping to lower BP. Rarely used in the UK but widely used elsewhere. Has also been used as a **tocolytic drug**. Recently shown to decrease mortality in **myocardial infarction**. Acts peripherally at the **neuromuscular junction**, decreasing **acetylcholine** release and reducing end-plate sensitivity to acetylcholine; it may also cause cortical depression.

Magnesium chloride is also used.
- Dosage: 2–4 g initially, followed by 1–2 g/h iv.
- Side effects:
  –cardiac conduction defects, drowsiness, absent reflexes, hypoventilation and cardiac arrest may occur with increasing **hypermagnesaemia**.
  –may augment non-depolarizing and depolarizing neuromuscular blockade. Neonatal hypotonia may also occur.
Overdosage may be treated with iv **calcium**.
- Therapeutic plasma levels: 2.0–3.5 mmol/l; side effects may occur above 4–5 mmol/l, with cardiac arrest above 12 mmol/l.
James MFM (1992) Anesth Analg; 74: 129–36

Magnesium trisilicate. Particulate **antacid**, used in dyspepsia. Has been used to increase gastric pH preoperatively in patients at risk from **aspiration of gastric contents**, but may itself cause pneumonitis if inhaled. Has also been used to reduce risk of peptic ulceration on **ICU**, e.g. by hourly nasogastric administration to keep pH above 3–4.

Magnetic resonance imaging (MRI; Nuclear magnetic resonance, NMR). Imaging technique, particularly useful for investigating CNS and pelvic disease, where tissue movement is minimal. Has also been used in other parts of the body, including the chest; accurate measurements of the heart's dimensions and movement have been obtained.

Involves placement of the patient within a powerful magnetic field, causing alignment of atoms with an odd number of protons or neutrons, e.g. hydrogen. Radiofrequency pulses are then applied, causing deflection of the atoms with absorption of energy. When each pulse stops, the atoms return to their aligned position, emitting energy as radiofrequency waves. Computer analysis of the emitted waves provides information about the chemical make-up of the tissue studied. MRI can provide graphic tissue slices in any plane, or may be used to analyse metabolic processes, e.g. distribution and alterations of intracellular phosphate (spectroscopy).

• Problems and anaesthetic considerations:
  –magnets used are very powerful but thought not to be directly harmful. Metal objects may become dangerous projectiles if they are placed near the magnet. All ferromagnetic metal equipment, including cylinders, needles, laryngoscope batteries, etc., must be kept away from the machine. Intracranial clips, pacemakers, heart valves, etc., may also be affected. Non-ferromagnetic anaesthetic equipment is increasingly available. Monitoring may be difficult; automatic BP devices using plastic connectors, capnography, oesophageal stethoscopes and non-magnetic oximeters have been used. Resuscitation equipment should be available, but similar restrictions apply. Risk of electric current induction by the magnetic field, e.g. causing VF, is minimized by limiting the allowed induced current density. Some magnets may be switched off in emergencies, but may require lengthy and expensive restarting procedures.
  –radiofrequency pulses may cause heating effects, thought to be relatively insignificant. These effects may be increased with metal prostheses.
  –sedation/anaesthesia is often required. Problems include those of **radiology** in general, apart from the above. Scans may take up to 2–3 hours but are quicker with newer machines.

Menon DK, Peden CJ, Hall AS, Sargentoni J, Whitwam JG (1992) Anaesthesia; 47: 240–55 and 508–17

Malaria. **Tropical disease** caused by the protozoan Plasmodium, transmitted by the Anopheles mosquito. Although not endemic in the UK, individual cases occur not uncommonly because of widespread air travel. In milder forms, periodic release of the organism from the liver and reticuloendothelial system into the bloodstream causes relapsing fever, rigors and malaise.

Severe illness and death are more likely with *Pl. falciparum*, particularly common in tropical Africa and South East Asia. Incubation period is 7–14 days. Many features are thought to result from sludging of damaged infected red blood cells within capillaries, with resultant ischaemia of organs.

• Features include:
  –rigors, fever, vomiting, headache.
  –confusion, **convulsions**, **coma**. 80% of deaths result from cerebral malaria.
  –**renal failure**.
  –**hypoglycaemia**; thought to be caused by increased **insulin** secretion; it may also result from quinine therapy.
  –bronchopneumonia, **ARDS**, **pulmonary oedema**.
  –diarrhoea, endotoxaemia from bowel bacteria.
  –**anaemia**, **thrombocytopenia**, intravascular **haemolysis**, **DIC**.

Diagnosis is made by examining blood films, or rarely bone marrow, for parasites.

• Treatment:
  –chloroquine, amodiaquine, primaquine for mild infections.
  –quinine; usually reserved for resistant organisms or severe falciparum infection.
  –severe infection:
    –chloroquine 10 mg base/kg iv over 8 hours, then 5 mg/kg 8 hourly × 3. Oral therapy is started when possible to a total dose of 25 mg/kg.
      Dizziness, visual disturbances, ECG abnormalities and hypotension may occur.
    –quinine salt 20 mg/kg iv over 4 hours, then 10 mg/kg over 4 hours repeated 8 hourly until able to swallow (reduced by a third after 72 hours if unable to swallow). Oral therapy (10 mg/kg) is continued until 7 days' treatment is completed.
      Hypotension, arrhythmias, dysphoria, hypoglycaemia, dizziness, tinnitus, tremor and blurred vision may occur.

Malaria may be transmitted by **blood transfusion**; those with infection are therefore excluded from being donors.

Malignancy. Second commonest cause of death in the UK after cardiovascular disease. Patients may present to anaesthetists for investigative, therapeutic or non-related procedures.

• Anaesthetic considerations:
  –effects of malignancy itself:
    –primary:
      –local, e.g. pressure effects, ulceration, haemorrhage, etc.
      –systemic, e.g. **anaemia**, cachexia, susceptibility to infection, electrolyte disturbances (e.g. **hypercalcaemia**), endocrine effects (e.g. **Cushing's syndrome** caused by **bronchial carcinoma**, **carcinoid syndrome**, **myasthenic syndrome**, etc.).
    –metastatic, e.g. lung, liver, bone.
  –effects of previous treatment:
    –surgery/**radiotherapy**, e.g. scarring, deformities.
    –**antimitotic drugs**, **steroid therapy**, **opioid analgesic drugs**, **antidepressant drugs**, etc.
  –possible effects of anaesthesia on the **immune system** and cancer, e.g. administration of blood during bowel cancer resection may decrease survival.
  –anxiety, depression.
  –**pain management**.

Malignant hyperthermia (MH). Condition first recognized in 1960 in Australia, consisting of increased temperature and rigidity during anaesthesia. Incidence is reported between 1:5000 and 1:200 000. Results from abnormal skeletal **muscle contraction** and increased metabolism affecting muscle and other tissues. Susceptibility shows autosomal dominant inheritance; the predisposing gene has recently been suggested as being on or near the ryanodine receptor gene (near that for **muscular dystrophy**).

MH follows exposure to triggering agents, particularly the volatile anaesthetic agents and **suxamethonium**, although it is thought that a single dose of the latter by itself will not cause the syndrome. It may occur in patients who have experienced previous anaesthetics without problem. In certain animals, e.g. landrace pigs, a similar response may be provoked by stress. This has also been reported in a susceptible patient. Thus patients may show different sensitivity to triggering agents at different times. Reactions have been reported up to 11 hours postoperatively after triggering anaesthetics.

Most common in young patients undergoing musculoskeletal surgery, including trauma surgery. Whether this reflects an underlying abnormality of muscle predisposing to trauma is unknown. Operations in the young are commonly for squints and orthopaedic problems, and increased incidence in this group may simply represent the first exposure to anaesthesia in susceptible patients. MH is also thought to be more common in patients with muscular dystrophies and related disorders.

- Features are related to muscle abnormality and hypermetabolism, but not all may be present:
  - sustained muscle contraction; results from breakage of the normal impulse/contraction sequence (excitation/contraction uncoupling) causing abnormal **calcium** ion mobilization, and is unrelieved by neuromuscular blocking drugs. **Masseter spasm** may be an early sign.
  - muscle breakdown with release of potassium, myoglobin and muscle enzymes e.g. creatine kinase. **Hyperkalaemia** may cause cardiac **arrhythmias**.
  - increased O_2 consumption leading to **cyanosis**.
  - increased CO_2 production and **hypercapnia**. Hyperventilation may occur in the spontaneous breathing patient.
  - increased body temperature and sweating. Other causes of **hyperthermia** should be considered.
  - tachycardia and unstable BP.
  - metabolic **acidosis**.
- Management:
  - discontinuation of the triggering agent, and abandonment of surgery if feasible. Changing the anaesthetic machine, tubing and soda lime has been suggested if possible.
  - **dantrolene** is the only available specific treatment. 1 mg/kg is given iv, repeated as required up to 10 mg/kg.
  - supportive treatment:
    - hyperventilation with 100% O_2. Boluses of e.g. **thiopentone** iv will maintain anaesthesia.
    - correction of acidosis with **bicarbonate**, e.g. 0.5–1.0 mmol/kg until blood gas results are available.
    - cooling with cold iv fluids, fans, sponging, irrigation of body cavities, etc.
    - treatment of hyperkalaemia if severe.
    - **diuretic** therapy to reduce renal damage caused by

myoglobin. **Mannitol** or **frusemide** have been recommended.
  - treatment of any arrhythmias as they occur.
  - **steroid therapy**, e.g. dexamethasone 4 mg, has been advocated.
  - close monitoring in an ICU for 36–48 hours postoperatively, including of temperature. Blood should be taken 12 hourly for 36–48 hours, for measurement of creatinine kinase, and the first urine voided should be analysed for myoglobin.
  - **renal failure** and **DIC** are treated as neccessary.

Treatment should be instituted as soon as the diagnosis is suspected. Arterial blood gas analysis and measurement of plasma potassium should be performed early to detect acidosis and hyperkalaemia.

Prognosis is good if treated appropriately and early; mortality was 80% before dantrolene became available.

- Investigation:
  - serum creatine kinase elevation and **myoglobinuria** are suggestive but not diagnostic. The former is not reliable as a screening test. Creatine kinase and myoglobin may both increase after suxamethonium administration in normal patients.
  - muscle biopsy may appear normal histologically.
  - caffeine and halothane contracture tests are now accepted as investigations of choice. Biopsied muscle is exposed to caffeine and halothane, and tension in the muscle measured. Contractures are induced in susceptible muscle. Results are divided into positive, negative or equivocal. False positive results may occur. All suspected cases and immediate relatives should be tested for susceptibility.
- Management of known cases:
  - pretreatment with oral dantrolene 5 mg/kg over 24 hours preoperatively, or 1–2 mg/kg iv before induction, has been used, but this is rarely considered necessary now.
  - sedative **premedication** is sometimes given to reduce 'stress', but this is controversial.
  - avoidance of known triggering agents: volatile agents, **cyclopropane** and suxamethonium. N_2O is considered safe. Many other drugs have been implicated at some time, but the above are the only definite triggers. **TIVA** has been suggested as a useful technique. Local anaesthetic techniques may be used, but MH may still occur. All local anaesthetic agents are now considered as safe as each other. Some would avoid **phenothiazines** and **butyrophenones** because of the **neuroleptic malignant syndrome**, but there is no evidence that the two conditions are related.
  - use of an anaesthetic machine which has not previously been exposed to volatile agents has been suggested, but some consider a new breathing system to be sufficient, with flushing of the machine with fresh gas for 10–20 minutes prior to use.
  - **monitoring** should include temperature (rectal and axillary), expired CO_2 and oximetry. Some would consider arterial cannulation mandatory. Close monitoring should continue postoperatively.
  - dantrolene and supportive treatments should be readily available.
  - reactions have been reported following apparently 'trigger free' anaesthetics, but these have not been severe.

All patients should be questioned for family history of anaesthetic problems, since many susceptible patients give a positive family history. Susceptible patients should wear 'Medic Alert' bracelets.

Postgraduate Educational Issue (1988) Br J Anaesth; 60: 251–319

Malnutrition. Nutrient deficiency, usually of several dietary components. **Protein** depletion with near normal **energy** supply may lead to kwashiorkor, with **hypoproteinaemia** and **oedema**. Protein and energy depletion may lead to marasmus, with normal plasma protein concentration.

- Body reserves during total starvation under basal conditions:
    - **carbohydrate**: about 0.5 kg mainly as liver and muscle glycogen; lasts under 1 day.
    - protein: 4–6 kg mainly as muscle; lasts 10–12 days.
    - **fat**: 12–15 kg as adipose tissue; lasts 20–25 days.
    Protein breakdown is reduced by even small amounts of **glucose**, possibly by the effects of resultant **insulin** secretion, which prevents protein **catabolism**.
- Malnutrition is common to some degree in hospital patients. It may be associated with:
    - decreased intake, e.g. **vomiting**, malabsorption, anorexia, poor diet, nil-by-mouth orders.
    - decreased utilization, e.g. **renal failure**.
    - increased **basal metabolic rate**, e.g. **trauma**, **burns**, severe illness, pyrexia.
    Thus common perioperatively, especially in severe chronic illness, GIT disease/surgery, alcoholics, the elderly, immigrants and the mentally ill. May result in impaired healing, bedsores, increased susceptibility to infection, weakness, **anaemia**, hypoproteinaemia, electrolyte disturbances and **dehydration**, **vitamin deficiency** disorders, and predisposition to **hypothermia**. Respiratory muscle weakness may predispose to respiratory complications.
    Long-term **nutrition**, via enteral or parenteral routes, is thought to be beneficial preoperatively (at least 14 days). The place of short-term feeding is less certain. Progress may be monitored by weight or skin thickness measurements.

Mandatory minute ventilation (MMV). Ventilatory mode used to assist **weaning from ventilators**. The required mandatory minute ventilation is preset, and the patient allowed to breathe spontaneously, with the ventilator making up any shortfall in minute volume. Thus with the patient breathing adequately, the ventilator is not required. However, a minute ventilation made up of rapid shallow breaths will also 'satisfy' the ventilator, despite **alveolar ventilation** being inadequate. In addition, not all ventilators allow spontaneous minute ventilation to exceed the preset one (extended mandatory minute ventilation; EMMV). Thus MMV is less popular than **IMV**.

Cameron PD, Oh TE (1986) Anaesth Intensive Care; 14: 258–66

Mandibular nerve blocks. Performed for facial and intraoral procedures.
- Anatomy: the mandibular division (V³) of the trigeminal nerve passes from the **Gasserian ganglion** through the foramen ovale.
- Divisions:
    - motor nerves to the muscles of mastication and tensor muscles of the palate and eardrum.
    - sensory nerves (*See also, Fig. 65; Gasserian ganglion block*):
        - meningeal branch: passes through the foramen spinosum and supplies the adjacent dura.
        - buccal nerve: supplies the skin and mucosa of the cheek.
        - auriculotemporal nerve; supplies the anterior eardrum, ear canal, **temporomandibular joint**, cheek, temple, temporal scalp and parotid gland.
        - inferior alveolar nerve: enters the mandible at its ramus, supplying the lower teeth and gums; the central incisors are innervated bilaterally. Emerges through the mental foramen to supply the mucosa and skin of the lower lip, chin and gum.
        - lingual nerve: passes alongside the tongue to supply its anterior two-thirds, the floor of mouth and lingual gum.
    The supraorbital foramen, pupil, infraorbital notch, infraorbital foramen, buccal surface of the second premolar and mental foramen all lie along a straight line.
- Blocks:
    - mandibular: a needle is inserted at right angles to the skin between the coronoid and condylar processes, just above the bone. After contacting the pterygoid plate, it is redirected posteriorly until paraesthesiae are obtained, and 5 ml **local anaesthetic agent** injected (NB. the pharynx lies 5 mm internally).
    - inferior alveolar/lingual: with the mouth wide open, a needle is inserted parallel to the teeth and 1 cm above their occlusal surface, medial to the oblique line of the mandibular ramus. It is advanced 1.5–2.0 cm and the syringe barrel swung across to the opposite side. 1–1.5 ml solution is injected with a further 0.5 ml on withdrawal (to block the lingual nerve).
        May also be performed extraorally, by injecting 1.5–2.0 ml between the mandibular ramus and maxilla, level with the upper teeth gingival margins; the needle is inserted from the front with the mouth shut.
        Buccal infiltration is required for surgery to the molar teeth; 0.5–1.0 ml is injected into the cheek mucosa opposite the third molar. The incisors receive bilateral innervation.
    - mental/incisive branches of the inferior alveolar nerve (supplying from the incisors to the first premolar): 0.5–1.0 ml is injected at the mental foramen from behind the second molar intraorally, or extraorally.
    - buccal nerve: 0.5–1.0 ml is injected lateral and posterior to the last molar, by the anterior border of the mandibular ramus.
    - submucous infiltration on both sides of individual teeth, directed along its long axis, may also be used.
    - auriculotemporal nerve: 1.5–2.0 ml is injected in the anterior wall of the ear canal, at the junction of its bony and cartilaginous parts. Allows myringotomy to be performed.

1–2% **lignocaine** or **prilocaine** with **adrenaline** is most commonly used. Systemic absorption of adrenaline may cause symptoms, especially if high concentrations are used, e.g. 1:80 000. Immediate collapse following dental nerve blocks is thought to result from retrograde flow of

solution via branches of the external carotid artery, reaching the internal carotid; perineural spread to the medulla has also been suggested.
See also, Gasserian ganglion block; Maxillary nerve blocks; Nose; Ophthalmic nerve blocks

Mandragora (Mandrake). Plant, supposedly human-shaped, thought to hold magic powers including the ability to induce sleep and relieve pain. Contains **hyoscine** and similar alkaloids. According to legend, its scream on uprooting killed all who heard it, hence the supposedly 'safe' method of collection: a dog is tied to the plant at midnight, whilst its owner retreats to a safe distance with ears stopped with wax. The dog is enticed to run after food, pulling out the mandrake and dying in the process.

Mannitol. Plant-derived alcohol. An osmotic **diuretic**; it draws water from the extracellular and intracellular spaces into the vascular compartment, expanding the latter transiently. Not reabsorbed once filtered in the the kidneys, it continues to be osmotically active in the urine, causing diuresis. Used mainly to reduce the risk of perioperative **renal failure** (e.g. during vascular surgery, surgery in obstructive **jaundice**, etc.), and to treat **cerebral oedema**. Efficacy in the latter depends on integrity of the **blood–brain barrier** which may be altered in neurological disease, although some benefit is derived from the systemic dehydration produced. Has also been used to lower **intraocular pressure**. It may also act as a free radical scavenger.

Temporarily increases **cerebral blood flow**; **ICP** may rise slightly before falling, especially after rapid injection. Excessive brain shrinkage in the elderly may rupture fragile subdural veins. A rebound increase in ICP may occur if treatment is prolonged, due to eventual passage of mannitol into the brain; the effect is small after a single dose. A transient increase in vascular volume and CVP may cause **cardiac failure** in susceptible patients.

- Dosage: 0.5–1 g/kg by iv infusion of 10–20% solution over 20–30 minutes. Effects occur within 30 minutes, lasting 6 hours. 0.25–0.5 g/kg may follow 6 hourly for 24 hours, unless diuresis has not occurred, cardiovascular instability ensues or plasma **osmolality** exceeds 315 mosmol/kg.

Available in 10%, 15%, 20% and 25% solutions; osmolalities are 550, 825, 1100 and 1375 mosmol/kg respectively.

Mann–Whitney rank sum test, *see Statistical tests*

MAO, *see Monoamine oxidase*

MAOI, *see Monoamine oxidase inhibitors*

MAP, *see Mean arterial pressure*

Mapleson classification of breathing systems, *see Anaesthetic breathing systems*

Marey's law. Increased pressure in the aortic arch and **carotid sinus** causes bradycardia; decreased pressure causes tachycardia.
[EJ Marey (1830–1904), French physiologist]
See also, Baroreceptor reflex

Marfan's syndrome. Connective tissue disease, inherited as an autosomal dominant gene. Prevalence is 1:20 000.
- Features:
  –tall stature, with long thin extremities. Joint dislocations, **kyphoscoliosis**, pes excavatum, inguinal and diaphragmatic herniae are common.
  –subluxation of the ocular lens (50%).
  –cardiovascular:
    –**aortic regurgitation** (<90%).
    –ascending **aortic aneurysm**.
    –**mitral valve prolapse**.
    –conduction defects.
  –respiratory:
    –kyphoscoliosis.
    –emphysema.
    –**pneumothorax**.
  –tracheal intubation may be difficult (high arched palate).

Death usually results from aortic dilatation and its complications. Careful **preoperative assessment** and antibiotic prophylaxis are required as for **congenital heart disease**.
[Bernard J Marfan (1858–1942), French paediatrician]
Wells DG, Podolakin W (1987) Can J Anaesth; 34: 311–4

Masks, *see Facepieces; Oxygen therapy*

Mass. Amount of matter contained in a body. Under conditions of differing gravity, mass remains constant, whereas **weight** varies. SI **unit** is the **kilogram**.

Mass spectrometer. Device used to analyse mixtures of substances acording to mw. The sample passes through an ionizing chamber, and becomes charged by electrons arising from a cathode. The charged sample particles are then accelerated by an electric field which imparts a certain velocity. When they subsequently pass through a strong magnetic field, the particles are deflected to varying degrees depending on their mass and momentum. The electrical charge arriving at certain distances from the accelerating chamber is measured, and corresponds to the amount of differently-sized particles present in the original sample. Different ranges of particle size may be analysed by altering accelerator characteristics. Compounds of identical mw may be distinguished by identifying breakdown products.

Alternatively, in the quadrupole mass spectrometer, the accelerated beam passes longitudinally between four rods, of variable potential. Particles are removed from the beam unless of a certain mass, depending on the rods' potential.

Mass spectrometers may be used for on-line **gas analysis** during anaesthesia.

Masseter spasm. Increase in jaw tone occurring after **suxamethonium**. More common in children and after **halothane** induction, although the incidence is hard to determine because of difficulty in definition. 1:100–1:3000 incidence has been reported, but amidst controversy. A protective effect of **thiopentone** has been suggested. Spasm may represent a normal dose-related response to suxamethonium, but has been associated with **MH** susceptibility, especially if spasm is severe and prolonged, and associated with markedly raised serum creatine kinase and **myoglobinuria**.

Management of spasm is controversial: termination of anaesthesia, treatment with **dantrolene**, proceeding with caution or referral for muscle biopsy have all been recommended.

Saddler JM (1991) Br J Anaesth; 67: 515–16

MAST, Military antishock trousers, *see Antigravity suit*

Mast cells. Basophilic cells in connective and subcutaneous tissues, involved in inflammatory reactions and immune responses. Storage granules contain lytic **enzymes** and inflammatory mediators, e.g. **histamine**, **kinins**, **heparin**, **5–HT**, **hyaluronidase**, **leukotrienes**, **platelet** aggregating and leucocyte chemotactic factors. Release is caused by injury to tissues, **complement** activation, drugs e.g. **tubocurarine**, and cross-linkage of surface IgE molecules (e.g. in **anaphylactic reactions**) by antigen. Also involved in presentation of antigen to lymphocytes. Occur in excess (either in the circulation of as tissue infiltrates) in mastocytosis.

Maternal mortality, *see Confidential Enquiries into Maternal Mortality, Report on*

Maxillary nerve blocks. Performed for facial and intra-oral procedures.

- Anatomy: the maxillary division (V^2) of the trigeminal nerve passes from the **Gasserian ganglion** through the foramen rotundum into the pterygopalatine fossa, dividing into sensory branches and continuing as the infraorbital nerve (*see Fig. 65; Gasserian ganglion block*). Branches:
  - –via the pterygopalatine ganglion to the **nose**, nasopharynx and palate via nasal, nasopalatine, greater and lesser palatine and pharyngeal nerves.
  - –nasopalatine nerve: supplies the anterior third of the hard palate and palatal gingiva of the upper incisors.
  - –greater palatine: supplies the posterior hard palate and palatal gingiva of adjacent teeth.
  - –zygomatic nerve: supplies the temple, cheek and lateral eye.
  - –posterior superior alveolar nerve: supplies the molar/premolar teeth.
  - –infraorbital nerve: supplies the lower eyelid, conjunctiva, side of the nose, upper lip, cheek, and via its anterior superior alveolar branch, the upper canines and incisors, maxillary sinus and cheek mucosa.

  The supraorbital foramen, pupil, infraorbital notch, infraorbital foramen, buccal surface of the second premolar and mental foramen all lie along a straight line.
- Blocks:
  - –maxillary nerve: a needle is inserted extraorally 0.5 cm below the midpoint of the zygoma and directed medially until bone is contacted. It is redirected anteriorly and advanced a further 1 cm, anterior to the lateral pterygoid plate. 3–4 ml **local anaesthetic agent** is injected. May also be blocked via the intraoral route: the needle is inserted behind the posterior border of the zygoma and directed upwards, medially and posteriorly 3 cm. Up to 5 ml solution is injected within the pterygopalatine fossa.
  - –nasopalatine nerve: 0.5–1.0 ml is injected at the incisive foramen, 0.5–1.0 cm posterior to the upper incisors in the midline.
  - –greater palatine nerve: 0.5–1.0 ml is injected at the greater palatine foramen, marked by a depression in the palate opposite the second/third molar 1 cm above the gingival margin.
  - –infraorbital nerve: 1–2 ml is injected at the infraorbital foramen, 0.5–1.0 cm below the infraorbital notch. Injection may be performed intraorally or extraorally.
  - –superior alveolar nerve branches to individual teeth may be blocked by submucous infiltration above each tooth.
  - –for the Cadwell–Luc approach, the mucosa and periosteum above the upper premolars may be infiltrated with 5–10 ml solution, to block branches of the anterior superior alveolar nerve. Topical application of e.g. **lignocaine** may assist the block. Further solution may be injected into the mucosa of the maxillary sinus once opened. Alternatively, maxillary or infraorbital nerve blocks may be performed.

1–2% lignocaine or **prilocaine** with **adrenaline** are most commonly used. Systemic absorption of adrenaline may cause symptoms, especially if high concentrations are used, e.g. 1:80 000.

Immediate collapse following dental nerve blocks is thought to result from retrograde flow of solution via branches of the external carotid artery, reaching the internal carotid; perineural spread to the medulla has also been suggested

[George Caldwell (1834–1918), US ENT surgeon; Henri Luc (1855–1925), French ENT surgeon]

See also, Mandibular nerve blocks; Ophthalmic nerve blocks

Maximal breathing capacity, *see Maximal voluntary ventilation*

Maximal voluntary ventilation (Maximal breathing capacity). Maximal minute volume of air able to be breathed, measured over 15 seconds. Normally about 120–150 l/min. Equals approximately $35 \times \mathbf{FEV_1}$. Rarely used, since very tiring to perform.

See also, Lung function tests

MCH/MCHC/MCV, Mean cell haemoglobin/Mean cell haemoglobin concentration/Mean cell volume, *see Erythrocytes*

MEA syndrome, *see Multiple endocrine adenomatosis*

Mean (Average). Expression of the central tendency of a set of observations or measurements. Equals the sum of all the observations divided by the number of observations (n), i.e.

$$\bar{x} = \frac{\Sigma x}{n}$$

Population mean is denoted by μ; sample mean by $\bar{x}$.

Means of more than one sample group may be compared using **statistical tests**.

See also, Median; Mode; Standard error of mean; Statistical frequency distributions; Statistics

Mean arterial pressure (MAP). Average **arterial BP** throughout the **cardiac cycle**. The area contained within the **arterial waveform** pressure trace above MAP equals the area below it.

Equals approximately $\dfrac{(2 \times \text{diastolic}) + \text{systolic}}{3}$, or

diastolic + $\dfrac{(\text{systolic} - \text{diastolic})}{3}$.

Preferred by some clinicians to measures of systolic or diastolic pressures, since it is less liable to errors or differences due to measuring techniques. Also represents the mean pressure available for perfusion of tissues.

Mechanocardiography. Recording of the mechanical pulsations of the CVS; includes tracings of the **JVP** and **venous waveform**, **arterial waveform** and recordings at the apex using an externally applied transducer. Has been used to investigate cardiovascular disease, especially valvular disease, and to determine **systolic time intervals**.

Median. Expression of the central tendency of a set of measurements or observations.

Equals the $\dfrac{(n + 1)\text{th}}{2}$ measurement.

Half the population lies above it, half below. Equals the **mean** for a normal distribution.
See also, Statistical frequency distributions; Statistics

Median nerve (C6–T1). Arises from the medial and lateral cords of the **brachial plexus** in the lower axilla, lateral to the axillary artery. Passes down the front of the arm to the **antecubital fossa**, first lateral to the brachial artery, then crossing it anteriorly at mid-upper arm to lie medially. Entering the forearm, it crosses the ulnar artery anteriorly, separated from it by pronator teres' deep head. Passes between flexor digitorum superficialis and profundus; at the wrist it lies between the tendons of palmaris longus (medially) and flexor carpi radialis (laterally).
- Apart from branches to the joints of the wrist and hand, it supplies:
  - superficial flexor muscles (except flexor carpi ulnaris), abductor pollicis brevis, flexor pollicis brevis and opponens pollicis.
  - radial side of the palm and the palmar surface of the radial 3½ digits, extending to their dorsal surface at their tips.
  - via the anterior interosseus branch arising at the distal antecubital fossa: flexor pollicis longus, radial part of flexor digitorum profundus, and pronator quadratus.

May be blocked at the brachial plexus, elbow and wrist.
See also, Brachial plexus block; Elbow, nerve blocks; Wrist, nerve blocks.

Mediastinum. Region of the thorax between the two pleural sacs. It is in contact with the **diaphragm** inferiorly, and continuous with the tissues of the neck superiorly. Lies between the vertebral column posteriorly and sternum anteriorly. Contains the **heart**, great vessels, **trachea**, **oesophagus**, thoracic duct, vagi, **phrenic** and recurrent **laryngeal nerves**, sympathetic trunk, thymus and lymph nodes (Fig. 89).
- Divided into:
  - superior mediastinum: above a horizontal line level with T4/5 and the angle of Louis.
  - inferior mediastinum: below this line. Comprised of anterior (between heart and sternum), middle (containing **pericardium** and contents) and posterior (between heart and **vertebrae**) portions.

Thus mediastinal enlargement may be caused by:
- enlargement of any of the above constituent structures (central).
- spinal and vertebral masses (posterior).
- thymic, thyroid, teratoma and dermoid tumours (anterior).

Tumours, e.g. **bronchial carcinoma**, may involve local structures within the mediastinum, e.g. recurrent laryngeal or phrenic nerves, pericardium, etc. Bleeding from the aorta following **chest trauma** may cause widening of the superior mediastinum.

Patients with mediastinal enlargement may present for biopsy, e.g. via mediastinoscopy through a suprasternal incision, or resection.
- Main anaesthetic considerations:
  - preoperative state, e.g. related to the primary **malignancy**. Tracheal compression and **airway obstruction**, **superior vena caval obstruction**, phrenic and recurrent laryngeal nerve involvement and drug and radiotherapy effects may be present.
  - classically, **induction of anaesthesia** is inhalational, but some advocate iv induction. Reinforced tracheal/bronchial tubes are often preferable.
  - severe haemorrhage may occur. Fluid replacement via the femoral vein may be required if the superior vena cava and its tributaries are involved.
  - **one-lung anaesthesia** and even **extracorporeal circulation** may be required during resection.

[Antoine Louis (1723–1792), French surgeon]
See also, Chest X-ray

Medicolegal aspects of anaesthesia. In the UK, these usually concern matters of civil law (i.e. between individuals), e.g. negligence, breach of contract or assault; proof must be according to 'balance of probalities'. Criminal law is involved less commonly (e.g. involving murder or manslaughter), e.g. due to criminal neglect or reckless disregard of clinical duties; proof must be 'beyond reasonable doubt'. Leaving anaesthetized patients unattended has led to criminal prosecution.
- Usually related to:
  - **consent** for surgery, procedures, taking of blood for tests (e.g. for police), etc.
  - negligence: the following must be proved:
    - duty of care owed to the patient by the anaesthetist, including knowing when one is out of one's depth and when to call a more senior colleague.
    - failure in that duty.
    - harm suffered as a result of that failure.

Comparison is made with doctors of similar experience/training/skill; expert opinion is obtained and clinical notes scrutinized.

Individual doctors are responsible privately; responsibilty is shared by the employing Health Authority in the National Health Service (NHS). Defence organizations provide advice and indemnity; the latter has been provided by the employer for NHS work from 1990.

Claims commmonly involve:
- faulty equipment, incorrect drugs or blood, etc.
- consent.
- wrong operation etc.
- poor **preoperative assessment** and preparation.
- absence of the anaesthetist.

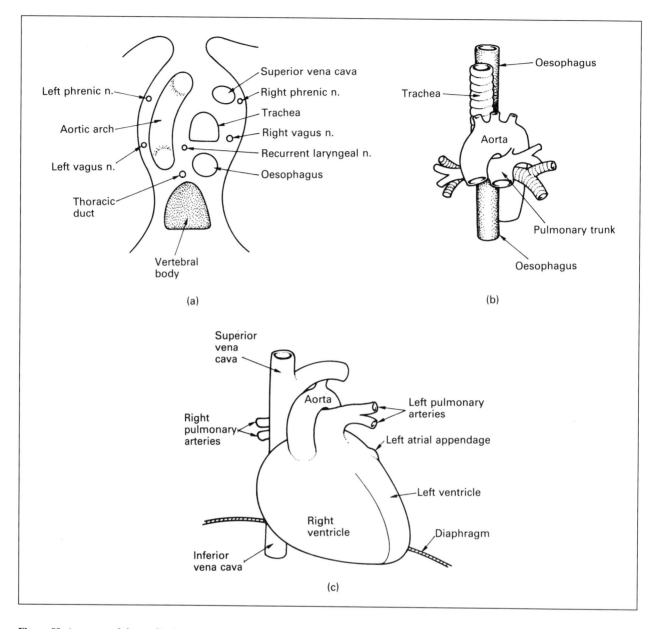

Figure 89 *Anatomy of the mediastinum: (a) transverse section through T4; (b) trachea and relations; (c) heart and great vessels*

–**nerve damage**, broken **teeth**, etc.
–**awareness**.
–**hypoxia**, **cardiac arrest**, etc.
Anaesthesia is considered a high risk specialty because of common minor claims and very expensive major claims. Risks are reduced by:
–**checking of anaesthetic equipment**, drugs, drips, allergies, patients' names and operation sites.
–adequate preoperative assessment and preparation, including warning patients of risks, e.g. to teeth, of dural tap, etc.
–consultation with senior colleagues when appropriate.
–adherence to generally accepted techniques, including adequate **monitoring**.
–careful writing of clinical notes and anaesthetic **record-keeping**, with copies kept for later use. Informing defence bodies early is encouraged,

should mishaps occur.
–full and honest explanation with patients and/or relatives when anything goes wrong.
–perioperative deaths: those occurring within 24 hours of anaesthesia are reported to the coroner, who may order an inquiry or inquest, although the time interval is not specified by law. Once reported, organs may not be harvested for transplantation.
–**Misuse of Drugs Act**.
–fitness to practise.
Postgraduate Educational Issue (1987) Br J Anaesth; 59: 813–927
See also, Abuse of anaesthetic agents; Anaesthetic morbidity and mortality; Sick doctor scheme

Membrane potential. Results from the differential distribution of charged particles across cell **membranes**.

The distribution of each particle is related to its permeability across the membrane, the distribution of other particles (e.g. **Donnan effect**), and to **active transport** systems, e.g. **sodium/potassium pump**. Membranes are impermeable to protein (negatively charged) which thus remains intracellular; membranes are poorly permeable to **sodium** ions and moderately permeable to chloride ions.

Concentration and electric gradients exist across membranes for each ion; the membrane potential at equilibrium for each is calculated by the **Nernst equation**. Membrane potentials at given intracellular/extracellular concentrations of sodium, chloride and **potassium** ions together are calculated by the **Goldman constant-field equation**.

Potential is conventially written as negative; i.e. the inside is negative relative to the outside. The potential's magnitude varies between tissues, e.g. –70 mV for nerves and –90 mV for muscle.

Changes in membrane permeability may alter, or be altered by, membrane potential, e.g. during **action potentials**.

Membranes. Biological membranes share certain features:
- –phospholipid bilayer; the hydrophilic end of each phospholipid molecule faces the membrane surface and the hydrophobic end lies within the membrane substance.
- –protein molecules at intervals within the membrane; they may traverse it or project on one side only, according to the water/lipid solubility of the protein subunits. Proteins are able to 'float' within the lipid molecules.
- –proteins may function as enzymes, receptors, pumps or channels for ions. They also have antigenic properties.
- –resting **membrane potential** is created by differential permeability for certain ions, together with **active transport** pumps. Most membranes are relatively permeable to chloride and **potassium** ions, less so to **sodium** ions, and relatively impermeable to proteins and anions. Non-charged substances, e.g. CO_2 and non-ionized drugs, are able to cross freely, as is water.
- –function of cells is dependent on the features of their membrane proteins, which may be altered by electrical signals or chemicals, e.g. drugs, hormones, **neurotransmitters**. The action of anaesthetic agents is thought to involve alteration of membrane configuration within the nervous system.

See also, Action potential; Anaesthesia, mechanisms of

Memory. Classically divided into short and long-term memory; the latter is subdivided into procedural (not requiring conscious retrieval, e.g. driving a car) and declarative (either requiring conscious retrieval of specific events (episodic) or related to information about the world and language (semantic)). The hippocampus, amygdala, frontal lobes, and thalamic and hypothalamic nuclei are thought to be concerned with memory storage and retrieval.

Anaesthetic agents are thought mainly to impair acquisition of short-term memory, although transfer into long-term memory may also be affected.

Griffiths D, Jones JG (1990) Br J Anaesth; 65: 603–6
See also, Amnesia

Mendelson's syndrome, *see Aspiration pneumonitis*

Meninges. Tissue layers surrounding the **brain** and **spinal cord**, comprised of:
- –pia mater: delicate vascular layer, closely adherent to the brain and cord, following their surfaces into clefts, sulci etc. Surrounded by **CSF** within the arachnoid. Thin projections of the latter cross the subarachnoid space to the pia. Blood vessels lie within the space.
  Within the **vertebral canal**, the denticulate ligament passes laterally from the pia along its length and attaches at intervals to the dura. The subarachnoid septum lies posteriorly, attaching to the arachnoid intermittently. The pia terminates as the filum terminale which passes through the caudal end of the dural sac and attaches to the coccyx.
- –arachnoid mater: delicate membrane, containing CSF internally. Does not project into clefts and sulci, apart from the longitudinal fissure. Applied to the dura externally; the potential subdural space lies between them, containing vessels. Fuses with the dura at S2. Arachnoid granulations project into the venous sinuses, for drainage of CSF.
- –dura mater: comprised of two fibrous layers: the outer is adherent to the periostial lining of the **skull**; the inner attaches to the outer but is separated by venous sinuses. The inner layer forms sheets within the skull:
  - –vertical: falx cerebri and falx cerebelli between the cerebral and cerebellar hemispheres respectively.
  - –horizontal: tentorium cerebelli above the cerebellum and the diaphragma sellae above the pituitary gland.
  The dura also forms two layers within the vertebral canal: the external adherent to the inner periostium of the **vertebrae** and the internal lying against the outer surface of the arachnoid. The space between the two dura layers is the **extradural space**. Projections and fibrous bands have been demonstrated from the dural within the extradural space, especially in the midline. Dura projects intermittently to the posterior longitudinal ligament of the vertebrae, especially lumbar. Dura ends at about S2.

All layers donate a thin covering 'sleeve' to **cranial nerves** and **spinal nerves** as they leave the CNS. These dural cuffs, which contain CSF, may accompany spinal nerves through the intravertebral foramina.
- Blood supply:
  - –intracranial:
    - –from ascending pharyngeal, occipital and maxillary branches of the external **carotid artery**. The maxillary artery gives rise to the middle meningeal artery (the largest artery), which enters the skull through the foramen spinosum.
    - –from branches of the internal carotid and vertebral arteries.
  - –spinal: as for the spinal cord.

See also, Meningitis; Vertebral ligaments

Meningitis. Inflammation of the **meninges**. Usually infective (rarely inflammatory, e.g. caused by malignancy):
- –viral: usually coxsackie, echo and mumps viruses. Usually has good prognosis, unless associated with generalized encephalitis.
- –bacterial: *Neisseria meningitidis, Streptococcus pneu-*

moniae and *Haemophilus influenzae* are the most common organisms. Mortalilty is high unless treated; adhesions, **hydrocephalus** and **cranial nerve** damage are still possible after treatment.

–others, e.g. **TB**, fungi.

- Features:
  –fever, nausea, vomiting, headache, photophobia, convulsions, coma.
  –neck stiffness, with muscle resistance to passive knee extension from the flexed position with the thigh flexed (caused by stretching of inflamed sciatic nerve roots (Kernig's sign)).
  –cranial nerve lesions or signs of **cerebral oedema** may be present.
  –meningococcal septicaemia is associated with petechial rash, shock, and possibly digital necrosis.
  –CAT scan may be required to exclude space-occupying lesions.
  –**CSF**:
    –viral: typically, increased lymphocytes, slightly raised protein and normal glucose.
    –bacterial: typically, increased polymorphs and protein, and reduced glucose. Bacteria may be visible on staining.

Treatment is directed at the underlying organism. If meningococcus is suspected, iv/im benzylpenicillin should be given before definitive microbiological diagnosis is obtained. Chloramphenicol is often given as it is active against all the most likely bacteria.

[Vladimir M Kernig (1840–1917), Russian neurologist]

Meperidine, *see Pethidine*

Mephentermine sulphate. Vasopressor drug, no longer available. Related to **amphetamine**; causes cerebral stimulation in addition to a rather variable increase in BP.

Mepivacaine hydrochloride. Amide **local anaesthetic agent**, first used in 1956. Similar to **lignocaine**, but more protein-bound. Does not cause vasodilatation. Not available in the UK. Used in 1–2% solutions for **extradural anaesthesia** and 4% solution for **spinal anaesthesia**, in the same doses as lignocaine. Maximal safe dose is 5 mg/kg; toxic plasma level is about 6 µg/ml. Rarely used in obstetrics because of greater fetal protein binding and longer fetal **half-life** than alternative drugs.

MEPP, Miniature end-plate potential, *see End-plate potentials*

Meptazinol hydrochloride. Synthetic **opioid analgesic drug**, first investigated in 1971. Has partial agonist properties, and therefore antagonizes respiratory depression caused by **morphine**. Causes less respiratory depression or sedation than morphine. Analgesic effects are almost completely reversed by **naloxone**. 100 mg is equivalent to 10 mg morphine or 100 mg **pethidine**.

- Dosage: 1–2 mg/kg 2–4 hourly as required, iv/im.; 200 mg 3–6 hourly, orally

Mesmerism. Treatment of various maladies by 'animal magnetism', the transmission between individuals of healing force derived from the ubiquitous magnetic fluid that pervaded the universe. Named after Mesmer, who originally passed magnets over his patients' bodies to treat them. He later used only his touch, and then speech, to achieve the same effects. Investigated in Paris by a French Royal Commission in 1784, which included Benjamin Franklin and **Lavoisier**; mesmerism was declared to have no scientific foundation, relying on suggestion alone. It continued to be popular until the 1840s, when the importance of psychological suggestion by the therapist was emphasized, leading to the concept of hypnotism.

[Franz A Mesmer (1734–1815), Swiss-born French physician; Benjamin Franklin (1706–1790), US statesman and scientist]

See also, Hypnosis

Metabolism. Physical and chemical changes occurring in an organism, including alteration in molecules and **energy** transformation. Involves anabolism (building-up; i.e. incorporation of substrate into living cells) and **catabolism** (breaking-down; usually concerned with energy production). Metabolic pathways and steps are controlled by **enzymes**, subject to hormonal and other control. Basic pathways are related to intake of foodstuffs:

  –**carbohydrates**: digested to monosaccharides, absorbed and passed to **liver** and **muscle**. Glucose is converted to **glycogen** for storage or broken down via **glycolysis**, **tricarboxylic acid cycle** and **cytochrome oxidase system** to CO_2 and water with production of energy, stored by **ATP** and other compounds.
  –**fats**: digested to fatty acids and glycerol, which pass to the liver. Stored as adipose tissue or oxidized to CO_2, water and energy.
  –**proteins**: digested to **amino acids**; form new proteins e.g. enzymes, secretions, cellular components e.g. **muscle**. Subsequently broken down to **urea**.

Carbohydrate, fat and protein subunits are interchangeable via many pathways, and are interlinked with other substances e.g. purines, nucleic acids, etc.

See also, Basal metabolic rate; Inborn errors of metabolism

Metaraminol tartrate/bitartrate. Vasopressor drug, acting directly via α-**adrenergic receptors**, and indirectly via **adrenaline** and **noradrenaline** release. Increases **cardiac output** and **SVR**, and thus **arterial BP**. Used to raise BP following **extradural/spinal anaesthesia** and **cardiogenic shock**. May cause excessive hypertension in hyperthyroidism and **monoamine oxidase inhibitor** therapy, and **myocardial ischaemia** in **ischaemic heart disease**.

- Dosage:
  –2–10 mg sc or im; acts within 10 minutes and lasts 1–1.5 hours.
  –1–5 mg iv; acts within 1–2 minutes, lasting for 20–30 minutes.

Methadone hydrochloride. Synthetic **opioid analgesic drug**, prepared in 1947. Used mainly for chronic **pain management** because of its prolonged duration of action (up to 24 hours). Also used as maintenance in opioid addicts, and to relieve cough in terminal care. Has been administered epidurally with good effect but its duration of action is shorter than that of **morphine**. Has similar actions and side effects to morphine, but is generally milder with less sedation. Elimination **half-life** exceeds 18 hours. Cumulation may be problematic.

- Dosage: 5–10 mg orally, im or sc, 6–8 hourly (12 hourly in chronic use).

See also, Spinal opioids

Methaemoglobinaemia. Increased circulating **haemoglobin** in which the iron atom of haem is in the ferrous (Fe^{3+}) state (normally <1%).

- May be:
  - –congenital:
    - –deficiency of reducing **enzymes**, which normally convert naturally formed methaemoglobin to haemoglobin. Usually autosomal recessive inheritance.
    - –abnormal haemoglobin chains, with fixation of iron in Fe^{3+} state; autosomal dominant inheritance.
  - –acquired: drugs and chemicals, e.g. **prilocaine**, chlorate, quinones, nitrites, phenacetin, sulphonamides, aniline dyes.
- Effects:
  - –because methaemoglobin is dark, patients appear to have **cyanosis**. Inaccurate readings of haemoglobin saturation may occur with pulse **oximetry**.
  - –affected haem portions of haemoglobin are less able to bind O_2. However, the **oxyhaemoglobin dissociation curve** of the unaffected haem is shifted to the left, reducing O_2 delivery to tissues. Dyspnoea and headache are common at above 20% methaemoglobin, although rate of formation is also important.
- Treatment: reducing agents, e.g. methylene blue iv, if acute and severe: 1–2 mg/kg over 5 minutes, repeated as necessary. Oral therapy with methylene blue or ascorbic acid may suffice in chronic methaemoglobinaemia.

See also, Sulphaemoglobinaemia

Methionine and methionine synthase. Methionine (an **amino acid**) is the main source of methyl groups in the body, and is involved in many biochemical reactions including myelination. It is also the precursor of glutathione, depleted in the liver by toxins e.g. **paracetamol poisoning**, hence its use in the latter. Formation from homocysteine by methionine synthase is involved in folate metabolism, and thymidine and DNA synthesis.

Methionine synthase containing **vitamin B_{12}** as a cofactor is inhibited by N_2O, which interacts directly with the vitamin. Prolonged exposure to N_2O may result in features of folate/vitamin B_{12} deficiency, e.g. subacute combined degeneration of the cord and megaloblastic **anaemia**. Myelination may also be affected. Significant effects are thought to be minimal up to 8 hours' normal anaesthetic use, but biochemical changes have been found after a few hours. Megaloblastic changes have been found in dentists who use N_2O. Effects on DNA synthesis are thought to be involved in teratogenesis following prolonged exposure of experimental animals to N_2O, but risk during anaesthesia in early pregnancy is generally considered negligible.

Methohexitone sodium. IV anaesthetic drug, first used in 1957. A methyl **barbiturate** (Fig. 90), presented as a white powder with 6% anhydrous sodium carbonate. Once mixed with water, it is stable for about 24 hours. pH of 1% solution is 10–11. pK_a is 7.9; thus a greater proportion is unionized in plasma than is **thiopentone**. The cheapest of the iv agents in common use. Mainly used for short procedures and **day case surgery**.

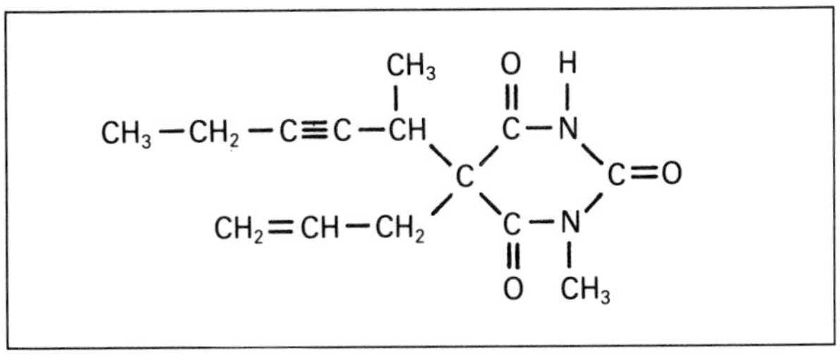

- Effects:
  - –induction:
    - –similar to thiopentone but with greater incidence of pain, involuntary movement, hiccup, laryngo-

Figure 90 *Structure of methohexitone*

spasm, etc., reduced by sedative premedication. Movements may be increased by phenothiazine premedication. Pain is reduced by mixing with 1–2 ml 1% lignocaine. Adverse effects of intra-arterial injection are less than with thiopentone, due to the more dilute solution.
  - –recovery within 3–4 minutes after a single dose.
  - –CVS/RS: less cardiovascular and respiratory depression than with thiopentone.
  - –CNS:
    - –may cause convulsions in epileptic patients. Considered by many to be the drug of choice for **electroconvulsive therapy**.
    - –similar other effects to thiopentone.
  - –other: as for thiopentone. **Adverse drug reactions** are less common.
- Metabolism: faster clearance than thiopentone, with **half-life** 2–4 hours. Remains within the body for at least 12 hours after administration.
- Dosage:
  - –1.0–1.5 mg/kg iv.
  - –3–6 mg/kg/h by iv infusion.
  - –may be given rectally (15–25 mg/kg), or im (6–10 mg/kg), with slower and smoother onset of action (up to 15 minutes).

Methoxamine hydrochloride. Vasopressor drug, acting via selective α_1-**adrenergic receptor** stimulation. Slows the heart rate by reflex **baroreceptor**-mediated inhibition secondary to raised BP, and possibly via a direct effect on the heart. Used to raise BP, e.g. during **extradural** or **spinal anaesthesia**, and to treat **SVT**. In obstetric patients, it causes uteroplacental vasoconstriction, and is therefore unsuitable before delivery. May cause excessive hypertension in **hyperthyroidism** and **monoamine oxidase inhibitor** therapy, and **myocardial ischaemia** in **ischaemic heart disease**.

- Dosage: 1–2 mg iv, repeated as required. Acts within 1–2 minutes; effects last for 1–1.5 hours. **Atropine** is usually administered concurrently to prevent severe bradycardia. May also be given im.

Methoxyflurane. $CHCl_3CF_2OCH_3$ **Inhalational anaesthetic drug**, first used in 1960. Withdrawn because of high output **renal failure** caused by **fluoride ion** production following its administration. Has high boiling point (105°C) and therefore difficult to vaporize; the Pentec **vaporizer** required the double-release of its safety catch to enable higher concentrations to be delivered, following which the whole of the fresh gas flow passed through the vaporizing chamber. Very soluble in blood (blood/gas **partition coefficient** of 13); induction and recovery are therefore slow.

Extremely potent (**MAC** 0.2) and a powerful analgesic. Formerly used for general anaesthesia and draw-over analgesia, e.g. during labour, using the Cardiff fixed output (0.35%) inhaler. Cheap and non-explosive.

α-Methyldopa. Antihypertensive drug. Originally thought to act via uptake into **catecholamine** synthetic pathways and formation of a 'false transmitter', α-methyl-noradrenaline. The latter is now thought to have a direct antihypertensive action of its own, possibly via stimulation of central inhibitory α-**adrenergic receptors**, or reduction of plasma renin activity. Use has been supplanted by more modern drugs, but it is still occasionally used, e.g. in **pre-eclampsia** (shown to be non-teratogenic).
- Dosage:
  –250 mg orally, 8–12 hourly, adjusted according to response.
  –250–500 mg iv over 30–60 minutes (as methyldopate hydrochloride). Onset of action is 4–6 hours, lasting up to 16 hours.
- Side effects:
  –leucopenia, hepatitis, haemolytic anaemia. 10–20% of patients have a positive direct Coombs' test which may interfere with **blood cross-matching** (*see Haemolysis*). A systemic lupus-like syndrome has been reported.
  –sedation, confusion.
  –bradycardia, hypotension, oedema.
  –GIT disturbances.
  –paradoxical hypertension has occurred after iv use.
[Robin RA Coombs, Cambridge immunologist]

Methylmethacrylate. Acrylic cement used in **orthopaedic surgery** for fixation of prostheses. Thought to be the cause of **hypotension, hypoxaemia** or cardiovascular collapse upon prosthesis insertion, although the mechanism is unclear.
- Possible mechanisms:
  –direct cardiotoxicity of the monomer.
  –allergic reaction.
  –peripheral vasodilatation.
  –activation of the **coagulation** cascade within the pulmonary vasculature.
  –**fat** or **air embolism** resulting from insertion of lipid-soluble cement into the bone cavity under pressure.
  –combination of the above, exacerbated by the high temperatures generated (over 90°C) as the cement hardens.
Risks are reduced by washing out the bone cavity with saline before cement insertion, and retrograde insertion avoiding air trapping within the cavity.
Duncan JAT (1989) Anaesthesia; 44: 149–52

α-Methyl-*p*-tyrosine (Metyrosine). **Antihypertensive drug**; inhibits conversion of tyrosine to dopa and thus blocks **catecholamine** synthesis. Has been used to reduce the incidence and severity of hypertensive episodes in **phaeochromocytoma**, e.g. before or instead of surgery.
- Dosage: 2–4 g/day orally.
- Side effects include sedation, extrapyramidal movements, renal stones and diarrhoea.

Metoclopramide hydrochloride. Antiemetic drug, acting via **dopamine receptor** antagonism at the **chemoreceptor trigger zone**. Also increases **gastric emptying** and

lower oesophageal sphincter pressure via a peripheral cholinergic action, but will not reverse the effects of **opioid analgesic drugs** in this respect unless given iv. It also decreases the sensitivity of visceral afferent nerves to local emetics and irritants. Metabolized in the liver and excreted via the kidneys; thus the dose should be reduced in renal or hepatic impairment.
- Dosage:
  –10 mg iv, im or orally, repeated 8 hourly. Total daily dose: 0.5 mg/kg.
  –has been used in very high doses (up to 5 mg/kg iv) to treat **vomiting** caused by cytotoxic therapy; thought to antagonize central **5–HT** receptors.
- Side effects: **dystonic reactions** (particularly affecting the face), especially following iv administration and in children or young adults.

Metocurine, *see Dimethyl tubocurarine chloride/bromide*

Metoprolol, *see β-Adrenergic receptor antagonists*

Metre. SI **unit** of length. Originally defined according to the length of a platinum-iridium bar kept near Paris, but redefined in 1960 according to the speed of light in a vacuum, following doubts as to the bar's constant length over time: 1 metre = the distance occupied by 1 650 763.73 wavelengths of a specified orange-red light from gaseous krypton-86.

Meyer–Overton rule. States that **inhalational anaesthetic agents** act via the lipid-rich cells of the CNS; thus anaesthetic potency increases with lipid solubility. Can be seen if **MAC** is plotted against oil/gas **partition coefficients** at 37°C for various agents, using logarithmic scales (Fig. 91).
[Hans Meyer (1853–1939), German pharmacologist; Charles Overton (1865–1933), English-born German pharmacologist]
See also, Anaesthesia, mechanism of

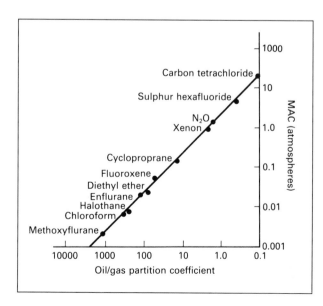

Figure 91 *Meyer–Overton rule*

Mexiletine hydrochloride. Class Ib **antiarrhythmic drug**; reduces fast sodium entry and shortens the refractory period. Chemically related to **lignocaine**, but active orally. **Half-life** is about 10 hours. Used to treat ventricular **arrhythmias**.

- Dosage:
  - –400 mg orally, followed by 200–250 mg 6–8 hourly.
  - –100–250 mg iv over 10 minutes, followed by 250 mg over 1 hour, then 250 mg over 2 hours, then 30 mg/h thereafter.
- Side effects:
  - –hypotension, bradycardia.
  - –confusion, ataxia, nystagmus, tremor, convulsions.
  - –hepatitis, jaundice, GIT disturbances.

MH, *see Malignant hyperthermia*

MI, *see Myocardial infarction*

Michaelis–Menten kinetics. Refers to the reaction between a single substrate S and an **enzyme** E, via an intermediate complex ES to give a single product P:

S + E = ES = P.

As the concentration of S ([S]) increases from zero, rate of reaction increases, until the enzyme binding sites become saturated, and maximal rate of reaction is reached. Thus initally, velocity of reaction (V) is proportional to [S]; i.e. first order kinetics apply. Eventually, V does not increase as [S] increases; i.e. zero order kinetics apply (Fig. 92).

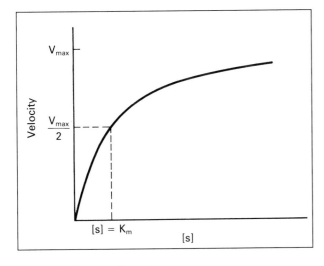

Figure 92 *Michaelis–Menten kinetics*

Michaelis–Menten equation: $V_i = \dfrac{V_{max}\,[S]}{K_m + [S]}$

where V_{max} = maximal reaction velocity;

K_m = Michaelis constant, the concentration of S at which $V = \dfrac{V_{max}}{2}$.

V_{max} and K_m are found by plotting $1/V$ against $1/[S]$ to obtain a straight line; the x-intercept is $-1/K_m$, the y-intercept is $1/V_{max}$, and the slope is K_m/V_{max}.

May also be applied to pharmacology, to describe absorption, distribution, elimination, etc. of drugs.
[Leonor Michaelis (1875–1945), German-born US chemist; Maud Menten (1879–1960), US physician]
See also, Pharmacokinetics.

Microshock, *see Electrocution and electrical burns*

Midazolam hydrochloride. Benzodiazepine, used mainly for **sedation**; has also been used for **premedication** and **induction of anaesthesia**. Water-soluble because of the open imidazole ring (five-membered ring containing carbon and nitrogen atoms); it becomes highly lipid-soluble at body pH due to ring closure, resulting in rapid onset of action following iv administration (usually under 90 seconds). Also rapidly absorbed after im injection. **Half-life** is about 2 hours. Metabolized to inactive compounds. Anterograde **amnesia** is marked.

Has slow onset when used for induction, with prolonged recovery. Effects may be antagonized by **flumazenil**.

- Dosage:
  - –premedication: 0.07–0.1 mg/kg im, 30–60 minutes preoperatively. Has been administered orally to children: 0.5–0.75 mg/kg 30 minutes preoperatively.
  - –sedation: 0.5–2 mg increments iv. By infusion: 0.05–0.2 mg/kg/h.
  - –induction: up to 0.3 mg/kg.

Respiratory and cardiovascular depression may occur, especially in elderly and sick patients, in whom reduced dosage is required.
Reves JG, Fragen RJ, Vinik HR et al (1985) Anesthesiology; 62: 310–24
See also, Intravenous anaesthetic agents

Midwives, administration of drugs by. Approved hospital midwives in the UK are usually permitted to administer certain drugs on the labour ward without individual prescription by doctors, according to agreement with the local health authority and obstetricians. Specified drugs thus vary between hospitals, but usually include:

- –**opioid analgesic drugs**, usually **pethidine** 100–150 mg, repeated once.
- –**Entonox** and O_2.
- –oxytocics, e.g. **oxytocin** and **ergometrine** separately or combined.
- –**antiemetic drugs/H_2 receptor antagonists**, e.g. **metoclopramide/ranitidine**.
- –**lignocaine** 0.5% 10–20 ml for local perineal infiltration.
- –**vitamin K** and **naloxone** for the **neonate**.

Others include hypnotics, traditionally **chloral hydrate** or **trichlofos. Temazepam** and alternative opioids, e.g. **pentazocine**, are sometimes given. Community midwives usually have freedom to prescribe iron, **antacids**, etc., in addition.

Midwives may give extradural solutions (but not the first injection) according to written instructions; responsibility for administration lies with the prescribing doctor. They may also administer **TENS**.

Military antishock trousers, *see Antigravity suit*

Milrinone lactate. Phosphodiesterase inhibitor, used as an **inotropic drug**. Increases **cardiac output** and reduces **SVR** without increasing **heart rate** or myocardial O_2

demand, although rate of atrioventricular conduction may increase slightly. Elimination **half-life** is about 2–2.5 hours. Excreted mainly via urine.

- Dosage:
  - –50 μg/kg over 10 minutes iv, followed by 0.3–0.75 μg/kg/min up to 1.1 mg/kg/day; doses should be reduced in renal impairment.
- Side effects: hypotension, ventricular and supraventricular arrhythmias, angina, headache.

Minaxolone. Water-soluble steroid **iv anaesthetic agent** derived from **Althesin**, investigated in the late 1970s/early 1980s. Causes rapid induction with involuntary muscle movement, anaesthesia lasting up to 20 minutes. Development was terminated because of reported toxicity in rats.

Miniature end-plate potential, *see End-plate potentials*

Minimal alveolar concentration (MAC). Minimal alveolar concentration of **inhalational anaesthetic agent** that prevents movement in response to skin incision in 50% of subjects studied. Thus inversely related to anaesthetic potency. Useful as a means of comparing different agents, and may be used to guide clinical dosage if end-tidal concentration of agent is monitored. Defined in terms of percentage of one atmosphere; therefore not influenced by altitude.

- MAC is reduced by:
  - –other depressant drugs (e.g. opioids, sedatives, other inhalational agents, etc.),
  - –CNS depletion of catecholamines, e.g. by **α-methyl-dopa**, **reserpine**.
  - –**hypothermia**.
  - –**hypoxaemia**/hypotension.
  - –extremes of age.
- MAC is increased in:
  - –children.
  - –**hyperthermia**.
  - –**hyperthyroidism**.
  - –chronic alcoholism.

It is unaffected by duration of anaesthesia, sex, acidaemia/alkalaemia, hypercapnia or hypocapnia.
Quasha AL, Eger EI, Tinker JH (1980) Anesthesiology; 53: 315–34
For values of MAC, see Table 18; Inhalational anaesthetic agents

Minimal blocking concentration (C_m). Lowest concentration of **local anaesthetic agent** that will block a nerve *in vitro* within (usually) 10 minutes. Temperature, pH, electrolyte composition, etc., are specified. Higher concentrations are required clinically, in order to achieve C_m at the axons. Dependent on the size of axon, not the site (although important clinically because of diffusion across membranes, drug absorption, etc.).

Minimal infusion rate (MIR). Application of the **MAC** concept to infusions of **iv anaesthetic agents**, e.g. in **TIVA**. Equals the minimal infusion rate of agent that prevents movement in response to skin incision in 50% of subjects studied. More complex than MAC of inhalational agents, because of the influence of pharmacokinetic factors associated with the use of iv infusions.

Minitracheotomy. Commercially available device, enabling easy **cricothyrotomy** in emergencies. Also useful

as a route for tracheobronchial suction when sputum retention is a problem, e.g. respiratory infection, impaired coughing, or postoperatively. May thus avoid tracheal intubation or formal **tracheostomy**, e.g. in ICU.

The pack includes a blade, 4 mm internal diameter tube and introducer, standard 15 mm connector, suction catheter and securing tapes. The introducer is inserted through a small incision in the cricothyroid membrane and the minitracheotomy tube railroaded over it into the trachea. Complications include haemorrhage, subcutaneous emphysema and misplacement.
Ryan DW (1990) BMJ; 300: 958–9

Minivent, *see Ventilators*

Minoxidil. Antihypertensive drug causing peripheral vasodilatation. Reserved as third-line treatment after **diuretics** and **β-adrenergic receptor antagonists**, because of tachycardia and water and salt retention. Also causes increased hair growth. Taken orally, 5–25 mg once–twice daily.

Minute ventilation (Minute volume). Volume of air breathed per minute. Equals tidal volume × respiratory rate; i.e. includes **alveolar ventilation** and **dead space** ventilation. Normally 5–7 litres.

Minute volume dividers, *see Ventilators*

MIR, *see Minimal infusion rate*

Misuse of Drugs Act, 1971. Introduced in the UK as a replacement for the obsolete Dangerous Drugs Act. Defined three classes of drugs, according to the penalties for offences:

- –class A:
  - –**opioid analgesic drugs** e.g. **morphine**, **pethidine**, **fentanyl**, **alfentanil**, **diamorphine**, **methadone**.
  - –**cocaine**, lysergide (LSD), phencyclidine.
  - –parenteral forms of Class B drugs.
- –class B:
  - –opioids e.g. **codeine**, **pentazocine**.
  - –**amphetamines**, **barbiturates**, cannabis.
- –class C: includes **benzodiazepines** and certain amphetamine-related drugs.
- Misuse of Drugs Regulations 1985: specified the requirements for handling, storage, record-keeping, etc.:
  - –Schedule 1: drugs not used therapeutically, e.g. cannabis.
  - –Schedule 2: opioids including codeine, pentazocine, morphine, etc. and cocaine (controlled drugs). To be kept in locked cupboards; details of patients are recorded in registers with practitioners' signatures and kept for 2 years.
  - –Schedule 3: barbiturates, **nalbuphine**, **buprenorphine**. Registers and locked cupboards are not required (except the latter for buprenorphine, from 1989), but special prescription requirements are required.
  - –Schedule 4: benzodiazepines.

Mitral regurgitation. About 50% of cases are due to **rheumatic fever**; **mitral stenosis** usually coexists. May be due to a floppy valve or papillary muscle dysfunction secondary to **MI** or degeneration; rare causes include left ventricular dilatation in **cardiac failure**, **cardiomyopathy**, bacterial **endocarditis**, and ruptured chordae tendinae.

- Effects:
  - left atrial dilatation; **pulmonary oedema** especially if acute. Rugurgitant fraction increases if SVR rises.
  - left ventricular hypertrophy and increased stroke volume.
  - **AF** if severe. Ventricular filling is less reliant on atrial contraction than in mitral stenosis; thus cardiac output is usually maintained.
- Features:
  - left ventricular hypertrophy, with pansystolic murmur usually at the apex, loudest on expiration and sitting forward, and radiating to the axilla. A thrill, third **heart sound** and diastolic flow murmur may be present. AF, left and later right ventricular failure may be present.
  - systemic embolism.
  - endocarditis.
  - **ECG** may reveal P mitrale, ventricular hypertrophy, and ventricular ectopics. **Chest X-ray** features may include cardiac enlargement, particularly of the left atrium, and pulmonary oedema. **Echocardiography** and **cardiac catheterization** are useful.
- Anaesthetic management:
  - prophylactic antibiotics as for **congenital heart disease**.
  - main principles are as for congenital and **ischaemic heart disease**. Drugs taken may include **diuretics**, **digoxin** and **anticoagulant drugs**. The following should be avoided: myocardial depression, **hypovolaemia**, bradycardia (which increases regurgitation; mild tachycardia is preferable), and vasoconstriction, e.g. due to sympathetic hyperactivity (pain, light anaesthesia), cold, etc. **Pulmonary artery catheterization** is useful; large V waves are typically seen in the pulmonary **venous waveform**.

See also, Heart murmurs; Valvular heart disease

Mitral stenosis. **Rheumatic fever** is by far the most common cause; others include congenital, infective and inflammatory causes. Symptoms are usually present if the valve area is reduced from the normal 4–6 cm^2 to about 1–3 cm^2.

- Effects:
  - reduced left ventricular filling, with left atrial hypertrophy and dilatation.
  - increased pulmonary vascular pressures, with pulmonary congestion and reduced pulmonary compliance. Work of breathing is increased.
  - if prolonged, it may cause **pulmonary hypertension**, with right ventricular overload and or tricuspid or pulmonary regurgitation. Progression may be rapid in 25–30%; the reason is unknown.
  - **AF** occurs in up to 50%; ventricular filling is reliant on atrial contraction, thus AF may lead to **pulmonary oedema**.
- Features:
  - **cardiac failure** and dyspnoea. Haemoptysis may be caused by recurrent chest infection, pulmonary oedema or infarction, or blood vessel rupture.
  - AF and systemic embolism.
  - malar flush (mitral facies), parasternal heave and features of tricuspid valve regurgitation may be present.

- 'tapping apex' (palpable first **heart sound**). The first sound is loud, with opening snap following the second sound. Low-pitched rumbling diastolic murmur, heard best at the apex on expiration with the stethoscope bell, leaning forward and to the left. Presystolic accentuation is heard before the first heart sound, due to atrial contraction; it disappears in AF. The opening snap may disappear if the valve is calcified.
  - **ECG** may reveal P mitrale, AF, and right ventricular hypertrophy. **Chest X-ray** features may include cardiac enlargement, particularly of the left atrium, and pulmonary oedema. Mitral calcification and features of pulmonary hypertension may be present. **Echocardiography** and **cardiac catheterization** are useful.
- Anaesthetic management:
  - prophylactic antibiotics as for **congenital heart disease**.
  - main principles are as for congenital and **ischaemic heart disease**. Drugs taken may include **diuretics**, **digoxin**, **anticoagulant drugs**. The following should be avoided: myocardial depression, tachycardia (which reduces left ventricular filling time), **hypovolaemia** and vasodilatation (reduce atrial and thus ventricular filling), and increased **pulmonary vascular resistance**, e.g. due to **hypoxaemia**. **Pulmonary artery catheterization** is useful, but **left ventricular end-diastolic pressure** estimation is inaccurate due to stenosis. Percutaneous catheter ballon valvuloplasty is sometimes performed in poor-risk patients.
  - postoperative IPPV may be required.

See also, Heart murmurs; Valvular heart disease; Tricuspid valve lesions

Mitral valve prolapse. Thought to occur in up to 15% of the population, sometimes associated with autosomal dominant inheritance. Also associated with **Marfan's syndrome** and possibly other disorders of collagen formation. Often asymptomatic, but may lead to **mitral regurgitation**, **cardiac failure**, bacterial **endocarditis** and systemic emboli.

- Signs:
  - mid-diastolic click, occurring at the onset of the carotid pulsation.
  - late systolic **heart murmur**, not always present.

Diagnosis is usually aided by **echocardiography** or angiography.

Prophylactic antibiotics as for **congenital heart disease** are usually advised preoperatively. Complications are unlikely unless mitral regurgitation is severe or left ventricular dysfunction is present.

Kowalski SE (1985) Can Anaesth Soc J; 32: 138–41

See also, Heart sounds

Mivacurium chloride. Non-depolarizing **neuromuscular blocking drug**, introduced in the UK in 1993. Tracheal intubation is possible approximately 2 minutes after a dose of 0.07–0.15 mg/kg. Effects last 10–20 minutes. Supplementary dose: 0.1 mg/kg. May be given by iv infusion at 0.2–0.5 mg/kg/h. Causes little or no cardiovascular instability, although **histamine** release may accompany high doses. Metabolized by plasma **cholinesterase** to highly water-soluble metabolites, excreted rapidly via the urine; **half-life** is 2–5 minutes. Also undergoes some hepatic metabolism. More easily reversed than atracurium or **vecuronium**. Has been suggested as an alternative to **suxamethonium**, especially in children, in whom onset and recovery are faster than in adults.

Mixed venous blood. Truly mixed venous blood is obtained from the right ventricle or pulmonary artery, since superior and inferior vena caval blood is different in composition, and mixes during passage through the heart.

Mixed venous O_2 saturation (S_vO_2) is related to arterial O_2 content, O_2 consumption and cardiac output; it may be monitored continuously via a fibreoptic bundle on a pulmonary artery catheter. S_vO_2 has been used as an indicator of O_2 supply/demand in critically ill patients, and as an early indicator of imminent haemodynamic failure; tissue **O_2 delivery** is considered critical at S_vO_2 of under 50% (normally 75%). The measurement is non-specific, however, and is increased by peripheral shunting, e.g. in **septic shock**.

Vincent JL (1992) Intensive Care Med; 18: 386–7
See also, Arteriovenous oxygen difference

MMV, *see Mandatory minute ventilation*

Mode. Expression of the central tendency of a set of observations or measurements. Equals that observation, or group of observations, which occurs the most often. Equals the **mean** for a normal distribution.
See also, Median; Statistical frequency distributions; Statistics

Molality. Number of **moles** of solute per kilogram of solvent. A molal solution contains 1 mole/kg.

Molarity. Number of **moles** of solute per litre of solution. A molar solution contains 1 mole/l.

Mole. SI **unit** of amount of substance. Defined as that quantity containing the same number of particles as there are atoms in 12 g of carbon-12. This number (**Avogadro's number**) equals 6.022×10^{23}.

Molecular weight (mw). Mass of a molecule, equal to the sum of atomic weights of its constituent atoms.

Monitoring. Adequate monitoring during anaesthesia and recovery is now generally accepted as improving patient safety and helping to reduce **anaesthetic morbidity and mortality**. Standards of minimal monitoring have been published in many countries, e.g. in the USA in 1986 and the UK in 1988. Failure to employ appropriate monitoring equipment is increasingly considered negligent. Devices should warn of adverse changes in the state of the patient, and of altered functioning of anaesthetic equipment.
- Most monitors involve electrical equipment. Technical considerations:
  - signal from patients may be:
    - primary electrical signals, e.g. **ECG, EEG**.
    - electrical signals derived from other energy forms, e.g. via pressure **transducers**.
    - evoked signals, e.g. **neuromuscular blockade monitoring, evoked potentials**.
  - skin electrodes are usually made of silver/silver chloride to reduce alterations in **impedance**, and to reduce the creation of interfering potentials within the electrode.

  - amplification/processing of the signal via intermediate components. Accuracy of reproduction is related to:
    - signal:noise ratio: improved by filtering, and averaging the signal so that background noise is cancelled out. Recording between two recording leads (differential input) also cancels out background noise, since the noise is in phase in both the leads.
    - baseline drift: may be random or due to the effect of temperature on semiconductors.
    - sensitivity of the amplifier: related to the voltage of the original signal (i.e. appropriate **gain**).
    - linearity of the response: distortion causes non-linear response characteristics.
    - **damping**.
    - frequency range: related to the **harmonics** of the measured signal.
    - matched output/input voltage, current, etc. of components.
    - interference; may be caused by:
      - **capacitance** between the patient and electrical equipment.
      - **inductance** of current in the patient, monitor wires, etc. by electrical equipment.
      - other electrical equipment, e.g. **diathermy**, other monitors, etc.
  - display of the signal, as e.g. a waveform on **oscilloscopes**, numerical display, galvanometer and/or paper strip, etc.
  - alarms are usually incorporated into monitors; limits are set to minimize inappropriate warnings without compromising sensitivity. Alarms of different devices are often of random pitch and frequency; standardization of alarms has been suggested.
  - risk of **electrocution and electrical burns** from electrical equipment.
- UK recommendations (**Association of Anaesthetists**):
  - presence of the anaesthetist is mandatory during the whole procedure, with adequate **record-keeping** and hand-over.
  - monitoring is instituted before induction and continued until **recovery**.
  - equipment monitoring: **O_2 failure warning device**, output O_2 analyser, and disconnection detection by expired tidal volume measurement, **capnography** and **airway pressure** measurement.
  - patient monitoring: continuous clinical observation of colour, respiration, pulse and response to surgery, and chest auscultation. ECG, **arterial BP measurement**, pulse **oximetry**, capnography, expired tidal volume, airway pressure and **temperature measurement** 'where appropriate'.
  - heart rate and BP recorded at regular intervals as appropriate.
  - nerve stimulator readily available.
  - direct BP measurement, **CVP** measurement, pulmonary artery pressures, **urine** output, **blood loss**, arterial blood gas analysis and blood tests as appropriate.
  - the same standards to apply for **sedation**, **regional anaesthesia** and short procedures, in any location.
  - clear instructions to be given to recovery staff, and appropriate monitoring used during recovery and transfer.

- USA recommendations (**American Society of Anesthesiologists**) for any general, regional or iv technique (extradural anaesthesia provision for labour or pain management was specifically excluded from the original standards, introduced first at Harvard):
  –presence of the anaesthetist during the whole procedure.
  –arterial BP and heart rate measured at least every 5 minutes.
  –ECG.
  –continuous monitoring: at least one of each for:
    –ventilation: palpation/observation of reservoir bag, auscultation of breath sounds, expired gas flow or capnography (the last is preferred).
    –circulation: palpation of pulse, auscultation of heart sounds, intra-arterial pressure trace, **pulse detector** or oximetry.
  –disconnection alarm for IPPV.
  –O_2 analyser.
  –temperature measurement readily available.
Monitoring in ICU is usually more complicated, but similar principles are employed.
Symposium Issue (1988) Anaesth Intensive Care; 16: 5–116
See also, Anaesthesia, depth of; Blood flow; Carbon dioxide measurement; Cardiac output measurement; Echocardiography; Gas analysis; Oxygen measurement; Pulmonary artery catheterization; Pulmonary wedge pressure; Respirometer

Monoamine oxidase (MAO). **Enzyme** present in mitochondria of most tissues, especially liver, intestinal mucosa, lung, kidney and central and peripheral **catecholamine** secreting nerve endings. Catalyses oxidative deamination of amines to aldehyde derivatives, e.g. $R\text{-}CH_2\text{-}NH_2 \rightarrow R\text{-}CHO$. Inactivates active amines including catecholamines, whether circulating, absorbed from the gut, or at adrenergic/**5–HT** nerve endings. Many products are subsequently metabolized by **catechol-*O*-methyl transferase** (COMT), and many products of COMT metabolism are subsequently metabolized by MAO.

Two distinct types have been identified: type A, mainly inactivating **noradrenaline** and 5HT, and type B, mainly inactivating tryptamine and phenylethylamine. **Dopamine** and tyramine are inactivated by both. Both are present in liver and brain; type B is thought to be predominant in certain CNS regions e.g. basal ganglia.

Non-specific **MAO inhibitors** are used to treat depression. Selegiline, used in **Parkinson's disease**, selectively inhibits type B, increasing central dopamine levels without exhibiting exaggerated response to dietary amines.

Monoamine oxidase inhibitors (MAOIs). Antidepressant drugs, developed in the 1950s from anti-**TB** drugs. Recently increasing in use following a period of unpopularity. Interact with **monamine oxidase** irreversibly, resynthesis of the enzyme taking at least 3 weeks.
- Anaesthetic importance:
  –interaction with **opioid analgesic drugs**: may be:
    –excitatory: may cause agitation, **hypertension**, tachycardia, hyperreflexia, hypertonus, pyrexia, **convulsions, coma**. Thought to be caused by excessive central **5-HT** activty, and only reported with **pethidine**, which reduces 5-HT uptake from nerve endings. Treatment includes α-**adrenergic receptor**

antagonists, vasodilator drugs and **chlorpromazine**. Steroids have been used.
  –depressive: may cause **hypoventilation, hypotension**, coma. Thought to be caused by impaired hepatic metabolism of opioid. **Naloxone** and directly acting vasopressors, e.g. **noradrenaline**, have been used for treatment.
  Morphine has been suggested as the opioid of choice, titrated carefully against effect. Although **fentanyl** and **phenoperidine** are related to pethidine, the former has been safely used; however experience is limited. **Pentazocine** has also been used safely.
  –**sympathomimetic drugs** may produce exaggerated hypertensive responses, especially those acting indirectly via **catecholamine** release, e.g. **ephedrine, metaraminol**. Directly acting drugs, e.g. noradrenaline, **adrenaline** and **isoprenaline** should be used in small amounts, if required. Catecholamines and drugs increasing catecholamine levels should be avoided, e.g. **pancuronium, ketamine, cocaine**, and adrenaline in local anaesthesic solutions (the last is controversial).
  –other iv and inhalational agents, **benzodiazepines** and non-depolarizing neuromuscular blocking drugs are considered safe; **doxapram** is considered unsafe.
  –phenelzine may decrease plasma **cholinesterase** levels.
Crises may also follow oral ingestion of active amines or precursors, e.g. in tyramine-rich food such as cheese and red wine, because of inhibition of the enzyme in the gut wall.

Traditional advice, to stop taking MAOIs 2–3 weeks preoperatively, is rarely given now, because of risks of worsening depression, and possible inadequacy of this interval.
Stack CG, Rogers P, Linter SPK (1988) Br J Anaesth; 60: 222–7

Monro–Kellie doctrine. The cranial cavity is a rigid closed container; thus any change in intracranial blood volume is accompanied by the opposite change in **CSF** volume, if **ICP** is maintained.
[Alexander Monro (1733–1817) and George Kellie (1700s), Scottish anatomists]

Morbidity and mortality, *see Anaesthetic morbidity and mortality*

Morphine hydrochloride/sulphate/tartrate. Opioid analgesic drug, in use for thousands of years as **opium** derived from poppy seeds. Isolated in 1803, and synthesized in 1952, although still obtained from poppies. The standard drug against which other opioids are compared.

Used for **premedication** and as an **analgesic drug**. Also useful in **pulmonary oedema**. Peak effect occurs 15–20 minutes after iv, and 60–90 minutes after im injection; action lasts 4–5 hours. Undergoes significant **first pass metabolism** if given orally. Undergoes hepatic dealkylation, oxidation and conjugation to morphine 3– and 6–glucuronide, excreted in urine. The latter compound has analgesic properties, and may be responsible for prolonged action, e.g. in renal impairment or chronic administration.
- Actions:
  –CNS:

–depression of:
  –respiratory centre; rate is reduced more than tidal volume. **Neonates** and the **elderly** are particularly susceptible.
  –**cough** reflex.
  –**pain** sensation, especially dull continuous pain. Most effective if given before the painful stimulus. Interpretation of painful stimuli is altered as well as pain sensation itself.
  –anxiety; morphine causes sedation and euphoria.
  –**ACTH** and prolactin secretion.
  –metabolic rate.
  –**vasomotor centre**; depression is now thought to be minimal, if it occurs at all.
–stimulation of:
  –**chemoreceptor trigger zone**.
  –parasympathetic nucleus of the 3rd **cranial nerve**, causing miosis.
  –**vasopressin** release.
  –vagus nerve; thought to result in occasional bradycardia.
  –higher centres; may cause dysphoria.
–muscle rigidity following high doses; thought to be caused by central interference with motor function, although the mechanism is unclear.
–may cause addiction.
–peripheral:
  –**histamine** release; may cause vasodilatation, bronchoconstriction, itching (typically of the nose), flushing. Hypotension may occur (partly a central effect).
  –constipation, delayed **gastric emptying** and reduced **lower oesophageal sphincter** tone. Increases the tone of biliary and genitourinary smooth muscle, including sphincters.
  –increases **catecholamine** release from the adrenal medulla.
• Dosage:
  –standard im, iv or sc dose: 0.1–0.15 mg/kg.
  –orally: 10 mg increased slowly up to 200 mg, 4 hourly. Sustained release preparation: from 10 mg 12 hourly.
  –has been given via buccal and rectal routes.
  Doses should be reduced in renal or hepatic failure.
[Morpheus, Greek God of Dreams]
See also, Spinal opioids

Mortality/survival prediction on intensive care unit.
Scoring systems may allow estimation of prognosis for individual patients, and comparison of different treatment regimens and between centres. Resource allocation depending partially on survival scores has been suggested, as a means of improving efficiency. Specific scoring systems exist, e.g. **coma scales** (e.g. **Glasgow coma scale** (GCS)), **trauma scales**, for **burns**, etc.
• Methods of assessing patients on ICU include:
  –simple five-point scale according to clinical judgement, e.g. certain to die; likely to die, etc. May correlate with outcome better than complicated scoring systems.
  –Therapeutic Intervention Scoring System (TISS): 80 therapeutic and monitoring variables, each scored 1–4; totals are added per 24 hours.
  –Acute Physiology Score (APS) and Simplified Acute Physiology Score (SAPS): comprised of 34 and 13 physiological variables respectively. The former has

been adapted to a statistical model to indicate mortality probability.
  –**APACHE scoring system** (Acute Physiology and Chronic Health Evaluation): derived from APS. The most widely used scoring system. Originally applied immediately on admission to ICU; serial measurements have also been used.
  –Mortality Prediction Models (MPMs): variables derived from multiple regression analysis applied to patient data. Each variable is assigned a coefficient for calculation of mortality probability immediately on admission, and thus is independent of treatment.
Civetta JM (1990) Crit Care Med; 18: 1487–90

Morton, William Thomas Green (1819–1868). US dentist, considered the founder of anaesthesia despite being pre-dated by **Clarke**, **Long** and **Wells**. Briefly practised with Wells in Boston in 1842–3, before entering Harvard Medical School in 1844, although he never completed his medical studies. Present at Wells' unsuccessful demonstration of N_2O at Harvard in 1844. Morton approached **Jackson** for advice on supplies of N_2O for further experiments. Jackson's suggestion of **diethyl ether** as a topical analgesic led to Morton's use of ether for inhalational anaesthesia for dental extraction on September 30th 1846. At the Massachusetts General Hospital on October 16th, he successfully anaesthetized Gilbert Abbott, whilst **Warren** excised a mass from the latter's jaw. Became demoralized by subsequent battles against Jackson's claim to the discovery, and against widespread infringement of his patent. His contribution was recognized only posthumously.
[Edward Gilbert Abbott (1825–1855), US printer]
See also, Letheon

Motor neurone disease (Amyotrophic lateral sclerosis). Progressive degenerative disorder of unknown aetiology, affecting spinal **motor neurones**, lower **cranial nerves** and motor cortex. More common in older men. Causes lower motor neurone-type weakness, typically with fasciculations, combined with increased reflexes of upper motor neurone lesions. Progressive bulbar palsy may occur, with dysarthria and dysphagia. Usually fatal within 5 years.
• Anaesthetic problems are related to:
  –possible laryngeal incompetence.
  –muscle weakness (including respiratory) and sensitivity to **neuromuscular blocking drugs**. Respiratory depressant effects of drugs are thus more pronounced. An exaggerated hyperkalaemic response to **suxamethonium** is theoretically possible but has not been reported.

Motor neurone, lower. Term used to describe motor neurones that directly innervate **muscle**, i.e. without other neurones interposed. Lesions of these neurones (lower motor neurone lesions) therefore result in complete cessation of neural input to the muscle, resulting in characteristic clinical features:
  –flaccid paralysis.
  –visible **fasciculations**, thought to be caused by spontaneous firing of neighbouring **motor units** that have taken over the affected muscle.
  –absent reflexes.
  –muscular atrophy.
  –**denervation hypersensitivity**. Thought to be the cause

of invisible fibrillation of muscle fibres. An increased hyperkalaemic response to **suxamethonium** may occur from 4 days to 7 months after injury.
See also, Motor neurone, upper

Motor neurone, upper. Term used to decribe neurones of the **motor pathways** excluding lower motor neurones. Thus include neurones of the motor cortex, cerebellar and extrapyramidal pathways, although the term commonly refers to the former only. Upper motor neurone lesions may thus occur at any level above the lower neurone cell bodies, producing characteristic features, after initial flaccid paralysis:
  –increased tone and spastic paralysis. Typically, muscle exhibits 'clasp-knife' rigidity, possibly due to activity of **muscle spindles** without inhibitory higher input.
  –increased reflexes and upwards plantar responses (Babinski reflex).
  –no **fasciculation**.
  –no atrophy.
  –an increased hyperkalaemic response to **suxamethonium** may occur from 10 days to 7 months after injury, although the mechanism is unclear.
[Joseph Babinski (1857–1932), French neurologist]
See also, Motor neurone, lower

Motor pathways. Consist of the following systems:
  –pyramidal pathways (Fig. 93): fibres arise from pyramidal cells of the motor cortex of the precentral gyrus and premotor area. Legs are represented uppermost, with the head at the lower part of the gyrus. Regions of greatest importance (e.g. face,

hands) have a disproportionately greater representation. Fibres then pass via the internal capsule (legs represented behind, face anteriorly), and via the cerebral peduncle and pons to the medulla, forming the pyramids. Most of the fibres decussate in the lower medulla and pass within the lateral corticospinal tract of the **spinal cord**. Some pass within the anterior corticospinal tract without decussating; these cross within the spinal cord at their spinal levels. Some fibres pass to **cranial nerve** motor nuclei. Most of the fibres synapse with intermediate **neurones**.
  –extrapyramidal pathways: less well-defined than the above system. Fibres arise from the premotor area and corpus striatum, and pass via the basal ganglia, substantia nigra and nuclear masses of the midbrain and hindbrain. They descend within the rubroreticulospinal and vestibulospinal tracts. Other pathways pass from the tectum of the midbrain and olives of the medulla. Concerned with control of movement.
  –cerebellar pathways: involve the **thalamus**, red nucleus, pons, medulla and cerebral cortex.
  –pathways of the **autonomic nervous system**.
See also, Motor neurone, lower; Motor neurone, upper; Spinal cord lesions

Motor unit. One lower **motor neurone** and the **muscle** fibres it innervates. In muscles for fine movement, e.g. of the eye and hand, motor units are small, i.e. under ten fibres per neurone. Muscles involved in posture may have up to 1000 fibres per neurone. All fibres of a motor unit are of the same type, i.e. fast or slow; the type is thought to be determined by characteristics of the nerve itself.

Mouth, *see Larynx; Pharynx; Teeth; Tongue*

Mouth gags. Devices used to hold open the patient's mouth, e.g. during **dental surgery** (Fig. 94). Held by the anaesthetist from behind the patient's head, they are grasped at the blades' pivot to ensure control of the blades during insertion. The blades' tips are usually covered with plastic or rubber to prevent dental damage, and are placed at the molars.
[Eugene L Doyen (1859–1916), French surgeon; Sir William Fergusson (1808–1877), Scottish-born London surgeon; Francis Mason (1837–1886), London surgeon]

MRI, *see Magnetic resonance imaging*

Multiple endocrine adenomatosis (MEA; Multiple endocrine neoplasia, MEN). Syndrome of multiple endocrine tumours; may occur in three groups:
  –type I: parathyroid adenoma, pancreatic adenoma or carcinoma, and anterior pituitary adenoma.
  –type II: medullary thyroid carcinoma, **phaeochromocytoma**, and parathyroid adenoma.
  –type III: medullary thyroid carcinoma, phaeochromocytoma, and mucosal neuromas or generalized **neurofibromatosis**.
Patients presenting for endocrine surgery may thus have other tumours and associated syndromes.
  May be inherited by autosomal dominant transmission.
See also, Apudomas; Hyperparathyroidism

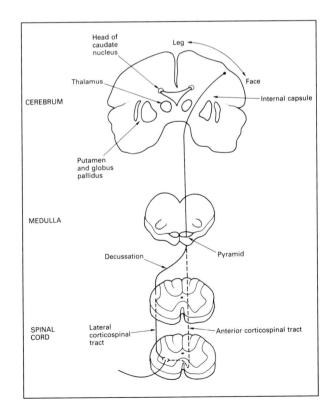

Figure 93 *Pyramidal motor system*

Multiple sclerosis, *see Demyelinating diseases*

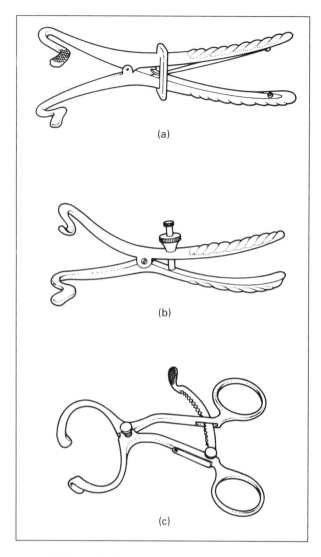

Figure 94 *Examples of mouth gags: (a) Fergusson; (b) Mason; (c) Doyen*

Murphy eye, *see Tracheal tubes*

Muscarine and muscarinic receptors. Muscarine, an alkaloid extracted from certain mushrooms, mimics certain actions of **acetylcholine** (hence it is a **parasympathomimetic drug**) and was used to investigate the physiology of the **autonomic nervous system**. It stimulates postganglionic **acetylcholine receptors** (muscarinic receptors) at effector organs of the **parasympathetic nervous system**, and at sweat glands of the **sympathetic nervous system**. It also causes Parkinsonian tremor, ataxia and rigidity; thus muscarinic receptors are thought to exist in the CNS. Other receptors may be involved in an inhibitory role at adrenergic nerve endings, e.g. in the heart, and at autonomic ganglia.

Division of receptors into subtypes is suggested by experimental work: M_1 (stimulation of gastric acid secretion; may be present at sympathetic ganglia), M_2 (heart), and M_3 (causes smooth muscle contraction, and lacrimal and salivary gland secretion). Pirenzepine is thought to antagonize M_1 receptors.

Muscle. Contractile tissue; may be:
- skeletal (striated; voluntary):
    - the most abundant form.
    - normally contracts only when stimulated.
    - no connections between individual fibres.
    - comprised of elongated cylindrical fibres, each surrounded by its sarcolemma (muscle cell membrane). Each fibre contains myofibrils, containing **actin** and **myosin** filaments and surrounded by sarcoplasmic reticulum and mitochondria. The T-tubule system invaginates from the sarcolemma to connect all myofibrils with the extracellular space.
    - microscopically visible striations are due to myosin and actin arrangements, labelled for historical reasons (Fig. 95). The sarcomere (portion between adjacent Z lines) shortens during **muscle contraction**.

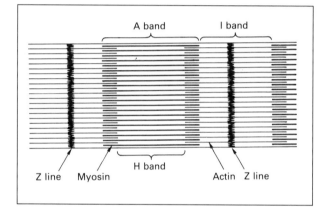

Figure 95 *Microscopic appearance of myofibril*

- different types of fibres:
    - type I: red muscle; responds slowly with slow metabolism and high oxidative capacity (high **myoglobin**, mitochondria and capillary content). Suitable for prolonged contraction, e.g. postural muscles.
    - type IIB: white muscle, short contracting with low oxidative capacity. Suitable for rapid skilled movement, e.g. eye and hand muscles.
    - type IIA: as for IIB but with high oxidative capacity, i.e. red. Uncommon in humans.
- cardiac:
    - similar to slow striated muscle, but fibres are branched, and joined end-to-end by intercalated discs; also connected to adjacent fibres by gap junctions. Requires continuous O_2 supply.
    - has spontaneous pacemaker activity, due to slow depolarization between **action potentials**.
    - cannot exhibit **tetanic contraction**, due to a prolonged **refractory period**.
- smooth:
    - no striations; actin and myosin filaments arranged randomly.
    - occurs in sheets of interconnecting cells (e.g. visceral) or multiunits (e.g. iris).
    - exhibits slow spontaneous activity; also responsive to stimulation of the **autonomic nervous system**. Visceral muscle contracts if stretched.

See also, Motor unit; Muscle spindles; Neuromuscular junction

Muscle contraction. Involves the following steps:
- –depolarization of the postsynaptic **membrane** at the **neuromuscular junction**.
- –area of depolarization spreads across the **muscle** membrane and into the muscle bulk via the T-tubule system.
- –depolarization causes release and mobilization of intracellular **calcium** ions from sarcoplasmic reticulum.
- –calcium ions bind to the troponin component of the **actin** complex, causing displacement of the tropomyosin component from **myosin** binding sites.
- –myosin can now bind to actin, with hydrolysis of **ATP**, structural alteration of myosin and shortening of muscle fibres. ATPase is present on myosin molecule heads. The process repeats with further muscle shortening.
- –further hydrolysis of ATP allows uptake of calcium, and muscle relaxation.

A single twitch caused by an **action potential** of 1 ms lasts up to 200 ms. Contraction may be isometric (force increases but muscle length remains constant) or isotonic (force is constant and muscle shortens). Repeated fast stimulation results in summation of contraction, since there is inadequate time for relaxation between stimuli. Above a certain frequency, **tetanic contraction** occurs.

ATP is derived from **glycolysis** and from dephosphorylation of phosphorylcreatine, stored during rest. Anaerobic **glycolysis** and metabolism of free fatty acids are also used. During severe exercise, anaerobic glycolysis predominates, incurring an O_2 debt which is paid back during recovery.

Muscle relaxants, *see Neuromuscular blocking drugs*

Muscle spindles. Encapsulated structures present in and parallel to skeletal **muscle**. Contain up to ten specialized muscle (intrafusal) fibres, attached to the ordinary muscle (extrafusal) fibres or to their tendons. **Muscle contraction** thus results in shortening of the spindles. Sensory **nerve** fibres from the spindles end on the motor **neurones** supplying the extrafusal muscle fibres of that muscle. They transmit impulses when stretched; thus passive muscle stretching causes reflex contraction, e.g. knee jerk **reflex arc**. Discharge in some afferent fibres is proportional to degree of stretch; discharge in others is also proportional to speed of stretch. Muscle contraction reduces tension within the spindle, reducing the afferent discharge. Activation of the reflex also inhibits contraction of opposing muscle groups (reciprocal innervation) via an inhibitory spinal interneurone.

Small γ-motor fibres innervate the ends of the intrafusal fibres, causing them to contract. This stretches the central portions, with reflex extrafusal fibre contraction as before, and increases the sensitivity of the spindles to passive stretching. γ-Motor activity is controlled by descending pathways in the spinal cord; thus muscle tone and posture is controlled at both spinal and supraspinal levels. Increased muscle tone and clonus seen in upper **motor neurone** lesions may result from overactive γ-activity due to interruption of inhibitory descending pathways. γ-Activity is also increased in anxiety, resulting in exaggerated tremor.

Increased passive stretching of a muscle eventually causes sudden relaxation, due to stimulation of Golgi tendon organs within the muscle tendons. This inverse stretch reflex is exaggerated in upper motor neurone lesions (clasp-knife effect).
[Camillo Golgi (1843–1926), Italian physician]

Muscular dystrophies. Rare (up to 30:100 000 live births) hereditary disorders of **muscle**, involving progressive destruction of mainly skeletal, but also cardiac, muscle. Mechanism is unknown but thought to involve abnormal muscle **membrane** function. Plasma creatine kinase levels may be increased. Classified according to inheritance: may be sex-linked (e.g. Duchenne's, Becker's), autosomal dominant (e.g. facioscapulohumeral, ocular, pharyngeal) or recessive (e.g. limb girdle):
- –Duchenne's: most common form. Affects boys usually from 3 to 5 years old; usually fatal by the early twenties. A similar autosomal recessive form may occur in girls.
- –Becker's, facioscapulohumeral, limb girdle: less severe, with later onset and death. Cardiac involvement is less common.
- **Orthopaedic surgery** is common for limb contractures, etc. Severe forms may present significant anaesthetic risk:
  - –weak respiratory muscles: impaired ventilation, sputum clearance, etc. Pre-existing and postoperative chest infection is more likely. Patients may be more sensitive to respiratory depressant drugs and neuromuscular blocking drugs.
  - –rhabdomyolysis may follow **suxamethonium** or volatile anaesthetic agents, typically following prolonged exposure to the latter. Severe **hyperkalaemia** and **myoglobinuria** may result. **MH** may also be commoner.
  - –cardiac involvement, with risk of failure, arrhythmias, hypotension, etc.

[Guillaume Duchenne (1806–1875), French neurologist; PE Becker, German geneticist]
Smith CL, Bush GH (1985) Br J Anaesth; 57: 1113–18

MVV, Maximal voluntary ventilation, *see Lung function tests*

Myasthenia gravis. **Autoimmune disease** characterized by skeletal **muscle** weakness and increased fatigability. Incidence is 1:20 000–30 000; most common in young women (female:male 3:2). May also occur in neonates born to affected mothers, and may be caused by drugs, e.g. penicillamine.

Caused by an immune response directed against **acetylcholine receptors** at the **neuromuscular junction**. Receptors are reduced in number, with abnormal turnover and loss of synaptic folds. Antireceptor antibodies are present in up to 90% of patients, but their level is unrelated to severity. Hyperplasia of the thymus gland is present in 65% of cases, thymoma in 12%. The role of the thymus is unclear, but it may involve initiation of the acetylcholine receptor antibody response, or secretion of immunogenic factors.
- Features:
  - –weakness typically worse on exertion and improving with rest. Has been classified according to the muscles affected:
    - –ocular, with/without symptomless peripheral involvement.

303

–generalized, with/without bulbar involvement.

–acute fulminating: rapid and progressive with respiratory and bulbar involvement.

–late severe: slow (over 2 years) progression of the ocular group.

–myasthenic crises (suddenly worsening and spreading weakness) may be provoked by drug omission, infection, stress, etc.

–other autoimmune diseases may be associated.

–increased sensitivity to non-depolarizing **neuromuscular blocking drugs**. The effects of a small dose of **tubocurarine** administered systemically or into an isolated (by tourniquet) limb have been used to aid diagnosis; this is rarely performed now.

–marked improvement following iv **edrophonium** 2 + 8 mg (Tensilon test).

–**EMG** reveals **fade** in muscle **action potentials** and twitch height on repeated stimulation.

–antibody testing may be used in diagnosis.

● Treatment:

–**acetylcholinesterase inhibitors**, e.g. **pyridostigmine** 30–180 mg 6 hourly, **neostigmine** 15–30 mg 4 hourly. Muscarinic side effects include miosis, colic, lacrimation, diarrhoea, salivation; **atropine** may be given to reduce these. May cause **cholinergic crisis** in overdosage; distinguished from myasthenic crises by injection of edrophonium 2 mg. Myasthenic crises improve transiently, cholinergic crises do not.

–immunosuppressive therapy:

–**steroid therapy**, e.g. prednisolone 1 mg/kg on alternate days. Often used in severe cases. Usually started in hospital because of possible deterioration.

–azathioprine 1–2 mg/kg/day; cyclophosphamide 1–2 mg/kg/day.

–**plasmapheresis**, especially combined with immunosuppressive therapy. Used in severe cases.

–thymectomy: indications are controversial. Some improvement is claimed in most patients. Anaesthetic management:

–preoperatively: assessment of respiratory function is important. Pyridostigmine is usually withheld on the morning of surgery. Preoperative plasmapheresis and steroids have been used. Potassium abnormalities increase muscle weakness and should be corrected.

–peroperatively: tracheal intubation and IPPV are usually performed without neuromuscular blocking drugs, using a volatile agent and **lignocaine** spray. **Atracurium** in small doses has been suggested over other drugs. **TIVA** has also been used. Resistance to **suxamethonium** has been reported, although the response is usually normal. Surgery is performed via a suprasternal or trans-sternal route. Haemorrhage and pneumothorax may occur. The tracheal tube may be left *in situ* and ventilation monitored on ICU or HDU; tracheal extubation is usually possible within a few hours postoperatively, although 24–48 hours' intubation is preferred in some centres. Extubation may be possible immediately postoperatively.

–postoperatively: pyridostigmine may be restarted, usually in reduced dosage. Close monitoring of respiration and **physiotherapy** are required. Postoperative **atelectasis** and infection are common.

Anaesthetic management of patients with myasthenia gravis for other surgery should follow the above guidelines. Regional techniques, where feasible, have been suggested as being safer.

Baraka A (1992) Can J Anaesth; 39: 476–86

See also, Myasthenic syndrome

Myasthenic syndrome (Eaton-Lambert syndrome; Pseudomyasthenia). Rare syndrome of peripheral **muscle** weakness associated with underlying carcinoma (usually bronchial) or rarely **autoimmune disease** (e.g. thyroiditis). May precede clinical evidence of carcinoma by up to 2 years.

● Distinguished from **myasthenia gravis** thus:

–classically improves on repetitive muscle use.

–usually affects proximal limb muscles.

–tendon reflexes are depressed or absent.

–power is only slightly improved by **neostigmine**, despite possible improvement following **edrophonium**.

–caused by defective release of **acetylcholine** from presynaptic nerve endings, with normal postsynaptic receptors.

EMG may aid diagnosis.

May improve with oral guanidine hydrochloride 30–50 mg/kg thrice daily or **aminopyridine**; **steroid therapy** and **plasmapheresis** have been tried.

General anaesthetic considerations are as for myasthenia gravis. There is increased sensitivity to non-depolarizing and depolarizing **neuromuscular blocking drugs**. **Atracurium** has been suggested as the drug of choice. Postoperative respiratory complications are more likely with severe weakness.

[LM Eaton (1905–1958), US neurologist; Edward H Lambert, US neurophysiologist]

Myelin. Lipoprotein derived from multiple layers of cell **membranes**, encasing the axons of myelinated **neurones**. Arises from Schwann cells in the peripheral nervous system (one cell to one axon portion), and from oligodendrocytes in the CNS (one cell to up to 40 axon portions). Deficient at 1 mm intervals (nodes of Ranvier). Unmyelinated peripheral nerves are merely encased in Schwann cell cytoplasm. Acts as an insulating sheath, increasing speed of **nerve conduction** in myelinated nerves by restricting membrane depolarization to the nodes of Ranvier; depolarization 'jumps' from node to node (saltatory conduction) instead of slower, smooth progression along unmyelinated nerves.

[Theodor Schwann (1810–1882), German physiologist; Louis Ranvier (1835–1922), French physician and pathologist]

Myocardial contractility. Force with which the myocardium contracts; thus a major determinant of **stroke volume** and **cardiac output**, and myocardial O_2 demand.

● Increased by:

–intrinsic mechanisms:

–**Starling's law**.

–**Anrep effect**.

–**Bowditch effect**.

–extrinsic factors:

–**sympathetic nervous system** activity.

–**catecholamines** via β1–**adrenergic receptors**.

–**inotropic drugs**.

- Decreased by:
  - –reduced filling (Starling's law).
  - –**parasympathetic nervous system** (slight effect).
  - –**hypoxaemia** and **hypercapnia** (via direct effects; also cause increased sympathetic activity).
  - –**acidosis** and **alkalosis**.
  - –cardiac disease, e.g. **ischaemic heart disease, cardiomyopathy**, myocarditis, etc.
  - –electrolyte disturbances, e.g. **hyperkalaemia, hypocalcaemia**.
  - –drugs, e.g. most **iv** and **inhalational anaesthetic agents, antiarrhythmic drugs**.
- Assessment is difficult; indirect methods include measurement of:
  - –stroke volume and **stroke work**.
  - –speed of contraction.
  - –cardiac output.
  - –ratio of **left ventricular end-diastolic pressure** to **left ventricular end-diastolic volume**.
  - –peak left ventricular pressure.
  - –**ejection fraction**.

Myocardial infarction (MI). Consequence of unrelieved **myocardial ischaemia**. Usually starts at the endothelium, spreading outwards. The left ventricle is usually affected, but it may involve the right ventricle or atria. Most acute MIs are associated with coronary vessel thrombosis.

- Features:
  - –pain as for ischaemia, but more severe and persistent (MI may be silent, especially in the elderly and possibly perioperatively).
  - –**arrhythmias. Cardiac arrest** may occur.
  - –sweating, pallor, dyspnoea.
  - –**hypertension** or **hypotension**.
  - –**cardiac failure** and **cardiogenic shock**.
  - –may lead to:
    - –ventricular rupture, usually 5–8 days later.
    - –ventricular aneurysm.
    - –interventricular septum rutpure, usually 4–6 days later.
    - –papillary muscle damage and **mitral regurgitation**.
    - –mural thrombus formation and systemic embolism.
    - –**PE**.
  - –Dressler's syndrome: **pericarditis**, pleurisy and pneumonitis, typically 4–6 weeks later.
- Investigations:
  - –**ECG** changes: typically **T wave** changes and **S–T segment** elevation with **Q waves** in leads overlying the infarct. S–T elevation usually lasts for for under 2 weeks, T wave inversion for several months, and Q waves for at least several years (Fig. 96). Persistent S–T elevation may indicate ventricular aneurysm or an area of dyskinetic myocardium. Q waves may be absent in subendocardial infarction. Other changes include abnormalities of the **P wave** and **P–R interval** in atrial infarction, conduction defects, e.g. **bundle branch block** and **heart block**, and arrhythmias.
  - –**cardiac enzymes** may show characteristic changes.
  - –**nuclear cardiology** may reveal areas of infarcted muscle. **Echocardiography** and other imaging techniques may reveal areas of reduced or absent contraction.
- Differential diagnosis: pain and ECG changes may occur with lesions of:
  - –heart/great vessels, e.g. **aortic dissection**, pericarditis.
  - –lung, e.g. PE, **chest infection**.
  - –oesophagus, e.g. spasm, inflammation, rupture.
  - –abdominal organs, e.g. **peptic ulcer disease, pancreatitis**, cholecystitis.
- Medical management:
  - –analgesia, e.g. iv **opioid analgesic drugs**.
  - –systemic **fibrinolytic drugs** within 24 hours. Oral **aspirin** therapy is usually commenced but use of **heparin** is associated with increased risk of bleeding.
  - –monitoring, bed rest and O_2 therapy, usually within a **coronary care unit**. Management of the above complications. **Pulmonary artery catheterization** and use of **inotropic** and **vasodilator drugs** may be required.
  - –nitrates and β-**adrenergic receptor antagonists** are used in some units to restrict infarct size. **Magnesium sulphate** has recently been shown to reduce mortality; 8 mmol is given over 15 minutes, followed by 65 mmol over 24 hours.
  - –consideration for **cardiac surgery** if angina or surgical complications develop post infarct.
- Perioperative MI has been investigated by several studies. Summary of findings:
  - –with previous MI, overall reinfarction rate is 6–7% (if no previous MI, infarction rate is 0.1–0.2%).
  - –reinfarction rate is related to the time since the MI:
    - –within 3 months of surgery: 20–30%.
    - –within 4–6 months: 10–20%.
    - –greater than 6 months: 4–5%.
  - –aggressive management, e.g. **pulmonary artery catheterization**, use of **inotropic** and **vasodilator drugs**, admission to ICU, etc., has been reported to lower the overall infarction rate to 2%, and the reinfarction rates as follows:
    - –MI within 3 months: under 6%.
    - –within 4–6 months: 2–3%.
    - –greater than 6 months: 1–2%.
  - However, the statistical analysis used has been criticized, and the value of routine intensive monitoring and treatment remains controversial, especially when the increased cost is considered.
  - –perioperative reinfarction carries increased mortality (up to 70%), and is commonest on the 3rd postoperative day.
  - –incidence of silent MI may be higher.
  - –unstable angina, peroperative hypotension, prolonged surgery, and upper abdominal/thoracic or vascular surgery have been identified as risk factors.
  - –risk is not increased by previous cardiac surgery.
  - –risk is not associated with the type of anaesthetic or drugs used.
  - –**cardiac risk index** has been developed for assessment of risk of death or severe perioperative cardiovascular complications. Presence of cardiac failure is the

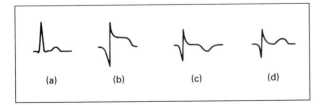

Figure 96 *Typical changes in ECG following MI: (a) normal; (b) immediate; (c) few weeks; (d) few months*

most important risk factor. Other factors are related to arrhythmias, age and general condition of the patient.

–reinfarction is often associated with peroperative myocardial ischaemia detected by S–T depression. It is not always associated with hypertension or hypotension.

• Risk of perioperative MI is thus reduced by:

–postponment of elective surgery until at least 6 months after MI.

–treatment of preoperative risk factors where possible.

–avoidance of myocardial ischaemia as for **ischaemic heart disease**.

[William Dressler (1890–1969), US cardiologist]

Maille JG, Boulanger M, Dyrda I, Tremblay N (1986) Can Anaesth Soc J; 33: 808–19

Myocardial ischaemia. Inadequate blood supply to the myocardium. Effects are related to myocardial O_2 supply/demand balance; largely dependent on:

–supply:

  –**coronary blood flow**:

    –aortic end-distolic pressure minus left ventricular end-diastolic pressure.

    –length of diastole.

    –coronary vessels: calibre is usually maintained by **autoregulation**. Stenosis may be caused by atheroma, thrombosis and spasm. Collateral vessels are important (e.g. **coronary steal**). The subendocardial region is most at risk of ischaemia.

    –blood **viscosity**.

  –O_2 content.

–demand:

  –**myocardial contractility** and wall tension.

  –**heart rate**.

• Effects:

–reversible increases in **hydrogen ion**, **potassium**, phosphate, **lactate**, **adenosine**, etc. Unless ischaemia is corrected within about 30 minutes, permanent damage ensues, with release of **cardiac enzymes** and **myoglobin**, i.e. **MI** occurs.

–**ECG** changes: thought to be caused by ion leakage across the ischaemic myocardial membrane, altering membrane potentials and causing current flow between normal and ischaemic areas. **S–T segment** changes are most common; depression is due to subendocardial ischaemia, elevation due to transmural ischaemia. **Arrhythmias** may occur.

–impaired myocardial contraction: first depressed, then absent, then myocardial lengthening with worsening ischaemia.

–pain (angina): possibly due to increased in potassium or **substance P**. Pain is typically steady, crushing and midsternal, radiating across the chest, to the neck or arms. Related to exertion, cold or emotion and relieved by rest, it may be absent (silent ischaemia). Unstable angina is thought to be caused by repeated small thromboses, with infarction following if vessel patency is not maintained. Dyspnoea, sweating, etc. may occur.

• Detection:

–symptoms and signs as above.

–detection of reduced supply/increased demand. Indices of supply include **diastolic pressure time index**. Indices of demand include **rate–pressure**

product and **tension time index**. **Endocardial viability ratio** has been used to indicate the ratio between supply and demand.

–ECG. Preoperative 'silent' ischaemia (i.e. without symptoms) has been found in up to 15% of patients over 40 years old; the significance of this in terms of outcome is unknown. The figure is higher for patients presenting for vascular surgery.

–**pulmonary capillary wedge pressure** monitoring.

–**echocardiography**.

–**nuclear cardiography**.

–**coronary sinus catheterization**.

Mangano DT (1990) Anesthesiology; 72: 153–84

See also, Monitoring; Myocardial metabolism

Myocardial metabolism. Myocardial O_2 consumption is normally about 30 ml/min (10 ml/100 g/min). **Coronary blood flow** is directly proportional; the mechanism is unclear but may involve **adenosine**, CO_2, **potassium** ions, **prostaglandins**, **hydrogen ions** and **lactate**. O_2 extraction from blood is about 70%; thus increased demands are met mainly by increasing blood flow. The main energy substrate is free fatty acids; other substrates include glucose, pyruvate and lactate. Utilization of the latter compounds increases in ischaemia.

O_2 requirements are reduced by volatile anaesthetic agents and other negative inotropes, e.g. **β-adrenergic receptor antagonists**. Effects on other factors determining myocardial O_2 supply/demand may be important, e.g. possibility of **coronary steal** and tachycardia with **isoflurane**. **Etomidate** and **propofol** may decrease demand; other iv agents may increase it if tachycardia occurs.

Myofascial pain syndromes. Dysfunction and usually **pain** in one or more muscle/muscle groups, associated with **trigger point** activity. May follow acute strain or repeated use. Typically associated with patterns of **referred pain**, e.g. trigger points in the neck with facial pain, trigger points in the shoulder with arm pain, etc. Identified trigger points may be injected with local anaesthetic, treated with **acupuncture**, ultrasound, pressure, etc., or the muscles passively stretched using a cold spray to allow adequate relaxation.

Myoglobin. Iron-containing molecule with mw 17 000. Similar to **haemoglobin**, but binds only one molecule of O_2 per molecule. Its O_2 dissociation curve is to the left of that of haemoglobin, being a rectangular hyperbola with a steep rise to a plateau. The **Bohr effect** does not occur. 95% saturated at Po_2 of 5.3 kP_a (40 mmHg), falling below 65% saturation only at Po_2 below 1 kP_a (7.5 mmHg). Found in skeletal and heart **muscle**, where it binds O_2 from arterial haemoglobin, releasing it at O_2 tensions close to zero. Thus it acts as an O_2 transporter and reservoir for contracting muscle.

See also, Oxyhaemoglobin dissociation curve

Myoglobinuria. Presence of **myoglobin** in the urine, colouring it red. Results from skeletal muscle breakdown (rhabdomyolysis) due to:

–crush injury (**crush syndrome**).

–prolonged immobility/**hypothermia** from any cause, especially **poisoning and overdoses** (and particularly **opioid overdose**).

–extreme exertion.

–polymyositis, myopathies, e.g. alcoholic, deficiency states, congenital conditions, or associated with viral infections.
–toxins, e.g. of sea snakes, multiple wasp stings.
–**MH**.
–**neuroleptic malignant syndrome**.
–**carbon monoxide poisoning**.
–heatstroke.
–paroxysmal myoglobinuria: rare disorder of muscle pain, weakness, paralysis and myoglobinuria. Most common in young men/children.

Affected muscles are classically painful and oedematous. Creatine kinase levels may be markedly raised. Myoglobin is readily filtered by the kidneys because of its small size. May be associated with **renal failure**, possibly due to tubular obstruction; myoglobin itself is not thought to be directly nephrotoxic. Maintenance of good hydration and **urine** output is thought to prevent renal impairment.

Myosin. Muscle protein (mw 460 000), consisting of two heavy and four light chains. Globular portions of the molecules contain ATPase and **actin** binding sites, and project sideways from myosin filaments.
See also, Muscle contraction

Myotomes. Inner parts of embryonic somites, differentiating into skeletal muscle and related to their corresponding **dermatomes**. Although the origins of certain skeletal muscle groups are controversial, they tend to retain their original somatic nerve supply; thus particular **spinal nerves** may be assessed clinically by testing specific muscles or groups (Table 23). Used to assess neurological lesions and the extent of **spinal/extradural anaesthesia**, etc.

Myotonia congenita. Autosomal dominant disorder of skeletal muscle. No systemic symptoms occur other than myotonia (involuntarily sustained muscle contraction

Table 23. Segmental innervation of limb muscles

Movement	Muscle(s)	Level
Shoulder		
Abduction	Supraspinatus	C4–5
External rotation	Infraspinatus	C4–5
Adduction	Pectoralis	C6–8
Elbow		
Flexion/supination	Biceps	C5–6
Pronation	Pronators	C6–7
Extension	Triceps	C7–8
Wrist		
Extension/radial flexion		C6–7
Ulnar flexion		C7–8
Fingers		
Extension	Long extensors	C7
Flexion	Long flexors	C8
Spreading and closing	All short muscles of the hand	T1
Hip		
Flexion	Iliopsoas	L1–3
Extension	Gluteal	L5–S2
Knee		
Extension	Quadriceps	L3–4
Flexion	Hamstrings	L5–S2
Ankle		
Extension	Anterior tibial	L4–5
Flexion	Calf muscles	S1–2

following stimulation) exacerbated by cold and rest, and relieved by exercise. A more common, milder form is inherited as autosomal recessive. Anaesthetic management is as for **dystrophia myotonica**. Hypothermia should be avoided.

Myxoedema, *see Hypothyroidism*

N

Nalbuphine hydrochloride. Opioid analgesic drug and **opioid receptor antagonist**, synthesized in 1968. Partial agonist at kappa and sigma **opioid receptors**, and antagonist at mu receptors. Used for **premedication**, anaesthesia and treatment of pain. Active within 2–3 minutes of iv, or 15 minutes of im, injection. **Half-life** is about 5 hours. Undergoes hepatic metabolism and excreted renally. Side effects such as vomiting are thought to be less than with **morphine**, although maximal analgesia attainable is also less. Psychomimetic effects are less problematic than with **pentazocine**.
- Dosage: 0.1–0.3 mg/kg iv/im/sc. Up to 1.0 mg/kg iv has been used during anaesthesia.

Nalorphine hydrochloride/hydrobromide. Opioid analgesic drug and **opioid receptor antagonist**, synthesized in 1941. Partial agonist at kappa and sigma **opioid receptors**, and antagonist at mu receptors. Psychomimetic effects are common at analgesic doses (5–10 mg). No longer available.

Naloxone hydrochloride. Opioid receptor antagonist, synthesized in 1961. *N*-allyl derivative of **oxymorphone**. Has no agonist properties. Used to reverse unwanted effects of **opioid analgesic drugs**, e.g. sedation, respiratory depression, spasm of the biliary sphincter. Also reverses opioid-mediated analgesia. Reverses the effects of **pentazocine** but not **buprenorphine**. Has been used to reverse ventilatory depression and pruritus following **spinal opioids**, without reversing analgesia. Has also been used in **poisoning and overdose** due to other depressant drugs, e.g. **alcohol, benzodiazepines, barbiturates**, although its efficacy is disputed. Reportedly useful in **septic shock**, increasing BP and cardiac output; the mechanism is unclear but may involve increase of endogenous **catecholamine** secretion. Effective within 1–2 minutes of iv injection, with a **half-life** of 1–2 hours; thus depressant effects of opioid analgesic drugs may recur after a few hours. Metabolized in the liver and excreted renally.
- Dosage:
  - –opioid poisoning: 0.4–2.0 mg iv/im/sc, repeated after 2–3 minutes to a total of 10 mg. Administration by infusion (3–10 µg/kg/h) may be required.
  - –postoperatively: 1.5–3 µg/kg iv, followed by 1.5 µg/kg repeated every 2 minutes as required. Infusion or im injection may be used to prevent later resedation.
  - –neonatal resuscitation: 10 µg/kg im, iv or sc repeated every 2–3 minutes or 60 µg/kg im as a single injection.
- Side effects: **hypertension, arrhythmias, pulmonary oedema** and **cardiac arrest** have followed sudden iv injection, possibly due to sudden catecholamine release secondary to reversal of sedation and analgesia.

Acute withdrawal may be precipitated in patients addicted to opioids.

Naltrexone hydrochloride. Opioid receptor antagonist, synthesized in 1965. Derived from **naloxone**, with similar actions but longer duration (24 hours after a single dose). Use is restricted to treatment of opioid dependence.
- Dosage: 25–50 mg/day orally.

Narcotic drugs. Strictly, drugs which induce sleep, but the term usually refers to **morphine**-like drugs. Preferred terms include **opiates, opioids** and **opioid analgesic drugs**.

Nasal inhalers. Used instead of **facepieces** for **dental anaesthesia**. Designed to fit over the nose, leaving the mouth free. During **induction of anaesthesia**, the patient is instructed not to 'mouth breathe'. During anaesthesia, a mouth pack prevents mouth breathing.
- Different types:
  - –Goldman's: black rubber, with an inflatable rim as for facepieces. Incorporates an **adjustable pressure-limiting valve**, and attaches to the breathing system over the patient's forehead. It should be held from behind the patient's head using both thumbs whilst the other fingers support the jaw. May also be held with a head **harness** using two studs incorporated into the sides.
  - –McKesson's: made of malleable black rubber, thus adjustable. Connected to the breathing system via two tubes which pass around the sides of the head to meet behind, helping to hold the inhaler in place. Incorporates an expiratory valve.
  - –newer types are made of plastic, and may incorporate unidirectional gas flow, e.g. through inspiratory and expiratory tubes passing around the head. **Scavenging** of exhaled gases is thus aided.

[Victor Goldman, London anaesthetist]

Nasal positive pressure ventilation. An alternative to **IPPV** via **tracheostomy** in patients who require nocturnal IPPV, e.g. central **sleep apnoea**, severe respiratory muscle weakness and skeletal deformities. Has been suggested for end-stage **COAD** or during **weaning**. Applied via a tightly-fitting nasal mask attached with a harness. Requires a ventilator capable of delivering twice-normal tidal volumes, since **dead space** is very high and the facial tissues very compliant.

BIPAP (Bi-level positive airway pressure) is the trade name for a technique in which two levels of positive pressure are provided. During exhalation, pressure is variably positive or near atmospheric; during inspiration pressure is variably positive. Airflow in the patient circuit is sensed by a **transducer** and augmented to a preset level of ventilation even if leaks occur around the mask. Cycling between inspiratory and expiratory modes may be triggered by the patient's spontaneous breaths, or timed according to preset controls (cycling either fully automatically or only if the patient fails to take a spontaneous breath within a certain time period). **CPAP** may also be delivered in either mode. BIPAP may also be administered via an oral mask.

Wedzicha W (1992) Br J Hosp Med; 47; 257–61

Nasogastric intubation. Performed for enteral **nutrition**, or gastric drainage. Fine bore tubes are used for the former, usually inserted using a wire stilette which is removed after placement. Larger tubes (e.g. 10–16 Ch) are used for gastric drainage, e.g. following abdominal surgery or in intestinal obstruction. They may be placed in the awake patient (who aids placement by swallowing or sipping water) or unconscious patient (e.g. after induction of anaesthesia, either before or after tracheal intubation). Placement can often be performed blindly, and may be aided by passage through a plain nasal tracheal tube placed into the pharynx. Placement may require direct vision using a laryngoscope and **forceps** (the oesophagus lies posterior to the **larynx** and to the left of the midline). Correct placement is confirmed by aspiration of gastric contents (may be tested for acidity), auscultation over the left hypochondrium during injection of air, palpation by the surgeon during surgery or abdominal X-ray. If already in place, withdrawal of the tube prior to induction of anaesthesia has been suggested, to avoid increasing gastro-oesophageal reflux or rendering **cricoid pressure** inefficient. However, this practice is controversial.

National Halothane Study, *see Halothane hepatitis*

Natriuretic hormone, *see Atrial natriuretic peptide*

Nausea, *see Vomiting*

Near-drowning. Defined as initial survival following immersion in liquid, usually water; death at the time of immersion may be due to anoxia (drowning), or **cardiac arrest** caused by sudden extreme lowering of temperature (immersion syndrome). May eventually lead to death from other causes, e.g. **ARDS**.

Autopsy following drowning reveals little or no lung water in 15% of cases (dry drowning); **laryngospasm** following initial laryngeal contamination has been suggested. In 85% of cases, pulmonary aspiration of water occurs (wet drowing) this may involve:
- –fresh water: systemic absorption may cause **haemolysis**, **haemodilution** and electrolyte distubances.
- –salt water: draws water into the lungs.

Both types cause **pulmonary oedema** and **hypoxaemia**. Haemodynamic changes due to fluid shifts are rare.

Other adverse factors include **hypothermia**, **aspiration of gastric contents**, and predisposing conditions, e.g. **alcohol** or drug abuse, **trauma**, **epilepsy**, **MI**, **CVA**, etc.

Complications include ARDS, **cerebral oedema**, **renal failure**, **acidosis** and **shock**. Sepsis is especially likely if the water is contaminated.
- Management:
  - –**CPR**.
  - –treatment of complications as appropriate.
  - –rewarming.
  - –antibiotics as approriate. Use of steroids is controversial and declining.
  - –nasogastric aspiration to remove gastric water.

Recovery has been reported after up to 60 minutes' immersion followed by prolonged CPR, especially in children and if hypothermic. Cerebral damage may occur.

Taylor MES (1990) Hosp Update; 16: 419–31

Nebulizers. Devices used to provide a suspension of droplets in a gas, for administration of inhaled drugs or **humidification**. Droplets of 5 μm are deposited in the trachea and bronchi; those of 1 μm pass to alveoli and may impair gas exchange. Thus the ideal droplet size is between 1 and 5 μm.
- Nebulizers may be:
  - –gas-driven: water is entrained by the gas flow (**Venturi principle**) and broken into a spray; this may be directed against an anvil which breaks up the drops into smaller droplets. May be combined with a heater.
  - –ultrasonic: droplets are formed from water lying on a vibrating plate, or from water dropped on to the plate. Water overload may occur, since the droplets are very small and the water content of the gas is high.
  - –mechanical: water is dispersed into a mist by a spinning disc.

Gas-driven devices are used for drug delivery; all types may be used for humidification.

Neck, cross-sectional anatomy. At the level of C6, major anatomical structures within the layer of skin, fat and subcutaneous tissue are related to fascial layers (Fig. 97):
- –superficial fascia: encloses platysma muscle and deep fascial layers.
- –deep fascia: comprised of three layers:
  - –investing fascia: lies posterior to the anterior and external **jugular veins**. Splits to enclose sternohyoid, sternothyroid, omohyoid, sternomastoid and trapezius muscles.
  - –prevertebral fascia: extends laterally on scalenus anterior and medius to form the floor of the posterior triangle of the neck, and passes downwards to form the axillary sheath. Separated from the oesophageal/pharyngeal junction in the midline by the retropharyngeal space.
  - –pretracheal fascia: contains the trachea, oesophagus and **thyroid gland**.

See also, Carotid arteries; Tracheobronchial tree

Needles. Christopher Wren described injection via a quill and bladder in 1659. Metal tubes and stylets were subsequently used, but the hypodermic cannula and trocar were first described by Rynd in 1845. Different sizes and types are available for different uses, e.g. for iv/hypodermic use, **extradural** and **spinal anaesthesia**. Short-bevelled needles are traditionally preferred for **regional anaesthesia**. Internal lumina are not required for needles used for **acupuncture** or electrical stimulation/recording.

Needle size is described by a wire gauge classification (G; Stubbs Gauge; Birmingham Gauge) which originally referred to the number of times the wire was drawn through the draw plate (Table 24). It differs slightly from the American and Standard Wire Gauges. Inside diameter varies according to different materials and needle strengths. The system is also used for iv cannulae. For hypodermic needles, colour-coding is mandatory in the UK for certain sizes: 26 G brown; 25 G orange; 23 G blue; 22 G black; 21 G green; 20 G yellow; 19 G cream.

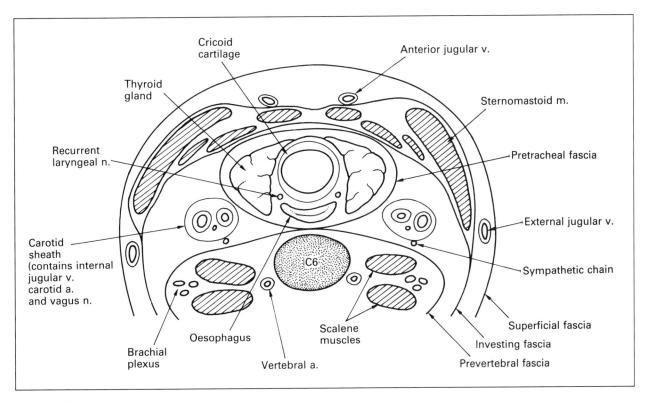

Figure 97 *Cross-section of neck at C6*

Table 24. Diameter of needles of different gauge number

Gauge number (G)	Outside diameter (mm)
36	0.10
30	0.30
29	0.33
28	0.36
27	0.41
26	0.46
25	0.51
24	0.56
23	0.64
22	0.71
21	0.81
20	0.90
19	1.08
18	1.27
17	1.50
16	1.65
15	1.83
14	2.11
13	2.41
12	2.77
11	3.05
10	3.40
9	3.76
8	4.19
7	4.57
6	5.16
1	7.62

[Sir Christopher Wren (1633–1723), English scientist and architect; Francis Rynd (1801–1861), Irish surgeon; Peter Stubbs (described 1843), English engineer]

NEEP, *see Negative end-expiratory pressure*

Nefopam hydrochloride. Analgesic drug, unrelated to **opioid analgesic drugs** and **NSAIDs.** Peak action occurs 1–2 hours after im injection. Drowsiness and respiratory depression may occur, but less than with opioids.
- Dosage:
    - 30–90 mg orally, 8 hourly.
    - 20 mg im, 6 hourly.
- Side effects: nausea, headache, confusion, anticholinergic effects. Avoidance with **monoamine oxidase inhibitors** is suggested by its manufacturers.

Negative end-expiratory pressure (NEEP). Adjunct to **IPPV,** popular in the 1960s–1970s as a method of reducing the adverse cardiovascular effects of IPPV by maintaining a subatmospheric **airway pressure** at end-expiration. However, NEEP increases airway collapse, **alveolar-arterial O_2 difference** and **dead space,** whilst reducing **FRC.** Thus no longer used.

Neonatal resuscitation, *see Cardiopulmonary resuscitation, neonatal*

Neonate. Child within 28 days of birth. Usually weighs 3–4 kg, with body surface area approximately 0.19 m².
- Major changes at birth include the following:

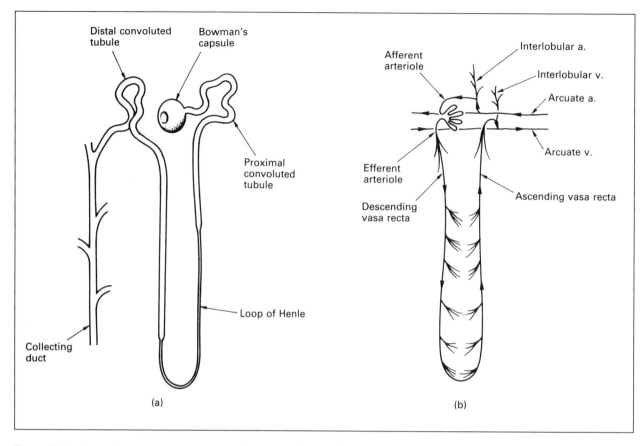

Figure 98 *Structure of nephron: (a) glomerulotubular system; (b) vascular system*

–change from **fetal circulation** to adult circulation via transitional circulation. The fibrous left ventricle, which is of similar size to the right ventricle at birth, gradually increases in compliance and contractility.

–expansion of fluid-filled alveoli; requires negative intrapleural pressures exceeding 70 cmH$_2$O. Increasing numbers of alveoli are expanded in successive breaths. Most fluid is rapidly expelled via the upper airway, with the remainder drained via capillary and lymphatic vessels over 1–3 days.

Anatomical and physiological features, and principles of anaesthesia are as for **paediatric anaesthesia**. Perioperative risks are higher than for older children, especially in premature neonates; surgery is usually deferred if possible.

See also, Cardiopulmonary resuscitation, neonatal; Fetal haemoglobin, Fetal wellbeing, during labour; Neurobehavioural testing of neonates; Obstetric analgesia and anaesthesia; Surfactant

Neostigmine methylsulphate/bromide. **Acetylcholinesterase inhibitor**, synthesized in 1931. Used to increase **acetylcholine** concentrations at the **neuromuscular junction**, e.g. reversal of **non-depolarizing neuromuscular blockade** and **myasthenia gravis**. Also has a direct stimulatory effect on skeletal muscle **acetylcholine receptors**. May cause **depolarizing neuromuscular blockade** in overdosage. Other effects are those of muscarinic stimulation, e.g. bradycardia, increased GIT motility and bladder contractility, sweating, salivation, miosis, bronchospasm. Has been used to treat urinary retention

and ileus, e.g. postoperatively. Effects on autonomic ganglia are small, consisting of stimulation at low doses and depression at high doses. A quaternary ammonium compound, it crosses the **blood-brain barrier** poorly and has few CNS effects. Routinely given with **atropine** or **glycopyrronium** when administered iv to prevent muscarinic effects. Active within 1 minute of iv injection, with action lasting 20–30 minutes. Active for up to 4 hours after oral administration. Excreted mainly renally, mostly unchanged. Elimination **half-life** is 50–90 minutes. May be administered parenterally (as methylsulphate) or orally (as bromide).

● Dosage:
  –reversal of non-depolarizing blockade: 0.04–0.08 mg/kg iv with 0.02–0.04 mg/kg atropine or 10–20 µg/kg glycopyrronium.
  –myasthenia gravis: 15–30 mg orally or 1.0–2.5 mg sc/im, 2–4 hourly.
  –other uses: as for myasthenia gravis.
● Side effects: as above; nystagmus, agitation and weakness may occur in overdosage.

Neosynephrine, *see Phenylephrine*

Nephron. Basic renal unit; each **kidney** contains about 1.3 million.
● Structure (Fig. 98a):
  –glomerulus: formed by a 200 µm diameter invagination of capillaries into the blind end of the nephron (Bowman's capsule). Water is filtered from the blood

across the glomerular membrane, together with substances under 4–8 nm in diameter. **GFR** equals about 120 ml/min (180 l/day).

–tubule: 45–65 mm long. The site of reabsorption/secretion of substances from/into the filtrate, giving rise to the eventual composition of **urine**. Consists of:

–proximal convoluted tubule: 15 mm long. Lies within the renal cortex. Lined by a brush border. Site of active reabsorption of **sodium** and **potassium** ions, **bicarbonate**, phosphate, **glucose**, uric acid and **amino acids**. Water moves passively from the tubule by **osmosis**. Up to 80% of filtered water and solutes are reabsorbed.

–loop of Henle: about 15–25 cm long; length depends on whether the glomerulus lies within the outer or inner renal cortex (short in the former, long in the latter). A further 15% of filtered water is reabsorbed. 15% of loops extend into the medulla, where interstitial osmolality is very high (up to 1200 mosmol/l). Water moves out of the descending limb, followed by sodium ions along a concentration gradient as the tubular fluid becomes more concentrated. In the ascending limb, which is impermeable to both water and sodium ions, sodium and chloride ions are actively cotransported from the tubule. The fluid thus becomes more dilute as it ascends. **Urea** is relatively free to pass across the tubular membranes. The solutes remain in the region of the medulla because of the countercurrent multiplier mechanism whereby the blood vessels supplying the loop pass close to those draining it. Solutes pass down concentration gradients from ascending vessels to descending vessels, and thus recirculate at the tip of the loop. Water passes from the descending vessels to the ascending vessels, and is thus removed from the area. This maintains the high osmolality in the medullary region. The thick ascending segment forms part of the **juxtaglomerular apparatus** where it passes near the glomerulus.

–distal convoluted tubule: 5 mm long. A further 5% of filtered water is reabsorbed. Sodium ions are reabsorbed in exchange for potassium or **hydrogen ions**, under the influence of **aldosterone**.

–collecting ducts: 20 mm long. Each receives several tubules. Pass through the cortex and medulla, opening into the renal pelvis at the medullary pyramids. Some sodium/potassium/hydrogen ion exchange occurs at the cortical part. Water is reabsorbed depending on the amount of **vasopressin** present, which increases tubular permeability to water and thus increases urine concentration.

● Blood supply (Fig. 98b):

–afferent and efferent arterioles supply and drain the capillaries to the glomerulus respectively.

–efferent arterioles subsequently divide to form peritubular capillaries or vasa recta (long loops which accompany the loop of Henle).

–peritubular capillaries and ascending vasa recta drain into interlobular veins.

[Sir William P Bowman (1816–1892), English surgeon; Friedrich GJ Henle (1809–1885), German anatomist]
See also, Acid–base balance; Clearance; Diuretics; Renin/angiotensin system

Nernst equation. Equation for calculating the **membrane potential** at which individual ions are at equilibrium across the **membrane**. For ion X:

$$E = \frac{RT}{FZ} \ln \frac{[X]_o}{[X]_i}$$

where E = equilibrium potential

R = **universal gas constant**

T = absolute temperature

F = Faraday constant (coulombs per mole of charge)

Z = valence of the ion

$[X]_o$ = extracellular concentration of X

$[X]_i$ = intracellular concentration of X.

For chloride, potassium and sodium, E = –70 mV, –90 mV and +60 mV respectively. Since the normal resting membrane potential is about –70 mV, other factors must affect potassium and especially sodium distribution (i.e. the **sodium/potassium pump**).

[Hermann W Nernst (1864–1941), German physicist; Michael Faraday (1791–1867), English scientist]

Nerve. Excitable tissue whose function is the transmission of nerve impulses. Typical peripheral nerves consist of several groups of **neurones**. The axon of each neurone has its own connective tissue covering (endoneurium). Each group of axons is covered by a second layer (perineurium), and an outer layer (epineurium) invests the whole nerve.

Peripheral nerves originate in the **spinal cord**, and may be sensory, motor or mixed. Some also carry **autonomic nervous system** fibres.

See also, Motor pathways; Sensory pathways

Nerve conduction. Passage of an **action potential** along **neurones**; involves waves of depolarization and repolarization that move longitudinally across the nerve **membrane**.

In unmyelinated **nerves**, impulses spread at up to 2 m/s. Positive charge flows into the depolarized area from the membrane just distally, altering the distal permeability to ions (especially sodium and potassium) as for action potential generation. When the threshold potential is reached, depolarization occurs. Retrograde conduction is prevented by the **refractory period** of the membrane proximally.

The **myelin** sheath of myelinated nerves acts as an insulator that prevents the flow of ions across the nerve membrane. Breaks in the myelin (nodes of Ranvier), approximately 1 mm apart, allow ions to flow freely between the neurone and the ECF at these points. Depolarization 'jumps' from node to node (saltatory conduction), a process that increases conduction velocity (up to 120 m/s) and conserves energy.

[Louis A Ranvier (1835–1922), French pathologist and physician]

Nerve injury during anaesthesia. May occur during general, local or regional anaesthesia.

● Causes of neuronal injury include:

–general anaesthesia:

–poor **positioning of the patient**; thought to cause local **nerve** ischaemia.

–ischaemia caused by **hypotension** or use of **tourniquets**.

–**hypothermia**.
–extravasation of drugs into perineural tissue.
–toxicity of degradation products of anaesthetic agents, classically **trichloroethylene** with **soda lime**.
–local/**regional anaesthesia**:
  –direct trauma from a **needle** or catheter.
  –intraneural injection of **local anaesthetic agent**.
  –infection.
  –haematoma formation.
  –chemical contamination of local anaesthetic, or injection of the wrong solution.
  –poor positioning of the part rendered anaesthetic with ischaemia as above.
–other:
  –**central venous cannulation**.
  –tracheal intubation.

- Classic division of nerve injuries:
  –neurapraxia: caused by compression. Typically incomplete, affecting motor more than sensory components (when present, touch and proprioception predominate). Usually recovers within 6 weeks. Damage during general anaesthesia is usually of this nature, and associated with positioning.
  –axonotmesis: axonal and **myelin** loss within the intact connective tissue sheath. Typically there is complete motor and sensory loss, with slow recovery due to nerve regeneration from proximal to distal nerve.
  –neurotmesis: partial or complete severence. Recovery is rare.
Electromyographic and conduction studies may aid differentiation between types of injury, and are most useful 1–3 weeks after injury.

- Many specific neuropathies have been described, including lesions of the following:
  –**brachial plexus**: usually stretched, typically by shoulder abduction and extension, with supination. Stretch is exacerbated by bilateral abduction. Upper roots are usually affected; weakness lasts up to several months, although recovery usually occurs within 2–3 months. Compression may also occur.
  –**ulnar nerve**: may be compressed between the humeral epicondyle and the operating table, or injured by the stretcher poles during transfer of the patient.
  –**radial nerve**: caused by the patient's arm hanging over the side of the operating table.
  –**median nerve**: may be damaged by direct needle trauma, or drug extravasation in the **antecubital fossa**.
  –facial nerve: compressed between the anaesthetist's fingers and the patient's mandible during mask anaesthesia.
  –abducens nerve: temporary lesions may follow **spinal** or **extradural anaesthesia**.
  –trigeminal nerve: typically damaged by the trichloroethylene/soda lime interaction.
  –supraorbital nerve: compressed by the tracheal tube connector, catheter mount, head **harness** or ventilator tubing.
  –common peroneal nerve: compressed between lithotomy pole and fibular head.
  –saphenous nerve: compressed between lithotomy pole and medial tibial condyle.
  –sciatic nerve: damaged by im injections or compressed against the operating table in emaciated patients.

–pudendal nerve: compressed between a poorly padded perineal post and the ischial tuberosity.
Nerve injury may also be caused by surgical trauma/compression.
Dawson DM, Krarup C (1989) Arch Neurol; 46: 1355–60
See also, Cranial nerves

Nerve stimulator, *see Neuromuscular blockade monitoring; Regional anaesthesia; Transcutaneous electrical nerve stimulation*

Neuralgia. Pain in distribution of nerve(s).

Neuritis. Inflammation of nerve(s).

Neurobehavioural testing of neonates. Investigation of the effects of **obstetric analgesia and anaesthesia** on the **neonate** is difficult because of many variables, e.g. obstetric details, fetal distress, method of delivery, type and route of drugs administered, methods of analysis of data, etc. In many early studies, **aortocaval compression** was not avoided.

- Tests used:
  –neonatal behavioural assessment scale (NBAS): very detailed, taking up to 1 hour to perform. More sensitive than the others.
  –early neonatal neurobehavioural scale (ENNS): directed more towards disorders of tone. Quicker and easier to perform.
  –neurological and adaptive capacity score (NACS): even more directed towards tone. Takes a few minutes to perform. The least sensitive test of subtle effects.
- Summary of results:
  –**pethidine**: reduces alertness and responsiveness before respiratory depression is evident. Greatest effect is at 2 days. Rapid placental transfer follows maternal iv injection.
  –anaesthetic agents: **thiopentone** causes more neonatal depression than **ketamine** (but tone is increased by ketamine, giving higher scores). Low concentrations of volatile **inhalational anaesthetic agents** produce little, if any, effects. Regional techniques produce consistently higher scores.
  –**local anaesthetic agents**: initial fears of hypotonia following **lignocaine** have now been dispelled. All local anaesthetic drugs have similar effects, lowering scores only when very sensitive testing is employed. The significance of this is unknown.

Neurofibromatosis (von Recklinghausen's disease). Autosomal dominant condition, with incidence of 1:3000, characterized by multiple tumours derived from the neurilemmal sheath of peripheral **nerves**/nerve roots. Flat, brown 'café au lait' spots occur in almost all sufferers, over six spots larger than 1.5 cm being diagnostic. Neurofibromata may be subcutaneous/cutaneous, or may occur in deeper peripheral nerves or autonomic nerves supplying viscera. They may also occur at the foramen magnum or within the theca, causing nerve root or **spinal cord** compression. **Pulmonary fibrosis** occurs in 20% of cases, **phaeochromocytoma** in 1%, intracranial tumours in 5–10%, and skeletal abnormalities (including **kyphoscoliosis**) in 2%. May be part of the **multiple endocrine adenomatosis** syndrome.

Potential anaesthetic problems result from the distribution of neurofibromata and may include difficulty with tracheal intubation or regional blocks. Increased sensitivity to non-depolarizing **neuromuscular blocking drugs** has been reported in some sufferers.
[Friedrich D von Recklinghausen (1833–1910), German pathologist]

Neurolepsis, *see Neuroleptanaesthesia and analgesia*

Neuroleptanaesthesia and analgesia. Use of very potent **opioid analgesic drugs** (e.g. **fentanyl** and **phenoperidine**) combined with **butyrophenones** (e.g. **droperidol** and haloperidol) to produce a state of reduced motor activity and passivity (neurolepsis). Introduced in 1959. The term neuroleptanaesthesia is usually restricted to the combination of opioid, butyrophenone and **N₂O**. Characterized by profound analgesia, **sedation** and antiemesis, with cardiovascular stability (although mild hypotension may occur). Used for **premedication**, sedation and as the sole anaesthetic technique for surgical procedures, with/without neuromuscular blocking drugs. Recovery may be prolonged.
See also, Lytic cocktail

Neuroleptic malignant syndrome (NMS). Rare condition described in 1968, characterized by **hyperthermia**, extrapyramidal dysfunction and autonomic disturbances. Follows medication with **butyrophenones** (especially haloperidol), **phenothiazines** and other antipsychotic drugs. Thought to be related to the antidopaminergic activity of the drugs, caused by receptor blockade in the basal ganglia and **hypothalamus**. Occurs in under 1% of patients, mostly young males. Increased by dehydration, CNS disease and exhaustion.
- Features develop over 1–3 days:
   –hyperthermia and tachycardia (thought to be caused mostly by increased muscle metabolism, although a central component may be present).
   –extrapyramidal dysfunction: rigidity, dystonia, tremor.
   –autonomic dysfunction: labile BP, sweating, salivation, urinary incontinence.
   –increased creatine kinase and white cell count.
Differential diagnosis is as for hyperthermia (in particular **MH**), **Parkinson's disease**, catatonia, **central cholinergic syndrome**, **monoamine oxidase inhibitor** reaction, and infection including **tetanus**. Although similar to MH, NMS is generally considered an entirely separate entity.
- Management:
   –supportive: O₂, cooling, hydration, **DVT** prophylaxis.
   –increased central dopaminergic activity, e.g. with bromcriptine (dopamine agonist) 2.5–20 mg 8 hourly (orally only). Amantidine and L-dopa have also been used.
   –**dantrolene** and non-depolarizing **neuromuscular blocking drugs** have been used to treat the peripheral muscle effects, reducing fever, rigidity and tachycardia. The latter drugs are effective in NMS, in contrast to MH.
   –**anticholinergic drugs** have also been suggested.
Mortality is 20–30%, from **renal failure**, **arrhythmias**, **PE** or **aspiration pneumonitis**.
Kellam AMP (1987) Br J Psych; 150: 752–9

Neuromuscular blockade monitoring. Ideally, this should be undertaken whenever non-depolarizing **neuromuscular blocking drugs** are used. Performed using a nerve stimulator, with assessment of the appropriate muscle response to stimulation of a peripheral nerve via surface or needle electrodes.
- Assessment may be:
   –visual.
   –tactile.
   –mechanical: reflects both **neuromuscular transmission** and muscle contractility. Assessed by:
      –measurement of tension developed in a muscle with a strain gauge or pressure **transducer**.
      –accelerometry: the transducer consists of a piezo-electric ceramic wafer with electrodes on both sides. Following changes in velocity, an electrical voltage proportional to the acceleration is generated between the electrodes. Force = mass × acceleration; thus the muscle tension response may be evaluated.
   –electrical: registers the **EMG** response via two surface/needle electrodes. Only monitors transmission across the **neuromuscular junction**, and thus is more specific than mechanical assessment.
- Stimulation:
   –unipolar square waveform lasting 0.2–0.3 ms.
   –in order to eliminate variation in muscle response caused by partial depolarization of the nerve, supra-maximal stimulation is required, which results in simultaneous depolarization of all nerve fibres within the nerve. Required current may vary between 20 and 60 mA, and is minimized by placing the positive electrode proximally.
   –direct stimulation of the muscle should be avoided, since any response will be independent of neuromuscular blockade.
   –commonly used sites:
      –ulnar nerve: electrodes are placed along the ulnar border of the forearm, with assessment of thumb adduction. More sensitive than the diaphragm and vocal cords to neuromuscular blocking drugs.
      –facial nerve: electrodes are placed anterior to the tragus of the ear, with assessment of facial muscle contraction. Underestimation of the degree of blockade is common, because of direct muscle stimulation and relative insensitivity of the facial muscles to neuromuscular blocking drugs.
      –tibial nerve: electrodes are placed behind the medial malleolus, with assessment of big toe plantarflexion.
      –common peroneal nerve: electrodes are placed lateral to the neck of the fibula, with assessment of foot dorsiflexion.
   –patterns of stimulation:
      –single pulses (0.1–1.0 Hz).
      –tetanic stimulation (50–100 Hz) for 3–5 seconds. Painful in the awake patient. May be repeated every 5–10 minutes.
      –post-tetanic stimulation using single pulses.
      –train-of-four (TOF; four pulses at 2 Hz). TOF count is the number of palpable muscle twitches; TOF ratio is force of the first twitch divided by force of the fourth. May be repeated every 10–15 seconds.
      –post-tetanic count: used to assess intense blockade.

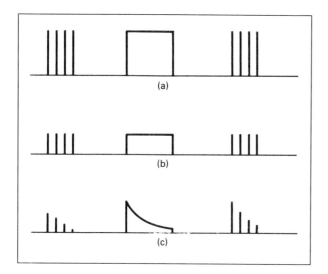

Figure 99 *EMG responses to peripheral nerve stimulation in a train-of-four, tetanus, train-of-four pattern: (a) normal; (b) partial depolarizing block; (c) partial non-depolarizing block*

Following 5 seconds' tetanus at 50 Hz, the number of twitches produced by single pulses at 1 Hz is counted. Should not be performed more than once in 5 minutes.

  –double-burst stimulation: used to assess recovery from non-depolarizing blockade. Two short tetanic stimulations, e.g. 50 Hz for 60 ms, are applied 750 ms apart. The second response is weaker than the first in non-depolarizing blockade. More sensitive at detecting **fade** than TOF.

• Observed responses:
  –normal neuromuscular function:
    –equal twitches in response to single pulses.
    –sustained **tetanic contraction**, with **post-tetanic potentiation** (PTP) revealed by mechanical assessment only.
  –**depolarizing neuromuscular blockade**:
    –equal but reduced twitches in response to single pulses and TOF (Fig. 99b). TOF ratio thus equals unity.
    –sustained but reduced tetanic contraction, with neither fade nor PTP.
    –**dual block** may supervene if large amounts of **suxamethonium** are administered.
  –**non-depolarizing neuromuscular blockade**.
    –progressively decreasing twitches in response to single pulses (Fig. 99c), with eventual disappearance.
    –tetanic contraction exhibits fade and PTP.
    –TOF: successive decrease in the four responses, with eventual disappearance of the 4th, 3rd, 2nd and 1st twitches at 75%, 80%, 90% and 100% blockade respectively. During recovery, the twitches reappear in the reverse order. Suggested suitable values during anaesthesia:
      –TOF count of 1 for tracheal intubation.
      –TOF count of 1–2 for maintenance; deeper levels may be required for complete diaphragmatic paralysis.
      –TOF count of 3–4 before attempting reversal of blockade, especially with long-acting drugs.

      –TOF ratio of 0.7–0.8 for adequate maintenance of spontaneous ventilation, if no fade follows tetanic stimulation.
      –post-tetanic count and double-burst stimulation as above.
      –sustained head-lift for 5 seconds is the most useful clinical indicator of adequate neuromuscular function (under 30% blockade). Other suggested indicators include the ability to open the mouth, protrude the tongue, cough, maintain sustained hand-grip, and achieve adequate tidal volume, vital capacity (15 ml/kg) and inspiratory pressure (–20 cmH$_2$O). However, these may all be possible at 50–80% blockade.

Beemer GH, Reeves JH, Bjorksten AR (1990) Anaesth Intensive Care; 18: 490–6

Neuromuscular blocking drugs. Drugs used to impair **neuromuscular transmission** and provide skeletal **muscle** relaxation during anaesthesia or critical care.

• May be one of two types:
  –non-depolarizing: include **tubocurarine** (first used as **curare** in 1912), **gallamine** (1948), **dimethyl tubocurarine** (1948), **alcuronium** (1961), **pancuronium** (1967), **fazadinium** (1972), **atracurium** (1980) and **vecuronium** (1983). **Doxacurium**, **pipecuronium**, **mivacurium** and **rocuronium** are the latest to be investigated. Non-depolarizing agents are competitive **antagonists** at postsynaptic **acetylcholine** (ACh) **receptors** of the **neuromuscular junction**. They are highly ionized at body pH, containing two quaternary ammonium groups (tubocurarine and vecuronium contain one each, but acquire a second following injection). Poorly lipid-soluble and poorly protein-bound. Following injection, the drugs are rapidly redistributed from blood to the **ECF** and other tissues, e.g. kidney, liver. The clinical effect depends on individual drug characteristics and drug concentration at the neuromuscular junction which depends on the drug's pharmacokinetics.
  –depolarizing: cause depolarization by mimicking the action of ACh at ACh receptors, but without rapid hydrolysis by **acetylcholinesterase**. An area of depolarization around the ACh receptor–drug complex results in local currents which open sodium channels before the continuing current flow inactivates them. Propagation of an **action potential** is prevented by the area of inexcitability that develops around the ACh receptors. Thus **fasciculations** occur before paralysis. Examples are **suxamethonium** (1951) and **decamethonium** (1948); only the former is available for clinical use in the UK.

Apart from the presence or absence of fasciculation, **non-depolarizing** and **depolarizing neuromuscular blockade** may be distinguished by **neuromuscular blockade monitoring**.

In general, suxamethonium is used for paralysis of rapid onset and short duration, e.g. to allow rapid tracheal intubation. The non-depolarizing drugs are traditionally used for prolonged paralysis when rapid intubation is not required, although atracurium and vecuronium (and more recently, mivacurium) have bridged the gap to some extent between these drugs and suxamethonium (Table 25).

See also, Interonium distance; Nicotine and nicotinic receptors

Table 25. Properties of neuromuscular blocking drugs

Drug	Onset time (min)	Half-life (min)	Vol. of distribu-tion (l/kg)	Clearance (ml/kg/min)	Clinical duration of action (min)	Route of elimination	Hista-mine release	Autonomic effects
Alcuronium	3–5	180–200	0.1–0.3	1.5	20–40	Renal	±	—
Atracurium	1.5–2	20	0.16–0.18	5.5–6.0	20–30	Hofmann degrada-tion + plasma hydrolysis	+	—
Dimethyl tubocurarine (metocurine)	3–5	345	0.5	1.0	90–120	Renal	+	Weak ganglion blockade
Doxacurium	4–5	85–100	0.2	2.2–2.6	100–200	Renal + hepatic	−	—
Fazadinium	0.5–1.5	40–80	0.2	4.0	40–60	Renal	−	Muscarinic + ganglion blockade
Gallamine	1–2	160	0.25	1.2	20–30	Renal	−	Muscarinic blockade
Mivacurium	1.5–2	2–5	—	—	10–15	Plasma cholin-esterase + hepatic	±	—
Pancuronium	2–3	120–140	0.25–0.3	1.8	40–60	Renal + hepatic	−	Weak muscarinic blockade + sympathomimetic action
Pipecuronium	2.5–3	140	0.3	2.5	90–120	Renal + hepatic	−	—
Tubocurarine	3–5	150–190	0.5–0.6	2–3	30–50	Renal + hepatic	++	Ganglion blockade
Vecuronium	1.5–2	55–70	0.27	5.2	20–30 (at usual dose)	Renal + hepatic	−	—
Suxa-methonium	0.5–1.5	2.5	—	—	2–5	Plasma cholin-esterase	+	Muscarinic + ganglionic stimulation

Neuromuscular junction. Synapse between the presynaptic motor **neurone** and the postsynaptic **muscle** membrane. On approaching the junction, the axon divides into terminal buttons that invaginate into the muscle fibre. The synaptic cleft is 50–70 nm wide and filled with ECF. The muscle **membrane** is folded into longitudinal gutters, whose ridges conceal orifices to secondary clefts. The orifices lie opposite the release points for **acetylcholine** (ACh) and contain high concentrations of **acetyl-cholinesterase** (Fig. 100).

● Three types of **acetylcholine receptor** have been identified at the neuromuscular junction:
  –postjunctional: involved in traditional **neuromuscular transmission**. Following activation of both α subunits, sodium and calcium move into the muscle and potassium exits, along specialized ion channels (*see Fig. 2b; Acetylcholine receptors*).
  –prejunctional: control an ion channel specific for sodium and essential for mobilization of ACh. **Non-depolarizing neuromuscular blockade** is thought to result in **fade**.
  –extrajunctional: normally present in small numbers, but proliferate over the muscle membrane in **dener-vation hypersensitivity**.
Standaert FG (1987) Can J Anaesth; 34: S21–9
See also, Neuromuscular blocking drugs

Neuromuscular transmission. Stages of transmission:
  –depolarization of the motor **nerve** leading to **action potential** propagation to the nerve endings at the **neuromuscular junction**.
  –increased permeability to **calcium** ions, causing release of **acetylcholine** (ACh) into the junctional gap.

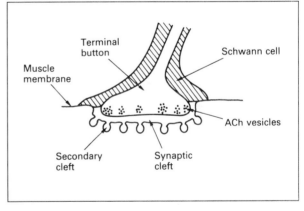

Figure 100 *Structure of a neuromuscular junction*

  –binding of ACh to nicotinic **ACh receptors**, causing an **end-plate potential**. If the latter is large enough, depolarization of the muscle membrane occurs.
  –resultant action potential causing **muscle contraction**.
  –hydrolysis of ACh by **acetylcholinesterase** within 1 ms.
● Transmission may be impaired by:
  –inhibition of ACh synthesis, storage or release, e.g. by **hemicholinium**, β-**bungarotoxin** and **botulism** respectively. Aminoglycoside antibiotics are also thought to impair ACh release.
  –blockade of ACh receptors, e.g. by **neuromuscular blocking drugs**, α-bungarotoxin, receptor destruction in **myasthenia gravis**.
  –**acetylcholinesterase inhibitors**.
See also, Synapse

Neurone. Basic unit of the nervous system. Consists of:
- –cell body: contains the nucleus and most of the cytoplasm. Usually at the dendritic end of the neurone. The dendritic zone is the site of integration of incoming impulses via dendrites, and of initiation of the **action potential**.
- –axon: may exceed 1 metre in length. May be myelinated or unmyelinated (*see Myelin; Nerve conduction*). Anterograde and retrograde flow of organelles and proteins occurs along the axon.
- –terminal buttons (**nerve** endings): situated near the cell body or dendrites of other neurones and contain **neurotransmitters**.
- Divided into classes in 1924 according to the compound action potential obtained when a mixed nerve is stimulated:
  - –A: 1–20 μm diameter myelinated fibres. Subdivided into:
    - –α: 70–120 m/s conduction; somatic motor and proprioception sensation.
    - –β: 50–70 m/s; touch and pressure sensation.
    - –γ: 30–50 m/s; motor fibres to **muscle spindles**.
    - –δ: <30 m/s; **pain**, cold, touch sensation.
  - –B: 1–3 μm diameter; <15 m/s conduction: myelinated preganglionic autonomic fibres.
  - –C: <1 μm diameter; <2 m/s conduction: unmyelinated post-ganglionic autonomic fibres, and pain and temperature sensation.

  Local anaesthetic agents block C fibres first, then B then A fibres. Pressure blocks A, B and C fibres in order, and hypoxia B, A and C fibres.
- An alternative classification has been suggested:
  - –I:
    - –a: muscle spindles.
    - –b: Golgi tendon organ.
  - –II: muscle spindles, touch, pressure.
  - –III pain, cold, touch.
  - –IV: pain, temperature, others.

[Camillo Golgi (1843–1926), Italian physician]
See also, Nociception

Neuroradiology. Most neuroradiological procedures are painless and do not require anaesthetic intervention; sedation or anaesthesia may be required in children, uncooperative or neurologically impaired patients or for prolonged procedures. Principles are as for **radiology** and **neurosurgery**.
- Specific techniques:
  - –cerebral angiography: injection of **radiological contrast media** via femoral or carotid puncture. Hyperventilation improves the arteriogram quality by increasing cerebrovascular resistance. Complications include **CVA** (1% of patients), haemorrhage, haematoma, thrombosis, arterial spasm and bradycardia (especially during vertebral angiography).
  - –myelography: injection of contrast into the thecal sac to examine the spinal cord. Usually performed via lumbar puncture but occasionally via a cervical approach. Steep tilting is often required to aid spread of the contrast. Complications include headache, **convulsions** and **arachnoiditis**.
  - –**CAT scanning**.
  - –**magnetic resonance imaging**.
  - –**positron emission tomography**.
  - –ventriculography and pneumoencephalography: injection of gas (usually air) into the ventricular system, with imaging in different positions. **N₂O** is usually avoided. Bradycardia may occur. Rarely performed now.

Panning B, Piepenbrock S (1991) Curr Opin Anaesth; 4: 645–8

Neurosurgery. Encompasses procedures involving the cranium, **brain**, **meninges**, **cranial nerves**, **spinal cord** and **vertebral column**, and those performed for **pain management**. Basic principles for intracranial surgery are related to maintenance of normal **cerebral perfusion pressure** and **cerebral blood flow**, with avoidance of **cerebral ischaemia**, **cerebral steal**, and increased **ICP**. **Cerebral protection** has been employed.
- Main considerations:
  - –preoperatively:
    - –**preoperative assessment** of neurological status, **hydrocephalus**, etc. Endocrine abnormalities may be present (e.g. pituitary tumours).
    - –fluid and electrolyte imbalance may be present, especially if associated with reduced oral intake and **vomiting**.
    - –**hypertension** may be present, especially in association with **subarachnoid haemorrhage**.
    - –drug therapy may include **anticonvulsant drugs** and **steroid therapy**.
    - –other injuries may accompany **head injury**.
    - –opioid **premedication** is usually avoided because of possible pre- or postoperative repiratory depression. **Benzodiazepines** are commonly used.
  - –peroperatively:
    - –iv **induction of anaesthesia** is usual; most **iv anaesthetic agents** are suitable apart from **ketamine**. Smooth induction avoiding **hypoxaemia**, **hypercapnia**, hypertension and tachycardia is required. **Hyperkalaemia** has followed **suxamethonium** in certain upper and lower **motor neurone** lesions. **β-Adrenergic receptor antagonists** may be given to reduce the hypertensive response to laryngoscopy, whilst **lignocaine** 0.5–1.5 mg/kg may be given iv to reduce the increase in ICP. Adequate time should be allowed for full paralysis before tracheal intubation is attempted. Lignocaine spray is usually employed during laryngoscopy. Use of a non-kinkable **tracheal tube** is usual, with thorough fixation. The eyes and face should be protected with padding.
    - –a large-bore iv cannula is necessary, since blood loss may be considerable. **CVP** measurement may be required, especially if the patient is to be positioned sitting. **Arterial cannulation** is usual. End-tidal CO_2 measurement, pulse **oximetry** and **temperature measurement** are usually considered mandatory in addition to **ECG**. **Neuromuscular blockade monitoring** is especially useful, since inadequate paralysis may have disastrous results. **ICP measurement**, **evoked potentials** and **EEG** derivatives are sometimes employed.
    - –peroperative problems include:
      - –those related to **positioning of the patient**. The supine position is common; others also used include:
        - –lateral/prone: vena caval obstruction and damage to the face, eyes, etc. may occur.

–sitting (for posterior fossa lesions): **air embolism**, hypotension, and obstruction of neck veins may occur. The first two may be reduced by the **antigravity suit**, **PEEP** and administration of iv fluids.

–inaccessibility of the airway.

–those of prolonged surgery, e.g. **heat loss**, fluid balance.

–acute control of ICP.

–**arrhythmias** and cardiovascular instability during manipulation of **brainstem** structures (posterior fossa lesions). Respiratory irregularity may occur during spontaneous ventilation, employed in some centres to monitor brainstem function.

–maintenance is usually with N_2O/O_2, supplemented by a volatile **inhalational anaesthetic agent** (**isoflurane** is usually preferred) with or without a short-acting opioid, e.g. **fentanyl**. **Naloxone** is administered routinely at the end of surgery in some centres. **TIVA** has been used. Hyperventilation to arterial P_{CO_2} of 3.5–4.0 kPa (23–30 mmHg) is usual.

–**hypotensive anaesthesia** is sometimes employed, especially for vascular lesions.

–bradycardia may follow application of suction to intracranial and extracranial drains.

–some procedures involving **CAT scanning** (e.g. stereotactic surgery) require moving the anaesthetized patient between operating and imaging rooms.

–local anaesthetic techniques may also be used. Once the skull and dura opened, there is usually little discomfort and the patient's neurological state is easily monitored.

–postoperatively:

–tracheal **extubation** is usually possible at the end of surgery; coughing or straining should be avoided. Elective IPPV may be required, e.g. following prolonged operations, in **cerebral oedema**, or when oedema is likely to affect vital centres (e.g. posterior fossa lesions). **Airway obstruction** caused by acute swelling of the tongue has been reported following posterior fossa surgery.

–close observation is required, in case of bleeding, vasospasm, increased ICP, **convulsions**, hypotension, hypertension, etc. The **Glasgow coma scale** is commonly employed to monitor progress. **ICP monitoring** may be used.

–analgesia is traditionally provided by im **codeine**.

–**diabetes insipidus** or the **syndrome of inappropriate antidiuretic hormone secretion** may occur.

–increased risk of **DVT** has been associated with cerebral malignancies. Mechanical methods of prophylaxis are usually preferred to **heparin**.

See also, Spinal surgery

Neurotransmitters. Substances secreted from presynaptic nerve endings, which act at the postsynaptic **membrane** to cause excitatory or inhibitory effects. Act via specific receptors, binding to which opens or closes membrane channels. The same neurotransmitter may be excitatory at one **synapse**, and inhibitory at another.

● Examples:

–**acetylcholine**.

–amines, e.g. **noradrenaline**, **adrenaline**, **dopamine**, **5–HT**.

–amino acids, e.g. **glycine**, **glutamate**, **GABA**, aspartate.

–polypeptides, e.g. **substance P, enkaphalins**. Substances active as circulating hormones may also function as neurotransmitters, e.g. **vasopressin, oxytocin, vasoactive intestinal peptide**.

More than one neurotransmitter may be secreted by one neurone, e.g. vasoactive intestinal peptide is often secreted with acetylcholine, and is thought to potentiate the latter's actions. Amines are often secreted with peptide neurotransmitters.

See also, Neuromuscular junction; Synaptic transmission

Neutral thermal range, *see Thermoneutral range*

Newton. Unit of **force**. 1 N is the force required to accelerate a mass of 1 kg by 1 m/s^2.

[Sir Isaac Newton (1643–1727), English physicist]

New York Heart Association classification. Method of assessment of cardiac disease, used e.g. in **preoperative assessment**:

–class I: no functional limitation.

–class II: slight functional limitation. Fatigue, palpitations, dyspnoea or angina on ordinary physical activity, but asymptomatic at rest.

–class III: marked functional limitation. Symptoms on less than ordinary activity, but asymptomatic at rest.

–class IV: inability to perform any physical activity, with or without symptoms at rest.

Nicotine and nicotinic receptors. Nicotine, a toxic alkaloid derived from tobacco, mimics certain actions of **acetylcholine**, and was used to investigate the physiology of the **autonomic nervous system**. At low doses, it stimulates postsynaptic nicotinic **acetylcholine receptors** of the **neuromuscular junction**, autonomic ganglia and adrenal medulla; at high doses, it blocks them. Also causes CNS stimulation, followed by depression. Neuromuscular and ganglionic nicotinic receptors have different properties, since **neuromuscular blocking drugs** and **ganglion blocking drugs each** act at one site predominantly, although some cross-over effect occurs. For example, **tubocurarine** causes some ganglion blockade.

Nifedipine. **Calcium channel blocking drug**, affecting coronary and peripheral vascular smooth muscle more than myocardial muscle. Negative inotropic effect is usually insignificant because of **baroreceptor**-mediated tachycardia. Has no antiarrhythmic action. Used in **hypertension**, **ischaemic heart disease** and Raynaud's phenomenon. Active within 20–30 minutes of oral administration, but a faster response follows sublingual retention of the capsule's contents. May thus be administered sublingually during anaesthesia. 95% protein-bound. **Half-life** is 3–5 hours. Metabolized in the liver and excreted renally.

● Dosage:

–5–20 mg orally, 8–12 hourly.

–100–200 µg may be infused into the coronary arteries, e.g. for spasm during coronary angiography.

● Side effects: headache, flushing, dizziness, GIT disturbance, peripheral oedema.

[Maurice Raynaud (1834–1881), French physician]

Nikethamide. **Analeptic drug**, formerly used as a respiratory and cardiovascular stimulant but rarely used now because of its non-specific actions. Dose: 0.25–1.0 g slowly iv. Side effects are common and included restlessness, **arrhythmias**, tremor and **convulsions**.

Nimodipine. Calcium channel blocking drug, preferentially affecting cerebral vascular smooth muscle. Increases **cerebral blood flow**, especially to poorly perfused areas, e.g. affected by arterial spasm following **subarachnoid haemorhage** (SAH).

- Dosage:
    - prophylactically following SAH: 60 mg orally, 4 hourly, for 21 days.
    - in established vasospasm: 15 μg/kg/h iv, doubled after two hours if BP is stable. Continued for 5–14 days.

Reacts with PVC infusion tubing; polypropylene and polyethylene are suitable. May be degraded by light.

- Side effects: hypotension, flushing. Should be used with care in raised **ICP**.

Nitrogen. Non-metallic element existing in the atmosphere as a colourless, odourless 'inert' gas (isolated in 1772). Forms 78.03% of atmospheric **air**. Atomic weight is 14; boiling point is –195°C. Obtained by fractional distillation of air. Reacts poorly with other substances. Blood/gas **solubility coefficient** is 0.014. Has anaesthetic properties at hyperbaric pressures (*see Inert gas narcosis*). Converted into organic compounds by nitrifying bacteria and plants, and present throughout the body in **amino acids** and **proteins**.

See also, Nitrogen balance; Nitrogen washout

Nitrogen balance. Difference between the amount of nitrogen ingested (as **amino acids** or **proteins**) and the amount of nitrogen exreted (mainly urinary). Usually measured within a 24 hour period. Negative if losses exceed intake, e.g. **catabolism**, starvation; positive if intake exceeds losses, e.g. during recovery from severe illness.

- Estimated thus:
    - intake = the nitrogen content of all foods/fluids taken.
    - output = the sum of nitrogen losses calculated from the following three components:
    - from urinary **urea**: nitrogen (g/24 h) =
    urea (mmol/24 hrs) × ⅚ because ⅙ is excreted as substances other than urea
        × 1/1000 to convert mmol to mol
        × 60 to convert mol urea to g
        × 28/60 to convert g urea to g nitrogen
    i.e. urea (mmol/24 h) × 0.0336.
    - from blood urea: nitrogen (g/24 h) =
    change in urea (mmol/l/24 h) × 1/1000
        × 60
        × 28/60 as above
        × 60% × body weight (kg) since urea is distributed amongst total body water
    i.e. change in urea (mmol/l/24 h) × 0.0168 × body weight
    - from other routes of loss, e.g. proteinuria:
    nitrogen loss (g/24 h) = protein loss (g/24 h)
        × 1/6.25 since 6.25 g protein contains 1 g nitrogen.
    Other losses occur from sweat and stools (e.g. 2–4 g per l GIT fistula fluid lost per 24 h).

Calculation is a useful guide to appropriate **nutrition** in critical illness.

Nitrogen, higher oxides of. Nitric oxide (NO), nitrogen dioxide (NO_2) and nitrogen trioxide (N_2O_3); the latter decomposes to form NO and NO_2. NO reacts with O_2 forming NO_2, which dissolves in water to form nitrous and nitric acids. The gases are produced during some fires, during manufacture of N_2O, and in the metal industry. Irritant if inhaled, they cause mild upper airway symptoms initially but **pulmonary oedema** several hours after initial recovery. Severe pulmonary fibrotic destruction may follow 2–3 weeks later. Formation of nitrates in the body may result in vasodilatation and hypotension, and cause **methaemoglobinaemia**. Treatment is supportive. Contamination of some N_2O cylinders in 1967 in the UK led to widespread recall of cylinders. May be tested for using moistened starch-iodide paper, which turns blue on exposure. NO is thought to be (or to be related to) **endothelium-derived relaxing factor**, involved in intercellular communication and control of vascular tone.

See also, Smoke inhalation

Nitrogen narcosis, *see Inert gas narcosis*

Nitrogen washout. Elimination of nitrogen from the lungs whilst breathing non-nitrogen-containing gas. During successive breaths, the concentration of nitrogen exhaled falls as an **exponential process**, falling to about 2.5% after 7 minutes in normal patients. During anaesthesia using **circle systems**, 7–10 minutes' high fresh gas flow is required to remove most body nitrogen. Elimination is prolonged if ventilation is distibuted unevenly (see below).

- Tests employing nitrogen washout:
    - measure of **FRC**.
    - single-breath nitrogen washout (**Fowler's method**).
    - multiple-breath nitrogen washout: the patient breathes 100% O_2, with nitrogen measurement at the lips. Log nitrogen concentration is plotted against number of breaths. If lung ventilation is uniform, expired nitrogen concentration decreases by the same

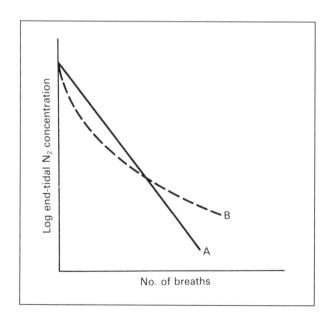

Figure 101 *Multiple-breath nitrogen washout. A, uniform ventilation; B, uneven ventilation*

fraction with each breath, as demonstrated by a straight line on the graph. A curved line is obtained if ventilation is uneven, as nitrogen is quickly washed out from well-ventilated alveoli but only slowly from poorly-ventilated ones (Fig. 101).

Nitroglycerin, *see Glyceryl trinitrate*

Nitroprusside, *see Sodium nitroprusside*

Nitrous oxide (N_2O). **Inhalational anaesthetic agent,** first isolated by **Priestley** in 1772. Suggested as being potentially useful for analgesia by **Davy** in 1799; first used for dental extraction by **Wells** in 1844 but superceded by **diethyl ether.** Reintroduced by **Colton** in 1863.

Manufactured by heating ammonium nitrate to 240°C, removing impurities, e.g. higher oxides of nitrogen, ammonia and nitric acid, by passage through scrubbers and washers. Water vapour is also removed.

- Properties:
  - –colourless, slightly sweet-smelling gas, 1.53 times denser than air.
  - –mw 44.
  - –boiling point –88°C.
  - –**critical temperature** 36.5°C.
  - –**partition coefficients**:
    - –blood/gas 0.47.
    - –oil/gas 1.4.
  - –**MAC** 105%.
  - –non-flammable but supports combustion, breaking down to O_2 and nitrogen at high temperatures.
  - –supplied as a liquid/gas in blue **cylinders**: pressure is 40 bar at 15°C and 54 bar at room temperature. Ice often forms on the cylinder during use because of **latent heat** of vaporization. Also supplied as gaseous **Entonox.**
- Effects:
  - –CNS:
    - –fast onset and recovery; strongly analgesic but weakly anaesthetic.
    - –increases **cerebral blood flow** and **ICP** slightly.
  - –RS:
    - –non-irritant. Depresses respiration slightly.
    - –may cause **diffusion hypoxia** at the end of surgery.
  - –CVS: little effect on heart rate and BP usually, although it decreases myocardial contractility, especially when combined with volatile agents or opioids.
  - –GIT: associated with postoperative nausea and vomiting; expansion of gas-containing bowel or inner ear cavities, or a direct central effect (possibly via **opioid receptors**), have been suggested as possible causes.
  - –other:
    - –does not affect hepatic or renal function, nor uterine or skeletal muscle tone.
    - –interacts with **methionine** synthase; prolonged use may cause bone marrow depression, megaloblastic **anaemia** and **peripheral neuropathy.** Implicated in causing fetal abnormalities and spontaneous abortion, but no direct evidence exists. Generally considered as being safe during pregnancy.
    - –expands air-filled cavities because it is over 40 times as soluble as nitrogen; thus passes from the blood into the cavity faster than the nitrogen can diffuse out. Can double the size of a **pneumotho-**rax in 10 minutes at 70%. Also expands **air embolism.**

Excreted unchanged from the lungs.

Commonly used for analgesia (above 20%) and as a carrier gas for other inhalational agents and O_2, usually in concentrations of 50–66%. Although weakly anaesthetic and rarely adequate alone, it reduces the requirement for other agents. Its adverse effects and cost have led to a small reduction in its use and replacement by air.

Also used in the **cryoprobe.**

See also, Environmental safety of anaesthetists; Nitrogen, higher oxides of; Relative analgesia

NMJ, *see Neuromuscular junction*

NMR, Nuclear magnetic resonance, *see Magnetic resonance imaging*

Nocioception. Sensation of noxious stimuli, i.e. associated with injury or threatened injury.

- Occurs via specialized **nerve** endings (nocioceptors) of certain **neurones**:
  - –C-fibres: respond to heat, mechanical and chemical stimuli, giving rise to **pain.**
  - –A-fibres:
    - –type I: respond to heat and mechanical stimuli, with high threshold. Thought to give rise to pain from long-standing stimuli.
    - –type II: respond to heat and mechanical stimuli, with fast response and low threshold. Thought to give rise to initial pain sensation.
  - –receptors responding to cold and mechanical stimuli, thought to give rise to pain associated with cold.

Other types may also exist. Although initially described and most abundant in skin, they also exist in other tissues, e.g. muscle, joints, teeth. Injury increases their response and sensitivity.

See also, Pain; Pain pathways

Nodal arrhythmias, *see Junctional arrhythmias*

Non-depolarizing neuromuscular blockade. Caused by competitive antagonism of **acetylcholine** (ACh) by non-depolarizing **neuromuscular blocking drugs** (NDNMBDs) at the **ACh receptors** of the **neuromuscular junction.** The end-plate potential produced by ACh diminishes as receptor occupancy by the NDNMBD increases; when it fails to reach the threshold value **neuromuscular transmission** fails. This occurs when 80–90% of ACh receptors are blocked, confirming the wide margin of safety of neuromuscular transmission.

- Features:
  - –absence of **fasciculation** following administration of drug.
  - –exhibits **fade** and **post-tetanic potentiation.**
  - –antagonized by **acetylcholinesterase inhibitors.**
  - –potentiated by aminoglycosides, volatile **inhalational anaesthetic agents, acidosis,** electrolyte disturbances (especially **hypokalaemia, hypermagnesaemia, hypocalcaemia**), **myasthenia gravis.**

    Blockade may also be potentiated by excess drug at the neuromuscular junction, e.g. caused by overdose, or reduced metabolism, excretion or muscle blood flow.

See also, Neuromuscular blockade monitoring

Non-parametric tests, *see Data; Statistical tests*

Non-rebreathing valves. Prevent exhaled gas from passing upstream from the patient in **anaesthetic breathing systems**, thus almost eliminating rebreathing (but reducing efficiency because **dead space** gas is wasted). Most commonly used in **draw-over techniques** and for **CPR** with **self-inflating bags**. Also used in **demand valves**. For use with a fixed fresh gas supply, a reservoir bag is required unless fresh gas flow rate exceeds peak inspiratory flow rate. Should be placed as near to the patient as possible, e.g. attached directly to the facepiece/tracheal tube.

- Valves may be designed for either spontaneous ventilation or IPPV; commonly used ones may be used for both, and include:
  - Ambu-E valve (Fig. 102a): contains silicone rubber flaps (mushroom valves) within a clear plastic housing. Those designed for CPR contain one mushroom valve; those for anaesthetic use contain a second distal one to prevent indrawing of room air.
  - Laerdal valve (Fig. 102b): contains a circular silicone rubber internal valve and a ring-shaped rubber expiratory valve.
  - Ruben valve (Fig. 102c): contains a bobbin which is held against the upstream port by a spring at rest and moved downstream by gas flow during inspiration.

Malfunction, e.g. due to condensation of water vapour, may cause sticking of the valve or rebreathing. **Barotrauma** may occur if high internal pressure holds the expiratory port closed, e.g. during apnoea with high fresh gas flow.

[Ambu: from ambulant, Danish for moveable; Asmund S Laerdal (1913–1981), Norwegian businessman and manufacturer; Henning M Ruben, Danish anaesthetist]

Non-steroidal anti-inflammatory drugs (NSAIDs). Group of chemically dissimilar compounds, mostly organic acids, with anti-inflammatory, antipyretic and analgesic actions. Thought to act via inhibition of **prostaglandin** synthesis. May be classified into salicylic acids (e.g. **aspirin**, benorylate, diflunisal), propionic acids (e.g. fenbufen, ibuprofen, naproxen), acetic acids (e.g. **diclofenac**, **indomethacin**), the fenamates (mefenamic acid, flufenamic acid), the pyrazolones (e.g. phenylbutazone, azapropazone) and the oxicams (e.g. piroxicam).

Widely used for mild pain (e.g. musculoskeletal disease, headache, dysmenorrhoea, etc.) and inflammatory disease (especially musculoskeletal). Increasingly used for **postoperative analgesia**. Individual responses to NSAIDs are variable and many drugs may have to be tried before achieving optimal benefit.

Side effects: GIT disturbance, rash, decreased **platelet** function and impaired coagulation, fluid retention, renal impairment, rarely hepatotoxicity.

Although platelet dysfunction has been shown after perioperative use, bleeding problems are rare.

Dahl JB, Kehlet H (1991) Br J Anaesth; 66: 703–12

Noradrenaline. Catecholamine, the immediate precursor of **adrenaline** (differing by one methyl group on the terminal amine). A **neurotransmitter** in the **sympathetic nervous system**, **ascending reticular activating system** and **hypothalamus**. Also a hormone, forming about 20% of the catecholamines released from the adrenal medulla.

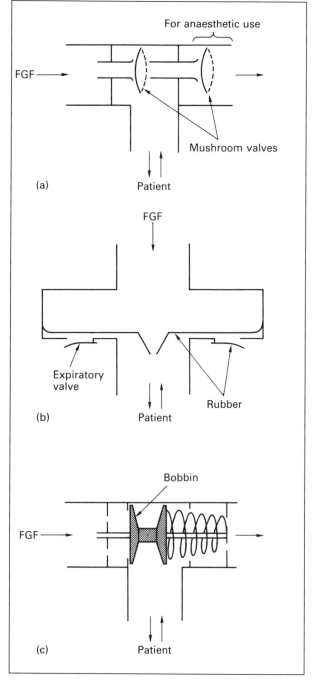

Figure 102 *Examples of non-rebreathing valves: (a) Ambu-E; (b) Laerdal; (c) Ruben. FGF, fresh gas flow*

Predominately stimulates α-**adrenergic receptors** (non-selectively), although with some β_1–receptor stimulation. After secretion, 80% is taken up by postganglionic sympathetic nerve endings for reuse (uptake$_1$); the remainder is metabolized by **catechol-O-methyltransferase** and **monoamine oxidase** or taken up by other cells, e.g. vascular smooth muscle (uptake$_2$).

Used as an **inotropic drug** when **SVR** is low, e.g. in sepsis. An extremely potent **vasopressor drug**, it increases both systolic and diastolic arterial BP via arterial and venous vasoconstriction. There may be compensatory bradycardia caused by **baroreceptor reflex** activation. Coronary perfusion is increased but with increased myocardial O_2 demand. **Cardiac output** may increase or decrease depending on clinical circumstances. **Cerebral blood flow** and O_2 demand may fall. Although hypotension may be corrected, renal and mesenteric vasoconstriction may reduce **renal blood flow**.

Supplied commercially as noradrenaline tartrate.

● Dosage: 0.03–0.2 µg/kg/min.

Tachyphylaxis may occur. Tissue necrosis may follow extravasation.

Norepinephrine, *see Noradrenaline*

Normal solution. One containing one gram equivalent weight of substance per litre. So-called 'normal' **saline solution** (0.9%) is incorrectly described, being less than ⅙ normal.

See also, Equivalence

Noscapine, *see Papaveretum*

Nose. Entrance to the **pharynx** and thence **larnyx** and **lungs**. Apart from its olfactory role, it filters, humidifies and warms inspired air with its extensive vascular surfaces (turbinates and septum). Filtering relies on the mucous lining which traps particles larger than 4–6 µm, sweeping them back to the pharynx. Sneezing also rids the nose of irritants.

● Divided into:
  –external nose:
    –bones:
      –nasal part of frontal bones.
      –frontal process of maxillae.
      –nasal bones.
    –cartilages (lower part and septum).
    –fibrofatty tissue (ala).
  –nasal cavity: subdivided by the septum into two separate compartments, opening anteriorly by the nares and posteriorly by the choanae. The small dilatation immediately within the nares (vestibule) is lined with stratified squamous epithelium bearing hairs and sebaceous and sweat glands. The remainder is lined with columnar ciliated cells and mucus-secreting goblet cells. Subdivided into:
    –roof: slopes upwards and backwards forming the bridge of the nose; it then has a horizontal part (cribriform plate of the ethmoid bone) and finally a downward sloping part (palatine bone).
    –floor: composed of the palatine process of the maxilla and horizontal plate of the palatine bone. A tissue flap (soft palate) extends into the nasopharynx, closing off the nasal passages during **swallowing**.
    –medial wall: nasal septum.
    –lateral wall: ethmoidal labyrinth, nasal surface of the maxilla and perpendicular plate of the palatine bone. The three scroll-like conchae hang down over the nasal meatus. The olfactory organ of the first **cranial nerve** lies above and beside the upper concha. The orifices of the maxillary, sphenoid, frontal and ethmoidal sinuses open on to the lateral nasal wall.

● Blood supply:
  –upper: anterior and posterior ethmoidal branches of the ophthalmic artery.
  –lower: sphenopalatine branch of the maxillary artery.
  –anteroinferior septum: septal branch of the superior labial branch of the facial artery.
  Venous drainage is via a submucous plexus which drains into the sphenopalatine, facial and ophthalmic veins.
● Nerve supply is from branches of the ophthalmic (V^1) and maxillary (V^2) divisions of the trigeminal nerve:
  –skin:
    –supratrochlear branch of the frontal nerve (V^1).
    –anterior ethmoidal branch of the nasociliary nerve (V^1).
    –infraorbital branch of V^2.
  –maxillary antrum: V^2 via sphenopalatine ganglion.
  –frontal sinus: frontal nerve (V^1).
  –ethmoid region: anterior and posterior branches of the nasociliary nerve (V^1).
  –nasal cavities:
    –anterior: anterior ethmoidal branch of the nasociliary nerve (V^1).
    –posterior: short sphenopalatine and posterior nasal branches of V^2 (septum); long sphenopalatine branch (lateral wall).

Trauma to the nose may result from passage of a tracheal or nasogastric tube, or nasal airway. Resultant **epistaxis** may be severe, and may be reduced by prior administration of **cocaine** spray or paste, or other vasopressor solutions, e.g. xylometazoline 0.1%.

● For topical anaesthesia of the nose, many techniques have been described. Moffett's method is one of the best known:
  –solution consists of 2 ml 8% cocaine, 2 ml 1% sodium **bicarbonate** and 1 ml 1:1000 **adrenaline**.
  –one-sixth of the solution is instilled into each nostril and retained for 10 minutes in each of the following positions: right lateral head down, face down, and left lateral head down.
  Other techniques involve application of 8–10% cocaine or other agent plus 1: 200 000 adrenaline swabs to the anterior septum and posterior nasal cavity.

Maxillary and **ophthalmic nerve blocks** may be used for operations on or around the nose.

[Arthur J Moffett, Birmingham otolaryngologist]

See also, Ear, nose and throat surgery

NPPV, *see Nasal positive pressure ventilation*

NSAIDs, *see Non-steroidal anti-inflammatory drugs*

Nuclear cardiology. Assessment of cardiac function using gamma cameras to trace **radioisotopes**, using data processors. Technetium-99m labelled blood may be followed through the heart during first pass of a bolus, or over many cardiac cycles linked to the ECG (multigated scintigraphy; MUGA). Individual chamber movement and valve function may be visualized, and **ejection fraction** calculated by recording the number of counts in systole and diastole. Alternatively, the uptake of thallium-201 by cardiac tissue may be observed (uptake by normal myocardium is proportional to blood flow). Recently-infarcted myocardium may be labelled with technetium-99m pyrophosphate. Other tracers used to identify areas of infarction, necrosis or inflammation include indium-111, gallium-67 citrate, and radiolabelled **myosin**-specific antibodies.

Cahalan MK, Litt L, Botvinick EH, Schiller NB (1987) Anesthesiology; 66: 356–72

Nuclear magnetic resonance, *see Magnetic resonance imaging*

Null hypothesis. In **statistics**, the assumption that the observed frequency of an event equals the expected frequency. It may state that any observations are due to chance alone, or that the groups studied come from the same population, etc.; **statistical tests** aid the acceptance or rejection of this hypothesis (i.e. whether an alternative hypothesis, that observed differences are statistically significant, can be accepted). Results are expressed in terms of the **probability** that the null hypothesis does not hold for the case concerned.

See also, Confidence intervals; Statistical significance

Nutrition. An adequately balanced daily supply of **carbohydrates**, **fats**, **proteins**, vitamins, electrolytes, trace elements and water is essential to maintain normal health.
- Average normal adult daily requirements:
  - water: 30–40 ml/kg.
  - nitrogen: 0.2 g/kg.
  - **energy** : 30–40 Cal/kg.
  - electrolytes:
    - **sodium**: 1 mmol/kg.
    - **potassium**: 1 mmol/kg.
    - chloride: 1.5 mmol/kg.
    - phosphate: 0.2–0.5 mmol/kg.
    - **calcium**: 0.1–0.2 mmol/kg.
    - **magnesium**: 0.1–0.2 mmol/kg.
  - trace elements:
    - iron: 0.2 mg/kg.
    - zinc: 0.2 mg/kg.
  - vitamins:
    - A: 15–20 µg/kg.
    - D: 0.1–0.2 µg/kg.
    - E: 0.1–0.2 mg/kg.
    - K: 1 µg/kg.
    - folate: 2–3 µg/kg.
    - B_{12}: 0.04–0.1 µg/kg.
    - C: 1 mg/kg.
    - thiamine: 0.02 mg/kg.
    - riboflavine: 0.02 mg/kg.
    - niacin: 0.4 mg/kg.
    - pyridoxine: 0.02 mg/kg.

Energy requirements depend on the particular circumstances for each individual, e.g. they increase after **trauma**, **burns**, etc. (*see Catabolism*), and with pyrexia (by about 10% for every °C above normal). Patients should be fed via the oral route if possible, preferably with normal food.

For critically ill patients, more precise estimation of nutritional requirements is necessary, whether administered parenterally or enterally, e.g.:
- calculation of **nitrogen balance**.
- calculation of energy requirement (150–200 Cal per g nitrogen).
- division of energy requirement into carbohydrate (4 Cal/g) and fat (9 Cal/g) components to accompany nitrogen. Carbohydrate should comprise 40–50% of energy requirements.

- selection of the appropriate solutions from commercially available products (some pharmacies make up their own solutions), satisfying requirements for energy, fluid and electrolytes. Vitamins, etc. may be added as required.

Willatts SM (1988) Br J Anaesth; 58: 201–22
See also, Malnutrition; Metabolism; Nutrition, enteral; Nutrition, total parenteral

Nutrition, enteral. Ingestion of foodstuffs via the GIT. In patients recovering from critical illness or major surgery, it is commonly performed via fine-bore nasogastric tubes. Percutaneous gastrostomy may be superior for long-term feeding. Principles are those of **nutrition** generally.

Carbohydrate is the usual energy source in most enteral feeds, but high concentrations increase osmolality, causing diarrhoea. The **protein** source is usually whole protein although preparations containing oligopeptides or **amino acids** are useful in pancreatic disease and malabsorption syndromes. Medium chain triglycerides are the usual source of **fat**.

Enteral feeds are usually delivered from a reservoir bag to the patient via a controllable pump, e.g. at low continuous infusion rates.
- Complications:
  - mechanical, e.g. tube blockage, passage of the tube into the trachea, regurgitation.
  - diarrhoea: may be caused by high osmolality feeds or the underlying bowel disorder.
  - electrolyte and liver function test disturbances.

Willatts SM (1988) Br J Anaesth; 58: 201–22
See also, Nutrition, total parenteral

Nutrition, total parenteral (TPN). Administration of total nutritional requirements by iv infusion; it may be required in patients who are hypercatabolic and/or have an abnormal GIT. Commonly required in critically ill patients on ICU with intra-abdominal conditions or multiorgan failure. Enteral **nutrition** should be considered before instituting TPN, since the latter is more costly and has more complications. IV nutrition may also be used to supplement enteral nutrition.

Principles are those of nutrition generally, i.e. calculation of **nitrogen balance**, energy and fluid requirements. Nitrogen and the energy source should be given together, preferably continuously. 5–6 mmol potassium and 1–2 mmol magnesium are required per gram of nitrogen.

The nitrogen component is given as mixtures of essential and non-essential **amino acids** (the nitrogen content varies considerably between different solutions). Some amino acid solutions contain electrolytes and most are hypertonic. Some contain energy sources, e.g. **glucose** and fructose. **Carbohydrate** is usually given as glucose 10–50%, and requires central venous infusion to avoid venous thrombosis. Other energy sources, e.g. sorbitol, xylitol and ethanol have also been used. **Insulin** is usually required to control **hyperglycaemia** associated with glucose-rich infusions. **Fat** is usually administered as 10 or 20% soya bean oil emulsions; allergic reactions may occur rarely with the 20% preparation. Trace elements and vitamins must be added.

Most solutions are administered from one large bag via a pump and a single dedicated central venous cannula, although a peripheral line is acceptable for temporary infusion of fat emulsion.

The patient should be encouraged to mobilize to prevent muscle breakdown.

- Complications:
  - those associated with **central venous cannulation**.
  - **septicaemia**.
  - metabolic disorders:
    - hyperglycaemia.
    - **hypophosphataemia**.
    - metabolic **acidosis**.
    - **hypernatraemia**.
    - lipaemia.
    - trace element or **vitamin deficiency**.
- Routine monitoring should include:
  - clinical signs, weight and fluid balance daily. Skinfold thickness and arm circumference have been used.
  - plasma urea, creatinine, electrolytes and osmolality daily. Glucose should be measured more frequently, e.g. by stick-testing. Liver function and plasma calcium, phosphate and magnesium should be assessed at least twice a week.
  - urine urea and osmolality daily.
  - full blood count every 1–3 days; prothrombin time once a week. Iron, folate and vitamin B_{12} should be measured at least weekly.

Willatts SM (1988) Br J Anaesth; 58: 201–22

O

Obesity. Common problem in the Western world. Body mass index (weight in kg divided by (height in m)^2) is sometimes used for definition, e.g.: <25 kg/m^2 = normal; 25–30 kg/m^2 = overweight; >30 kg/m^2 = obese. Morbid obesity is defined as twice ideal body weight; general mortality in this group is twice that of normal. Distribution of fat may be important; abdominal deposition is thought to be particularly detrimental.

- Effects:
  - RS:
    - increased body O_2 demand and CO_2 production, because of increased tissue mass. Minute ventilation required to maintain normocapnia is thus increased, which further increases O_2 demand.
    - reduced **FRC** because of the weight of the chest wall. FRC is especially reduced in the supine position, due to the weight of the abdominal wall and contents. Lung **compliance** is thus reduced, increasing work of breathing and O_2 demand. $\dot{V}/\dot{Q}$ **mismatch** results in **hypoxaemia**.
    - **hypoxic pulmonary vasoconstriction** increases work of the right ventricle, and may lead to **pulmonary hypertension** and right-sided **cardiac failure**.
    - obstructive **sleep apnoea** and **alveolar hypoventilation syndrome** may occur.
  - CVS:
    - cardiac output and blood volume increase, to increase **O_2 flux**.
    - **hypertension** is common; thus left ventricular work is increased. Left ventricular hypertrophy and ischaemia may occur, with resultant left-sided cardiac failure.
  - other diseases are more likely, e.g. non-insulin dependent **diabetes mellitus** (caused by insulin resistance and inadequate insulin production, the latter worsening with age), hypercholesterolaemia, gout and arthritis, gall bladder disease, hepatic impairment, **CVA**, certain malignancies.

Patients may require surgery for related or unrelated conditions, or for 'treatment', e.g. gastroplasty, jejunoileal bypass.

- Anaesthetic considerations:
  - preoperatively:
    - **preoperative assessment** for the above complications and appropriate management. Patients may be taking **amphetamines** for weight loss.
    - **heparin** prophylaxis is usual, because patients are less mobile and risk of **DVT** is increased.
    - im injection may be difficult because of subcutaneous fat.
  - peroperatively:
    - veins may be difficult to find and cannulate.
    - **hiatus hernia** is common, with risk of **aspiration of gastric contents**. Volume and acidity of gastric contents may be increased. In addition, tracheal intubation may be difficult: insertion of the laryngoscope blade into the mouth may be hindered, the neck may be short and movement reduced.
    - hypoxaemia may occur rapidly during **apnoea**, since FRC (hence O_2 reserve) is reduced, and O_2 utilization increased.
    - **airway** maintenance is often difficult, because of increased soft tissue mass in the upper airway. Spontaneous ventilation is often inadequate because of respiratory impairment, which worsens in the supine position (especially in the head-down position or with legs in the lithotomy position). Thus IPPV is usually employed; high inflation pressures may be required.
    - lifting and positioning the patient may be difficult.
    - monitoring may be difficult, e.g. BP cuff too small, ECG complexes small.
    - surgery is more likely to be difficult and prolonged, with increased blood loss.
    - drug use:
      - appropriate dosage may be difficult; e.g. **neuromuscular blocking drugs** are given according to lean body weight. Distribution of drugs is affected by the increase in adipose tissue mass.
      - increased metabolism of **inhalational anaesthetic agents** is thought to occur, e.g. increased **fluoride ion** concentrations after prolonged use of **enflurane**.
    - although regional techniques may have potential advantages over general anaesthesia, they are often technically difficult.
  - postoperatively:
    - **atelectasis** and **hypoventilation** are common, with increased risk of infection, hypoxaemia and **respiratory failure**. Patients are often best nursed sitting. Elective IPPV may be required.
    - **postoperative analgesia**, **O_2 therapy** and **physiotherapy** are especially important. **HDU** admission is useful.

Shenkman Z, Shir Y, Brodsky JB (1993) Br J Anaesth; 70: 349–59

Obstetric analgesia and anaesthesia. Pain during the first stage of labour is thought to be caused by cervical dilatation, and is usually felt in the T11–L1 **dermatomes**. Back and rectal pain may also occur. Pain often worsens at the end of the first stage. Pain during the second stage is caused by stretching of the birth canal and perineum.

Early attempts at pain relief included the use of abdominal pressure, **opium** and **alcohol**. **Simpson** administered the first obstetric anaesthetic in 1847, using **diethyl ether**. He used **chloroform** later that year, subsequently preferring it to ether. Moral and religious objections to anaesthesia in childbirth declined after **Snow's** administration of chloroform to Queen **Victoria** in 1853. Regional techniques were introduced from the early 1900s, and have become increasingly popular since the 1960s.

Choice of technique is related to the physiological effects of **pregnancy** (especially risk of **aortocaval compression** and **aspiration pneumonitis**), and effects of drugs and complications on the fetus, **neonate** and course of labour. Anaesthesia has consistently been a major cause of death during pregnancy as revealed in the Report on **Confidential Enquiries into Maternal Deaths**.

- Methods used:
  - non-drug methods, e.g. **TENS, acupuncture, hypnosis, psychoprophylaxis, white noise, abdominal decompression**: generally safe for mother and fetus, but of variable efficacy.
  - systemic **opioid analgesic drugs**:
    - **morphine** was used with **hyoscine** to provide **twilight sleep** in the early 1900s. However, it readily crosses the **placenta** to cause neonatal respiratory depression. **Pethidine** was first used in 1940 and approved for use by UK midwives in 1950; it is the most commonly used opioid (e.g. 50–150 mg im up to two doses), but 30–75% of women gain no benefit from its use. Nausea, vomiting, delayed **gastric emptying** and sedation may occur, with neonatal respiratory depression especially likely between 2 and 4 hours after im injection. Subtle changes may be detected on **neurobehavioural testing of the neonate**. Neonatal respiratory depression is marked after iv injection.
    - other opioids have been used with similar effects. A lower incidence of neonatal depression has been claimed for partial agonists and agonist/antagonists, e.g. **nalbuphine, pentazocine, meptazinol**, but they are not commonly used.
    - **patient-controlled** analgesia has been used, e.g. pethidine 10–20 mg iv, nalbuphine 2–3 mg iv (lockout time 10 minutes). Adverse effects may be less than following im injection, and analgesia better.
    - **opioid receptor antagonists**, e.g. **naloxone** may be given to the neonate if resiratory depression is marked.
  - sedative drugs: rarely used except in extreme anxiety or **pre-eclampsia**. Promazine, promethazine, benzodiazepines, chloral hydrate, chlormethiazole and chlordiazepoxide are most commonly used. All may cause neonatal depression.
  - **inhalational anaesthetic agents**:
    - ether and chloroform were first used in 1847. **Trichloroethylene** was used in the 1940s, and **methoxyflurane** in 1970; formerly approved for midwives' use with **draw-over techniques**, their use in the UK ceased in 1984.
    - **N$_2$O** was first used in 1880. **Intermittent flow anaesthetic machines** were developed from the 1930s, using N$_2$O with air or O$_2$. The Lucy Baldwin apparatus (funded by the Lucy Baldwin fund for supplying labour wards) was developed in the late 1950s, delivering preset N$_2$O/O$_2$ mixtures. **Entonox** was used in 1962 by Tunstall, and approved for midwives in 1965. It is usually self-administered using a facepiece or mouthpiece and **demand valve**, although continuous administration via nasal

cannulae has been described. Slow deep inhalation should start as soon as a contraction begins, in order to achieve adequate blood levels at peak pain. May cause nausea and dizziness; it is otherwise safe with minimal side effects. Useful in 50% of women but of no help in 30%.
    - **enflurane** and **isoflurane** have been used for draw-over inhalation.
  - general anaesthesia: no longer used for normal vaginal delivery. Problems are as for **Caesarean section**.
  - regional techniques: involve blockade of the nerve supply of:
    - **uterus**:
      - via sympathetic pathways in paracervical tissues and broad ligament to the **spinal cord** at T11–12, sometimes T10 and L1 also.
      - the cervix is possibly innervated via separate S2–4 pathways in addition.
    - birth canal and perineum: via pudendal nerves (S2–4), genitofemoral and ilioinguinal nerves and sacral nerves.
- Regional techniques used:
  - **extradural anaesthesia**:
    - **caudal analgesia** was first used in obstetrics in 1909 by Stoeckel; a continuous technique was introduced in the USA in 1942.
    - continuous lumbar techniques were used in 1946; they have become popular in the UK from the 1960s, with many units now providing a 24–hour service. Up to 30% uptake has been reported; 80% of women obtain complete relief, with 15% helped and 5% gaining no benefit.
    - advantages:
      - reduces maternal exhaustion, **hyperventilation**, ketosis, and plasma **catecholamine** levels.
      - avoids adverse effects of parenteral opioids.
      - reduces fetal **acidosis** and maintains or increases uteroplacental blood flow if hypotension is avoided.
      - may improve contractions in incoordinate uterine activity.
      - reduces morbidity and mortality in breech delivery, multiple delivery, premature labour, pre-eclampsia, maternal cardiovascular or respiratory disease, **diabetes mellitus**, forceps delivery and Caesarean section.
    - disadvantages:
      - risk of hypotension, extensive blockade, iv injection and other complications. **Postspinal headache** is more common following accidental dural tap (incidence of the latter is about 1% in teaching centres). **Shivering** is common, and urinary retention may occur.
      - motor block may be distressing, and is associated with delayed descent of the fetal head.
      - requires iv infusion, and 24–hour anaesthetic cover.
      - increased incidence of backache has been reported; this may be secondary to muscular relaxation and posture during labour, or may reflect selection of patients prone to backache (e.g. complicated labour, lower pain threshold, etc.).
    - effect on labour:
      - temporary reduction in uterine activity may follow injection of solution. Severe reduction

may occur if hypotension or aortocaval compression occur.

–incoordinate uterine activity may improve.

–forceps rate is increased, thought to occur because:

  –patients likely to require forceps delivery are more likely to receive extradural anaesthesia.

  –muscle tone is reduced as above.

Normal vaginal delivery rates are thought to occur if adequate time is allowed for the second stage. **Oxytocin** may be required. Perineal tears may occur if the second stage is very prolonged.

–technique:

  –standard techniques are used, but the dose of **local anaesthetic agent** is reduced by ⅓ because venous engorgement reduces the volume of the **extradural space**. Hypotension is common, especially in the presence of **hypovolaemia**; it is reduced by preloading with iv fluid. **Crystalloid** is usually administered (e.g. 0.9% **saline/ Hartmann's solution**, 500–1000 ml. Ketosis and **hyponatraemia** may occur with excess administration of **dextrose** solutions). L2–3 or L3–4 interspaces are usually chosen.

  –**bupivacaine** is usually preferred, since fetal transfer is least. Others have been used, e.g. **lignocaine, chloroprocaine. Prilocaine** is rarely used because of the risk of **methaemoglobinaemia**.

  –use of a **test dose** is controversial.

  –suitable dose regimens:

    –bupivacaine 0.25% 5–10 ml as boluses. More concentrated solutions provide analgesia lasting slightly longer, but with more motor blockade. 0.75% solution is contraindicated in obstetrics. Top-up injections are usually given by midwives. Aspiration through the catheter should precede top-ups, which should be given in divided doses. A maximum of 25 mg bupivacaine has been suggested for any single injection.

    –infusions: increasingly used. Provide more consistent analgesia, with less motor block and hypotension, and reduce the risk from accidental iv or subarachnoid injection. Bupivacaine 10–20 mg/h is usually employed, usually as a 0.1–0.2% solution. Large volumes of more dilute solutions have been used, supporting the concept of an 'extended sleeve' of anaesthetic solution over the appropriate segments. The height of the block must be regularly assessed, and the infusion adjusted accordingly.

    –patient-controlled extradural anaesthesia has also been used.

  –extradural opioids have been used, but with risk of maternal and neonatal respiratory depression (*see Spinal opioids*). **Fentanyl** has been added to bupivacaine infusions, e.g. 5–10 μg/h, reducing the requirement for local anaesthetic.

  –inadequate blockade: includes 'missed segment' (commonly in one groin, the cause is unclear), backache, rectal or perineal pain, and unilateral blocks. Remedial measures include further injection of 5 ml solution, with the unblocked part

dependent. Larger volumes of dilute solution, or a different local anaesthetic, may be helpful. Fentanyl 50–75 μg may be effective, but with risk of respiratory depression. Infiltration of the unblocked dermatome with local anaesthetic has been used. The catheter should be withdrawn 1–2 cm if unilateral block occurs. Resiting of the catheter may be required. Suprapubic pain may result from a full bladder, and may be relieved by urinary catheterization.

  –contraindications, complications and management are as for extradural anaesthesia. Care should be taken in antepartum haemorrhage (see below). Extensive blockade and accidental iv injection of local anaesthetic are possible following catheter migration. An anaesthetist should regularly assess all blocks and be readily available, with resuscitative drugs and equipment. Maximal doses of local anaesthetic agents should not be exceeded in a 4 hour period.

    Backache and neurological damage may be caused by labour itself, although extradural anaesthesia is often blamed by the patient and non-anaesthetic staff.

–**spinal anaesthesia** was first used in 1900. Popular in the USA in the 1920s, it only recently increased in popularity in the UK. Technique and management are as standard, but with more rapid onset of hypotension and greater incidence of postspinal headache and variable blocks (especially using plain bupivacaine) than in non-pregnant subjects. Dose requirement is reduced, possibly due to altered **CSF** dynamics, although changes in CSF pH, proteins and volume have been suggested. Effects are as for extradural anaesthesia. Mostly used for Caesarean section, forceps and ventouse delivery, removal of retained placenta, etc. Doses for vaginal procedures: 1.0–1.6 ml heavy bupivacaine 0.5%; 0.8–1.0 ml **amethocaine** or heavy **cinchocaine** 0.5%.

–**paravertebral block**: bilateral blocks are required at either L2 (for sympathetic block) or T11–12 (somatic block).

–**paracervical block**: rarely performed because of fetal arrhythmias.

–**pudendal nerve block** and perineal infiltration/spraying with local anaesthetic: only of use for the second stage. Pudendal block is used for forceps and ventouse delivery.

–local infiltration of the abdomen for Caesarean section.

• Particular problems in obstetric anaesthetic pratice:

  –obstetric conditions, e.g. **eclampsia**, antepartum haemorrhage due to placental abruption (hypovolaemia, **DIC**, renal impairment) or placenta praevia. Haemorrhage may follow any delivery, and facilities for urgent transfusion should be available, including a cut-down set and O negative uncrossmatched blood. DIC may also occur in septic abortion, intrauterine death, hydatidiform mole and severe **shock**.

  –maternal disease, e.g. cardiovascular, respiratory, diabetes, etc. Extradural blockade is usually preferred.

  –fluid overload associated with oxytocin administration; **pulmonary oedema** associated with **tocolytic drugs**.

–specific procedures/presentations:
  –premature labour: spinal/extradural anaesthesia is usually preferred, since it allows smooth controlled delivery with or without forceps. The immature fetus may be especially susceptible to drug-induced depression. Tocolytic drugs may have been used.
  –twin delivery: extradural anaesthesia is usually employed. The block should be adequate for Caesarean section, in case this is required for delivery of the second twin. Blood loss at delivery is greater than with a single fetus. The enlarged uterus is more likely to cause aortocaval compression.
  –breech presentation: similar considerations as for twin delivery.
  –manual removal of placenta: spinal/extradural anaesthesia is usually considered preferable to general anaesthesia, since the latter risks aspiration of gastric contents, and inhalational agents cause uterine relaxation.
–collapse on labour ward:
  –causes include: **shock** associated with abruption and DIC, postpartum haemorrhage, total spinal blockade, overdosage or iv injection of local anaesthetic, **amniotic fluid embolism**, **PE**, eclampsia, inversion of the uterus, and pre-existing disease.
  –**CPR** is hindered by aortocaval compression, relieved by tilting the patient to one side or manually displacing the uterus laterally. Caesarean section may be required.

[Lucy Baldwin (1859–1945), wife of the British Prime Minister; Walter Stoeckel (1871–1961), German obstetrician; Michael E Tunstall, Aberdeen anaesthetist]
See also, Cardiopulmonary resuscitation, neonatal; Ergometrine; Fetal wellbeing, during labour; Flying squad, obstetric; Labour, active managament of; Midwives, administration of drugs by

Obturator nerve block. Performed to accompany **sciatic nerve block** or **femoral nerve block**, or in the diagnosis and treatment of hip pain. The obturator nerve (L2–4), a branch of the **lumbar plexus**, passes down within the pelvis and through the obturator canal into the thigh, to supply the hip joint, anterior adductor muscles and skin of medial lower thigh/knee.

With the patient supine and the leg slightly abducted, an 8 cm needle is inserted 1–2 cm caudal and lateral to the pubic tubercle, and directed slightly medially to encounter the pubic ramus. It is then withdrawn and redirected laterally to enter the obturator canal, and advanced 2–3 cm. After careful aspiration to exclude intravascular placement, 10–15 ml **local anaesthetic agent** is injected.

Occipital nerve blocks, *see Scalp, nerve blocks*

Oculocardiac reflex. Bradycardia following traction on the extraocular muscles, especially medial rectus. Afferent pathways are via the occipital branch of the trigeminal nerve; efferents are via the **vagus**. The reflex is particularly active in children. Bradycardia may be severe, and may lead to **asystole**. Other **arrhythmias**, e.g. ventricular ectopics or junctional rhythm, may occur. Bradycardia may also follow pressure on or around the eye, fixation of facial fractures, etc. Reduced by **anticholinergic drugs** administered as **premedication** or on induction

of anaesthesia. If it occurs, surgery should stop, and **atropine** or **glycopyrronium** administered. **Retrobulbar block** does not reliably prevent it and is itself hazardous; local infiltration of the muscles has been used instead.
See also, Ophthalmic surgery

Oculogyric crises, *see Dystonic reactions*

Oculorespiratory reflex. Hypoventilation following traction on the external ocular muscles. Reduced respiratory rate, reduced tidal volume or irregular ventilation may occur. Thought to involve the same afferent pathways as the **oculocardiac reflex**, but with efferents via the respiratory centres. Heart rate may be unchanged, and the reflex is unaffected by **atropine**.

Odds ratio. Indicator of relative risk. For example, if a disease is suspected to be caused by exposure to a certain factor, a 2×2 table may be drawn for proportions of patients in the following groups:

	with disease	*without disease*
exposed	*a*	*c*
not exposed	*b*	*d*

Odds ratio = the ratio of *a/b* to *c/d*
         = *ad/bc*.

O'Dwyer, Joseph (1841–1898). US physician; regarded as the introducer of the first practical intubation tube in 1885, although the technique had been described previously. His short metal tube, used as an alternative to **tracheostomy** in **diphtheria**, was inserted blindly into the **larnyx** on an introducer; the flanged upper end rested on the vocal cords. He mounted his tube on a handle for use with Fell's resuscitation bellows in 1888; the Fell-O'Dwyer apparatus could be used for **CPR** or anaesthesia. Later modifications included addition of a **cuff**.
[George Fell (1850–1918), US ENT surgeon]

Oedema. Generalized or local excess **ECF**. Caused by:
  –**hypoproteinaemia** and decreased plasma **oncotic pressure**.
  –increased hydrostatic pressure, e.g. **cardiac failure**, venous or lymphatic obstruction; salt and water retention (e.g. renal impairment, drugs, e.g. **NSAIDs**, oestrogens, steroids).
  –leaky capillary endothelium, e.g. inflammation, allergic reactions, toxins.
  –direct instillation, e.g. extravasated iv fluids, infiltration.

Several causes often coexist, e.g. hypoproteinaemia, portal hypertension and fluid retention in **hepatic failure**. Characterized by pitting when prolonged digital pressure is applied, although fibrosis reduces this in chronic oedema. Generalized oedema occurs in dependent parts of the body, e.g. ankles if ambulant, sacrum if bed-bound. Treatment is directed at the cause. If localized, the affected part is raised above the heart.
See also, Cerebral oedema; Hereditary angioneurotic oedema; Pulmonary oedema; Starling's forces

Oesophageal contractility. Used as an indicator of anaesthetic depth and **brainstem** integrity. Skeletal muscle is present in the upper third of the oesophagus, smooth muscle in the lower third, and both types in the middle

third. Afferent and efferent nerve supply is mainly vagal via oesophageal plexuses, but also via sympathetic nerves.
- Normal pattern of contractions:
  - –primary: continuation of the **swallowing** process; propels the food bolus down the oesophagus.
  - –secondary (provoked): caused by presence of food, etc. within the oesophageal lumen. Unrelated to swallowing.
  - –tertiary (spontaneous): non-peristaltic; function is uncertain.

Measured by passing a double-ballooned probe into the lower oesophagus. The distal balloon is filled with water and connected to a pressure **transducer**; the other balloon (just proximal) may be inflated intermittently to study provoked contractions.
- Altered by:
  - –anaesthesia: provoked contractions diminish in amplitude as depth increases, and spontaneous contractions become less frequent. Oesophageal contractility index ((70 × spontaneous rate) + provoked amplitude) is used as an overall measure of activity. Thought to be analogous to BP, heart rate, lacrimation, sweating, etc., during anaesthesia; i.e. suggestive of anaesthetic depth but not reliable. Activity may be decreased by **atropine** and smooth muscle relaxants, e.g. **sodium nitroprusside**, and increased by **neostigmine**.
  - –brainstem death: spontaneous contractions disappear, and provoked contractions show a low amplitude pattern. Has been used to indicate the presence or absence of brainstem activity in ICU, but its role is controversial. Presently not included in UK brainstem death criteria.

See also, Anaesthesia, depth of

Oesophageal obturators and airways. Devices inserted blindly into the oesophagus of unconscious patients to secure the **airway** and allow **IPPV** when tracheal intubation is not possible, e.g. by untrained personnel. They have been used in failed intubation. Consist of a cuffed oesophageal tube, usually attached to a facepiece for sealing the mouth and nose and preventing air leaks. The cuff reduces gastric insufflation and regurgitation but may not prevent it.

The epiglottis is pushed anteriorly, creating an air passage for ventilation. An ordinary **tracheal tube** may be used to isolate the stomach and improve the airway in a similar way.
- Two main types are described:
  - –blind-ended cuffed tube, perforated level with the hypopharynx for passage of air. Inflation is through the tube and via the perforations to the lungs.
  - –open-ended tube, to allow gastric aspiration. Inflation is through a separate port of the facepiece. If accidental tracheal placement occurs, IPPV may be performed through the tube.

The above features have been combined in a double-lumen device (Combitube), which may be placed in either the oesophagus or trachea. A distal cuff seals the oesophagus or trachea, whilst a proximal balloon seals the oral and nasal airways. IPPV may be performed through either tube depending on the device's position.

Eichinger S, Schreiber W, Heinz T, et al (1992) Br J Anaesth; 68: 534–5

Oesophageal stethoscope, *see Stethoscope*

Ohm's law. Current passing through a conductor is proportional to the potential difference across it, at constant temperature. Thus: voltage = current × **resistance**. An analogous form exists for **flow** of a **fluid**: pressure = flow × resistance.
[Georg S Ohm (1787–1854), German physicist]

Old age, *see Elderly, anaesthesia for*

Oliguria. Reduced **urine** output; definition is controversial but usually described as under 0.5 ml/kg/h. Common after major surgery or in ICU.
- Caused by:
  - –**urinary retention**, blocked catheter, etc.
  - –poor renal perfusion, e.g. **hypotension**, **hypovolaemia**, low **cardiac output**. **Urine** formation usually requires MAP of 60–70 mmHg in normotensive subjects.
  - –increased intra-abdominal pressure: the mechanism is unknown but ureteric stents do not prevent it, suggesting mechanisms other than ureteric compression.
  - –**renal failure**.
- Management:
  - –exclusion of retention or blocked catheter.
  - –urinary and plasma chemical analysis, e.g. sodium, **osmolality**, etc., is useful in distinguishing renal from prerenal causes (*see Renal failure*). Management is as appropriate.

Sweny P (1991) Br J Anaesth; 67: 137–45

Omeprazole. Prodrug whose metabolite irreversibly inhibits the gastric proton pump (a **membrane** ATPase which exchanges luminal potassium ions for hydrogen ions). Used to reduce gastric acidity, e.g. in **peptic ulcer disease**, **oesophageal reflux**. Effects last for 24 hours after single dosage. 20 mg is given orally once a day; 40 mg has been given the night before and on the morning of surgery to reduce gastric acidity and volume. An iv form has been developed but is not yet generally available (40 mg iv 12 hourly).

Side effects are uncommon and mild, including nausea, diarrhoea and skin rash.
Dorman T, Reilly CS (1991) Curr Opin Anaesth; 4: 480–5

Omphalocele, *see Gastroschisis and exomphalos*

Oncotic pressure (Colloid osmotic pressure). **Osmotic pressure** exerted by plasma proteins, usually about 3.3 kPa (25 mmHg). Important in the balance of **Starling forces**, and movement of water across capillary walls, e.g. in **oedema**. Although related to plasma protein concentration, the relationship is thought to be an upwards curve, not a straight line, because of molecular interactions and effects of charge.
Bevan DR (1980) Anaesthesia; 35: 263–70
See also, Intravenous fluids

Ondansetron hydrochloride. Antiemetic drug, introduced in 1990. A **5-HT** type 3 receptor antagonist, it has no effect on **dopamine receptors** (i.e. does not cause **dystonic reactions**). Undergoes hepatic metabolism and renal excretion.

- Dosage:
    - postoperative nausea/vomiting:
        - prophylaxis: 4 mg slowly iv on induction, or 8 mg orally 1 hour preoperatively followed by two further oral doses of 8 mg at 8 hourly intervals.
        - treatment: 4 mg slowly iv.
    - nausea following radiotherapy or chemotherapy: 8 mg orally or iv, followed by 8 mg orally 12 hourly for up to 5 days.
- Side effects: headache, constipation, flushing sensation.

Robey PG, Rowbotham DJ (1992) Curr Opin Anaesth; 5: 477–80

Ondine's curse. **Hypoventilation** caused by reduced ventilatory drive, originally described following CNS surgery (classically to medulla/high cervical spine). Despite being awake, victims may breathe only on command, with apnoea when asleep. The term has also been applied to respiratory depression caused by **opioid analgesic drugs**, and a congenital form of hypoventilation. [Ondine, German mythological sea-nymph; the curse of having to remember when to breathe, and thus being unable to sleep for fear of dying, was inflicted on her unfaithful husband by her father, King of the Sea]

Wiesel S, Fox GS (1990) Can J Anaesth; 37: 122–6

One-lung anaesthesia. Deliberate peroperative collapse of one lung to allow or facilitate **thoracic surgery**, whilst maintaining ventilation and gas exchange on the other side. Requires the use of **endobronchial tubes** or blockers. Commmonly performed for surgery to the lungs, oesophagus, aorta and mediastinum, but most operations are possible without it (sleeve resection of the bronchus being a notable exception). Its main problem is related to **hypoxaemia** caused by the $\dot{V}/\dot{Q}$ **mismatch** produced, exacerbated by the lateral position used for most thoracic surgery.

- Effects of lateral positioning on gas exchange:
    - awake:
        - ventilation: **FRC** of the upper lung exceeds that of the lower lung, because of mediastinal movement to the other side, and pushing up of the lower hemidiaphragm by abdominal viscera. Thus the upper lung lies on a flatter part of the **compliance** curve, i.e. is less compliant, whilst the lower lung lies on the steep part of curve, i.e. is more compliant (Fig. 103a). In addition, the higher hemidiaphragm contracts more effectively. Thus most ventilation is of the lower lung.
        - perfusion: mainly of the lower lung because of gravity; i.e. is matched with ventilation.
    - anaesthetized:
        - FRC of both lungs is reduced; the upper lung now lies on the steep part of the curve and the lower lung on the flat part (Fig. 103b). Thus the upper (more compliant) lung, is ventilated in preference to the lower (less compliant) lung.
        - perfusion is still mainly of the lower lung, i.e. $\dot{V}/\dot{Q}$ mismatch occurs (usually of minor importance in normal patients, since both blood flow and ventilation usually differ by up to 10% between the two sides).
    - one-lung anaesthesia: all ventilation is of the lower lung, whereas considerable perfusion is still of the upper lung. Thus significant **shunt** occurs in the upper lung, with $\dot{V}/\dot{Q}$ mismatch usual in the lower lung.

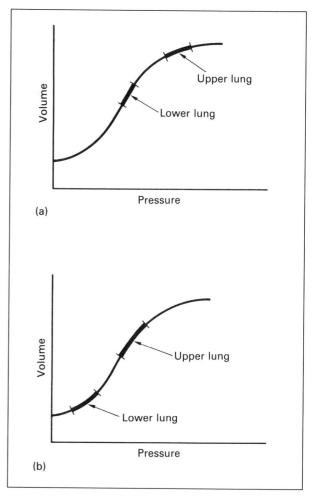

Figure 103 *Compliance curve for upper and lower lungs in the lateral position: (a) awake; (b) anaesthetized*

CO_2 exchange increases via the lower lung; thus CO_2 elimination is thought to be maintained if minute ventilation is unchanged. Degree of hypoxaemia is affected by:
- pre-existing state of the lungs: decrease in oxygenation is greatest in normal lungs, e.g. during non-pulmonary surgery. In abnormal lung, blood flow is usually already reduced preoperatively, thus the drop in arterial PO_2 is smaller.
- F_IO_2: increases above 0.5 may not improve oxygenation, since pure shunt is not corrected by raising F_IO_2.
- cardiac output: hypoxaemia worsens if cardiac output falls because of a decrease in the PO_2 of mixed venous blood passing through the shunt. The situation is complicated by altered distribution of pulmonary blood flow caused by changes in cardiac output.
- **hypoxic pulmonary vasoconstriction**: whether it is attenuated by use of anaesthetic agents, or whether it contributes any protection against shunt, is unclear.
- **PEEP** to the ventilated lung: may exacerbate hypoxaemia by reducing cardiac output, or by forcing more blood to flow through the uppermost lung.
- pattern of ventilation: 12 ml/kg tidal volume is thought to be optimal.

–content of the collapsed lung: hypoxaemia worsens after about 10 minutes as contained O_2 is absorbed. Arterial Po_2 is increased by application of O_2 at 5–7 cmH$_2$O positive pressure, or by intermittent inflation, e.g. every 10–15 minutes.

–surgery: e.g. leaning on mediastinum, reduction of venous return, etc. Tying the uppermost pulmonary artery stops shunt to the uppermost lung.

● Practical management:

–**preoperative assessment** as for thoracic surgery; patients particularly at risk during one-lung anaesthesia may be identified.

–close **monitoring** using **oximetry** and/or arterial blood gas analysis.

–F_iO_2 is usually increased to 0.4–0.5; further increases or use of PEEP may improve oxygenation.

–adminstration of O_2 to the uppermost lung (especially with positive pressure) or intermittent inflation.

–surgical ligation of the pulmonary artery is performed early.

–re-inflation and ventilation of both lungs should be performed if hypoxaemia is unacceptable.

–suction is applied to the collapsed lung before reinflation, to remove accumulated secretions.

–slow manual inflation is performed at the end of the procedure, to encourage expansion. The surgeon may request sustained pressures (e.g. 30–40 cmH$_2$O) to test the integrity of the bronchial suturing.

Benumof JL (1985) Anesth Analg; 64: 821–33

Open-drop techniques. Common and convenient technique of administering **inhalational anaesthetic agents** in the 1800s/early 1900s. The volatile anaesthetic agent, e.g. **chloroform, diethyl ether, ethyl chloride**, was dripped on to a cloth (originally a folded hankerchief) on the patient's face from a dropper bottle. Concentration of agent depended on the rate of drop administration. Specially designed bottles and masks were later developed; the best known mask is that of Schimmelbusch, although this was adapted from Skinner's earlier model. After covering the face with gauze wadding, with a hole for the mouth and nose, the wire mask was placed on the face, and further layers of wadding laid on it. Some masks had retaining clips or wire loops for securing the wadding. The eyes were usually covered to reduce irritation by liquid agent. Poor fitting of the mask allowed inhalation of air around it. Some incorporated channels for O_2 insufflation, or gutters around the edge to catch liquid anaesthetic. Freezing of exhaled water vapour on the wadding was problematic during prolonged procedures.

[Curt Schimmelbusch (1860–1895), German surgeon; Thomas Skinner (?-1906), Liverpool obstetrician]

Operant conditioning. Manipulation of behaviour by reinforcing wanted or unwanted behaviour with rewards or punishments respectively. Has been used in chronic **pain management**, with several weeks admission to hospital, involving reduction in drug therapy and encouragement of activity and independence. Thus concentrates on behaviour secondary to pain instead of pain itself.

Ophthalmic nerve blocks. Performed for procedures around the eye, **nose** and forehead, and certain intraoral procedures.

● Anatomy (*see* Fig. 65; *Gasserian ganglion block*):

–ophthalmic division of the trigeminal nerve (V^1) is entirely sensory and passes from the **Gasserian ganglion**, where it divides into branches which pass through the superior orbital fissure:

–lacrimal nerve; supplies the lateral upper eyelid and conjunctiva, and lacrimal gland.

–frontal nerve; supplies the upper eyelid, frontal sinuses and anterior scalp via the supraorbital branch; upper eyelid and medial forehead via the supratrochlear branch.

–nasociliary nerve; supplies the anterior dura, anterior ethmoidal air cells, upper anterior nasal cavity and skin of the external nose via the anterior ethmoidal branch; posterior ethmoidal and sphenoid sinuses via the posterior ethmoidal branch; medial upper eyelid, conjunctiva and adjacent nose via the infratrochlear branch; eyeball via the long ciliary nerves and branches to the ciliary ganglion.

–supraorbital foramen, pupil, infraorbital notch, infraorbital foramen, buccal surface of the second premolar and mental foramen all lie along a straight line.

● Blocks:

–supraorbital nerve: 1–3 ml **local anaesthetic agent** is injected at the supraorbital notch.

–supratrochlear nerve: 1–3 ml is injected at the superiomedial part of the opening of the orbit.

–both the above nerves may be blocked by subcutaneous infiltration above the eyebrow.

–frontal nerve: 1 ml is injected at the central part of the roof of the orbit.

–anterior ethmoidal nerve: 2 ml is injected at the superomedial side of the orbit, at a depth of 3–4 cm.

See also, Mandibular nerve blocks; Maxillary nerve blocks

Ophthalmic surgery. Historically, first performed without anaesthesia and then under topical anaesthesia, because of the eye's accessibility and the disastrous effects of coughing during general anaesthesia. Subsequently, increasingly performed under general anaesthesia because of patients' expectations and the ability to control **intraocular pressure** (IOP). More recently local anaesthesia has been favoured again, especially in the elderly. Children (for strabismus repair) and the elderly (for cataract extraction) form the largest groups of patients.

● Local anaesthesia:

–cornea and conjunctiva: 4% **lignocaine** (with or without **adrenaline**) or 2–4% **cocaine** is instilled into the conjunctival sac. Cocaine is not used in **glaucoma**, as it dilates the **pupil**.

–**retrobulbar** or **peribulbar blocks**; the latter has been introduced as a safer alternative to the former.

–prevention of blepharospasm: infiltration between the muscles and bone parallel to the lower and lateral orbital margins from a point 1 cm behind the orbit's lower lateral corner; alternatively local anaesthetic may be injected above the condyloid process of the mandible.

–**sedation** may be used, e.g. **benzodiazepines, neuroleptanaesthesia**. Close **monitoring** is required as the patient's head is covered by drapes. Supplementary O_2 should be delivered.

● General anaesthesia:

–preoperatively:

–**preoperative assessment** of children with strabismus for muscle disorders and **MH** susceptibility. Cataracts may occur in **dystrophia myotonica, inborn**

errors of metabolism, chromosomal abnormalities, **diabetes mellitus**, **steroid therapy** or following trauma. Lens subluxation may occur in **Marfan's syndrome** and inborn errors, e.g. homocystinuria. The elderly should be assessed for other diseases, e.g. diabetes, **hypertension** (*see Elderly, anaesthesia for*).

–drugs used in eye drops may be absorbed and active systemically, e.g. **ecothiopate**, timolol.

–opioid **premedication** is usually avoided because of its emetic properties. Benzodiazepines are popular.

–peroperatively:

  –procedures include the above operations, repair of retinal detachment, vitrectomy, repair of eye injuries (*see Eye, penetrating injury*) and operations on the lacrimal system.

  –the **airway** is usually not easily accessible to the anaesthetist.

  –for children, considerations include those for **paediatric anaesthesia**, the very active **oculocardiac** and **oculorespiratory reflexes**, and the increased incidence of **vomiting** after strabismus repair (thought also to be associated with traction on extra-ocular muscles). **Atropine** should be given to all patients; iv administration on induction of anaesthesia is often used. Standard techniques are employed, usually with tracheal intubation; spontaneous or controlled ventilation are acceptable.

  –for adults, standard agents and techniques are used. Control of IOP is usually achieved by iv induction, IPPV and **hyperventilation**, and use of a volatile **inhalational anaesthetic agent** (*for effects of specific drugs, use of suplhahexafluoride, etc., see Intraocular pressure*). Administration of iv **acetazolamide** may be required. Spontaneous ventilation is often used for extra-ocular procedures. The oculocardiac reflex may still occur in adults.

  –systemic absorption of topical solutions, e.g. **adrenaline**, cocaine, may occur.

  –coughing, straining, vomiting, etc. may increase IOP, especially undesirable if the globe is open.

–postoperatively: avoidance of straining and vomiting is desirable. Postoperative pain tends to be mild.

Opiates. Strictly, substances derived from **opium**. Formerly used to describe agonist drugs at **opioid receptors**; the terms **opioids** and **opioid analgesic drugs** are now preferred.

Opioid analgesic drugs. Opium and **morphine** have been used for thousands of years; morphine was isolated in 1803 and **codeine** in 1832. **Diamorphine** was introduced in 1898, **papaveretum** in 1909. Other commonly-used drugs include **pethidine** (1939), **phenoperidine** (1957), **fentanyl** (1960), **alfentanil** (1976) and **sufentanil** (1974). Drugs with **opioid receptor antagonist** properties include **pentazocine** (1962), **nalbuphine** (1968), **meptazinol** (1971) and **buprenorphine** (1968).

May be divided into naturally-occurring alkaloids (e.g. morphine, codeine), semisynthetic drugs (slightly modified natural molecules, e.g. diamorphine, **dihydrocodeine**), and synthetic opioids (e.g. pethidine, fentanyl, alfentanil). May also be classified according to their **opioid receptor** specificity and actions, or according to their onset and duration of action.

Each drug has slightly different effects on the body's systems, but their general effects are those of morphine.

The 'purer' drugs, e.g. fentanyl, alfentanil, sufentanil, do not cause **histamine** release, and may be used in very high doses with relative cardiostability, e.g. for **cardiac surgery**. In lower doses, they are used to provide intra- and **postoperative analgesia**, and to prevent the haemodynamic consequences of tracheal intubation and surgical stimulation. Also used as general **analgesic drugs** and for **premedication**, anxiolysis, cough suppression and chronic diarrhoea. *See also, Opioid...; Spinal opioids*

Opioid poisoning. Presents with nausea and **vomiting**, respiratory depression, **hypotension**, pinpoint **pupils** and **coma**. Depressant effects are exacerbated by **alcohol** ingestion. **Hypothermia**, **hypoglycaemia** and rarely **pulmonary oedema** and rhabdomyolysis may occur. **Convulsions** may occur with **pethidine**, **codeine** and **dextropropoxyphene**. Drug combinations containing opioids include **atropine**/diphenoxylate for diarrhoea and **paracetamol/ dextropropoxyphene** for pain. The former combination may cause convulsions, tachycardia and restlessness; the latter may cause delayed **hepatic failure**.

- Management:
  –supportive; includes **gastric lavage**, **iv fluids**, **O$_2$ therapy** and **IPPV**.
  –**naloxone** 0.4–2.0 mg iv repeated after 2–3 minutes as required to a total of 10 mg; infusion may be necessary as naloxone's duration of action is short. Respiratory depression due to **buprenorphine** may not be responsive.

Opioid receptor antagonists. Different types:

–pure antagonists, e.g. **naloxone**, **naltrexone**: antagonists at all **opioid receptor** subtypes.

–agonist–antagonists: agonists at some receptors but antagonists at others, e.g.:

  –**pentazocine**: agonist at kappa and sigma, antagonist at mu receptors.

  –**nalorphine**: partial agonist at kappa and sigma, antagonist at mu receptors.

  –**nalbuphine**: as for nalorphine, but a less potent sigma agonist.

–partial agonists, e.g. **buprenorphine**, **meptazinol** (mu receptors); may antagonize mu effects of other opioids, e.g. morphine, although not themselves antagonists.

Their main clinical use is to reverse effects of **opioid analgesic drugs**, e.g. in **opioid poisoning**. Those with agonist properties are also used as **analgesic drugs**; some have been used to reverse unwanted effects of other opioids, e.g. respiratory depression, whilst still maintaining analgesia. In practice, this is very difficult to achieve. Also used in diagnosis and treatment of opioid addiction. Receptor-specific compounds have been developed for research and identification of receptor subtypes.

Many result from modification or substitution of the side chain on the nitrogen atom of parent analgesic drugs, e.g. *N*-allyl group substitution for the *N*-methyl group (hence the name, nal...).

Edwards RE, Ghodse AH, Gould T (1992) Curr Opin Anaesth; 5: 545–8

Opioid receptors. Naturally-occurring receptors to **morphine** and related drugs, isolated in the 1970s. Distinction between sub-types was made from the late 1970s. Found mainly in the CNS but also GIT; thought to be involved in central mechanisms involving **pain** and emotion. Evidence for several different types now exists, but the picture is confused by different terminology used (e.g. **opioids**, **opiates**, **narcotics**), the use of different animal experiments (e.g. rat and guinea-pig in particular), and the effects of different drugs at the various receptors.

- Subtypes:
  - mu:
    - activation causes analgesia, respiratory depression, euphoria, hypothermia, miosis, bradycardia, physical dependence; i.e. the classic effects of morphine.
    - responsible for 'supraspinal analgesia'; i.e. drugs act at brain level.
    - have been subdivided into mu_1 and mu_2, the former causing supraspinal analgesia, the latter causing most of the other effects.
    - agonists: most **opioid analgesic drugs**.
    - partial agonists: **buprenorphine**, **meptazinol** (thought to be specific at mu_1 receptors).
    - antagonists: **nalorphine**, **nalbuphine**, **pentazocine**.
  - kappa:
    - activation causes analgesia, respiratory depression, miosis, sedation, different sort of dependence.
    - responsible for 'spinal analgesia'; i.e. drugs thought to act at spinal level.
    - agonists: pentazocine, **butorphanol**, **dynorphins**, morphine.
    - partial agonists: nalorphine, nalbuphine.
  - sigma:
    - now thought not to be a true opioid receptor subtype, since stimulation is not antagonized by naloxone. May bind to phencyclidines and its derivatives, e.g. **ketamine**.
    - activation causes mydriasis, tachycardia, tachypnoea, delirium and dysphoria.
    - agonists: pentazocine, butorphanol.
    - partial agonists: nalorphine, nalbuphine.
  - delta:
    - activation has been experimentally shown to produce analgesia, especially at spinal level, but their precise role is unclear.
    - agonists: **endorphins** and **enkephalins**.
  - epsilon:
    - found in rat vas deferens only. β-Endorphin is an agonist.

All subtypes are antagonized by **naloxone** and naltrexone (mu, kappa and sigma more than delta and epsilon).

Pleuvry BJ (1991) Br J Anaesth; 66: 370–80

Opioids. Substances which bind to **opioid receptors**; include naturally-occurring and synthetic drugs, and endogenous compounds.

Opium. Dried juice from the unripe seed capsules of the opium poppy *Papaver somniferum*. Contains many different alkaloids including **morphine** (9–20%), **codeine** (up to 4%) and **papaverine**. Used for thousands of years as a recreational drug and for analgesia, especially in the Far East. Use as a therapeutic drug is rare now, purer drugs and extracts being preferred.

Orbeli effect. Increase in strength of contraction of fatigued **muscle** following sympathetic nerve stimulation. [Leon A Orbeli (1882–1958), Russian physiologist]

Oré, Pierre-Cyprien (1828–1889). French physician; Professor of Physiology at Bordeaux. Investigated **blood transfusion** and the effects of iv injection of drugs. Produced general anaesthesia with iv **chloral hydrate**, thus becoming the first to employ **TIVA**.

Organ donation. Organs for **transplantation** may be donated by living subjects, e.g. kidney and bone marrow. The main issue concerns the undertaking of anaesthesia and surgery (with their attendant risks) by a healthy patient for altruistic reasons.

Many organs may be obtained from patients following diagnosis of **brainstem death**. They include kidney, heart, lung, liver, small bowel, pancreas, skin and cornea. Demand for organs outstrips supply.

- Brainstem-dead patients may be unsuitable for donation because of:
  - systemic infection.
  - age: e.g. approximately >40 years for hearts; >50 years for livers; >70 years for kidneys.
  - **malignancy**.
  - disease of the organ or organ system concerned.
  - direct **trauma** to the organ.
  - **poisoning or overdose**, until the drug is cleared from the body.

Maintenance of tissue oxygenation, organ function, and metabolic and cardiovascular stability should be pursued as for critically ill patients, until and during organ removal.

Timmins AC, Hinds C (1991) Curr Opin Anaesth; 4: 287–92

Organe, Geoffrey Stephen William (1908–1989). English anaesthetist, born in India. A major influence on the development of anaesthesia in the UK and abroad, and involved in much research, particularly into the newly introduced **neuromuscular blocking drugs**. Professor of Anaesthesia at Westminster Hospital, and knighted in 1968.

Organophosphorus poisoning. Organophosphorus compounds are **acetylcholinesterase inhibitors**, commonly used as insecticides but also manufactured as chemical warfare agents. One, **ecothiopate**, is used in glaucoma. Those used in insecticides are usually ester, amide or thiol derivatives of phosphoric or phosphonic acids, or their mixtures. They may be absorbed via the GIT, lungs or skin, and are rapidly distributed to all tissues, especially liver and kidney. **Half-lives** vary from minutes to hours, with metabolism by oxidation, ester hydrolysis and combination with glutathione, and excretion in faeces or urine.

- Toxic effects:
  - peripheral **enzyme** inhibition:
    - phosphorylation of **acetylcholinesterase**: may be irreversible depending on the compound involved. Features are those of **cholinergic crisis** and include muscarinic effects (bronchospasm, sweating, increased secretions, abdominal cramps, bradycardia, miosis) and nicotinic effects (muscle twitching, weakness, hypertension and tachycardia). Spontaneous enzyme 'reactivation' may occur; this process is induced by **pralidoxime** if administered within 24–36 hours.
    - phosphorylation of other enzymes, e.g. lipases, GIT enzymes.

–myopathic effects: predominantly shown in animals. Weakness may occur within 24 hours of poisoning, with recovery taking up to 3 weeks. Muscle paralysis in humans may occur after recovery from the initial cholinergic crisis, 24–96 hours after poisoning. Mainly affecting proximal muscles, it is thought to involve postsynaptic dysfunction at the **neuromuscular junction**.

–delayed polyneuropathy: usually follows poisoning with non-insecticide compounds. Develops 2–4 weeks after the cholinergic crisis, with weakness and paraesthesiae. Pyramidal signs may be present. Recovery is variable.

–CNS effects: anxiety, tremor, confusion, **coma** and **convulsions** may occur, with EEG abnormalities.

Respiratory failure may result from peripheral weakness, central depression and increased tracheobronchial secretions.

Diagnosis is based on history, tolerance to **atropine** therapy, **acetylcholine** assay and measurement of blood and urine organophosphorus and metabolite levels.

- Treatment:
  –supportive measures as for **poisoning and overdoses** in general. Care should be taken to avoid self-contamination.
  –drug therapy:
    –atropine 2–4 mg iv each 5–10 minutes as required (0.02–0.05 mg/kg in children).
    –pralidoxime 1 g slowly iv 12 hourly for 5–7 days (20–60 mg/kg in children).

Karalliedde L, Senanayake N (1989) Br J Anaesth; 63: 736–50

Orthopaedic surgery. Anaesthetic considerations may be related to:
–reasons for surgery:
  –**trauma**: presence of other injuries, risks of **emergency surgery** (e.g. **aspiration of gastric contents**). Adequate resuscitation is important preoperatively, especially in the **elderly**, e.g. following fractured neck of femur (NOF). Cases with risk of infection, ischaemia or nerve damage are particularly urgent.
  –musculoskeletal disease, e.g. **rheumatoid arthritis**, **connective tissue diseases**, muscular abnormalities, etc. There is a higher than normal incidence of **MH** susceptibilty in young patients with musculoskeletal abnormalities.
  –congenital malformations: may be accompanied by other system involvement, e.g. cardiac lesions.
  –risk of massive **hyperkalaemia** following **suxamethonium** if neurological or muscle lesions are present.
–surgical procedure:
  –may involve repeated anaesthesia.
  –use of **tourniquets**.
  –use of **methylmethacrylate** cement.
  –problems of specific procedures, e.g. **kyphoscoliosis**.
  –regional techniques are particularly useful, e.g. hip surgery (arthroplasty, fractured NOF). **Extradural** and **spinal anaesthesia** are associated with fewer postoperative complications (including **DVT**) than after general anaesthesia, although mortality after fractured NOF is the same at 1 year.

–DVT and **PE** are common, especially after hip surgery; prophylactic measures should always be taken. **Fat embolism** is common after trauma.

Oscilloscope. Device for displaying recorded signals, especially of high frequency and when analysis of their shape is required, e.g. **ECG** or **arterial waveform**.

An electron beam is produced by heating a cathode at one end of an evacuated glass tube (cathode ray tube) and accelerated by anodes along the tube's length. It is focused on to one edge of a fluorescent screen at the other end of the tube, and is visible as a bright dot. If a saw-tooth patterned potential is applied horizontally (transversely across the beam), the beam is deflected across the screen as the potential increases, flipping back to its original position as the potential returns to zero. The dot appears to sweep across the screen continuously from one side to the other.

The signal potential is applied vertically across the beam, causing vertical deflection; a spatial reconstruction of the signal against time is seen on the screen. The pattern may be made to persist by altering the characteristics of the fluorescent material, or by using a second cathode system. It may also be achieved using rapid computer-controlled repeated movements of the electron beam. Further manipulation allows the frozen pattern to track across the screen, e.g. by storing the signal as a series of digital values, and displaying each in turn for a predetermined period.

May also be used without the time-base to plot two signals applied at right angles to each other, e.g. **flow–volume loops**.

Oscillotonometer. Device for indirect **arterial BP measurement**, using one cuff for occluding the brachial artery and a second cuff for detecting pulsations. Modern devices contain a double cuff with separate tubing, attached to a circular chamber containing aneroid gauges and a lever amplification system, with an indicator dial on its face.

- Principles of use:
  –the upper (occluding) cuff is about 5 cm wide; the lower (sensing) cuff is about 10 cm wide; they overlap by 2–3 cm.
  –with the control lever in its normal (up) position, both cuffs are inflated by hand to above systolic BP; the dial indicates the pressure within both cuffs.
  –moving the lever down connects the sensing cuff to a more sensitive aneroid gauge, and connects both cuffs to atmosphere via an adjustable screw-valve. The cuffs are allowed to deflate slowly, whilst observing the pointer needle for changes in sensing cuff pressure.
  –as pressure falls, small oscillations of the needle may occur, representing transmitted pulsations from the occluding cuff. At systolic BP, the oscillations suddenly increase in amplitude, representing pulsations reaching the sensing cuff under the occluding cuff.
  –the lever is released to the up position, and systolic pressure read from the dial.
  –the lever is pressed down and the process continued until the oscillations diminish suddenly, representing diastolic BP, which is read as before. Peak amplitude may occur between systolic and diastolic pressure, and is thought to represent **MAP**.

Automated devices employ similar principles.

May be used for continuous measurement, by keeping the cuffs inflated at around systolic BP, and the control lever held down: rising BP is indicated by increasing amplitude of oscillations, falling BP by decreasing amplitude. Periodic deflation allows circulation of the arm, e.g. for 1 minute out of every 5. Less accurate at high BP and low pulse pressure. Accuracy is decreased if the cuffs are reversed.

Hutton P, Prys-Roberts C (1982) Br J Anaesth; 54: 581–91

Osmolality and osmolarity. Expressions of concentration of osmotically active particles in solution:
  –osmolality = the number of osmoles per kilogram solvent.
  –osmolarity = the number of osmoles per litre solution.
  –osmoles = the mw of a substance divided by the number of freely moving particles liberated in solution.
Thus 1 mmol of a salt which dissociates completely into two ions provides 2 mosmol. In the body, the solvent is water, with density 1 kg/l; thus osmolality and osmolarity are often used interchangeably, although proteins and fats in plasma give rise to a small difference.

Osmolality of plasma is maintained at 280–305 mosmol/kg. Regulatory mechanisms include stimulation of thirst by **osmoreceptors**, **baroreceptors** and the **renin/angiotensin system**. Osmoreceptors also stimulate **vasopressin** release. Most contribution to plasma osmolality arises from **sodium** and its anions, **glucose** and **urea**; thus plasma osmolality may be estimated thus:

mosmol/kg = glucose + urea + (2 × Na⁺) (all in mmol/l).

Alcohol, **proteins**, triglycerides, **mannitol**, etc., are not accounted for. Proteins usually contribute little since, despite their high concentration, few particles are liberated in solution because of their high mw.

Osmolality/osmolarity is determined by measuring ionic concentration with a flame photometer, measuring **osmotic pressure** or by employing the **colligative properties of solutions** (e.g. depression of freezing point, lowering of vapour pressure).

Urinary and plasma osmolality measurement is useful in investigating **oliguria** and **renal failure**.

Bevan DR (1978) Anaesthesia; 33: 794–814
See also, Fluid balance; Hyperosmolality; Hypo-osmolality; Osmolar gap; Tonicity

Osmolar gap (Osmolality gap). Difference between calculated and measured plasma **osmolality**. Normally under 10 mosmol/kg; increased by high levels of osmotically active substances, e.g. **alcohol**, methanol, **mannitol**, **glycine** (in the **TURP syndrome**), etc. May also be applied to **urine** osmolality, e.g. to indicate the presence of osmotically active substances such as ammonium ions.

Osmoreceptors. Cells in the anterior **hypothalamus**, outside the **blood–brain barrier**; respond to changes in plasma **osmolality**. Control thirst and secretion of **vasopressin**, possibly via separate groups of osmoreceptors.

Bevan DR (1978) Anaesthesia; 33: 801–8

Osmosis. Movement of solvent molecules across a semipermeable **membrane** from a dilute solution to a concentrated one, so as to equalize the concentrations on both sides. Thus water moves across cell membranes from the **ECF** following **dextrose** infusion, once the dextrose has been metabolized. Similarly, water in very hypotonic **iv fluids** may move into red blood cells after infusion, causing **haemolysis**.

Osmotic clearance, *see Clearance, osmotic*

Osmotic diuretics, *see Diuretics*

Osmotic pressure. Pressure required to prevent movement of solvent molecules by **osmosis** across a semipermeable **membrane**.

Equals $\frac{nRT}{V}$, as for the **ideal gas law**,

where n = number of particles,
  R = **universal gas constant**,
  T = absolute temperature,
  V = volume.
Thus proportional to the number of particles per volume, not mw. Ideal ionic solutions dissociate completely in solution, whereas in the body incomplete dissociation and interactions between ions result in lower osmotic pressure than predicted. Plasma osmotic pressure is approximately 7.3 atmospheres.
See also, Oncotic pressure; Osmolality and osmolarity; Tonicity

Ouabain. **Cardiac glycoside**, poorly absorbed from the GIT and administered iv. Faster acting than **digoxin**; thus used when rapid action is required. 5% protein bound, with **half-life** about 24 hours, and excreted via kidneys and liver.
● Dosage: 100–250 µg by iv infusion. Not commercially available in the UK.

Overdoses, *see Poisoning and overdoses*

Oximetry. Determination of arterial **O₂ saturation** of **haemoglobin** (S_aO_2) by measuring absorbance of light by blood. Described in 1934 using open blood vessels, and in 1940 using ear/hand probes, but the technique was cumbersome and difficult to perform. Modern pulse oximeters became widespread from the 1980s following advances in microchip technology, allowing manipulation of the recorded signal.

Relies on the principle that absorbance of light by a substance depends on the substance's concentration and the distance the light travels through it (**Beer–Lambert law**). Oxygenated and deoxygenated haemoglobin (HbO and Hb respectively) have different absorbance spectra (Fig. 104). **Isobestic points** occur where the lines cross. Thus comparison of absorbances at different wavelengths allows estimation of the relative concentrations of HbO and Hb (i.e. S_aO_2). Earlier machines used two wavelengths including one isobestic point as a reference; modern pulse oximeters may use two or more wavelengths, not necessarily including an isobestic point.

Blood gas machines estimate S_aO_2 from arterial samples, whereas pulse oximeters read from ear or finger probes measuring light passing through tissue. Analysis of reflected light has also been used to determine S_aO_2; surface probes have been developed which may be stuck on to skin at any site, e.g. the head of a fetus.

Oxpentifylline

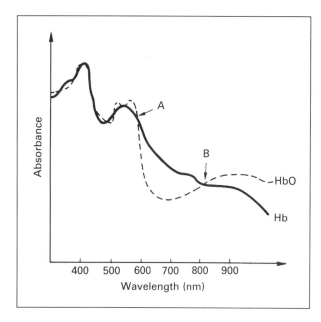

Figure 104 *Absorbance of light by oxygenated (HbO) and deoxygenated (Hb) haemoglobin. A and B are isobestic points*

- Method of measurement (pulse oximeter):
    - diodes within the probes produce light of the required wavelengths, usually in the red/infrared range as absorbance by body tissue is small. Emitted light may alternate between wavelengths at several hundred Hz.
    - a photodetector on the opposite side of the probe detects transmitted light.
    - the signal is converted to a DC component representing tissue background, venous blood and the constant part of arterial blood flow, and a AC component representing pulsatile arterial blood flow. The former is discarded, the latter amplified and averaged over a few seconds.
    - the signal is displayed ideally as a continuous trace, showing quality of signal and a numerical value of S_pO_2 (suggested as appropriate notation of S_aO_2 measured by a pulse oximeter). Some machines automatically adjust gain to maintain a constant size of trace.

Used in routine **monitoring**, e.g. during and after anaesthesia and on ICU, but particularly useful during **one-lung anaesthesia**, poor-risk cases, **paediatric anaesthesia**, or where observation of **cyanosis** is difficult, e.g. dark skin, darkened room or poor access to the patient. Oximetry has also been used to monitor **sleep apnoea**, in cardiac and respiratory function testing, **CPR** and assessment of peripheral circulation. It has been shown to detect desaturation in patients when clinical assessment reveals no abnormality, e.g. during anaesthesia, **recovery** and transport of patients.
- Inaccuracy may result from movement, electrical interference, venous congestion, and when S_aO_2 is less than 50%. Coloured nail polish may produce inaccuracies. Effects of other pigments, etc.:
    - carboxyhaemoblogin: most is counted as HbO, thus S_pO_2 is falsely high.
    - methaemoglobin and bilirubin: counted as Hb, thus S_pO_2 is falsely low.

- methylene blue, indocyanine green, etc.: may temporarily decrease S_pO_2 for a few minutes after iv injection.
    - **fetal haemoglobin, polycythaemia**: no effect.
Machines are calibrated during manufacture. Some are preset for low values of carboxyhaemoglobin and methaemoglobin. Others have specific filters.

Burns have been reported following prolonged use, especially with finger probes on children.
Severinghaus JW, Kelleher JF (1992) Anesthesiology; 76: 1018–38

Oxpentifylline. Xanthine used in peripheral vascular disease. Reduces blood **viscosity**. Also inhibits **tumour necrosis factor** production by macrophages; has thus been studied as a potential therapeutic agent in **septicaemia**.
Zabel P, Schonharting MM, Wolter DT et al (1989) Lancet; ii: 1474–7

Oxycodone hydrochloride. Opioid analgesic drug derived from **morphine**, with which it is equipotent. Described in 1916. Available in the USA for oral use, and in the UK for rectal administration as the pectinate. Action lasts 4–7 hours.

Oxygen. Non-metallic element existing as a colourless odourless diatomic gas (O_2) in the lower atmosphere, and as triatomic oxygen (O_3, ozone) and monoatomic oxygen (O) in the upper atmosphere. The most plentiful element in the Earth's crust (as opposed to nitrogen, the most plentiful in the atmosphere), it makes up 21% of **air** by volume. Discovered independently in 1771 by Scheele and **Priestley**, the latter calling it 'dephlogisticated air'. Recognized as a gas by **Lavoisier** who named it and explained the process of combustion. Combines with many other elements and molecules, and most abundant as water.

Essential for cellular respiration in animals and lower plants; higher plants take in CO_2 and release O_2 during photosynthesis. Boiling point is –183°C; melting point is –218°C; **critical temperature** is –118°C. Atomic weight is 16; **specific gravity** is 1.1 for liquid O_2 and 1.4 for gaseous O_2.

Commercial O_2 is supplied in liquid form, manufactured by the fractional distillation of air. Available in hospitals by **piped gas supply**, **O_2 concentrators** or in **cylinders** at 137 bar.
[Carl W Scheele (1742–1786), Swedish chemist]
See also, Oxygen....; Vacuum insulated evaporator

Oxygen cascade. Series of steps of Po_2 from atmospheric **air** to mitochondria in cells:
    - dry atmospheric gas: 21 kPa (160 mmHg)
    - humidified tracheal gas: 19.8 kPa (150 mmHg)
    - alveolar gas: 14 kPa (106 mmHg)
    - arterial blood: 13.3 kPa (100 mmHg)
    - capillary blood: 6–7 kPa (45–55 mmHg)
    - mitochondria: 1–5 kPa (7.5–40 mmHg)
Reduction in Po_2 at any stage, e.g. due to **hypoventilation**, lung disease, etc., causes reduction in subsequent steps, risking inadequate mitochondrial Po_2 for aerobic metabolism (below the **Pasteur point**).
See also, Oxygen transport

Oxygen concentrator. Device for extracting **O_2** from atmospheric **air**. Air is passed under pressure through a

338

column of **zeolite** which acts as a molecular sieve, trapping nitrogen and water vapour whilst leaving O_2 and trace gases. Nitrogen is removed by depressurizing the column. Two columns are used, each alternatively adsorbing or expelling nitrogen. Produces a continuous supply of over 90% O_2, suitable for most medical uses. Range in size from small units to large ones supplying whole hospitals.
Howell RS (1985) Br J Hosp Med; 40: 221–3

Oxygen delivery ($\dot{D}O_2$). Calculated **O_2 flux**. Used with O_2 consumption ($\dot{V}O_2$) to optimize treatment in critical illness.

$\dot{D}O_2$ = **cardiac output** (CO) × arterial O_2 content
= 850–1200 ml/min (500–700 ml/min/m^2)

$\dot{V}O_2$ = CO × (arterial O_2 content - mixed venous O_2 content)
= 240–270 ml/min (120–160 ml/min/m^2)

May be used to supplement traditional measurement of cardiovascular variables, e.g. BP, CVP, CO, etc. As $\dot{D}O_2$ falls, a critical point is reached after which $\dot{V}O_2$ also falls, representing tissue anaerobic respiration. Maintenance of $\dot{D}O_2$ above 600 ml/min/m^2, and $\dot{V}O_2$ above 170 ml/min/m^2, is thought to increase survival in critical illness. It has been suggested that patients with severe **trauma**, **burns** and **septicaemia** may require supramaximal values of $\dot{D}O_2$ and $\dot{V}O_2$.

O_2 extraction ratio has also been used (normally 22–30%):

$$\frac{\text{arterial – mixed venous } O_2 \text{ contents}}{\text{arterial } O_2 \text{ content}}$$

Vincent JL (1991) Can J Anaesth; 38: R44–7
See also, Shock

Oxygen failure warning device. Device attached to the **anaesthetic machine**; designed to alert anaesthetists to failure of the **O_2** supply. Earlier models were often unreliable, e.g. Bosun device (required batteries to power a warning light which could be switched off, and only operated when the N_2O supply was connected).

- Features of modern devices:
  - audible warning activated when O_2 pressure falls below a certain value; powered by O_2 itself.
  - warning continues when O_2 is exhausted; powered by N_2O.
  - delivery of N_2O turned off.
  - breathing system opened to atmosphere, allowing inhalation of air.
  - cannot be switched off.

Most consist of a spindle, kept at one end of its casing by the normal working O_2 pressure; a spring moves the spindle towards the other end as O_2 pressure falls, allowing O_2 to pass to a whistle via a port previously blocked by the spindle. Further movement as O_2 pressure continues to fall allows N_2O to flow to a whistle, stops N_2O delivery to the patient, and opens the system to air. Many have a visual indicator too, e.g. producing a colour change.

Oxygen flux. Amount of O_2 delivered to the tissues per unit time.

Equals: CO × arterial **O_2** content
= (CO × O_2 bound to **haemoglobin** + O_2 dissolved in plasma)
= CO × [(10 × Hb × S_aO_2 × 1.34) + (10 × P_aO_2 × 0.0225)]

where CO = **cardiac output**
Hb = haemoglobin concentration in g/dl
S_aO_2 = arterial **O_2 saturation** of haemoglobin
1.34 = **Hüfner's constant**
P_aO_2 = arterial PO_2
0.0225 = ml of O_2 dissolved per 100 ml plasma per kPa (0.003 ml per mmHg).

Normally 850–1200 ml/min; or 500–700 ml/min/m^2 if **cardiac index** is used.

The tissues cannot utilize all of the transported O_2: the last 20–25% remains bound to haemoglobin. Tissue O_2 supply can increase during times of extra demand, e.g. exercise, via increases in cardiac output. If the O_2 carrying capacity of blood is reduced, e.g. in **anaemia**, cardiac output must increase at rest in order to maintain O_2 flux, and reserves are less. Cardiac depression during anaesthesia in this situation is thus particularly hazardous.
See also, Oxygen delivery; Oxygen transport

Oxygen, hyperbaric. O_2 therapy at greater than atmospheric pressure, usually 2–3 atmospheres. Increases the amount of dissolved O_2 in blood according to **Henry's law**. In 100 ml blood, 0.3 ml O_2 dissolves at PO_2 of 13.3 kPa (100 mmHg). Thus for 100% O_2 at three atmospheres, dissolved O_2 = 5.7 ml. Since **haemoglobin** is always saturated, even in venous blood, its binding capacity for CO_2 and buffering capacity are reduced, and pH falls. The resultant **hyperventilation** may result in **hypocapnia**.

Used in the treatment of **carbon monoxide poisoning**, **air embolism**, **gas gangrene**, **decompression sickness**, and has been investigated as an adjunct to **radiotherapy** and in multiple sclerosis. Single-patient chambers filled with 100% O_2 may be used, or large pressurized chambers containing patient and attendants, with a tightly-fitting mask applied to the patient.
Grim PS, Gottlieb LJ, Boddie A, Batson E (1990) JAMA; 263: 2216–20
See also, Oxygen transport

Oxygen measurement. Methods include:
- **gas analysis**:
  - chemical, e.g. conversion to non-gaseous compounds, with reduction in overall volume of gas mixture (**Haldane apparatus**).
  - physical:
    - O_2 electrode (Clark electrode; polarographic cell): silver/silver chloride anode and platinum cathode in potassium chloride solution inside a cylinder, with a gas-permeable plastic membrane covering its end. 0.6 V potential is applied across the electrodes. O_2 diffuses to the cathode, picking up electrons with water present to become hydroxide ions and causing current flow proportional to the O_2 concentration. May be used with gas or liquid samples. Maintained at 37°C. Falsely high readings caused by **halothane** are prevented by using a membrane impermeable to halothane.
    - fuel cell: similar to the O_2 electrode but produces its own potential. Consists of lead anode and gold mesh cathode within potassium hydroxide solution. Hydroxide ions are produced at the cathode as above; they combine with lead at the anode to form lead oxide and give up electrons. Thus current flows, proportional to the number

of O_2 molecules diffusing through the plastic membrane. No external power source is required, but lifespan is limited. May be affected by **N₂O** unless special cells are used.

–paramagnetic cell: most gases are diamagnetic, i.e. repelled by magnetic fields. O_2 and nitric oxide are paramagnetic, i.e. attracted. The cell contains two nitrogen-filled glass spheres joined by a bar which is suspended on a vertical wire within a magnetic field. O_2 introduced into the cell is attracted into the magnetic field, displacing the spheres and rotating the bar against the torque of the wire. Degree of rotation is proportional to the number of O_2 molecules. It may be measured by observing the deflection of a beam of light reflected by a mirror mounted on the wire, or by measuring the current required to prevent rotation when passing through a coil mounted on the bar. Alternatively, an alternating magnetic field is applied to the gas, producing a sound wave; its amplitude is proportional to the concentration of O_2 (magnetoacoustic technique). Accuracy of these techniques is high.

–non-specific methods, e.g. **mass spectrometer**, ultra-violet light absorption.

–measurement of arterial P_{O_2}:

–O_2 electrode as above. Tiny intravascular probes have been developed for continuous arterial measurement.

–transcutaneous electrode: similar to the O_2 electrode, but with a heating coil to cause vasodilatation, increase rate of O_2 diffusion, and reduce the difference between arterial and skin P_{O_2}. Inaccurate, especially in adults, and with slow response time; they may also cause burns.

–fibreoptic sensor placed intravascularly; measures intensity or wavelength of reflected light.

–measurement of arterial O_2 content:, e.g. liberation of gas from blood with chemical analysis (**van Slyke apparatus**) or use of an O_2 electrode.

–measurement of **oxygen saturation** of haemoglobin.

[Leland C Clark, US biochemist]

Oxygen radicals, *see Free radicals*

Oxygen saturation. Refers to percentage saturation of **haemoglobin** with O_2; equals

$$\frac{O_2 \text{ content of haemoglobin}}{O_2 \text{ capacity of haemoglobin}}$$

May be calculated for whole blood, and the dissolved O_2 component subtracted, or measured using **oximetry**.

Oxygen therapy. Used to:

–correct **hypoxaemia** due to $\dot{V}/\dot{Q}$ **mismatch, hypoventilation** or impaired alveolar gas **diffusion**. Only partially corrects hypoxaemia due to **shunt**.

–increase pulmonary O_2 reserves, e.g. in case of **apnoea, hypoventilation**, etc.

–increase the amount of dissolved oxygen, e.g. in **anaemia, cyanide poisoning** and **carbon monoxide poisoning** (also increases rate of carboxyhaemoglobin dissociation).

–other uses include reduction of **pulmonary hypertension**, reduction of air-filled cavities (e.g. subcutaneous

Table 26. Effects of breathing 100% O_2 or air

	Air	*100% O_2*
Alveolar P_{O_2} (kPa (mmHg))	14 (106)	88 (667)
Arterial blood		
P_{O_2} (kPa (mmHg))	13.3 (100)	84 (638)
O_2 saturation (%)	99	100
O_2 content: (ml/100 ml blood)		
bound to haemoglobin	19.7	20.1
dissolved	0.3	1.9
Venous blood		
P_{O_2} (kPa (mmHg))	5.3 (40)	7 (53.2)
O_2 saturation (%)	75	85
O_2 content: (ml/100 ml blood)		
bound to haemoglobin	14.9	17.2
dissolved	0.1	0.2

emphysema, **pneumothorax**, **air embolism**, intestinal distension), and special uses of hyperbaric O_2 (*see Oxygen, hyperbaric*).

The effects of breathing 100% O_2 compared with air are shown in Table 26.

● Methods of administration:

–fixed performance devices; i.e. F_1O_2 is constant despite changes in inspiratory flow rate:

–O_2 tent.

–**anaesthetic breathing system**.

–high air flow O_2 enrichers (HAFOE): the feed connector to a plastic mask incorporates holes designed to allow entrainment of atmospheric air into the O_2 stream by **jet mixing**.

Specific connectors produce set F_1O_2 values at certain O_2 flow rates, assuming the patient's peak inspiratory flow rate does not exceed 30 l/min. For total gas flow of 30 l/min, calculations are as follows:

–O_2 flow rate = a.

–entrained air flow rate = b.

–$a + b = 30$.

–volume of O_2 delivered per minute $= (a \times 100\%) + (b \times 21\%)$.

–but volume of O_2 delivered also = 30 × required %.

–therefore $100a + 21b = 30 \times$ required %, and $a + b = 30$.

–thus the values for a and b may be determined.

–variable performance devices; i.e. actual F_1O_2 depends on inspiratory flow rates:

–nasal cannulae.

–plastic masks, e.g.:

–moulded hard plastic.

–Edinburgh: soft plastic.

–MC: soft plastic with foam-padded edges.

All perform similarly, delivering approximately 25–30% O_2 at 2 l/min O_2 flow, and 30–40% at 4 l/min flow.

–other means of administration include **IPPV** and its variations, **CPAP, apnoeic oxygenation** and hyperbaric therapy. Transtracheal administration has also been used in chronic lung disease requiring continuous O_2 therapy, via a narrow bore catheter inserted above the sternal notch.

- Problems of O_2 therapy:
    - –reduction of hypoxic ventilatory drive in a small group of patients who have chronic CO_2 retention, e.g. **COAD**. Apnoea may result if chronic hypoxaemia is reversed, thus necessitating controlled O_2 therapy. 24% O_2 is administered initially; if arterial P_{CO_2} has not risen by more than 1–1.5 kPa (7.5–10 mmHg), and P_{O_2} has not improved adequately, 28% O_2 is administered, then 30%, etc., until satisfactory P_{O_2} and P_{CO_2} have been achieved.
    - –pulmonary and CNS **O_2 toxicity**.
    - –absorption **atelectasis**.
    - –increased risk of **explosions and fires**.

[MC: Mary Catterall, London physician]

Oxygen toxicity. May be:
- –respiratory: pulmonary toxicity is related to actual P_{O_2}, not concentration. Tracheobronchial irritation and substernal discomfort is noticed by healthy volunteers after 12–24 hours' breathing 100% O_2. Reduced **vital capacity**, **compliance** and **diffusing capacity**, and increased arteriovenous **shunt** and **dead space** may occur after 24–36 hours. Changes include endothelial damage, with reduced mucus clearance and infiltration by inflammatory cells including macrophages and neutrophils. **Surfactant** may decrease and capillary permeability increase. Eventually fibrosis may occur, although maximal safe concentrations and duration of O_2 therapy are unclear. Up to 48 hours' breathing 100% is thought not to be associated with permanent damage; up to 50% is thought to be safe for any period. Certain **antimitotic drugs** increase the incidence and severity of fibrosis, e.g. bleomycin. Mechanisms are uncertain, but **free radical** formation is thought to be most likely. Neutrophil involvement is controversial. **Arachidonic acid** metabolites may also be involved. Free radical scavengers, surfactant and **leukotriene** blocking drugs have been studied as possible protective or therapeutic treatments, but prevention is considered more important at present. The lowest F_IO_2 that produces an acceptable arterial P_{O_2} should be used whenever O_2 is administered.
- –neurological:
    - –depression of respiratory drive in patients with chronic hypercapnia, e.g. **COAD**. Ventilation relies on hypoxic drive that is abolished by high F_IO_2; controlled **O_2 therapy** is employed in this situation.
    - –at above 2–3 atmospheres, **convulsions** may occur (**Bert effect**).
    - –**retrolental fibroplasia**.

Oxygen transport. In a normal person breathing air, arterial blood carries approximately 20 ml O_2 per 100 ml:
- –19.7 ml combined with **haemoglobin**.
- –0.3 ml dissolved in plasma.

In venous blood, 15 ml is carried per 100 ml blood:
- –14.9 ml combined with haemoglobin.
- –0.1 ml dissolved.

Normally, the amount carried by haemoglobin is only slightly increased with **O_2 therapy**, since haemoglobin is already over 97% saturated; the dissolved O_2 is increased in proportion to the arterial P_{O_2}: 0.0226 ml per kPa per 100 ml blood (0.3 ml per 100 mmHg).

See also, Oxygen flux

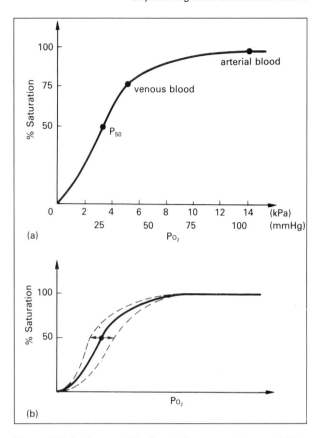

Figure 105 *Oxyhaemoglobin dissociation curve: (a) normal; (b) shift to right or left*

Oxygenators, *see Cardiopulmonary bypass*

Oxyhaemoglobin dissociation curve. Plot of **oxygen saturation** of **haemoglobin** against P_{O_2}, for normal haemoglobin and P_{CO_2} at 37°C (Fig. 105a). The curve is sigmoid-shaped because of the increasing affinity of haemoglobin for successive O_2 molecules after the first.
- Important points on the curve:
    - –P_{50}: P_{O_2} at which saturation is 50%; normally about 3.5 kPa (27 mmHg).
    - –venous blood: normally corresponds to 75% saturation and P_{O_2} of 5.3 kPa (40 mmHg).
    - –arterial blood: normally corresponds to 97% saturation and P_{O_2} of 13.3 kPa (100 mmHg).

Thus a small drop in P_{O_2} from normal levels causes only slight reduction in arterial saturation, because the curve is flat at this point. If P_{O_2} is already reduced, e.g. in lung disease, the same small drop may cause significant desaturation, corresponding to the steep part of the curve.

The curve is shifted to the right (i.e. P_{50} >3.5 kPa) by **acidosis, hyperthermia, hypercapnia (Bohr effect)** and increased **2,3–DPG** levels (Fig. 105b). Saturation becomes lower for any given P_{O_2}; i.e. O_2 is bound less avidly. Thus O_2 unloading to the tissues is favoured.

The curve is shifted to the left (i.e. P_{50} < 3.5 kPa) in the opposite situations, and in **fetal haemoglobin, methaemoglobinaemia** and **carbon monoxide poisoning**. Saturation becomes greater for any given P_{O_2}; i.e. O_2 is bound more avidly. Thus fetal haemoglobin can bind O_2 from maternal haemoglobin, but with reduced tissue liberation.

Oxymorphone hydrochloride. Opioid analgesic drug, derived from **morphine** and 6–8 times as potent. Prepared in 1955. Available in the USA for parenteral and rectal use. Action lasts 4–5 hours.

Oxytocin. Hormone secreted by the posterior **pituitary gland**, causing smooth muscle contraction in the **uterus** and milk ducts. Used to stimulate uterine contraction, e.g. during labour, postpartum or postabortion. Less effective in early pregnancy. Acts within 2–3 minutes of iv injection. Synthetic preparation (Syntocinon) is free of **vasopressin**, and thus preferable to pituitary extract.

Does not cause nausea/vomiting, and with minimal CVS effects; transient reduction in SVR and BP has been reported, and CVP may increase (by 1–2 cmH$_2$O for up to 30 minutes following iv injection) due to autotransfusion from the uterus to systemic circulation. CVS effects are least with iv infusion. Thus oxytocin has fewer side effects than **ergometrine**, although the latter is still widely used. Oxytocin is available as 5 units in combination with ergometrine 500 μg.

Dosage: 5–10 U iv. 1–5 mU/min is used during labour; much higher rates are used in postpartum haemorrhage and after abortion.

Severe **hyponatraemia** has followed prolonged infusion if diluted in **dextrose solutions**, exacerbated by a direct antidiuretic effect of the hormone itself.

P

P_{50}, see Oxyhaemoglobin dissociation curve

P wave. Component of the **ECG** representing atrial depolarization. Normally positive (i.e. upwards) in lead I, and best seen in leads II and V_1 (*see Fig. 49b; Electrocardiography*). Maximal amplitude is normally 2.5 mm in lead II, and its duration 0.12 seconds (three small squares). In right atrial enlargement, the P wave is tall and peaked (P pulmonale); in left atrial enlargement, it is wide and notched (P mitrale).
See also, P–R interval

Pacemaker cells. Cardiac muscle cells which undergo slow spontaneous depolarization to initiate **action potentials**. Their activity results from a slow decrease in **membrane** potassium ion permeability, resulting in gradual increase in intracellular potassium concentration. Rate of discharge depends on the slope of phase 4 depolarization, resting **membrane potential** and threshold potential. Pacemaker cells exist in the sinoatrial (SA) node, atrioventricular (AV) node, bundle of His, and ventricular cells. Spontaneous rates of discharge for the different sites: SA node 70–80/min, AV node 60/min, His bundles 50/min and ventricular cells 40/min. Impulses from the faster SA node usually reach and excite the slower pacemaker cells before the latter can discharge spontaneously.
See also, Heart, conducting system

Pacemakers, *see Cardiac pacing*

Packed cell volume, *see Haematocrit*

PAD, Pulmonary artery diastolic pressure, *see Pulmonary artery pressure*

Paediatric anaesthesia. Main considerations are related to the anatomical and physiological differences between adults and children, especially **neonates** (defined as up to 1 month old; infants are defined as up to 1 year old).
- Thus in children compared with adults:
  - RS:
    - the **tongue** is large and the **larynx** is situated more anteriorly and more cephalad (C3–4). The epiglottis is large and U-shaped. Airway management and tracheal intubation may thus be difficult, compounded by the large size of the head compared with the body. A straight **laryngoscope blade** is often preferred.
    - the cricoid cartilage is the narrowest part of the upper airway (cf. glottis in adults). A small decrease in diameter (e.g. caused by oedema or stricture formation following prolonged tracheal intubation) may lead to **airway obstruction**.

- the left and right main bronchi arise at equal angles from the trachea. At birth, the **tracheobronchial tree** is developed as far as the terminal bronchioles. Alveoli number 20 million, increasing to 300 million by 6–8 years.
- respiration is predominantly diaphragmatic, and sinusoidal and continuous instead of periodic. Neonates are obligatory nose breathers. Respiratory rate is increased. **Tidal volume** is about 7 ml/kg as in adults. The infant lung is more susceptible to **atelectasis** because the chest wall is more compliant and therefore pulled inwards by the lungs, decreasing **FRC**. **Closing capacity** may exceed FRC during normal respiration in neonates and infants. **Surfactant** may be deficient in premature babies.
- response to CO_2 is reduced at birth, and irregular breathing may also occur. Premature babies may suffer from apnoeic episodes; they may be at risk from postoperative apnoea up to about 50 weeks postconceptual age. **Gasp** and **Hering-Breuer reflexes** are active.
- **basal metabolic rate** and O_2 consumption are high (the latter is 5–6 ml/kg/min, compared with about 3–4 ml/kg/min in adults). **Hypoxaemia** thus occurs more rapidly than in adults.
- the **oxyhaemoglobin dissociation** curve of **fetal haemoglobin** is shifted to the left (P_{50} of 2.4 kPa (18 mmHg)). **Haemoglobin** concentration falls from 18 g/dl (1–2 weeks of age) to 11 g/dl (6 months–6 years).
- CVS:
  - **cardiac output** is 30–50% higher than in adults, largely due to increased **heart rate** (since **stroke volume** is able to increase only slightly). **Arterial BP** is lower (Table 27).
  - left and right ventricles are similar at birth, the former fibrous and non-compliant.
  - **blood volume** at birth is up to 90 ml/kg (or 50 + **haematocrit**). It falls to 80 ml/kg for children and 70 ml/kg by 14 years.
  - veins are more difficult to cannulate.
  - reversion to **fetal circulation** may occur in severe hypoxaemia.

Table 27. Normal heart rate and BP at different ages

Age	Heart rate (beats/min)	BP (mmHg)
0–6 months	120–180	80/45
3 years	95–120	95/65
5 years	90–110	100/65
10 years	80–100	110/70

–CNS:
  –the **spinal cord** ends at L3 at birth, receding to L1–2 by adolescence.
  –the immature **blood–brain barrier** results in increased sensitivity to centrally depressant drugs, particularly **opioid analgesic drugs**. These drugs have traditionally been avoided in children because of the fear of respiratory depression and the theory that neonates do not feel pain because their nervous system is insufficiently developed. This theory is now generally disbelieved, and opioids are widely used to provide analgesia for children.
  –vagal reflexes are particularly active in children. Bradycardia readily occurs in hypoxaemia.
  –subependymal vessels are fragile in premature neonates, with risk of rupture if BP and **ICP** increase.
–**temperature regulation** is impaired. Ratio of body **surface area** to body weight is greater than in adults. Thus **heat loss** is rapid, compounded by impaired shivering and increased metabolic rate. **Brown fat** is metabolized to maintain body temperature. **Insensible water loss** is increased in premature babies.
–prolonged fasting may cause **hypoglycaemia** in small children, and oral fluids are usually allowed up to 2–4 hours preoperatively. IV administration of dextrose may be required.
–**fluid balance** is delicate, since a greater proportion of body water is exchanged each day. Thus **dehydration** readily occurs in illness. Total body water is normally increased, with a higher ratio of **ECF** to **intracellular fluid** (ECF exceeds intracellular fluid in premature babies). The kidneys are less able to handle a water or solute load, or to conserve water or solutes.

  Appropriate maintenance fluid requirements (using dextrose/saline) may be calculated thus:
  4 ml/kg/h for each of the first 10 kg, plus
  2 ml/kg/h for each of the next 10 kg, plus
  1 ml/kg/h for each kg thereafter.

  Other losses, e.g. blood, must be added. Blood is traditionally given above 10% of blood volume loss, but larger blood losses are increasingly allowed if starting haemoglobin concentration is high. In **hypovolaemia**, 10 ml/kg **colloid** is a suitable starting regimen.
–actions of drugs may be affected by the above factors, or by lower plasma **albumin** levels (up to 1 year of age), resulting in greater amounts of free drug. Renal and hepatic immaturity may contribute to delayed excretion. **MAC** of **inhalational anaesthetic agents** is increased in neonates, but may be reduced in premature babies. Neonates are more sensitive to non-depolarizing **neuromuscular blocking drugs**, probably due to altered **pharmacokinetics**. They may be resistant to **suxamethonium**, requiring up to twice the adult dose.
● Practical conduct of anaesthesia:
  –children are placed first on the operating list, to interfere minimally with feeding, etc.
  –most standard drugs are used, administered according to weight. As a rough guide the following scheme may be useful:
    –14 years: adult dose.
    –7 years: ½ adult dose.
    –4 years: ⅓ adult dose.
    –1 year: ¼ adult dose.
    –newborn: ⅛ adult dose.
    –premature: ¹⁄₁₀ adult dose.
  –**premedication** is often given orally, to avoid injections, but standard im drugs are also given. Rectal administration has also been used. **Atropine** is often given to reduce excessive secretions and vagal reflexes.
  –**induction of anaesthesia**:
    –**cyclopropane** has been popular but its use is declining because of its flammability and cost. **Halothane** is also popular; **halothane hepatitis** is extremely rare in children but has been reported. Other **inhalational anaesthetic** agents are also suitable. Inhalational induction is rapid because of increased alveolar ventilation.
    –standard **iv anaesthetic agents** are suitable. Administration im (e.g. **ketamine**, **methohexitone**) or rectally (e.g. methohexitone) may also be used. **EMLA** cream is increasingly used before iv induction.
  The presence of parents at induction is controversial but is increasingly allowed.
–awake tracheal intubation is traditionally used in neonates, but fears have been expressed over adverse effects, e.g. raised ICP. However, ICP has been shown to rise markedly during normal crying, and awake intubation is often felt to be the safest technique, especially in inexperienced hands. Small **laryngoscope** handles and blades are usually employed. Uncuffed **tracheal tubes** are employed usually until puberty, to avoid subglottic stenosis. The approximate size may be calculated thus:
  –diameter = age/4 + 4.5 mm.
  For neonates:
    –under 750 g/26 weeks gestation: 2.0–2.5 mm.
    –750–2000 g/26–34 weeks: 2.5–3.0 mm.
    –over 2000 g/34 weeks: 3.0–3.5 mm.
  –length = age/12 + 12 cm.
A small air leak should be present at 15–20 cmH$_2$O airway pressure.
–**dead space** and resistance should be minimal in **anaesthetic breathing systems**; adult forms are suitable if the child weighs over 20–25 kg but the Bain system is often avoided because of increased resistance to expiration. Ayre's T-piece is suitable up to 25 kg. Spontaneous ventilation via a **facepiece** is usually suitable for short procedures in children older than 3 months. Below this, tracheal intubation and IPPV is usually performed.
–for IPPV using a T-piece, the following fresh gas flows have been suggested, producing slight hypocapnia:
  –10–30 kg: 1000 ml + 100 ml/kg per minute.
  –>30 kg: 2000 ml + 50 ml/kg per minute.
Set minute volume should equal twice fresh gas flow.
–**monitoring** should include praecordial or oesophageal stethoscope, and **temperature measurement**. Pulse **oximetry** is especially useful.
–anaesthetic rooms and operating theatres should be warmed. Warming blankets, reflective coverings, etc. should also be used, with **humidification** of inspired gases.
–tracheal **extubation** is usually performed with the child awake, to reduce the risk of aspiration or **laryngospasm**.

–regional techniques are popular for per- and **postoperative analgesia**, e.g. **caudal analgesia, inguinal field block, penile block**. Local wound infiltration is also effective. **Spinal** and **extradural anaesthesia** have also been used.

–**paracetamol** and **codeine** are often used for postoperative analgesia, with **pethidine** or other opioids for severe pain. **Antiemetic drugs** are usually avoided, since **dystonic reactions** are more common in children.

• Other problems are related to the procedure performed, e.g.:

–repair of congenital defects, e.g. **tracheo-oesophageal fistula, gastroschisis, diaphragmatic hernia, congenital heart disease**, etc.

–related to **trauma**.

–**ENT**, **dental** and **ophthalmic surgery**, etc.

The National **Confidential Enquiry into Perioperative Deaths** focused for its first year on paediatric anaesthesia. It concluded that general care was good, although outcome was related to clinicians' experience.

Pain. Usually defined as an unpleasant sensory and emotional experience resulting from a stimulus causing, or likely to cause, tissue damage (**nocioception**), or expressed in terms of that damage. Thus affected by subjective emotional factors, making **pain evaluation** difficult. Chronic pain may arise from nervous system dysfunction rather than tissue damage (neurogenic pain, e.g. **trigeminal neuralgia, postherpetic neuralgia, causalgia, phantom limb pain, central pain**), and may be associated with damage to **pain pathways**. Substances released from damaged tissues, and/or reorganization of somatic and sympathetic spinal reflex pathways are thought to be involved in the aetiology of chronic pain. Chronic pain is usually more difficult to diagnose and treat than acute pain, and psychological and emotional factors are more important.

See also, Allodynia; Dysaesthesia; Hyperaesthesia; Hyperalgesia; Hyperpathia; Hypoalgesia; Myofascial pain syndromes; Pain clinic; Pain management; Postoperative analgesia

Pain clinic. Outpatient clinic run by consultants (usually anaesthetists) with a special interest in the management of chronic **pain**. Developed from the 1950s. Requires appropriate facilities for consultation, and performance of nerve blocks and surgical procedures. Anaesthetists, physicians, psychologists and neurologists may be involved. Primary referrals to the clinic are usually from general practitioners or hospital consultants.

Swerdlow M (1992) Anaesthesia; 47: 977–80

See also, Pain management

Pain evaluation. Difficult to perform, because **pain** is a subjective experience.

• Methods used depend on the setting and whether the pain is acute or chronic:

–experimental methods (e.g. assessing analgesic effects of new drugs):

–animals: tail-flick response to pinching; pedal withdrawal response to pinching the foot; head shaking response to ear pinching.

–humans: degree of tolerated digital pressure; tolerated duration of immersion of the forearm into icy water.

–acute pain, e.g. postoperative: **linear analogue scale**;

using numbers or words to rate the degree of pain (patient and observer assessment may be used); demand for analgesia. Babies have been studied by recording and analysing their cries.

–chronic pain: the pain is characterized by noting its type, duration, location, quality, intensity, modifying factors (e.g. food, exercise, etc.), time relations, and associated symptoms and mental changes. Full clinical examination is performed, with investigations as appropriate. Linear analogue and rating scales may be used as above. Complicated psychological questionnaires for analysis of personality and pain have been used.

Pain, intractable, *see Pain; Pain clinic; Pain management; individual conditions*

Pain management. Acute **pain**, e.g. postoperative, is usually treated with systemic analgesics and regional techniques (*see Postoperative analgesia*).

• Chronic pain management may involve the following, after full **pain evaluation**:

–simple measures, e.g. rest, exercise, heat and cold treatment, vibration, etc.

–systemic drug therapy:

–**analgesic drugs**: different drugs, dosage regimens and routes of administration may be chosen, depending on the severity and temporal pattern of the pain, and efficacy and side effects of the drugs. Drugs used range from mild **NSAIDs** to **opioid analgesic drugs**. The latter are usually reserved for severe pain of short duration, or pain associated with malignancy; they may require concurrent antiemetic and aperient therapy. Implantable devices may be used for intermittent iv, extradural or subarachnoid injection or continuous infusion of opioids.

–other drugs used include:

–psychoactive drugs, e.g. **antidepressant drugs** (especially tricyclics), **anticonvulsant drugs** (e.g. **carbamazepine, phenytoin, clonazepam), phenothiazines, butyrophenones**. Thought to have a direct analgesic effect in addition to their other actions.

–**steroid therapy**, either by local injection or oral therapy. Particularly useful in **neuralgia** or pain associated with oedema, e.g. malignancy. Often injected with **local anaesthetic agents**, e.g. extradurally for back pain.

–muscle relaxants, e.g. baclofen, **dantrolene, benzodiazepines**; may be useful if muscle spasm is problematic.

–others, e.g. **antimitotic drugs**, calcitonin in bony pain, **β-adrenergic receptor antagonists, clonidine**.

–local anaesthetic nerve blocks: may be diagnostic, prognostic (to allow assessment prior to destructive lesions) or therapeutic. Include:

–injection of **trigger points** in **myofascial pain syndromes**.

–**facetal injection**.

–**caudal analgesia, extradural anaesthesia, spinal anaesthesia**.

–**paravertebral nerve blocks**.

–**sympathetic nerve blocks**, e.g. **stellate ganglion, coeliac plexus** and **lumbar sympathetic blocks**, iv **guanethidine** block.

–destructive procedures: usually reserved for severe pain associated with malignancy, since relief may not be permanent and unacceptable side effects may be produced (e.g. **anaesthesia dolorosa**). X-ray control is increasingly used to aid correct positioning before percutaneous destruction. Methods include:

 –regional techniques as above, using phenol or absolute alcohol. The former is hyperbaric compared to **CSF**, the latter hypobaric. Thus for intrathecal neurolysis the required posterior sensory roots may be selectively destroyed with appropriate positioning of the patient. Pituitary ablation has also been used.

 –extremes of temperature, e.g. **cryoprobe**, radiofrequency probe. The latter delivers a high frequency alternating current, producing up to 80°C heat. It is used at peripheral nerves, facet joints, dorsal root ganglia and trigeminal ganglion, and for percutaneous **cordotomy**.

 –surgery: includes peripheral neurectomy, dorsal rhizotomy or lesions in the dorsal root entry zones (DREZ), commissurotomy (sagittal division of the **spinal cord**), mesencephalotomy and thalamotomy.

 –electrical stimulation:

 –**TENS** and electroacupuncture.

 –**dorsal column stimulation**.

 –stimulation of deep brain structures has also been used, e.g. via electrodes implanted in the periventricular grey matter or thalamus.

 –**acupuncture**.

 –psychological techniques, e.g. psychotherapy, **operant conditioning**, **hypnosis**, **biofeedback**, relaxation techniques.

Pain pathways. Most **pain** arises in pain receptors (nociceptors) widely distributed in the skin and musculoskeletal system. Those responding to pinprick and sudden heat (thermomechanoreceptors) are related to myelinated Aδ fibres, and are responsible for rapid pain sensation and reflex withdrawal. Receptors responding to pressure, heat, chemical substances (e.g. **histamine**, **prostaglandins**, **acetylcholine**, etc.) and tissue damage (polymodal receptors) are associated with unmyelinated C fibre endings, and are responsible for slow pain sensation and immobilization of the affected part.

• Afferent impulses pass centrally thus:

 –first order neurones have cell bodies within the dorsal root ganglia of the **spinal cord**. Aδ fibres synapse with cells in laminae I and V of the cord, whilst C fibres synapse with cells in laminae II and III (substantia gelatinosa).

 –most second order neurones synapse with Aδ fibres in the posterior horn, crossing to the opposite side immediately or within a few segments. They ascend within the anterolateral columns (spinothalamic tract) to the thalamus and periaqueductal grey matter.

 The substantia gelatinosa does not project directly to higher levels, but contains many interneurones involved in modification of pain transmission (e.g. described by the **gate control theory of pain**). Some fibres are projected to deeper layers of the spinal grey matter, from which arises the spinoreticular tract to the **ascending reticular activating system** (ARAS). Fibres are then relayed to the thalamus and **hypothalamus** (some fibres reach the thalamus without

passing to the ARAS, via the palaeospinothalamic tract).

 –fibres are relayed from the thalamus to the somatosensory cortex.

Pain sensation may thus be modified by ascending or descending pathways at many levels.

See also, Nerves; Nociception; Sensory pathways

Pain, postoperative, *see Postoperative analgesia*

Pancreatitis. Acute pancreatitis is an autodigestive process in which pancreatic proteolytic **enzymes** are activated and cause haemorrhagic necrosis of the pancreatic parenchyma. The gland may be destroyed by haemorrhage, oedema and fat necrosis, releasing serosanguinous exudate into the peritoneal cavity causing peritonitis. There is also local and systemic release of toxins. Mortality may be high because of resulting **septicaemia**, **respiratory failure**, **shock** and **renal failure**.

 Commonly associated with biliary tract disease or excessive **alcohol** intake. May occasionally follow upper abdominal surgery, pancreatic ductal obstruction (e.g. by carcinoma), **trauma**, mumps, **hypothermia**, **hypercalcaemia**, hyperlipidaemia, **diuretic** or **steroid therapy**.

• Features:

 –severe epigastric pain (typically radiating through to the back), nausea and vomiting, fever, occasionally mild jaundice.

 –epigastric tenderness on palpation, progressing to features of peritonitis.

 –**hypotension, oliguria, respiratory failure**.

Investigations reveal raised serum amylase (secondary to leakage from the pancreas), leucocytosis, **hyperglycaemia**, **hypocalcaemia** (secondary to calcium sequestration in areas of fat necrosis), **hypoproteinaemia** and hyperlipidaemia. Abdominal X-ray may reveal a 'sentinel loop' of small bowel overlying the pancreas. **Chest X-ray** may show a raised hemidiaphragm, **pleural effusion**, **atelectasis** or **ARDS**.

 Poor prognosis may be indicated by: age >55 years; systolic BP <90 mmHg; white cell count >15 $\times$ 10^9/l; temperature >39°C; blood glucose >10 mmol/l; arterial Po_2 <8 kPa (60 mmHg); plasma urea >15 mmol/l; serum calcium <2 mmol/l; haematocrit reduced by over 10%; abnormal **liver function tests**.

• Management:

 –supportive, e.g. **O$_2$ therapy**, **iv fluid administration**, analgesia, nasogastric drainage, **insulin** therapy where indicated, **TPN**. Multiple organ failure is treated along conventional lines.

 –**aprotinin**, peritoneal lavage, **glucagon**, **calcitonin** and **somatostatin** have been used, but with little evidence of efficacy.

 –surgery may be required for drainage of an abscess or pseudocyst. Resection of necrotic pancreas has been performed but mortality from surgery in early disease is high.

Chronic pancreatitis usually occurs in alcoholics, and is characterized by pancreatic calcification and impaired enzyme secretion with malabsorption, and repeated episodes of pain. Surgery may be required; anaesthetic considerations are related to alcohol abuse, and the consequences of malabsorption and **malnutrition**.

Reynaert MS, Dugernier T, Kestens PJ (1991) Intensive Care Med; 16: 352–62

Pancuronium bromide. Synthetic non-depolarizing **neuromuscular blocking drug**, first used in 1967. Bisquaternary amino-steroid, but with no steroid activity. Initial dose is 0.05–0.1 mg/kg, with tracheal intubation possible after 2–3 minutes. Effects last 40–60 minutes. Supplementary dose: 0.01–0.02 mg/kg. **Histamine** release is extremely rare. May cause increases in heart rate, BP and cardiac output, caused by vagolytic and sympathomimetic actions. The latter may be due to release of **noradrenaline** from sympathetic nerve endings or blockade of its uptake. Pancuronium is strongly bound to plasma gamma-globulin after iv injection, and metabolized mainly by the kidney but also by the liver. Elimination is delayed in renal and hepatic impairment.

Traditionally used in shocked patients requiring anaesthesia, because of its cardiovascular effects. Formerly commonly used in ICU, but superseded by **atracurium** and **vecuronium**.

Papaveretum. Opioid analgesic drug preparation, first prepared in 1909. Contains **opium** alkaloids: **morphine** 47.5–52.5%, **codeine** 2.5–5.0%, noscapine (narcotine) 16–22%, **papaverine** 2.5–7.0% and others, e.g. thebaine <1.5%. 20 mg is approximately equivalent to 12.5 mg morphine. Said to have greater sedative power than morphine, but generally its effects are similar. Indications and use are as for morphine.
● Dosage: 0.2 mg/kg.
Also available in combination with **hyoscine** (20 mg papaveretum and 0.4 mg hyoscine/ml).
The **Committee on Safety of Medicines** issued a warning in 1991 that noscapine (an alkaloid with similar effects to papaverine) induces polyploidy in mammalian cell lines *in vitro* and may be genotoxic. Administration of the original formulation to women of child-bearing age is thus contraindicated. A noscapine-free preparation was made available in 1992.

Papaverine. Benzylisoquinolone **opium** alkaloid, without CNS activity. Used for its non-specific relaxant effect on smooth muscle, especially vascular. May be injected iv or applied directly during surgery. Its use is advocated following intra-arterial injection of **thiopentone**.
● Dosage: up to 30 mg slowly iv (may cause **histamine** release). Also used in combination oral preparations to relieve GIT spasm.

Paracelsus (1493–1541). Swiss philosopher and physician; his real name was Theophrastus Bambastus von Hohenheim. Lectured at the University of Basle. Revolutionized the theory of medicine, encouraging the science of research and experimentation. Described the effects of **diethyl ether** on chickens in 1540.

Paracervical block. Used to provide analgesia during the first stage of labour, or for gynaecological procedures, e.g. dilatation and curettage. First performed in 1926.

With the patient's legs apart, a special sheathed needle (with tip protected) is directed into the lateral vaginal fornix by the operator's fingers. The needle tip is advanced 0.5–1 cm to point cranially, laterally and dorsally, and 5–10 ml **local anaesthetic agent** injected into the parametrial tissue on either side, blocking the uterine nerves which form a plexus at the base of the broad ligament. Vaginal, vulval and perineal sensation is unaffected.

Seldom used in modern obstetrics, because of the high incidence of fetal arrhythmias (especially bradycardia), thought to be caused by alterations in uteroplacental blood flow or absorption of local anaesthetic.
See also, Obstetric analgesia and anaesthesia

Paracetamol (Acetaminophen). **Analgesic drug**, derived from para-aminophenol; introduced in the 1950s. Inhibits central **prostaglandin** synthesis; has a central antipyretic action with minimal peripheral anti-inflammatory effects. Does not cause gastric irritation or alter **platelet** adhesiveness. Used to treat minor pain.

Minimally protein-bound in plasma. Conjugated with glucuronide and sulphate in the liver; under 10% is oxidized to form *N*-acetyl-*p*-benzoquinoneimine, a potential cellular toxin. Normally, this is safely conjugated with glutathione, but it may cause hepatic necrosis in **paracetamol poisoning**, when the glucuronide and sulphate pathways are saturated and glutathione stores are depleted. **Half-life** is about 2 hours, but its effects last longer.
● Dosage:
–0.5–1.0 g 4 hourly, up to 4 g maximum daily.
–10 mg/kg in children 4 hourly, up to four doses/day.
Available in combination with other analgesics, e.g. **dextropoxyphene**, **codeine**.

Paracetamol poisoning. Hepatocellular necrosis may occur if more than about 7.5 g (15 tablets) are taken, due to saturation of the normal metabolic pathways for **paracetamol** and exhaustion of hepatic glutathione stores.

Patients may be asymptomatic for 24 hours after ingestion. Early features include nausea and vomiting, anorexia and right upper quadrant pain. Early impaired consciousness suggests concurrent depressive drug ingestion, e.g. **alcohol, opioid analgesic drugs. Liver function tests** become abnormal after about 18 hours, with prolonged prothrombin time and raised bilirubin at 36–48 hours. Hepatotoxicity peaks at about 3–4 days, with **hepatic failure** if severe. **Lactic acidosis, hypoglycaemia** and **renal failure** may also occur. Overall mortality is about 5% if untreated.
● Treatment:
–as for **poisoning and overdoses**; e.g. **gastric lavage** or ipecacuanha within 4 hours of ingestion, plus supportive treatment. Ingestion of opioid/paracetamol combinations (e.g. containing **codeine, dextropropoxyphene**) should be considered if level of consciousness is depressed on presentation to hospital, and **naloxone** given.
–replenishment of hepatic glutathione stores with glutathione precursors:
  –methionine: 2.5 g orally, followed by 2.5 g 4 hourly for 12 hours. Vomiting is common.
  or
  –*N*-acetylcysteine: 150 mg/kg in 200 ml 5% dextrose iv over 15 minutes, followed by 50 mg/kg in 500 ml dextrose over 4 hours, then 100 mg/kg in 1 litre dextrose over 16 hours.

Treatment is traditionally thought to be effective only if started within 16 hours, being possibly harmful thereafter; it should ideally be started within 10 hours. Recent evidence suggests that it is safe and may improve outcome even if given later.
Risk of hepatic failure may be predicted from a single measurement of plasma paracetamol levels (if more than

4 hours after ingestion); treatment is recommended if it is above a line drawn between 200 mg/ml (1.32 mmol/l) at 4 hours and 30 mg/ml (0.2 mmol/l) at 15 hours.
Anon (1988) Drug and Ther Bull; 26: 97–9

Paraesthesiae. Abnormal positive sensation similar to 'pins and needles', occurring when neural tissue is irritated (e.g. peripheral nerve, **spinal cord**, sensory cerebral cortex). May be produced accidentally or intentionally during **regional anaesthesia**. Elicitation of paraesthesiae may increase the chances of successful nerve block but also of neurological damage.

Paraldehyde. Hypnotic and **anticonvulsant drug**, introduced in 1882. Has an offensive smell, and is irritant and flammable (but not explosive). Decomposes with heat and light to acetic acid, and dissolves plastic. Used in the treatment of psychiatric disturbance and persistent **convulsions**. Has been used for **premedication**. Metabolized in the liver; 10–30% is excreted in the breath. Duration of action is about 8 hours.
• Dosage: 5–10 ml im or rectally, given with a glass syringe. Sterile abscesses may occur following im administration. May also be given iv, diluted several times in saline. Cardiovascular depression may occur.

Paramagnetic oxygen analysis, *see Oxygen measurement*

Parametric tests, *see Data; Statistical tests*

Paraplegia. Paralysis of the lower body secondary to a **spinal cord** lesion. Causes include **spinal cord injury**, tumours, infective or inflammatory myelitis, and vascular and skeletal disorders. Effects of acute lesions are as for spinal cord injury, i.e. initial flaccid paralysis and **spinal shock**, followed by development of **autonomic hyperreflexia**.
• Anaesthetic considerations in chronic paraplegia:
  –danger of severe **hyperkalaemia** following administration of **suxamethonium** (from 10 days to 6 months after injury).
  –autonomic hyperreflexia and impaired **temperature regulation**.
  –chronic infection, especially urinary tract (renal function may be impaired).
Care must be taken during moving and positioning.

Parasympathetic nervous system. Part of the **autonomic nervous system**. Myelinated preganglionic efferent fibres emerge with **cranial nerves** III, VII, IX and X, and **spinal nerves** S2–4. They pass directly to their target organs, where they synapse with short non-myelinated postganglionic fibres (cf. **sympathetic nervous system**). The **vagus nerves** carry about 75% of all parasympathetic fibres and innervate the **heart**, **lungs**, oesophagus, stomach, other viscera, and GIT as far as the splenic flexure. The sacral nerves run directly as the pelvic splanchnic nerves to the pelvic viscera (*see Fig. 16; Autonomic nervous system*). Afferent fibres travel in cranial nerves IX and X and in the sacral nerves.
• Effects of parasympathetic stimulation:
  –pupillary and ciliary muscle contraction, increased lacrimal secretion.
  –bradycardia, reduced velocity of cardiac conduction.

Vasodilatation occurs in skeletal muscle, abdominal viscera, and coronary, pulmonary and renal circulations.
–bronchoconstriction and increased secretions.
–increased GIT motility, relaxation of sphincters and increased secretions (profuse watery secretion from salivary glands). Increased **insulin** and **glucagon** secretion.
–bladder contraction and relaxation of sphincter.
–variable effect on the **uterus**.
–penile erection.
–generalized sweating.
Acetylcholine is the **neurotransmitter** at all synapses. Its actions are divided into nicotinic (at ganglia) and muscarinic (at postganglionic synapses).
See also, Acetylcholine receptors; Muscarine and muscarinic receptors; Nicotine and nicotinic receptors

Parasympathomimetic drugs. Drugs producing the effects of stimulation of the **parasympathetic nervous system**. Include:
  –drugs which stimulate **acetylcholine receptors**:
    –**acetylcholine**: has diffuse actions, therefore not used therapeutically.
    –synthetic choline esters, e.g. carbachol, methacholine: the former has nicotinic and muscarinic actions, the latter mainly muscarinic. Both are resistant to hydrolysis by cholinesterases. Carbachol is used in **glaucoma** and urinary retention. Bethanechol is a similar drug, and used in urinary retention and as a laxative.
    –cholimimetic alkaloids, e.g. pilocarpine: used in glaucoma.
  –**acetylcholinesterase inhibitors**.

Paravertebral nerve block. Used to block the **lumbar plexus**, e.g. in abdominal or leg surgery. May also be used in the thoracic region. Blocks nerves as they pass through the intervertebral foramina into the paravertebral space; solution may track medially through the foramina into the **extradural space**, or laterally into the **intercostal space**.
With the patient in either the lateral or prone position, with a soft pillow between the iliac crest and costal margin, a skin wheal is raised 3–5 cm lateral to the cephalic end of the L1–4 spinous processes. An 8 cm needle is inserted approximately 3–4 cm perpendicular to the skin until the transverse process is encountered, then walked off the cephalad border and advanced a further 1–2 cm. 5 ml **local anaesthetic agent** is then injected. Must be performed at both sides for bilateral blockade.
A loss-of-resistance technique has been used to confirm correct needle placement, as for **extradural anaesthesia**. A catheter may be passed into the paravertebral space for prolonged analgesia. Complications include extradural, subarachnoid and iv injection.

Parenteral nutrition, *see Nutrition, total parenteral*

Parkinson's disease. Degenerative disorder of the CNS involving the basal ganglia and extrapyramidal motor system, with loss of **dopamine** in the striatum and substantia nigra. Causes abnormal control of movement, which normally depends on the balance between cholinergic and dopaminergic activity within the basal ganglia. Usually idiopathic, it may follow encephalitis, CVA, heavy metal

poisoning, or drugs which antagonize **dopamine receptors** (e.g. **phenothiazines**). Prevalence is about 1:1000; up to 1:200 in the elderly. A viral aetiology, and more recently an environmental toxin, have been proposed.
- Features:
    - bradykinesia, rigidity ('lead-pipe' or 'cogwheel'), rest tremor (4–6 Hz). Initiation, speed, strength and precision of movement are impaired. The face is typically expressionless and the gait shuffling.
    - autonomic dysfunction is characterized by salivation, postural hypotension and abnormal control of breathing.
    - a restrictive ventilatory defect may occur.
- Treatment is aimed at restoring the dopaminergic/cholinergic balance, and includes:
    - increasing brain levels of dopamine by administering its precursor levodopa (dopamine itself does not cross the **blood–brain barrier**). Conversion of levodopa to dopamine outside the CNS with resultant side effects is prevented by concurrent administration of carbidopa or benserazide. These inhibit dopa decarboxylase peripherally, but do not cross into the brain themselves. Bradykinesia and rigidity are improved more than tremor. Side effects include involuntary movements, nausea, vomiting, and psychiatric disturbances. Improvement may be intermittent (on–off effect).
    - **anticholinergic drugs, e.g.** benztropine, benzhexol, orphenadrine: improve tremor and rigidity more than bradykinesia.
    - other drugs: bromocriptine and lysuride (dopamine agonists), selegiline (type B **monoamine oxidase inhibitor**), amantadine.
    - stereotactic surgery has been performed. Fetal tissue implantation has been performed experimentally.
- Anaesthetic considerations:
    - pre-existing restrictive lung disorders and postural hypotension. Excessive salivation and dysphagia may result in tracheal aspiration of secretions.
    - levodopa is continued up to surgery, since its **half-life** is short. It has been given iv.
    - symptoms may be exacerbated by dopamine antagonists, e.g. phenothiazines and **butyrophenones** (including **antiemetic drugs**).
    - the risk of massive **hyperkalaemia** following **suxamethonium** is controversial.
    - postoperative **sleep apnoea** has been reported, especially in the postencephalitic disease.

[James Parkinson (1755–1824), London physician]
Severn A (1988) Br J Anaesth; 61: 761–70

Paroxysmal nocturnal haemoglobinuria. Rare acquired chronic haemolytic **anaemia**, resulting from blood cell **membrane** abnormality and increased sensitivity to lysis by **complement**. Haemoglobinuria is classically noticed on waking. **Platelet** destruction may lead to bleeding, or abnormal function may lead to venous thrombosis. Renal impairment is common. Drugs causing complement activation should be avoided, and red blood cells washed before **blood transfusion** to reduce risk of complement activation. **Haemolysis** may be precipitated by surgery, infection and cold.

Partial pressure. Pressure exerted by each component of a **gas** mixture. For a gas dissolved in a liquid, e.g. blood,

the term '**tension**' is used, although denoted by the same symbol (*P*).
See also, Dalton's law; Respiratory symbols

Partial thromboplastin time, *see Coagulation studies*

Partition coefficient. Ratio of the amount of substance in one phase to the amount in another phase at stated temperature, with the two phases being of equal volume and at equilibrium with each other. Depends on the relative **solubility** of the substance in the two phases. May refer to solids, liquids or gases; when the phases are liquid and gas it equals the Ostwald **solubility coefficient**. Blood/gas and oil/gas partition coefficients of **inhalational anaesthetic agents** are related to speed of uptake and potency respectively.

Pascal. SI **unit** of **pressure**. 1 pascal (Pa) = 1 N/m^2.
[Blaise Pascal (1623–1662), French physicist]

Pasteur point. Critical mitochondrial Po_2 below which aerobic **metabolism** cannot occur. Thought to be 0.15–0.3 kPa (1.4–2.3 mmHg).
[Louis Pasteur (1822–1895), French scientist and microbiologist]
See also, Oxygen cascade

Patent ductus arteriosus, *see Ductus arteriosus, patent*

Patient-controlled analgesia (PCA). Technique whereby small doses of analgesic drugs (usually **opioid analgesic drugs**) are administered (usually iv) by patients themselves according to their pain. Widely used for **postoperative analgesia**. Systems usually consist of sophisticated infusion devices which allow on-demand bolus injections, with or without continuous background infusions. Size and rate of bolus injection may be altered. Inadvertent overdosage is avoided by limiting the size of individual boluses and total dose administered within a set period; the minimal time between boluses can also be preset (lock-out interval). The controls must be inaccessible to the patient (or relatives), and the infusion connected downstream from a non-return valve if attached to another iv infusion (to prevent retrograde flow into the second infusion set with subsequent overdosage when the latter is flushed).

PCA has been shown to provide more consistent plasma drug levels when compared with standard im techniques, with less sedation, fewer pulmonary complications and reduced total drug usage. Background infusions may increase risk of overdosage without improving analgesia, although this is controversial. Patients may 'save up' their drug allowance for potentially painful procedures, e.g. **physiotherapy**. Preoperative explanation of the technique is desirable but not vital.

Drugs with relatively short **half-lives** are usually employed. Widely varying dosage regimens have been described; individual adjustment is usually required (Table 28). Complications may be related to incorrect programming and setting-up, patients' misunderstanding of the technique, and equipment malfunction. Patients require adequate **monitoring**, since respiratory depression may still occur. Has also been used with **extradural anaesthesia**, e.g. postoperatively, or in **obstetric analgesia and anaesthesia**.
White PF (1988) JAMA; 259: 243–7

349

Table 28. Dosage regimens for different opioids for patient-controlled analgesia

Drug	Bolus dose (mg)	Lock-out interval (min)
Pethidine	5–20	5–15
Diamorphine	0.5–1.5	3–5
Morphine	0.5–2.0	5–15
Fentanyl	0.02–0.1	3–10
Nalbuphine	1–5	5–15

PAV, *see Proportional assist ventilation*

PCA, *see Patient-controlled analgesia*

PCV, Packed cell volume, *see Haematocrit*

PCWP, *see Pulmonary capillary wedge pressure*

PDA, Patent ductus arteriosus, *see Ductus arteriosus, patent*

PE, *see Pulmonary embolism*

Peak expiratory flow rate (PEFR). Maximal rate of air flow during a sudden **forced expiration**. Most conveniently measured with a **peak flowmeter**; may also be measured from a **flow–volume loop**, or with a **pneumotachograph**. Highly dependent on patient effort. Reduced by obstructive airways disease, e.g. **asthma**, **COAD**. Normal values: 450–700 l/min (males), 250–500 l/min (females).

Peak flowmeters. Simple and inexpensive hand-held **flowmeters** for measuring **peak expiratory flow rate** (PEFR). The Wright peak flowmeter is a constant pressure, variable orifice device, able to measure peak flow rates of up to 1000 l/min. It has a flat circular body, with a handle and mouthpiece. Exhaled air is directed by a fixed baffle within the body on to a moveable vane, which is free to rotate around a central axle against the force of a small spiral spring. There is a circular slot in the base of the chamber, through which expired air escapes to the atmosphere. As the vane moves, the slot is uncovered, thus increasing the effective orifice size. The vane reaches its furthest excursion according to PEFR, and is held there by a ratchet. PEFR is read from a dial on the face of the meter, according to a pointer attached to the vane. It slightly underreads in comparison with a **pnemotachograph**.

A simpler, cheaper version consists of a cylindrical tube, employing a piston which is blown along its length. As it does so, it uncovers a linear slot along the tube. A ratchet mechanism operates as before. PEFR is read from a scale at the top of the cylinder.
[Basil M Wright, London physician]

PEEP, *see Positive end-expiratory pressure*

PEFR, *see Peak expiratory flow rate*

Pendelluft. Phenomenon originally believed to cause the **hypoxaemia** occurring in **flail chest**. The theory suggested that air is drawn from the affected side into the unaffected lung during inspiration, due to the disrupted chest wall integrity on the damaged side. During expiration, air passes from the normal lung back into the affected lung; thus air moves to and fro between the two sides, instead of in and out of the chest via the trachea. **Hypoventilation** and $\dot{V}/\dot{Q}$ **mismatch** due to pain, lung contusion and sputum retention are now thought to be more important. [German: 'oscillating breath']

Penicillin, *see Antibacterial drugs*

Penile block. Used to provide per- and **postoperative analgesia** for circumcision and other procedures on the penis, especially in children.

The dorsal nerves of the penis (terminal branches of the pudendal nerves, S2–4) travel medial to the ischiopubic rami into the deep perineal pouch, and pierce the perineal membrane to pass to the penis. They may be blocked within a triangular space bounded by the symphysis pubis above, corpora cavernosa below, and superficial fascia anteriorly. The penile vessels lie in the midline. Some innervation of the skin at the base of the penis arises from the genital branch of the genitofemoral nerve.

A needle is introduced at right angles through a skin wheal in front of the symphysis, and passed below its caudal edge. It is inserted up to 3–5 mm deeper than the symphysis (a click may be felt). After careful aspiration, 1–2 ml **local anaesthetic agent** is injected for children up to 3 years old, 3–5 ml for older children, and 5–10 ml for adults. **Adrenaline** may cause ischaemia and necrosis and must not be used. Solution diffuses to block both sides following midline injection, but risk of haematoma is greater; therefore the needle may be tilted to each side and solution injected in two halves. 1–5 ml solution is also injected around the base of the penis.
See also, Lumbar plexus; Sacral plexus

Pentastarch. Synthetic **colloid**, related to **hetastarch** but with 45% of glucose subunits substituted with hydroxyethyl groups (70% for hetastarch). Mean mw is 250 000 and median mw 63 000. Administration increases plasma volume by 1.5 times the volume infused, lasting 18–24 hours. Pattern of excretion is as for hetastarch, but 70% is cleared within 24 hours and 80% within a week. Presented as a 10% solution in 0.9% saline; pH is about 5.0 and osmolarity 320 mosmol/l.
See also, Intravenous fluids

Pentazocine hydrochloride/lactate. Agonist–antagonist **opioid analgesic drug** described in 1962. Benzomorphan derivative, with agonist activity at kappa and sigma **opioid receptors**, and antagonist activity at mu receptors. Used for moderate to severe pain; has been used to reverse the respiratory depression caused by **morphine** or **fentanyl** whilst maintaining analgesia.

Undergoes extensive **first-pass metabolism**; conjugated with glucuronides and excreted renally. **Half-life** is about 2–3 hours.
- Dosage: 0.5–1.0 mg/kg, iv/im/sc.
  50–100 mg orally, 3–4 hourly; 50 mg rectally.
- Side effects:
  –sedation, dizziness.
  –hallucinations and dysphoria, especially in the elderly.
  –sweating, hypertension, tachycardia.

–precipitation of withdrawal reactions in opioid addicts.

Its side effects have contributed to its unpopularity.
See also, Opioid receptor antagonists

Pentolinium tartarate. Ganglion blocking drug, no longer commercially available. More potent and longer-lasting than **hexamethonium**. Previously used orally in **hypertension**, and iv in **hypotensive anaesthesia** (0.1–0.15 mg/kg). Maximal hypotensive effect occurs in about 30 minutes; actions may last up to 4 hours. Pupillary dilatation and postural hypotension may occur.

PEP, Pre-ejection period, *see Systolic time intervals*

Peptic ulcer disease. May occur at any site where peptic acid digestion occurs, e.g. oesophagus, stomach, duodenum. Thought to be due to imbalance between gastric acid digestion and the normal protective mechanisms of the upper GIT mucosa. Abnormal **gastric emptying, gastro-oesophageal reflux**, drugs (e.g. **NSAIDs, steroid therapy, alcohol**), psychological and epidemiological factors are thought to contribute. Infection with Helicobacter has also been implicated.

More common in men; duodenal ulceration is more common than gastric ulceration. Usually presents with epigastric pain, typically relieved by food. Complications include haemorrhage, perforation, or stenosis following chronic ulceration. Investigations include endoscopy and barium meal.

- Treatment:
    –neutralization of existing acid with **antacids**.
    –increased surface protection (postulated mechanism):
        –**sucralfate**.
        –bismuth compounds.
        –carbenoxolone.
    –reduction of acid production:
        –**H$_2$ receptor antagonists**.
        –omeprazole.
        –**anticholinergic drugs**, e.g. pirenzepine.
    –surgery: indications include failed medical treatment, malignant change, or complications as above. Surgery may involve highly selective vagotomy or vagotomy and drainage procedure (duodenal ulcer), or partial gastrectomy (gastric ulcer).

Anaesthesia in chronic disease requires no special precautions unless gastro-oesophageal reflux or **anaemia** is present. Acute haemorrhage or perforation may present with vomiting, **shock** and **hypovolaemia**.

Percentile. Value which indicates the percent of a distribution equal to or below it; e.g. 97% of measurements are equal or less than the 97th percentile. Often used in charts, e.g. of children's height against age. The 3rd, 50th and 97th percentiles plotted on the chart indicate the heights which includes 3%, 50% and 97% of the population respectively, at each age. May thus be used to follow a child's growth, since height would be expected to remain within the same percentile during normal development. The 3rd and 97th percentiles approximate to ± two **standard deviations** from the **mean**.

Often used to indicate variability (scatter) around the **median** for ordinal **data**.

Percutaneous transluminal coronary angioplasty (PTCA). Non-surgical technique, first described in 1977, for treating obstructive coronary **arteriosclerosis**. Under X-ray control, a catheter is threaded via a peripheral artery into the stenosed or occluded vessel, and a small balloon at the tip inflated using contrast medium at 4–6 atmospheres for a few seconds. The narrowed portion of the artery is thus dilated; effects may be confirmed by pressure measurements and angiography. Best results are obtained in single vessel disease. Complications include **MI**, the need for urgent **coronary artery bypass graft**, restenosis and death. PTCA is considerably cheaper than bypass surgery. The technique has been used for dilatation of occluded vessels throughout the body. It may be combined with fibrinolytic therapy, microlaser ablation, revolving cutting devices and insertion of rigid stents.
Baim DS (1992) New Engl J Med; 326: 56–7

Perfusion pressure. Represents the pressure head for **blood flow** to an organ or tissues. Equals **MAP** minus mean venous pressure. **Cerebral perfusion pressure** equals MAP minus **ICP**.

Peribulbar block. Used in **ophthalmic surgery** as an alternative to **retrobulbar block**, since risk of complications (e.g. retrobulbar haemorrhage) is minimal. **Facial nerve block** is not required. Involves injection of **local anaesthetic agent** outside the muscle cone.

A needle is inserted through the lid margin between the superior orbital notch and the medial canthus, and directed upwards between the globe and orbital roof. 3–4 ml solution is injected at a depth of 2.0–2.5 cm. The needle is then inserted through the lid margin at the junction of the outer ⅓ and inner ⅔ of the lower orbital rim, and directed downwards between the globe and orbital floor. 4–5 ml solution is injected at a depth of 2.0–2.5 cm. Gentle pressure is applied to the eye for 10 minutes. A mixture of **lignocaine** 2% and **bupivacaine** 0.5–0.75% in equal proportions, together with **hyaluronidase** 5 units/ml, is a suitable solution, with or without **adrenaline** 1:400 000.
Fry RA, Henderson J (1990) Anaesthesia; 45: 14–7

Pericarditis. Inflammation of the **pericardium**. May be:
    –acute:
        –caused by infections, **connective tissue diseases, renal failure, hypothyroidism, MI, trauma**, drugs, radiation and tumours. Postviral pericarditis is the most common form.
        –features include sudden central chest pain, worse lying down or on moving, often with fever and tachycardia. Auscultation reveals a pericardial friction rub. **ECG** reveals **S–T segment** elevation, possibly with **T wave** inversion later.
        –**NSAIDs** are often effective in providing analgesia.
        –pericardial fluid may accumulate, with disappearance of the rub. Slow accumulation may cause little cardiovascular disturbance, whereas rapid accumulation may cause **cardiac tamponade**.
    –chronic constrictive:
        –the pericardium becomes fibrous or calcified, and thus rigid.
        –usually follows radiation, chronic renal failure, **rheumatoid arthritis, TB**, or is idiopathic.
        –resembles cardiac tamponade, with restriction of diastolic cardiac filling. A sharp drop in right atrial pressure ('y' descent) occurs just before right

ventricular filling, due to rapid blood flow across the tricuspid valve (cf. tamponade, where atrial pressures remain high throughout diastole). The **heart sounds** may be quiet, and ECG complexes small. Pericardial calcification may be present on the **chest X-ray**.
–management: as for cardiac tamponade. Surgery may be required.

Lake CL (1983) Anesth Analg; 62: 431–43

Pericardium. Sac enclosing the **heart** and roots of the great vessels. The outer fibrous pericardium fuses below with the central tendon of the **diaphragm**, and above and superiorly with the adventitia of the great vessels. The inner serous pericardium has visceral and parietal layers, enclosing the pericardial cavity. The visceral layer covers the heart and is termed the epicardium.
See also, Pericarditis

Peridural..., *see Extradural...*

Peripheral neuropathy. Term encompassing any disorder affecting the peripheral nerves (both motor and sensory).
• Divided into:
–polyneuropathy: generalized process characterized by widespread and symmetrical degeneration of the:
–axon, e.g. drugs, metabolic disorders.
–**myelin** sheath, e.g. **diphtheria**, **Guillain–Barré syndrome**.
–**neurone** cell body, e.g. **motor neurone disease**.
–focal and multifocal neuropathies: asymmetrical involvement of one or more peripheral nerves, e.g. by ischaemia, trauma (including **nerve injury during anaesthesia**), vasculitis, infiltration (e.g. by tumour).
Diabetes mellitus is the most common cause of peripheral neuropathy (causing both polyneuropathy and focal neuropathy), followed by carcinoma, vitamin B_1 and B_{12} deficiency, and drug therapy (e.g. isoniazid). Other causes include **renal failure**, **hypothyroidism**, **connective tissue diseases**, leprosy, severe sepsis, amyloidosis, **porphyria** and heavy metal poisoning.
Clinical features include weakness and sensory disturbance, usually initially distal in polyneuropathies. **Autonomic neuropathy** may occur.
• Anaesthetic considerations:
–underlying disease.
–bulbar involvement.
–autonomic involvement.
–risk of exaggerated increase in plasma **potassium** following administration of **suxamethonium** in motor neuropathy.

Peripheral vascular resistance, *see Systemic vascular resistance*

Peroneal nerve block, *see Ankle, nerve blocks; Knee, nerve blocks*

Perphenazine. **Phenothiazine**, used as an **antiemetic drug** and tranquillizer. More potent than **chlorpromazine**, with fewer side effects. **Dystonic reactions** are common.
• Dosage: 2–5 mg orally/im, 6–8 hourly.

PET, Pre-eclamptic toxaemia, *see Pre-eclampsia*

PET scanning, *see Positron emission tomography*

Pethick's test, *see Checking of anaesthetic equipment*

Pethidine hydrochloride. Synthetic **opioid analgesic drug**, developed in Germany in 1939 whilst **atropine**-like compounds were being investigated. One-tenth as potent as **morphine**, with duration of action of 2–4 hours and **half-life** of about 3–4 hours. Approximately 60% protein-bound in plasma. 5–10% is excreted unchanged in urine, more if the urine is acidic. 90% undergoes hepatic metabolism to norpethidine, an active substance (half-life 20–40 hours) which may cause hallucinations and **convulsions**.
Has similar effects to morphine, but also has local anaesthetic and anticholinergic actions. May cause bronchodilatation, but may also cause **histamine** release. May relax contracted GIT and urinary smooth muscle. High doses may cause convulsions and myocardial depression.
Indications for use are as for morphine.
• Dosage: 1 mg/kg. Also used in **obstetric analgesia and anaesthesia** (100–150 mg im, up to 200 mg/patient), and has been given by subarachnoid injection (50–100 mg).
Has been used as a component of the **lytic cocktail**.
Should be avoided in patients taking **monoamine oxidase inhibitors**.

pH. Negative logarithm to base 10 of **hydrogen ion** concentration; i.e. pH = –log $[H^+]$. Used as an indication of acidity; the more acid a solution, the lower the pH (Table 29). pH of normal arterial blood is 7.34–7.46, corresponding to $[H^+]$ of 34–46 nmol/l.
See also, Acid–base balance

Table 29. Corresponding values for pH and hydrogen ion concentrations

pH units	$[H^+]$ (nmol/l)
6.8	158
6.9	126
7.0	100
7.1	79
7.2	63
7.3	50
7.4	40
7.5	32
7.6	25
7.7	20
7.8	16
7.9	13
8.0	10

pH measurement. Performed using a glass electrode, which responds specifically and quantitatively to **hydrogen ions** and not to O_2 or CO_2. The potential difference across the inner and outer surfaces of a glass capillary tube depends on the difference between **pH** inside and pH outside the tube. pH outside is kept constant by a **buffer** solution, and blood is passed along the inside of the capillary tube. Potential difference is measured with a silver/silver chloride electrode in the buffer outside the tube, and a mercury/potassium chloride electrode system making contact with the blood. The system is maintained

at 37°C. Potential output is linear: approximately 60 mV per pH unit at 37°C.
See also, Blood gas tensions

Phaeochromocytoma. Rare tumour secreting **catecholamines** developing in chromaffin tissue, usually in the **adrenal gland**. 6% occur at other sites within the **sympathetic nervous system**. 10% are bilateral and 10% malignant. May occur as part of **multiple endocrine adenomatosis** or in association with **neurofibromatosis**.

Usually presents with headache, psychosis, palpitations, sweating and **hypertension** (episodic or sustained). Tumours secreting mainly **adrenaline** cause tachyarrhythmias; those secreting **noradrenaline** cause vasoconstriction, ischaemia and hypertension. Some tumours secrete both these **catecholamines**, and also **dopamine**. **Glucose** intolerance and **cardiomyopathy** may occur.
- Diagnosis is confirmed by:
  - measuring plasma catecholamines or urinary catecholamine metabolites (e.g. metanephrine, hydroxymethylmandelic acid; HMMA).
  - suppression tests (e.g. using **pentolinium**, **clonidine**) with measurement of plasma catecholamines.
  - provocation tests (e.g. using **histamine**, tyramine or **glucagon**). Rarely used now, since dangerous hypertension may occur.

Tumours may be located using selective venous catheterization and catecholamine assays, arteriography (may provoke hypertensive crises), CAT scanning, and radioactive *meta*-iodobenzyl guanidine (MIBG) scintigraphy.
- Anaesthetic considerations:
  - preoperatively:
    - preparation includes oral therapy with **α-adrenergic receptor antagonists** (e.g. **phentolamine** or **phenoxybenzamine** up to 100 mg/day, **prazosin** up to 12 mg/day). When α-receptor blockade is complete, **β-adrenergic receptor antagonists** (e.g. **propranolol** up to 120 mg/day) are administered. Initiation of β-receptor blockade before α-receptor blockade may exacerbate hypertension because of antagonism of β_2–mediated vasodilatation in muscle. **Labetalol** has been used, as has **α-methyl-*p*-tyrosine**.
    - fluid therapy may be required; this may be aided by **central venous cannulation** or possibly **pulmonary artery catheterization**.
  - peroperatively:
    - drugs causing minimal cardiovascular disturbance are used for anaesthesia, e.g. **etomidate, fentanyl, alfentanil, vecuronium, N_2O, enflurane** and **isoflurane**.
    - direct **arterial BP measurement** and CVP with or without **pulmonary capillary wedge pressure** monitoring are required.
    - catecholamines may be released in response to surgical stress, anaesthetic drugs and handling of the tumour. **Sodium nitroprusside**, phentolamine, **glyceryl trinitrate**, prazosin and **magnesium sulphate** have been used to control peroperative hypertension. β-Receptor antagonists or other **antiarrhythmic drugs** may be used to control tachycardia.
    - following the tumour's removal, **iv fluids** and occasionally **phenylephrine** or dopamine may be required to maintain BP.

  - postoperatively:
    - ICU care is required.
    - **hypoglycaemia**, cardiovascular instability and fluid imbalance may occur.

Rarely, phaeochromocytoma may present for the first time during incidental surgery, pregnancy or labour. Morbidity and mortality are high.
Hull CJ (1986) Br J Anaesth; 58: 1453–68

Phantom limb. Sensation of the continued presence of an amputated limb. More common after arm amputation, and when amputation is delayed after the original injury. May be associated with tingling or **pain**, which is severe in 15% of cases and usually described as burning or throbbing. The 'limb' may be felt to be in an abnormal position. Thought to be a state of **central pain**, due to abnormal afferent activity in the interrupted intermediate neurones. Treatment has included **phenytoin, carbamazepine**, local somatic and **sympathetic nerve blocks**, injection of **trigger points, TENS, dorsal column stimulation** and **cordotomy**. **Spinal anaesthesia** is reputed to exacerbate the pain.

Pharmacodynamics. Describes the effects of drugs on the body. Drugs may act by physical interactions (e.g. **antacids**, general anaesthetics), or by interacting with receptors (**receptor theory**) or **enzymes**.
Stanski DR (1988) Can J Anaesth; 35: S42–5
See also, Dose–response curves; Pharmacokinetics

Pharmacokinetics. Describes the absorption, distribution, metabolism and elimination of drugs, i.e. effects of the body on drugs. These factors determine the concentration of a drug at its effector site, and its temporal effect. Population differences in pharmacokinetic data may arise from general individual variations and genetic factors (e.g. plasma **cholinesterase** abnormalities, fast or slow acetylation of many drugs).
- Absorption:
  - may be via oral, sublingual, buccal, inhalational, iv, im, sc, rectal or topical routes.
  - rate of absorption determines the intensity and duration of drug action. Most drugs are absorbed by simple **diffusion**; i.e. rate depends on drug **solubility**, tissue permeability, surface area of the absorption site, and blood supply to the site of absorption. Permeability depends on the degree of **ionization** of the drug, which depends on **pH**. Some drugs are absorbed by **active transport**, e.g. L-dopa, **α-methyl-dopa**.
  - absorption from the GIT also depends on drug characteristics, gut motility, vomiting, destruction of drug by digestive enzymes, interaction with food or other drugs, GIT disease, and intestinal microflora. **First-pass metabolism** reduces the **bioavailability** of many orally-administered drugs, e.g. **opioid analgesic drugs**. Other routes may avoid this.
  - absorption occurs via the lungs for **inhalational anaesthetic agents**.
- Distribution:
  - related to lipid solubility, **pK**, body fluid pH, **protein-binding**, regional blood flow, and specific properties of the drug (e.g. iodine taken up by thyroid tissue).
  - protein-binding limits both the amount of drug free to cross **membranes**, and redistribution of drugs from

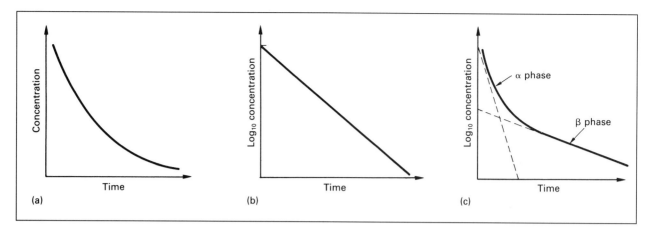

Figure 106 *Drug concentration against time: (a) and (b) one-compartment model; (c) two-compartment model*

the blood. **Volume of distribution** and **clearance** of a drug are inversely proportional to its protein-binding.
–initial redistribution may reduce blood levels of a drug with recovery from its effects, although the total amount in the body has hardly changed, e.g. **thiopentone** and other **iv anaesthetic agents**.
–compartment models have been devised to explain the distribution of drugs in the body:
  –one-compartment model: plasma concentration declines as a simple negative **exponential process** after a bolus injection (first-order kinetics; Fig. 106a), i.e.:

$$C_t = C_0 e^{-kt}$$

where C_t = concentration at time t,
C_0 = concentration at time zero,
k = a constant.
A straight line is obtained when the graph is plotted on semilogarithmic paper (Fig. 106b).

The slope of the line $= \dfrac{k}{2.303}$,

and **half-life** $= \dfrac{0.693}{k}$.

Clearance $= k \times$ volume of distribution
$= \dfrac{C_0}{\text{AUC}}$

where AUC = area under the plasma concentration/time curve.
  –two-compartment model: bi-exponential decline in plasma level; an initial rapid α distribution phase is followed by a slower β elimination phase (Fig. 106c). Each component of the curve may be analysed separately.
    Drug is thought to be distributed from a central compartment (i.e. blood, brain, lungs, etc.) to a peripheral one (e.g. **ECF**, tissues). The central compartment does not necessarily correspond to an anatomical volume, but is defined in terms of its apparent volume. Elimination occurs from the central compartment.
  –three-compartment distribution: one central and two peripheral compartments are assumed.
● Metabolism:
  –drug activity may be enhanced (e.g. **chloral hydrate**

converted to trichloroethanol), decreased (most drugs) or unaltered (e.g. certain **benzodiazepines**).
–usually occurs in two phases in the **liver**. Phase I involves oxidation, reduction or hydrolysis, often involving the cytochrome P_{450} enzyme system. Phase II reactions involve conjugation with glucuronic acid, glycine, glutamine, sulphate, etc., increasing water solubility. Rate of metabolism may be altered by **enzyme induction/inhibition**.
–other sites may be involved, e.g. plasma cholinesterase (**suxamethonium**), kidney (e.g. **dopamine**).
● Elimination:
  –may occur via lungs, bile, urine, GIT, saliva or breast milk. Renal excretion depends on **GFR**, water solubility and extent of active tubular secretion and resorption.
  –most drugs are eliminated by first-order kinetics, whereby rate of elimination is proportional to the amount of drug in the body (i.e. simple exponential decay).
  –in zero-order kinetics, a constant amount of drug is eliminated per unit time (e.g. **alcohol**, **phenytoin**). Zero-order kinetics may replace first-order kinetics when elimination pathways are saturated, i.e. at high drug concentrations.
These analyses allow prediction of drug kinetics, and calculation of appropriate dosage regimens for achieving desired plasma concentrations. For a continuous drug infusion, 50% of steady-state levels are reached after one half-life, 75% after two half-lives, 87.5% after three, 93.75% after four, 96.875% after five, etc. A loading dose achieves steady-state levels more quickly, but is limited by adverse effects if a large dose is given, depending on the drug's **therapeutic ratio/index**. The BET (bolus, elimination, transfer) regimen is often used: a bolus loading dose is followed by an infusion which equals rate of drug elimination, with extra drug infused to allow for transfer between compartments. Alternatively, two or three sequential infusion rates are used. At steady-state, the infusion rate equals the rate of elimination of drug for a one-compartment model, or the rate of transfer to a peripheral compartment for a multi-compartment model.
Stanski DR (1988) Can J Anaesth; 35: S42–5
See also, Drug interactions; Michaelis–Menten kinetics

Pharynx. Common upper end of the respiratory and alimentary tracts, extending from the base of the **skull** to the level of C6.
- Divided into:
  - nasopharynx: lies behind the nasal cavities, above the soft palate. Contains the adenoids, and the eustachian tube orifice on its side wall.
  - oropharynx: lies behind the mouth and **tongue**, below the soft palate. Bounded anteriorly by the anterior pillars of the fauces (with buccal cavity anteriorly), superiorly by the palate and inferiorly by the tip of the epiglottis. Contains the tonsils, lying between the anterior and posterior pillars (containing palatoglossus and palatopharyngeus muscles respectively).
  - laryngopharynx: lies behind and around the **larynx**, extending from the level of the epiglottic tip to the C6 level. The larynx projects into the laryngopharynx, leaving a deep recess (piriform fossa) on each side.

Composed of mucosa (ciliated columnar type in the nasopharynx; stratified or squamous elsewhere), submucosa, muscle layer and loose areolar sheath. The muscles (superior, middle and inferior constrictors) are arranged so that the upper parts of each overlap the lower fibres of the muscle above. They arise thus:
  - superior: from the pterygomandibular raphe, and bony points at either end.
  - middle: from the hyoid bone and stylohyoid ligament.
  - inferior: from the thyroid and cricoid cartilages.

Their anterior borders are open to form the nasal, buccal and laryngeal cavities. Their posterior borders insert into a median raphe along the length of the pharynx.
- Blood supply:
  - arterial: via superior thyroid and ascending pharyngeal branches of the external **carotid artery**.
  - venous: via pharyngeal plexus to the internal **jugular vein**.
- Nerve supply: 9th and 10th **cranial nerves**, with additional nasal innervation via the 5th nerve.

[Bartolomeo Eustachi (1513–1574), Italian physician]
See also, Nose

Phase II block, *see Dual block*

Phase shift. Delay between the arrival of a signal at a **monitoring** device, e.g. **transducer**, and the latter's output. Distortion of the signal is minimized by applying the same delay to all components of the **waveform**, thus maintaining the phase relationship between **harmonics**. This is achieved by adjusting the **damping** of the system to about ⅔ critical damping, at which there is a linear relationship between phase lag and the frequency of the wave.

Phenazocine hydrobromide. Synthetic **opioid analgesic drug** related to **morphine**, but causing less sedation. Has less effect on sphincter of Oddi tone than other opioids. May be administered sublingually. 5 mg is equivalent to 25 mg morphine.
- Dosage: 5 mg orally, 4–6 hourly; up to 20 mg may be given.

[Ruggero Oddi (1845–1906), Italian physiologist]

Phenobarbitone/phenobarbitone sodium. Long-acting **barbiturate**, introduced in 1912; mainly used now in **epilepsy**. Absorbed slowly after oral administration, with duration of action up to 16 hours. Elimination **half-life** is about 90 hours. 40–60% protein-bound, and 75% metabolized by hepatic microsomal enzymes; 25% is normally excreted unchanged in urine.
- Dosage:
  - 60–180 mg orally once daily (5–8 mg/kg/day in children);
  - 50–200 mg may be given im or iv 6 hourly, up to 600 mg/day.
- Side effects include sedation and ataxia. Paradoxical excitement may occur in children.

Hepatic **enzyme induction** may reduce the effectiveness of other drugs, e.g. **warfarin**, oral contraceptives, corticosteroids.

Phenol. Neurolytic agent used for nerve blocks in chronic **pain management**. Thought to spare large myelinated fibres whilst damaging unmyelinated C pain fibres by protein denaturation. Hyperbaric 5% solution in glycerin is used for subarachnoid neurolysis of posterior nerve roots; 0.5–2.0 ml has an effect lasting up to 14 weeks. 6–7% solution in water is used for **sympathetic nerve blocks**.

Also used for sclerotherapy of haemorrhoids, and as a throat gargle. 1–5% solution (carbolic acid) is also used for disinfection of equipment. Irritant to the skin. Used for antisepsis in surgery by Lister in Glasgow in 1865.
[Joseph Lister (1827–1912), English surgeon]

Phenoperidine hydrochloride. Synthetic **opioid analgesic drug** related to **pethidine**, developed in 1957. Has potent analgesic and respiratory depressant properties, and may cause vasodilatation and hypotension. Increased **ICP** has been reported. Used during anaesthesia, and for **sedation** in ICU. Acts within 2–3 minutes of iv injection, with duration of action about 45–60 minutes. Approximately 50% is excreted unchanged in urine; the remainder is metabolized to pethidine and norpethidine.
- Dosage:
  - spontaneous ventilation: 0.5–1 mg in adults; 30–50 µg/kg in children.
  - IPPV: 2–5 mg iv in adults; 100–150 µg/kg in children. 1–4 mg/h by infusion.

Phenothiazines. Group of drugs used as antipsychotic and sedative drugs. Also have antimuscarinic, antiemetic, antihistamine, antidopaminergic and α-**adrenergic receptor** antagonist properties. Some may potentiate the effects of **opioid analgesic drugs**. Different drugs have varying degrees of these properties, depending on the side chains of the molecule. Act mainly on the **ascending reticular activating system**, **limbic system**, basal ganglia, **hypothalamus** and **chemoreceptor trigger zone**. Cause sedation, with reduced muscular, GIT and cardiovascular activity. Effect on respiration is variable. Central temperature regulatory mechanisms, shivering, and peripheral vasoconstriction are impaired, but metabolic rate is unaffected. Highly lipid soluble and extensively protein-bound. Metabolized in the liver to mostly inactive metabolites.
- Side effects:
  - extrapyramidal symptoms, e.g. tardive dyskinesia, tremor, facial grimacing, etc.
  - drowsiness, insomnia, depression, hypothermia, prevention of shivering.

–anticholinergic effects, e.g. tachycardia, **arrhythmias**, dry mouth, urinary retention, blurring of vision.

–galactorrhoea, menstrual irregularity, gynaecomastia, weight gain.

–blood dyscrasias, **haemolysis**.

–photosensitivity, contact dermatitis, rash.

–obstructive **jaundice**.

–hypotension.

–**neuroleptic malignant syndrome**.

–potentiation of other depressant drugs.

Chlorpromazine is the standard phenothiazine; others include **trimeprazine**, **promethazine**, **perphenazine**, promazine, thioridazine, fluphenazine and trifluoperazine.

Phenoxybenzamine hydrochloride.

α-**Adrenergic receptor antagonist**, chemically related to the nitrogen mustards; forms covalent bonds with α-**adrenergic receptors**. Used mainly to control **hypertension** caused by **phaeochromocytoma**. More active at α_1–receptors than at α_2–receptors. Onset of action may be up to 1 hour after iv injection, due to conversion to an active form. Effects last for several days, although its elimination **half-life** is about 24 hours.

- Dosage: 10 mg orally daily, increased by 10 mg/day as required.
- Side effects: postural hypotension, tachycardia, retrograde ejaculation, nasal congestion, miosis, rarely GIT disturbances.

See also, Vasodilator drugs

Phentolamine mesylate.

Non-selective α-**adrenergic receptor antagonist**, with an additional direct relaxant action on vascular smooth muscle. Used to control **hypertensive crises**, e.g. caused by **phaeochromocytoma**, **monoamine oxidase inhibitor** interactions and **clonidine** withdrawal, and in **hypotensive anaesthesia**. Previously used for diagnosing phaeochromocytoma. Acts within 2 minutes of iv injection, with duration of action 10–15 minutes.

- Dosage: 5–10 mg iv repeated as required; 0.1–2.0 mg/min by infusion.
- Side effects: postural hypotension, tachycardia, abdominal pain, diarrhoea, nasal congestion.

See also, Vasodilator drugs

Phenylephrine hydrochloride.

Directly-acting synthetic **sympathomimetic drug**, used as a **vasopressor drug**, e.g. in acute hypotension. Has been administered topically to the nasal mucosa and eye to cause vasoconstriction and mydriasis respectively, and as a vasoconstrictor agent for local anaesthesia. Has also been used to treat **SVT**. Of similar structure to **adrenaline**, lacking only the 4-hydroxyl group. Acts at α-**adrenergic receptors**, causing intense vasoconstriction and compensatory bradycardia.

- Dosage:
  –5 mg im or sc.
  –100–500 µg iv (5–10 µg/kg in children); 20–50 µg/min by infusion.
  –2.5–5 mg added to 100 ml local anaesthetic solution.
- Side effects: hypertension, palpatations, vomiting.

Phenytoin/phenytoin sodium.

Anticonvulsant drug, introduced in the late 1930s. Used to treat all types of **epilepsy** except petit mal, in chronic **pain management**, and as a class Ib **antiarrhythmic drug** (especially for **digoxin**-induced arrhythmias). Thought to act centrally via activation of **GABA** receptors. Has membrane stabilizing effects on all neuronal cells including peripheral nerves and cardiac muscle, thought to involve decreased **sodium** and **calcium** flux during depolarization.

A poorly water-soluble weak acid, with **pK_a** of about 8.3. Variably absorbed from the GIT, it may cause gastric irritation. Erratically absorbed after im injection, probably due to local precipitation. About 90% protein-bound, and metabolized in the liver to inactive metabolites which are excreted renally. Elimination follows first order kinetics at plasma levels below 10 mg/l; zero order kinetics occur above 10 mg/l, due to saturation of enzyme systems (*see Pharmacokinetics*). Elimination **half-life** is about 24 hours but varies. Susceptible to hepatic **enzyme induction**, and is itself an enzyme inducer.

- Dosage:
  –3–4 mg/kg daily as one or two oral doses, increased up to 600 mg/day.
  –for **convulsions**: 10–15 mg/kg iv slowly, with ECG monitoring, followed by 100 mg 6 hourly. Plasma levels should be monitored.
  –for arrhythmias: 3.5–5.0 mg/kg iv slowly, repeated once if required.

  IV administration should be via a large vein at no more than 50 mg/min. Flushing with saline should follow as the solution is strongly alkaline and irritant. Arrhythmias and hypotension may occur.
- Plasma therapeutic range is 10–20 mg/l (40–80 µmol/l).
- Side effects:
  –headache, vomiting, confusion, tremor. Ataxia, nystagmus and blurred vision may indicate overdosage.
  –skin eruptions, lymphadenopathy, hirsutism, fever, hepatitis, gingival hyperplasia.
  –osteomalacia.
  –rarely, megaloblastic anaemia (due to impaired folate absorption and storage), other blood dyscrasias.
  –fetal abnormalities and neonatal bleeding may follow its use in pregnancy.

Chronic usage may increase **fluoride ion** production from **enflurane**, and cause resistance to non-depolarizing **neuromuscular blocking drugs**.

Phlogiston.

Imaginary substance proposed in the 1720s, thought to separate from combustible material during burning. Following experiments in the 1770s, **Priestley** concluded that 'dephlogisticated air' (O_2) and 'dephlogisticated nitrous air' (N_2O) were deficient in phlogiston and could thus support combustion, whereas 'nitrous air' (NO_2) was saturated with it and was unable to do so. The phlogiston theory was subsequently disproved by **Lavoisier**.

Phonocardiography.

Technique employing contact microphones placed on the chest, for amplification and recording of **heart sounds**. Used to obtain an objective record of heart sounds and **heart murmurs**. May be performed simultaneously with **ECG** and **arterial waveform** recording, allowing calculation of **systolic time intervals**. A similar technique is employed to monitor **fetal wellbeing during labour**.

See also, Cardiac cycle

Phosphate.

Total body content is about 25 000 mmol, most of which is intracellular. 80% is in bone, 15% is in soft tissues and only 0.1% is in **ECF**. Most intracellular phosphate is in the organic form. Normal plasma inorganic phosphate levels: 0.8–1.45 mmol/l.

Involved in cell **membranes** (phospholipids), **enzyme** regulation, **energy** storage (**ATP**), O$_2$ transport (**2,3-DPG**) and acid–base buffering.

Levels are controlled by renal excretion; most of the filtered phosphate is reabsorbed in the proximal tubule of the **nephron**. Excretion is increased by parathyroid hormone, calcitonin, **adrenaline** and increased phosphate intake. Decreased excretion occurs when intake is low or in response to thyroxine or **growth hormone**. Hyperphosphataemia causes no specific clinical sequelae but may disturb **calcium** metabolism. **Hypophosphataemia** is uncommon but may occur during **TPN**, **ketoacidosis**, etc.

Phosphodiesterase inhibitors. Substances which prevent conversion of 3',5'-adenosine monophosphate (**cAMP**) to 5'-adenosine monophosphate, or 3',5'-guanosine monophosphate (cGMP) to 5'-guanosine monophosphate by the **enzyme** phosphodiesterase (PDE). Both cAMP and cGMP are important intracellular messengers. Many isoenzymes of PDE exist:
- PDE I: stimulated by **calcium**/calmodulin.
- PDE II: stimulated by cGMP.
- PDE III: inhibited by cGMP.
- PDE IV: cAMP specific.
- PDE V: cGMP specific.

PDE inhibitors have antithrombotic, anti-inflammatory, vasodilator, inotropic and bronchodilator properties. **Amrinome**, **milrinone** and **enoximone** are examples of PDE III inhibitors. **Aminophylline** is a non-specific inhibitor and dipyridamole is a PDE V inhibitor.

Torphy TJ, Undem BJ (1991) Thorax; 46: 512–23

Phrenic nerve pacing. Intermittent electrical stimulation of the **phrenic nerves** (usually bilaterally), to pace the **diaphragm** in chronic **hypoventilation** due to brainstem, medulla or upper cervical cord lesions. Has also been used in **COAD**. Described in the 1960s, it requires intact phrenic nerves and diaphragm function, thus excluding its use in lower **motor neurone** lesions and myopathies.

Platinum electrodes are implanted around the nerves in the neck or thorax and connected to a subcutaneous radio receiver, which is triggered by an external power source. Respiratory rate, inspiratory time, sighs, etc., may be adjusted. Neck electrodes risk inadvertent stimulation of the brachial plexus. Nerve trauma at surgery, infection and poor contacts may cause failure. Diaphragmatic fatigue may also occur. Obstructive apnoea may be precipitated in some cases of central alveolar hypoventilation.

Tibballs J (1991) Anaesth Intensive Care; 19: 597–601

Phrenic nerves. Originate from the ventral rami of C3–5 on each side, supplying the motor innervation of the **diaphragm**. Also convey sensory fibres from the diaphragm, hence the shoulder-tip **referred pain** caused by diaphragmatic irritation. Sensory fibres from the mediastinal **pleura**, fibrous **pericardium** and parietal serous pericardium are also conveyed.

Descend vertically on the scalenus anterior muscles, which they cross from lateral to medial sides. Each nerve passes to the root of the neck beneath the sternomastoid muscle, inferior belly of omohyoid, internal **jugular vein** and (on the left) the thoracic duct. The right phrenic nerve enters the thorax behind the subclavian/internal jugular venous junction, descending subpleurally next to the right brachiocephalic vein, superior and inferior venae cavae and pericardium. Some of its branches pass through the caval foramen of the diaphragm, spreading over its peritoneal surface. The remainder pierce the diaphragm just lateral to the caval orifice. The left nerve enters the thorax between the subclavian artery and vein. It passes superficially to the aortic arch, to pierce the diaphragm anteriorly and to the left of the caval opening. Some of the divisions of each nerve cross to the other side.

Local anaesthetic block has been advocated as a cure for chronic **hiccups**. 10 ml **local anaesthetic agent** is injected 1–2 cm deep at a point 2 cm above the sternoclavicular joint and for 5 cm laterally.

Phrenic paralysis may complicate **brachial plexus block**, trauma, tumour, etc. Paradoxical abdominal movement may occur on inspiration, with a raised hemidiaphragm on **chest X-ray**.

See also, Phrenic nerve pacing

Physiotherapy. Treatment and prevention of disease using passive and active movement, vibration, massage and application of heat. Used for neurological, musculoskeletal and respiratory disorders. Chest physiotherapy aims to maintain clear airways, increase lung expansion and thus reduce **atelectasis** and sputum retention. It is thought to be most useful when excessive sputum production is present; its place in uncomplicated **COAD**, **chest infection** without sputum production, and routine postoperative management has recently been questioned. It is thought to have little place if disease is mainly peripheral; thus it is most efficient if secretions are within the bronchi.

- Techniques include:
  - postural drainage: positioning according to the anatomy of the **tracheobronchial tree**, with or without breathing excercises, etc.
  - breathing exercises, e.g. **incentive breathing**, coughing, etc. **Forced expirations** may be more effective than cough alone, especially if combined with postural drainage.
  - intermittent lung inflations using **ventilators**, to increase lung expansion.
  - chest wall percussion and vibration: their efficacy has also been questioned.
  - upper airway suction: usually combined with the above.

Administration of nebulized **bronchodilator drugs** before physiotherapy may produce a better sputum yield. Nebulized saline, humidified O$_2$ and mucolytics are also commonly used.

May be painful, especially postoperatively, and may require administration of **N$_2$O/Entonox**, **ketamine** or even **opioid analgesic drugs**.

Often beneficial pre- and postoperatively in patients with respiratory disease, helping to optimize respiratory function. It is also valuable in the ICU management of patients with **respiratory failure**, before, during and after **IPPV**.

Selsby D, Jones JG (1990) Br J Anaesth; 64: 621–31

Physostigmine salicylate/sulphate. **Acetylcholinesterase inhibitor**, derived from the West African calibar bean. Causes reversible inhibition of **acetylcholinesterase**

by binding to its esteratic site, lasting 1–2 hours. Readily crosses the **blood–brain barrier** because of its tertiary amine structure. Used to treat the **central anticholinergic syndrome**, and topically in **glaucoma**. Formerly used as a general CNS stimulant, e.g. in **tricyclic antidepressant drug** poisoning and to reverse opioid-induced respiratory depression.

- Dosage: 0.04 mg/kg slowly iv.
- Side effects: nausea, hypertension, tachycardia.

Pickwickian syndrome, *see Alveolar hypoventilation syndrome*

Pierre Robin syndrome, *see Facial deformities, congenital*

Pin index system. International system introduced in 1952, preventing accidental connection of the wrong gas **cylinder** to the wrong **anaesthetic machine** yoke. The cylinder valve block bears holes into which fit pins protruding from the yoke. A flush connection is only achieved if the holes and pins align correctly. The positions of the holes on the valve block (and corresponding pins on the yoke) are specified by an international standard (Fig. 107):

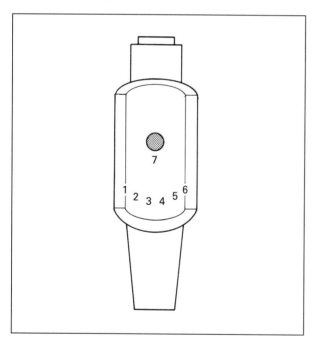

Figure 107 *Position of holes (1–7) in pin index system*

- **O₂**: positions 2 and 5.
- **N₂O**: positions 3 and 5.
- **cyclopropane**: positions 3 and 6.
- **air**: positions 1 and 5.
- **CO₂**: positions 1 and 6.
- **Entonox**: position 7.

The system may be circumvented, e.g. by removing pins, or using several **Bodok seals**. When **piped gas supplies** were first introduced, pin-indexed fittings were attached to the pipelines; these could be inserted upside-down into the cylinder yokes, allowing incorrect gas connection.

Pipecuronium bromide. Non-depolarizing **neuromuscular blocking drug**, synthesized in Hungary in the late 1970s and made available in the USA in 1990. A more potent analogue of **pancuronium**, which it resembles in its clinical action but with less CVS side effects. 40% excreted by the kidneys, it accumulates in renal failure. Reversibly inhibits plasma **cholinesterase**, and does not release **histamine**. A 0.07–0.08 mg/kg intubating dose acts within 2.5–3 minutes, lasting for 1.5–2 hours.

Piped gas supply. Networks of pipes and socket outlets that distribute medical gases from a central source to points of use. In the UK, only **O₂, N₂O, Entonox, CO₂** (rarely) and compressed **air** may be distributed by such systems. All are supplied at 4 bar except air which may be required at 7 bar for orthopaedic instruments, etc. Medical vacuum is also supplied by a pipeline system.

- Essential features include:
  - indexing system to prevent cross-connection.
  - prevention of contamination of gases.
  - automatic function, especially when switching over supplies.
  - anticombustion and antiexplosion controls.
- Systems consist of:
  - central gas source: either a large primary source and small reserve supply, or large primary and secondary sources used alternatively with a small reserve supply. The primary source may be a manifold of **cylinders, vacuum insulated evaporator**, air compressor or **O₂ concentrator**.
  - pipeline distribution network: made of phosphorus deoxidized non-arsenical copper, greased and specially cleaned with steam, shot and medical air. Joints are usually made with a silver alloy although some are threaded. They should be colour-coded and marked with the name of the gas contained. Isolation valves should be supplied.
  - terminal distribution system: includes self-closing sockets, probes, **flowmeters**, and hoses and their connections with **anaesthetic machines**. The probes and sockets should be specific for the service supplied, the probe of one gas fitting only the socket for the same gas. Some probes (e.g. for ward use) may incorporate flowmeters. Connections between hoses and probes should only be possible if specialized equipment is used, reducing the risk of misconnection. Hose connections to anaesthetic machines are made specific for each service by non-interchangeable screw-thread connectors. UK colour-coding of hoses:
    - N₂O: French blue.
    - O₂: white.
    - air: black/white.
    - Entonox: French blue/white.
    - vacuum: yellow.
  - system failure alarms: predominantly low pressure alarms, they sound when secondary and reserve systems are in use. Usually situated at hospital telephone switchboards.

Howell RS (1980) Anaesthesia; 35; 676–98
See also, Suction equipment

Pirbuterol. β-Adrenergic receptor agonist, available for the treatment of **asthma** but also investigated as an orally active **inotropic drug**. Active at β₁–**adrenergic receptors**, with some activity at β₂–receptors. Thus increases cardiac output and causes vasodilatation; BP may fall. Tachycardia is uncommon.

Piritramide. Opioid analgesic drug, developed in 1960. 20 mg is equivalent to 15 mg **morphine**. Of faster onset than morphine, with similar duration of action. Causes less hypotension, nausea and vomiting, but with greater hypnotic effect.

Pirogoff, Nicholai Ivanovich (1810–1881). Russian surgeon at St Petersburg, best known for introducing rectal **diethyl ether** for surgery in 1847. Also studied the effects of ether, designed apparatus for its rectal and inhalational administration, and published a book on the subject in 1847.
Secher O (1986) Anaesthesia; 41: 829–37

Pituitary gland. Lies in the pituitary fossa of the sphenoid bone, above the sphenoid air sinuses and below the optic chiasma. Composed of anterior and posterior lobes, connected to the **hypothalamus** by the infundibular stalk which contains nerve fibres and the hyophyseal portal blood system. The infundibulum pierces the diaphragma sellae, a dural sheet, which covers the gland.
- Function:
  - anterior lobe:
    - contains different cells distinguishable by their staining properties (thus formerly labelled chromophobe, eosinophil and basophil cells):
      - somatotrophs: secrete **growth hormone**.
      - lactotrophs: secrete prolactin.
      - corticotrophs: secrete **ACTH**.
      - thyrotrophs: secrete thyrotrophin.
      - gonadotrophs: secrete luteinizing and follicle-stimulating hormones.
    - secretion is controlled by hypothalamic inhibitory or releasing factors, carried to the anterior pituitary by the portal blood system.
  - posterior lobe: secretes **vasopressin** and **oxytocin**.

Pituitary gland disease may be associated with over- or undersecretion of hormones (usually the latter). Enlargement may cause visual field defects, optic atrophy and raised **ICP**.
See also, Acromegaly; Cushing's disease; Diabetes insipidus; Hypopituitarism

pK. Negative logarithm (to base 10) of the dissociation constant for a chemical reaction. The law of mass action states that for the reaction $HA \rightleftharpoons H^+ + A^-$:

dissociation constant $K_a = \dfrac{[H^+][A^-]}{[HA]}$

Thus $-\log [H^+] = -\log K_a + \log \dfrac{[A^-]}{[HA]}$

Substituting **pH** for $-\log [H^+]$, and pK_a for $-\log K_a$:

$pH = pK_a + \log \dfrac{[A^-]}{[HA]}$

The pK represents the pH value at which the solute is 50% dissociated; i.e. $[A^-] = [HA]$.

Whilst pK_a strictly refers to an acidic substance and pK_b to a basic one, by convention pK_a is used to refer to both acids and bases.

The stronger an acid, the lower its pK_a, and the stronger a base, the higher its pK_a. Thus important when considering **ionization of drugs** and passage of drugs or other substances across **membranes**.

Placenta. Structure dividing the fetal and maternal circulations. Approximately 5–6 days after conception the fertilized egg (now a mass of uniform cells) attaches to the endometrium. The endometrium is invaded by the outer layer of the trophoblast of the egg, the syncytiotrophoblast. Further proliferation of the trophoblast forms finger-shaped masses of tissue, the chorionic villi, between which spaces (lacunae) appear. The tips of the villi erode the walls of the endometrial spiral arteries so that the lacunae expand to form large spaces filled with maternal blood within which float the villi. Primitive blood vessels appear in the villi from about 18 days after fertilization, eventually joining the fetal umbilical vessels. Densely packed masses of fetal villi (fetal cotyledons) are supplied by branches of the umbilical arteries, distributed radially as end-arteries. Several cotyledons form a single placental lobe. Thus the barrier between fetal and maternal circulations is two cells thick, consisting of the fetal capillary endothelium and its covering of syncytial trophoblast.
- Blood supply:
  - fetal: blood arrives via two umbilical arteries and leaves by a single umbilical vein. Umbilical blood flow is up to 100 ml/min at 22 weeks and 300 ml/min at term, of which about 20% does not participate in exchange with maternal blood.
  - maternal: delivered via the uterine arteries. Uterine blood flow (UBF) at term is 500–700 ml/min, 80% of which passes to the placenta. It is directly related to mean uterine perfusion pressure and inversely related to uterine vascular resistance. UBF may be reduced by maternal hypotension, hyperventilation and stress, and by **vasopressor drugs**, e.g. **methoxamine** and **metaraminol**.

Placental function is related to its total surface area and UBF. Impaired function causes fetal **hypoxaemia** and **acidosis** if acute, and may lead to delayed fetal growth if chronic.
- Functions:
  - gas exchange: O_2 and CO_2 exchange is favoured by **fetal haemoglobin** and the double **Bohr effect**, respectively.
  - nutrient exchange: all energy substrates, water, minerals, electrolytes, etc. enter the fetus via the placenta by facilitated or **active transport**.
  - hormonal synthesis and release: hormones include chorionic gonadotrophin, oestrogens, progesterone, prolactin, somatomammotrophin and renin. Several steroid hormones are synthesized by the fetoplacental unit, e.g. placental pregnenolone is metabolized by the fetus before further placental metabolism to form oestrogens.

See also, Fetus, effect of anaesthetic agents on; Obstetric analgesia and anaesthesia

Plasma. Non-cellular portion of **blood**; represents the **ECF** component within the vascular space. A clear, yellowish fluid.
- Normal composition:
  - water.
  - **proteins**:
    - **albumin** (35–50 g/l).

–globulins including **immunoglobulins** (25–35 g/l).
–electrolytes:
  –main cations:
    –**sodium** (135–145 mmol/l).
    –**potassium** (3.5–5.5 mmol/l).
    –**calcium** (2.12–2.65 mmol/l).
    –**magnesium** (0.75–1.05 mmol/l).
  –main anions:
    –chloride (95–105 mmol/l).
    –**bicarbonate** (24–33 mmol/l).
    –**phosphate** (0.8–1.45 mmol/l).
    –**lactate** (0.6–1.8 mmol/l).
–others, e.g. **urea** (2.5–7.0 mmol/l), **creatinine** (60–130 μmol/l), **fats**, **carbohydrates**, e.g. **glucose** (4.0–6.0 mmol/l), **amino acids**, **enzymes**, vitamins, hormones, bilirubin.
Osmolality is 280–305 mosmol/kg.

Plasma clots on standing; the supernatant solution is termed serum. Plasma volume is about 3.5 litres in adults (5% of body weight), and measured by **dye dilution techniques**, using dyes or radioactive markers.

Available for transfusion as fresh frozen plasma.

See also, Blood products; Coagulation

Plasma exchange, *see Plasmapheresis*

Plasma expanders. IV fluids which increase plasma volume by an amount greater than that infused, because of indrawing of water from the extracellular and intracellular spaces by **osmosis**. The term is usually reserved for **colloids**, although **hypertonic iv solutions** act as short-term plasma expanders.

Plasma, fresh-frozen, *see Blood products*

Plasma substitutes, *see Colloids*

Plasmapheresis. Selective removal of small volumes (up to 600 ml) of **plasma** from the body. Replacement with **iv fluids** is not required. Removal of larger volumes with fluid replacement is termed plasma exchange. Used to remove plasma constituents associated with disease, e.g. antibodies, antigens, immune complexes, drugs, etc. Rate of removal must exceed that of renewal. Not always beneficial, and usually reserved for disease resistant to conventional therapy.

● Often beneficial in:
  –**myasthenia gravis**.
  –**Guillain–Barré syndrome**.
  –multiple myeloma.
  –Goodpasture's syndrome.
  –thrombotic thrombocytopenic purpura.
  –poisoning with mushrooms and **digoxin**.
● May be beneficial in:
  –bullous pemphigoid.
  –**rhesus** haemolytic disease.
  –systemic lupus erythematosus.
  –**rheumatoid arthritis**.

Requires extracorporeal centrifugation or filtration. Removal of over 1000 ml requires replacement with **albumin** to prevent a fall in plasma **oncotic pressure**. Partial substitution with **colloids** or **crystalloids** is often used. A single volume exchange (40 ml/kg) reduces plasma components by 50–60%, usually lasting 24–48 hours. Usually, 1.5 plasma volumes are exchanged during each session, repeated every 1–2 days according to clinical response.

Practical considerations and complications are as for **extracorporeal circulation** and **iv fluid administration**.
[Ernest W. Goodpasture (1886–1960), US pathologist]
Reimann PM, Mason PD (1991) Intensive Care Med; 16: 3–10

Plasmin and plasminogen, *see Fibrinolysis*

Plastic surgery. Anaesthetic considerations:
  –related to the reason for surgery, e.g. **burns**, **trauma**, **facial deformities**, etc. (*See also, Ear, nose and throat surgery*).
  –possible requirement for **hypotensive anaesthesia**.
  –problems of prolonged surgery, e.g. **heat loss**, **blood loss**, **positioning of the patient**.
  –skin grafts may be taken from trunk or limbs, reducing sites of access to the patient.
  –regional techniques may be useful for graft donor sites, e.g. **femoral nerve block**, **lateral cutaneous nerve of the thigh block**.
  –a low **haematocrit** is thought to improve perfusion and healing of grafts. **Dextran** solutions may be used to improve perfusion of grafted areas.
  –**tourniquets** may be required.

Platelets. Non-nucleated, smooth, disc-shaped **blood** cells derived from cytoplasmic fragments of megakaryocytes (bone marrow stem cells). Maturation of megakaryocytes, and thus platelet production, is controlled by a feedback mechanism involving the humoral agent thrombopoietin. Measure 2–4 μm in diameter and 5–8 fl in volume, with a circulatory life span of 8–14 weeks. Normal adult count is $150–400 \times 10^9$/l blood; 10–20% of the total platelet population lies within the spleen. Platelet deficiency and excess are termed **thrombocytopenia** and thrombocytosis respectively.

Essential for normal **coagulation**, spontaneous haemorrhage occurring at counts below $20–30 \times 10^9$/l. Cytoplasmic granules within platelets contain many substances including **ATP**, ADP, **5–HT**, **adrenaline**, **calcium**, fibronectin, fibrinogen, β-thromboglobulin and thrombospondin, which contribute to platelet aggregation, blood coagulation, local vasoconstriction, chemotaxis and vessel repair. Also present is an enzyme, **thromboxane** synthetase, which is activated when platelets contact damaged vascular endothelium. Release of thromboxane stimulates platelet aggregation via increased ADP levels. Aggregation leads to further ADP release and release of the other substances, eventually resulting in formation of a plug. During this process, the platelets become more spherical and extend pseudopodia. Conversely **prostacyclin**, present in the vascular endothelium, stimulates production of platelet cAMP and reduces release of ADP, inhibiting aggregation. Thus a fine balance exists between the two processes.

Apart from **coagulation disorders** arising from abnormal platelet numbers, prolonged bleeding may arise from abnormal function despite apparently normal counts, e.g. **renal failure**, **hepatic failure**, **pre-eclampsia**, and use of **antiplatelet drugs**. Platelet function may be assessed using the bleeding time.
Gibbs NM (1991) Anaesth Intensive Care; 19: 495–505
See also, Coagulation studies

Plethysmography. Recording of volume changes of an organ, part of the body or the whole body.

- Clinical applications:
  - **body plethysmograph**.
  - photoelectric plethysmography, used for **arterial BP measurement** (Finapres device).
  - **impedance plethysmography**.
  - measuring limb blood flow:
    - recording pressure changes in a circumferential cuff or strain gauges.
    - inflating a proximal cuff to between venous and arterial pressures, and recording volume changes by immersing the limb in water.

Pleura. Double-layered sac enclosing the **lungs**. The outer parietal layer attaches to the **diaphragm**, **mediastinum** and chest wall. The inner visceral layer is closely applied to the lung surface and enters its fissures. The layers meet at the lung hila. They are held together by the negative **intrapleural pressure** within the pleural cavity which normally contains a small amount of serous fluid.

- Surface markings:
  - apex: 3.5 cm above the clavicular midpoint.
  - medial border: passes behind the sternoclavicular joint, meeting the opposite pleura level with the 2nd costal cartilage. Descends to the costoxiphoid angle on the right; deflects laterally to the lateral sternal edge on the left.
  - inferior border: lies level with the 8th rib in the midclavicular line, 10th rib in the midaxillary line, and passes up to the spine of T12 posteriorly.

Pleural effusion. Serous fluid between the parietal and visceral layers of **pleura** (interpleural pus and blood are called empyema and haemothorax respectively). May be unilateral or bilateral. Divided according to the protein content into:

- transudates (<30 g/l):, e.g. **cardiac failure, hypoproteinaemia**.
- exudates (>30 g/l):, e.g. tumours, inflammatory disease (e.g. **connective tissue diseases**), infection (e.g. **TB**), **PE**, abdominal disease (e.g. subphrenic abscess, **pancreatitis**, ovarian carcinoma).

Features include dyspnoea, usually related to the size of the effusion. Chest wall movement and breath sounds are reduced over the effusion, with percussion typically 'stony dull'. Large unilateral effusions may displace the mediastinum (and thus the trachea) towards the opposite side. Confirmed by **chest X-ray**; examination of the fluid aids diagnosis.

Treatment includes **chest drainage** and is otherwise directed towards the cause.

Large pleural effusions may hinder lung expansion and should be drained preoperatively. Other anaesthetic considerations are related to the underlying cause.

Pneumatics, *see Fluidics*

Pneumonia, *see Chest infection*

Pneumonitis. Inflammation of the lung caused by physical or chemical agents, e.g. inhalation of toxic or irritant substances and fumes, **radiation**, etc. Clinical features vary from slight **dyspnoea** to those of **ARDS**. Inflammation caused by infection is termed pneumonia; that caused by an allergic reaction is termed alveolitis.
See also, Aspiration pneumonitis

Pneumotachograph. Constant orifice, variable pressure **flowmeter**, used widely in anaesthetic and respiratory research. Senses the pressure difference across a fixed resistance using pressure **transducers**; if **flow** is laminar, the pressure difference is proportional to flow. The resistance is produced by winding strips of corrugated foil into spiral tubes 1–2 mm in diameter, the number of tubes being matched for the desired flow range. Enclosing the resistor within an electrical coil prevents condensation when moist gases are used. Alternatively, the resistance consists of a layer of metal or plastic gauze, the latter less likely to cause condensation.

The instrument head should be appropriately sized to avoid turbulence, and the gas flow spread evenly over the resistance unit. The pressure gradient depends not only on the gas flow but also on its composition, viscosity and temperature; thus difficulties may arise if gas composition varies throughout breaths.

Pneumothorax. Free gas, usually air, within the pleural cavity.

- Has been classified as:
  - simple: the gas is not under tension. May be:
    - open: continuing communication between the source of the gas and the pleural cavity. Intrapleural and atmospheric pressures are equal and lung expansion is poor, causing marked **hypoxaemia**. **Pendelluft** may occur. Mediastinal shift may occur in phase with respiration, causing cardiovscular collapse. Gas exchange may improve with **IPPV**, which increases expansion of the collapsed lung (but tension pneumothorax may develop if gas is forced into the pleural cavity and unable to return).
    - closed: no continuing communication with the gas source; lung collapse is proportional to the volume of gas introduced into the pleural cavity, usually via the bronchi. Gas exchange is unaltered by IPPV, if there is no risk of further gas leakage.
  - tension: gas flow into the pleural cavity is unidirectional and a 'valve' mechanism prevents its escape. The pressure within the pleural cavity increases, with worsening pulmonary collapse, hypoxaemia, **hypercapnia**, mediastinal shift and obstruction to venous return. Tension is increased by IPPV.
- May occur by three mechanisms:
  - intrapulmonary rupture: retrograde perivascular dissection of gas towards the lung hilum, which may result in mediastinal emphysema. May follow use of high inflation pressures during IPPV, or severe cough or **Valsalva manoeuvre**. May also occur spontaneously if the alveolar septum is weakened by infection or chronic lung disease.
  - injury to the visceral **pleura**: air escapes through the hole into the pleural cavity; the lung collapses and the hole may seal or act as a valve. Causes include spontaneous rupture of an emphysematous bulla, fractured **ribs**, regional anaesthetic techniques or **central venous cannulation**, **tracheostomy** and lung biopsy.
  - injury to the parietal pleura: gas enters from the atmosphere (e.g. open chest wound, during central venous cannulation, etc.) or from adjoining structures:

–peritoneal cavity: gas passes upwards through the retroperitoneal tissue and ruptures through the mediastinal parietal pleura, or passes through defects in the **diaphragm**.

–mediastinum: gas ruptures through the pleura as above; it may arise following oesophageal perforation and procedures such as tracheostomy and thyroidectomy.

- Features:
  –range from mild dyspnoea and chest pain to respiratory distress. If the pneumothorax is very large or under tension, severe hypoxaemia and cardiovascular collapse may occur.

  –clinical signs may be absent in small pneumothoraces, but there may be subcutaneous emphysema and ipsilateral reduction of chest wall movement and breath sounds, and increased resonance to percussion. There may be audible wheezing, or a 'crunch' caused by air in the mediastinum (Hamman's sign). Inflation pressures may rise during anaesthesia with IPPV.

  –erect **chest X-ray** in expiration may reveal absent lung markings beyond the edge of the collapsed lung, with the characteristic lung edge usually visible. Diagnosis may be difficult from a supine film. Pleural gas under tension causes marked lung collapse, hyperexpansion of the ipsilateral lung and mediastinal shift.

Treatment depends on the size of the pneumothorax; small ones often resolve spontaneously. If symptomatic, or if IPPV is planned, **chest drainage** should be performed. A tension pneumothorax may be life-threatening and requires urgent relief, e.g. with a needle or iv cannula. **N₂O**, being more soluble than atmospheric nitrogen, may rapidly expand a pneumothorax (by 100% in 10 minutes at inspired concentration of 70%); it should therefore not be used unless a chest drain has been placed.

[Louis Hamman (1877–1946), US physician]

See also, Chest trauma; Flail chest

Poise. Unit of **viscosity** in the **cgs system of units**. 1 P = 1 dyne s/cm^2.

[Jean Poiseuille (1797–1869), French physiologist]

Poiseuille's equation, *see Hagen–Poiseuille equation*

Poisoning and overdoses. May be deliberate, or may follow accidental exposure or ingestion. Substances responsible include those found in the home, industrial or agricultural chemicals, plant or animal toxins, and therapeutic drugs.

- Principles of management:
  –removal of the patient from the source of the toxic substance, e.g. from scene of a fire, chemical spillage, etc. Medical staff should be adequately protected, since absorption through skin and lungs may occur.

  –**CPR** and standard management of the unconscious patient, including **monitoring**.

  –blood analysis for drug, glucose and electrolyte levels, specific organ function tests, etc.

  –prevention of further absorption of ingested substances, e.g. using activated **charcoal**, **gastric lavage**, **emetic drugs**.

  –specific antidotes and treatments, e.g. **naloxone**, **flumazenil**, **chelating agents**, **digoxin** antibody fragments, thiosulphate in **cyanide poisoning**.

–increasing elimination of ingested substances, e.g. **forced diuresis**, **haemoperfusion**, **dialysis**, activated charcoal.

Common problems include respiratory depressiom, **hypotension**, **arrhythmias**, **coma**, **convulsions** and disturbances of **temperature regulation**. **Pulmonary oedema**, **ARDS**, **hepatic failure** and **renal failure** may also occur.

Regional or national poisons units provide information and advice.

Henry JA (1986) Br J Anaesth; 58: 223–33

See also, Alcohol; Barbiturate poisoning; Carbon monoxide poisoning; Opioid poisoning; Organophosphorus poisoning; Paracetamol poisoning; Salicylate poisoning; Smoke inhalation; Tricyclic antidepressant drugs

Polarographic oxygen analysis, *see Oxygen measurement*

Poliomyelitis. Disease caused by one of three small RNA enteroviruses transmitted by the respiratory or faecooral routes. Now uncommon in the West following successful immunization programmes. Following 7–14 days incubation period, an acute febrile illness occurs, with upper respiratory or GIT symptoms lasting a few days. Over 90% of cases of infection are subclinical. Pyrexia may recur with features of acute viral **meningitis**. Asymmetrical lower **motor neurone** weakness develops in 0.1% of cases of infection, caused by destruction of the anterior horn cells of the **spinal cord** and **cranial nerve** nuclei. Ventilatory support is required during the acute illness in approximately 30% of cases, because of intercostal or diaphragmatic involvement. Bulbar involvement may impair swallowing, cough reflexes and vocal cord function. Rarely, medullary involvement may cause cardiovascular instability or **sleep apnoea**.

Most patients have residual disability, but improvement may continue for up to 2 years after the acute episode. Progressive weakness may occur 20–30 years later (postpolio syndrome). 10–30% of those requiring ventilatory support acutely require long-term support.

Pollution, *see Environmental safety of anaesthetists; Scavenging*

Polyarteritis nodosa, *see Connective tissue diseases*

Polycythaemia. General term for a **haemoglobin** concentration above 16–17 g/dl, red cell count above 5.6–6.4 × 10^{12}/l, or **haematocrit** above 0.47–0.54 (all values female-male respectively).

- May be:
  –relative (reduced plasma volume, e.g. **burns**, **dehydration**).

  –absolute (increased red cell volume):
    –primary (polycythaemia rubra vera, PRV): myeloproliferative disorder, occurring mainly in men over 50 years. Features are caused mainly by hypervolaemia and hyperviscosity (headaches, plethora, pruritus, dyspnoea, visual disturbances, reduced cardiac output, thrombotic and haemorrhagic episodes) and a high metabolic rate (night sweats, weight loss). Hepatosplenomagaly may occur. White cell and **platelet** counts may also be increased; platelet function may be abnormal.

    The main perioperative risks are haemorrhage (caused by abnormal platelets) and thrombosis.

Elective surgery should be delayed to allow treatment; **emergency surgery** should proceed only after venesection and volume replacement. Treatment is directed at keeping the haematocrit below 0.5, usually with repeat venesection, radioactive phosphorus or myelosuppressive drugs (busulphan). PRV progresses to myelosclerosis in 20–30% of cases.

–secondary to raised **erythropoietin** levels, e.g. in response to chronic **hypoxaemia** (e.g. pulmonary disease, cyanotic heart disease, high **altitude**) or inappropriate secretion (e.g. renal carcinoma, hepatocellular carcinoma, haemangioblastoma). Risks are related to increased blood viscosity and thrombosis as above.

Barabas AP (1980) Br J Hosp Med; 23: 289–94

Polymyositis. Group of idiopathic autoimmune inflammatory diseases including dermatomyositis, affecting muscle and skin. May involve multiple systems. Usually presents with myalgia, muscle tenderness and weakness (mainly proximal). Bulbar weakness may lead to dysphagia, dysphonia and regurgitation. Intercostal and diaphragmatic weakness may result in **respiratory failure**, exacerbated by interstitial pneumonitis which is also a feature of the disease. In dermatomyositis, there is a characteristic erythematous rash of the face and neck. **Malignancy** is common, especially in older men.

Creatine kinase is raised; muscle biopsy is confirmatory. Treatment includes **steroid therapy** and other **immunosuppressive drugs**.

An abnormal sensitivity to **neuromuscular blocking drugs** has been suggested but is unproven.

Ganta R, Campbell IT, Mostafa SM (1988) Br J Anaesth; 60: 854–8

Polyneuropathy, acute post-infection, *see Guillain–Barré syndrome*

Popliteal fossa. Diamond-shaped space behind the knee joint, bounded inferiorly by the two heads of gastrocnemius muscle and superiorly by biceps femoris (laterally) and semimembranosus/semitendinosus muscles (medially).

● Contents (medially to laterally):
  –popliteal artery; continues from the femoral artery, and divides into anterior and posterior tibial arteries at or below the lower part of the fossa. The popliteal vein lies superficially.
  –tibial nerve: arises from the sciatic nerve, usually at the upper pole of the fossa. Lies superficial to the popliteal vessels. The common peroneal nerve passes laterally around the fibular head, lateral to the fossa.
  –fat pad.

See also, Knee, nerve blocks

Pop-off valve, *see Adjustable pressure-limiting valve*

Populations. In **statistics**, any group of similar objects, events or observations. Usually contains too many individuals to be studied as a whole, thus **samples** are studied and any conclusions drawn are applied to the whole population. A population may be described by its:
  –shape i.e. **statistical distribution curve**, e.g. normal, binominal.
  –central tendency, e.g. **mean**, **median**, **mode**.
  –scatter, e.g. **standard deviation**, **percentiles**.

Porphyria. Group of diseases characterized by overproduction and excretion of porphyrins (intermediate compounds produced during haemoprotein synthesis) and their precursors. Caused by specific **enzyme** defects within the haem metabolic pathway. Several forms exist, divided into hepatic and erythropoietic varieties. Only three forms, all of them hepatic varieties transmitted by autosomal dominant inheritance, affect the conduct of anaesthesia:
  –acute intermittent porphyria (AIP): results in increased amounts of urinary porphobilinogen and δ-aminolaevulinic acid (D-ALA) during attacks. May present with acute abdominal pain, vomiting, motor and sensory **peripheral neuropathy**, autonomic dysfunction, **cranial nerve** palsies, mental disturbances and coma. Common in Sweden. Diagnosed by urinalysis.
  –variegate porphyria: may present with similar features to AIP. Photosensitivity is common. Common in South African Afrikaners. Diagnosed by stool examination for copro- and protoporphyrin.
  –hereditary coproporphyria: photosensitivity may occur.

Acute attacks may be precipitated by drugs, stress, infection, **alcohol** ingestion, menstruation, **pregnancy** and starvation, although not at every exposure. Information about drugs is obtained from case reports, animal studies and analysis of drug effects on cell cultures.

● Effects of drugs:
  –definite precipitants: include **barbiturates**, **phenytoin** and sulphonamides.
  –implicated in laboratory or animal studies but not in humans: **etomidate**, **lignocaine**, chlordiazepoxide.
  –considered safe to use: **opioid analgesic drugs**, N_2O, **suxamethonium**, **tubocurarine**, **gallamine**, **atropine**, **neostigmine**, **bupivacaine**, **prilocaine**, **procaine**, **propranolol**, **chlopheniramine**, **droperidol**, **chlorpromazine**, **chloral hydrate**, **aspirin**, **paracetamol**, **insulin**.
  –controversial: **diazepam**, **halothane**, steroids, **ketamine**, **propofol**. All have been used safely despite conflicting evidence.

Moore MR, Disler PD (1988) Adverse Drug Reaction Bull; 129: 484–7
See also, Inborn errors of metabolism

Poseiro effect. Decrease in arterial BP during uterine contraction; thought to be caused by exacerbations of **aortocaval compression**.

[JJ Poseiro (described 1967), Uruguayan obstetrician]
See also, Obstetric analgesia and anaesthesia

Positioning of the patient. Undertaken to:
  –facilitate surgery, imaging, etc.
  –encourage venous drainage (for surgery) or distension (for **central venous cannulation**).
  –allow the performance and control the extent of **regional anaesthesia**.
  –protect the **airway** (e.g. **recovery** position).

Often performed when the patient is anaesthetized; damage to limbs, joints, pressure areas and nerves may occur unless care is taken. Tracheal tube, iv lines, etc. may be displaced during movement.

● Specific problems associated with certain positions:
  –supine: $\dot{V}/\dot{Q}$ mismatch may occur, especially if **closing capacity** exceeds **FRC**. **Regurgitation** of **gastric**

contents may occur. The calves should be raised off the bed to reduce risk of **DVT**. In **pregnancy**, **aorto-caval compression** may occur.

–prone: similar considerations to the supine position apply. Chest wall and abdominal movement during respiration may be hindered. **Venous return** may be impeded if the abdomen is compressed. Supports should be positioned under the iliac crests and shoulders, leaving the abdomen free. The face and eyes should be carefully padded.

–lateral: $\dot{V}/\dot{Q}$ mismatch occurs (*see One-lung anaesthesia*). The lower arm may be compressed and its venous drainage impaired.

–Trendelenburg: originally described as supine with steep head-down tilt, with the knees flexed over the 'broken' end of the table. Diaphragmatic movement is limited by the weight of the abdominal viscera, reducing FRC and increasing **atelectasis**. Risk of regurgitation is increased. Venous engorgement of the head and neck may be accompanied by raised **ICP** and **intraocular pressure**. **Brachial plexus** injury may occur if shoulder supports are used.

–reversed Trendelenburg: hypotension may occur if the head-up tilt is achieved rapidly.

–lithotomy position: similar considerations to the Trendelenburg position. Injury to the lower back, hips and knees may occur. Common peroneal or saphenous nerves may be compressed against the lithotomy poles. DVT may follow calf compression against the poles.

–sitting: difficult to position the unconscious patient. Hypotension and **air embolus** may occur (*see Dental surgery; Neurosurgery*).

[Friedrich Trendelenburg (1844–1924), German surgeon]
Healy TEJ, Wilkins RG (1984) Ann R Coll Surg Engl; 66: 56–8
See also, Nerve injury during anaesthesia

Positive end-expiratory pressure (PEEP). Adjunct to **IPPV**, introduced in 1967. Produced by maintaining a positive airway pressure during expiration: usually 5–20 cmH$_2$O, although higher levels have been used ('super-PEEP'). Minimizes airway and alveolar collapse and increases **compliance**, by increasing **FRC**. Thus improves oxygenation and reduces pulmonary **shunt**. High levels may increase **dead space**. Also, the adverse effects of IPPV related to intrathoracic pressure are increased. Thus **barotrauma** and reduced cardiac output are more likely. Urine output is reduced, and **vasopressin** secretion and **ICP** increased.

Has been used to reduce O$_2$ requirement and improve oxygenation in **respiratory failure** of any cause, except where its adverse effects are especially dangerous, e.g. **asthma**. The following terms have been used to describe the adjustment of PEEP:

–best PEEP: produces the least shunting without significant reduction of cardiac output.

–optimum PEEP: produces maximal **O$_2$ delivery** with the lowest dead space/tidal volume ratio.

–appropriate PEEP: that with the least dead space.

Duncan AW, Oh TE, Hillman DR (1986) Anaesth Intensive Care; 14: 236–50

Positron emission tomography (PET). Technique for imaging the distribution of inhaled or injected positron-emitting **radioisotopes**, e.g. ^{15}O, ^{13}N, ^{11}C and ^{18}F.

Tomographic techniques similar to those used for **CAT scanning** are used. Usually restricted to brain imaging, providing information about **cerebral blood flow**, O$_2$ and glucose metabolism, etc.

Postherpetic neuralgia. Persistent **pain** in the distribution of one or more peripheral nerves following shingles (herpes zoster). Usually defined as pain lasting for over one month. Shingles is caused by infection with the varicella-zoster virus which also causes chicken-pox. It usually affects adults and occurs spontaneously although predisposing factors include old age and **immunodeficiency**. The virus lies dormant in the dorsal root ganglia but may multiply and invade the corresponding sensory nerves. Pain usually precedes the appearance of cutaneous vesicles on an inflamed base, which last 2–4 weeks. In 10% of cases, scarring and pain persist; the latter may be severe and intractable, triggered by contact, draughts and stress.

Treatment may be disappointing, but includes **tricyclic antidepressant drugs**, **anticonvulsant drugs**, local counterirritants, **TENS**, **acupuncture**, **local anaesthetic agent** creams, repeated **extradural anaesthesia**, peripheral or **sympathetic nerve blocks**, and dorsal root entry zone coagulation. Modification with acyclovir or steroids is unproven.

Postoperative analgesia. Recognized as an area where improvement is required, since the traditional on-demand im administration of **opioid analgesic drugs** is widely accepted as often being inadequate. Acute pain services are increasingly being set up: duties include education of medical and nursing staff, **audit**, research, and visiting postoperative patients specifically to monitor and adjust analgesia regimens.

Analgesic requirements vary according to the type of surgery, fitness of the patient, psychological factors and interpatient differences.

- Techniques available:
  –opioid analgesic drugs:
    –im: painful to administer, and result in variable plasma drug levels. The time from the patient's expressing pain to the drug's administration depends on the patient's persistence, the level of nursing staffing and the procedures for obtaining and checking controlled drugs. Commonly used, however, because of its convenience and low cost.
    –iv: more reliable; methods include:
      –incremental small boluses titrated against effect; reduces accidental overdosage but still may allow windows of inadequate analgesia.
      –continuous infusion: may be adjusted to the minimal effective rate with minimal side effects. Steady-state plasma levels may be slow to achieve, and overdosage may still occur.
      –**patient-controlled analgesia**: may reduce the total amount of drug required, and the patient's sense of being in control may be beneficial.
  –**spinal opioids**: usually administered via extradural catheters which remain *in situ* for a few days. Although analgesia is usually extremely good, large interpatient variability exists. Side effects include urinary retention, nausea, pruritus and respiratory depression; careful monitoring is required to detect the latter.

–sc: useful if iv access is limited but confers no advantage over iv administration.

–oral: generally not useful immediately postoperatively, because of inability to drink, nausea and **vomiting**, delayed **gastric emptying** and **first-pass metabolism**.

–transdermal: slow-release patches are stuck to the skin; does not require cannulae or catheters, but adjustment of the release rate is impossible. **Fentanyl** has been studied for transdermal administration.

–sublingual/buccal: avoids injection but suffers the disadvantages of intermittent administration. **Buprenorphine** is administered in this way.

–rectal: drug absorption may be variable; the technique is less common in the UK.

–**NSAIDs**: popular as a method of reducing opioid requirements, particularly after **day-case surgery**, **dental surgery** and **orthopaedic surgery**. **Ketorolac** and **diclofenac** may be given parenterally and may be powerful enough to obviate the need for opioids; others are administered orally or rectally. They may cause GIT upset and impair renal and **platelet** function. Increased perioperative bleeding has been reported, but this has not been clnically significant even if statistically significant.

–**local anaesthetic agents**: provide excellent analgesia but with motor blockade, risk of toxicity of local anaesthetics and variable duration of action (depending on the technique and drug chosen). Duration may be prolonged by the use of repeated injections or infusions via catheters.

–infiltration or nerve block: performed before or after surgery.

–**caudal analgesia**, **extradural anaesthesia** or **spinal anaesthesia**: limited by hypotension and motor paralysis. May be combined with opioids.

–**inhalational anaesthetic agents**: some postoperative benefit is derived from the agents used peroperatively. **Entonox** is the only agent widely used postoperatively, e.g. for **physiotherapy** or changes of dressings, and is limited by its adverse effects on the haematological system.

–nerve destruction, e.g. using **cryoanalgesia** is commonly used in **thoracic surgery**, but has limited application elsewhere.

–other methods less widely used include **TENS**, **acupuncture** and **hypnosis**.

Mitchell RWD, Smith G (1989) Br J Anaesth; 63: 147–58
See also, Analgesic drugs; Pain; Pain evaluation; Pain management; Pre-emptive analgesia

Postspinal headache. Headache occurring after dural puncture, e.g. **spinal anaesthesia** or investigative lumbar puncture. First described by **Bier** in 1899. May rarely develop after **extradural anaesthesia** without an obvious dural tap. Thought to be due to **CSF** leaking through the dural hole, with settling of the **brain** and stretching of intracranial nerves, dura and blood vessels. The incidence is increased by using large gauge needles, especially if the longitudinal dural fibres are cut transversely by the needle bevel instead of being split longitudinally. More common in obstetrics and in young patients. Reported incidence varies but is approximately 1–3% for 25–29 G needles in non-pregnant patients, and up to 75% with 16 G

extradural needles in **obstetric analgesia and anaesthesia**.

Headaches usually occur within 1–3 days of dural puncture, normally lasting for 1–2 weeks but occasionally for months. They are classically severe, frontal or occipital, and exacerbated by sudden movement, getting up from the supine position, and coughing and straining. Neck stiffness may occur. The incidence is reduced by careful technique and use of small needles, probably by using non-cutting needles. Prophylactic bed rest after dural puncture is now thought to be unnecessary. If cutting needles are used, they should be inserted with the bevel aligned with the longitudinal dural fibres.

● Treatment:
–simple analgesics, e.g. **paracetamol**. **Caffeine** has been reported to be effective.
–maintenance of good hydration.
–extradural **blood patch** if headache is persistent. The use of prophylactic extradural injection of saline or blood at the time of dural puncture is controversial.

Reid JA, Thorburn J (1991) Br J Anaesth; 67: 674–7

Post-tetanic potentiation (PTP; Post-tetanic facilitation). Increased response to a single pulse stimulus following **tetanic contraction**. Seen during **non-depolarizing neuromuscular blockade**; thought to be caused by increased presynaptic mobilization and release of **acetylcholine** in response to the tetanus. Absent in **depolarizing neuromuscular blockade**. Mechanical PTP occurring in normal subjects without neuromuscular blockade is thought to be caused by **calcium** ion accumulation resulting in increased **muscle** strength. **EMG** recording does not exhibit PTP in unblocked muscle.
See also, Neuromuscular blockade monitoring

Potassium. Principal intracellular cation, present at 135–150 mmol/l. Present in the **plasma** at 3.5–5.0 mmol/l. Total body content is about 3200 mmol, of which 90% is intracellular, 7.5% within bone and dense connective tissue, and 2.5% in **interstitial fluid**, transcellular fluid and plasma. About 90% is exchangeable. Essential for maintenance of the cell **membrane potential** and generation of **action potentials**.

Filtered potassium is reabsorbed mainly at the proximal convoluted tubule of the **nephron**. It is secreted at the distal tubule, in effect in exchange for **sodium** and **hydrogen ions** under the influence of **aldosterone**.
● Daily requirement: about 1 mmol/kg/day.
Vitez T (1987) Can J Anaesth; 34: S30–1

Potency. Ability of a drug to produce a certain effect. Influenced by the drug's absorption, distribution, metabolism, excretion and **affinity** for its receptor. Very potent drugs are effective in very small doses.
See also, Dose–response curves

Potentiation, post-tetanic, *see Post-tetanic potentiation*

Power. Rate of performing **work**. SI **unit** is the **watt**:

$$1 \text{ W} = 1 \text{ J/s.}$$

Also refers to the ability of **statistical tests** to reveal a difference of a certain magnitude. Power analysis is performed before a **clinical trial** to determine the sample size required to show a certain difference, or retrospectively when analysing a statistically insignificant result.

Increased if groups are equally sized and large, and if the difference between them is large. Power equals 1–β, where β = type II **error**; power of 80% (β = 0.2) is usually considered acceptable.

Power spectrum analysis. Fourier analysis of 2–16 second sections (epochs) of the **EEG**, with graphical representation of the distribution of frequencies within each epoch. The frequency distribution of successive epochs may be plotted consecutively on continuous paper as a series of peaks and troughs (compressed spectral array) representing frequencies of high and low activity respectively. Has been used to monitor depth of anaesthesia.
See also, Anaesthesia, depth of

Poynting effect. Dissolution of gaseous **O₂** when bubbled through liquid **N₂O**, with vaporization of the liquid to form a gaseous O_2/N_2O mixture.
[John H Poynting (1852–1914), English physicist]
See also, Entonox

PPF, Plasma protein fraction, *see Blood products*

P–R interval. Represents atrial depolarization. Measured from the beginning of the **P wave** to the beginning of the **QRS complex** of the **ECG**, irrespective of whether the QRS complex starts with a **Q wave** or an **R wave** (*see Fig. 49b; Electrocardiography*). Normally 1.2–2.0 ms. Shortened in **junctional arrhythmias, Wolff–Parkinson–White syndrome** and **Lown–Ganong–Levine syndrome**. Prolonged in **heart block** and **hypothermia**.

Pralidoxime mesylate. Acetylcholinesterase reactivator, used with **atropine** to treat **organophosphorus poisoning**. Has three main actions:
  –converts the **acetylcholinesterase inhibitor** to a harmless compound.
  –protects acetylcholinesterase transiently against further inhibition.
  –reactivates the inhibited acetylcholinesterase.
Does not reverse the muscarinic effects of organophosphorus compounds, but highly active at nicotinic sites. Must be given within 24–36 hours of poisoning to be effective. Its effects usually occur within 10–40 minutes of administration.
• Dosage: 1 g im or slowly iv (20–60 mg/kg in children), repeated once or twice if required. The initial dose may be doubled in very severe poisoning. Up to 12 g may be given in 24 hours.
• Side effects: drowsiness, visual disturbances, nausea, tachycardia, muscle weakness.

Prazosin hydrochloride. α-Adrenergic receptor antagonist, highly selective for α_1-**adrenergic receptors**. Used as a **vasodilator drug**, e.g. in **hypertension** and **cardiac failure**, and as a bladder smooth muscle relaxant in outflow obstruction. Rarely causes compensatory tachycardia, presumably because of its α_1-receptor specificity. 97% protein-bound, with a **half-life** of 2–3 hours. Excreted mainly via bile and faeces.
• Dosage: 0.5–5.0 g orally, 6–12 hourly.
• Side effects: postural hypotension (especially after the first dose), nausea, drowsiness, headache.

Predictive value. In **statistics**, the ability of an abnormal test result to predict true abnormality.

Equals

$$\frac{\text{number with abnormal test and the condition tested for}}{\text{total number with an abnormal test}}$$

See also, Errors; Sensitivity; Specificity

Prednisolone, *see Steroid therapy*

Pre-eclampsia (Pre-eclamptic toxaemia, PET; Pregnancy-induced hypertension, PIH). Defined as the following occurring after the 20th week of **pregnancy**:
  –**hypertension**: systolic, mean or diastolic BP >140, 105 or 90 mmHg respectively, or an increase in systolic or diastolic BP greater than 30 and 15 mmHg respectively.
  –peripheral **oedema**.
  –proteinuria >0.3 g/l.
Represents a multisystem disease with many other manifestations. Occurs in 3–12% of pregnancies. More common in first pregnancies, **diabetes mellitus**, polyhydramnios and multiple pregnancy. Improves rapidly following delivery of the fetus. Aetiology is unknown but may be related to **prostaglandin** metabolism, since **aspirin** has been reported to have a preventative role. An increase in the **thromboxane/prostacyclin** ratio has been suggested, with **platelet** aggregation within the placental vascular bed causing release of vasoactive substances and intravascular fibrin deposition. Apart from maternal effects, placental perfusion is decreased, and secondary trophoblastic invasion at 16 weeks is absent. Perinatal mortality is increased.
• Maternal features:
  –cardiovascular: thought to involve increased sensitivity to angiotensin II (sensitivity is normally decreased in pregnancy) and **catecholamines**, with vasoconstriction, reduced plasma volume, **oedema** and increased arterial BP.
  –renal: **renal blood flow**, **GFR** and **urine** output are decreased, with proteinuria.
  –haematological: fibrinogen, fibrin and platelet turnover is increased. HELLP syndrome (ḥaemolysis, ẹlevated ḷiver enzymes, ḷow ṗlatelets) may occur. Platelet function may be impaired.
  –neurological: hyperexcitability and hyperreflexia; visual symptoms and headache may forewarn of impending **convulsions (eclampsia)**.
Severe PET is heralded by BP >160/110, severe proteinuria or oliguria <500 ml/24 h, **DIC, pulmonary oedema**, neurological symptoms and epigastric (hepatic) pain.
Consistently one of the most common causes of maternal mortality; death may result from **aspiration of gastric contents, CVA**, hepatorenal failure or **cardiac failure**.
• Treatment includes bed rest, control of hypertension, prevention of convulsions, and delivery of the fetus if possible:
  –**antihypertensive drugs** used include α-**methyldopa, labetalol, hydralazine** and **calcium channel blocking drugs** orally. Severe PET may require iv treatment with:
   –labetalol 5–10 mg increments, or 10–200 mg/h infusion.
   –hydralazine 5–10 mg increments, or 5–50 mg/h infusion.

–**sodium nitroprusside** or **glyceryl trinitrate** 0.1–5.0 μg/kg/min.

Concurrent administration of **iv fluids** is important; **central venous cannulation** or **pulmonary artery catheterization** may be required (the latter because myocardial dysfunction may be present).

–**anticonvulsant drugs** include **diazepam** 2–5 mg orally or iv in the UK; **magnesium sulphate**, 2–4 g then 1–2 g/h iv, is widely used in the USA. Other drugs, e.g. **chlormethiazole**, **phenytoin**, have also been used.

Anaesthetic involvement may be required for analgesia during labour, **Caesarean section** or assistance with fluid management.

● Anaesthetic techniques:
–**extradural anaesthesia**:
–prevents the increases in catecholamines associated with pain, thus increasing placental blood flow.
–avoids the risks of general anaesthesia.
–contraindicated if there is a coagulopathy or low platelet count (below 50 000 × 10⁹/l constitutes an absolute contraindication; 50–100 000 × 10⁹/l has been suggested as acceptable if the bleeding time is under 10 minutes, depending on clinical circumstances). Measurement of bleeding time has also been suggested in patients taking aspirin.
–careful fluid management and local anaesthetic administration is required to avoid cardiovascular instability following blockade. Sensitivity to **sympathomimetic drugs** is increased.
–use of relatively large doses of **local anaesthetic agents** has been questioned in patients with neurological symptoms.
–avoidance of **adrenaline** in local anaesthetic solutions has been suggested but this is controversial.
–**spinal anaesthesia** is usually avoided because sudden severe hypotension is more common.
–general anaesthesia:
–risks include difficult intubation because of laryngeal oedema, the hypertensive response to intubation and cardiovascular instability. Administration of antihypertensive drugs or **opioid analgesic drugs** (e.g. **alfentanil** 10 μg/kg or **fentanyl** 2.5 μg/kg) before intubation has been used.
–the anticonvulsant effect of **thiopentone** may be beneficial.
–magnesium sulphate may result in increased sensitivity to **neuromuscular blocking drugs**.

Careful **monitoring** should continue after delivery.

Brown MA (1989) Anaesth Intensive Care; 17: 185–97

See also, Obstetric analgesia and anaesthesia

Pre-ejection period, *see Systolic time intervals*

Pre-emptive analgesia. Concept that administering an **analgesic drug** before a painful stimulus results in more effective pain relief than when the same dose of drug is given after the stimulus. Modification of the memory of pain has been suggested as a possible mechanism. Supported by animal studies, although clinical relevance has yet to be proven.

McQuay HJ (1992) Br J Anaesth; 69: 1–3

Pregnancy. Usually lasts 40 weeks. Most physiological changes occur in response to the increased metabolic demands of the **uterus**, **placenta** and fetus, and include alterations in the following systems:

–cardiovascular:
–increased intravascular volume from the first trimester, returning to normal within 2 weeks of delivery. Plasma expansion (50%) exceeds red cell expansion (20%), resulting in the 'physiological **anaemia**' of pregnancy. **Haemoglobin** concentration is usually about 12 g/dl at term.
–increased **heart rate**, peaking at 28–36 weeks when it may exceed normal rate by 10–15 beats/min.
–increased **cardiac output** from 10 weeks, reaching 140% of normal at term with further increases during labour. **Stroke volume** increases by 30%. Ejection systolic **heart murmurs** are common, and 3rd or 4th **heart sounds** may occur.
–decreased **SVR** as a result of the smooth muscle relaxation caused by progesterone. Sites of venous engorgement include cutaneous and extradural vessels, the latter affecting height of block in **extradural anaesthesia**.
–reduced **MAP**, being lowest at the time of maximal cardiac output.
–**aortocaval compression** in the supine position.
–**ECG** changes caused by cephalad displacement of the diaphragm by the uterus include left axis deviation and inverted **T waves** in leads V_2 and V_3.
–respiratory:
–increased minute ventilation (by 50% in the first trimester), mainly caused by increased **tidal volume** (thought to be a central effect of progesterone).
–reduced arterial $P\text{CO}_2$ to about 4 kPa (30 mmHg) by the 12th week of pregnancy; arterial $P\text{O}_2$ increases by about 1.3 kPa (10 mmHg). Arterial pH remains normal due to renal retention of **bicarbonate**.
–reduced **FRC** (both **expiratory reserve volume** and **residual volume** decrease) from the 20th week onwards, caused by the upward displacement of the **diaphragm** by the uterus.
–increased O_2 consumption throughout pregnancy, but especially in the third trimester (up to 20%).
–increased risk of **hypoxaemia** during anaesthesia results from reduced FRC and increased O_2 demand.
–venous engorgement of the upper **airway**, which may lead to spontaneous epistaxis or haemorrhage on instrumentation.
–gastrointestinal: delayed **gastric emptying**, caused by the uterus pushing the stomach into a horizontal position, and by progesterone. During labour, gastric stasis is increased further by pain, anxiety and opioids. Gastric acidity is increased because of gastrin secretion by the placenta, and gastric volumes are increased. **Gastro-oesophageal reflux** and heartburn are common. The time after conception at which the GIT effects occur, and the time after delivery at which they revert to normal, are unknown. 16–20 weeks has been suggested as the time of onset; progesterone levels fall to non-pregnant levels by 24 hours of delivery, and reflux usually resolves by 36 hours.
–**coagulation**: increased levels of fibrinogen and factors VII, IX, X and XII, predisposing towards thromboembolism. Platelet count increases slightly.

Systemic fibrinolytic activity is depressed, but localized activity (i.e. ability to lyse clots from within) is maintained. Thus the level of **fibrin degradation products** increases as pregnancy progresses. However, in normal pregnancy neither bleeding nor clotting times are increased.

–renal: dilatation of the renal pelvices and ureters from the end of the first trimester. **Renal blood flow** and **GFR** increase by 40%. Sodium and water reabsorption increase, with falls in serum creatinine and urea; glycosuria may occur.

–hepatic: blood flow is unaltered. Serum **albumin** and **cholinesterase** levels fall, whilst hepatic enzyme levels may increase.

Non-urgent surgery is usually delayed until the second trimester, because of the possible risk (although never proven) of teratogenic effects on the fetus. Conditions requiring abdominal surgery are associated with increased risk of miscarriage or premature labour.

Camann WR (1992) Curr Opin Anaesth; 5: 319–23

See also, Fetus, effect of anaesthetic agents on; Obstetric analgesia and anaesthesia

Pregnenolone. Steroid metabolite of progesterone, presently being studied as an **iv anaesthetic agent**. Formulated in a soya bean emulsion. Produces smooth rapid onset of anaesthesia of short duration, with cardiovascular stability. Has a higher **therapeutic ratio** than other iv anaesthetic agents.

Powell H, Morgan M, Sear JW (1992) Anaesthesia; 47: 287–90

Preload. End-diastolic ventricular wall tension. Usually inferred from ventricular end-diastolic pressure, itself approximating to **pulmonary capillary wedge pressure** (left) or **CVP** (right). Related to **myocardial contractility** and **cardiac output** by Starling's law.

Also refers to prophylactic administration of **iv fluids** to reduce hypotension, e.g. before **spinal** or **extradural anaesthesia**.

Premedication. Administration of medication prior to anaesthesia.

- Aims:
  –allay anxiety.
  –alleviate pain.
  –facilitate smooth **induction of anaesthesia** and reduce the amount of anaesthetic agents required.
  –reduce secretion formation.
  –reduce **awareness**.
  –reduce nausea and **vomiting**.
  –reduce the risks of specific complications associated with anaesthesia or the patient's pre-existing condition, e.g.:
    –bradycardia, e.g. in **ophthalmic surgery**.
    –hypertensive response to tracheal intubation.
    –**aspiration pneumonitis**.
    –**adverse drug reactions**.
    –bronchospasm.
    –DVT.
- Drugs commonly used for premedication include:
  –**opioid analgesic drugs**, e.g. morphine, papaveretum, pethidine.
  –**benzodiazepines**, e.g. **diazepam, temazepam, lorazepam**.

–**barbiturates**, e.g. pentobarbitone.
–**butyrophenones**, e.g. **droperidol**.
–**phenothiazines**, e.g. **trimeprazine, promethazine**.
–**anticholinergic drugs**, e.g. **atropine, hyoscine, glycopyrronium**.
–other **antiemetic drugs**, e.g. **metoclopramide**.
–**H₂ receptor antagonists**, e.g. **ranitidine, cimetidine**.
–**antacids**, e.g. sodium citrate.

In addition, certain drugs already taken regularly by the patient are usually continued up to and including the day of surgery, e.g. **antiarrhythmic drugs, antihypertensive drugs**, drugs used in **ischaemic heart disease** and **asthma, anticonvulsant drugs**, etc.

Oral premedication (e.g. with benzodiazepines) has become more popular recently, in place of traditional im injection of opioid and anticholinergic drugs.

- Many anaesthetists do not routinely prescribe premedication because of disadvantages such as:
  –excessive sedation.
  –difficulty with timing of drug administration.
  –pain from im injections.
  –nausea and vomiting (with opioids).
  –dry mouth with anticholinergic drugs.
  –unnecessary drug administration.
  –**antanalgesia** and restlessness.
  –delayed **recovery**.

Madej TH, Paasuke RT (1987) Can J Anaesth; 34: 259–73

Preoperative assessment. Main objectives include assessment of:

–the risks to the patient of suffering perioperative deterioration in health.
–whether the patient's condition may be improved prior to surgery, e.g. by changing medication, treating pre-existing disease, administering fluids, etc.
–how otherwise to minimize the perioperative risk, e.g. by enlisting more experienced help, rescheduling the time of surgery, using special anaesthetic or analgesic techniques, booking a bed on ICU or HDU, etc.

- Assessment is directed towards the individual patient's circumstances but in general is divided into:
  –history:
    –medical and surgical history, including the nature of the proposed surgery.
    –previous anaesthetic history including adverse reactions, nausea and vomiting, other problems, etc.
    –family history of medical or anaesthetic problems.
    –drug history (past and present).
    –**smoking** and **alcohol** intake.
    –known allergies and **atopy**.
    –weight of the patient (especially children).
    –presence of capped, crowned, chipped or loose **teeth**.
    –anxiety.
    –time of last oral intake.
    –systems review, in particular:
      –CVS: **hypertension**, features of **ischaemic heart disease, cardiac failure, arrhythmias**.
      –RS: recent **chest infection**, features of **COAD** or **asthma**.
      –GIT: **hiatus hernia** or other risk factors for **aspiration of gastric contents**.
      –CNS: **epilepsy**, pre-existing neurological lesions.
  –examination:

–**airway**, teeth, **cervical spine** (including assessment for possible difficult tracheal intubation).

–CVS: for **hypovolaemia**, **dehydration**, **cyanosis** and **anaemia**; **pulse**, BP, **JVP**, cardiac impulse, **heart sounds**, lung bases, periphery (for **oedema**).

–RS: for clubbing and cyanosis, position of the trachea, chest expansion, air entry, nature of breath sounds.

–CNS: **cranial nerves**, **spinal cord** and peripheral nerves including **dermatomes** and **myotomes**.

–suitable veins for cannulation.

–suitability for regional techniques where intended.

–preoperative **investigations**.

Scoring systems may be used for classifying patients according to preoperative status, e.g. **ASA physical status**, **cardiac risk index**, **New York Heart Association classification**, **Glasgow coma scale**, **subarachnoid haemorrhage** and **hepatic failure** scoring systems.

The need for blood cross-matching and **premedication** is also assessed. The forthcoming anaesthesia is explained and the patient's **consent** confirmed.

See also, individual diseases and drugs; Emergency surgery

Preoxygenation. Administration of 100% O_2 prior to **induction of anaesthesia**. Increases the O_2 reserve in the lungs and thus the time to **hypoxaemia** during subsequent **apnoea**, e.g. during tracheal intubation. Also increases arterial Po_2, although O_2 content and saturation may not increase by much. Particularly useful when difficulties are anticipated, or in patients at risk from **aspiration of gastric contents**. Thus a vital part of 'rapid sequence induction'. The optimal technique is uncertain; 3 minutes administration is thought to be as effective as 5 minutes administration, or even four **vital capacity** breaths.

Anon (1992) Lancet; 339: 31–2

See also, Induction, rapid sequence

Pressure. **Force** per unit area. SI **unit** is the **pascal**: 1 Pa = 1 N/m^2.

Pressure generators, *see Ventilators*

Pressure measurement. May be:

–direct:

–liquid manometers which measure:

–absolute pressure, e.g. mercury barometer.

–pressure relative to atmospheric pressure (gauge pressure), e.g. U tube. The sensitivity may be increased by using liquid of low density, inclining the manometer tube or using a different non-miscible liquid in each of the limbs of the U tube (differential liquid manometer).

–aneroid gauge (one in which there is no liquid). In one form a sealed metal bellows changes size with changes in external or applied pressure, moving a pointer on a scale (e.g. aneroid barometer). In the Bourdon gauge used in anaesthesia, a coiled tube of oval cross-section uncoils as it becomes circular on cross-section, due to the high pressure of the gas inside it, and this moves the pointer.

–pressure **transducers**.

–indirect, e.g. in **arterial BP measurement**.

[Eugene Bourdon (1808–1884), French engineer]

Pressure regulators. Formerly called reducing valves, devices for reducing the high pressures delivered by **cylinders** to **anaesthetic machines**, and maintaining the reduced pressure at a constant level which is easier to use. Also reduce the requirement for high-pressure tubing.

● May be:

–direct: cylinder pressure tends to open the valve.

–indirect: cylinder pressure tends to close the valve (Fig. 108).

The diaphragm moves according to *p* and the tension in the springs. As *p* falls, the diaphragm bulges into the regulator, allowing more gas flow into the upper half and thus maintaining *p*. If *p* increases, the diaphragm is pushed upwards, decreasing gas flow and again maintaining *p*.

The regulators are specific for the different gases, and should be labelled accordingly. Pressure relief valves are incorporated in case of excessive pressures. Pressure gauges may also be incorporated.

Two-stage regulators are often used, to reduce wear and tear on the diaphragm and reduce pressure fluctuations, especially if high gas flows are required. The output of one stage is the input of the second. **Demand valves** may be based on this principle.

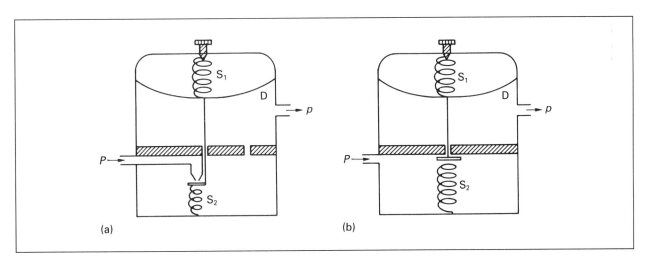

(a)　　　　　　　　　　　　　(b)

Figure 108 *Diagram of pressure regulators: (a) direct; (b) indirect. P, cylinder pressure; p, reduced pressure; S_1, main spring; S_2, sealing spring; D, diaphragm*

Slave regulators are those whose output depends on the output of another regulator. For example, the output of an O_2 regulator may be applied above the diaphragm of a N_2O regulator, keeping the latter's valve open. If the O_2 pressure fails, the N_2O valve closes.

Pressure support, *see Inspiratory pressure support*

Priestley, Joseph (1733–1804). English scientist, best known for his work on various gases. A major protagonist of the **phlogiston** theory, he isolated ammonia (as 'alkaline air'), sulphur dioxide ('vitriolic acid air'), O_2 ('dephlogisticated air'), N_2O ('dephlogisticated nitrous air'), nitrogen dioxide ('nitrous acid air'), and methane. Also investigated electrical conduction. Emigrated to the USA in 1794 because of his unpopular religious and political views.

Prilocaine hydrochloride. Amide **local anaesthetic agent**, introduced in 1959. Slower in onset than **lignocaine**, but lasts about 1.5 times as long and less toxic. pK_a is 7.9. 55% protein-bound. Undergoes hepatic and renal metabolism. Maximal safe dose: 5 mg/kg alone, 8 mg/kg with **adrenaline**. Used as 0.5–1.0% solutions for infiltration, 1–2% for nerve blocks and 0.5% for **IVRA**. Also available as a 4% plain or 3% solution with **felypressin** for dental infiltration, and in **EMLA** cream. May cause **methaemoglobinaemia** in doses above about 600 mg in adults, due to its metabolite *ortho*-toluidine.

Priming principle. Shortening of the time of onset of **non-depolarizing neuromuscular blockade** by administration of a non-depolarizing **neuromuscular blocking drug** in divided aliquots. The priming dose (15–20% of the usual intubating dose) is followed by the remainder of the intubating dose 4–8 minutes later, depending on the drug used.
- Suggested explanatory theories:
  –the priming dose occupies a proportion of postsynaptic receptors at the **neuromuscular junction**; the main dose can thus occupy more rapidly the critical mass of receptors for neuromuscular blockade.
  –the priming dose occupies presynaptic receptors, reducing mobilization and release of acetylcholine; the main dose thus acts faster.

Initially thought to answer the need for rapid tracheal intubation without using **suxamethonium**. However, the priming dose itself may cause unpleasant symptoms, e.g. diplopia and weakness, and may risk dangerous events, e.g. **hypoventilation** and **aspiration of gastric contents**.

Jones RM (1989) Br J Anaesth; 63: 1–3

Proarrhythmias. **Arrhythmias** caused by or exacerbated by **antiarrhythmic drugs**. May occur even with standard dosage and normally therapeutic plasma drug levels. Common examples include **VT** and **torsade de pointes**.

Probability (*P*). Used to describe the likelihood of a type I **error** in **statistics**. **Statistical significance** is usually denoted by a *P* value <0.05; i.e. the observed event might be expected to occur by chance alone, no more than once in 20 times.

Probability limits, *see Confidence intervals*

Procainamide hydrochloride. Class Ia **antiarrhythmic drug**, chemically related to **procaine**. Effective against ventricular and supraventricular arrhythmias. 15% protein-bound. Undergoes hepatic metabolism (largely via acetylation to *N*-acetylprocainamide) and renal excretion, although 40–50% is excreted unchanged.
- Dosage:
  –up to 50 mg/kg/day orally in 4–8 doses.
  –25–50 mg/min slowly iv up to 1 g, with ECG monitoring for widened **QRS complex** or **P–R interval** prolongation. 2–6 mg/min may follow.
- Side effects: hypotension with iv usage, GIT upset, rash, agranulocytosis, systemic lupus-like syndrome (especially in slow acetylators).

Procaine hydrochloride. Ester **local anaesthetic agent**, introduced in 1904. The first synthetic local anaesthetic. Less lipid soluble than **lignocaine**, with slower onset of less intense anaesthesia, and shorter duration of action. pK_a is 8.9. 6% protein-bound. Poorly absorbed from mucous membranes; thus not useful as a surface anaesthetic. Used in 0.25–1.0% solutions for infiltration anaesthesia, and 1–2% for nerve blocks, usually with **adrenaline** 1:200 000. Maximal safe dose: 12 mg/kg.

Prochlorperazine maleate/mesylate. Piperazine **phenothiazine** with antiemetic, α-adrenergic agonist and weak sedative properties. Used mainly as an antipsychotic and **antiemetic drug**. Active within 10–20 minutes of im administration and 30–40 minutes of oral administration. Action lasts 3–4 hours.
- Dosage:
  –5–20 mg orally/im, 6–12 hourly. Not licensed for iv use in the UK, although it has been safely given by that route. A buccal preparation is also available: dose 3–6 mg.
  –25 mg rectally 6 hourly.
- Side effects: as for phenothiazines. Extrapyramidal reactions are more likely than following **chlorpromazine**, especially in children.

Prodrug. Inactive substance metabolized to active drug within the body, e.g. **chloral hydrate** (converted to trichloroethanol).

Prolonged Q–T syndromes, *see Q–T interval*

Promethazine hydrochloride/theoclate. **Phenothiazine** and **antihistamine drug**, with sedative, anticholinergic and antiemetic properties. Used for antiemesis, allergic reactions, sedation and **premedication**, especially in children. Also used topically to relieve pruritus, etc. One component of the **lytic cocktail**. Well absorbed orally but undergoes extensive **first-pass metabolism**. Excreted renally following hepatic metabolism.
- Dosage:
  –25–75 mg orally/day; 0.5–1.0 mg/kg for paediatric premedication.
  –25–50 mg im/iv.
- Side effects are those of phenothiazines and **anticholinergic drugs**.

Propafenone hydrochloride. Class IC **antiarrhythmic drug**, affecting atria, conducting system and ventricles. Has slight β-adrenergic antagonist properties. Used for treating and preventing ventricular arrhythmias. Undergoes hepatic metabolism and renal excretion.

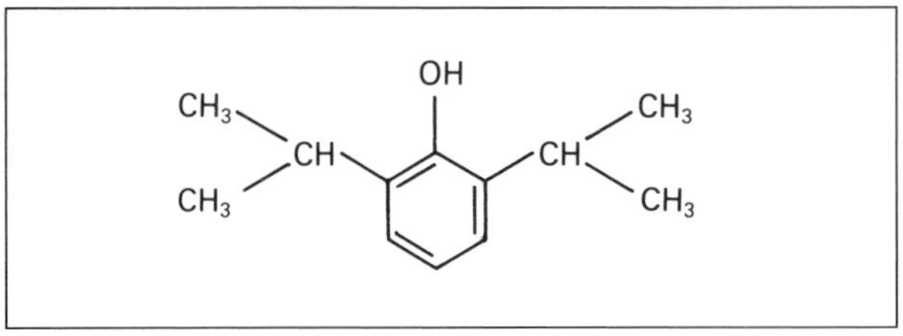

Figure 109 *Structure of propofol*

- Dosage: 150–300 mg orally, 8 hourly.
- Side effects are usually mild and include dizziness, GIT disturbances, blurred vision and bradycardia.

Propofol. 2,6–Diisopropylphenol (Fig. 109). **IV anaesthetic agent**, first used in 1977 and introduced into clinical practice in 1986. Originally prepared with **Cremophor EL**, but reformulated before commercial release because of fears about allergic reactions. Now presented in a 1% oil-water emulsion containing 10% soya bean oil, 1.2% egg phosphatide and 2.25% glycerol. Available in 20, 50 and 100 ml vials for single-use only. pK_a is 11. 98% protein-bound after iv injection. Distribution and elimination **half-lives** are 1–2 minutes and 1–5 hours respectively, with hepatic metabolism and renal excretion. Extrahepatic metabolism is suggested by a plasma **clearance** (25–30 ml/kg/min) which exceeds hepatic blood flow. There are no known active metabolites. Thus recovery is rapid with minimal residual effects, making it a popular agent in short cases, e.g. in **day-case surgery**. These properties also make it suitable for **TIVA** and iv **sedation**.
- Effects:
  - induction:
    - smooth and rapid, with only occasional movements.
    - pain on injection is common; it may be reduced by prior injection of, or mixing with, lignocaine.
  - CVS/RS:
    - hypotension is common, although whether caused by direct myocardial depression, reduced SVR or both, is controversial. Normo- or bradycardia is common; resetting of the **baroreceptor reflex** has been suggested. Reduces the hypertensive response to tracheal intubation.
    - respiratory depression is marked.
    - tends to obtund upper airway reflexes, thus allowing manipulation/instrumentation more readily than **thiopentone**. Thus particularly useful when a **laryngeal mask** is used.
  - CNS:
    - **antanalgesia** has not been reported.
    - has an antiemetic effect. Increased appetite has been suggested but may reflect the excellent quality of recovery rather than a direct effect.
    - convulsions have been reported following propofol, but its causative role is controversial. Has been used successfully in intractable epilepsy.
    - reduces **cerebral blood flow**, **ICP** and **intraocular pressure**.
    - dreams may occur. Claims by patients of sexual assault whilst anaesthetized have been made.
  - other: allergic phenomena and delayed recovery, in addition to convulsions, have been reported to the **Committee on Safety of Medicines**.

- Dosage:
  - 1.5–2.5 mg/kg for induction.
  - for maintenance, several regimens have been suggested, based on pharmacokinetic studies. The following (Bristol regimen) is commonly used:
    - 10 mg/kg/h for 10 minutes.
    - 8 mg/kg/h for 10 minutes.
    - 6 mg/kg/h thereafter, adjusted if required according to clinical response.
  This applies to concurrent use of 66% **N₂O**, or infusion of **alfentanil** 30–50 µg/kg/h.
  - 1.0–4.0 mg/kg/h for sedation (licensed for up to 3 days).

Contamination during preparation for infusion has led to iatrogenic septicaemia.

Contains the same energy content as 10% fat emulsion (900 Cal/l).

Not licensed for use in children under 3 years. Not licensed for sedation of children of any age (neurological, cardiac, renal and hepatic impairment have been reported after sedation of children with propofol in ICUs).

Proportional assist ventilation (PAV). Mode of ventilatory support in which the pressure provided to the airway increases as inspiratory effort increases. Continuous adjustment of support is made throughout inspiration, with switching to expiration when flow falls below a set level at end-inspiration. Has been used in **respiratory failure** and **weaning from ventilators**.
Anon (1992) Lancet; 339: 1085–6

Propanidid. IV anaesthetic agent, first used in 1956 and withdrawn in 1984. Eugenol (oil of cloves) derivative, prepared in **Cremophor EL** or polyoxyethylated castor oil. Hydrolysed by plasma and liver esterases. Rapidly acting, with rapid recovery. Hypotension, apnoea following initial hyperventilation, venous thrombosis and **adverse drug reactions** were common.

Propranolol. β-Adrenergic receptor antagonist (the first to be introduced, in 1964). Non-selective, and without **intrinsic sympathomimetic activity**. Still widely used, although increasingly superseded by newer agents. 90–95% protein-bound. Its primary metabolite, 4–hydroxypropanolol, has β-blocking activity.
- Dosage:
  - 10–40 mg orally 6–12 hourly. Up to 320 mg/day may be required in **hypertension** and angina.
  - 1 mg increments iv.

Prostacyclin. Prostaglandin produced by the intima of blood vessels via the cyclooxygenase limb of the **arachidonic acid** metabolism pathway. The most potent inhibitor of **platelet** aggregation known, via an increase in **cAMP** levels. At high doses, may disperse circulating platelet aggregates. Thought to have vital importance in preventing coagulation within normal blood vessels. Also a potent **vasodilator** drug. Increases renin production and blood glucose levels.

Provided commercially as synthetic epoprostenol sodium, which is reconstituted in saline and glycerine to produce a clear colourless solution of pH 10.5. Used to prevent platelet aggregation during renal **dialysis** or other forms of **extracorporeal circulation**; has also been used in **pre-eclampsia**, **pulmonary hypertension**, haemolytic uraemic syndrome and **septic shock**. **Half-life** is 2–3 minutes, with cessation of platelet effects within 30 minutes of stopping an infusion. Its main metabolite is 6–keto-prostaglandin $F_{1\alpha}$.

- Dosage: 2–35 ng/kg/min iv.
- Side effects: flushing, headache, hypotension.

Prostaglandins (PGs). Unsaturated fatty acids containing 20 carbon atoms and a five-membered carbon ring (cyclopentane ring) at one end. Derived from **arachidonic acid**, and thought to be synthesized in most tissues, although originally isolated from the prostatic glands in the 1930s. Named according to the configuration of the cyclopentane ring (e.g. PGA, B, C, etc. to PGI (**prostacyclin**)), with subscript numbers denoting the number of side-chain double bonds. Involved in many processes throughout the body including immunological and inflammatory responses, temperature regulation, exocrine and endocrine glandular secretion, renal blood flow and renin production, reproductive function, fat metabolism and CNS neurotransmitter activity. They have been implicated in pain perception and local sensitization of tissues to inflammatory mediators.

Have varying effects on smooth muscle; thus PGE_2, PGI_2 and PGA_2 cause arteriolar dilatation, whilst $PGF_{2\alpha}$ causes vasodilatation in some vascular beds and vasoconstriction in others. $PGF_{2\alpha}$ and PGD_2 cause bronchoconstriction, whereas PGE_2 causes bronchodilatation. PGE_2 and $PGF_{2\alpha}$ cause uterine contraction and are used to induce abortion or labour, e.g. administered vaginally. They may also be given by intra- or extra-amniotic routes for abortion. Oral and iv administration is rarely used, the latter because of side effects including vomiting, diarrhoea, dizziness, pyrexia and rash.

PGE_1 is used iv to maintain patency of the **ductus arteriosus** in **congenital heart disease** before corrective surgery. Tachy- or bradycardia, hypotension, pyrexia, DIC and convulsions may occur. It has been studied in the treatment of **ARDS**. An analogue is available for oral use, to prevent gastric ulcers associated with **NSAIDs**.

Half-life is at most a few minutes, with local destruction and metabolism of circulating PGs via the pulmonary, hepatic and renal circulations.

Many of the effects of NSAIDs are thought to involve inhibition of PG synthesis.

PGE_2 and $PGF_{2\alpha}$ are given as dinoprostone and dinoprost trometamol respectively; PGE_1 is given as alprostadil.

Protamine sulphate. Mixture of low molecular weight, cationic, basic proteins prepared from the sperm of salmon and other fish. Used as a **heparin** antagonist, and in the preparation of protamine zinc **insulin**. Has an anticoagulant effect when given alone in high doses, via inhibition of formation and action of thromboplastin. Binds and inactivates anionic, acidic heparin, forming a stable salt.

- Dosage: 1 mg iv neutralizes 100 U mucous heparin if given within 15 minutes of the latter's administration; less is required after longer intervals. Dosage is usually adjusted according to the patient's coagulation status. Should be given slowly; individual doses should not exceed 50 mg.
- Side effects: myocardial depression, bradycardia, pulmonary hypertension, **histamine** release, **comple-**ment activation, **anaphylactic reaction**. These effects are more likely following rapid administration. Chronic exposure in diabetics, previous vasectomy or allergy to fish may predispose to allergic reactions.

Protein-binding. Occurs for many blood-borne substances, e.g. bilirubin, mineral ions, hormones, and many drugs. Important in drug **pharmacokinetics** because only the free unbound fraction is available to cross membranes, produce its effects, or be metabolized or excreted. Free fraction of drug is affected by plasma protein levels, drug concentration, pH and presence of other substances which compete for the same binding sites. Thus one substance may be displaced from protein binding sites by another. The drug–protein complex may act as an **antigen** in **adverse drug reactions**.

- The main proteins involved are:
  - **albumin**: binds acidic drugs, e.g. **thiopentone, phenytoin, warfarin, salicylates**.
  - α_1–acid glycoprotein: binds basic drugs, e.g. **local anaesthetic agents, propranolol**, quinidine.
  - globulins: bind e.g. **tubocurarine**.

Protein-binding within the CNS may be involved in the mechanism of action of anaesthetic agents.

Wood M (1986) Anesth Analg; 65: 786–804
See also, Anaesthesia, mechanism of; Drug interactions; Hypoproteinaemia

Proteins. Polypeptide chains (usually defined as over 50–500) of **amino acids**. May incorporate **carbohydrates** or **fats**. Present in all cell protoplasm and required for growth and healing. Involved in:
  - structure, e.g. collagen, **myosin, actin, membranes**.
  - **enzymes**.
  - hormones and precursors.
  - blood components, e.g. **immunoglobulins, haemoglobin, albumin**.

See also, Nitrogen balance; Nutrition

Prothrombin time, *see Coagulation studies*

Pseudocholinesterase, *see Cholinesterase, plasma*

Pseudocritical temperature. Temperature at which gas mixtures separate into their component parts. Varies with pressure: for **Entonox**, highest (–5.5°C) at 117 bar, and decreases above and below this pressure. Thus equals –7°C for Entonox cylinders (135 bar) and –30°C for pipelines (4 bar).

Psoas compartment block. Used to block the **lumbar plexus** and part of the **sacral plexus**, which lie between psoas major anteriorly and quadratus lumborum posteriorly, e.g. for leg surgery.

With the patient in the lateral position with hips flexed, a skin wheal is raised 5 cm lateral to the lower border of the spinous process of L5. A 15 cm needle is inserted perpendicular to the skin until it contacts the transverse process, then withdrawn and redirected slightly cranially to pass the process. A syringe is attached and a loss-of-resistance technique used to identify the psoas compartment (usually at 10–12 cm) as for **extradural anaesthesia**. 30–40 ml **local anaesthetic agent** is injected.

Complications include subarachnoid, extradural and iv injection.

Psychoprophylaxis. Technique used in **obstetric analgesia and anaesthesia** to increase comfort and relaxation during labour. Requires preparation during pregnancy, with education about pregnancy and labour, and training in relaxation and breathing techniques. During labour, deep breathing during contractions, and the concentration this requires, helps to distract attention from the pain.

PT, Prothrombin time, *see Coagulation studies*

PTT, Partial thromboplastin time, *see Coagulation studies*

Pudendal nerve block. Used bilaterally to provide analgesia in **obstetric analgesia and anaesthesia**, especially for forceps and ventouse delivery. The pudendal nerve (S2–4) arises from the **sacral plexus** and leaves the pelvis through the greater sciatic foramen, passing behind the ischial spine and sacrospinal ligament to re-enter the pelvis through the lesser sciatic foramen. It supplies the perineum, vulva and lower vagina.
- Techniques:
  - transvaginal approach: with the patient in the lithotomy position, two fingers palpate the ischial spine from within the vagina. A 12.5 cm guarded needle is introduced 1.2 cm beyond the spine, into the sacrospinal ligament, and the needle point extended. After negative aspiration for blood, 10 ml **local anaesthetic agent** is injected.
  - transperineal approach: a needle is introduced through a point midway between the anus and ischial tuberosity, and directed as above by a finger in the vagina.

Local infiltration of the labia is required to block cutaneous branches of the genitofemoral and ilioinguinal nerves.

Has a high failure rate in obstetrics, exacerbated by inadequate time between performance of the block and attempted delivery.

Pulmonary artery catheterization. Performed using flow-directed balloon-tipped pulmonary artery catheters, introduced into clinical practice in the early 1970s by Swan and Ganz (after whom one commercial device is named) amongst much controversy.
- Catheters may have some of the following features:
  - 70 cm long, marked every 10 cm.
  - channels/lumina:
    - distal (opens at the tip).
    - proximal (opens 30 cm from the tip).
    - for inflating the balloo n (1–1.5 ml air used).
    - connections to a thermis tor, a few cm from the tip.
    - fibreoptic bundles for continuous **oximetry**.
    - others include those for pacing, Doppler imaging, etc.
- Insertion:
  - all lumina are prefilled with heparinized saline, and the balloon checked.
  - aseptic technique is used. The catheter is usually passed through a sterile plastic protective sleeve to allow manipulation without contamination after insertion.
  - insertion is as for **central venous cannulation**, usually employing the **Seldinger technique**. The right internal jugular vein is most commonly used. The catheter is threaded down an 8 G introducer sheath, with continuous visible pressure monitoring from the

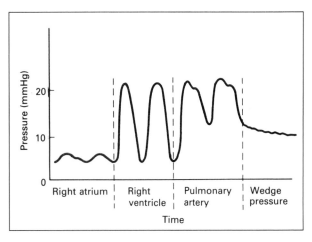

Figure 110 *Pressure trace obtained during placement of a pulmonary artery catheter*

distal lumen. The balloon is inflated in the right atrium and directed by the flow of blood into the pulmonary artery via the right ventricle. **Pulmonary capillary wedge pressure** is displayed when the balloon occludes a pulmonary vessel; the catheter tip is now separated from the left atrium by a continuous column of blood. Placement is confirmed by the changes in the pressure trace obtained (Fig. 110).
  - coiling and/or knotting of the catheter within the heart may occur if excessive length of catheter is inserted without a change in the pressure trace.
  - once inserted, the balloon is left deflated until wedge pressure measurement is required, to reduce risk of pulmonary artery damage and infarction. The distal lumen pressure should always be displayed, to alert to accidental wedging.
  - use of a catheter is often limited to 2–3 days to reduce risk of complications.
- Information gained:
  - mixed venous, right atrial and ventricular gas tensions and O_2 saturations; e.g. for estimation of cardiac **shunt**, etc. Continuous monitoring of mixed venous O_2 saturation is possible via fibreoptic bundles.
  - measurement of right atrial and ventricular pressures, **pulmonary artery pressure** and pulmonary capillary wedge pressure. By convention, measured at end-systole and end-expiration.
  - measurement of right ventricular ejection fraction.
  - **cardiac output measurement**.
  - derived data:
    - **systemic** and **pulmonary vascular resistance**.
    - **cardiac index**, **stroke volume** and index.
- Uses, e.g. perioperatively and in ICU:
  - investigating cardiac shunts.
  - monitoring the above pressures and optimizing fluid therapy; particularly useful when right atrial pressures do not reflect left heart function; e.g. left ventricular failure or infarction, severe **bundle branch block**, **pulmonary hypertension**, **cardiac tamponade** and constrictive **pericarditis**, valvular heart disease (*for interpretation, etc., see Pulmonary capillary wedge pressure*).
  - measuring cardiac output and derived data.

373

–monitoring mixed venous O_2 saturation as a continuous indicator of cardiac output and tissue perfusion, e.g. in ICU.
- Complications:
  –as for central venous cannulation.
  –arrhythmias.
  –infection.
  –catheter knotting.
  –damage to valves, myocardium, etc.
  –pulmonary artery rupture or damage.
  –pulmonary infarction.
  –incorrect positioning, measurement and interpretation.

Although widely used in critically ill patients, absolute indications for the use of pulmonary artery catheters are controversial.

[Harold JC Swan and William Ganz, Los Angeles cardiologists]

Finegan B (1992) Can J Anaesth; 39: R71–5

Pulmonary artery pressure (PAP). Typically one-fifth of systemic circulatory pressure; normal ranges are 15–30 mmHg systolic, 0–8 mmHg diastolic and 10–15 mmHg mean. Usually measured by right-sided cardiac catheterization. Changes may indicate changes in **pulmonary capillary wedge** pressure and **pulmonary vascular resistance**.

Pulmonary capillary wedge pressure (PCWP; Pulmonary wedge pressure; PWP; Pulmonary artery occlusion pressure; PAOP). Pressure measured within the pulmonary arterial system during **pulmonary artery catheterization**, with the catheter's tip 'wedged' in a tapering branch of one of the pulmonary arteries. In most patients, represents left atrial filling pressure and thus **left ventricular end-diastolic pressure** (LVEDP). Thus an indirect indicator of left ventricular end-diastolic volume and myocardial fibre length (*see Starling's law*). Also indicates the likelihood (with measurement of plasma colloid **osmotic pressure**) of **pulmonary oedema** formation, assuming normal pulmonary capillary permeability.
- Normal range: 6–12 mmHg; usually 1–4 mmHg less than pulmonary artery diastolic pressure (PADP). Traditionally measured at end-expiration.
- Values should be interpreted with caution in:
  –left ventricular failure: LVEDP may exceed PCWP.
  –mitral valve disease: in stenosis PCWP may exceed LVEDP; in regurgitation large 'v' waves interfere with the PCWP waveform.
  –raised intrathoracic pressure, e.g. **PEEP**: LVEDP may exceed PCWP.
  –non-compliant left ventricle: LVEDP may exceed PCWP.
  –aortic regurgitation: LVEDP may greatly exceed PCWP.

Gradients between PADP, PCWP and LVEDP may be increased in tachycardia and increased **pulmonary vascular resistance**. The position of the catheter tip is also important; a continuous column of blood between the catheter and the left ventricle only occurs if the tip lies in zone 3 of the lung (*see Pulmonary circulation*). Although the catheter usually flows to zone 3, especially in the supine position, repositioning of the patient may alter the zonal distribution.

The waveform resembles the **venous waveform**, with 'a', 'c' and 'v' waves, and swings with respiration. PCWP should not exceed PADP.

As with **CVP** interpretation, trends are more useful than single values. Response of PCWP to drug or iv fluid administration may be used to indicate intravascular volume status and cardiac function, and guide therapy. Pulmonary oedema is likely at PCWP above 18–20 mmHg, with normal colloid osmotic pressure.

Pulmonary circulation. Low pressure/low resistance system in series with the systemic circulation; it receives the whole cardiac output. The pulmonary artery divides after about 4 cm into right and left main pulmonary arteries. Pulmonary arteries are thin-walled and easily distensible, and lie close to the corresponding airways in connective tissue sheaths, eventually dividing to form capillaries with a total gas exchange interface of about 70 m^2. Venules run close to the septa which separate the **lung** segments and finally drain into four main pulmonary veins which deliver oxygenated blood into the left atrium.

The separate bronchial circulation supplies the airways down to the respiratory bronchioles, local connective tissue and the visceral pleura; it arises from the aorta and eventually drains via the azygos system into the pulmonary veins, i.e. representing an anatomical **shunt**.

The diameter of 'extra-alveolar' vessels (those running through lung parenchyma) is affected by lung volume, via the pull of lung parenchyma on their walls. That of 'alveolar' pulmonary vessels (predominantly capillaries) depends on the difference between arterial (P_a), venous (P_v) and alveolar (P_A) pressures, and thus on gravity. Four zones have been described by West, from above downwards:
  –zone 1: lung apex; P_A exceeds both P_a and P_v; thus no flow occurs. Does not occur at normal BP in normal lungs.
  –zone 2: $P_a > P_A > P_v$: thus flow depends on the difference between P_a and P_A, and not on P_v.
  –zone 3: $P_a > P_v > P_A$; i.e. flow depends on the difference between P_a and P_v, as usually occurs in other tissues.
  –zone 4: suggested as existing at lung bases; pulmonary interstitial pressure exceeds P_a, thus impairing blood flow.

The vessels are supplied by sympathetic vasoconstrictor (α-receptors) and vasodilator (β_2–receptors) fibres, and by parasympathetic vasodilator fibres. However, resting vascular tone is minimal, with vessels almost maximally dilated in the resting state. Other factors affecting vessel calibre include vascular responses to local changes, e.g. **hypoxic pulmonary vasoconstriction** and other factors affecting **pulmonary vascular resistance**.

The pulmonary circulation contains about 10–20% of the total blood volume (i.e. 0.5–1.0 litre). It changes during respiration (especially **IPPV**) and may increase by 25–40% in moving from the erect to the supine postition.

[John B West, Californian physiologist]

See also, Starling resistor; Ventilation/perfusion mismatch

Pulmonary embolism (PE). Mechanical obstruction of a pulmonary artery/arteriole; usually refers to blood-borne thrombus. The most common cause of death within the first ten postoperative days. Thrombus usually arises from a **DVT** in the legs/pelvis, although the venae cavae and right side of the heart are sometimes sources. The effects depend on the size and distribution of the PE; release of vasoactive mediators, e.g. **prostaglandins** may contribute to resultant vasospasm. Massive PEs cause rapid respiratory and cardiovascular collapse, and death. Smaller PEs may cause few haemodynamic effects, but may result in infarction of a section of lung tissue if collateral blood flow is inadequate. Multiple PEs may cause widespread pulmonary vascular obstruction and lead to **pulmonary hypertension**.

- Features:
  - pleuritic chest pain, haemoptysis, dyspnoea and mild pyrexia in small PEs.
  - cyanosis, tachypnoea, hypotension, tachycardia, raised JVP and bronchospasm. 3rd and 4th **heart sounds** may be present. A pleural rub may develop.
  - arterial blood gas analysis reveals hypoxaemia and hypocapnia, with subsequent metabolic acidosis in severe PE. During anaesthesia, end-tidal CO_2 concentration may fall dramatically because of increased **dead space** and reduced cardiac output.
  - right axis deviation, right bundle branch block and T inversion in leads V_{1-4} may occur in the **ECG**; the 'classic' $S_1Q_3T_3$ pattern is rarely seen.
  - **chest X-ray** may show enlarged proximal pulmonary arteries with peripheral oligaemia, but is usually non-specific. Wedge-shaped infarcts, elevation of the ipsilateral diaphragm and **pleural effusion** may subsequently develop.

Definitive diagnosis is by pulmonary angiography or ventilation–perfusion scan, with simultaneous inhalation and iv injection of **radioisotopes** to demonstrate areas of adequate ventilation but absent perfusion. Perfusion-only scans may also be useful.

Features of DVT may be present.

- Management:
  - immediate **CPR** if required. A praecordial thump may break up a large PE and improve circulation.
  - O_2 therapy, **iv fluids**, **inotropic drugs**, analgesia.
  - anticoagulation: **heparin** is usually given initially, with substitution by **warfarin** as for DVT. **Fibrinolytic drugs** have also been used.
  - pulmonary embolectomy may be required for large PEs. Ligation of the inferior vena cava/superficial femoral vein, or insertion of a vena caval umbrella may be required for recurrent PEs.

Dehring DJ, Arens JF (1990) Anesthesiology; 73: 146–64
See also, Air embolism; Amniotic fluid embolism; Fat embolism

Pulmonary fibrosis. Thickening and inflammatory infiltration of alveolar walls and perialveolar tissue.
- May result from:
  - localized loss of lung parenchyma, e.g. following infection or infarction. Causes decreased movement and breath sounds, dullness to percussion and increased vocal resonance. Neighbouring structures, e.g. trachea, may be pulled towards the affected portion.
  - interstitial lung disease (interstitial fibrosis). Feature of several diseases, e.g.:
    - caused by chemical/physical agents, e.g. asbestos, fumes, radiation, **aspiration of gastric contents**, drugs, e.g. **antimitotic drugs**, paraquat.
    - idiopathic fibrosis (fibrosing alveolitis).
    - **connective tissue diseases**, **rheumatoid arthritis**, **sarcoidosis**, amyloidosis, residual **ARDS**.
    Features include dyspnoea, dry cough, cyanosis,

clubbing and fine crepitations, typically end-expiratory and in the middle/lower lung fields.

Loss of the pulmonary vascular bed may lead to **pulmonary hypertension** and **cor pulmonale**. Typically, there is hypoxaemia with hypocapnia due to hyperventilation. $\dot{V}/\dot{Q}$ **mismatch** is now thought to be responsible for the hypoxaemia, rather than alveolar membrane thickening as previously suspected. **Diffusing capacity**, **compliance** and lung volumes are reduced, with normal **FEV_1/FVC** ratio. Work of breathing is increased; patients usually take small breaths at rapid rates. **Chest X-ray** may reveal diffuse nodular/reticular shadowing, with local contraction in focal disease.

Treatment is of the underlying cause; steroids are often used.
- Anaesthesia: although the pulmonary defect is restrictive instead of obstructive, principles are as for **COAD**.

Pulmonary function tests, *see Lung function tests*

Pulmonary hypertension. Definitions vary, but it has been defined as mean **pulmonary artery pressure** (PAP) above 15 mmHg, or systolic PAP above 30 mmHg, at rest. May be primary, but is usually secondary to:
  - pulmonary venous/capillary hypertension, e.g. in left ventricular failure, **mitral stenosis**.
  - increased pulmonary blood flow caused by right-to-left cardiac **shunts**, e.g. **ASD**, **VSD**, patent **ductus arteriosus**.
  - increased **pulmonary vascular resistance** (PVR), e.g. in **COAD**, recurrent **PE**, **pulmonary fibrosis**.

Chronic hypoxaemia, acidosis, polycythaemia and other factors which increase PVR may be involved in development of pulmonary hypertension.

The pulmonary arteries show medial hypertrophy and intimal thickening. The right ventricle becomes hypertrophied and dilates when right ventricular failure supervenes.
- Features:
  - fatigue, dyspnoea, angina, syncope, haemoptysis.
  - low cardiac output, cyanosis, features of right ventricular enlargement/failure, e.g. sternal heave, peripheral oedema. On auscultation: reduced splitting of the second **heart sound**, with loud pulmonary component.
  - **ECG** findings: right axis deviation, right **bundle branch block**, right atrial and ventricular hypertrophy. **Chest X-ray**: right atrial and ventricular enlargement, large pulmonary arteries with peripheral pruning.

Usually progressive and fatal in primary disease, which is more common in young women. Treatment may include heart–lung transplantation. Treatment of secondary disease is directed towards the underlying cause.

Anaesthetic management is based on avoidance of factors which further increase PVR. Monitoring of **pulmonary capillary wedge pressure** is more informative than **CVP** measurement, but risk of pulmonary artery rupture is increased. **Vasodilator drugs** have been used, e.g. **tolazoline**, **sodium nitroprusside**, **glyceryl trinitrate** and **phentolamine**, but none are specific to the pulmonary circulation; thus systemic hypotension may occur. **Prostacyclin**, **prostaglandin** PGE_1 and **calcium channel blocking drugs** have recently been studied.

See also, Cor pulmonale

Pulmonary irritant receptors. Receptors situated between airway epithelial cells, responsible for initiating bronchospasm and hyperpnoea in response to inhaled noxious gases, smoke, dust and cold air. Afferent impulses pass via the vagi to the medulla. May be involved in initiating **asthma** attacks.

Pulmonary oedema. Increased pulmonary **ECF** (normally minimal). Small amounts of fluid normally pass through the capillary wall into the interstitial space of the lung. The junctions between alveolar epithelial cells are relatively resistant to fluid, which is removed by the lymphatic system at about 10 ml/h. Lymphatic removal may increase dramatically if transudation into the interstitial space increases. Net flux into the interstitial space is governed by **Starling forces**.
- Mechanisms of formation of pulmonary oedema:
  - alteration of Starling forces:
    - increased hydrostatic pressure, e.g. hypervolaemia, left ventricular failure, **mitral stenosis**.
    - decreased plasma **oncotic pressure**, e.g. **hypoproteinaemia**.
    - acute severe subatmospheric airway pressure, e.g. upper **airway obstruction**.
  - damage to the alveolar-capillary membrane, e.g. **ARDS**.
  - impairment of lymphatic drainage, e.g. lymphangitis carcinomatosis, silicosis.
  - causes of uncertain aetiology:
    - neurogenic: thought to involve sudden **catecholamine** release following **head injury**, with vasoconstriction increasing lung capillary pressures and capillary permeability.
    - following **naloxone** administration: also thought to involve catecholamine release.
    - in **opioid poisoning**, possibly related to decreased vascular permeability.
    - following pulmonary surgery or re-expansion of a **pneumothorax**: probably involves local changes in capillary pressures and permeability.
    - after exposure to high altitude, possibly via pulmonary vasoconstriction.

As fluid clearance mechanisms are overwhelmed, interstitial oedema increases, until alveolar oedema occurs. Eventually, frothy oedema fluid fills the airways, impairing gas exchange. Airways and pulmonary vessels become narrowed by interstitial oedema, and **FRC** and **compliance** decrease.
- Features:
  - dyspnoea, tachypnoea, cough with pink frothy sputum, and tachycardia. Respiratory distress is worse lying flat (orthopnoea).
  - wheeze and basal crepitations on auscultation.
  - features of **respiratory failure**.
  - arterial blood gas analysis usually reveals **hypoxaemia**, with hypocapnia secondary to hyperventilation. Metabolic acidosis may be present in severe cases.
  - **chest X-ray** features include those of the underlying condition. Lung oedema itself appears as fluffy shadowing, typically perihilar (bat's wing) in left ventricular failure and patchy (cotton-wool) and peripheral in ARDS. Bronchial and vascular markings may appear thickened due to interstitial oedema. **Kerley** B **lines** and fluid in the transverse fissure may be present.

Differentiation between hydrostatic and other causes may be aided by measurement of **pulmonary capillary wedge pressure**. Alveolar fluid protein content may also be measured. Total lung water content has been measured using radioactive or dye dilution techniques.
- Treatment of severe acute pulmonary oedema:
  - of the underlying condition.
  - O_2 therapy. **CPAP** may be useful.
  - sitting the patient, with the legs over the edge of the bed.
  - **diuretics, e.g. frusemide** 20–120 mg iv (causes vasodilatation and diuresis).
  - opioids, e.g. **morphine**, **diamorphine** 1–5 mg iv (reduce anxiety and cause vasodilatation).
  - **inotropic** and **vasodilator drugs**.
  - **IPPV** may be required. Gas exchange is usually improved by **PEEP**.
  - traditionally, venesection has been performed for cardiogenic pulmonary oedema, with removal of 200–500 ml blood. Placing tourniquets on each limb in turn has also been used.

Pulmonary stretch receptors. Mechanoreceptors within the airway smooth muscle; transmit impulses via the vagi to the dorsal medulla. Excitation limits inspiration during pulmonary overinflation (**Hering–Breuer reflex**). Sensitivity is increased by decreased arterial $P\text{CO}_2$ and increased pulmonary venous pressure. May also be involved in other pulmonary reflexes, e.g. **gasp** and **deflation reflexes**.

Pulmonary valve lesions. Include:
- pulmonary stenosis (PS): may occur at the valve (90%), infundibulum or within the artery. Almost always congenital, accounting for 5–10% of **congenital heart disease**. Other causes include **rheumatic fever** and **carcinoid syndrome**. Usually asymptomatic; if severe, PS may cause fatigue, dyspnoea and angina secondary to decreased cardiac output. Right ventricular (and later atrial) hypertrophy may occur. May be associated with right-to-left **shunt** and cyanosis, e.g. **Fallot's tetralogy**.

   Features: ejection systolic murmur at the upper left sternal edge, heard best during inspiration. Splitting of the second **heart sound** is increased, with a quiet pulmonary component in severe PS. Right ventricular and atrial enlargement may be shown on the **ECG** and **chest X-ray**; a prominent pulmonary artery and pulmonary oligaemia may appear on the latter.

   During anaesthesia, increased right ventricular O_2 consumption (e.g. caused by tachycardia and increased contractility) should be avoided.
- pulmonary regurgitation (PR): usually a feature of **pulmonary hypertension**, and results from dilatation of the valve ring. Other causes include congenital absence of the valve, **endocarditis**, and surgical valvotomy. Causes right ventricular hypertrophy, but usually with little clinical effect.

   Features: high-pitched blowing diastolic murmur at the upper left sternal edge.

Pulmonary vascular resistance (PVR). **Resistance** in the **pulmonary circulation**, analogous to **SVR**. May be calculated using the principle of **Ohm's law**:
PVR (**dyne** s/cm^5) =

$$\frac{\text{mean pulmonary artery pressure} - \text{left atrial pressure}}{(\text{mmHg}) \times 80}$$
$$\text{cardiac output (l/min)}$$

where 80 is a correction factor.

Normally 20–120 dyne s/cm^5. (NB. 1 dyne s/cm^5 = 100 N s/m^5).

Resistance is distributed more evenly than in the systemic circulation, with approximately 50% residing in the arteries and arterioles, 30% in the capillaries and 20% in the veins. The pulmonary arteries are thin-walled, large in diameter and easily distensible. The pulmonary circulation is therefore more dependent on gravity, posture and the relationship between alveolar and intravascular pressures than on vascular muscular tone.

- PVR is affected by:
  - passive factors:
    - lung expansion: at lung volumes below FRC, the radial forces acting on the extra-alveolar vessels and holding them open are reduced; thus increasing PVR. However, at high lung volumes, the increased airway pressures associated with hyperexpansion may compress the vessels, also increasing PVR. PVR is lowest at lung volumes around FRC.
    - intravascular pressures: PVR falls when either pulmonary artery pressure or pulmonary venous pressure increase, because of recruitment of previously closed vessels or distension of individual capillary segments.
    - cardiac output: as pulmonary blood flow increases, vessel diameter increases, thus reducing PVR.
    - **haematocrit** and blood **viscosity**.
  - active factors via changes in muscle tone:
    - **hypoxia** (*see Hypoxic pulmonary vasoconstriction*), **hypercapnia** and **acidosis** increase PVR, especially in combination, whilst their opposites decrease PVR.
    - drugs and hormones, e.g. **vasoconstrictor drugs, 5–HT** and **histamine** increase PVR whilst **vasodilator drugs** and **acetylcholine** decrease it. Drugs may also affect PVR via changes in cardiac output and lung volumes.
    - nervous control: **sympathetic nervous system** supplies vasoconstrictor (α-**adrenergic receptor**) and vasodilator (β-adrenergic receptor) fibres to the pulmonary vessels, whilst the **parasympathetic nervous system** supplies cholinergic vasodilator fibres.

In addition, local vascular resistance may be increased by **PE**, **atelectasis**, **pleural effusions**, surgery, etc.

PVR may be corrected for differences in body size by multiplying by body **surface area** (PVR index).

See also, Lung; Pulmonary artery catheterization; Pulmonary hypertension

Pulse. Traditionally palpated at the wrist, but commonly palpated at the head and neck during anaesthesia (*see Carotid arteries*).

- Should be assessed for:
  - **heart rate**: speed, rhythm, regularity.
  - volume and character, i.e. reflecting **pulse pressure** and **arterial waveform**. **Pulsus alternans** and **pulsus paradoxus** are two specific abnormalities.
  - simultaneous pulsation at upper and lower limb arteries; femoral delay occurs in **coarctation of the aorta**.

Pulse deficit. Difference between the auscultated heart rate and palpated pulse rate. Occurs when one heart beat follows another so quickly that ventricular filling is insufficient for a palpable pulsation, e.g. in **ventricular ectopic beats** and **AF**.

Pulse detector. Several devices have been used to detect the **pulse**, e.g. to monitor heart rate or to aid in **arterial BP measurement**. Each utilizes a small **transducer** positioned over a peripheral artery or attached to a digit. Commonly used methods:

- microphone or **Doppler** probe.
- finger probe containing a light source and photocell which detects changes in reflected or transmitted light due to arterial pulsation.

Simple devices emit a noise or flashing light in time with the pulse, or register the pulse rate on a meter. More sophisticated devices display a waveform, e.g. pulse oximeter.

Pulse oximeter, *see Oximetry*

Pulse pressure. Difference between systolic and diastolic blood pressures, normally about 35–45 mmHg. Depends on:

- **stroke volume**.
- compliance of the arterial tree; e.g. increased in the elderly, because of arterial calcification and reduced compliance.
- duration and speed of ventricular ejection.
- aortic valve function.
- site of measurement; increased as the **arterial waveform** moves peripherally.

See also, Pulse

Pulsus alternans. Alternating weak and strong **pulses** reflecting similar alterations in left ventricular filling and output. Common in left ventricular failure.

See also, Arterial waveform

Pulsus paradoxus. Usually defined as a decrease in **arterial BP** greater than 10 mmHg on inspiration, caused by reduced left ventricular output secondary to increased negative intrathoracic pressure. May be marked when large negative intrathoracic pressures are generated, e.g. upper or lower **airway obstruction**, or when diastolic cardiac filling is reduced, e.g. **cardiac tamponade**, constrictive **pericarditis**.

See also, Pulse

Pupil. Central orifice of the iris; normally 1–8 mm in size. Contraction (miosis) is caused by parasympathetic stimulation, drugs including **opioid analgesic drugs** and anaesthetic agents, and pontine lesions. Dilatation (mydriasis) is caused by sympathetic stimulation and **anticholinergic drugs**. Dilated pupils may occur during **awareness** or **hypercapnia** during anaesthesia.

- Abnormal pupils and **pupillary reflex** may occur in particular lesions, e.g.:
  - ipsilateral fixed dilatation in **head injury**, followed by bilateral dilatation due to stretching of the 3rd **cranial nerve**.
  - **Horner's syndrome**.
  - Argyll–Robertson pupil: small and irregular, fixed to light but responsive to accommodation. Classically

occurs in tertiary **syphilis** but may occur in **diabetes mellitus** and brainstem encephalitis.

–Holmes–Adie pupil: large and regular, with sluggish light reflex. Often associated with loss of knee reflexes but no other pathology.

[Douglas Argyll Robertson (1837–1909), Scottish surgeon; Gordon M Holmes (1876–1965), Irish-born English neurologist; William J Adie (1886–1935), Australian-born English neurologist]

Pupillary reflex. Easily tested reflex arcs involving the **pupils**:

–light reflex: pupillary constriction normally follows direct or contralateral (consensual) illumination. Occasionally, phasic contraction and dilatation occurs (hippus). Pathway: from retina via optic nerve to the optic chiasma, thence to both lateral geniculate bodies via the optic tracts. Fibres then pass to the Edinger–Westphal nuclei of the 3rd **cranial nerve**. Efferent parasympathetic fibres pass to the ciliary ganglia, then via oculomotor and short ciliary nerves to the iris sphincter muscles of both sides. The cerebral cortex is not involved in the reflex.

–accommodation reflex: constriction normally occurs when the eyes converge. Fibres from the lateral geniculate bodies pass to the visual areas of the cerebral cortex; impulses then pass via superior longitudinal fasciculus and internal capsule to the oculomotor nuclear mass next to the Edinger-Westphal nucleus. When both medial recti are adducted, the pupils constrict.

Impaired reflexes are caused by lesions anywhere along their paths.

[Ludwig Edinger (1855–1918) and Karl FO Westphal (1833–1890), German neurologists]

Pyloric stenosis. Stenosis of the gastric outflow. May be:

–congenital:

–hypertrophy of the circular pyloric muscle; cause is unknown. Occurs in 1:500 births, 80% in males (usually first-born).

–usually presents within 4–6 weeks of age, with persistent projectile vomiting, failure to gain weight and hunger. A 'tumour' may be palpable in the right hypochondrium.

–marked **dehydration** and metabolic **alkalosis** may be present. Resultant **aldosterone** secretion causes exchange of potassium and hydrogen ions for sodium in the urine, resulting in **hypokalaemia** and hypochloraemia with paradoxical acid urine.

–treated initially by nasogastric drainage and restoration of electrolyte/fluid balance, e.g. using 0.9% saline followed by dextrose–saline with potassium supplementation according to plasma electrolyte analysis.

–corrective surgery (pyloromyotomy; Ramstedt's procedure) should only be performed following adequate resuscitation, as indicated by absent clinical features of dehydration, good urine output, and normal acid–base and electrolyte status. Anaesthetic management is as for **paediatric anaesthesia**, taking measures to avoid **aspiration of gastric contents**. Rapid sequence induction is usual, but awake intubation and inhalational induction have been used.

–acquired: usually results from gastric carcinoma or ulcer. Metabolic features are similar to those above. Residual gastric contents may be voluminous.

[Wilhelm C Ramstedt (1867–1963), German surgeon]

Pyridostigmine bromide. Acetylcholinesterase inhibitor. Pyridine analogue of **neostigmine**, with slower onset and longer duration of action. Also has weaker nicotinic action on voluntary muscle and less muscarinic action on viscera. Used in **myasthenia gravis** but less useful than neostigmine for reversing **non-depolarizing neuromuscular blockade**. **Half-life** is 3–4 hours.

• Dosage: 30–120 mg orally 4–12 hourly, up to 3.0–1.2 g/day.
• Side effects: as for neostigmine.

Q

Q wave. Initial downward deflection of the **QRS complex** of the **ECG** (*see Fig. 49b; Electrocardiography*). Small (q) waves are normal in leads aVL and I when left axis deviation is present, and in leads II, III and aVF with right axis deviation. They may be large in aVR. Pathological (Q) waves are wide (greater than 0.04 seconds) and deep (greater than 4 mm, or more than a quarter of the height of the R wave in the same lead); in the absence of left **bundle branch block** they suggest **MI**.

QRS complex. Represents ventricular depolarization; normally follows the **P wave** of the **ECG** (*see Fig. 49b; Electrocardiography*). Upper case letters are used if a particular wave is considered large, lower case if small. The initial deflection is termed the **q** (Q) **wave** if downward, and **R wave** if upward. The downward **S wave** follows an R wave. The QRS complex may be used to calculate electrical axis. Normally has rS pattern in V_1, qR pattern in V_6. The initial small deflection represents left to right septal depolarization; the larger subsequent deflection represents (mainly left) ventricular depolarization. Normal duration: <0.12 seconds. Abnormalities may represent **arrhythmias**, **heart block**, **bundle branch block**, **MI**, etc.

Q–T interval. Represents the duration of ventricular systole; varies with age, sex and heart rate. Measured from the beginning of the **QRS complex** to the end of the **T wave** of the **ECG** (*see Fig. 49b; Electrocardiography*). Corrected for heart rate by dividing by the square root of the preceding R–R interval (seconds). Normally <0.44 seconds.

Shortened in **hypercalcaemia**, **hyperkalaemia** and **digoxin** therapy. May be prolonged congenitally, or in myocardial disease, **rheumatic fever**, **hypocalcaemia** and with various drugs, e.g. **antiarrhythmic drugs**, **phenothiazines** and **tricyclic antidepressant drugs**. Prolonged Q–T syndromes may be associated with recurrent syncope or sudden death due to ventricular arrhythmias including **VT** and **torsade de pointes**. Drugs, e.g. **β-adrenergic receptor antagonists**, **phenytoin**, **verapamil** and **bretylium**, **cardiac pacing**, sympathectomy and implanted defibrillators have been used for treatment.

Galloway PA, Glass PSA (1985) Anesth Analg; 64: 612–20

Quantal theory. Widely accepted theory proposed in the 1960s to explain miniature **end-plate potentials** recorded from the **neuromuscular junction** postsynaptic membrane, at approximately 2 Hz. Postulates that small 'quanta' (packets) of **acetylcholine** are released randomly from the nerve cell membrane even in the absence of motor nerve activity. Each quantum is thought to be one vesicle's content, about 10 000 acetylcholine molecules. During single motor nerve activation about 200 quanta are released into the synaptic cleft.

Quantiflex apparatus. Continuous flow **anaesthetic machines**, which can deliver preset mixtures of O_2 and N_2O, adjusted by a percentage control (minimum of 30% O_2). A single dial adjusts total gas flow delivered. Individual **flowmeters** indicate flow of O_2 and N_2O; the O_2 flowmeter is usually on the right, and N_2O flowmeter on the left. They are sometimes used in **dental surgery**.

Quincke, Heinrich Irenaeus (1842–1922). German physician; described and standardized lumbar puncture in 1891. Used the paramedian approach, and suggested 24 hours bed rest afterwards. His bevelled needle design is still used for lumbar puncture and **spinal anaesthesia**.

Quinidine. Class Ia **antiarrhythmic drug**. An isomer of quinine. Used to treat supraventricular and ventricular arrhythmias, but rarely used now. **Half-life** is 5 hours; 40% is excreted unchanged in urine.
- Dosage: 200–400 mg orally, 6–8 hourly.
- Side effects are common due to a low **therapeutic ratio**; they include ventricular arrhythmias, CNS and GIT disturbances and hypersensitivity reactions. May potentiate non-depolarizing neuromuscular blockade.

R

R on T phenomenon. Arises when the **R wave** of a **ventricular ectopic beat** falls on the **T wave** of the preceding beat. At the middle of the T wave, the myocardium is partly depolarized and partly repolarized, and thus vulnerable to establishment of re-entry and circulatory conduction, leading to **VF** or **VT**.

R wave. First upward deflection of the **QRS complex** of the **ECG** (*see Fig. 49b; Electrocardiography*). Tends to increase in size from V_1 to V_6. In V_{1-6}, at least one normally exceeds 8 mm, but none exceeds 27 mm.

Rabies. Infection caused by a rhabdovirus, eradicated from Britain in 1902. Spread mainly via domestic dogs and cats, but also by foxes, bats and other wildlife. Transmitted via infected saliva penetrating broken skin or intact mucosa; the virus replicates in local muscle then migrates proximally along peripheral nerves to dorsal root ganglia and the CNS. Incubation period is usually 20–90 days in man, but may be 4 days to several years.

Malaise, fever, depression and psychosis may be followed by laryngeal spasm, and terror and arousal on drinking fluids. Respiratory failure occurs early and cardiac abnormalities, including myocarditis, are common.

Treatment of established rabies includes injection of human antirabies immunoglobulin, early IPPV, sedation and paralysis, with careful maintenance of acid–base and fluid balance. Almost inevitably fatal once established, but may be prevented by wound cleaning and active and passive immunization.

Radford nomogram. Diagram showing the relationship between **tidal volume**, patient's weight and respiratory frequency. Used to aid appropriate selection of ventilator settings for children and adults. Now rarely used.
[Edward P Radford, US physiologist]

Radial artery. Terminal branch of the brachial artery. Arises in the **antecubital fossa**, level with the radial neck, and passes downwards on the tendons and muscles attached to the radius (biceps tendon, supinator, pronator teres, flexor digitorum superficialis, flexor pollicis longus, pronator quadratus). Lies deep to brachioradialis muscle in the upper forearm, but subcutaneous in the lower forearm and easily palpable, especially over the distal quarter of the radius. Runs deep to abductor pollicis longus and extensor pollicis brevis tendons at the radial styloid, entering the anatomical snuffbox. Then enters the palm between the 1st and 2nd metacarpals. Branches include a superficial palmar branch (enters the palm superficial to the flexor retinaculum). At the wrist, it is a common site for palpation of the **pulse** and for **arterial cannulation**.

Radial nerve (C5–T1). Terminal branch of the posterior cord of the **brachial plexus**. Descends in the posterior upper arm, passing laterally behind the middle of the humerus in the radial groove. Crosses the **antecubital fossa** anterior to the elbow joint, between brachialis and brachioradialis. Descends under brachioradialis lateral to the **radial artery** in the forearm, passing posteriorly proximal to the wrist to end on the dorsum of the hand as digital branches.
● Branches:
  –axillary: to triceps and skin of the posteromedial upper arm.
  –upper arm:
    –to triceps, brachioradialis and extensor carpi radialis longus.
    –skin of the lower posterolateral arm.
  –forearm:
    –to the elbow joint.
    –posterior interosseous nerve arising at the elbow joint: passes posteriorly round the radial neck to supply the elbow, wrist and intercarpal joints, and all extensor muscles of the forearm apart from extensor carpi radialis longus.
    –via digital branches to the lateral side of the dorsum of the hand and posterior aspects of the lateral 2.5 digits up to the distal phalanx.
May be blocked at the elbow, wrist, and at midhumerus with the elbow flexed (the nerve is palpable in the radial groove).
See also, Brachial plexus block; Elbow, nerve blocks; Wrist, nerve blocks

Radiation. Emission of **energy** in the form of waves or particles. Includes emission of electromagnetic waves, e.g. light, most of which is non-ionizing (does not have sufficient energy to overcome electron binding energy). Ionizing radiation may result in displacement of electrons in organic material with the potential for tissue damage, and includes:
  –α particles: helium nuclei consisting of two protons and two neutrons. Have high energy but penetrate matter poorly.
  –β particles: electron or positrons with variable energy and velocity. Those with high energies are more penetrative than α particles but much less than γ-rays and X-rays.
  –γ-rays and X-rays: electromagnetic waves emitted from (γ-rays) or outside (X-rays) the nuclei of excited atoms. Have extremely high penetration of matter and thus pose a health hazard requiring radiation safety precautions. γ-Rays are used in **radiotherapy** and imaging, and X-rays in imaging.
Exposure to ionizing radiation is kept to a minimum with appropriate storage and handling of **radioisotopes**,

minimal use of X-rays and appropriate use of shielding. Recent regulations require those performing or directing radiology procedures to have attended a course.

See also, Environmental safety of anaesthetists

Radioisotopes. Isotopes of elements that undergo disintegration; i.e. the nucleus emits α, β or γ **radiation** either spontaneously or following a collision. Used clinically as labels to determine fluid compartments, blood flow, pulmonary $\dot{V}/\dot{Q}$ distribution, etc. Technetium-99m and xenon-133 are often suitable because they are easy to use and their **half-lives** are short. Also used to label metabolically active substances which are taken up by certain tissues, allowing imaging of the tissue concerned, e.g. fibrinogen labelled with iodine-123 accumulates in clot and may be used to detect **DVT**. Therapeutic use includes **radiotherapy**.

Radiological contrast media. Contain large molecules which absorb X-rays; e.g. most enteral media contain barium or iodine; most iv media contain iodine. Adverse reactions may follow iv injection:
- related to high **osmolality** (up to approximately 7 times that of plasma):
  - initial hypervolaemia followed by osmotic diuresis and hypovolaemia.
  - damage to red blood cells and vascular endothelium.
- immunological:
  - direct **histamine** release is thought to be most likely; **complement** activation may be involved. True **anaphylactic reactions** are not thought to occur.
  - reactions range from mild symptoms to cardiovascular collapse and death.
- direct toxicity: myocardial depression and systemic vasodilatation.

Thus initial hypertension may be followed by prolonged hypotension. Vagally mediated bradycardia may be due to central effects.

Incidence of reactions is decreased by using low osmolar, non-ionic media and low doses. Risk of subsequent immune reactions is low, especially with use of antihistamines and steroid therapy. Resuscitation equipment and drugs must always be available when contrast medium is injected.

Goldberg M (1984) Anesthesiology; 60: 46–56

See also, Adverse drug reactions

Radiology, anaesthesia for. Most radiological procedures require neither general anaesthesia nor **sedation**. Anaesthesia may be required for the very young, confused or agitated patients and those with movement disorders. Procedures for which the anaesthetist may be required include **CAT scanning**, **magnetic resonance imaging**, angiography, and invasive procedures, e.g. embolization of vascular lesions (e.g. in **neuroradiology**).
- Main anaesthetic considerations:
  - underlying disease process.
  - often cramped conditions, with poor lighting.
  - anaesthetic/**monitoring** equipment may be incomplete or old.
  - poor access to the patient.
  - adverse effects of **radiological contrast media**.

Preoperative assessment and preparation should be as for any anaesthetic procedure.

Radiotherapy. Use of ionizing **radiation** to treat neoplasms. May involve:
- external radiation.
- implantation of internal sources (interstitial radiotherapy), e.g. in gynaecological or CNS tumours.
- administration of radioactive **radioisotopes**, e.g. iodine-131 in hyperthyroidism, phosphorous-32 in polycythaemia.

- General anaesthesia is rarely required except when patients are uncooperative, e.g. children, patients with movement disorders, etc. Anaesthetic considerations:
  - general condition of the patient: features of **malignancy**, site and nature of the neoplasm, drug therapy, etc. Haematological abnormalities are common.
  - repeated anaesthetics: multiple treatments are required, e.g. daily for several weeks. Considerations include fear of injections, risk of **halothane hepatitis**, and repeated periods of starvation (especially important in children). IV cannulation may be difficult, although long-term catheters are often sited.
  - immobilization of the head may be required, e.g. for CNS tumours; clear plastic masks are often used, with risks of airway obstruction. Head-down positioning may be required. Problems also exist when moulding and making the mask.
  - treatments usually consist of short periods of radiation (e.g. a few minutes), during which time the anaesthetist cannot be present. Monitoring is usually visible via remote-control cameras, but may be restricted.

Techniques available include **sedation**, **neuroleptanaesthesia** and formal general anaesthesia. **Ketamine** is often used, especially in children. Repeated doses may be given as required during positioning and therapy.

Patients formerly treated by radiotherapy may have inflammatory or fibrotic changes in the irradiated area. Pulmonary, cardiac, renal and hepatic involvement may be present. Tissue fibrosis around the airway may make tracheal intubation difficult.

Randomization. Technique for allocating subjects, e.g. patients to treatment groups in **clinical trials**, thus overcoming bias when **samples** are compared. Ensures that factors such as age, sex, weight, etc. are randomly distributed amongst the groups; i.e. any difference in these factors is due to chance alone.
- Randomization may be:
  - simple: no restriction on allocation. Groups may be unequally sized.
  - block: allocation is performed in blocks, so that groups are equally sized within each block.
  - stratified: factors such as age, sex, etc. are randomized separately, so that they are equally distributed amongst the groups.

Computer-generated random numbers are usually employed. Use of coins or dice is tedious and presents the temptation to repeat an allocation if the result is not liked. Other methods, e.g. allocation of alternate patients, or according to patients' birthdays or record numbers have also been used. However, these methods cannot always be guaranteed free of hidden bias.

Ranitidine hydrochloride. H₂ **receptor antagonist**; better absorbed and more potent than **cimetidine**, with fewer side effects. Does not inhibit hepatic enzymes, nor interfere with metabolism of other drugs. Plasma levels peak within 15 mins of im injection; effect lasts about 8 hours. **Half-life** is about 2 hours. Excreted via urine, hence the dose is reduced in **renal failure**.

- Dosage:
    - –50 mg iv/im 8 hourly. Effective if given 45–60 minutes preoperatively. If administered iv, 50 mg should be diluted into 20 ml and injected over at least 2 minutes, since severe bradycardia may occur.
    - –150 mg orally 12 hourly. 150 mg the night before surgery and 2 hours preoperatively has been used.
- Side effects: blood dyscrasias, impaired liver function and confusion; all are rare.

Ranking, *see Statistical tests*

Raoult's law. The degree of lowering of vapour pressure of a solvent, due to addition of a solute, is proportional to the molar concentration of the solute.
[Francois M Raoult (1830–1901), French scientist]
See also, Colligative properties of solutions

RAP, Right atrial pressure, *see Cardiac catheterization; Central venous pressure*

Rate–pressure product (RPP). Product of heart rate and systolic BP, used as an indicator of myocardial workload and O_2 consumption. It has been suggested that RPP should be maintained below 15 000 in patients with **ischaemic heart disease** during anaesthesia. Its usefulness has been questioned, since a proportional increase in rate may increase myocardial O_2 demand more than the same increase in BP. Rate–pressure quotient has been suggested as being a better predictor of **myocardial ischaemia**: MAP/rate. If under 1, it may indicate ischaemia.

RBBB, Right bundle branch block, *see Bundle branch block*

RDS, *see Respiratory distress syndrome*

Reactance. Portion of **impedance** to flow of an alternating current not due to **resistance**; e.g. due to **capacitance** or **inductance**. Given the symbol X, and measured in ohms.
[Georg S Ohm (1787–1854), German physicist]

Rebreathing techniques, *see Carbon dioxide measurement*

Receptor theory. States that receptors are specific proteins or lipoproteins within cell **membranes** that interact selectively with extracellular compounds (**agonists**) to initiate biochemical events within the cell. The structures of the agonist and receptor determine the selectivity and quantitative response. Drugs which interact with the receptor but do not produce the effect of an agonist are **antagonists**. Degree of binding to receptors is **affinity**; ability to produce a response is **intrinsic activity**.

Initial assumptions that the degree of response is proportional to the number of receptors occupied are not universally accepted. Other suggestions include:
    - –reduced occupancy is required for a potent agonist compared with a less potent agonist, to produce the same response.
    - –degree of response is proportional to the rate of receptor–agonist interaction and dissociation.

Interaction of drug and receptor may resemble **Michaelis–Menten kinetics**. Covalent, ionic and hydrogen bonding, and **Van der Waals forces** may be involved.
Berkowitz DE, Schwinn DA (1991) Curr Opin Anaesth; 4: 486–96
See also, Dose–response curves; Pharmacodynamics

Record-keeping. The first anaesthetic chart was devised by Codman and **Cushing** in 1894 at the Massachusetts General Hospital, for recording of respiration and pulse rate. BP charting was included in 1901 at Cushing's insistence. Respiration and F_1O_2 were included by **McKesson** in 1911.

Careful record-keeping is now recognized as essential to chart preoperative risk factors and the peroperative course of anaesthesia. Particularly useful when taking over another anaesthetist's anaesthetic, and for providing information for subsequent anaesthetics. Also important for teaching, research and **audit**, and becoming increasingly important in **medicolegal aspects of anaesthesia**. Although tending to include similar information, different charts from different hospitals are not yet standardized, although this has been suggested.

Automated anaesthetic record systems are increasingly used, sometimes incorporated into anaesthetic machines. They provide accurate, legible and complete documents for data acquisition and subsequent scrutiny. Data from **monitoring** devices are incorporated with information provided by the anaesthetist, e.g. drug or other interventions, although lack of familiarity with keyboards or computers may be a hindrance.

Postoperative **recovery** and progress may be recorded on separate charts, or on the anaesthetic chart.
[Ernest A Codman (1869–1940), US surgeon]

Recovery. Period from the end of surgery to when the patient is alert and physiologically stable. Definition is difficult because some drowsiness may persist for many hours. **Recovery testing** is used for more precise investigation. Time to recovery depends on the patient's condition, drugs given, their doses, and the patient's ability to eliminate them. For **inhalational anaesthetic agents**, similar considerations to uptake are involved, plus length of operation and degree of redistribution to fat. Thus blood gas **solubility** is the most important factor initially, but more potent agents, e.g. **halothane** are more extensively bound to fat after prolonged anaesthesia than less potent ones, e.g. **enflurane**. For **iv anaesthetic agents**, initial recovery is due to drug redistribution from vessel-rich to vessel-intermediate tissues; subsequent course is related to the rate of clearance from the body. Thus **propofol** characteristically results in rapid clear-headed wakening, whereas **thiopentone** is more likely to produce drowsiness lasting several hours, especially after repeated dosage.

Dedicated **recovery rooms** are used whenever possible. Staff must be fully informed of anaesthetic techniques used and any difficulties. All patients unable to maintain their airway should be nursed with appropriate **monitoring** by at least one member of staff. Heart rate, BP and respiratory rate are usually recorded every 15 minutes for at least 1 hour, with other observations, e.g. neurological, if indicated. O_2 should be administered until awake, and patients placed in the recovery position, with uppermost

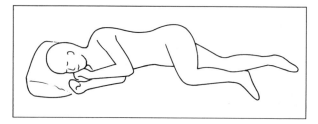

Figure 111 *Recovery position*

hand supporting the jaw (Fig. 111). In the tonsillar position, the pillow is placed under the loin and the trolley tipped head down.

Postoperative analgesia is an essential task during the recovery period.

- Problems during recovery:
  - –respiratory, e.g. **hypoventilation, hypercapnia, hypoxaemia, airway obstruction, bronchospasm, aspiration of gastric contents**.
  - –cardiovascular, e.g. **hypotension, hypertension, arrhythmias**.
  - –**confusion**, agitation, etc. Pain and bladder distension are common causes of restlessness and hypertension postoperatively. The above causes must also be excluded.
  - –related to anaesthetic drugs, e.g. inadequate reversal of **neuromuscular blockade, adverse drugs reactions, MH, dystonic reactions, emergence phenomena, central anticholinergic syndrome**, etc.
  - –**hypothermia**, nausea and **vomiting, shivering**.
  - –related to surgery, e.g. bleeding.

See also, Anaesthetic morbidity and mortality

Recovery room. An area reserved for postoperative care was described by Florence Nightingale in 1863, but the first dedicated recovery room was opened in the USA in 1923. Many more were introduced there after experiences in World War II and the Korean War. First introduced in the UK in 1955.

- Features:
  - –placed near the operating suite, if possible near ICU.
  - –open ward, allowing good patient observation; an isolation room may be required.
  - –1.5 bays per operating theatre are usually sufficient, with continuous one-to-one nursing care until the patient is able to maintain his or her airway.
  - –each bay is equipped for monitoring (ECG, BP, temperature, etc.) and patient care (suction, O_2, etc.), also electrical outlets, etc.
  - –a full supply of iv equipment and fluids, blankets, airways, etc. should be available.
  - –resuscitation equipment, ventilator and drugs should be readily available, with an emergency call system.
  - –discharge criteria: awake patient, maintaining his or her airway with adequate breathing, colour, cardiovascular status and analgesia, without surgical complications.
- Drugs available should include:
  - –analgesics, antiemetics, sedatives, anticonvulsants, naloxone, flumazenil.
  - –doxapram, bronchodilators, steroids, antihistamines.
  - –anticholinergics, antiarrhythmics, antihypertensives, diuretics, heparin.
  - –antibiotics, anticholinesterases, neuromuscular blocking drugs, insulin, dextrose, dantrolene.
  - –local anaesthetics.

[Florence Nightingale (1820–1910), English nurse]
van der Walt JH, Mackay P (1988) Anaesth Intensive Care; 16: 77–80
See also, Recovery

Recovery testing. Ranges from simple clinical assessment to more sophisticated methods, e.g. used for comparison between anaesthetic techniques, drugs, etc. Routine testing is usually limited to assessment of general alertness and orientation, and ability to respond, drink, dress and walk where appropriate (e.g. **day-case surgery**).

- Sophisticated techniques used include tests of:
  - –psychomotor function:
    - –assessing speed and number of errors made whilst performing set tasks:
      - –moving pegs from one set of holes in a board to another set.
      - –'posting' pieces of paper through a slot.
      - –deleting every letter 'p' from a page of text.
      - –following outlines of shapes with a pen without drawing over their edges, drawing a line from the centre of a maze to the outside, or moving a metal hoop along a tortuous wire without touching it.
      - –connecting dots on a page.
    - –reaction testing:
      - –being faced with four light sources, and pressing the correct switch (out of four choices) when one of them flashes.
      - –tracking moving targets with a pen or light.
      - –driving simulators.
  - –perception:
    - –noting the frequency at which a flashing light appears to be continuous (critical flicker–fusion threshold).
    - –perception of auditory stimuli in a similar fashion, including discrimination between left and right ears.
  - –memory:
    - –recall or recognition of objects, pictures, words or word associations shown a short time before.
    - –recall of pre- and postoperative events.
    - –orientation in person, time and space.
  - –cognitive function, e.g. adding/subtracting numbers, or adding values of different coins.
  - –intelligence: standard tests are used.
  - –physiological function, e.g. divergence of eyes caused by reductions in extraocular muscle tone.

Problems are related to the time taken, cumbersome equipment required, fatigue, boredom and learning if tests are repeated. Critical flicker fusion, reaction testing, letter deletion and memory tests are most widely used and thought to be reasonably efficient, the first two especially so. General advice to patients is usually to avoid potentially dangerous activities, e.g. driving, cooking, using machinery, etc., for 24 hours following day-case anaesthesia, although subtle changes may persist beyond this period. 48 hours has been suggested.

Rectal administration of anaesthetic agents. Results in effective absorption of drugs because of a rich blood supply provided by communicating plexuses formed by the superior, middle and inferior rectal arteries and veins. Drugs undergo less **first pass metabolism** than when orally administered, because the plexuses represent anastomoses between portal and systemic circulations. The technique is usually restricted to children. Traditionally used more in Continental Europe, e.g. France. Drugs used include **diazepam** 0.4–0.5 mg/kg (widely used for treatment of convulsions in children), **methohexitone** 15–25 mg/kg and **thiopentone** 40–50 mg/kg as 5–10% solutions. Opioids and **ketamine** have also been given in this way. **Diethyl ether** was administered rectally by **Pirogoff**. **Bromethol** and **paraldehyde** were used in the 1920s to produce unconsciousness (basal narcosis).

Rectus sheath block. Performed as part of **abdominal field block**, or to reduce pain from midline incisions (using bilateral blocks). Abdominal contents remain unanaesthetized.

   With the patient supine, a short-bevelled needle is introduced 3–6 cm above and lateral to the umbilicus. A click is felt as the tough anterior layer of the sheath is punctured. The needle is advanced up to the resistance offered by the posterior layer of the sheath, and 15–20 ml **local anaesthetic agent** injected after negative aspiration. Deposition of solution between rectus muscle and posterior layer allows spread up and down, blocking the lower 5–6 intercostal nerves within the sheath. Spread between the muscle and anterior layer is limited by the tendinous intersections along its length. Multiple injections have been suggested between intersections, to improve spread, but the posterior layer is deficient below a point half way between the umbilicus and pubis, and peritoneal puncture is more likely below this level.

Recurarization. Recurrence of **non-depolarizing neuromuscular blockade** after apparent reversal with **acetylcholinesterase inhibitors**. Originally described with **tubocurarine** in patients with impaired renal function, where the duration of action of the neuromuscular blocking drug exceeds that of the acetylcholinesterase inhibitor. Has been described with other neuromuscular blocking drugs.

Red-cell concentrates, *see Blood products*

Reducing valve, *see Pressure regulators*

Referred pain. Pain felt in a somatic site remote to the source of pain, usually visceral; e.g. diaphragmatic pain is felt in the shoulder tip. The aetiology is obscure, but is thought to be related to the embryological segment from which the organ arose, e.g. diaphragm from the neck region, and heart from the same region as the arm.
- Theories include:
   –convergence: somatic and visceral afferents converge on the same spinothalamic tracts. The brain assumes that neural activity in a particular pathway arises from somatic input, rather than visceral, since the former is far more common than the latter.
   –facilitation: input from visceral afferents increases sensitivity of neurones receiving somatic afferents, thus encouraging somatic sensation.
Effects of local anaesthetic injected at referred areas are inconstistent, supporting both theories (should ease the pain if facilitation is responsible, but not if convergence is responsible).

Reflex arc. Involves predictable, repetitive stereotypic responses to a particular sensory stimulus. Consists of sense organ, afferent **neurone**, one or more **synapses**, efferent neurone and effector. The afferent neurones enter the **spinal cord** via dorsal roots or **brain** via **cranial nerves**; the efferent neurones leave via ventral nerve roots or corresponding motor cranial nerves. Also involved in autonomic functions. The simplest reflex arc is monosynaptic, e.g. knee jerk and other stretch reflexes involving **muscle spindles**. Polysynaptic reflex arcs (two or more synapses) include the withdrawal reflex. Widespread effects may result from activation of a single reflex arc because of ascending, descending, excitatory and inhibitory interneurones.

Reflex sympathetic dystrophy. Continuous **pain** in part of an extremity after trauma including fractures, but not involving a major nerve. Worse with movement. Associated with sympathetic hyperactivity, with cool clammy skin; it may proceed to a pale, cold extremity with tissue atrophy and stiffness. Usually occurs within weeks of trauma, which may be mild. In Sudeck's atrophy, osteoporosis is also present. Treatment includes mobility, physiotherapy, rehabilitation and **sympathetic nerve blocks**.
[Paul HM Sudeck (1866–1945), German surgeon]

Reflux, *see Gastro-oesophageal reflux*

Refractometer, *see Interferometer*

Refractory period. Period during and following the **action potential** during which the neurone is insensitive to further stimulation. Subdivided thus:
   –absolute: excited by no stimulus however strong.
   –relative: excitation may follow stronger stimuli than normal.

Refrigeration anaesthesia. Use of cold to reduce pain sensation. Used by **Larrey** in 1807, although the effect of cold on pain has been recognized for centuries. Up to 3 hours packing in ice was recommended for operations through the thigh. The principle is still used today, e.g. **ethyl chloride** spray.

Regional anaesthesia. Term originally coined by **Cushing** to describe techniques of abolishing pain using **local anaesthetic agents** as opposed to general anaesthesia. Pioneers included **Corning** and **Labat** in the USA and **Bier**, **Braun** and **Lawen** in Europe.
- Techniques include:
   –**topical anaesthesia**.
   –**infiltration anaesthesia** and **Vishnevskiy technique**.
   –peripheral nerve blocks: plexus and single nerve blocks.
   –central neural blockade: **extradural** and **spinal anaesthesia**.
   –**IVRA** and **intra-arterial regional anaesthesia**.
   –**sympathetic nerve blocks**.
   –others, e.g. **interpleural analgesia**.
- Advantages of regional anaesthesia:
   –conscious patient, able to assist in positioning, etc. and warn of adverse effects (e.g. in **carotid artery surgery** and **TURP**). There is less interruption of oral intake, especially beneficial in **diabetes mellitus**.

–good **postoperative analgesia.**
–reduction of certain postoperative complications, e.g. **atelectasis** and **DVT.**
- Contraindications:
 –absolute: patient refusal, anaesthetist's inexperience and localized infection.
 –relative: abnormal anatomy or deformity, **coagulation disorders,** previous failure of the technique, and neurological disease or other medicolegal considerations.
Specific contraindications may exist for specific techniques.
- Management:
 –preoperatively:
  –**preoperative assessment** and preparation as for general anaesthesia.
  –full explanation of the procedure, and **consent.**
  –preparation of drugs and equipment for general anaesthesia and resuscitation, in addition to those required for the regional technique chosen.
 –peroperatively:
  –monitoring should be applied as for general anaesthesia, i.e. before starting the procedure and continued throughout it.
  –aseptic technique should be observed.
  –for nerve or plexus blocks, short-bevelled **needles** are traditionally used to minimize nerve contact, although nerve damage may be greater should the nerve be impaled. Nerve stimulators (using 0.3–1.0 mA current lasting 1–2 ms and delivered at 1–3 Hz) increase the success of many blocks and may reduce damage further. A distant ground electrode is required. The needle (preferably sheathed) is placed near the target nerve and stimulated until paraesthesiae or twitches are elicited; the output is reduced, the needle repositioned, and the process repeated.
  –a single injection of local anaesthetic, repeated boluses (using repeated injections or an indwelling catheter) or continuous infusions may be used.
  –the extent of the block should be assessed (e.g. by response to pinprick or cold) before allowing surgery to start.
  –if **sedation** is used, care should be taken to ensure that respiratory and cardiovascular depression do not occur. Analgesic drugs (e.g. **N$_2$O** or **opioid analgesic drugs**) may be used to supplement incomplete blockade. General anaesthesia may be used as a planned part of the technique, or if the technique is unsuccessful.
 –postoperatively:
  –close monitoring and supervision should continue as for general anaesthesia.
  –neurological complications may only become apparent once the block has worn off.
- Complications:
 –technical: direct trauma to nerves, blood vessels, pleura, etc., breakage of needles or catheters.
 –associated with **positioning of the patient,** e.g. compression of an anaesthetized limb.
 –local anaesthetic toxicity: intravascular injection or systemic absorption.
 –excessive spread, e.g. total spinal block during extradural anaesthesia, or phrenic nerve block during **brachial plexus block.**
 –failure of the technique.

–those of specific techniques, e.g. hypotension following spinal anaesthesia.
–others, e.g. injection of the wrong solution through catheters.
Symposium on Local Anaesthesia (1986) Br J Anaesth; 58: 691–800
See also, specific blocks; Nerve injury during anaesthesia

Regression, *see Statistical tests*

Regurgitation. Passive passage of **gastric contents** into the pharynx. Silent, thus **aspiration of gastric contents** may occur unnoticed. Normally prevented by the **lower oesophageal sphincter**; however, swallowed dyes have been found to stain areas of the pharynx and larynx during anaesthesia in normal patients.

Relative analgesia. Technique used in **dental surgery** involving nasal administration of subanaesthetic concentrations of **N$_2$O,** e.g. 10% in O$_2$ slowly increased to 30–50%. Verbal contact is maintained at all times, and the concentration of N$_2$O reduced if excessive drowsiness occurs. Performed by the dentist, it depends partly on suggestion.

Renal blood flow (RBF). Normally 1200 ml/min (400 ml/100 g/min); i.e. 22% of **cardiac output.**
- Measurement:
 –direct: circumferential **electromagnetic flow measurement, Doppler** or thermodilution techniques.
 –indirect:
  –**clearance** methods: a substance neither metabolized nor taken up by the kidney, and completely cleared, is required, e.g. *para*-amino hippuric acid (PAH). Clearance then equals renal plasma flow. RBF = plasma flow divided by (1–haematocrit). Continuous iv infusion of PAH is required; inaccuracies may occur since clearance of PAH is only 90% in man. Radioactive markers have been used; almost 100% cleared, they require only a single injection.
  –digital subtraction angiography and radioactive inert gas washout techniques have also been used, the latter indicating regional blood flow.
- Affected by:
 –arterial BP: maintained by **autoregulation** at MAP between 60–160 mmHg in normal subjects.
 –**sympathetic nervous system**: stimulation causes vasoconstriction and reduction of RBF, and also increases release of renin and **prostaglandins. Dopamine** is thought to increase RBF by vasodilatation via **dopamine receptors.**
 –**renin/angiotensin system**: angiotensin II decreases RBF via vasoconstriction, and increases **aldosterone** secretion. The latter increases fluid retention which reduces further renin release.
 –**vasopressin**: causes renal vasoconstriction, especially cortical.
 –intravascular volume: in **haemorrhage,** autoregulation is overridden, with vasoconstriction and intrarenal redistribution of blood away from the cortex.
 –prostaglandins: increase cortical blood flow, and reduce medullary blood flow.
 –**atrial natriuretic peptide**: causes vasodilatation, although effects on RBF are unclear. May alter blood flow distribution.

RBF and **GFR** are reduced by most anaesthetic agents, mainly via reduced cardiac output and BP. Volatile agents are also thought to interfere with autoregulation, although some benefit may arise from the vasodilatation they cause, maintaining blood flow. **Urine** output therefore often falls peroperatively.

Other factors include pre-existing renal disease or conditions predisposing to **renal failure** or impairment, e.g. vascular surgery, toxic drugs, **trauma**, **jaundice**, **hypovolaemia**, etc.

Renal failure. Loss of renal function causing increases in plasma **urea** and **creatinine**. Divided into acute and chronic renal failure.

- Acute renal failure (ARF):
  - often reversible, and occurs over a few days.
  - may develop with or without pre-existing renal impairment. ARF may follow major surgery (especially involving the heart and great vessels), surgery in the presence of hepatic impairment, trauma, obstetric emergencies, and any condition involving hypotension.
  - classically divided thus:
    - prerenal: caused by renal hypoperfusion, e.g. **shock**, **hypovolaemia**, **cardiac failure**, renal artery stenosis.
    - renal: caused by renal disease:
      - glomerular, e.g.:
        - **glomerulonephritis**.
        - **diabetes mellitus**.
        - amyloid.
      - tubulointerstitial, e.g.:
        - acute tubular necrosis (ATN): accounts for 75% of hospital ARF. Caused by renal hypoperfusion or ischaemia and/or chemical toxicity, trauma or sepsis. Nephrotoxins include analgesics (e.g. chronic **aspirin** therapy), aminoglycoside **antibacterial drugs**, **immunosuppressive drugs**, **radiological contrast media** and heavy metals. Usually associated with **oliguria** (caused by tubular cell necrosis, tubular obstruction and cortical arteriolar vasoconstriction).
        - acute cortical necrosis: typically associated with placental abruption, eclampsia and septic abortion, but also with factors causing ATN. Confirmed by renal biopsy. Usually irreversible.
        - tubulointerstitial nephritis/pyelonephritis.
        - polycystic renal disease.
        - tubular obstruction, e.g. in myeloma, **myoglobinuria**.
      - vascular, e.g. **hypertension**, **connective tissue disease**.
    - postrenal: caused by obstruction in the urinary collection system, e.g. bladder tumour, prostatic hypertrophy.

  Distinction between renal and pre- or postrenal failure is important since the latter two are potentially treatable before renal failure becomes established.
  - features:
    - oliguria.
    - **uraemia** and accumulation of other substances (e.g. ammonia): nausea, vomiting, malaise, increased bleeding and susceptibility to infection, decreased healing.

Table 30. Investigations used to differentiate between prerenal oliguria and acute renal failure

Investigation	Prerenal oliguria	Renal failure
Specific gravity	>1.020	<1.010
Urine osmolality (mosmol/kg)	>500	<350
Urine sodium (mmol/l)	<20	>40
Urine/plasma osmolality	>2	<1.1
Urine/plasma urea	>20	<10
Urine/plasma creatinine	>40	<20
Fractional sodium excretion	<1	>1
Renal failure index	<1	>1

Fractional sodium excretion =
$$\frac{\text{urine/plasma sodium ratio}}{\text{urine/plasma creatinine ratio}} \times 100\%$$

and renal failure index =
$$\frac{\text{urine sodium}}{\text{urine/plasma creatinine ratio}}$$

  - reduced sodium and water excretion and **oedema**, **hypertension**, **hyperkalaemia**, **acidosis**.
  - the following may aid diagnosis:
    - examination of **urine**: e.g. tubular casts may be seen in ATN.
    - plasma and urine indices (Table 30).
    - assessment of cardiac and fluid volume state to exclude hypovolaemia.
    - effect of a fluid challenge of, e.g. 200–300 ml: increased urine output may occur in incipient prerenal failure.
    - diuretic administration, e.g. **frusemide** followed by **mannitol**: increased urine output may occur in incipient ATN but there is no evidence of a prophylactic or therapeutic effect.
  - management:
    - directed at the primary cause, e.g. increasing renal blood flow.
    - monitoring of weight, cardiovascular status including JVP/CVP/pulmonary capillary wedge pressure as appropriate, urea and electrolytes, and acid–base status. Accurate fluid charts are vital.
    - fluid restriction to, e.g. previous hour's urine output + 30 ml/h whilst oliguric.
    - **H$_2$ receptor antagonists** are commonly administered since GIT haemorrhage is common.
    - treatment of hyperkalaemia.
    - **dialysis**.
    - adequate **nutrition**.
- Chronic renal failure (CRF):
  - irreversible, and often follows ARF.
  - glomerulonephritis is the most common cause, with others including pyelonephritis, diabetes, polycystic disease, vascular disease and hypertension, drugs and familial causes.
  - features (may not be present until **GFR** falls below 15 ml/min):
    - malaise, anorexia, confusion leading to convulsions and coma. Peripheral and **autonomic neuropathy** may occur.
    - oedema, **pericarditis**, hypertension (in 80%;

thought to result from increased **renin/angiotensin system** activity, sodium and water retention, and secondary **hyperaldosteronism**), peripheral vascular disease, **cardiac failure**.

–nausea, vomiting, diarrhoea.

–osteomalacia, muscle weakness, bone pain, **hypocalcaemia**, **hyperparathyroidism**.

–amenorrhoea, impotence.

–pruritus, skin pigmentation, poor healing, increased susceptibilty to infection.

–normocytic normochromic **anaemia**: caused by reduced **erythropoietin** production, shortened red cell survival and bone marrow depression. Reduced **platelet** function may cause bruising and bleeding.

–**hypernatraemia** or **hyponatraemia** may occur. Hyperkalaemia is usual, but **hypokalaemia** may follow diuretic therapy. Acidosis is common.

  –management:

  –reduction of dietary protein.

  –control of hypertension and cardiac failure.

  –erythropoietin is increasingly used for anaemia.

  –dialysis.

  –**renal transplantation**.

● Anaesthesia in renal failure:

  –preoperatively:

  –assessment for the above features, in particular cardiovascular complications, fluid and electrolyte and acid-base derangements. Dialysis may be required. Anaemia rarely requires transfusion because of its chronicity with compensatory mechanisms. Patients may be at risk from **aspiration of gastric contents** if autonomic neuropathy is present.

  –drugs taken commonly include antianginal and **antihypertensive drugs**, **insulin** and **steroid therapy**.

  –pre-existing arteriovenous fistulae should be noted.

  –**premedication** as required.

  –peroperatively:

  –iv cannulae should not be sited near arteriovenous fistulae.

  –potassium-containing iv fluids should be avoided.

  –preferred drugs are those that are not primarily excreted renally. Thus a common technique consists of any iv anaesthetic agent followed by **atracurium** and **isoflurane**.

  –drugs which accumulate in renal failure, e.g. **morphine**, should be used with caution. Patients are thought to be more sensitive to many iv agents including opioids because of smaller volumes of distribution and reduced plasma albumin levels.

  –**suxamethonium** is not contraindicated unless there is pre-existing peripheral neuropathy or hyperkalaemia.

  –drugs which may impair renal function should be avoided. **Enflurane** has been avoided because of **fluoride ion** formation, although the need for this is controversial since plasma levels attained are low.

  –regional techniques are often suitable, e.g. **brachial plexus block** for fistula formation.

  –postoperatively: close attention to fluid balance is required.

Byrick RJ, Rose DK (1990) Can J Anaesth; 37: 457–67

Renal failure index, *see Renal failure*

Renal transplantation. First performed in 1950, and now widespread but limited mainly by the supply of kidneys. Cadaveric graft survival is up to 80% at 2 years. Previously considered an emergency and performed on unprepared patients, but the importance of proper **preoperative assessment** and preparation is now generally accepted. **Dialysis** is usually performed within 24 hours before surgery.

● Anaesthetic problems and techniques are as for chronic **renal failure** and **transplantation**. Additional points:

  –general anaesthesia is preferred, although **extradural** and **spinal anaesthesia** have been successfully used.

  –direct arterial monitoring is not necessarily required, but **CVP** monitoring is usual, to guide per- and postoperative fluid therapy. Optimal hydration is vital to encourage graft function.

  –**mannitol**, **frusemide** or low-dose **dopamine** are sometimes given before the vessels to the new kidney are unclamped, in order to stimulate urine production.

  –transient hypertension may follow unclamping of the renal vessels.

Both live and cadaveric donors should be well hydrated to maintain urine output before harvesting.

Rudge CJ (1992) Curr Anaesth Crit Care; 3: 156–61
See also, Organ donation

Renal tubular acidosis. Group of conditions characterized by decreased ability of each **nephron** to excrete **hydrogen ions** (cf. **renal failure**, where the overall number of functioning nephrons is reduced, but those that remain excrete more hydrogen ions than normal). May be associated with distal tubule dysfunction (type 1), proximal tubule dysfunction (type 2; usually associated with other abnormalities of proximal tubule function, e.g. Fanconi's syndrome), or **aldosterone** deficiency or resistance (type 4). **Acidosis** may be severe, and accompanied by marked **hypokalaemia**. Treatment includes alkali (e.g. oral sodium bicarbonate) in types 1 and 2, thiazides in type 2, and mineralocorticoid therapy in type 4.

[Guido Fanconi (1892–1979), Swiss paediatrician]

Renin/angiotensin system. Renin, a glycoprotein hormone (mw 37 326), is synthesized and secreted by the **juxtacapillary apparatus** of the renal tubule. Formed from two prehormones, prorenin and preprorenin, its **half-life** is about 80 minutes. Secretion increases in **hypovolaemia**, **cardiac failure**, cirrhosis and renal artery stenosis. Secretion is decreased by angiotensin II and **vasopressin**. Renin acts upon the circulating glycoprotein angiotensinogen with subsequent production of the peptides angiotensin I, II and III, involved in **arterial BP** control and **fluid balance** (Table 31). Angiotensin I functions as a precur-

Table 31. Peptides of the renin/angiotensin system

Substance	Converted to	By the action of	Site
Angiotensinogen	Angiotensin I	Renin	Plasma
Angiotensin I	Angiotensin II	Angiotensin converting enzyme	Mainly in lungs
Angiotensin II	Angiotensin III	Aminopeptidase	Many tissues

sor only. Angiotensin II is a powerful vasoconstrictor with a half-life of a few minutes. It causes aldosterone release from the adrenal cortex, and **noradrenaline** release from sympathetic nerve endings. It also stimulates thirst and release of vasopressin, and acts directly on renal tubules resulting in sodium and water retention. Some may also be produced in the tissues. Angiotensin III also causes aldosterone release and some vasoconstriction.

Angiotensin converting enzyme inhibitors are used to treat hypertension.

Angiotensin II has been used as a **vasopressor drug** when α-agonists are unable to correct severe hypotension, e.g. during surgery for hepatic tumours secreting vasodilator substances.

Mirendon JV, Grissom TE (1991) Anesth Analg; 72: 667–83

Reptilase time, *see Coagulation studies*

Reserpine. Antihypertensive drug of the Rauwolfia alkaloid family, first used in the 1950s and rarely used now. Depletes postganglionic adrenergic neurones of **noradrenaline** by preventing its reuptake from axoplasm into storage granules. Crosses the **blood–brain barrier** and depletes central amine stores. Effects may last 1–2 weeks.

Side effects include bradycardia and postural hypotension, depression, sedation, extrapyramidal signs, diarrhoea and weight gain. Directly acting **sympathomimetic drugs** should be used in preference to indirectly acting ones, if required.

[Leonhard Rauwolf (1535–1596), German botanist]

Reservoir bag. Usually 2 litre capacity in most adult **anaesthetic breathing systems** and 0.5–1.0 litre for paediatric use; its volume must exceed tidal volume. Movement indicates ventilation, but estimation of tidal volume from the amount of movement is inaccurate. Made of rubber, distending when under pressure; maximal pressure is thus prevented from rising above about 60 cmH$_2$O (**Laplace's law**) unless the bag is particularly stiff or enclosed by string mesh (as required for certain ventilating vents/**ventilators**). Such bags should not be used in routine breathing systems.

Residual volume (RV). Volume of gas remaining in the lungs after maximal expiration. About 1.5 litres in the average 70 kg male; measured as for **FRC**. Increased RV accounts for most cases of increased FRC.

Resistance. In electrical terms, the ratio between potential difference across a conductor to the current flowing through it (**Ohm's law**). Measured in ohms (Ω). Resistance to **flow** of a fluid through a circular tube is analogous to this; it equals the ratio between the pressure gradient along the tube to the flow through it.

Resistance vessels. Term given to those blood vessels involved in regulation of **SVR**. 50% of resistance to blood flow is due to arterioles, which are thus the main regulators of SVR and therefore distribution of cardiac output.

Resonance. Situation in which an oscillating system responds with maximal amplitude to an alternating external driving force. Occurs when the driving force frequency coincides with the natural oscillatory frequency (resonant frequency) of the system. May occur in pressure transducer systems if long, compliant tubing is used. May give rise to artefacts in the **arterial waveform** during direct **arterial BP measurement**.

Respiration, *see Breathing...; Lung...; Metabolism*

Respirators, *see Ventilators*

Respiratory centres, *see Breathing, control of*

Respiratory depression, *see Hypoventilation*

Respiratory distress syndrome (RDS; Hyaline membrane disease). Occurs in approximately 1% of all live births, almost exclusively in premature babies. Caused by deficiency of **surfactant**. Surfactant is normally detectable in the fetal lung at 24 weeks gestation, although reversal of amniotic fluid lecithin/sphingomyelin ratio (related to fetal lung maturity) only occurs at 30 weeks. Decreased lung **compliance**, increased work of breathing and alveolar collapse may lead to **respiratory failure**, with characteristic granular appearance of the chest X-ray. Treatment is directed towards preventing **hypoxaemia**, e.g. with IPPV, whilst trying to avoid **O$_2$ toxicity** and **retrolental fibroplasia**. Surfactant administration and **extracorporeal membrane oxygenation** have been used.

Respiratory exchange ratio. Estimation of **respiratory quotient** derived from expired CO_2/inspired O$_2$ measurements, thus dependent on ventilation.

Respiratory failure. Defined as an arterial PO$_2$ at sea level, breathing air and at rest, below 8 kPa (60 mmHg), without intracardiac shunting.
- Divided into:
  - type I failure: **hypoxaemia** accompanied by normal or low arterial PCO$_2$. Usually due to $\dot{V}/\dot{Q}$ **mismatch**, with intrapulmonary right-to-left **shunt** if severe. Causes include **chest infection, pulmonary oedema, PE, ARDS, aspiration pneumonitis,** etc. O$_2$ **therapy** often improves $\dot{V}/\dot{Q}$ mismatch but not shunt; the response to breathing 100% O$_2$ may indicate the degree of shunt. PCO$_2$ is often low because of hyperventilation in response to hypoxaemia.
  - type II failure (ventilatory failure): hypoxaemia accompanied by arterial PCO$_2$ exceeding 6.5 kPa (49 mmHg). Causes are as for **hypoventilation**. Acute exacerbation of **COAD** is a common cause.

Diagnosis is made by arterial blood gas analysis, but may be suspected clinically by signs of hypoxaemia and **hypercapnia**, with tachypnoea and use of accessory **respiratory muscles**.
- Treatment:
  - of underlying cause.
  - **O$_2$ therapy.** Should be used cautiously in type II failure if chronic hypercapnia is suspected.
  - respiratory stimulant drugs, e.g. **doxapram,** have been used to avoid **IPPV,** e.g. in COAD.
  - **CPAP** may improve oxygenation and avoid requirement for IPPV.
  - **IPPV** may be required if PCO$_2$ is rising or the patient is exhausted. Criteria similar to those used in **weaning** have been suggested for institution of IPPV. Tracheal intubation is usually performed to allow IPPV,

although **nasal positive pressure ventilation** and IPPV via a facepiece have been used as alternatives.

–**extracorporeal oxygenation** and **extracorporeal CO_2 removal** have been used.

Respiratory function tests, *see Lung function tests*

Respiratory muscle fatigue.
Inability of the respiratory muscles to sustain tension with repeated activity. May be caused by:

–decreased central drive, e.g. caused by CNS depressant drugs (e.g. **opioid analgesic drugs**).

–increased ventilatory load caused by increased **airway resistance** and reduced **compliance** (e.g. **asthma**, **COAD**, etc.), or increased demand (e.g. exercise, fever, hypoxaemia, etc.).

–respiratory muscle weakness (e.g. following prolonged IPPV, malnutrition, electrolyte imbalance, thyroid disorders, hypoxaemia, sepsis, etc.).

Thought to be involved in hypercapnic **respiratory failure** and difficulty in **weaning from ventilators**. Treatment is directed at the underlying cause.

Moxham J (1990) Br J Anaesth; 65: 43–53

Respiratory muscles.
Muscle actions during:

–quiet inspiration :

–**diaphragm** (the most important muscle of respiration) flattens and moves 1–2 cm caudally.

–external intercostal muscles (pass downwards and forwards) lift the upper ribs and sternum up and forwards, and the lower ribs mainly up and outwards. The first rib remains fixed.

–forced inspiration: as above, with the diaphragm descending up to 10 cm, plus accessory muscles:

–scalene muscles.

–sternomastoid.

–serratus anterior.

–pectoralis major.

–ala nasi.

–quiet expiration: passive recoil of chest and abdomen.

–forced expiration: as above, plus:

–abdominal muscles.

–internal intercostal muscles (pass downwards and backwards); opposite action to the external intercostals, and prevent intercostal bulging.

Lumb A (1991) Curr Opin Anaesth; 4: 845–7

Respiratory quotient
(RQ). Ratio of the volume of CO_2 produced by tissues to the volume of O_2 consumed per unit time. Depends on the type of substrate being utilized: RQ of carbohydrate is 1, RQ of fat 0.7 and that of protein about 0.82. Whole body RQ calculated by measurement of expired CO_2 and inspired O_2 approximates to true RQ, since these volumes are affected by respiration. The term **respiratory exchange ratio** (R) is therefore becoming more commonly used for this measurement.

Respiratory stimulant drugs, *see Analeptic drugs; Opioid receptor antagonists*

Respiratory symbols.
By convention, standardized thus:

–general variables:

V = gas volume ⎱ with a dot above, =
Q = volume of blood ⎰ volume per unit time
P = pressure or tension

F = fractional concentration in dry gas mixture
f = respiratory frequency
C = concentration of gas in blood phase
D = **diffusing capacity**
R = **respiratory exchange ratio**
S = saturation of haemoglobin with O_2 or CO_2

A dash above a symbol indicates mean value.

–localization (in subscript):

I = inspired gas
E = expired gas
A = alveolar gas
T = tidal gas
D = dead space gas
B = barometric
a = arterial blood
c = pulmonary capillary blood
v = venous blood

e.g. F_IO_2 = inspired fractional concentration of O_2; P_aO_2 = arterial O_2 tension.

S_pO_2 has been suggested as representing haemoglobin saturation as measured by pulse **oximetry**.

Respirometer.
Device for measuring expiratory gas volumes. Wright's anemometer is most commonly used. Exhaled air is passed into its chamber through oblique slits, creating circular gas flow, and causing rotation of a double-vaned rotor within the chamber. Rotation is measured and displayed as the volume of gas passing through the device, using an indicator needle attached to the vane, and a dial. Electrical versions are also available; rotations of a disc attached to the vane interrupt passage of light between an emitter and photosensitive cell mounted astride the disc.

Wright's respirometer measures gas volume passing in one direction only; thus it may be placed in the 'to and fro' portion of a breathing system. It tends to underestimate at low volumes and overestimate at high volumes, due to inertia/momentum of the vane.

Other respirometers include **flowmeters** whose signals may be integrated to indicate volume.

[Basil M Wright, London physician]

See also, Spirometer

Resuscitation, *see Cardiopulmonary resuscitation*

Resuscitators, *see Self-inflating bags*

Reticular formation/activating system, *see Ascending reticular activating system*

Retrobulbar block.
Performed to allow surgery to the globe of the eye, e.g. cataract extraction, when combined with **facial nerve block** and conjunctival anaesthesia. The long and short ciliary nerves are blocked within the cone formed by the extraocular muscles.

With the patient supine and looking upwards and to the opposite side, a 3.5 cm needle is introduced through the lower eyelid at the inferolateral edge of the orbit, and advanced along the orbital floor until its tip lies at the tip of the orbit. After aspiration, 2–4 ml **local anaesthetic agent**, e.g. 2% **lignocaine**, is slowly injected. Produces extraocular muscle paralysis, pupillary dilatation and reduced **intraocular pressure**.

Complications include retrobulbar haemorrhage causing proptosis, intravascular and subarachnoid injec-

tion, the latter causing apnoea and cardiovascular collapse. **Peribulbar block** has been suggested as a safer alternative.
See also, Ophthalmic surgery

Retrolental fibroplasia (Retinopathy of prematurity). Abnormal proliferation of retinal vessels in response to high arterial P_O_2 for long periods. Very premature infants of low birth weight are the most susceptible, remaining so until 44 weeks postconceptual age. O_2 therapy should therefore be monitored closely. Precise mechanisms are unclear, as it may occur in infants who have not received additional O_2. The role of O_2 administered during anaesthesia is controversial, but F_IO_2 is generally thought to be best restricted to 0.3 unless higher concentrations are required to maintain arterial P_O_2 of 8.5–11 kPa (60–80 mmHg).
Phelps DL (1992) New Engl J Med; 326: 1078–80

Retzius cave block. Used to supplement anaesthesia for prostatectomy and bladder surgery. The cave of Retzius is the space between the bladder and pubic symphysis, containing nerves of the **sacral plexus** and a venous plexus. After subcutaneous infiltration 2–3 cm above the pubis, an 8 cm needle is directed to the back of the symphysis. After careful aspiration, 10 ml **local anaesthetic agent** with adrenaline is injected in the midline, with a further injection on each side.
[Anders Retzius (1796–1860), Swedish anatomist]

Reuben valve, *see Non-rebreathing valves*

Reye's syndrome. Rare condition of unknown aetiology, characterized by vomiting, depression of consciousness and **hepatic failure**. **Jaundice** is typically absent or minimal. Usually occurs in children, typically following a viral illness; **aspirin** has been implicated in epidemiological studies and is thus contraindicated in children. Thought to be due to an acquired mitochondrial abnormality. Treatment is mainly supportive, with correction of metabolic disturbances, **cerebral oedema** and raised **ICP**. Thought to be improved by administering up to a third of the fluid intake as 10% dextrose.
[Ralph Reye (1912–1977), Australian pathologist]
Glasgow JFT, Hicks EM, Jenkins JG et al (1985) Br J Hosp Med; 34: 42–5

Reynolds' number (*Re*). Dimensionless number predicting when **flow** of a **fluid** becomes turbulent:

$$Re = \frac{\text{density} \times \text{velocity} \times \text{diameter of tube}}{\textbf{viscosity}}$$

Turbulent flow occurs at *Re* >2000, laminar flow at <2000.
[Osborne Reynolds (1842–1912), Irish-born English engineer]

Rhabdomyolysis, *see Myoglobinuria*

Rhesus blood groups. System of **blood group** antigens first described in 1939 following work on rhesus monkeys. Includes many antigens (agglutinogens) but the terms Rhesus (Rh) positive and negative usually refer to the D agglutinogen, as it is the most antigenic. Rh negative individuals have no D antigen, and form anti-D antibodies when injected with Rh positive blood. 85% of Caucasians are Rh positive, 99% of Orientals.

- Clinical importance:
  - **blood transfusion** reactions: administration of Rh positive blood to Rh negative individuals with anti-D antibodies following previous exposure to Rh positive blood.
  - haemolytic disease of the newborn: occurs in Rh positive fetuses of Rh negative mothers. Passage of fetal blood cells into the maternal circulation during labour causes formation of maternal anti-D antibodies. These may pass into subsequent Rh positive fetuses, causing haemolysis which may be fatal. Incidence of primary immunization in primigravidae is about 15%. Uncommon now with widespread availability of anti-Rh immunoglobulin which is administered to Rh negative mothers at delivery, and after abortion, amniocentesis, etc.

Rheumatic fever. Acute disease, thought to be caused by an abnormal immune reaction to certain serotypes of group A Streptococcus. Most common between 5 and 15 years of age; now rare in the West but still common in developing countries. Typically occurring 1–3 weeks after a sore throat, features include fever, flitting arthritis, carditis, chorea and erythema marginatum (erythema speading out from a central macule whilst the centre returns to normal). Subcutaneous nodules may occur over pressure areas. Epistaxis and abdominal pain are common. Diagnosed clinically and by evidence of recent streptococcal infection. Traditionally treated with rest, aspirin and steroids, but the effect of drugs on valve disease is controversial. 50% of patients with carditis progress to valvular heart disease, which may not present until later in life. Mitral and aortic valves are most commonly affected.

Anaesthetic management of patients previously affected is directed towards any existing valve disease, with prophylactic antibiotics as for **congenital heart disease**.
See also, individual valve lesions

Rheumatoid arthritis (Rheumatoid disease). Systemic inflammatory disease with many features of **connective tissue diseases**. Characterized by symmetrical polyarthropathy, but affects other organs too. More common in females; peak incidence is at ages 30–50 years. Up to 5% of females over 60 years are affected in the UK. Aetiology is obscure but may involve an immunological process triggered by infectious agents.

- Anaesthetic considerations:
  - systemic effects:
    - skeletal: **temporomandibular joint** involvment, atlantoaxial subluxation, reduced mobility of the lumbar/**cervical spine**.
    - neuromuscular: nerve entrapment, sensory/motor neuropathy, myopathy.
    - respiratory: restrictive defect due to **pulmonary fibrosis** and costochondral disease, pulmonary nodules, pleural effusions, cricoarytenoid arthritis.
    - cardiovascular: **pericarditis**, conduction defects, coronary arteritis, peripheral vasculitis.
    - haematological: **anaemia** (usually normochromic normocytic), leucopenia. Felty's syndrome consists of rheumatoid arthritis, splenomegaly and leucopenia; **thrombocytopenia**, malaise and fever may occur.

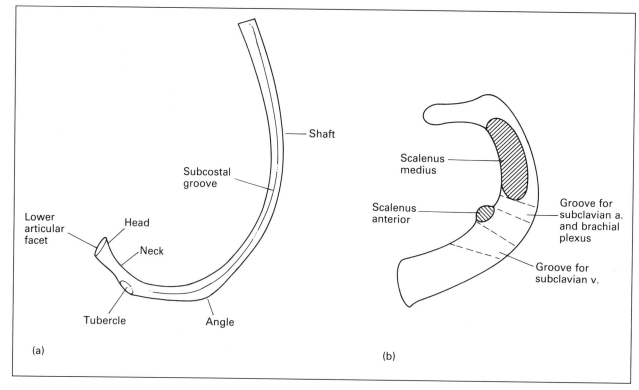

Figure 112 *Anatomy of (a) a typical rib, seen from undersurface; (b) the first rib, seen from above*

–renal: amyloidosis, pyelonephritis, drug-related impairment.
–others: ophthalmic complications including Sjögren's syndrome, and atrophic skin and subcutaneous tissues.
–drug therapy: may include **NSAIDs, steroid therapy** and **immunosuppressive drugs**. Gold may cause blood dyscrasias, peripheral neuritis, pulmonary fibrosis, hepatic and renal impairment. Penicillamine may cause blood dyscrasias, renal impairment, neuropathy and a **myasthenia gravis**-like syndrome.
–practical considerations:
   –drug administration whilst nil by mouth; rectal or im NSAIDs are useful.
   –venous cannulation may be difficult; skin and veins are fragile, and joints may have reduced mobility.
   –discomfort lying flat; skeletal involvement may make regional techniques unsuitable. Careful positioning and padding are required. Skin is easily damaged.
   –airway maintenance difficulties: caused by involvement of the temporomandibular joint, cervical spine and larynx.
[Augustus Felty (1895–1963), US physician; Henrik Sjögren, Swedish ophthalmologist]
See also, Intubation, difficult

Rib fractures. Middle ribs are most commonly affected. Fracture usually occurs at the posterior axillary line, the point of maximal stress. If the first three ribs are affected, injury to the aorta and tracheobronchial tree should be considered. If the lower ribs are involved, damage to liver, spleen and kidneys may occur. **Pneumothorax** and haemothorax may be present.

Rib fractures cause pain on breathing, with splinting of the chest wall, inability to cough and **atelectasis**. Multiple fractures may cause **flail chest**. The mainstay of treatment is good analgesia; this may involve systemic analgesics, **extradural anaesthesia** or **intercostal nerve block**.
General management is as for **chest trauma**.

Ribs. Exist in 12 pairs, with occasional additional cervical or lumbar ribs. Attached to thoracic vertebrae posteriorly and costal cartilage anteriorly. Ribs 2–8 are typical (Fig. 112a), consisting of:
   –head: bears two facets for articulation with adjacent vertebrae.
   –neck.
   –tubercle: articulates posteriorly with the transverse process of the corresponding vertebra.
   –shaft: flattened in the vertical plane. Curves forwards and inwards from the angle, lying lateral to the tubercle. The intercostal neurovascular bundle runs in the subcostal groove at the inferior border.
● The first rib is of particular anaesthetic importance because of its relationship to the **brachial plexus** and other structures (Fig. 112b). Features:
   –short, wide and flattened in the horizontal plane.
   –lower surface is smooth and lies on pleura.
   –upper surface is grooved for the subclavian vessels and brachial plexus.
   –sympathetic chain, superior intercostal artery and upper branch of the first intercostal nerve lie anterior to its neck, between it and the pleura.
   –scalenus anterior and medius attach to the scalene tubercle and body of the rib respectively.
See also, Intercostal nerve block; Intercostal space

Right atrial pressure, *see Cardiac catheterization; Central venous pressure*

Ringer's solution. Developed as an *in vitro* medium for tissues and organisms, emphasizing the importance of inorganic ions in maintaining cellular integrity. Exact constitution varies between laboratories, but approximates to sodium 137 mmol/l, potassium 4 mmol/l, calcium 3 mmol/l and chloride 142 mmol/l. Modifications include Ringer-lactate (**Hartmann's solution**).
[Sydney Ringer (1834–1910), English physician]

Rocuronium (Org 9426). Non-depolarizing **neuromuscular blocking drug**, currently being evaluated. Chemically related to **vecuronium**, with similar lack of cardiovascular effects. Initial studies suggest that its onset of action is faster than with other non-depolarizing agents, with duration of action comparable to vecuronium and **atracurium**.
Booij LHDJ, Knape HTA (1991) Anaesthesia; 46: 341–3

Ropivacaine hydrochloride. Amide **local anaesthetic drug**, currently being evaluated. Chemically related to **bupivacaine**, but thought to be 50% less cardiotoxic. Has been used in 0.5–1% solutions; onset seems quicker than bupivacaine, with possibly longer duration of action.
Reynolds F (1991) Anaesthesia; 46: 339–40

Rotameter. Refers to the trade name of a type of **flowmeter** commonly used on **anaesthetic machines**; first fitted in the 1930s.
• Features include:
–constant pressure, variable orifice.
–consists of a needle valve, below a bobbin within a tapered tube. Gas flow rates are marked along the tube's length. Readings are taken from the top of the bobbin. Tubes are arranged in banks at the back of the anaesthetic machine, traditionally for O_2, CO_2, cyclopropane and N_2O, from left to right in the UK (see below).
–accurate to within 2%.
–bobbins are made of light metal alloy; each is individually matched to its particular tube, and specific for a certain gas.
–the tube's taper is narrower at the bottom to allow accurate measurement of low flow rates, and wider above to measure higher flows.
–the space between the bobbin and walls of tube is narrow at the bottom of the tube; gas **flow** behaves as through a tube, i.e. is largely laminar. Thus gas **viscosity** is important at low flow rates. Higher up the tube, the space between the bobbin and tube is wide compared with the length of the bobbin, because of the tube's taper. Gas flow behaves as through an orifice, i.e. is turbulent. Thus gas density is important at high flow rates.
–inaccuracies may result from sticking of the bobbin against the sides of the tube. This is reduced by:
–keeping the tube vertical to reduce friction between bobbin and tube.
–angular notches in the bobbin, causing it to rotate when gas flows.
–regular cleaning to prevent dirt accumulating within the tube.

–reduction of static charge building up within the tube. Many are internally coated with a thin layer of gold. Alternatively, regular spraying with antistatic solution may be performed.
–the O_2 control knob is larger than the others and differently shaped to aid recognition. All are colour-coded as for **cylinders**.
–the CO_2 rotameter on older machines may be left open by mistake, with the bobbin hidden at the top of the tube. This is less likely in newer versions.
–with the traditional arrangement of rotameters, i.e. O_2 upstream, O_2 may be lost if there is a leak from a tube downstream. This may be prevented by placing the O_2 inlet downstream from the others, e.g. by fitting a baffle across the top of the rotameter tubes so that N_2O enters first, and O_2 last.
–in newer machines, N_2O and O_2 rotameters are connected such that less than 25% O_2 cannot be delivered.

Rowbotham, Edgar Stanley (1890–1979). English pioneer of anaesthesia. With **Magill**, developed tracheal intubation including blind nasal intubation, and endotracheal anaesthesia. Also pioneered **basal narcosis** with rectal **paraldehyde**, and local and intravenous techniques. The first anaesthetist in the UK to use **cyclopropane**. Designed several pieces of apparatus, including a **vaporizer**, airway, local anaesthetic needles and other equipment. Latterly worked at Charing Cross, London. Particularly interested in anaesthesia for thyroid surgery.
Condon HA, Gilchrist E (1986) Anaesthesia; 41: 46–52

Royal College of Anaesthetists. Arose from the granting of a Charter to the **College of Anaesthetists** by Queen Elizabeth II in March 1992.
Spence AA (1992) Br J Anaesth; 68: 457–8

R–R interval. Time between successive **R waves** on the **ECG**. Thus heart rate =

$$\frac{60}{R–R\ interval\ (s)}$$

Normally varies by less than 0.16 seconds at rest (**sinus arrhythmia**). Useful in the diagnosis of **autonomic neuropathy**.

RT, Reptilase time, *see Coagulation studies*

Rule of nines. Guide to the percentage of body **surface area** represented by various parts of the body; used in assessment and treatment of **burns**:
–head: 9%.
–arms: 9% each.
–trunk: 18% front; 18% back.
–legs: 18% each.
–perineum: 1%.
For small areas, the patient's palmar surface represents about 1% of surface area.
• For children, proportions of body parts are different:
–head: 15%.
–arms: 10% each.
–trunk: 20% front; 20% back.
–legs: 12% each.

S

S wave. Downward deflection following the **R wave** of the **ECG** (*see Fig. 49b; Electrocardiography*). Its size usually decreases from V_2 to V_6; the deepest wave is normally less than 30 mm. Prominence in standard leads I, II and III ($S_1S_2S_3$ pattern) may be normal in young people but may be associated with right ventricular hypertrophy. May also be seen in **MI** along with other changes. *See also, QRS complex*

SA node, Sinoatrial node, *see Heart, conducting system*

Sacral canal. Cavity, 10–15 cm long and triangular in section, running the length of the sacrum, itself formed from five fused sacral **vertebrae** (Fig. 113). Continuous cranially with the lumbar **vertebral canal**. The anterior wall is formed by the fused bodies of the sacral vertebrae, and the posterior walls by the fused sacral laminae. Due to failure of fusion of the fifth laminar arch, the posterior wall is deficient between the cornua, forming the sacral hiatus which is covered by the sacrococcygeal membrane (punctured during **caudal analgesia**). Congenital variants of fusion are common, e.g. deficient fusion of several laminae; this is thought to be a contributing cause of unreliability of caudal analgesia. The canal contains the termination of the dural sac at S2, the sacral nerves and coccygeal nerve, the internal vertebral venous plexus and fat. Its average volume in adults is 32 ml in females and 34 ml in males.

Sacral nerve block, *see Caudal analgesia*

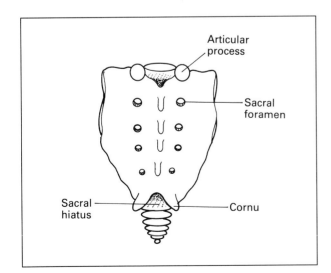

Figure 113 *Anatomy of the sacrum (posterior view)*

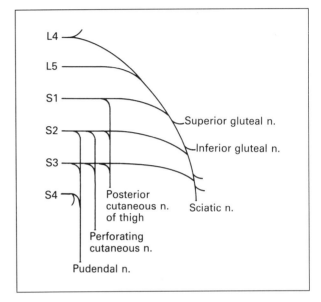

Figure 114 *Plan of the sacral plexus*

Sacral plexus. Supplies the pelvic and hip muscles, and the skin of the buttock and posterior thigh. Lies in front of the sacrum deep to the pelvic fascia, and formed from the anterior primary rami of L4–S4. Its major branch is the **sciatic nerve** (Fig. 114).

Saddle block, *see Spinal anaesthesia*

Salbutamol. β-Adrenergic receptor agonist, used mainly as a **bronchodilator drug**. Selective for $β_2$–receptors, although it does cause slight $β_1$–receptor stimulation. Undergoes extensive **first-pass metabolism** if given orally, thus usually administered by inhalation or iv. Produces bronchodilatation within 15 minutes; effects last 3–4 hours. May also reduce the release of **histamine** and inflammatory mediators from **mast cells** sensitized with IgE, hence its particular use in **asthma**.

Also used as a **tocolytic drug** in premature labour and to improve cardiac output in low perfusion states, via $β_2$–receptor mediated smooth muscle relaxation in the **uterus** and blood vessels respectively.
- Dosage:
    - –2–4 mg orally, 6–8 hourly.
    - –500 µg im/sc, 4 hourly as required.
    - –250 µg iv slowly, repeated as required. 3–20 µg/min infusion may be used. IV injection has been claimed to be more effective than inhalation in severe asthma, but this is controversial. Up to 45 µg/min may be required in premature labour.

–1–2 puffs by aerosol (100–200 µg) 6–8 hourly. 200–400 µg is recommended for dry powder inhalation, since **bioavailability** for the latter is lower.
–2.5–5 mg by nebulized solution, 4–6 hourly.
- Side effects: tachycardia, tremor, headache. **Hypokalaemia** may occur with prolonged use. **Pulmonary oedema** may occur after use for tocolysis.

Salicylate poisoning. **Salicylates** are the most commonly ingested drugs in self-poisoning, accounting for about 10% of cases. Poisoning is usually acute but may be chronic, especially in children.
- Features:
  –nausea, vomiting, sweating, tinnitus, deafness, confusion. Loss of consciousness is uncommon unless in severe poisoning.
  –**hyperventilation** results from direct respiratory centre stimulation, possibly via central uncoupling of oxidative phosphorylation. Respiratory **alkalosis** results. Compensatory renal excretion of **bicarbonate** results in urinary water and potassium loss with **dehydration** and **hypokalaemia**.
  –metabolic **acidosis** is caused by the salicylic acid, and its metabolic effects (increased production of **ketone bodies**, **lactic acid** and pyruvic acid, **hyperglycaemia** or **hypoglycaemia**). Thus the urine, initially alkaline, becomes acid.
  –**convulsions**, **pulmonary oedema**, **hyperthermia** and **renal failure** may occur.
  –impaired **coagulation** is rarely significant.
- Treatment:
  –general measures as for **poisoning and overdose**, e.g. **O$_2$ therapy**, **iv fluid administration**. Gastric lavage may be effective up to 12–24 hours after ingestion, as gastric absorption after high dosage is slow. Activated **charcoal** may be useful.
  –increased elimination may be indicated if plasma levels exceed 500 mg/l (3.6 mmol/l) in adults or 300 g/l (2.2 mmol/l) in children. Techniques include forced alkaline diuresis, **dialysis** and **haemoperfusion**.
See also, Forced diuresis

Salicylates. Group of **NSAIDs** derived from salicylic acid. **Aspirin** (acetylsalicylic acid) is the most commonly prescribed; others, e.g. sodium salicylate, are also available but less potent. Have anti-inflammatory and antipyretic effects; they act via inhibition of synthesis and release of **prostaglandins**. Thought to act (at least partly) centrally, since they are effective when injected into the brains of experimental animals. Inhibit **platelet** and vascular endothelial cyclooxygenase; at low dosage, they selectively inhibit platelet cyclooxygenase. They are thus used as **antiplatelet drugs**. Effects on platelets are irreversible, lasting until new platelets are synthesized (7–10 days).

Used for mild to moderate **pain**, pyrexia, **rheumatic fever**, **rheumatoid arthritis**, and peripheral and coronary artery disease including after coronary artery bypass graft. They are contraindicated in gout because urinary excretion of uric acid may be decreased.

Absorbed rapidly from the upper GIT after therapeutic dosage, with peak plasma levels within 2 hours of ingestion. Absorption is determined by the composition of tablets, intestinal pH and **gastric emptying**. About 90% protein bound, they compete with other substances for protein binding sites, e.g. thyroxine, penicillin, phenytoin. Biotransformation occurs in hepatic endoplasmic reticulum and mitochondria. Excreted mainly in the urine, especially if the latter is alkaline. **Half-life** is about 15 minutes, but is very dependent on the dose taken.
- Side effects: as for NSAIDs and **salicylate poisoning**. They have been implicated in causing **Reye's syndrome** in children.

Salicylates should not be given to children under 12 years, patients with **peptic ulcer disease** or **coagulation disorders**, or those taking **anticoagulant drugs**.

Saline solutions. **IV fluids** containing sodium chloride, used extensively to replace **sodium** and **ECF** losses, e.g. in **dehydration**, and perioperatively. A 0.9% solution is most commonly used ('physiological saline', often erroneously called 'normal saline'); other saline-containing solutions include **Hartmann's solution** and dextrose/saline mixtures. Twice 'normal' saline (0.18%) is used in **hyponatraemia**, and up to 7.5% solutions have been used (largely experimentally) in hypovolaemic **shock**.
See also, Hypertonic intravenous solutions; Normal solution

Samples, statistical. Parts of **populations**, selected for **statistical tests** or analysis. In order to represent the true population, samples should be as large as possible, and free of bias; i.e. should be random. Paired samples refer to groups matched for possible confounding variables, allowing better comparison of the desired measurements. Optimum pairing occurs when subjects act as their own controls.
See also, Clinical trials; Randomization; Statistics

Sanders oxygen injector, *see Injector techniques*

Saphenous nerve block, *see Ankle, nerve blocks; Knee, nerve blocks*

Sarcoidosis. Systemic disease, possibly caused by an infective agent or immunological derangement. The lungs or hilar lymph nodes are affected in over 80% of patients, but the disease may involve the eyes, skin, musculoskeletal system, abdominal organs, heart or nervous system. Often acute in onset and self-limiting.

Diagnosed on clinical grounds, supported by tissue biopsy, chest X-ray, raised angiotensin converting enzyme levels and positive Kveim test (granuloma formation following intradermal injection of sarcoid tissue suspension).

Anaesthetic considerations include the possibility of **pulmonary fibrosis**, **cardiac failure**, **heart block**, laryngeal fibrosis, **renal failure** and **hypercalcaemia**. **Steroid therapy** is often prescribed.
[Morten A Kveim (1892–1967), Norwegian pathologist]

Saturated vapour pressure (SVP). Pressure exerted by the vapour phase of a substance, when in equilibrium with the liquid phase. Indicates the degree of volatility; e.g. for **inhalational anaesthetic agents**, **diethyl ether** (SVP 59 kPa (425 mmHg)) is more volatile and easier to vaporize than **halothane** (SVP 32 kPa (243 mmHg)). SVP increases with temperature, therefore SVPs of volatile agents are quoted at standard temperature (usually 20°C). At **boiling point**, SVP equals atmospheric pressure.
See also, Vapour pressure

Scalp, nerve blocks. Local anaesthetic infiltration is usually performed with added vasoconstrictor, e.g. **adrenaline**, because of the rich vascular supply of the scalp. Injection is performed first in the subcutaneous tissue above the aponeurosis (where nerves and vessels lie), then below. Infiltration in a band around the head, above the ears and eyebrows, provides anaesthesia of the scalp. Individual branches of the **maxillary nerve** may also be blocked. The occipital nerves supplying the posterior scalp may be blocked by infiltrating between the mastoid process and occipital protuberance on each side.

Scavenging. Removal of waste gases from the expiratory port of **anaesthetic breathing systems**; thought to be desirable because of the possible adverse effects of chronic and short-term exposure to **inhalational anaesthetic agents**. Adsorption of volatile agents using activated **charcoal** (Aldasorber device) has been used but is ineffective at removing N_2O.
- Scavenging systems consist of:
  - collecting system: usually a shroud enclosing the **adjustable pressure limiting valve**. For paediatric breathing systems, several attachments have been described, including various connectors and funnels.
  - tubing: standard plastic tubing is usual; all connections should be 30 mm to avoid accidental connection to the breathing system.
  - receiving system: incorporates a reservoir to enable adequate removal of gases even if the volume cleared per minute is less than peak expiratory flow rate. May use rubber bags or rigid bottles, etc. If the system is closed, a **dumping valve** and pressure-relief valve are required to prevent excess negative or positive pressure, respectively, being applied to the patient's airway. Vents are often present in rigid reservoirs. Requirements:
    - negative pressure: maximum 0.5 cmH$_2$O at 30 l/min gas flow.
    - positive pressure: maximum 5 cmH$_2$O at 30 l/min gas flow, and 10 cmH$_2$O at 90 l/min. Ideally, the relief valve should be as near to the expiratory valve as possible.
  - disposal system: may be:
    - passive: no external energy supply; the gases pass through wide bore tubing to the roof of the building, terminating in a ventile. Maximal resistance should be 0.5 cmH$_2$O at 30 l/min. The least efficient system, since it depends on wind direction. Requires a water trap to remove condensed water vapour.
    - assisted passive: employs the air-conditioning system's extractor ducts.
    - active: uses a dedicated fan system or **ejector flowmeter**. Requires a low-pressure high-volume system (able to remove 75 l/min with a peak flow of 130 l/min); thus hospital **suction apparatus** is unsuitable.

USA maximal levels of inhalational agents: 2 ppm volatile agent or 25 ppm N_2O.

Gray WM (1985) Br J Anaesth; 57: 685–95

See also, COSHH regulations; Environmental safety of anaesthetists

Schimmelbusch mask, *see Open-drop techniques*

Sciatic nerve block. Used for surgery to the lower leg, usually combined with **femoral nerve block**, **obturator nerve block** and **lateral cutaneous nerve of the thigh block** (*see Fig. 57; Femoral nerve block*). May also be performed to provide analgesia after fractures, or **sympathetic nerve block** of the foot.

The sciatic nerve (L4–S3) arises from the **sacral plexus**, leaving the pelvis through the greater sciatic foramen beneath piriformis muscle, and between the ischial tuberosity and the greater trochanter of the femur. It becomes superficial at the lower border of gluteus maximus, and runs down the posterior aspect of the thigh to the **popliteal fossa**, where it divides into tibial and common peroneal nerves. It supplies the hip and knee joints, posterior muscles of the leg, and skin of the leg and foot below the knee except for the medial calf. The posterior cutaneous nerve of the thigh runs close to it and is usually blocked with it.
- Three different approaches are commonly used:
  - posterior: with the patient lying with the side to be blocked uppermost, and the uppermost knee flexed, a line is drawn between the greater trochanter and posterior superior iliac spine. At the line's midpoint, a perpendicular is dropped 3 cm, and a 12 cm needle introduced at this point, at right angles to the skin. The nerve lies on the ischial spine, and is identified by its feel and by elicitation of paraesthesiae (a nerve stimulator is particularly useful). 15–30 ml **local anaesthetic agent** is injected. Onset of blockade may take 30 minutes.
  - anterior: with the patient lying supine, a line is drawn between the pubic tubercle and anterior superior iliac spine, and divided into thirds. A perpendicular is dropped from the junction of the medial and middle thirds. Another line, parallel with the original line, is drawn from the greater trochanter; its intersection with the perpendicular marks the site of needle insertion. A 12 cm needle is directed slightly laterally to encounter the femur, then withdrawn and directed medial to the femur to a depth of 5 cm from the femur's anterior edge. 15–30 ml solution is injected. This approach is particularly useful if movement is painful, e.g. fractured femur.
  - lithotomy: with the hip and knee on the side to be blocked flexed to 90°, a needle is inserted perpendicular to the skin at the midpoint of a line between the greater trochanter and the ischial tuberosity. 15–20 ml solution is injected at a depth of 5–6 cm. The posterior cutaneous branch (supplying the posterior thigh) may be missed.

A lateral approach has also been described.

Scleroderma, *see Connective tissue diseases*

Scoliosis, *see Kyphoscoliosis*

Scopolamine, *see Hyoscine*

SDD, *see Selective decontamination of the digestive tract*

Second. SI **unit** of time; defined according to the frequency of radiation emitted by caesium-133 in its lowest energy (ground) state.

Second gas effect. Increased alveolar concentration of a less soluble **inhalational anaesthetic agent**, e.g. N_2O, following rapid uptake of an accompanying soluble agent, e.g. **halothane**. Thus the uptake of the N_2O is increased. Analogous but opposite to the **Fink effect** at the end of anaesthesia.

Second messenger. Intracellular substance, e.g. **cAMP**, **calcium** ions, linking extracellular chemical messengers (first messengers) with the physiological response.
Michell RH (1987) BMJ; 295: 1320–3

Sedation. State of reduced consciousness in which verbal contact with the patient may be maintained. Used to reduce discomfort during unpleasant procedures, e.g. **regional anaesthesia, dental surgery**, endoscopy, **cardiac catheterization**, etc., and on **ICU**. For short procedures, drugs of short duration of action and causing minimal cardiorespiratory depression are preferable. Best control is usually achieved with iv administration, although other routes may be used, e.g. oral **premedication**. Full **monitoring** should be employed during procedures as for general anaesthesia. Drugs may be given by small bolus repeated as necessary, or by continuous infusion; the latter is easier to titrate. The level of sedation required depends on the individual patient and the procedure performed.

On ICU, sedative and analgesic drugs are given to reduce pain, distress and anxiety, and to aid toleration of tracheal tubes, IPPV, tracheal suction, physiotherapy, etc. Cardiovascular depression is particularly undesirable, although respiratory depression may be an advantage if IPPV is required. Long-term administration is often required; thus side effects not seen after brief administration may occur, and drugs with long **half-lives** may cumulate. The desired end-point is usually a peaceful, cooperative patient who can respond to commands, with deeper levels of sedation provided for stimulating procedures, e.g. physiotherapy. Scoring systems have been devised to assist titration of drugs.

- Although described for iv use in ICU, the following drugs may also be used for short procedures:
  - **opioid analgesic drugs**: commonly used on ICU. Provide analgesia and euphoria, and aid toleration of IPPV. All produce respiratory depression; thus they should be used cautiously in patients breathing spontaneously. Hypotension is particularly likely if **hypovolaemia** is present and following rapid iv injection. GIT motility is reduced. Drugs used include:
    - **morphine** 2.5–5 mg boluses (20–60 µg/kg/h infusion), or **papaveretum** 5–10 mg boluses (40–100 µg/kg/h). Cumulation of metabolites may occur after prolonged infusion, especially in renal failure. Increased susceptibility to infection has been shown in experimental animals receiving very large doses.
    - **pethidine** 0.5–2 mg/kg/h. Myocardial depression may occur at high levels. Cumulation is particularly likely in hepatic failure, and cumulation of norpethidine (has convulsant properties) in renal failure.
    - **fentanyl** 1–5 µg/kg/h; cumulation readily occurs after prolonged infusion, since its short duration of action initially is due to redistribution, and **clearance** is slower than that of morphine.
    - **alfentanil** 30–60 µg/kg/h; increasingly used since cumulation is less likely.
    - **phenoperidine** 10–50 µg/kg/h. Hypotension is common. Increased **ICP** has been reported.

  - **benzodiazepines**: often used in conjunction with opioids. Widely used for short procedures. May produce cardiorespiratory depression, and may cumulate in impaired hepatic/renal function and after prolonged administration. Verbal contact with the patient may be impaired. **Flumazenil** has been used to reverse sedation. Commonly used drugs:
    - **diazepam** 2.5–10 mg boluses. It and its metabolites have long duration of action.
    - **midazolam** 2–5 mg boluses (50–200 µg/kg/h infusion). Particularly likely to cause hypotension.
  - **iv anaesthetic agents**, e.g.:
    - **ketamine** 5–10 mg boluses (1–2 mg/kg/h infusion). Has been used during regional anaesthesia, but rarely used in ICU except in **asthma**.
    - **thiopentone** 1–3 mg/kg/h; mainly used in neurological disease. Recovery may be prolonged.
    - **propofol** 1.0–4.0 mg/kg/h; allows rapid recovery. Convulsions have been reported after its use, but its role in this respect is unclear. Hypotension may be marked. Licensed for 3 days' sedation of adults (but should be avoided in children).
    - **etomidate**: no longer used because of adrenal suppression.
  - **inhalational anaesthetic agents**:
    - **N_2O** up to 70% is commonly used during regional anaesthesia, but haematological side effects preclude prolonged or frequent use.
    - **isoflurane** has been used on ICU with good results, although high plasma levels of **fluoride ions** have been reported after prolonged use.
  - others, e.g.:
    - **chlormethiazole** 30–60 ml/h of 0.8% solution. Water intoxication may occur with prolonged use.
    - **droperidol, chlorpromazine**; rarely used.
    - **chloral hydrate** 30–50 mg orally/rectally repeated as required; may be useful in children.

Neuromuscular blocking drugs are sometimes used in ICU to facilitate IPPV, especially if chest compliance is reduced or ICP is raised. Their use has declined in recent years because of the risk of paralysis with concurrent inadequate sedation, increased risk from accidental disconnection, possible increased incidence of **DVT** and **PE**, and impaired communication. **Atracurium** and **vecuronium** are most commonly used.

NSAIDs, etc. and regional techniques may also be used to provide analgesia in ICU.
Aitkenhead AR (1989) Br J Anaesth; 63: 196–206

Seebeck effect, *see Temperature measurement*

Seldinger technique. Method of percutaneous cannulation of a blood vessel, described in 1953. A needle is inserted into the vessel, and a guidewire passed through it. After removal of the needle, the cannula is introduced into the vessel over the wire, which is then removed. Refinements include the use of a dilator, passed over the wire to enlarge the hole made by the needle, before the cannula is inserted. Widely used for **central venous cannulation**; favoured by many as being safer and more reliable than using cannula-over-needle techniques, although more costly.
[Sven-Ivar Seldinger, Swedish radiologist]

Selective decontamination of the digestive tract (SDD; selective parenteral and enteral antisepsis regimen;

SPEAR). Technique for preventing endogenous infections in patients requiring ventilatory support on **ICU**. SDD aims to prevent colonization of the GIT by potentially pathogenic organisms, based on the premise that most infections on ICU are endogenous.

Non-absorbable **antibacterial drugs** (e.g. tobramycin, polymixin E, amphotericin B) are administered to the pharynx/mouth/upper GIT, whilst another (e.g. cefotaxime) is administered iv. Sparing of the normal anaerobic GIT organisms prevents overgrowth by pathogens. SDD significantly reduces nosocomial infection, although it has not consistently decreased mortality. Its place in ICU is therefore yet to be determined.
Vandebroucke-Grauls CMJE, Vandebroucke JP (1991) Lancet; 338: 859–61

Self-inflating bags. Rubber or silicone bags used for IPPV, which reinflate when released after compression. Thus may be used for IPPV without requiring an external gas supply, e.g. during **draw-over anaesthesia**, transfer of ventilated patients, or **CPR**. May be thick-walled or lined with foam-rubber. Usually assembled with a **non-rebreathing valve** at the outlet and a one-way valve at the inlet; thus fresh air is drawn in during refilling. O_2 may be added through a port at the inlet; a reservoir bag may also be added to the inlet to increase F_1O_2. Available in adult and paediatric sizes. **Bellows** may be used in a similar way, but are less convenient to use.

Sellick's manoeuvre, *see Cricoid pressure*

Semon's law, *see Laryngeal nerves*

Sengstaken–Blakemore tube. Double-cuffed gastric tube designed to compress gastro-oesophageal varices, thereby controlling bleeding. Passed via the mouth into the stomach; the distal cuff is then inflated with 150–250 ml air, preventing accidental removal. The proximal cuff is then inflated to 30–40 mmHg (4–5 kPa), compressing

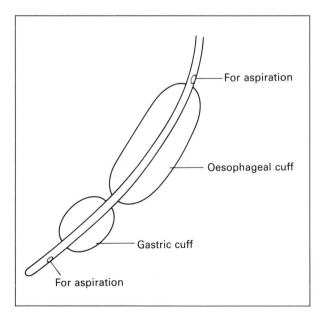

Figure 115 *Distal end of Sengstaken–Blakemore tube*

the varices. Traction has been advocated but is rarely used. Newer versions include channels for aspiration of gastric and oesophageal contents (Fig. 115); the latter may be aspirated continuously to reduce pulmonary soiling. Thus four lumina may be present:
–for aspiration above the oesophageal cuff.
–for aspiration from the stomach.
–for inflation of each cuff.
Usually kept inflated for 12–24 hours; the oesophageal cuff is deflated first. Careful placement is essential to avoid airway obstruction, pulmonary aspiration, ischaemic necrosis of gastric mucosa, oesophageal rupture, etc. The tubes are very uncomfortable.
[Robert W Sengstaken and Arthur H Blakemore (1879–1970), US surgeons]
McCormick PA, Burroughs AK, McIntyre N (1990) Br J Hosp Med; 43: 274–7

Sensitivity. In **statistics**, the ability of a test to exclude false positives. Equals

$$\frac{\text{the number tested as positive}}{\text{total with the condition.}}$$

See also, Errors; Predicitve value; Specificity

Sensory evoked potentials, *see Evoked potentials*

Sensory pathways. The sensory system includes the special senses, visceral sensation and general somatic sensation. The latter is divided into:
–exteroreceptive sensation: provides information about the external environment and includes modalities such as touch, pressure, temperature and **pain**.
–proprioceptive sensation: provides information about body position and movement.
Free nerve endings may be associated with **nociception**. Some nerve endings are 'specialized', e.g. Meissner's corpuscles (touch), Pacinian corpuscles (vibration and joint position) and Ruffini corpuscles (joint position). The last two may be involved with **muscle spindles**.
● The sensory fibres enter the **spinal cord** through the dorsal root, their cell bodies lying in the dorsal root ganglia. Subsequent pathways (Fig. 116):
–proprioception, vibration and ½ touch sensation:
–first order **neurones** turn medially and ascend in the ipsilateral posterior columns to the lower medulla, where they synapse with cells in the cuneate or gracile nuclei.
–second order neurones cross the contralateral side of the medulla and ascend in the medial lemniscus to the ventral posterolateral nucleus of the **thalamus**.
–third order neurones project to the sensory cortex.
–pain, temperature and the remainder of touch sensation:
–first order neurones synapse in the dorsal horn of the spinal cord (mainly in laminae VI and VII).
–most of the second order neurones cross (either at the same level or 1–2 segments higher) to reach the spinothalamic tracts. In the medulla, the latter form the spinal lemniscus, which ascends to the thalamus.
–third order neurones project to the sensory cortex.
The primary somatosensory area of the cerebral cortex is in the postcentral gyrus, although there is a large distrib-

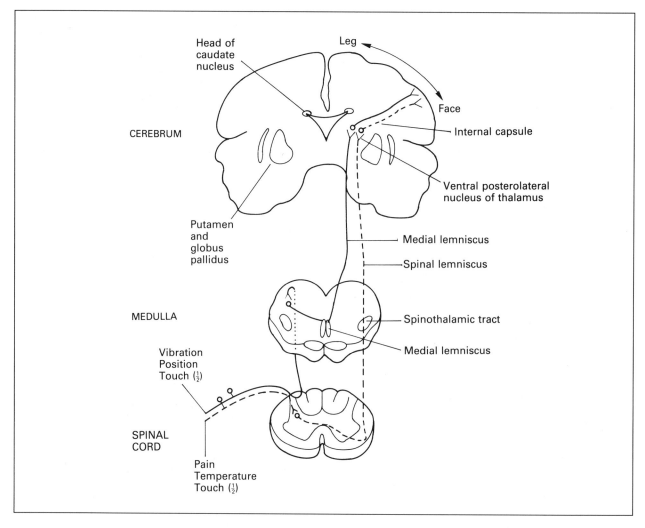

Figure 116 *Anatomy of sensory pathways*

ution of sensory fibres in other areas. Regions of greatest importance (e.g. face, mouth, hands) have a disproportionately greater representation than other areas.

- Signs of sensory pathway loss:
  – peripheral nerve lesion: complete loss of sensation in the nerve's distribution (although the zone of loss may be limited because of overlap between nerves).
  – posterior root lesion: pain and paraesthesiae are experienced in the dermatomal distribution. If the root involves a **reflex arc**, the reflex will be diminished or lost.
  – posterior column lesion: ipsilateral loss of position and vibration sense with preservation of pain, touch and temperature sensation.
  – spinothalamic tract lesion: contralateral loss of pain and temperature sensation.
  – **brainstem** and thalamus lesions: upper brainstem or thalamic lesions may cause complete hemisensory disturbance with loss of postural sense, light touch and pain sensation. 'Pure' thalamic lesions may result in **central pain**.
  – sensory cortex lesions: paraesthesiae may be felt, with or without disturbed appreciation of sensation, e.g.

inability to distinguish between heat and pain, or inability to identify objects by touch, etc.

[Georg Meissner (1829–1905), German anatomist; Filippo Pacini (1812–1883), Italian anatomist; Angelo Ruffini (1864–1929), Italian histologist]

See also, Dermatomes; Spinal cord lesions

Sepsis syndrome. Describes the systemic host response to infection with microorganisms. May include hypothermia or **hyperthermia**, tachycardia, hypotension, reduced **SVR**, tachypnoea, leucocytosis and deteriorating organ function. Features may be affected by the severity of infection, age, **immunodeficiency** and other diseases. Sepsis may be associated with positive blood culture (**septicaemia**) or cardiovascular collapse (**septic shock**).

- The means by which bacteria produce their pathophysiological effects are controversial but probably involve:
  – exotoxins: high mw proteins which act locally (e.g. cholera) or remotely (e.g. **botulism**).
  – **endotoxins**: lipopolysaccharides present in bacterial cell walls.

Bone RC (1991) Ann Intern Med; 114: 332–3

Septicaemia. Sepsis syndrome associated with circulating microorganisms (i.e. with positive blood culture). **Septic shock** is present when cardiovascular collapse occurs. A major cause of organ failure and death in **ICU**, severe sepsis is directly or indirectly responsible for 75% of all ICU deaths.

Most ICU infections are endogenous, caused by colonization of the patient's GIT by pathogenic organisms. Gram-negative bacteria (e.g. *Escherichia coli*, Klebsiella, Psuedomonas and Proteus species) are most commonly responsible, because of their widespread presence, their tendency to acquire resistance to **antibacterial drugs** and their resistance to drying and disinfecting agents. Gram-positive bacteria (e.g. Streptococci, Staphylococci) and other organisms (e.g. fungi) may also be responsible. Septicaemia may arise from any localized site of infection; it may also occur in the absence of an obvious source.

- Critically ill patients are susceptible to infection because of:
  - impaired local defences, e.g. anatomical barriers, **ciliary activity**, coughing, gastric pH. Presence of tracheal tubes and indwelling catheters and cannulae provide routes for infection.
  - impaired neutrophil function, humoral immunity (especially following splenectomy) and cell-mediated immunity. Contributory factors include drugs, **malnutrition**, old age, **malignancy**, organ failure and infection itself.
- Methods of reducing sepsis in ICU include:
  - hygiene, e.g. washing hands between touching patients.
  - isolation of infective and at-risk patients.
  - minimal intervention (e.g. vascular lines), employing aseptic techniques when procedures are performed.
  - regular changing of lines, tubing, etc., and removal as soon as they are no longer required.
  - antibacterial drug policies to reduce resistance.
  - **selective decontamination of the digestive tract**.
  - improving host defences, e.g. adequate **nutrition**.
  - surgical drainage of abscesses, etc.
- Management of septicaemia:
  - supportive, e.g. **iv fluids, O₂ therapy, inotropic drugs, etc.** Nutrition is important since hypercatabolism is common.
  - antibacterial drugs, **antifungal drugs**, etc. Initial choice of drug is based on the most likely infective organisms in each particular situation. Samples of urine, sputum, blood, CSF, etc. should be taken before starting therapy.
  - **anti-endotoxin antibodies** have until recently been used in Gram-negative septicaemia.
  - surgical drainage, debridement, etc.

Complications include septic shock and multiple organ failure including **ARDS, renal failure, hepatic failure, pancreatitis** and **diabetes mellitus, DIC, cardiac failure** and **coma**. GIT haemorrhage is common; preventative measures include **H₂ receptor antagonists, antacids** and **sucralfate**.

Septic shock. Shock associated with **sepsis syndrome**. Mortality is about 50% although it varies with age and the nature of sepsis. Initially, features include **hyperthermia**, tachycardia, tachypnoea, hypotension and vasodilatation with a hyperdynamic circulation and increased cardiac output. In later stages or if **hypovolaemia** or poor myocardial function are present, hypotension with vasoconstriction supervene. Urine output is then often reduced.

- Cardiovascular features include:
  - reduced **SVR** with relative hypovolaemia.
  - increased **pulmonary vascular resistance**.
  - increased capillary permeability.
  - reduced **myocardial contractility** caused by circulating depressant factors, **acidaemia** and **hypoxaemia**.
  - O₂ consumption may be normal but O₂ extraction and utilization are reduced.
- Management:
  - as for septicaemia.
  - **steroid therapy** does not improve outcome and may increase the incidence of secondary infection.
  - **prostaglandins, naloxone** and thyrotrophin releasing hormone have been used but their benefit has not been proven.
- Complications: as for septicaemia.

Rackow EC, Astiz ME (1991) JAMA; 266: 548–54

Sequential analysis, *see Statistical tests*

Serotonin, *see 5-Hydroxytryptamine*

Servomechanisms. Control systems involving continuous assessment of output and its automated modification, to maintain constancy. Used in **ventilators** and other computerized equipment. Have also been used to control iv infusions, e.g. of **sodium nitroprusside** to reduce BP; continuous measurement of BP is used as input for a **computer**-controlled infusion device.

Sevoflurane. CH(CF₃)₂OCH₂F, 1,1,1,3,3,3–hexafluoroisopropyl fluoromethyl ether. **Inhalational anaesthetic agent**, currently under investigation in the West. First reported in 1971 but not developed further in the USA until recently. Available in Japan from 1990. Non-flammable, with blood/gas **partition coefficient** of 0.6, and **MAC** of 1.7–2%. Has similar clinical effects to **isoflurane**, but non-irritant and pleasant smelling, with less hypotension and tachycardia. Induction of anaesthesia and recovery are rapid. Hydrolysed in water and degraded slightly by **soda lime**, although adverse effects have not been reported. Undergoes biotransformation to a similar extent to **enflurane**. Renal and hepatic toxicity have not been demonstrated. Has been suggested as the best agent for induction in children.

Jones RM (1990) Br J Anaesth; 65: 527–36

Shivering, postoperative. Tremors were first described after **barbiturate** administration, but they may occur following all types of general anaesthesia. Said to be most common following **halothane** ('halothane shakes'). May increase metabolic rate and O₂ requirement by up to 10 times, and may damage teeth and wounds.

EMG studies suggest that postoperative shivering differs from shivering due to cold. It has been suggested that anaesthetic agents suppress descending pathways which normally inhibit spinal reflexes; this may be more likely than a response to intraoperative hypothermia, although the latter may be of importance if severe.

- Suggested treatment:
  - O₂ administration.
  - **pethidine** 10–25 mg iv has been successfully used, as has **pentazocine** 30 mg or **doxapram** 1 mg/kg.

Shivering after **extradural anaesthesia** is common, and is thought to be caused by differential nerve blockade, either suppressing descending inhibition of spinal reflexes, or allowing selective transmission of cold sensation. Shivering is rare in **spinal anaesthesia**, where blockade is more dense. Warming of extradural injectate has produced conflicting results. Extradural administration of **opioid analgesic drugs**, e.g. **sufentanil** 50 µg, **fentanyl** 25 µg, pethidine 25 mg, may be an effective remedy.
Crossley AWA (1992) Anaesthesia; 47: 193–5

Shock. Syndrome in which tissue perfusion is inadequate for the tissues' metabolic requirements. Sympathetic compensatory mechanisms may preserve organ perfusion initially, but subsequent organ dysfunction may lead to irreversible organ damage and death.
- Classically divided into:
    - hypovolaemic shock, e.g. following **haemorrhage, burns, dehydration**, etc.
    - **cardiogenic shock**, e.g. following **MI**.
    - **septic shock**.
    - others, e.g. **anaphylactic reaction, adrenocortical insufficiency**, neurogenic shock (e.g. in high **spinal cord injury**).

Division into myocardial failure and peripheral vascular failure has been suggested as being more indicative of underlying mechanisms. Thus shock may arise from inadequate **cardiac output** or maldistribution of blood flow; the latter has been increasingly implicated by studies of **O_2 delivery** ($\dot{D}O_2$) and total body O_2 consumption ($\dot{V}O_2$). A decrease in $\dot{V}O_2$ is thought to represent maldistribution rather than an absolute decrease in blood flow. In cardiogenic shock both $\dot{V}O_2$ and cardiac output are reduced; in septic shock they may both increase initially. Features depend on the aetiology but include hypotension, tachycardia, oliguria and metabolic **acidosis**. Multiple organ failure may follow, with **renal failure** and **ARDS** common. Hepatic, gastrointestinal and pancreatic impairment, and **DIC** may occur.
- Management:
    - directed at the primary cause.
    - support of the cardiovasvular system. Haemodynamic monitoring has traditionally relied on measurement of BP, pulse rate, **CVP**, **urine** output, **pulmonary capillary wedge pressure** and **cardiac output**. **Lactate** has also been measured. Recently, $\dot{D}O_2$, $\dot{V}O_2$ and **gastric intramucosal pH** have been used to guide therapy. Cardiovascular support is achieved with **iv fluids, inotropic drugs** and **vasodilator drugs**.
    - support of other organs: as for renal failure, ARDS, etc. O_2 therapy is mandatory.
    - **steroid therapy** was advocated in the past but has been associated with increased mortality, and should now be reserved for proven adrenocortical insufficiency.

Mortality exceeds 50% for cardiogenic and septic shock.

Shock lung, *see Adult respiratory distress syndrome*

Shunt. One extreme form of $\dot{V}/\dot{Q}$ **mismatch**, causing **hypoxaemia**. Refers to the actual amount of venous blood bypassing ventilated alveoli and mixing with pulmonary end-capillary blood (cf. **venous admixture**, the calculated amount of shunt required to produce the observed arterial PO_2).

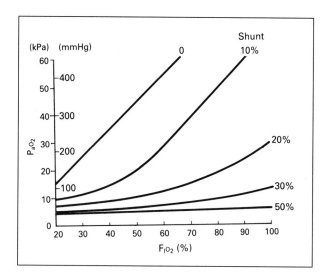

Figure 117 *P_aO_2 at varying F_IO_2 for different percentages of shunt*

- May be:
    - intrapulmonary, e.g. **atelectasis, chest infection**, etc.
    - extrapulmonary, e.g. **congenital heart disease**.

Physiological shunt (venous admixture) = shunt-like effect of $\dot{V}/\dot{Q}$ mismatch + anatomical shunt (actual shunt). The latter includes pathological shunt and normal mixing of bronchial and Thebesian venous blood with oxygenated pulmonary venous blood.

Hypoxaemia due to shunt responds poorly to increased F_IO_2, since the O_2 content of pulmonary end-capillary blood is already near maximum, because of the shape of the **oxyhaemoglobin dissociation curve**. Some benefit is derived from increased dissolved O_2. Thus the amount of shunt may be estimated from the response to breathing high concentrations of O_2, assuming a haemoglobin concentration of 10–14 g/100 ml, arterial PCO_2 of 3.3–5.3 kPa (25–40 mmHg), and arteriovenous O_2 difference of 5 ml/100 ml (Fig. 117). Amount of shunt may also be estimated from the **shunt equation**.
[Adam Thebesius (1686–1732), German physician]

Shunt equation.

$$\frac{\dot{Q}_S}{\dot{Q}_T} = \frac{(C_cO_2 - C_aO_2)}{(C_cO_2 - C_vO_2)}$$

Allows calculation of **shunt**. Derived thus:
Total pulmonary blood flow equals $\dot{Q}_T$, made up of blood flow to unventilated alveoli ($\dot{Q}_S$) and blood flow to ventilated alveoli ($\dot{Q}_T - \dot{Q}_S$; Fig. 118).

In unit time, the volume of O_2 leaving the lungs equals the volume of O_2 in blood draining ventilated alveoli plus the volume of O_2 in shunted blood. Or,

$$\dot{Q}_T \times C_aO_2 = [(\dot{Q}_T - \dot{Q}_S) \times C_cO_2] + [\dot{Q}_S \times C_vO_2],$$

where C_aO_2 = arterial O_2 content,
C_cO_2 = end-capillary O_2 content,
C_vO_2 = mixed venous O_2 content.

Thus $\dot{Q}_T \times C_aO_2 = (\dot{Q}_T \times C_cO_2) - (\dot{Q}_S \times C_cO_2) + (\dot{Q}_S \times C_vO_2)$, or $(\dot{Q}_S \times C_cO_2) - (\dot{Q}_S \times C_vO_2) = (\dot{Q}_T \times C_cO_2) - (\dot{Q}_T \times C_aO_2)$, or $\dot{Q}_S (C_cO_2 - C_vO_2) = \dot{Q}_T (C_cO_2 - C_aO_2)$.

Therefore

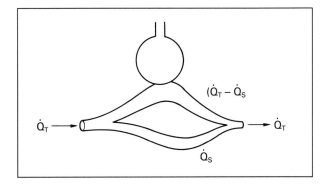

Figure 118 *Calculation of shunt equation*

$$\frac{Q_S}{Q_T} = \frac{(C_cO_2 - C_aO_2)}{(C_cO_2 - C_{\bar{v}}O_2)} = \text{shunt fraction.}$$

Arterial and venous O_2 contents may be estimated thus:

$$C_aO_2 = (P_aO_2 \times S) + (Hb \times 1.34 \times S_aO_2),$$

$$C_{\bar{v}}O_2 = (P_{\bar{v}}O_2 \times S) + (Hb \times 1.34 \times S_{\bar{v}}O_2),$$

where P_aO_2 and S_aO_2 = arterial PO_2 and haemoglobin saturation respectively,

$P_{\bar{v}}O_2$ and $S_{\bar{v}}O_2$ = venous PO_2 and haemoglobin saturation respectively,

S = volume of O_2 dissolved in 100 ml blood per kPa applied O_2 tension (0.0225), or per mmHg (0.003),

Hb = haemoglobin content in g/100 ml,

1.34 = **Hüfner's constant**.

End-capillary O_2 content cannot be measured directly, but is estimated from calculation of the **alveolar air equation**:

$$C_cO_2 = (P_AO_2 \times S) + (Hb \times 1.34),$$

where P_AO_2 = 'ideal' alveolar PO_2, and saturation is assumed to be 100%.

Shy–Drager syndrome, *see Autonomic neuropathy*

SI units, Units of the Système International d'Unités, *see Units*

SIADH, *see Syndrome of inappropriate antidiuretic hormone*

Siamese twins, *see Conjoined twins*

Sick doctor scheme. Scheme set up in 1981 in the UK by the **Association of Anaesthetists** and Royal College of Psychiatrists, to encourage voluntary reporting of sick doctors practising anaesthesia and thus potentially putting patients at risk. The anonymous reporter, having contacted the Association, is given the name and telephone number of a referee. The latter contacts an appointed psychiatrist from another Region, who in turn contacts the sick doctor. Intended as an alternative to the more formal schemes available via the Department of Health (a panel of senior staff is set up by the District; appropriate action is taken via a subcommittee ('three wise men' procedure)) and General Medical Council (offers medical examination/counselling, etc.; appropriate action may be taken via the GMC Health Committee).

A similar Competence to Practise scheme has recently been set up, to protect patients from anaesthetists practising unsafe anaesthesia.

Helliwell PJ (1985) Anaesthesia; 40: 221–2

Sick euthyroid syndrome. Abnormal thyroid function tests occurring in critically ill patients. Low triiodothyronine (T_3) with normal or raised thyroxine (T_4) is the most common pattern. Low T_3 and T_4 are generally associated with more severe disease and worse prognosis. Most patients are clinically euthyroid. Thought to result from reduced thyroid stimulating hormone secretion, reduced peripheral conversion of T_4 to T_3 and reduced plasma protein binding.

Sick sinus syndrome. Syndrome caused by impaired sinoatrial node activity or conduction; may lead to periods of severe bradycardia with intermittent loss of **P waves** or sinus arrest, and may alternate with periods of **SVT** or **AF** (bradycardia–tachycardia syndrome; bradytachy syndrome). Usually occurs in elderly patients with **ischaemic heart disease**. May be precipitated by anaesthesia. Requires **cardiac pacing** if diagnosed preoperatively or if it occurs peroperatively.

See also, Heart, conducting system

Sickle cell anaemia. Haemoglobinopathy, first described in 1910 in Chicago. Caused by substitution of glutamic acid by valine in the sixth amino acid from the N-terminal of **haemoglobin** β chains. Inherited as an autosomal gene; heterozygotes (genotype HbAS; sickle cell trait) possess both normal (HbA) and abnormal (HbS) haemoglobins, whilst homozygotes (HbSS) contain only abnormal haemoglobin. Thought to have originated from spontaneous genetic mutation, with subsequent selection owing to the relative resistance conferred by sickle cell trait against **malaria**. Most common in West Central Africa, North-East Saudi Arabia and East Central India, but has been described in Southern Mediterranean populations. Incidence of HbSS in US Blacks is under 1%; incidence of HbAS is 8–10%.

Deoxygenated HbS polymerizes and precipitates within red blood cells, with distortion and increased rigidity. Sickle-shaped red cells are characteristic. The distorted cells increase blood **viscosity**, impair **blood flow** and cause capillary and venous thrombosis and organ infarction. They have shortened survival time. O_2 affinity of dissolved HbS is normal, but overall affinity is reduced if some of the HbS is polymerized. HbS polymerizes at PO_2 of 5–6 kPa (40–50 mmHg); thus HbSS patients are continuously sickling. HbAS patients' red cells contain both HbS and HbA and sickle at 2.5–4.0 kPa (20–30 mmHg).

- Features:
  - HbSS:
    - **haemolysis** causing **anaemia** and hyperbilirubinaemia. Gallstones may occur. Enlargement of the skull and long bones is common, due to compensatory bone marrow hyperplasia. Acute aplastic crises may occur, and sequestration crises in children.
    - impaired tissue blood flow may result in **CVA**, papillary necrosis of the kidney, ulcers, pulmonary infarcts, priapism, and avascular necrosis of bone. Crises are caused by acute vascular occlusion, and

may feature neurological lesions and severe pain, e.g. abdominal, back, chest, etc. They may be precipitated by **hypothermia**, **dehydration**, infection, exertion and **hypoxaemia**. Treatment is with analgesia, O_2 and rehydration. Exchange **blood transfusion** may be required.

–increased susceptibility to infection. Osteomyelitis is typically caused by unusual organisms, e.g. Salmonella.

–HbAS: usually asymptomatic, since arterial Po_2 is unlikely to reach the level required to induce sickling.

–combinations of HbS with other haemoglobins usually produce mild disease. In heterozygotes for HbS and haemoglobin C (HbC), red cells may sickle at around 4 kPa (30 mmHg) because HbC itself is less soluble then HbA, and makes red cells more rigid.

Diagnosis is by detection of HbS in the blood. The Sickledex test involves addition of reagent to blood, with observation for turbidity. It detects HbS but provides no information about other haemoglobins. A sodium metabisulphite test induces sickling in susceptible cells, which are then counted. Haemoglobin electrophoresis is the only method of determining the nature of the haemoglobinopathy.

Sickle cells are usually present in peripheral blood in HbSS.

● Anaesthetic considerations:
  –preoperatively:
    –all races at risk should be screened for HbS, ideally by electrophoresis. In the UK, Sickledex testing is usual initially, with progression to electrophoresis if positive. In emergencies, if the Sickledex test is positive, the diagnosis is made on history/examination, blood counts and peripheral film. If the history does not suggest HbSS, and haemoglobin/reticulocyte count and peripheral film are normal with no red cell fragments, HbAS is likely. Management ultimately depends on the nature of the surgery, availability of blood, etc.
    –**preoperative assessment** is directed towards the above complications, especially impairment of pulmonary and renal function. Preoperative folic acid has been suggested. Exchange transfusion is often used in HbSS patients before major surgery, to achieve HbS concentrations of 30–40%.
    –hypoxaemia, dehydration, hypothermia and **acidosis** should be prevented at all times perioperatively. Prophylactic antibiotics are often administered.
  –peroperatively:
    –standard techniques may be used, apart from **tourniquets** which cause tissue ischaemia (**IVRA** is contraindicated). **Heat loss** should be prevented and cardiovascular stability maintained. **Preoxygenation** and F_iO_2 of 50% reduces the risk of hypoxaemia by increasing arterial Po_2 and pulmonary O_2 reserve. IV hydration should be maintained. Frequent analysis of acid–base status is required in HbSS patients. Prophylactic **bicarbonate** administration has been suggested, but administration according to acid–base analysis is usually preferred.
    –intraoperative crises may present with changes in breathing pattern or BP, acidosis and hypoxaemia. Detection may be difficult.
  –postoperatively: the precautions already instituted should continue, since complications may occur postoperatively. Patients are not suitable for **day-case**

surgery. O_2 administration for at least 24 hours is usually advocated.

Esseltine DW, Baxter MRN, Bevan JC (1988) Can J Anaesth; 35: 385–403

Siggaard-Andersen nomogram. Diagram derived from analysis of many blood samples, showing the plot of log arterial Pco_2 against plasma **pH**, with **base excess**, **standard bicarbonate** and **buffer base** illustrated as additional lines (Fig. 119). Allows determination of Pco_2 by equilibrating a blood sample with two known concentrations of CO_2, and measuring the sample pH at each concentration. The points are plotted on the diagram and joined by a line, and the Pco_2 read from the vertical scale according to the pH of the original sample. Alternatively, if Pco_2 can be measured directly, a single measurement of pH and Pco_2, together with **haemoglobin** concentration (since haemoglobin is a major blood **buffer**) allows determination of the derived data. Modern blood-gas machines automatically perform the required calculations, making such plotting unnecessary.

[Ole Siggaard-Andersen, Danish biochemist]

Sigh, see *Intermittent positive pressure ventilation*

Significance, see *Statistical significance*

Simpson, James Young (1811–1870). Scottish obstetrician; Professor of Midwifery at Edinburgh. The first to administer an anaesthetic for obstetrics in 1847, using **diethyl ether**. Following a suggestion by Waldie later that year, he used **chloroform** for the same purpose. Encountered stiff opposition from the clergy and others, who maintained that painful childbirth was either God's will, beneficial to the patient, or both; this continued until **Snow**'s administration of chloroform to Queen **Victoria** in 1853. Helped popularize chloroform as the replacement for ether. Created baronet in 1866.

[David Waldie (1813–1889), Scottish-born Liverpool doctor and chemist]

SIMV, Synchronized intermittent mandatory ventilation, see *Intermittent mandatory ventilation*

Sinoatrial node, see *Heart, conducting system*

Sinus arrhythmia. Normal phenomenon (especially in young people) characterized by alternating periods of slow and rapid **heart rates**. The **ECG** shows **sinus rhythm** with irregular spacing of normal complexes. Most commonly related to respiration, with a rapid rate at end-inspiration and a slower rate at end-expiration. Thought to be caused by activation of **pulmonary stretch receptors** during inspiration, causing inhibition of the **cardioinhibitory centre** via vagal afferents, with resultant speeding of heart rate; the opposite occurs during expiration. May also involve direct impulse conduction between medullary respiratory and cardiac neurones. Also seen in patients treated with **digoxin**. Abolished by **atropine**.

Sinus bradycardia. Usually defined as **sinus rhythm** at less than 60 beats/min. The **ECG** shows normal P waves and QRS complexes occurring at a slow rate.

● Caused by:
  –physiological slowing, e.g. in athletes, or during **sleep**.

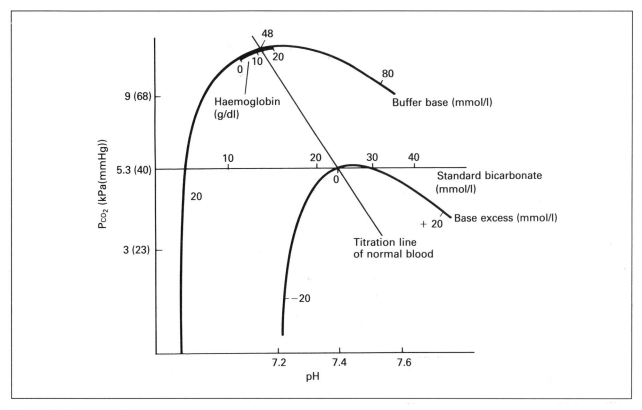

Figure 119 *Siggaard-Andersen nomogram*

–disease states, e.g. **hypothyroidism**, raised **ICP**, acute **MI**, **sick sinus syndrome**, **jaundice**.

–activation of vagal reflexes, e.g. **carotid sinus massage**, **Valsalva manoeuvre**. During anaesthesia, it may follow skin incision, stretching or dilatation of the anus, cervix, mesentery and bladder (**Brewer–Luckhardt reflex**), pulling on the ocular muscles (**oculocardiac reflex**), etc.

–**hypoxaemia**, especially in children. Thought to be caused by central depression of the **vasomotor centre**.

–blockade of the cardiac sympathetic innervation during high **spinal** or **extradural anaesthesia**.

–drugs, e.g. **halothane**, **neostigmine**, **digoxin**, **opioid analgesic drugs**, **β-adrenergic receptor antagonists**.

If it occurs, the stimulus should be stopped. It may be treated with **anticholinergic drugs** (e.g. **atropine**), **β-adrenergic receptor agonists** or **cardiac pacing,** but treatment is only required if accompanied by symptoms, hypotension or **escape beats**.

Sinus rhythm. Normal heart rhythm in which each **P wave** is followed by a **QRS complex** on the ECG; i.e. each impulse originates in the sinoatrial node, which has the fastest inherent rhythmicity of all cardiac **pacemaker cells**. Normal **heart rate** is usually defined as 60–100 beats/min. *See also, Cardiac cycle; Heart, conducting system; Sinus arrhythmia; Sinus bradycardia; Sinus tachycardia*

Sinus tachycardia. Usually defined as **sinus rhythm** at over 100 beats/min. The **ECG** shows regular normal P waves and QRS complexes at a rapid rate.

● Caused by:

–increased sympathetic activity, e.g. fear, anxiety; during anaesthesia, it may represent **hypoxaemia**, **hypercapnia**, and inadequate anaesthesia or neuromuscular blockade. It may also occur as a compensatory mechanism, e.g. in **anaemia**, **hypovolaemia**, **air embolism/PE**, etc.

–increased metabolic rate, e.g. **hyperthyroidism**, fever, **pregnancy**, **MH**.

–drugs, e.g. **enflurane**, **isoflurane**, **pancuronium**, **sympathomimetic drugs**, **anticholinergic drugs**.

Reduces the time available for ventricular filling and **coronary blood flow**; it may precipitate **myocardial ischaemia** if severe. Treatment is usually directed at the cause; **β-adrenergic receptor antagonists** may be required if the patient is at risk of myocardial ischaemia.

Skin diseases. Anaesthetic considerations may be related to:

–diseases with cutaneous and systemic manifestations, e.g. **connective tissue diseases**, **porphyria**, **polymyositis**, **neurofibromatosis**, severe skin disease with **anaemia** and **malnutrition**, etc.

–scarring or fibrosis of tissues around the face, mouth or neck causing difficulty with tracheal intubation, e.g. systemic sclerosis, epidermolysis bullosa dystrophica. In the latter, bullous lesion formation may follow instrumentation (e.g. laryngoscopy), and may be followed by scarring.

–involvement of the immune system causing **airway obstruction** (e.g. **hereditary angioneurotic oedema**) or severe manifestations of **histamine** release (e.g. urticaria pigmentosa). Histamine-releasing drugs should be avoided.

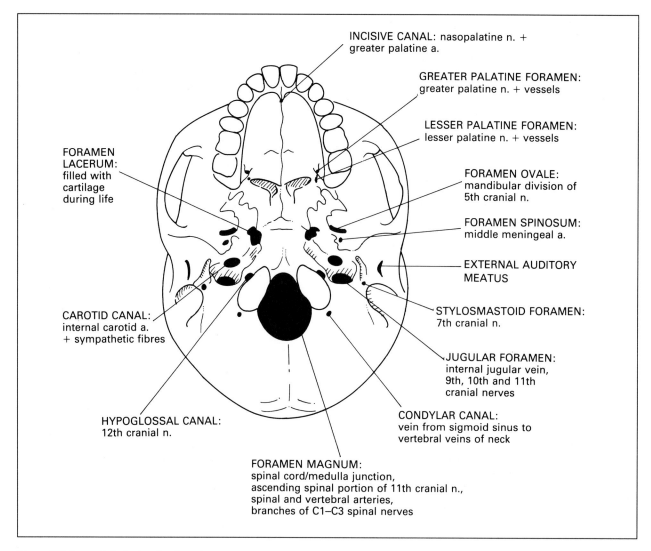

INCISIVE CANAL: nasopalatine n. + greater palatine a.

GREATER PALATINE FORAMEN: greater palatine n. + vessels

LESSER PALATINE FORAMEN: lesser palatine n. + vessels

FORAMEN LACERUM: filled with cartilage during life

FORAMEN OVALE: mandibular division of 5th cranial n.

FORAMEN SPINOSUM: middle meningeal a.

EXTERNAL AUDITORY MEATUS

CAROTID CANAL: internal carotid a. + sympathetic fibres

STYLOSMASTOID FORAMEN: 7th cranial n.

JUGULAR FORAMEN: internal jugular vein, 9th, 10th and 11th cranial nerves

HYPOGLOSSAL CANAL: 12th cranial n.

CONDYLAR CANAL: vein from sigmoid sinus to vertebral veins of neck

FORAMEN MAGNUM: spinal cord/medulla junction, ascending spinal portion of 11th cranial n., spinal and vertebral arteries, branches of C1–C3 spinal nerves

Figure 120 *Base of skull, showing foramina*

–increased **heat loss during anaesthesia** if large areas of erythema are present.
–susceptibility to skin trauma following handling, laryngoscopy, and use of sticking plaster, ECG electrodes, etc.
–effect of drug therapy, e.g. **steroid therapy**, **immunosuppressive drugs**.

In addition, anaesthetic agents may precipitate cutaneous lesions (e.g. in **adverse drugs reactions**, bullous eruption following **barbiturate poisoning**, porphyria).

Smith GB, Shribman AJ (1984) Anaesthesia; 39: 443–55

Skull. The upper part contains the **brain**, whilst the lower anterior portion forms the facial skeleton:

–superior aspect: divided from left to right by the coronal suture, separating the frontal bone anteriorly and the parietal bones posteriorly. The sagittal suture separates the two parietal bones in the midline, and the lambdoid suture separates the parietal bones and occipital bone posteriorly. The anterior fontanelle closes at about 18 months of age.

–lateral aspect: consists of parietal and occipital bones posteriorly, temporal and sphenoid bones inferiorly, and frontal bone, with the zygomatic and maxillary bones below, anteriorly. The mandible articulates with the temporal bone at the **temporomandibular joint**.

–anterior aspect: consists of frontal bone superiorly, zygomatic bones at the inferolateral edges of the orbits, and maxilla centrally, with the mandible inferiorly. Important nerves and vessels are transmitted by the following:

–optic canal: 2nd **cranial nerve** and ophthalmic artery.

–superior orbital fissure: 3rd, 4th, 5th (nasociliary, frontal and lacrimal branches of the ophthalmic division) and 6th cranial nerves.

–foramen rotundum (below and medial to the superior orbital fissure's medial end): maxillary division of the 5th cranial nerve.

–supraorbital, infraorbital and mental foramina: supraorbital, infraorbital and mental nerves (branches of the ophthalmic, maxillary and mandibular divisions of the 5th cranial nerve respectively).

–the inferior aspect is especially important because of the structures transmitted by its foramina (Fig. 120). In addition, branches of the 1st cranial nerve pass through the cribriform plate's perforations.

See also, Mandibular nerve blocks; Maxillary nerve blocks; Ophthalmic nerve blocks

Sleep. Naturally-occurring state of unconsciousness; the response to external stimuli is decreased, but the subject may usually be readily roused. Two patterns are described:

–non-rapid eye movement (NREM) sleep, divided into four stages according to **EEG** activity:

–stage 1: occurs as the subject falls asleep; characterized by low amplitude high frequency activity.

–stage 2: sleep spindles occur (alpha-like bursts of 10–14 Hz and 50 µV).

–stage 3: frequency slows and amplitude increases.

–stage 4: represents deep sleep, with rhythmic slow waves.

–rapid eye movement (REM) sleep (paradoxical sleep): rapid, irregular, low amplitude waves occur, similar to those seen in awake subjects. Dreaming occurs. The eyes make rapid movement, accompanied by tachycardia, tachypnoea, skeletal muscle relaxation and penile erection.

In a typical night's sleep, a young adult rapidly passes through stages 1 and 2, spending about 60–90 minutes in stages 3 and 4. A period of REM sleep follows, lasting 60–90 minutes. This cycle repeats, thus providing about five episodes of REM sleep per night (25% of total sleep time). REM sleep is inhibited by **barbiturates, antidepressant drugs** and **amphetamines**; following cessation of therapy, REM sleep increases on subsequent nights.

Sleep apnoea. Disorder characterized by temporary cessation of breathing during **sleep**, usually in males. Prevalence in adult men is about 1%. Apnoeic episodes may last up to 2 minutes; the resultant **hypoxaemia** causes arousal from deeper stages of sleep. May be central (loss of respiratory drive, e.g. **Ondine's curse**) or, more commonly, obstructive (obstructive sleep apnoea; OSA).

OSA is caused by passive collapse of the pharyngeal airway during sleep, and is associated with **obesity** (e.g. **alveolar hypoventilation syndrome**), pharyngeal anatomical abnormalities (e.g. retrognathia, tonsillar hypertrophy) and other conditions (e.g. **hypothyroidism**). Features include loud snoring, restless sleep, morning headaches and daytime somnolence. Diagnosis involves **oximetry** during sleep. Treatment includes weight loss, nasal **CPAP** and uvulopharyngopalatoplasty.

● Anaesthetic implications:

–of any predisposing cause.

–**premedication** may precipitate complete **airway obstruction** and should be avoided.

–maintenance of the airway during **induction of anaesthesia** and tracheal intubation may be difficult.

–airway obstruction may readily occur postoperatively; patients should be nursed in an ICU or HDU.

Hanning CD (1989) Br J Anaesth; 63: 477–88

Slow reacting substance-A, *see Leukotrienes*

Smoke inhalation. Resultant pulmonary insufficiency is the commonest cause of death in patients admitted to hospital with **burns**.

● Problems are related to:

–low F_1O_2 of inspired gas, and inhalation of carbon monoxide, cyanide, nitrogen oxides and other substances. All may result in **hypoxaemia**.

–inhaled carbon particles coated with irritant substances, e.g. aldehydes, which may cause **laryngospasm, bronchospasm** and inhibition of **ciliary activity**.

–$\dot{V}/\dot{Q}$ mismatch, **shunt** and **pulmonary oedema** may occur.

–thermal injury to the airway may be followed by upper **airway obstruction**, bronchospasm, tracheal and bronchial oedema and sloughing.

Further respiratory impairment may occur if infection and **ARDS** supervene.

● Management: as for burns, **carbon monoxide poisoning, cyanide poisoning, respiratory failure**.

Langford RM, Armstrong RF (1989) BMJ; 299: 902–5

See also, Nitrogen. higher oxides of

Smoking. Common cause of cardiovascular and respiratory pathology in surgical and non-surgical patients.

● Effects:

–cardiovascular:

–nicotine is an adrenergic agonist; it increases heart rate, SVR and thus BP. It also increases myocardial O_2 demand, and possibly decreases **coronary blood flow**.

–carbon monoxide combines with up to 15% of **haemoglobin** to form carboxyhaemoglobin, reducing the O_2-carrying ability of blood.

–increased risk of **ischaemic heart disease**.

–increased risk of **DVT** (this is disputed).

–pulmonary:

–impaired **ciliary activity**.

–reduced immunological defence mechanisms, e.g. neutrophil and lymphocyte activity.

–increased risk of **bronchial carcinoma**.

–increased bronchial reactivity and **COAD**.

Smokers are more likely to suffer increased sputum production and retention, **bronchospasm**, coughing, **atelectasis** and **chest infection** perioperatively.

Stopping smoking is thought to be beneficial preoperatively, in order to minimize its acute adverse effects. Effects of carbon monoxide and nicotine are significantly reduced after 12–24 hours' abstinence; up to 6–8 weeks is thought to be necessary for restoration of ciliary and immunological activity.

Jones RM, Rosen M, Seymour L (1987) Anaesthesia; 42: 1–2

See also, Carbon monoxide poisoning

Snow, John (1813–1858). Pioneer of English anaesthesia, born in York. Moved to London in 1836. Developed the science and art of anaesthesia, describing five stages of anaesthesia in 1847. Designed inhalers for **diethyl ether** and **chloroform**, and wrote two famous textbooks on the use of these agents (his book on chloroform was published posthumously). Widely regarded as the expert in his field, he administered chloroform to Queen **Victoria** during chilbirth in 1853 and 1857. Also famous for demonstrating that cholera was spread by contaminated drinking water, not by foul air as previously believed. Removal of the Broad Street water pump handle on his suggestion is said to have stopped the London epidemic of 1854.

Soda lime. Mixture used for **CO₂ absorption in anaesthetic breathing systems**, composed of calcium hydroxide (94%), sodium hydroxide (5%), potassium hydroxide (1%), silicates (for binding; less than 1%) and indicators. Used with 14–19% water content. CO_2 in solution reacts with sodium and potassium hydroxides to form the respective carbonates, which then react with calcium hydroxide to produce calcium carbonate, replenishing sodium and potassium hydroxides. Heat is produced during the reaction. Exhaustion of its activity is indicated by dyes; several have been used but the most common one changes from pink to white.

Provided in granules of size 4–8 mesh (will pass through a mesh of 4–8 strands per inch in each axis; i.e. pore size of ¹⁄₁₆–¹⁄₆₄ square inch). Cannisters should be tightly packed to reduce channelling of gases through large gaps. The total volume of space between granules should equal the volume of the granules themselves. Dust may be inhaled, especially using the 'to-and-fro' system. Large cannisters containing up to 2 kg soda lime are commonly employed.

Decomposes certain **inhalational anaesthetic agents**, e.g. **trichloroethylene**, which may lead to neurological damage. Also decomposes **sevoflurane** (slightly) and **halothane** (very slightly), but without clinical significance.

Sodium (Na⁺). Principal cation in the **ECF**, accounting for 90% of the osmotically active solute in **plasma** and **interstitial fluid**. Thus the prime determinant of ECF volume. Total body content is about 4000 mmol, of which 50% is in bone, 40% in ECF, and 10% intracellular. About 70% is available for exchange. Normal plasma levels: 135–145 mmol/l. Of central importance in the function of excitable cells, e.g. concerning **membrane potentials** and **action potentials**.

Actively absorbed from the small intestine and colon, facilitated by **aldosterone** and the presence of **glucose** in the gut lumen. The kidney filters approximately 26 000 mmol Na⁺/day, of which 99.5% is reabsorbed by passage through the **nephron** (mostly at the proximal convoluted tubule). Reabsorption is influenced by renal tubular hydrostatic and oncotic gradients, aldosterone, adrenocortical hormones, **atrial natriuretic hormone**, and the rate of secretion of hydrogen and potassium ions.
- Daily losses: about 150 mmol in the urine, with 10 mmol via each of faeces, sweat and skin. Saliva contains 10 mmol/l, sweat 50 mmol/l, gastric secretions 60 mmol/l, and the rest of the GIT about 130 mmol/l.
- Daily requirement: about 1 mmol/kg/day.
- Regulated via changes in:
  –ECF sodium concentration and **osmolality** via **osmoreceptors**, affecting the **renin/angiotensin system** and aldosterone secretion.
  –ECF volume changes: via **baroreceptors**, affecting atrial natriuretic peptide secretion in addition to the above hormones.

See also, Hypernatraemia; Hyponatraemia

Sodium bicarbonate, *see Bicarbonate*

Sodium citrate. Non-particulate **antacid**, widely used preoperatively to increase gastric pH in patients at risk of

aspiration of gastric contents, e.g. in obstetrics. Thought to be less harmful than **magnesium trisilicate** if inhaled. Effective for 30–50 minutes following oral intake of 30 ml 0.3 molar solution.

Also used to relieve discomfort from urinary tract infection by raising urinary pH.

Sodium nitroprusside (SNP). **Vasodilator drug**, used as an **antihypertensive drug, e.g.** in **hypotensive anaesthesia** and **hypertensive crises**. Also used in **cardiac failure**. Presented as a powder for reconstitution in 5% dextrose. Unstable in solution, with decomposition to highly coloured products. Solutions require protection from light and should be used within 24 hours of preparation.

Acts mainly on arterial smooth muscle, although veins are also affected. Thus reduces **SVR**, maintaining **cardiac output** and tissue perfusion. Also reduces myocardial O_2 consumption whilst increasing **coronary blood flow**, although **coronary steal** has been reported. Compensatory tachycardia is common. Hepatic blood flow remains constant, whilst **renal blood flow** and **cerebral blood flow** increase. Active within 30 seconds of administration. Broken down non-enzymatically within red blood cells (catalyzed by **haemoglobin**) to produce five cyanide ions from each molecule, most of which are released slowly into the plasma. Plasma **half-life** of SNP is about 2 minutes.
- Dosage: usually 0.1–5 µg/kg/min iv, to a maximum of 8 µg/kg/min (maximal total dose of 1 mg/kg over 2–3 hours). **Tachyphylaxis** may occur.
- Side effects:
  –rebound hypertension following its abrupt withdrawal. Caused by activation of the **renin/angiotensin system** and increased plasma **catecholamine** levels.
  –raised **ICP** may occur.
  –**platelet** aggregation may be inhibited.
  –pulmonary **shunt** may be increased in normal lungs via impairment of **pulmonary hypoxic vasoconstriction**.
  –cyanide toxicity (hence limitation of dose). More likely in **vitamin B₁₂** deficiency. May present with metabolic **acidosis**, and reduced **arteriovenous O₂ difference**. Treated as for **cyanide poisoning**. Combination of SNP with **trimetaphan**, and prophylactic administration of thiosulphate have been suggested as methods for reducing risk of cyanide toxicity.
  –thiocyanate may cumulate after more than 3 days' infusion, with possible interference with thyroid function.

Sodium/potassium pump. Protein pump system present in every cell **membrane**, responsible for **active transport** of **sodium** out of cells and **potassium** into cells. The protein is an **enzyme** which catalyses hydrolysis of **ATP** to ADP, providing the energy required for the transport. Consists of two α subunits (mw 95 000) which extend through the membrane and provide the binding site for ATP, and two β subunits (mw 40 000). Three sodium ions are transported for every two potassium ions, creating a net negative charge within the cell. Required for maintenance of body fluid and cell volumes and composition. Inhibited by **cardiac glycosides**.

Sodium valproate. Anticonvulsant drug used for all forms of **epilepsy**. Thought to act via enhancement of **GABA**. Rapidly absorbed by mouth and largely protein

bound. Recently made available for parenteral administration. **Half-life** is 15 hours.
- Dosage:
  - –20–30 mg/kg/day orally.
  - –5–10 mg/kg iv over 3–5 minutes; the dose may be repeated up to 2.5 mg/day.
- Side effects: GIT disturbances, transient hair loss, rarely **thrombocytopenia** and impaired **platelet** function, **pancreatitis** and severe **hepatitis**. Platelet function should be assessed prior to surgery.

Solubility. Extent to which a substance dissolves in another substance.
- Examples of clinical relevance:
  - –**inhalational anaesthetic agents**: uptake depends on their solubility in blood, and **potency** depends on their solubility in lipids (**Meyer–Overton rule**). The ability of N_2O to expand gas-containing cavities depends on its greater blood solubility than nitrogen. For a gas dissolving in a liquid, solubility depends on the temperature (solubility decreases as temperature increases), and the properties of the gas and liquid (expressed by the **solubility coefficient**). Volatile agents may also dissolve in rubber anaesthetic tubing, producing significant concentrations even when the vaporizer is turned off.
  - –non-gaseous drugs: solubility in water determines requirements for other solvents, e.g. **Cremaphor EL** or propylene glycol for parenteral injection. Solubility in lipid **membranes** affects the extent to which a drug crosses membranes, e.g. GIT wall, **blood–brain barrier**.

See also, Partition coefficient

Solubility coefficients. Expression of **solubility**. Two coefficients are commonly used:
- –Bunsen solubility coefficient: volume of gas measured at **STP** which dissolves in unit volume of liquid at the stated temperature and pressure.
- –Ostwald solubility coefficient: volume of gas dissolved in unit volume of liquid at the stated temperature and pressure, i.e. equals the **partition coefficient** between liquid and gas phases. If measured at 0°C, it equals the Bunsen solubility coefficient.

For solubility of **inhalational anaesthetic agents**, the Ostwald solubility coefficient (at 37°C) is usually used as it is independent of pressure.
[Robert WE Bunsen (1811–1899) and Wilhelm Ostwald (1853–1932), German chemists]

Solvent abuse. Common in young people. Solvents may include toluene (glues and spray paints), butane (lighter fluid), fluorocarbons (spray propellants), and trichloroethane/trichloroethylene (typewriter correction and dry-cleaning fluids). Inhalation may cause hallucinations and loss of consciousness; chronic abuse may cause impairment of all major organ systems. Severe **arrhythmias** have been reported during anaesthesia.
Boon NA (1987) BMJ; 294: 722

Somatostatin (Growth hormone inhibiting hormone). Hormone secreted by the median eminence of the **hypothalamus**. Exists in two forms, with either 14 or 28 amino acid residues. Thought to be a **neurotransmitter** in the brain and spinal cord (especially substantia gelatinosa, where it may be involved in **pain** transmission). Also secreted by the D cells of the pancreatic islets; secretion is stimulated by the presence of glucose and amino acids. Somatostatin inhibits **insulin** and **glucagon** release, gastric acid secretion and gallbladder contraction.

Analogues have been used to control diarrhoea and flushing in the **carcinoid syndrome**, possibly via inhibition of **5-HT** release. Somatostatin has been shown to produce analgesia when injected extradurally.

Sore throat, postoperative. Reported in up to 90% of cases in some studies, and up to 25% of patients following spontaneous breathing via a facepiece.
- May be related to:
  - –**tracheal intubation**:
    - –use of **suxamethonium**.
    - –shape and type of **tracheal tube** and **cuff**.
    - –trauma on laryngoscopy, intubation and extubation.
    - –use of stylets or bougies.
    - –pharyngeal suction.
    - –use of throat packs.
    - –use of lubricating/local anaesthetic gel or spray.
    - –use of nasogastric tubes.
  - –anticholinergic **premedication**.
  - –use of oro-/nasopharyngeal **airways** or **laryngeal mask**.
  - –use of unhumidified gases.

Sotalol, *see β-Adrenergic receptor antagonists*

SPEAR, Selective parenteral and enteral antisepsis regimen, *see Selective decontamination of the digestive tract*

Specific dynamic action. Energy required to assimilate food into the body, manifested as an increase in metabolic rate following intake. Thus the net total amount of energy obtained from foodstuffs is reduced (by 30% for protein, 6% for carbohydrates and 4% for fats).
See also, Nutrition

Specific gravity (Relative density). The **density** of a substance divided by that of water. Still used to indicate urinary concentration because measurement is easy (using a hydrometer), although not as useful clinically as **osmolality**. Depends on the nature and number of solute particles, whereas osmolality depends only on number of particles. Thus heavy molecules, e.g. radiographic contrast media, greatly increase specific gravity with only small increases in osmolality. Normal values: for urine, 1.002–1.035; for plasma, 1.010.

Glucose 2.7 g/l and protein 4 g/l each increase specific gravity by 0.001.

For a gas, the ratio of substance to that of **air** is used. Most anaesthetic gases and vapours are heavier than air, e.g. **isoflurane** and **enflurane** ($\times$ 7.5), **halothane** ($\times$ 6.8), N_2O ($\times$ 1.53), CO_2 ($\times$ 1.5), **cyclopropane** ($\times$ 1.4), O_2 ($\times$ 1.1).

Specific heat capacity, *see Heat capacity*

Specific latent heat, *see Latent heat*

Specificity. In **statistics**, the ability of a test to exclude false negatives. Equals

$$\frac{\text{the number tested as negative}}{\text{total without the condition.}}$$

See also, Errors; Predictive value; Sensitivity

Spinal anaesthesia (Subarachnoid/intradural anaesthesia). Probably first performed by **Corning** in 1885, but first performed for surgery by **Bier** in 1899. Initial use of **cocaine** was associated with tremor, headache and muscle spasms. The less toxic **procaine** was first used by **Braun** in 1905 and was soon used widely. Hyperbaric solutions were introduced by **Barker** in 1907. Further refinements were related to new **local anaesthetic agents**. Continuous spinal techniques were described in the 1940s, initially via rubber tubing connected to the **needle** left *in situ*.

Popularity waned in the late 1940s following reports of neurological damage and the introduction of **neuromuscular blocking drugs** for general anaesthesia (GA). In the classic Woolley and Roe case in the UK, two cases of paraplegia during the same operating list followed spinal anaesthesia. Phenol contamination via cracks in the **cinchocaine** ampoules was blamed at the time, although contamination of the syringes and needles with acidic descaler solution from the sterilizer has been suggested as being more likely.

Increasing popularity over the last 30–40 years has followed better understanding of the technique, and acceptance that the incidence of side effects is low when spinal anaesthesia is correctly performed (e.g. a classic paper by Dripps and Vandam in 1954, reporting the results of over 10 000 cases).

• Indications: surgical procedures to the lower body, especially perineum and legs. Considered the method of choice (with **extradural anaesthesia**) by many anaesthetists for **TURP**, **Caesarean section** and **orthopaedic surgery**, e.g. of the hip. Has been used for upper abdominal surgery. Deliberate high or total spinal anaesthesia was formerly used for **hypotensive anaesthesia**, and to provide abdominal muscle relaxation.

• Anatomy:
  – the **spinal cord** ends at L1–2 in adults, lower levels in children. The dura ends at S2; therefore lumbar puncture is usually performed at the L3–4, L4–5 or L5–S1 interspaces.
  – the L4 or L4–5 interspace is crossed by a line drawn between the iliac crests. The spinous process of T12 has a notched lower edge.
  – the course taken by the needle is as for reaching the **extradural space**, plus the dura (*See also, Meninges; Vertebrae; Vertebral canal; Vertebral ligaments*).

• Technique:
  – **preoperative assessment**, preparation and **premedication is** as for GA. Facilities for resuscitation and progression to GA must be available.
  – **monitoring** is as for GA. An iv cannula must be placed. Preloading with fluid is controversial unless for Caesarean section (see below).
  – the patient is placed in the lateral position, with chin on the chest and knees drawn up, or sitting on the edge of the trolley. Back flexion opens the intervertebral spaces. An assistant is required to steady the patient.
  – the back is cleaned, avoiding contamination of gloves and needles with cleaning solution (implicated in

causing **arachnoiditis**). Use of gown and drapes is controversial; they are usually employed in the UK, but less so in the USA.
  – median approach:
    – the chosen interspace is infiltrated with local anaesthetic.
    – the spinal needle is inserted in the midline, aiming slightly cranially. The **Quincke** needle point is often used, with a short-bevelled cutting tip. Non-cutting needles, e.g. Sprotte (smooth-sided pointed tip, with wide lateral hole proximal to the tip), Whitacre (pencil-tip-shaped, with the hole just proximal to the tip) or Greene (oblique bevel, with bevel edges rounded) have been claimed to cause a lower incidence of **postspinal headache** (Fig. 121). 22–29 G needles are commonly used; the

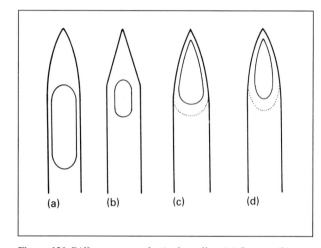

Figure 121 *Different types of spinal needles: (a) Sprotte; (b) Whitacre; (c) Greene; (d) Quincke*

larger are easier to use but increase the risk of postspinal headache. Thinner needles are often inserted through a 19 G iv needle or introducer, e.g. Sise introducer. The bevel is faced laterally to reduce the risk of headache.
    – resistance increases as the ligamentum flavum is entered and when dura is encountered, with a sudden give as the dura is pierced. Correct location is confirmed by CSF at the needle hub; aspiration may be required with very fine needles. Rotation of the needle in 90° steps may produce CSF if none is obtained initially.

      Hanging drop and other techniques have been used to identify the extradural space prior to dural puncture.
    – with the other hand securing the needle against the patient's back to avoid dislodgement, the solution is injected, with aspiration before, during and after injection to confirm correct placement. Injection should cease if pain is experienced.
  – paramedian approach: requires less back flexion, and is easier if the vertabral ligaments are calcified:
    – infiltration is performed 1.5 cm lateral to the cranial border of the spinous process at the selected interspace.
    – the needle is inserted, aiming medially and cranially until the resistance of the ligamentum

flavum is felt. If the lamina is encountered, the needle is walked off its cranial edge.
 –dural puncture and injection as before.
–a continuous catheter technique may be used as for extradural anaesthesia; it has been unpopular because of fears over infection and CSF leak, although it is used more widely in Europe. 32 G catheters have recently been introduced in the UK; although they have been used with success they are difficult to handle and have been associated with cauda equina syndrome (although their role in the latter's aetiology is unclear).
- Solutions used:
 –only hyperbaric **bupivacaine** 0.5% + 8% glucose is available specifically for spinal anaesthesia in the UK; plain bupivacaine and **lignocaine** have been used but blockade is less reliable, especially with lignocaine. Hyperbaric cinchocaine 0.5% + 6% glucose was previously available. In the USA, hyperbaric 0.75% bupivacaine + 8.25% glucose, **amethocaine** (tetracaine) 1% + 10% glucose, and lignocaine 5% + 7.5% glucose are available (Table 32).

Table 32. Doses (mg) of local anaesthetics required for spinal blockade of different heights

Agent	L4	T10	T4–6	Duration (h)
Bupivacaine 0.5% (heavy)	5–10	10–15	15–20	1.5–2.5
Amethocaine 1.0% (heavy; mixed with equal volumes of CSF)	4–6	8–12	14–16	1.5–2.5
Cinchocaine 0.5% (heavy)	4–6	6–8	10–12	2–3
Lignocaine 5% (heavy)	25–50	50–75	75–100	1–1.5

–larger volumes are required for plain solutions than for heavy ones. Duration of block may be extended by addition of vasopressors; **adrenaline** 0.2–0.5 ml 1:1000 and **phenylephrine** 0.5–5 mg have been used. Fears have been expressed concerning possible cord ischaemia provoked by their use. L5–S2 segments remain blocked for the longest.
–spread of solution and extent of blockade are affected by many factors, including:
  –dose: thought to be the most important; increased variability may occur with altered concentration and volume.
  –site of injection.
  –baricity of solution and position: thus hyperbaric solutions affect dependent parts, hypobaric solutions, e.g. amethocaine 0.1%, affect upper parts. Plain bupivacaine 0.5% is slightly hypobaric; amethocaine 1% is isobaric.
   Use of hyper- or hypobaric solutions relies on lateral/supine positioning and head-up/down tilt, combined with the normal curvature of the spine:
   –thoracic curve is concave anteriorly; T4 is the most posterior part (most dependent in the supine position).
   –lumbar curve is convex anteriorly; L3 is the most anterior part (uppermost in the supine position). This curve may be abolished by flexing the hips in the supine position.
In addition, the greater width of females' hips compared with their shoulders tends to tip their spinal canal head down, in the lateral position; in males, the opposite occurs.
   Thus slow injection of 1 ml hyperbaric solution at L5–S1 with the patient sitting produces saddle block suitable for perineal surgery, with minimal hypotension. Blocks may be restricted to one side by injection in the lateral position, although 'fixing' of local anaesthetic may require up to 40 minutes. Injection of hyperbaric solution in the lateral position with immediate turning into the supine position usually produces blockade to T4–6.
–patient factors, e.g. weight, height, sex, age, are not thought to be as critical as previously suspected, but they have a small influence. Large variability of blockade between patients is normally found. Reduced volumes are required in **obstetric analgesia and anaesthesia**.
–technical factors, e.g. speed of injection, barbotage (repeated aspiration of CSF into syringe, mixing it with local anaesthetic before reinjection), direction of the needle, etc., tend to affect variability of blocks; thus slow injection without barbotage produces the most reliable results.
–other drugs have been used, e.g. opioids (*see Spinal opioids*), **ketamine**, **midazolam** and **clonidine**.
- Effects:
 –results in rapid onset of block (usually within 3–5 minutes), although maximal effect may take up to 30 minutes. Vasodilatation in the feet is usually seen first, with flushing and increased warmth.
 –thought to act mainly at **spinal nerve** roots, although some effect is possible at the **spinal cord** itself. Differential blockade of different motor and sensory modalitites is traditionally thought to be related to the size and therefore sensitivity of different **neurones** to local anaesthetics. Thus the smaller sympathetic preganglionic fibres are more easily blocked than larger sensory and motor fibres, with the sympathetic 'level' higher than the sensory level. Assessment of the sympathetic level is difficult; the **galvanic skin response** has been used. The level of blockade for touch sensation is two segments below that for pinprick, whilst that for motor innervation is two segments lower than that for sensory innervation.
 –CVS:
  –sympathetic blockade causes vasodilatation below the level of block. Reductions in cardiac output and BP are thought to be caused mainly by reduced venous return consequent on venous dilatation, although the fall in SVR contributes. Increased or unaltered cardiac output has also been reported. Reflex vasoconstriction occurs above the level of block. Hypotension is particularly likely in **hypovolaemia**, since cardiac output in this case is dependent on resting vasoconstriction.
  Hypotension is also more likely in obstetrics, when **aortocaval compression** may occur. Hypotension may be exacerbated by bradycardia and sedative

drugs (depressant effects of local anaesthetic are minimal). The drop in BP may be greater with higher levels of blockade, but this is not always so.

–bradycardia may be due to block of sympathetic cardiac innervation (T1–4), vagal stimulation during surgery, or a reflex response to decreased venous return. **Cardiac arrest** has been reported.

–cardiac work and O_2 demand are reduced.

–renal, hepatic, cerebral and coronary blood flows are maintained if marked hypotension does not occur.

–reduction in peroperative bleeding is thought to be due to reduced BP, lack of venous hypertension secondary to venoconstriction, and pooling of blood in dependent vessels.

–reduction of postoperative **DVT** is thought to be due to vasodilatation, **haemodilution** and reduced **viscosity** secondary to iv fluid administration, increased **fibrinolysis**, and possible effects of local anaesthetics themselves.

–absorbed adrenaline may have systemic effects, if used.

–RS: intercostal and abdominal weakness may impair active exhalation and coughing, although tidal volume and inspiratory pressure are maintained by intact diaphragmatic innervation (C3–5). **FRC** is reduced when supine, and hypoventilation may follow sedation; thus O_2 is usually administered via a facepiece as a precaution, and to allow concurrent N_2O administration if required.

–GIT: bowel contraction results from dominant parasympathetic tone following sympathetic blockade. Sphincters relax and peristalsis increases.

–**urinary retention** may occur.

–**stress response to surgery** is attenuated.

Injected drug is eliminated via absorption by subarachnoid and extradural vessels.

● Management:

–assessment: level of sensory blockade is usually determined by testing for temperature (e.g. using ice or **ethyl chloride** spray) or pinprick sensation. Knowledge of appropriate **dermatomes** is required. Motor block is assessed by testing muscle groups of appropriate **myotomes**. The Bromage scale is commonly used for assessment of motor block:

–0: full flexion possible at knees and feet.

–1: cannot raise extended leg, but can move knees and feet.

–2: cannot flex knee, but can move feet.

–3: cannot move any part of leg or foot.

–positioning of the patient may be used to extend or reduce spread of the block as required, until fixed.

–a high level of block may produce feelings of impaired breathing and nasal stuffiness, plus impaired sensation or power in the arms. Total spinal blockade results in apnoea and loss of consciousness, with fixed dilated pupils. Treatment is as for hypotension, plus tracheal intubation and IPPV. Recovery is complete if BP and oxygenation are maintained.

–preloading with iv fluid prior to performing spinal anaesthesia is controversial (except in obstetrics, when the benefit of preloading is undisputed), since the incidence of hypotension may be similar whether preloaded or not. In addition, fears have been expressed concerning fluid overload, especially in the elderly.

A drop in systolic BP to one-third normal value is usually considered acceptable in healthy patients. Management of larger decreases:

–positioning the patient head-down: increases venous return but risks higher level of block unless the head is raised.

–**iv fluid administration. Crystalloids** are usually acceptable initially.

–use of **vasopressor drugs**. May increase myocardial work and O_2 demand secondary to increases in SVR. **Ephedrine** (3–6 mg iv repeated as required) is commonly used; effects on venous tone may be greater than with other drugs, e.g. **methoxamine**, phenylephrine, **metaraminol** (all of which may be given in 1–2 mg iv increments).

–**atropine** 0.3–0.6 mg if bradycardia occurs.

–nausea: may be related to vagal stimulation, e.g. during handling of the bowel. Hypotension is an important cause.

–**sedation** is commonly administered, by infusion or bolus. **Benzodiazepines** are commonly used; **ketamine** provides some analgesia, e.g. whilst positioning for injection in trauma cases. **Propofol** infusions may also be used. Advantages include unawareness, and a smoother procedure if unpleasant sensations are not completely abolished. Disadvantages include respiratory and cardiovascular depression and confusion, especially if sedation is excessive. General and spinal anaesthesia may be combined, not necessarily with increased risk of hypotension.

● Complications:

–hypotension and high blockade as above.

–postspinal headache.

–neurological damage:

–direct trauma is extremely rare. Injection should stop immediately if pain is felt.

–haematoma formation with spinal cord compression is extremely rare with normal coagulation. It may be masked by regional blockade. Permanent neurological damage may occur if surgical decompression is delayed.

–cord ischaemia, e.g. **anterior spinal artery syndrome**, thought usually to occur with severe hypotension. Vasopressor drugs have been implicated but their role is unclear.

–infection/aseptic meningitis.

–arachnoiditis.

–backache: thought to be caused by muscular relaxation with possible stretching of ligaments, etc., rather than direct trauma.

–**anaphylactic reaction** to local anaesthetics (extremely rare).

● Contraindications:

–non-acceptance by the patient.

–infection, both generalized and local.

–hypovolaemia/shock.

–neurological disease: raised **ICP** is an absolute contraindication because of the risk of **coning**. Other disease is controversial; medicolegal implications are usually quoted (e.g. fear of being blamed if a naturally progressive lesion becomes worse).

–abnormal coagulation: full anticoagulation or coagulation disorders are considered absolute contraindications. Low dose **heparin** therapy is controversial; the decision usually depends on consideration of

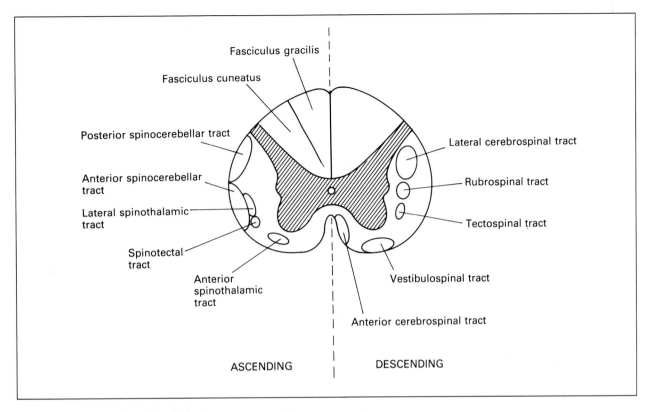

Fasciculus gracilis

Fasciculus cuneatus

Posterior spinocerebellar tract

Anterior spinocerebellar tract

Lateral spinothalamic tract

Spinotectal tract

Anterior spinothalamic tract

Lateral cerebrospinal tract

Rubrospinal tract

Tectospinal tract

Vestibulospinal tract

Anterior cerebrospinal tract

ASCENDING

DESCENDING

Figure 122 *Anatomy of spinal cord showing ascending and descending tracts*

individual risks and benefits, and immediately preoperative **coagulation studies**. A platelet count of $100 \times 10^9/l$ is usually taken as the lower safe limit, but the true safe value is unknown. Platelet function is also important, but effects of **antiplatelet drugs, e.g. salicylates** are unclear. A bleeding time of 10 minutes has been suggested as the lower safe limit. Spinal anaesthesia has been claimed to be safer than extradural anaesthesia, since the needles are finer.

–emergency abdominal surgery, especially intestinal obstruction: hypovolaemia may be present, and increased GIT activity following spinal anaesthesia may increase the risk of perforation. The patient may also be actively vomiting.

[Albert Woolley and Cecil Roe, English labourers; Robert D Dripps (1911–1974), Leroy D Vandam, Nicholas Greene and Lincoln F Sise (1874–1942), US anaesthetists; G Sprotte, German anaesthetist; RJ Whitacre (described 1951), US anaesthetist; Philip R Bromage, Canadian anaesthetist]
Greene NM (1985) Anesth Analg; 64: 715–30

Spinal cord. Cylindrical structure beginning superiorly at the foramen magnum and terminating inferiorly level with L1–2 (L3 at birth, rising to the adult level by 20 years). May rarely end at T12 or L3. Continuous superiorly with the medulla oblongata, it tapers inferiorly to form the conus medullaris. The filum terminale, an extension of the pia mater, attaches the lower end to the back of the coccyx. Lies within the **vertebral canal**, surrounded by the **meninges** and bathed in **CSF**. The anterior median fissure is a deep longitudinal fissure and the posterior median

sulcus is a shallow furrow. Gives off 31 pairs of **spinal nerves** throughout its length. On cross-section, consists of central H-shaped grey matter surrounded by white matter. The grey matter is composed of anterior and posterior horns, with lateral horns (sympathetic columns) in the thoracic region. The two halves are joined across the midline by the grey commissure which contains the central canal (Fig. 122).

● Main ascending tracts:
  –posterior columns: convey ipsilateral touch and vibration/proprioception sensation, from the lower body via the fasciculus gracilis and upper body via the fasciculus cuneatus.
  –posterior and anterior spinocerebellar tracts: convey proprioception sensation to the cerebellum via inferior and superior cerebellar peduncles respectively.
  –lateral and anterior spinothalamic tracts: the former conveys contralateral pain and temperature sensation; the latter conveys contralateral touch and pressure sensation.
  –spinotectal tract: conveys information to the brainstem involved in spinovisual reflexes.
● Main descending tracts:
  –lateral and anterior cerebrospinal tracts: convey motor innervation from the cerebral cortex; the former via crossed (pyramidal) fibres and the latter via uncrossed (extrapyramidal) fibres.
  –rubrospinal, tectospinal and vestibulospinal tracts: contain extrapyramidal fibres passing from brainstem nuclei to lower motor neurones.
● Blood supply:

–anterior spinal artery: formed from two branches of the vertebral arteries, and descends in the anterior median fissure. Supplies the anterior 2/3 of the cord.

–posterior spinal arteries: arise from the vertebral arteries, each dividing into two branches which descend along the side of the cord, one anterior and one posterior to the dorsal nerve roots.

–radicular branches: arise from local arteries, e.g. intercostal, lumbar, and feed the spinal arteries. The most important are at T1 and the lower thoracic/upper lumbar level (artery of Adamkiewicz). The cord at T3–5 and T12–L1 is thought to be most at risk from ischaemia.

[Albert Adamkiewicz (1850–1921), Polish pathologist]
See also, Motor pathways; Sensory pathways; Spinal cord injury

Spinal cord injury. Most common in males aged 15–35, mostly caused by motor vehicle accidents. C5–6 and T12–L1 levels of the **spinal cord** are affected most often. Associated injuries (especially **head injury**) occur in 25–65% of cases.

- Features of acute injury:
  –initial hypertension and peripheral vasoconstriction. **Arrhythmias** are common. Hypotension and brady-cardia may occur in lesions above T6 and T1 respec-tively, caused by sympathetic disruption (**spinal shock**). **Autonomic hyperreflexia** may occur after 4–6 weeks if the lesion is above T5–6.
  –neurogenic **pulmonary oedema** is common with cervi-cal lesions.
  –initial flaccid paralysis is followed after 2–3 weeks by spastic paralysis. Paralytic ileus is common for 2–3 weeks.

- Certain clinical syndromes may occur:
  –complete injury, with loss of motor or sensory function below a certain level.
  –incomplete injury syndromes:
    –central cord: arms paralysed more than legs, with bladder dysfunction and variable sensory loss.
    –anterior cord: paralysis below the level of lesion, with proprioception, touch and vibration sense preserved.
    –posterior cord: only touch and temperature sensa-tion impaired.
    –hemisection of cord (Brown-Séquard): ipsilateral paralysis and loss of proprioception, touch and vibration sensation, with loss of contralateral pain and temperature sensation.

Primary damage is from the initial injury; the following have been suggested as causing secondary damage: ischaemia, compression, **oedema**, release of **free radicals**, **arachidonic acid** metabolites and excitatory amino acids, and leakage of **calcium** into cells and **potassium** out of cells. Thus initial treatment is aimed at reducing ischaemia, inflammation and oedema formation.

- Management:
  –as for any **trauma**, with particular emphasis on the **airway**, maintenance of cardiac output and oxygena-tion, and stabilization of the spine.
  –high dose methylprednisolone (30 mg/kg iv, followed by 5.4 mg/kg/h for 23 hours) within 8 hours of injury has recently been shown to reduce the incidence and severity of long-term sequelae.
  –IPPV is required in lesions above C3–5.
  –prevention of **DVT**, **stress ulcers**, bedsores, etc.

Mortality is about 45%, being highest in patients under 1 year and over 70 years. Pulmonary complications (e.g. **hypoventilation**, **aspiration pneumonitis**, **chest infection**, **PE**) are the commonest causes of death within the first 3 months of injury. Other complications are related to **nutri-tion**, urinary function and sepsis, osteoporosis, psycholog-ical problems and **pain** syndromes.

- Anaesthetic management is related to:
  –other injuries and cardiorespiratory impairment.
  –potential difficult intubation and risk of aspiration.
  –hyperkalaemic response to **suxamethonium** within 10 days–6 months of injury.
  –**positioning of the patient**.
  –impaired **temperature regulation**.
  –requirement for postoperative IPPV.
  –impaired cardiovascular responses and autonomic hyperreflexia.

[Charles E Brown-Séquard (1818–1894), Mauritius-born US, English and French physician]
Fraser A, Edmonds-Seal J (1982) Anaesthesia; 37: 1084–98

Spinal headache, *see Postspinal headache*

Spinal nerves. Consist of pairs of **nerves** (8 cervical, 12 thoracic, 5 lumbar, 5 sacral and 1 coccygeal). Formed within the **vertebral canal** from anterior (ventral) and posterior (dorsal) roots, themselves formed from rootlets which emerge from the antero- and posterolateral aspects of the **spinal cord**. The anterior roots convey efferent motor fibres from the cord, and the posterior roots convey afferent sensory fibres to the cord. Each spinal nerve leaves the vertebral canal through an intervertebral foramen. The posterior (dorsal) root ganglia lie within the foramina except for C1 and C2 (lie on the posterior verte-bral arches) and the sacral and coccygeal ganglia (lie within the canal). The first cervical nerve emerges between the occiput and the arch of the atlas; C2–7 emerge above their respective **vertebrae** and C8 emerges between C7 and T1. Below this, each spinal nerve emerges below its corresponding vertebra. After giving off a small meningeal branch, each divides into a large anterior and smaller posterior primary ramus (Fig. 123).

- Anterior primary rami:
  –supply cutaneous and motor innervation of the limbs, and front and sides of the neck, thorax and abdomen.

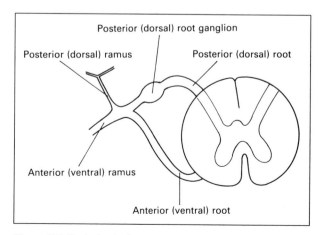

Figure 123 *Typical spinal nerve*

–cervical: C1–4 form the **cervical plexus**, C5–8 the **brachial plexus**.

–thoracic: termed the **intercostal nerves**.

–lumbar: L1–4 form the **lumbar plexus**.

–sacral and coccygeal: contribute to the **sacral plexus**.

- Posterior primary rami:

  –supply motor and sensory innervation to the muscles and skin of the back.

  –do not contribute to limb innervation or plexus formation.

  –divide into medial and lateral branches (except for C1, S4, S5 and coccygeal rami). Cutaneous innervation of T6 and above is contained in the medial branch, below this in the lateral branch.

  –cervical:

  –C1: entirely motor, supplying the muscles of the upper neck.

  –C2: supplies the skin of the back of the head via the greater occipital nerve; motor supply to the neck muscles.

  –C3–8: sensory supply to the lower occiput and neck; motor fibres to the neck muscles.

  –thoracic, lumbar, sacral and coccygeal: unremarkable.

Embryonic segmental distribution of nerves to the skin and muscles is represented by the segmental distribution of cutaneous and motor innervation (**dermatomes** and **myotomes** respectively).

Spinal opioids. Spinal or extradural administration of **opioid analgesic drugs** has become widespread since the first report of extradural **morphine** administration in man in 1979. Opioids given in this way are thought to bind to **opioid receptors** in the substantia gelatinosa of the **spinal cord**, interfering with **pain pathways**. Although systemic absorption of opioid may contribute to the analgesia, selective spinal block is suggested by high CSF/plasma drug levels and the low doses required compared with those used for parenteral administration. A segmental effect has been reported, i.e. maximal analgesia is related to the site of injection, although lumbar administration has been used for analgesia after **thoracic surgery**. This may be related to the lipid solubility of the opioid used; thus morphine diffuses further in the CSF than less soluble drugs.

The main advantage of spinal opioids over systemic opioids is profound analgesia which lasts longer. Advantages over spinal or extradural **local anaesthetic agents** are the lack of sympathetic, motor or sensory blockade, and the ability to provide analgesia distant to the level of injection (e.g. lumbar injection is effective for pain following thoracotomy).

Onset and duration of action are closely related to the lipid solubility of the drug. Highly lipid soluble drugs, e.g. **fentanyl** and **methadone**, cross the **CSF** and bind to the spinal cord rapidly (molecular shape is also important). Only a small amount is thus available to diffuse throughout the CSF. However, their duration of action is short since they are more rapidly absorbed into the bloodstream. They are more likely to act (at least partially) via systemic absorption. Poorly lipid soluble drugs, e.g. morphine have slower onset time (up to 1 hour) and their actions last for up to 24 hours. There is great variability in effective dose and duration of action between patients (Table 33).

- Extradural infusions are commonly used, e.g. postoperatively:

Table 33. Extradural doses of commonly used opioids

Drug	Extradural dose	Duration (h)
Morphine	1–8 mg	12–18
Fentanyl	100–200 µg	3–6
Pethidine	25–100 mg	6–8
Diamorphine	0.5–10 mg	5–8
Sufentanil	10–75 µg	4–10
Methadone	4–6 mg	4–6
Buprenorphine	60–300 µg	8–10

–morphine 0.5 mg/h.

–fentanyl 50–100 µg/h.

–**pethidine** 10–15 mg/h.

–**diamorphine** 0.25–2.0 mg/h.

–**sufentanil** 25–50 µg/h.

–methadone 0.5 mg/h.

Infusions of opioid/local anaesthetic mixtures may also be used, e.g. for **postoperative analgesia**: a common combination is diamorphine 2.5–5.0 mg added to 50 ml of 0.1–0.2% **bupivacaine**; the solution is run at 2–10 ml/h.

Intrathecal administration is less commonly used, because of the greater incidence of side effects. Morphine 0.1–2.0 mg has been described most commonly. Pethidine 50–100 mg has been used as sole anaesthetic agent for procedures on the lower body, possibly related to its local anaesthetic properties.

- Side effects:

  –respiratory depression:

  –early (within an hour of administration): thought to be related to high plasma levels of the drug; thus more common if highly soluble drugs are used.

  –late (4–15 hours after administration, depending on the drug used): thought to be caused by rostral spread of the drug within the CSF to the medullary respiratory centre. More likely with poorly lipid soluble drugs (e.g. morphine), after intrathecal administration, in the elderly, and if other parenteral opioids are administered at the same time. Highly lipid soluble drugs, e.g. fentanyl, bind more avidly to the spinal cord, with less drug available to spread within the CSF. Although uncommon (0.5–3.0%), late respiratory depression may occur when the patient is unattended, e.g. at night, hence the requirement for close monitoring for up to 24 hours after administration, especially if morphine is used. Respiratory rate alone is a poor indicator of the degree of depression; arterial oxygen saturation and level of sedation may be more useful. **Naloxone** may reverse respiratory depression without affecting analgesia; prophylactic low dose infusion has been used.

  –urinary retention: occurs in 30–40% of cases, although its occurrence in up to 90% of males has been reported. Presence of vesical opioid receptors has been suggested.

  –pruritus: affects up to 70% of patients after morphine, 10% after fentanyl. More common after intrathecal administration. May be helped by **antihistamine drugs** and naloxone. The cause is unknown.

  –nausea and vomiting: similar incidence to that after parenteral administration, although more common after intrathecal opioids.

–Herpes simplex virus reactivation has been described in obstetric patients.

Spinal opioids are used widely for **postoperative analgesia** following major surgery, and in chronic **pain management**. Their use alone in **obstetric analgesia and anaesthesia** is associated with a relatively high incidence of side effects. In obstetrics, fentanyl is most commonly used in small doses or by extradural infusion together with local anaesthetics (and may reduce requirements for the latter).

Morgan M (1989) Br J Anaesth; 63: 165–88

Spinal shock. Syndrome following sudden **spinal cord injury**, characterized by hypotension (if the level of injury is above T6) and bradycardia (if the level is above T1). Hypotension arises from interrupted sympathetic vasoconstrictor tone, and is greatest in the upright position. Usually replaced by **autonomic hyperreflexia** after 4–6 weeks. Hypotension may be dramatic on **induction of anaesthesia** and institution of **IPPV**.

See also, Valsalva manoeuvre

Spinal surgery. May be required for **kyphoscoliosis**, **trauma**, laminectomy, tumours, abscess, etc.

- Anaesthetic management is as for kyphoscoliosis and **neurosurgery**; main points:
  - **preoperative assessment** for associated disease, ventilatory impairment, neurological damage, etc.
  - traction and impaired movement may hinder access and tracheal intubation, especially for **cervical spine** surgery.
  - severe **hyperkalaemia** may follow **suxamethonium** if neurological damage is present. Period of risk: 10 days – 6 months.
  - surgery may be prolonged with risk of excessive **blood loss**, **hypothermia**, etc. Damage to inferior cava, aorta and iliac arteries may lead to rapid exsanguination without obvious bleeding from the operation site.
  - **hypotensive anaesthesia** reduces blood loss but may risk **spinal cord** ischaemia. Infiltration with vasopressors has been used.
  - **extradural anaesthesia** has been used, e.g. for laminectomy, with good results.
  - cord function may be assessed by the **wake-up test** or by monitoring **evoked potentials**.
  - **airway obstruction** may follow anterior cervical spine surgery if extensive. **Ondine's curse** may also occur.

Spirometer. Device for measuring **lung volumes**. The wet spirometer consists of a lightweight cylinder suspended over a breathing chamber with a water seal (Fig. 124). Vertical movement of the cylinder corresponding to respiratory movements is recorded on a rotating drum via a pen attached to the cylinder.

May be used to measure volumes directly, or using **dilution techniques**. Also used to calculate flow rates and **basal metabolic rate**. Inaccuracies may arise from inertia of the system at high respiratory rates, and the dissolution of small amounts of gas into the water of the seal.

Dry spirometers, e.g. the Vitalograph, are more convenient for bedside use. It contains bellows attached to a pen, with a sheet of recording paper automatically moved by a motor during expiration. The best results from three attempts are usually recorded.

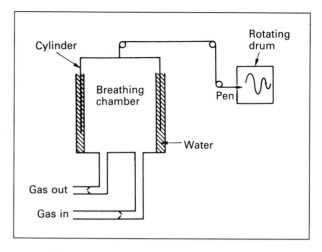

Figure 124 *Wet spirometer*

Spironolactone. Diuretic, acting via competitive antagonism of **aldosterone**. Inhibits sodium/potassium exchange in the distal renal tubule, with retention of potassium and hydrogen ions. Used to treat oedema due to secondary **hyperaldosteronism**, e.g. associated with **hepatic failure** and **cardiac failure**; and in primary hyperaldosteronism. Diuresis occurs 2–3 hours after oral administration.

- Dosage: 100–400 mg daily, orally.
- Side effects: GIT disturbances, gynaecomastia, hyperkalaemia.

Splitting ratio. Ratio of gas flow bypassing an anaesthetic **vaporizer** to the gas flow entering it. At a splitting ratio of zero, the total gas flow passes through the vaporizer; at a ratio of infinity, none passes through (i.e. the vaporizer is switched off).

Sprays. In anaesthesia, usually employed to deliver **local anaesthetic agent** (usually 4% **lignocaine**) to the **larynx** and trachea, e.g. for awake tracheal intubation, and to reduce stimulation during positioning and tracheal extubation. Spraying the cords at laryngoscopy does not attenuate the hypertensive response to laryngoscopy itself. Common laryngeal sprays include the Forrester, **Macintosh** and Swerdlow sprays (Fig. 125). A metered-dose aerosol is also available, delivering 10 mg of 10% lignocaine per spray; its nozzle may be too short to reach the larynx. Syringes with long perforated nozzles are also available.

Sprays may also be used to spray **cocaine** into the nose, to produce anaesthesia and vasoconstriction.

Other sprays used in anaesthesia include the **ethyl chloride** spray for **refrigeration anaesthesia** and testing **regional anaesthesia**, and disinfectant sprays, dressings, etc.

Problems include blockage, bacterial contamination of the local anaesthetic agent, parts of the spray becoming detached and entering the airway (e.g. the tip of the Macintosh spray), and excessive administration of local anaesthetic agent.

[Alexander C Forrester, Glasgow anaesthetist; Mark Swerdlow, Manchester anaesthetist]

SRS-A, Slow reacting substance-A, *see Leukotrienes*

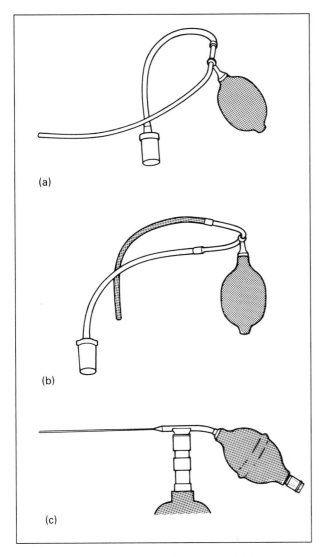

Figure 125 *Commonly used anaesthetic sprays: (a) Forrester; (b) Macintosh; (c) Swerdlow*

S–T segment. Portion of the **ECG** between the end of the **QRS complex** and the beginning of the **T wave** (*see Fig. 49b; Electrocardiography*). Represents ventricular repolarization. Average duration is 0.32 seconds. Normally within 1 mm of the height of the isoelectric line (between the T wave and following P wave). Elevated following acute myocardial damage, e.g. **MI** and **pericarditis**. Depressed by **myocardial ischaemia**, **hypokalaemia** and **digoxin** therapy, the latter typically producing a 'reverse tick' pattern. May also be depressed in reciprocal leads following MI.

Stages of anaesthesia, *see Anaesthesia, stages of*

Standard bicarbonate. Plasma concentration of **bicarbonate** when arterial P_{CO_2} has been corrected to 5.3 kPa (40 mmHg), with **haemoglobin** fully saturated and at a temperature of 37°C. Thus eliminates the respiratory component of **acidosis** or **alkalosis**. Normally 24–33 mmol/l.
See also, Acid–base balance

Standard deviation (SD). Expression of the variability of a **population** or **sample**. Equals the square root of **variance**, i.e.:

$$SD = \frac{\sqrt{\Sigma(x - \bar{x})^2}}{n-1}$$

Squaring $(x - \bar{x})$ eliminates any minus signs, i.e. for those values of x less than $\bar{x}$

In a sample of normal distribution, a range of 1 SD on either side of the **mean** includes about 68% of all observations, 2 SDs on either side include about 95%, and 3 SDs on either side include about 99.7%.
See also, Statistical frequency distributions; Statistics

Standard error of the mean (SE). Indication of how well the **mean** of a **sample** represents the true **population** mean.

$$SE = \frac{\textbf{standard deviation} \ (SD)}{\sqrt{n}}$$

where n = number of values.
SE is large when n is small, i.e. the sample mean is less likely to represent the population mean.

May also be used to calculate the likelihood of two samples being part of the same population; i.e. whether the difference between them is statistically significant (only applicable when each sample contains more than 30 values).

Often presented with the mean in statistical **data**, because the data appears tidier, and mean ± SE has a smaller spread than mean ± SD. Apart from this, SE has no advantage over SD.
See also, Statistical tests; Statistics

Starling forces. Factors determining the movement of fluid across the capillary wall endothelium. Movement into the interstitial space is encouraged by the hydrostatic pressure gradient (capillary hydrostatic pressure (P_c) – interstitial fluid hydrostatic pressure (P_i)). This flow is counteracted by the colloid osmotic gradient (capillary colloid osmotic pressure (π_c) – interstitial fluid colloid osmotic pressure (π_i)):

$$Q = K \left[(P_c - P_i) - \sigma(\pi_c - \pi_i) \right]$$

where Q = net flow of fluid for a given surface area,
  K = permeability or filtration coefficient (flow rate per unit pressure gradient across the endothelium),
  σ = reflection coefficient (represents permeability of the endothelium to plasma proteins).

The equation does not account for **active transport** of solutes, and effects of **surface tension** in the lung.

In health, the volumes of fluid leaving and entering the capillaries are equal. Capillary hydrostatic pressure falls from about 30 mmHg at the arteriolar end (favouring net flow of fluid out of the capillary) to 15 mmHg at the venous end (favouring net flow in). Imbalance may result in **oedema**.
[Ernest H Starling (1866–1927), London physiologist]

Starling resistor. Model consisting of a length of collapsible tubing passing through a rigid box (Fig. 126). The effects of different upstream pressures (P_1), pressures in the chamber (P_2) and downstream pressures (P_3) on

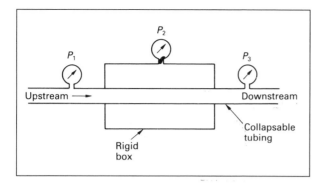

Figure 126 *Starling resistor (see text)*

flow through the tubing can be studied. Used to illustrate the effect of gravity on regional **pulmonary circulation**, P_1, P_2 and P_3 representing arterial, alveolar and venous pressures respectively.
See also, Starling forces; Ventilation/perfusion mismatch

Starling's law (Frank–Starling law). Intrinsic regulatory mechanism of the heart stating that force of myocardial contraction is proportional to initial fibre length, up to a point (Fig. 127). Neither variable is easily measured; hence myocardial contraction is often represented by **cardiac output**, **stroke volume**, **stroke index** or **stroke work** (*y*-axis) and initial fibre length is represented by **left ventricular end-diastolic volume**, **left ventricular end-diastolic pressure** or **pulmonary capillary wedge pressure** (*x*-axis).

Changes in **myocardial contractility** shift the curve's position; e.g. in **cardiac failure** and **MI** it is moved downwards and to the right. Cardiac dilatation compensates initially, by moving along the curve to the right. The curve is shifted upwards and to the left by exercise, **inotropic drugs**, etc.

The (Starling) curves may be plotted for individual patients, and have been used to guide management of reduced output states.

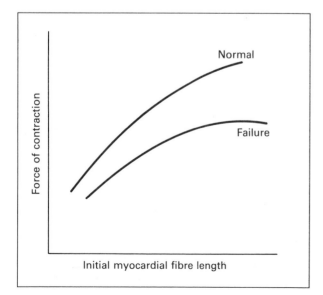

Figure 127 *Starling's law*

[Freidrich WF Frank (1865–1944), German physiologist]
O'Rourke MF (1984) Aust NZ J Med; 14: 879–87
See also, Starling forces

Starvation, *see Malnutrition*

Static electricity, *see Antistatic precautions; Explosions and fires*

Statistical frequency distributions. In **statistics**, relationships between measured variables and the frequency with which each value occurs. For continuous **data**, the resultant curve may often be described by a mathematical equation, allowing **statistical tests** and other analyses to be performed. Many types of biological data have a 'normal' (Gaussian) distribution (Fig. 128). Such

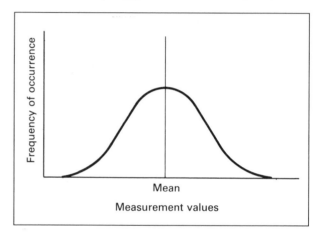

Figure 128 *Normal frequency distribution curve*

data are described by the **mean** and **standard deviation** (SD). The standard normal deviate (z) describes any individual value by relating it to the mean and SD, and can be used to calculate the **probability** that such a value lies within the 'normal' range. Parametric statistical tests may be used to test the hypothesis that different **samples** of normally-distributed data are in fact taken from the same **population** (**null hypothesis**). They compare within-group variability with between-group differences; e.g. two samples are likely to represent different populations if the scatter (SD) of each is small and their means are very different.

Data which are not normally distributed (e.g. skewed) may often be 'normalized', e.g. by logarithmic transformation, allowing application of parametric tests which are more sensitive than non-parametric tests.

Other types of distribution include the binomial (in which there are two possibilities for each measurement, e.g. yes or no, dead or alive, etc.), multinomial, and Poisson distribution (which describes random events where non-events cannot be counted, e.g. radioactive decay).
[Karl F Gauss (1777–1855), German mathematician; Simeon D Poisson (1781–1840), French mathematician]
See also, Samples, statistical

Statistical significance. Term denoting a **probability** of less than 0.05 ($P < 0.05$) for a **statistical test** or a result of

inferential **statistics**. Represents an arbitrary cut-off without reference to practical or clinical significance, but widely used by convention. More stringent 'levels' of probability are sometimes used (e.g. $P < 0.01$), e.g. to account for the increased likelihood of a significant result due to chance alone when large numbers of comparisons are made. The terms 'very' or 'highly' significant to describe very small P values should no longer be used when presenting data, but the P value itself should be provided.
See also, Errors

Statistical tests. Methods of comparing or extrapolating **data** in inferential **statistics**, e.g. in **clinical trials**. Involve mathematical calculations depending on the descriptive statistics of **each** sample group. Results are traditionally expressed as the **probability** that any observed differences between groups are due to chance alone, i.e. the likelihood that the samples are taken from the same **population** (**null hypothesis**). Increasingly, **confidence intervals** are being used to indicate the range within which a real difference is likely to lie.

- Many different tests have been described, applicable to specific types of data and situations, e.g.:
  - comparing groups consisting of:
    - different subjects with different treatments:
      - two groups:
        - parametric (for normally-distributed interval data): unpaired t test (Student's t test). Compares the **mean** and **standard deviation** for each group. Two-tailed tests allow for either an increase or a decrease in the variable measured.
        - non-parametric:
          - nominal data: chi-squared test (contingency table) with Yates's correction for continuity. Compares the observed frequency of events with the expected frequency. Fisher's exact test is used if any expected frequency is less than 5.
          - ordinal data: Mann–Whitney rank sum test. Ranks all the results in ascending order and compares the group's distributions within the ranking.
        - all types of data: sequential analysis. Subjects are treated in pairs, each receiving one of the treatments. Each pair is analysed following treatment to determine which treatment achieved better results for that pair. The results are plotted on a graph which indicates any overall superiority of one treatment over the other by the direction of the line (e.g. up or down). The study is stopped when the line crosses 'significance lines' previously marked on the graph. Thus involves the minimal number required to achieve a significant result.
      - more than two groups:
        - parametric: analysis of **variance** (ANOVA). Similar basis to the t test. Only indicates that a significant difference exists, not between which groups it exists. Student–Neuman–Keuls, Tukey's and other tests are used to indicate which of the comparisons achieve **statistical significance**.
        - non-parametric:
          - nominal data: chi-squared test as above (Yates's correction is not required).
          - ordinal data: Kruskal–Wallis test. Similar basis to the Mann–Whitney test.
    - same subjects before and after a treatment:
      - two groups:
        - parametric: paired t test. More powerful than the unpaired test because intersubject variability is reduced, since each subject acts as his or her own control.
        - non-parametric:
          - nominal data: McNemar's test.
          - ordinal data: Wilcoxon signed-rank sum test. Ranks the differences between the paired results.
      - more than two groups:
        - parametric: repeated-measure ANOVA.
        - non-parametric:
          - nominal data: Cochrane's test.
          - ordinal data: Friedman statistic.
  - comparing two variables for association:
    - parametric: linear regression analysis and Spearman correlation. Regression analysis determines the magnitude of change of one variable produced by the other variable. Expressed as the slope of the line of best fit, the equation relating the two variables, indicators of scatter, or statistical differences from the line of no association. Correlation indicates the degree of association only and is expressed as the correlation coefficient (r). An r of $+1$ or -1 indicates complete positive or negative association respectively, whilst an r of 0 indicates no association. For comparison of two methods of measurement (e.g. invasive and non-invasive **arterial BP measurement**), the difference between the two values obtained at each measurement is calculated. Bias and precision (mean and standard deviation respectively of the differences) indicate the degree of agreement between the two methods.
    - non-parametric:
      - nominal data: contingency coefficient.
      - ordinal data: Spearman rank correlation.

Non-normally distributed interval data may be transformed and normalized before application of parametric tests, otherwise weaker non-parametric tests must be applied.

- Inappropriate study design or tests may result in **errors** and incorrect conclusions. Common examples include:
  - multiple testing without correction. With a probability (P) of 0.05 taken as representing **statistical significance**, one test in 20 would be expected to produce a 'significant' result by chance. The Bonferroni correction is commonly used to account for multiple comparisons between groups.
  - insufficient **power**.
  - application of the incorrect test, e.g. use of the t test to compare ordinal data.

The tests and modifications are usually named after the mathematicians that described or developed them (apart from Student's t test).
[Student: pseudonym of William S Gosset (1876–1937), English chemist]
See also, Statistical frequency distributions

419

Statistics. Collection, analysis and interpretation of numerical **data**, used to describe and compare **samples** and **populations**. May be:
  –descriptive; i.e. describes sample data without extrapolation to the whole population. Descriptive terms vary according to the type and distribution of data but include measures of:
    –central tendency, e.g. **mean**, **mode**, **median**.
    –scatter, e.g. **standard deviation**, **percentiles**.
  Thus normally distributed data are described by their mean and standard deviation, ordinal data by the median and percentiles, and nominal by the mode and a list of possible categories.
  –inferential (analytical); i.e. used to relate sample data to the whole population. Applications include the use of clinical or laboratory measurements to define disease, and determining whether different samples are from the same population (**null hypothesis**). The latter is commonly performed in **clinical trials**, using **statistical tests**.
See also, Confidence intervals; Predictive value; Sensitivity; Specificity; Standard error of the mean; Statistical frequency distributions

Status asthmaticus. Has been variously defined as acute severe **asthma** which is refractory to medical treatment, or which persists for 12, or 24 hours. Acute severe asthma is now the preferred term.

Status epilepticus. Epileptic seizures so prolonged or frequent that there is no break interval them. Usually refers to tonic–clonic **convulsions**. May result in permanent neurological damage, with mortality of up to 15%.
● Causes and management: as for convulsions.

Status lymphaticus. 'Syndrome' supposedly occurring in children who died unexpectedly under anaesthesia; said to have characteristic associated pathological findings. Now thought not to exist, and merely an excuse for poor management.

Stellate ganglion block. Performed for painful arm conditions, e.g. **reflex sympathetic dystrophy**, herpes zoster, **phantom limb**, shoulder/hand syndrome, and to improve circulation, e.g. in Raynaud's syndrome, postembolectomy. Has formerly been performed in quinine poisoning, angina and **asthma**.
  The ganglion represents the fused inferior cervical and first thoracic sympathetic ganglions, and is present in 80% of subjects. It usually lies on or above the neck of the first **rib**. Some sympathetic fibres may leave the sympathetic chain below the ganglion of T1, and run directly to the **brachial plexus**, bypassing the ganglion. The precise site of action of the block is controversial, since studies using dye have shown that the ganglion itself may not be affected by injected solution.
  With the patient supine and the neck extended, **Chassaignac's tubercle** (transverse process of C6) is palpated level with the cricoid cartilage. The carotid sheath is retracted laterally with the fingers, and a skin wheal raised over the tubercle. A 5 cm needle is inserted directly posteriorly to contact the tubercle, passing medial to the retracted carotid sheath. It is withdrawn 1–2 mm and 5–10 ml **local anaesthetic agent** is injected after careful aspiration. A 2 ml test dose has been suggested

before injection of the main dose. Successful block is signalled by **Horner's syndrome**.
  Complications include intravascular injection (including into the vertebral artery), recurrent laryngeal nerve and brachial plexus blocks, pneumothorax, subarachnoid and extradural injection, and haematoma formation.
[Maurice Raynaud (1834–1881), French physician]
See also, Sympathetic nerve blocks; Sympathetic nervous system

Sterilization of anaesthetic equipment, *see Contamination of anaesthetic equipment*

Steroid therapy. Used in **adrenocortical insufficiency**, and to suppress inflammatory and immunological responses, e.g. in **connective tissue diseases**, raised **ICP** due to tumours, etc., skin diseases, blood dyscrasias, allergic reactions, **asthma**, **myasthenia gravis**, and following organ **transplantation**. Has been used in **ARDS** but its efficacy is disputed. Use in severe sepsis is now thought to increase mortality.
● Uses:
  –treatment of disease processes, e.g. hydrocortisone, prednisolone (4 times as potent as hydrocortisone), methylprednisolone (5 times as potent) and dexamethasone (30 times as potent). The last three have little mineralocorticoid activity.
  –replacement therapy: hydrocortisone and fludrocortisone are usually administered, for **glucocorticoid** and mineralocorticoid (**aldosterone**-like) effects respectively. Fludrocortisone is also used in congenital adrenal hyperplasia and postural hypotension.
● Associated with many side effects:
  –related to mineralocorticoid activity: water and sodium retention, **hypokalaemia**, **hypertension**.
  –**hyperglycaemia** and **diabetes mellitus**, osteoporosis and pathological fractures, skeletal wasting with proximal myopathy.
  –GIT effects: dyspepsia, **peptic ulcer disease**.
  –mental changes: euphoria, depression.
  –spread of infection.
  –decreased wound healing.
  –cataract formation.
  –growth suppression in children.
  –**Cushing's syndrome** may occur with high dosage.
  –adrenal suppression, due to inhibition of **ACTH** release. Pituitary–adrenal axis function may take 6 months to recover following withdrawal of therapy; during this time patients are unable to mount a normal cortisone response to stress (secretion increases from 25 mg/day to 300 mg/day), and may develop circulatory collapse. Although this is thought to be rare, steroid therapy (e.g. hydrocortisone 100 mg 6–8 hourly, reduced by quarter/half every 24 hours) is usually given to patients who have:
    –received steroid therapy for longer than 2 weeks within the previous 2 months (up to 1 year has been suggested).
    –adrenocortical insufficiency, adrenalectomy, etc.
See also, Stress response to surgery

Stethoscope. Invented by Laennec in 1819. During anaesthesia, allows continuous auscultation of breath and heart sounds. May indicate **air embolism**. Two forms are commonly used in anaesthesia:

–praecordial stethoscope: often connected to a monoaural earpiece to allow the anaesthetist greater freedom.

–oesophageal stethoscope: a modified nasogastric tube. Widely used in the USA; less so in the UK, apart from paediatric anaesthesia. Addition of temperature probe, ECG electrodes and pacing wires have been described.

[Rene TH Laennec (1781–1826), French physician]

Stoichiometric mixture. Mixture of reactants in such proportions that none remain at the end of the reaction. Stoichiometric mixtures often react violently, and are thus more likely to be involved in **explosions and fires**.

Stokes–Adams attack. Syncope occurring in complete **heart block**; may be due to transient **asystole** or **VF**. Occurs suddenly, and may progress to **convulsions**. Recovery is typically rapid. Differential diagnosis includes vasovagal syncope, transient ischaemic attack, micturition and cough syncope, and postural hypotension. Requires **cardiac pacing**.

[William Stokes (1804–1878), Irish physician; Robert Adams (1791–1875), Irish surgeon]

Stovaine. Local anaesthetic drug, introduced in 1904, as a less toxic alternative to **cocaine**. Slightly irritant, and replaced in turn by **procaine**.

[Ernest Forneau (1872–1949), French chemist; *forneau* is French for stove]

STP/STPD. S̲tandard t̲emperature and p̲ressure (0°C; 101.3 kPa (760 mmHg)) and STP d̲ry. Used for standardizing gas volume measurements.

Streptokinase. Fibrinolytic drug produced by certain strains of haemolytic streptococci. Activates plasminogen to form plasmin, causing **fibrinolysis**. Used to treat severe **DVT** and **PE**, and in acute **MI**. Has also been used to treat intra-arterial thrombosis, e.g. in limbs.

- Dosage: 250 000 units iv over 30 minutes, then 100 000 units hourly. For MI, 1 500 000 units are given over 60 minutes.
- Side effects: allergic reactions, especially on subsequent administration; haemorrhage.

Stress response to surgery. Term used to encompass the metabolic and hormonal changes following surgery, although the same may occur after **trauma**, **burns**, **haemorrhage**, etc. The response has been suggested as being necessary for survival and recovery after trauma.

Tissue trauma (involving release of polypeptides from the wound site), **hypovolaemia** and **pain** initiate a neuroendocrine reflex involving secretion of **ACTH**, **endorphins**, **growth hormone**, **vasopressin** and prolactin. Stimulation of the **sympathetic nervous system** increases plasma **catecholamines**. Plasma cortisol and **aldosterone** increase, with increased **renin/angiotensin system** activity. Increase in these hormones produces a period of intense **catabolism**, the magnitude and duration of which are proportional to the extent of injury. Fatty acids are mobilized and utilized, **amino acids** are converted to **carbohydrate**, and negative **nitrogen balance** occurs. Plasma **glucose** is raised, with impaired **insulin** production. Metabolic rate, body temperature, O_2 consumption and

CO_2 production increase. Water and sodium retention occurs, with increased urinary potassium loss.

- Effects of anaesthesia:
  - **inhalational anaesthetic agents** have little effect.
  - **opioid analgesic drugs** in high dosage (e.g. 50–100 μg/kg **fentanyl**, 2–4 mg/kg **morphine**) attenuate the response to abdominal and pelvic surgery, but do not abolish the response to initiation of **cardiopulmonary bypass**.
  - **etomidate** infusion prevents the cortisol response, but with little other effect.
  - **spinal** and **extradural anaesthesia** with **local anaesthetic agents** abolish the response to surgery on the lower part of the body. The effect on upper abdominal and thoracic surgery is less clear, with suppression of the glucose response but not of the cortisol response. Block of autonomic and somatic afferent pathways is thought to be required for complete prevention. **Spinal opioids** do not prevent the response despite good analgesia, although slight modification may occur.

To be effective, the above require administration before the surgical stimulus; their effects last for several hours after single dosage.

The benefit of attenuating the stress response is controversial, although improved outcome has been claimed in critically ill patients.

Weissman C (1990) Anesthesiology; 73: 308–27

Stress ulcers. Acute gastric ulceration secondary to any severe medical or surgical illness, e.g. classically burns (**Curling's ulcers**) and head injury (**Cushing's ulcers**). Usually involve the fundus and may be multiple. Gastric mucosal ischaemia and acid production are thought to be involved, although the aetiology is unclear. Prophylaxis is usual in **ICU**.

See also, Peptic ulcer disease

Stridor. High-pitched sound occurring in upper **airway obstruction**. Inspiratory stridor suggests obstruction at or above the upper trachea (e.g. **epiglottitis**), since extrathoracic obstruction is exacerbated by the negative intrathoracic pressures generated during inspiration. Expiratory stridor suggests obstruction of the lower trachea or bronchi with exacerbation as the airways are compressed during forced expiration. Typically present on exertion initially, progressing to stridor at rest as obstruction worsens.

More common in children because of the smaller diameter of their airways. Slight narrowing thus has a proportionately greater effect.

Treatment is as for airway obstruction. **Helium**/O_2 mixtures may decrease work of breathing and improve oxygenation.

Stroke, *see Cerebrovascular accident*

Stroke index. Stroke volume divided by body **surface area**, thus accounting for the effect of body size. Normally 30–50 ml/m².

Stroke volume (SV). Volume of blood ejected by the ventricle per heart beat; i.e.

$$SV = \frac{\textbf{cardiac output}}{\textbf{heart rate}}$$

Also equals end-diastolic volume – end-systolic volume. Normally 70–80 ml for a 70 kg man at rest.

Affected by ventricular filling and **preload**, **myocardial contractility**, and outflow resistance and **SVR**.

Stroke work. Measurement of (usually left) ventricular performance, indicating the work done by the ventricle. Increased in **hypertension** and hypervolaemia, and decreased in **shock**, **cardiac failure** and **aortic stenosis**.

$$\text{Stroke work (g)} = \textbf{stroke volume (ml)} \times (\text{MAP} - \text{PCWP (mmHg)}) \times 0.0136,$$

where PCWP = **pulmonary capillary wedge pressure**
    0.0136 = correction factor for units.
Normally 60–80 g. Stroke work index = stroke work divided by body **surface area**; normally 40–80 g/m^2.

Stuffing box, *see Cylinders*

Stump pressure, *see Carotid artery surgery*

Subarachnoid block, *see Spinal anaesthesia*

Subarachnoid haemorrhage (SAH). Usually caused by rupture of an intracranial aneurysm (Berry aneurysm), most commonly arising from the anterior communicating artery of the circle of Willis (*see Cerebral circulation*). Occurs in approximately 15–20 per 100 000 population, 60% in women. Typically presents very suddenly.
- Features:
    –initial rupture: headache, meningeal irritation, unconsciousness.
    –neurological deficit, due to cerebral vasospasm with resultant ischaemia and infarction.
    –**hydrocephalus**, due to obstruction of **CSF** circulation by blood.
- Patients are classified thus:
    –grade I: asymptomatic or mild headache. Mortality 0–5%.
    –grade II: moderate/severe headache, neck stiffness, no neurological deficit other than cranial nerve palsy. Mortality 2–10%.
    –grade II: drowsiness, confusion, mild focal deficit. Mortality 8–15%.
    –grade IV: stupor, hemiparesis, early decerebrate rigidity. Mortality 60–70%.
    –grade V: deep coma, **decerebrate posture**. Mortality 70–100%.
Diagnosed by xanthochromic CSF on lumbar puncture and CAT scanning; the aneurysm may be revealed by angiography.
- Treatment:
 –maintenance of good hydration and control of severe **hypertension**. Unconscious patients are managed as for **coma**. **Nimodipine** has been used to relieve vasospasm both pre- and postoperatively.
    –surgery is usually delayed for 7–10 days to allow stabilization, despite risk of rebleeding. More recently, earlier surgery has been advocated, especially in low grade SAH.
    –percutaneous embolization of the aneurysm may be performed.
- Anaesthetic considerations:
    –as for **neurosurgery**.
    –**hypotensive anaesthesia** is traditionally employed but

cerebral perfusion may be further impaired if hypotension is profound.
[Sir James Berry (1860–1946), Canadian surgeon]
Archer DP, Shaw DA, Leblanc RL, Tranmer BI (1991) Can J Anaesth; 38: 454–70

Subclavian venous cannulation. The suclavian vein is the continuation of the axillary vein and arises at the lateral border of the first **rib** (*see Fig. 74; Internal jugular venous cannulation*). It passes over the first rib anterior to the subclavian artery, separated from it by scalenus anterior, to join with the internal **jugular vein** at the medial end of the clavicle. It receives the external jugular vein at the clavicle's midpoint. The right **phrenic nerve** lies between the vein and scalenus anterior, the left phrenic nerve between the vein and artery.
- Technique:
    –head-down position distends the vein and reduces risk of **air embolism**. The head is turned to the contralateral side. Aseptic techniques are used.
    –a finger is run medially in the subclavian groove until an 'obstruction' is felt (subclavius muscle), also marked by a notch on the under surface of the clavicle. This point lies between the midpoint of the clavicle and a point dividing its middle and medial thirds.
    –after local anaesthetic infiltration, a needle is introduced under the clavicle and directed towards the sternal notch, aspirating during advancement. When the vein has been entered, the cannula is advanced or a wire inserted (**Seldinger technique**).
The approach is contraindicated in patients with coagulopathy, since direct pressure cannot be applied to a bleeding vessel.
For complications and comparison with other techniques, see Central venous cannulation

Subdural haemorrhage. Haemorrhage between the pia and arachnoid. May be:
    –cranial:
        –acute: usually caused be acceleration–deceleration **head injury**. Patients usually present with confusion or loss of consciousness following a 'lucid interval'.
        –chronic: initial haematoma enlarges slowly, by continued slow bleeding, e.g. from subdural veins or by absorbing fluid from **CSF** by **osmosis**. Patients may present in many ways, from transient ischaemic attacks to progressive dementia.
    –spinal (very rare), e.g. following lumbar puncture.
Treated by surgical evacuation.
See also, Neurosurgery

Substance P. Peptide (11 amino-acids) involved in **pain pathways** (*see Gate control theory of pain*). High levels are found in axons and cell bodies of primary afferent fibres in the dorsal root ganglia, also in the superficial levels of the dorsal horn of the **spinal cord**.
- Evidence for its involvement in pain transmission includes:
    –distribution in the regions of pain pathways.
    –depletion by **capsaicin**, a red pepper extract, renders animals insensitive to noxious thermal and chemical stimuli, without affecting other sensory modalities.
Fleetwood-Walker S, Mitchell R (1989) Curr Opin Anaesth; 2: 645–8

Substantia gelatinosa, *see Sensory pathways; Spinal cord*

Succinylcholine, *see Suxamethonium*

Sucralfate. Ulcer-healing drug, a complex of aluminium hydroxide and sulphated sucrose. Thought to act via mucosal protection from acid. Has no antacid effect. Used in **peptic ulcer disease,** and has been used on **ICU** as prophylaxis against peptic ulceration; thought to be associated with fewer nosocomial infections than the **H₂ receptor antagonists.** 1 g is given orally 6 hourly, or 2 g 12 hourly. Side effects are rare and include constipation, nausea and vomiting.
McCarthy DM (1991) N Engl J Med; 14: 1017–25

Suction equipment. Consists of:
- –pump to generate a vacuum. Efficiency of the system is related to the degree of subatmospheric pressure generated, and the volume of air that can be moved in unit time (displacement). Pumps may employ pistons (usually low displacement), rotating fans (high displacement), foot-operated bellows and compressed gases using the **Venturi principle.** Piped suction systems use a high displacement pump connected to a large central reservoir, with traps to prevent contamination.
- –reservoir: must be large enough to enable aspiration of large volumes, but not so large that the desired vacuum takes too long to achieve. A filter and float valve prevent contamination of the pump with aspirated liquid.
- –delivery tubing; usually disposable, attached to rigid (Yankauer) or flexible catheters. Smooth-tipped catheters may reduce the mucosal damage following endotracheal suctioning. Prolonged endotracheal suction may cause lung collapse and hypoxaemia; bradycardia is common in critically ill patients. Preoxygenation should thus precede tracheal suction. Enclosed suction catheters which do not require detachment of the patient from the breathing system have recently been described; the catheter is handled through a plastic sleeve, maintaining sterility. Hypoxaemia and dispersal of infectious droplets have thus been reduced.

Minimal flow rate of 35 l/min air, and generation of at least 80 kPa (600 mmHg) negative pressure, have been suggested for apparatus for anaesthetic use.
[Sidney Yankauer (1872–1932), US surgeon]

Sudeck's atrophy, *see Reflex sympathetic dystrophy*

Sufentanil citrate. Synthetic **opioid analgesic drug,** developed in 1974. An analogue of **fentanyl,** with 5–7 times the latter's potency. Of shorter elimination **half-life** (about 2–3 hours) than fentanyl, with similar clearance and slightly smaller volume of distribution. Has similar clinical effects to fentanyl, including cardiovascular stability and lack of **histamine** release. Usual dose is 0.1–0.5 µg/kg for minor surgery, up to 8 µg/kg for longer procedures and up to 30 µg/kg as the sole agent for, e.g. **cardiac surgery.**
Available in the USA but not the UK.

Sulphaemoglobinaemia. Presence of an abnormal **haemoglobin** of uncertain chemical structure, but which may be produced by adding hydrogen sulphide *in vitro.*

Often coexists with **methaemoglobinaemia.** Reduces O₂–carrying capacity of blood and shifts the **oxyhaemoglobin dissociation curve** to the left, decreasing O₂ delivery to the tissues. Usually due to ingestion of phenacetin, sulphonamides or primaquine. Treatment includes O₂ therapy; normal haemoglobin cannot be regenerated from sulphaemoglobin.

Sulphonylureas. Group of oral hypoglycaemic drugs, used in non-insulin-dependent **diabetes mellitus.** Act by encouraging surviving β cells of the pancreas to secrete insulin, and possibly by increasing peripheral uptake of glucose. Several are available, e.g.:
- –chlorpropamide: **half-life** 35–45 hours.
- –glibenclamide, gliclazide and glibornuride: half-life 8–12 hours.
- –tolbutamide, tolazamide: half-life 5–8 hours.
- –glipizide: half-life 2–4 hours.
- –gliquidone: half-life 1–2 hours.

All of the above are excreted by the liver except chlorpropamide, which is excreted renally.

The shorter-acting drugs may be stopped on the day of surgery; perioperative **hypoglycaemia** is most likely with long-acting drugs, e.g. chlorpropamide, and in the elderly.

Superior vena caval obstruction (Superior vena caval syndrome). 80–90% of cases are caused by malignancy, especially **bronchial carcinoma** and lymphoma. Other causes include mediastinal fibrosis and thrombosis. Results in distended veins, oedema and cyanosis in the arm, head and neck, with prominent collateral vessels in the chest wall. Visual disturbances and headache may occur. Most patients have dyspnoea and orthopnoea. Emergency radiotherapy is required if malignancy is the cause. Steroids have also been used to reduce oedema.
- Anaesthetic considerations:
  - –patients should be nursed sitting up preoperatively, to minimize facial and neck swelling.
  - –induction of anaesthesia with iv agents may be prolonged if an arm vein is used.
  - –tracheal intubation may be difficult. Laryngeal oedema may be present.
  - –bleeding may be torrential, especially during median sternotomy.

Supine hypotension syndrome, *see Aortocaval compression*

Supraorbital nerve block, *see Ophthalmic nerve blocks*

Suprascapular nerve block. Performed for analgesia in painful shoulders. A needle is inserted 1–2 cm cranial to the scapular spine, on a line bisecting the inferior scapular angle. 5 ml **local anaesthetic agent** is injected when the scapular notch is identified.

Supraventricular tachycardia (SVT). Paroxysmal tachycardia with a rate of 140–250 beats/min, caused by a rapidly firing ectopic focus in the atria or atrioventricular node. Circular conduction of impulses via abnormal anatomical pathways or within the node itself result in re-entry and perpetuation of the **arrhythmia.** Occurs in otherwise healthy individuals although it may be associated with heart disease, **Wolff–Parkinson–White** and **Lown–Ganong–Levine syndromes, hyperthyroidism,** and

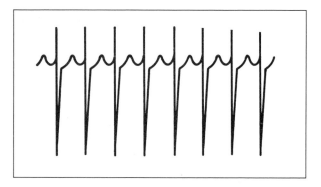

Figure 129 *SVT*

excessive consumption of **caffeine**, nicotine or **alcohol**. Typically sudden in onset. May cause palpitations, dyspnoea, lightheadedness, and polyuria if prolonged.

- Features: regular narrow **QRS complexes** on the **ECG** (Fig. 129), unless **bundle branch block** is also present. A degree of atrioventricular block may be present, especially when associated with **digoxin** toxicity. It may be difficult to distinguish SVT from **VT**.
- Treatmemt:
  - **carotid sinus massage**, **Valsalva manoeuvre**, and other methods of vagal stimulation (e.g. holding ice to the face); may abolish SVT or slow the rate if atrioventricular block is present.
  - **antiarrhythmic drugs**: verapamil is classically used but **adenosine** is increasingly employed. Others include β-**adrenergic receptor antagonists**, **disopyramide**,

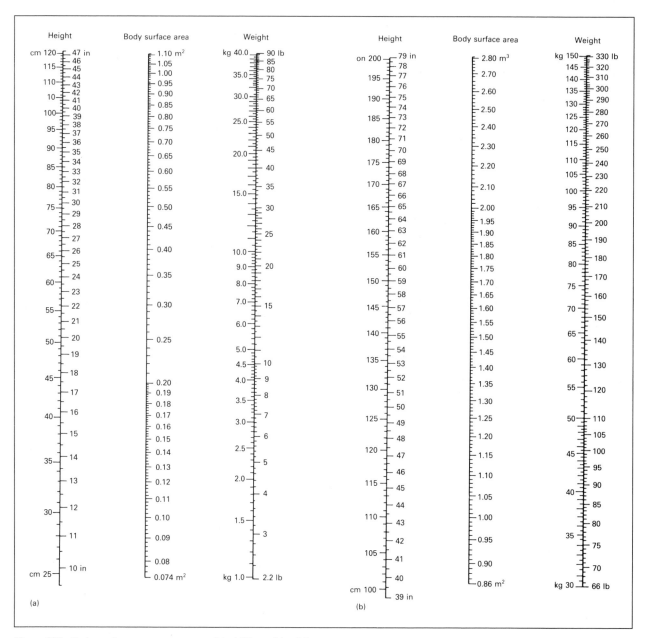

Figure 130 *Body surface area nomograms: (a) children; (b) adults*

amiodarone, etc. Digoxin has been used but is contra-indicated in Wolff–Parkinson–White syndrome.
   –**cardioversion** or **cardiac pacing** in resistant cases. Ablation therapy or surgery may be required.
See also, Atrial fibrillation; Atrial flutter

Sural nerve block, *see Ankle, nerve blocks; Knee, nerve blocks*

Surface area, body. Used to estimate drug doses, and in physiological calculations, e.g. **cardiac index**, **basal metabolic rate**, etc., since it reflects body requirements and activity more accurately than weight, height, etc.
   The **rule of nines** is used to estimate surface area of parts of the body. Nomograms for total surface area (Fig. 130) are based on the formula:

$$\text{surface area (m}^2) = \text{weight}^{0.425} \text{ (kg)} \times \text{height}^{0.725} \text{ (cm)} \times 0.007184$$

Surface tension. Tangential **force** in the surface of a liquid, defined in terms of the force acting perpendicularly across a line of unit length. Caused by attraction between the liquid molecules; whereas molecules in the bulk of the liquid are attracted in all directions, those at the surface are only attracted inwards. Thus the surface tends to contract to the smallest possible area, e.g. a free drop tends to be spherical. Has important implications in lung mechanics; normally reduced by pulmonary **surfactant**. Measured in N/m.
See also, Laplace's law

Surfactant. Complex material comprised of dipalmitoyl phosphatidyl choline (DPPC), protein and carbohydrate, which prevents alveolar collapse at lower lung volumes by reducing alveolar **surface tension**. Thought to do this by alignment of the hydrophilic parts of the DPPC molecules on the surface of the alveolar fluid lining, with repulsion between adjacent molecules. Repulsion increases as the molecules are pressed together at low volumes. **Compliance** is increased, **alveoli** are held open, and alveolar fluid is reduced.
   Produced by type II pneumocytes, partly under control of the hypothalamic–pituitary–adrenal axis. Appears at about 24 weeks gestation. Deficiency due to immaturity causes the **respiratory distress syndrome** (RDS). It may also be deficient in areas of lung affected by **PE**, bronchial obstruction, and in heavy smokers.
   Administration of synthetic surfactant has been used in neonatal RDS, and has been investigated in **ARDS**.
Morton NS (1989) Br J Hosp Med; 42: 52–8

Suxamethonium chloride (Succinylcholine). Depolarizing **neuromuscular blocking drug**, introduced in 1951. Formerly available as the bromide/iodide. Structurally composed of two **acetylcholine** molecules joined together

(Fig. 131). Stored at 4°C to prevent hydrolysis. Incompatible with **thiopentone**.
● Dosage:
   –0.5–1.5 mg/kg iv depending on the relaxation required. Usual initial dose is 1 mg/kg iv, producing paralysis within 30 seconds which lasts 2–5 minutes. Subsequent doses: 0.2–0.5 mg/kg.
   –has been used by infusion of 0.1% solution with 5% dextrose or 0.9% saline at 2–5 mg/min.
   –may also be given im (2 mg/kg) or sc.
Rapidly hydrolysed by plasma **cholinesterase** to succinyl monocholine and choline, then to succinic acid and choline. Succinyl monocholine has weak blocking properties.
   Hexafluorenium and tetrahydroaminocrine have been used to prolong suxamethonium's action.
● Side effects:
   –prolonged paralysis. May be caused by:
      –reduced cholinesterase activity (*see Cholinesterase, plasma*) due to:
         –inherited atypical cholinesterase.
         –reduced amount of cholinesterase.
         –inhibition of cholinesterase by drugs.
      –excessive dosage, cumulation of succinylcholine and production of **dual block**. The latter may occur after 400–500 mg in adults.
   Dual block may also develop with reduced enzyme activity. Management of prolonged paralysis:
      –maintenance of anaesthesia and oxygenation.
      –diagnosis of the nature of block using **neuromuscular blockade monitoring**. **Edrophonium** has been suggested to distinguish non-depolarizing from depolarizing blockade, but is less commonly used.
      –**neostigmine** has been used to reverse dual block.
      –in prolonged depolarizing blockade ('suxamethonium or Scoline apnoea'), recovery usually occurs within 4 hours. It may be speeded by administering plasma or blood, but spontaneous recovery is usually preferable.
      –blood may be analysed for cholinesterase activity, and screening of relatives performed.
   –muscle **fasciculations**, coinciding with initial depolarization of muscle fibres. They are painful if the patient is awake. Thought to contribute to:
      –postoperative muscle pains, typically around the neck, back and upper arms, and occurring on the 2nd–3rd day. Most common in young fit women and after early ambulation.
      –increased **intraocular pressure**. Suxamethonium causes contraction of the extraocular muscles, but may also cause choroidal vasodilatation; the response may still occur if the extrinsic muscles are cut. The increase usually lasts for under 10 minutes. Suxamethonium is usually avoided in penetrating eye injuries but this is controversial (*see Eye, penetrating injury*).

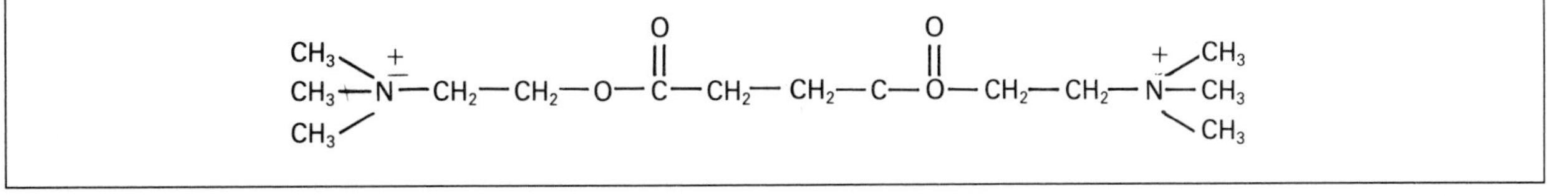

Figure 131 *Structure of suxamethonium*

–increased intragastric pressure. Formerly thought to increase risk of **aspiration of gastric contents**, but an accompanying increase in **lower oesophageal sphincter** tone maintains barrier pressure.

–increased plasma **potassium**. Although this arises mainly from depolarization (see below), leakage of potassium from damaged muscle fibres may contribute. Plasma **myoglobin** and creatine phosphokinase (normally intracellular) are increased after injection of suxamethonium.

Fasciculations and the resulting complications may be reduced by pretreatment with other drugs, although not consistently. Adverse effects may also still occur despite lack of fasciculations. Drugs used include:

–non-depolarizing neuromuscular blocking drugs (usually 1/10 usual intubating dose), given 2–3 minutes before suxamethonium, which may be required in increased dosage. **Tubocurarine** is the best studied, although others have been used. The possibility of **aspiration pneumonitis** precludes this technique in rapid sequence induction.

–**lignocaine** 1–2 mg/kg iv, given 2–3 minutes before suxamethonium.

–**diazepam** 10 mg iv.

–**dantrolene** 100–200 mg orally, 2 hours preoperatively.

–suxamethonium 0.1 mg/kg iv 1–2 minutes before the main dose.

–**calcium** 10 mmol iv. Arrhythmias may occur.

–**magnesium** sulphate 1–2 g iv.

–chlorpromazine 0.1 mg/kg.

–hexafluorenium.

–**hyperkalaemia**. Plasma potassium increases usually by 0.5 mmol/l in normal patients, and lasts for 3–5 minutes. This follows normal movement of potassium out of muscle cells during depolarization at the **neuromuscular junction**, with some leakage due to trauma following fasciculations as above. The increase may be dangerous in patients whose plasma potassium levels are already high (typically **renal failure**, although the response is of normal magnitude unless neuropathy is present). Increases of several mmol/l may occur if the **acetylcholine receptors** are not confined to the neuromuscular junction, but have spread along the whole length of the muscle fibres, as occurs in **denervation hypersensitivity**. This process is also thought to occur in other conditions in which massive hyperkalaemia may follow administration of suxamethonium for certain periods after the lesion:

–**burns**: 9 days–2 months.

–**spinal cord injury**, intracranial lesions (e.g. **CVA**, **subarachnoid haemorrhage**, **head injury**) and muscle trauma: 10 days–6–7 months.

–peripheral nerve injury: 4 days–6–7 months.

–peripheral neuropathy, tetanus and severe infection: uncertain period of risk.

Maximal risk occurs at 14–28 days. Severe arrhythmias and **cardiac arrest** may occur, usually responding well to **CPR**. The same drugs used to attenuate the fasciculations have been used to reduce the hyperkalaemic response, with varying success. **Salbutamol** has also been used.

The risk of hyperkalaemia in **disseminated sclerosis** and **Parkinson's disease** is unclear. It has been described in **muscular dystrophies** (related to massive

rhabdomyolysis and possibly **MH**), but not in **motor neurone disease**.

–bradycardia: common after the second dose, but may occur after the first dose, especially in children. Other muscarinic effects may occur, e.g. increased GIT motility and secretion.

–**adverse drug reactions**. Although rare, they may be severe. **Anaphylactic** and **anaphylactoid reactions** have been described.

–MH.

–**masseter spasm**.

–abnormal sustained contraction in **dystrophia myotonica** and **myotonia congenita**.

Resistance may occur in **myasthenia gravis**, and increased sensitivity in the **myasthenic syndrome**.

Its use has declined because of its many disadvantages and the introduction of short-acting alternative drugs, e.g. **atracurium** and **vecuronium**. However, the conditions suxamethonium provides for tracheal intubation are generally considered superior and occur faster than those attained by other drugs. Its short duration of action allows tracheal intubation with subsequent spontaneous ventilation, and is especially advantageous if intubation is difficult.

See also, Depolarizing neuromuscular blockade

Suxethonium bromide/iodide. Depolarizing **neuromuscular blocking drug**, introduced with **suxamethonium** in 1951. Similar to suxamethonium, but the quaternary ammonium group at each end of the molecule contains two methyl and one ethyl group instead of three methyl groups.

SVP, *see Saturated vapour pressure*

SVR, *see Systemic vascular resistance*

SVT, *see Supraventricular tachycardia*

Swallowing (Deglutition). Active passage of liquid or food bolus from mouth to stomach. Initiated voluntarily by the **tongue** pressing against the palate from the tip back, pushing food into the oropharynx. Continues by reflex activity, with afferent fibres in the 9th and 10th **cranial nerves**; impulses pass to the tractus solitarius and nucleus ambiguus of the medulla, with efferent fibres to pharyngeal and tongue muscles via 9th, 10th and 12th nerves. The nasopharynx is sealed by soft palate elevation and superior constrictor contraction, and the **larynx** by elevation and glottic closure. The epiglottis moves posteriorly but does not seal the glottic opening as formerly suspected. Respiration ceases. Food is propelled by the inferior constrictor into the upper oesophagus where it initiates peristalsis (*see Oesophageal contractility*).

Suppressed in plane 1 of surgical anaesthesia; its reappearance may herald the onset of **vomiting**.

Difficulty with swallowing (dysphagia) may be caused by anatomical (e.g. local tumours, inflammation, **achalasia**) or neurological (e.g. **myasthenia gravis**, bulbar palsies) factors; pulmonary aspiration of food and saliva may lead to repeated chest infection.

Swan–Ganz catheter, *see Pulmonary artery catheterization*

Sympathetic nerve blocks. Although blockade of sympathetic nerves commonly accompanies various regional techniques (e.g. **extradural** or **spinal anaesthesia**,

brachial plexus block), selective blockade of sympathetic fibres is used for:

-   **pain management**: certain pain syndromes are thought to involve abnormal sympathetic activity, e.g. **reflex sympathetic dystrophy**, **causalgia**, **phantom limb** pain. The underlying mechanism is unknown but may involve abnormal linkage between mechanoreceptors and sympathetic neurones.
-   improvement of blood flow, e.g. in peripheral ischaemia, Raynaud's disease, accidental intra-arterial injection of **thiopentone**.

Sympathetic ganglia may be blocked at three levels: the cervicothoracic ganglia (**stellate ganglion block**), coeliac plexus (**coeliac plexus block**) and lumbar ganglia (**lumbar sympathetic block**). Blockade may be short-term (using local anaesthetic agents) or permanent (chemical sympathectomy), when neurolytic agents such as phenol or alcohol are used. **IVRA** using **guanethidine** is also used. [Maurice Raynaud (1834–1881), French physician]

Sympathetic nervous system. Part of the **autonomic nervous system**. Myelinated preganglionic efferent fibres emerge from spinal segments T1–L2 into the corresponding primary ramus at each level, and pass via a white ramus communicans into the sympathetic trunk (*see Fig. 16; Autonomic nervous system*). They may then:

-   synapse in the corresponding ganglion and pass via a grey ramus communicans to the corresponding **spinal nerve** for distribution.
-   ascend or descend in the sympathetic chain, and synapse at a distant ganglion.
-   pass without synapsing to a peripheral ganglion, to synapse there.

The sympathetic trunk is a ganglionated nerve chain extending from the base of the skull to the coccyx, and lying about 2–3 cm lateral to the vertebral column. The portion above T1 does not receive any rami communicantes; i.e. the cervical sympathetic outflow must descend to T1, then into the sympathetic trunk and ascend to the cervical ganglia. The trunk descends in the neck behind the carotid sheath and enters the thorax anterior to the neck of the first rib. It passes over the heads of the upper ribs and overlies the sides of the lower four thoracic vertebrae. It enters the abdomen behind the medial arcuate ligament (*see Diaphragm*) and lies between the lumbar vertebral bodies and psoas major, passing into the pelvis anterior to the sacral ala. The two chains meet and terminate on the anterior surface of the coccyx.

-   Ganglia:
    -   cervical:
        -   superior:
            -   lies opposite C2–3.
            -   branches: superior cardiac nerve, and branches to the upper four cervical nerves, internal carotid plexus and **cranial nerves** VII, IX, X and XII.
        -   middle:
            -   lies opposite C6.
            -   branches: middle cardiac nerve, and branches to C5 and C6.
        -   inferior:
            -   lies opposite C7; often fused with the first thoracic ganglion to form the stellate ganglion on the neck of the first rib.
            -   branches: inferior cardiac nerve, and branches to C7 and C8.
    -   thoracic:
        -   usually 12 although variable.
        -   branches: to splanchnic and **intercostal nerves**.
    -   lumbar: usually four ganglia.
    -   sacral: usually four ganglia.
-   Sympathetic innervation of viscera is via the cardiac, coeliac and hypogastric plexuses. The sympathetic nervous system is concerned with the 'flight or fight' response to stress. Stimulation causes:
    -   pupillary dilatation and ciliary muscle relaxation.
    -   tachycardia and increased myocardial contractility and velocity of conduction of impulses.
    -   α-**adrenergic receptor**-mediated vasoconstriction ($β_2$–receptor-mediated vasodilatation in skeletal muscle, abdominal viscera, and coronary, pulmonary and renal circulations).
    -   bronchodilatation and reduced bronchial secretion.
    -   decreased GIT motility, contraction of sphincters and reduction of secretions (thick viscous secretion from salivary glands). Mixed effects on **insulin** and **glucagon** secretion (decreased by α-receptor stimulation, increased by $β_2$–receptor stimulation).
    -   bladder relaxation and sphincteric contraction. Increased renin secretion.
    -   variable effect on the **uterus**.
    -   ejaculation of semen.
    -   piloerection and sweating of palms.
    -   hepatic glycogenolysis and adipose lipolysis.

Acetylcholine is the **neurotransmitter** at ganglia and the adrenal medulla; **noradrenaline** is the neurotransmitter at postganglionic nerve endings (except for sweat glands, where acetylcholine is the transmitter). The adrenal medulla represents a sympathetic ganglion which secretes directly into the bloodstream.

Central control for sympathetic activity is from the medulla, pons and hypothalamus.
See also, Acetylcholine receptors; Sympathetic nerve blocks

Sympathomimetic drugs. Refer to drugs that stimulate **adrenergic receptors**. Actions of individual drugs vary depending on whether they affect predominantly α- or β-receptors, or both. Some stimulate receptors directly; others act indirectly via release of endogenous **catecholamines** (Table 34).

Used clinically as **vasopressor**, **inotropic**, and **bronchodilator drugs**. Amphetamine is used in narcolepsy for its CNS stimulant action.
See also, individual drugs

Table 34. Actions of sympathomimetic drugs

Drug	Direct stimulation		Indirect activity
	α	β	
Adrenaline	+	++	—
Noradrenaline	++	+	—
Isoprenaline	—	++	—
Phenylephrine	++	—	—
Methoxamine	++	—	—
Salbutamol	—	++	—
Ephedrine	+	+	+
Metaraminol	++	+	++
Amphetamine	+	+	++

Synapse. Junction between a **neurone** (presynaptic cell) and another (postsynaptic) cell, usually another neurone but also **muscle** or glandular cells. Allows unidirectional transmission of **action potentials** between cells (**synaptic transmission**), usually by **neurotransmitter** release although electrical transmission across gap junctions may also occur. One presynaptic neurone may contribute to over 1000 synapses. Most presynaptic nerve endings bear terminal buttons (synaptic knobs), with up to several thousand from different cells contacting each postsynaptic neurone. The terminal buttons contain many mitochondria and vesicles containing neurotransmitter, and are separated from the postsynaptic membrane by the synaptic cleft (30–50 nm wide). Neurotransmitter receptors are present in high concentrations in the postsynaptic membrane opposite the terminal buttons.
See also, Neuromuscular junction

Synaptic transmission. Usually involves release from presynaptic cells of a **neurotransmitter** which passes across the synaptic cleft and binds to specific receptors in the postsynaptic membrane. This initiates a change in **membrane potential** in the postsynaptic cell; the neurotransmitter is then broken down by a specific **enzyme** (e.g. acetylcholinesterase), diffuses into surrounding tissues, or is taken up by the presynaptic nerve ending (e.g. **noradrenaline**). Initiation of an **action potential** in the postsynaptic cell depends on the number and frequency of impulses arriving from different presynaptic cells; impulses may be excitatory or inhibitory. In addition, presynaptic inhibition and facilitation may occur, via neurones forming synapses at the presynaptic nerve ending.

Some **synapses** are electrical, with transmission across gap junctions; some are both electrical and chemical. A synaptic delay of at least 0.5 ms occurs at chemical synapses, but not at electrical ones.
See also, Neuromuscular transmission

Synchronized intermittent mandatory ventilation, *see Intermittent mandatory ventilation*

Syndrome of inappropriate antidiuretic hormone secretion (SIADH). Increased plasma **vasopressin** levels and water retention despite plasma hypo-osmolality and expanded or normal ECF.
- Caused by:
  –ectopic production of vasopressin, e.g by carcinoma of bronchus, pancreas, prostate, colon and other tissue, or lymphoma.
  –pulmonary disease, e.g. **chest infection**, TB, abscess.
  –CNS disorders, e.g. brain tumour, **CVA**, **head injury**, encephalitis, **meningitis**, surgery.
  –stress, e.g. **pain**, severe illness, **trauma**.
  –drugs, e.g. vasopressin overtreatment, **oxytocin**, indomethacin, antidepressants, chlorpropamide, **carbamazepine**.
- Features: those of **hyponatraemia**. Urinary sodium exceeds 20 mmol/l, and urinary/plasma osmolality ratio exceeds 1.
- Treatment:
  –of primary cause.
  –water restriction; demeclocylcine 600–1200 mg daily in divided doses if persistent (thought to block the renal effects of vasopressin).
  –as for hyponatraemia if severe.

Syphilis. Sexually transmitted infection caused by the spirochaete *Treponema pallidum*.
- Divided clinically into:
  –primary stage: appearance of chancre at site of infection, 10 days–10 weeks after inoculation.
  –secondary stage: faint macular rash, condylomata and lymphadenopathy.
  –tertiary stage: lesions in skin, subcutaneous tissue, bone, tongue, testes, liver and CNS (meningovascular syphilis, tabes dorsalis, general paralysis of the insane).

Carditis and aortitis may occur, leading to ascending or arch **aortic aneurysm** and **aortic regurgitation**. Angina may occur in 50% of patients with aortitis.

Serological tests are strongly positive after 3 months in untreated cases. Treatment is usually with penicillin. Anaesthetic considerations are mainly related to the CVS effects.

Blood donors are screened for syphilis before donation.

Syringes. First use is attributed to Wood in 1855, although parenteral administration of drugs had been described earlier. Disposable polystyrene or polypropylene syringes are now widely used. Glass syringes are used for injecting drugs which are incompatible with plastic, e.g. **paraldehyde**, and for location of the **extradural space**. Plastic 'loss of resistance devices' resemble syringes but do not meet the required standards to be termed as such.
[Alexander Wood (1817–1884), Scottish physician]

Systemic lupus erythematosus, *see Connective tissue diseases*

Systemic sclerosis, *see Connective tissue diseases*

Systemic vascular resistance (SVR; Peripheral vascular resistance, PVR; Total peripheral resistance, TPR). **Resistance** against which the heart pumps. May be calculated using the principle of **Ohm's law**:

$$SVR\ (\textbf{dyne}\ s/cm^5) = \frac{\textbf{MAP} - \textbf{CVP}\ (mmHg)}{\textbf{cardiac output}\ (l/min)} \times 80\ (correction\ factor)$$

Normally 1000–1500 dyne s/cm^5. (NB. 1 dyne s/cm^5 = 100 N s/m^5).

The above equation ignores the effects of blood **viscosity**, pulsatile **flow** and the different results of pressure changes on different vascular beds.
- SVR is mainly determined by the diameter of the arterioles, small changes in their calibre producing large changes in resistance. Arteriolar calibre may be affected by:
  –intrinsic contractile response of vascular smooth muscle to increased intravascular pressure (myogenic theory of **autoregulation**).
  –locally-produced substances causing vasodilatation (e.g. CO_2, **potassium** and **hydrogen ions**, **lactic acid**, **histamine**, nitric oxide, **adenosine**, **prostaglandins** and **kinins**; metabolic theory of autoregulation), or vasoconstriction, e.g. **5-HT**. **Hypoxia** causes vasodilatation peripherally and vasoconstriction in the lungs. Increased temperature causes vasodilatation, whilst cold causes vasoconstriction.

–neural innervation:

  –α-**adrenergic receptors**: the most important type, affecting most vessels. Stimulation causes vasoconstriction.

  –β_2–adrenergic receptors: stimulation causes vasodilatation of arterioles to muscle and viscera.

  –**dopamine receptors**: stimulation causes vasodilatation of renal and splanchnic vessels.

  –sympathetic cholinergic receptors: stimulation causes vasodilatation in skeletal muscle.

  –other **neurotransmitters** may be involved, e.g. **substance P, vasoactive intestinal peptide**, etc.

–circulating substances, e.g. **noradrenaline**, angiotensin II, **vasopressin, vasopressor drugs** (causing vasoconstriction); **vasodilator drugs, atrial natriuretic peptide** (causing vasodilatation). **Adrenaline** causes vasodilatation in skeletal muscle and the liver. Toxins released in **septic shock** may cause vasodilatation. The locally-produced substances above may also cause systemic effects.

SVR increases progressively with age. Chronically increased SVR is the hallmark of essential **hypertension**.

The product of SVR and body surface area (SVR index) adjusts for differences in body size between individuals.

Ebert TJ, Stowe DF (1991) Curr Opin Anaesth; 4: 3–11
See also, Arterial blood pressure; Renin/angiotensin system

Systole, *see Cardiac cycle*

Systolic time intervals. Measurements derived from the systolic phase of the **cardiac cycle**, obtained from simultaneous **phonocardiography** and recording of **ECG** and carotid artery tracing. Allow evaluation of left ventricular function.

● Include:

  –QS_2 (qA_2): interval between the ECG **QRS complex** and the aortic component of the second **heart sound**.

  –left ventricular ejection time (LVET): period from the beginning of the carotid upstroke to the dicrotic notch.

  –pre-ejection period (PEP): QS_2–LVET. Represents the rate of ventricular isometric pressure change,

  i.e. $\dfrac{dp}{dt}$

  –others, e.g. duration of mechanical systole, are less commonly measured. Ratios of the intervals have been calculated, e.g. $\dfrac{PEP}{LVET}$

T

$t_{1/2}$, *see Half-life*

T-piece breathing systems, *see Anaesthetic breathing systems*

t **tests,** *see Statistical tests*

T wave. Wave on the **ECG** representing ventricular repolarization (*see Fig. 49b; Electrocardiography*). Normally upright in leads I, II and V_{3-6}; the upper height limit is 5 mm in the standard leads and 10 mm in the chest leads.
- Abnormalities:
    - –may be inverted in **myocardial ischaemia**, ventricular hypertrophy, **bundle branch block** and **digoxin** toxicity.
    - –may be notched in **pericarditis**.
    - –tall peaked waves may occur in **hyperkalaemia**.

Tachycardias, *see Sinus tachycardia; Supraventricular tachycardia; Ventricular tachycardia*

Tachyphylaxis. Term usually referring to **tolerance** that develops rapidly.

Tacrine, *see Tetrahydroaminocrine*

Tamponade, *see Cardiac tamponade*

TB, *see Tuberculosis*

Teeth. Comprised of the crown (consisting of enamel, dentine and pulp from outside inwards) and root. All parts may be damaged during anaesthesia; the deeper the damage, the more extensive is the treatment required. Traumatic damage is involved in about 30% of malpractice claims against anaesthetists. Damage most commonly occurs during intubation or postoperatively when the patient bites on an oral airway. **Preoperative assessment** of the teeth is essential, noting any loose, chipped or false teeth. Patients with caries, prostheses and periodontal disease, and those in whom tracheal intubation is difficult, are at particular risk. Appropriate warnings should be given and noted on the anaesthetic chart preoperatively.

Dentures and removable bridges, etc. are traditionally removed before anaesthesia, in case they should become dislodged and obstruct or pass into the airway. However, the need for routine preoperative removal of dentures has been questioned since this may cause distress to many patients, especially women.

Clokie C, Metcalf I, Holland A (1989) Can J Anaesth; 36: 675–80

See also, Dental surgery; Mandibular nerve blocks; Maxillary nerve blocks

Temazepam. Benzodiazepine used in insomnia, and commonly used for **premedication**, especially in **day-case surgery**. Shorter acting than **diazepam**, with faster onset of action. **Half-life** is 8 hours.

10–40 mg given orally, 45–60 minutes preoperatively, is usually an effective anxiolytic. For children, 0.5 mg/kg may be given.

Temperature. Property of a system which determines whether **heat** is transferred to or from other systems. Three temperature scales are recognized: **Kelvin** (formerly Absolute) scale, Celsius (formerly Centrigrade) scale and Fahrenheit scale (Table 35). The SI **unit** of temperature is the kelvin.
[Anders Celsius (1701–1744), Swedish scientist; Gabriel D Fahrenheit (1686–1736), German scientist]

Table 35. Corresponding points on different temperature scales

	Kelvin (K)	Celsius (°C)	Fahrenheit (°F)
Absolute zero	0	–273	–459
Melting point of ice	273	0	32
Boiling point of water	373	100	212

Temperature measurement. Methods used may be:
- –electrical:
    - –thermocouple: relies on the Seebeck effect; i.e. the production of voltage at the junction of two different conductors, the magnitude of which is proportional to **temperature**. A circuit may consist of a measuring thermocouple junction (e.g. as a needle) and a reference junction, with measurement of the voltage produced at the measuring probe. Because voltage is also produced at the reference junction, electrical manipulation is required to compensate for changes in temperature at the latter.
    - –thermistor: resistance falls exponentially with temperature. Consists of a metal oxide semiconductor bead which may be small enough to be placed within body cavities. Calibration may be difficult.
    - –platinum resistance wire: resistance increases proportionally with temperature. Very accurate but fragile.
- –non-electrical:
    - –liquid thermometers: the liquid (usually mercury) expands as temperature increases, and moves out

of its glass bulb and up the barrel of the instrument. Temperature is read from a scale along its length. A constriction just above the bulb prevents the mercury from withdrawing back into the bulb. Alcohol is used for very low temperatures.

–gas expansion thermometers, e.g. an anaeroid gauge used for **pressure measurement** is calibrated in units of temperature.

–bimetallic strip, arranged in a coil. A pointer is moved by coiling or uncoiling of the strip as temperature changes.

Measured peroperatively to **monitor heat loss during anaesthesia** or to warn of **hyperthermia**.

- Sites of measurement:
  –tympanic membrane: correlates most closely with hypothalamic temperature, and has rapid response time. Carries risk of tympanic perforation. The aural canal may be used.
  –oesophageal: accurate if the lower third is used, otherwise measured temperature is influenced by the temperature of inspired gases.
  –nasopharyngeal and bladder: similar to oesophageal.
  –rectal: usually 0.5–1.0°C higher than core temperature, because of bacterial fermentation. Response time is slow because of insulation by faeces.
  –blood: thermistors incorporated into pulmonary artery catheters allow continuous measurement.
  –skin: does not reflect core temperature. The difference between core and skin temperatures gives some indication of peripheral perfusion.

[Thomas J Seebeck (1770–1831), Russian-born German physicist]

Temperature regulation. Man is homeothermic, maintaining body core **temperature** at 37°C ± 1°C. The core usually includes cranial, thoracic, abdominal and pelvic contents, and variable amounts of the deep portions of the limbs. Temperature is lowest at night and highest in midafternoon, also varying with the menstrual cycle.

Constant temperature is required for optimal **enzyme** activity. Denaturation of proteins occurs at 42°C. Loss of consciousness occurs at **hypothermia** below 30°C.

- Mechanisms of heat loss/gain:
  –heat gain:
    –from the environment.
    –from **metabolism** (mainly in the brain, liver and kidneys): approximately 80 W is produced in an average man under resting conditions. This would raise body temperature by about 1°C per hour if totally insulated. Vigorous muscular activity may increase heat production by up to 20 times. In babies, **brown fat** produces much heat.
  –heat loss:
    –radiation from the skin. May account for 40% of total loss.
    –convection: related to air flow (e.g. 'wind-chill'). Accounts for up to 40% of total loss.
    –evaporation from the respiratory tract and skin: the latter is increased by sweating, which normally accounts for 20% of total loss but this figure may increase markedly.
    –conduction: of little importance in air, but significant in water.

Temperature-sensitive cells are present in the anterior **hypothalamus** (thought to be the most important site), brainstem, **spinal** cord, skin, skeletal muscle and abdominal viscera. Peripheral temperature receptors are primary afferent nerve endings and respond to cold and hot stimuli via Aδ and C fibres respectively. Central control of thermoregulation is in the hypothalamus. Efferents pass via the **sympathetic nervous system** to blood vessels, sweat glands and piloerector muscles. Local reflexes are also involved. Efferents also pass to somatic motor centres in the lower brainstem to cause shivering, and to higher centres.

- Regulatory mechanisms:
  –behavioural, e.g. curling up in the cold, etc.
  –skin blood flow: may be altered by vasodilatation or vasoconstriction of skin vessels, and by opening or closing of arteriovenous anastomoses in the skin. Affects all routes of heat loss. Alteration alone is sufficient to maintain constant body temperature in environments of 20–28°C in adults and 35–37°C in **neonates (thermoneutral range)**.
  –shivering and piloerection (reduced or absent in babies, brown fat metabolism occurring instead).
  –sweating.

Imrie MM, Hall GM (1990) Br J Anaesth; 64: 346–54
See also, Heat loss during anaesthesia

Temporomandibular joint (TMJ). Synovial joint between the mandibular condyle and the articular surface of the squamous temporal bone. Protrusion, retraction and grinding movements of the lower jaw occur by a gliding mechanism whereas mouth opening and closing involves gliding and hinging movements. Joint stability is least when the mouth is fully open (e.g. during laryngoscopy) and forward dislocation may occur. Affected by **rheumatoid arthritis**, degenerative disease, **ankylosing spondylitis** and scleroderma. Mouth opening may be severely limited, hindering laryngoscopy.

Aiello G, Metcalf I (1992) Can J Anaes; 39: 610–6
See also, Intubation, difficult; Trismus

TENS, *see Transcutaneous electrical nerve stimulation*

Tension. In physics, another word for **force**, implying stretching (cf. compression). Also refers to the **partial pressure** of a **gas** in solution.

Tension time index. Area between tracings of left ventricular pressure and aortic root pressure during systole, multiplied by heart rate (*see Fig. 52; Endocardial viability ratio*). Represents myocardial workload and hence O_2 demand; when taken in conjunction with **diastolic pressure time index**, it may indicate the myocardial O_2 supply/demand ratio and the likelihood of **myocardial ischaemia**.

Terbutaline sulphate. β-Adrenergic receptor agonist, used as a **bronchodilator drug** and **tocolytic drug**. Has similar effects to **salbutamol**, but possibly has less cardiac effects.

- Dosage:
  –5 mg orally, 8–12 hourly.
  –250–500 μg im/sc, 6 hourly as required.
  –250–500 μg iv slowly, repeated as required. 1–5 μg/min infusion may be used (containing 3–5 μg/ml). Up to 25 μg/min may be required in premature labour.
  –1–2 puffs by aerosol (250–500 μg) 6–8 hourly.
  –5–10 mg by nebulized solution, 6–12 hourly.
- Side effects: as for salbutamol.

Test dose, extradural. In **extradural anaesthesia**, injection of a small amount of **local anaesthetic agent** through the catheter before injection of the main dose, in order to identify accidental subarachnoid or iv placement of the catheter. Less commonly performed before 'through the needle' extradural block, since leakage of CSF or blood should be more easily noticeable.

Controversial, since it is not always reliable. The volume and strength of the test solution is also controversial. 3 ml 2% **lignocaine** with **adrenaline** 1:200 000 has been suggested as the ideal solution; subarachnoid injection produces **spinal anaesthesia** within 2–3 minutes, and iv injection produces tachycardia within 90 seconds (requires ECG monitoring).
Scott DB (1988) Br J Anaesth; 61: 129–30

Tetanic contraction. Sustained **muscle contraction** caused by repetitive electrical stimulation of a motor nerve. About 25 Hz stimulation is required for frequent enough **action potentials** to produce it, although the necessary rate varies according to the muscle studied. The force produced exceeds that of single muscle twitches. During tetanic contraction, **acetylcholine** is mobilized from reserve stores to the readily-available pool.
Produced during **neuromuscular blockade monitoring**.
See also, Neuromuscular junction; Neuromuscular transmission; Post-tetanic potentiation

Tetanus. Rare in developed countries following immunization programmes, but common worldwide. Caused by infection with *Clostridium tetani*, a widely occurring spore-forming Gram-positive bacillus found in soil. Inoculation may be via minor injury. Clinical features are caused by a potent exotoxin, which moves along peripheral nerves to the **spinal cord**, where it blocks inhibitory neurones causing muscle spasm. Incubation period is under 14 days in 90% of cases, but it may be 1–54 days. Local infection may cause muscle spasm around the site of injury; generalized tetanus is characterized by **trismus**, irritability, rigidity and opisthotonos. Cardiac **arrhythmias** and **hypertension** may follow sympathetic hyperactivity.
- Treatment:
  –human antitetanus **immunoglobulin**.
  –surgical excision and debridement of the wound.
  –penicillin to eradicate existing organisms.
  –**sedation**, **neuromuscular blocking drugs** and **IPPV** may be required.
  –of cardiovascular complications.
Overall mortality is up to 55% (greater if age exceeds 50, and if generalized spasms rapidly follow initial symptoms).
Active immunization with tetanus vaccine should always be performed in **trauma** and **burns** unless within 5–10 years of previous administration. Anti-tetanus immunoglobulin is given to non-immune patients with heavily contaminated or old wounds.

Tetany. Increased sensitivity of excitable cells, manifested as peripheral muscle spasm. Usually facial and carpopedal, the shape of the hand in the latter termed *main d'accoucheur* (French: obstetrician's hand). Usually caused by **hypocalcaemia**; it also occurs in **hypomagnesaemia** and may be hereditary.

Tetracaine, *see Amethocaine*

Tetrahydroaminocrine hydrochloride (Tacrine). **Acetylcholinesterase inhibitor**, no longer available; formerly used to prolong the action of **suxamethonium**. Also used prophylactically to reduce muscle pains following suxamethonium, and as a central stimulant.

Tetrodotoxin. Toxin obtained from puffer fish which selectively blocks **sodium** channels. Useful experimentally, e.g. for investigating **neuromuscular transmission**.

Thalassaemia. Group of inherited disorders involving decreased production of the α or β chains of **haemoglobin** (Hb). More common in Mediterranean, African and Asian areas. Severity is related to the pattern of inheritance of the Hb genes (normally, one β gene and two α genes are inherited from each parent).
- Divided into :
  –β thalassaemia:
    –not apparent immediately as **fetal haemoglobinn** does not contain β chains.
    –heterozygous β thalassaemia (thalassaemia minor) produces mild **anaemia**, but may be associated with other types of Hb (e.g HbC, HbE, HbS); resultant anaemia may vary from mild to severe.
    –homozygous β thalassaemia (Cooley's anaemia; thalassaemia major) results in severe anaemia in infancy, with no production of HbA. Features include craniofacial bone hyperplasia, hepatosplenomegaly and **cardiac failure**. Haemosiderosis may occur due to repeated **blood transfusion**. Usually fatal before adulthood. Some genetic subtypes are associated with a milder clinical course (thalassaemia intermedia).
  –α thalassaemia: severity varies, depending on the number of gene deletions. Usually causes mild anaemia; deletion of all four α genes is incompatible with life.
[Thomas B Cooley (1871–1945), US paediatrician]

Theophylline. Bronchodilator drug, used alone or in combination with ethylenediamine as **aminophylline**. Actions and effects: as for aminophylline.
- Dosage:
  –125–250 mg orally, 6–8 hourly; 175–300 mg slow-release preparation 12 hourly.
  –4 mg/kg by slow iv infusion, followed by 0.4–0.5 mg/kg/h.

Therapeutic ratio/index. Relationship between the doses of a drug required to produce undesirable and desirable effects. A drug with a high therapeutic ratio has a greater margin of safety than one with low therapeutic ratio. Defined experimentally as the ratio of median lethal dose to median effective dose:

$$\frac{LD_{50}}{ED_{50}.}$$

Thermal conductivity detector, *see Katharometer*

Thermistor, *see Temperature measurement*

Thermocouple, *see Temperature measurement*

Thermodilution techniques, *see Dilution techniques*

433

Thermoneutral range. Temperature range in which **temperature regulation** may be maintained by changes in skin blood flow alone. Corresponds to the temperature which feels 'comfortable'. About 20–28°C in adults and 35–37°C in **neonates**. Neonatal metabolic rate and mortality is reduced if body temperature is kept within the thermoneutral range.

Thiamylal sodium. IV anaesthetic agent, with similar properties to **thiopentone**. Unavailable in the UK.

Thiazide diuretics. Group of **diuretics** used to treat mild **hypertension** and **oedema** caused by **cardiac failure**. Chlorothiazide was the first to be studied but many now exist, e.g. bendrofluazide, chlorthalidone. Act mainly at the proximal part of the distal convoluted tubule of the **nephron**, where they inhibit **sodium** resorption. They also act at the proximal tubule, causing weak inhibition of **carbonic anhydrase** and increasing **bicarbonate** and **potassium** excretion, and have a direct vasodilator action. Their antihypertensive action increases only slightly as dosage is increased. Rapidly absorbed from the GIT with onset of action within 1–2 hours, lasting 12–24 hours.

Side effects include **hypokalaemia**, **hyponatraemia**, hyperuricaemia, **hypomagnesaemia**, hypochloraemic **alkalosis**, **hyperglycaemia**, hypercholesterolaemia, exacerbation of renal and hepatic impairment, impotence, and rarely rashes and **thrombocytopenia**.

Thigh, lateral cutaneous nerve block. Provides analgesia of the anterolateral thigh/knee, e.g. for leg surgery (especially skin graft harvesting) and diagnosis of meralgia paraesthetica (numbness and paraesthesiae caused by lateral cutaneous nerve compression by the inguinal ligament, under which it passes).

With the patient supine, a needle is introduced perpendicular to the skin, 2 cm medial and caudal to the anterior superior iliac spine. A click is felt as the fascia lata is pierced. 10–15 ml **local anaesthetic agent** is injected in a fan shape laterally.

Thiopental, *see Thiopentone*

Thiopentone sodium (5–ethyl–5–(1–methylbutyl)–2–thiobarbiturate). Widely used **iv anaesthetic agent**, synthesized in 1932 and first used in 1934 by **Lundy** and **Waters**. Also used as an **anticonvulsant drug** in severe **convulsions**. The sulphur analogue of pentobarbitone (Fig. 132). Stored as the sodium salt, a yellow powder with a faint garlic smell,

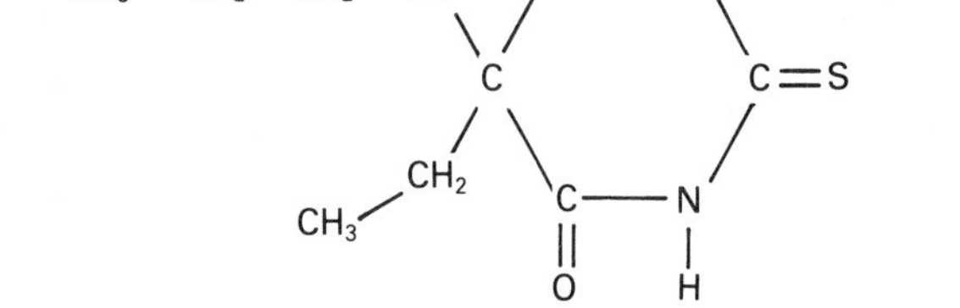

Figure 132 *Structure of thiopentone*

with 6% anhydrous sodium carbonate added to prevent formation of (insoluble) free acid when exposed to atmospheric CO_2. Presented in an atmosphere of nitrogen. Readily soluble in water; the solution is stable for 24–36 hours after mixing. Most commonly used as a 2.5% solution, with pH of 10.5. pK_a is 7.6; about 60% is non-ionized at a pH of 7.4. About 85% bound to plasma proteins after injection. Follows a multicompartmental pharmacokinetic model after a single iv injection, with redistribution from vessel-rich tissues (e.g. brain) to lean body tissues (e.g. muscle), with return of consciousness. Slower redistribution then occurs to vessel-poor tissues (e.g. fat).

- Effects:
  - induction:
    - smooth, occurring within one **arm–brain circulation time**. Involuntary movements and painful injection are rare.
    - recovery within 5–10 minutes after a single dose.
  - CVS:
    - causes dose-related direct myocardial depression, decreasing cardiac output and causing compensatory tachycardia with increased myocardial O_2 demand. Cardiovascular depression is related to speed of injection and is exacerbated by **hypovolaemia**.
    - has little effect on SVR but may decrease venous vascular tone, reducing venous return.
  - RS:
    - causes dose-related depression of the respiratory centre, decreasing the responsiveness to CO_2 and **hypoxia**. **Apnoea** is common after induction.
    - **laryngospasm** readily occurs following laryngeal stimulation.
    - has been implicated in causing **bronchospasm**, but this is disputed.
  - CNS:
    - anticonvulsant.
    - decreases pain threshold (**antanalgesia**).
    - reduces **cerebral perfusion pressure** and **ICP**.
  - other:
    - causes brief skeletal muscle relaxation at peak CNS effect.
    - reduces renal and hepatic blood flow secondary to reduced cardiac output. Causes hepatic **enzyme induction**.
    - reduces **intraocular pressure**.
    - has no effect on uterine tone.

Metabolized by oxidization in the liver (10–15% per hour), with under 1% appearing unchanged in the urine. Desulphuration to pentobarbitone may also occur following prolonged administration. Elimination **half-life** is 5–10 hours. Up to 30% may remain in the body after 24 hours. Cumulation may occur on repeated dosage.

- Complications:
  - extravenous injection causes pain and erythema.
  - intra-arterial injection causes intense pain, and may cause distal blistering, oedema and gangrene, traditionally attributed to crystallization of thiopentone within arterioles and capillaries, with local **noradrenaline** release and vasospasm. Endothelial damage and subsequent inflammatory reaction have been suggested as being more likely. Particularly hazardous with the 5% solution, now rarely used. Treatment: leaving the needle/cannula in the artery, the following may be injected:

 –saline, to dilute the drug.
  –vasodilators, e.g. **papaverine** 40 mg, **tolazoline** 40 mg, **phentolamine** 2–5 mg, to reduce arterial spasm.
  –local anaesthetic, e.g. **procaine** 50–100 mg (also a vasodilator), to reduce pain.
  –**heparin**, to reduce subsequent thrombosis.
Brachial plexus block and **stellate ganglion block** have been used to encourage vasodilatation (before heparinization). Postponement of surgery has been suggested. Injection of thiopentone should always stop after 1–2 ml, to ask whether there is any pain.
  –respiratory/cardiovascular depression as above.
  –**adverse drug reactions**. Severe **anaphylactic reactions** are rare (1:14 000–35 000), typically occurring after several previous exposures.
  Contraindicated in **porphyria**.
• Dosage:
  –3–6 mg/kg iv. Requirements are reduced in **hypoproteinaemia**, hypovolaemia, the elderly and critically ill patients. Injection should always proceed slowly, with a pause after the expected adequate dose before further administration.
  –Has also been given rectally: 40–50 mg/kg as 5–10% solution.
  –By infusion for convulsions: 2–3 mg/kg/h.

Third gas effect, *see Fink effect*

Third space. 'Non-functional' **interstitial fluid** compartment, to which fluid is transferred following **trauma**, **burns**, surgery and other conditions including infection, **pancreatitis**, etc. Most of the fluid originates from the **ECF**, but some movement from **intracellular fluid** also occurs. Includes fluid lost to the transcellular fluid compartment, e.g. ascites, bowel contents, etc. Although not lost from the body, fluid shifts to the third space are equivalent to functional ECF losses and must be accounted for when estimating **fluid balance**. Losses may exceed 10 ml/kg/h during abdominal surgery, and should be replaced initially with 0.9% **saline** or **Hartmann's solution**, although **colloids** may also be used.
See also, Stress response to surgery

Thoracic inlet. Kidney-shaped space about 10 cm wide and 5 cm anteroposteriorly. Slopes downward and forward at 60° to the horizontal. Bounded by the first thoracic vertebra posteriorly, the superior border of the manubrium anteriorly and the first rib and costal cartilages laterally. It transmits the oesophagus, trachea, brachiocephalic artery and veins, left carotid and subclavian arteries, vagus and phrenic nerves, cervical sympathetic chain and thoracic duct. Thoracic inlet views are useful in radiological assessment of lower neck and mediastinal lesions and **airway obstruction**.

Thoracic surgery. The first pneumonectomy was performed in 1911. Surgical and anaesthetic techniques improved with experience of treating chest injuries during World War II. The commonest indication for thoracic surgery was formerly **TB** and empyema but is now **malignancy**, especially **bronchial carcinoma**.
• Main anaesthetic principles:
  –preoperatively:
    –**preoperative assessment** of exercise tolerance, cough, haemoptysis, etc. **Ischaemic heart disease**

secondary to **smoking** is common. **Cyanosis**, tracheal deviation, **stridor**, abnormal chest wall movement, **pleural effusion** and systemic features of malignancy may be present.
  –investigations include **chest X-ray** and tomography, **CT scanning** and **magnetic resonance imaging**. Rarely, bronchography is performed, e.g. in **bronchiectasis**. Arterial blood gas analysis and **lung function tests** are routinely performed, e.g. spirometry, **flow–volume loops**, etc. A poor postoperative course following pneumonectomy is suggested by **FVC**, **FEV$_1$**, **maximal voluntary ventilation** or **residual volume**:total lung capacity ratio under 50% of predicted value. Poor outcome is also likely if resting **pulmonary arterial pressure** is raised, or **diffusing capacity** is low.
  –preparation includes antibiotic therapy, **physiotherapy** and use of **bronchodilator drugs** as appropriate. **Digoxin** is sometimes given prophylactically, especially in older patients.
  –**premedication** commonly includes **anticholinergic drugs** to reduce secretions.
  –peroperatively:
  –specific diagnostic procedures include **bronchoscopy**, mediastinoscopy, bronchography and oesophagoscopy.
  –**preoxygenation** is usually employed. IV **induction of anaesthesia** is usually suitable; difficulties may include cardiovascular instability, **airway obstruction**, difficult tracheal intubation, risk of **aspiration of gastric contents** in oesophageal disease, and problems of lesions affecting the **mediastinum**.
  –**endobronchial tubes** are often used, although standard **tracheal tubes** are usually acceptable unless isolation of lung segments is required. **Endobronchial blockers** may also be used.
  –large bore iv cannulae are vital, since blood loss may be severe.
  –standard **monitoring** is used; **arterial** and **central venous cannulation** are often employed. **Capnography** and pulse **oximetry** are especially useful.
  –maintenance of anaesthesia is usually with standard agents and techniques. Spontaneous ventilation is rarely allowed, since ventilation of the affected lung is poor once the chest is opened. **Pendelluft**, $\dot{V}/\dot{Q}$ mismatch and decreased venous return secondary to mediastinal shift may also occur. **Hypoxaemia** is common during **one-lung anaesthesia**. **Injector techniques** and **high frequency ventilation** have been used for tracheal resection.
  –**positioning of the patient**: the lateral position is usually employed, with the affected lung uppermost. The arm is placed over the head, displacing the scapula upwards. Drainage of secretions from the affected lung without soiling the unaffected lung may be achieved using the Parry Brown position (prone, with a pillow under the pelvis and a 10 cm rest under the chest. The arm on the operated side overhangs the table's edge with the head turned to the opposite side. The table is tipped head down so that the trachea slopes downwards).
  –at closure of the chest, the lung is re-expanded after endobronchial suction. Up to 40 cmH$_2$O airway pressure may be requested by the surgeon to test

bronchial sutures. Tubes are placed for **chest drainage**. After pneumonectomy, chest drains are often not used; air is introduced or removed to equalize the intrapleural pressures on both sides and centralize the mediastinum. The pleural space slowly fills with fluid postoperatively, with eventual fibrosis.
  –postoperatively:
    –IPPV is usually avoided if possible, as it risks leakage from the bronchial stump with possible fistula formation.
    –**postoperative analgesia** is vital to ensure adequate ventilation. Standard techniques are used, especially continuous iv opioid infusions (including **patient-controlled analgesia**), thoracic **extradural anaesthesia** and use of **spinal opioids**. **Cryoanalgesia** and **intercostal nerve block** may be performed by the surgeon whilst the chest is open.
    –physiotherapy is important postoperatively.
Specific procedures and conditions include removal of inhaled **foreign body**, **bronchopleural fistula**, **chest trauma**, **bronchopulmonary lavage**.
  Similar considerations apply to oesophageal surgery. Ivor Lewis oesophagectomy (performed for carcinoma of the middle third of the oesophagus) involves laparotomy to mobilize the stomach and duodenum, followed by turning of the patient and right thoracotomy. Patients are often malnourished.
[Arthur I Parry Brown (described 1948), London surgeon; Ivor Lewis (1895–1982), London surgeon]
See also, Pneumothorax

Three-in-one block, *see Femoral nerve block; Lumbar plexus*

Thrombelastograghy, *see Coagulation studies*

Thrombin time, *see Coagulation studies*

Thrombocytopenia. Defined as a **platelet** count below 100×10^9/l. Common in critically ill patients.
● Caused by:
  –decreased production:, e.g. bone marrow depression (by drugs, infection, etc.), vitamin B_{12}/folate deficiency, hereditary defects, **paroxysmal nocturnal haemoglobinuria**, **thiazide diuretics**, **alcohol** toxicity.
  –shortened survival:
    –immune, e.g. autoantibodies, alloantibodies (e.g. post-transfusion), immune complex disease, malignancy, drug-induced (e.g. quinine, **heparin**, **α-methyldopa**), infection.
    –non-immune, e.g. **DIC**, **cardiopulmonary bypass**.
  –abnormal distribution, e.g. hypersplenism, **hypothermia**.
Patients with platelet counts above 50×10^9) are usually asymptomatic. Bleeding time increases progressively as the count falls below 100×10^9. Counts below $20–30 \times 10^9$ are associated with spontaneous bleeding, e.g. mucocutaneous, gastrointestinal, cerebral. Diagnosis of the underlying condition requires examination of the blood film and bone marrow, **coagulation studies**, etc.
● Treatment: according to the underlying cause. Platelet transfusion is required for counts below $20–30 \times 10^9$ or if bleeding occurs; transfusion may be ineffective if increased platelet destruction is responsible.

Thromboembolism, *see Coagulation; Deep vein thrombosis*

Thrombolytic drugs, *see Fibrinolytic drugs*

Thromboplastin time, *see Coagulation studies*

Thromboxanes. Substances related to **prostaglandins**, derived from **arachidonic acid**. Thromboxane A_2 is released by **platelets** at sites of injury, causing vasoconstriction and platelet aggregation, and is opposed by **prostacyclin**. It is metabolized to thromboxane B_2 which has little activity.

Thymol. Aromatic hydrocarbon used as an antoxidant in **halothane** and **trichloroethylene**. May build up inside **vaporizers** unless cleaned regularly. Also used as a disinfectant and deodorant, e.g. in mouthwashes.

Thyroid crisis (Thyroid storm). Rare manifestation of severe **hyperthyroidism**. May be triggered by stress including surgery and infection. Features include tachycardia, **arrhythmias** (including **VT**, **VF** and **AF**) **cardiac failure**, fever, diarrhoea, sweating, hyperventilation, confusion and coma.
● Treatment:
  –supportive, e.g. cooling, sedation, rehydration, treatment of arrhythmias (**β-adrenergic receptor antagonists** are usually employed). **IPPV** may be required in **respiratory failure**.
  –hydrocortisone 100 mg iv 6 hourly.
  –antithyroid drugs:
    –200 mg potassium iodide orally/iv 6 hourly.
    –60–120 mg carbimazole or 600–1200 mg propylthiouracil orally/day.
  –**plasmapheresis** and exchange transfusion have been used in severe cases.

Thyroidectomy, *see Hyperthyroidism; Thyroid gland*

Thyroid gland. Largest endocrine gland, extending from the attachment of sternothyroid muscle to the thyroid cartilage superiorly, to the 6th tracheal ring inferiorly. The two lateral lobes lie lateral to the oesophagus and pharynx, with the isthmus overlying the 2nd–4th tracheal rings anteriorly. Arterial supply is via the superior and inferior thyroid arteries (branches of the external **carotid** artery, and thyrocervical trunk of the subclavian artery, respectively). The external and recurrent **laryngeal nerves** are closely related to the superior and inferior thyroid arteries respectively.
  Produces thyroxine (T_4) and triiodothyronine (T_3), which increase tissue metabolism and growth. They also increase the effects of **catecholamines** by increasing the number and sensitivity of β-**adrenergic receptors**. Iodine is absorbed from the GIT as iodide and actively transported into the thyroid gland, where it is oxidized by a peroxidase and bound to thyroglobulin. Iodination of tyrosine residues of thyroglobulin produces T_3 and T_4, which are cleaved from the parent molecule. Both hormones are more than 99% bound to plasma proteins including thyroxine-binding globulin (TBG) and albumin. T_3 is secreted in smaller amounts than T_4, is 3–5 times as potent, is faster-acting, and has a shorter **half-life.** T_4 is converted to T_3 peripherally.

Control of T_3 and T_4 production is by thyroid stimulating hormone (TSH), secreted by the **pituitary gland**. Secretion is inhibited by T_3, T_4 and stress, and stimulated by thyrotrophin releasing hormone (TRH), secreted by the **hypothalamus**. TRH secretion is also inhibited by T_3 and T_4.
● Tests of thyroid function:
  –radioactive iodine uptake.
  –total plasma T_3 and T_4 (normally 1–3 nmol/l and 60–150 nmol/l respectively). Increased in **hyperthyroidism**, and when TBG levels are raised, e.g. in **pregnancy**, **hepatitis**. Decreased in **hypothyroidism** and when TBG levels are reduced, e.g. **steroid therapy**, or when binding of T_3 and T_4 is inhibited, e.g. by **phenytoin** and **salicylates**.
  –free T_3 or T_4 index: obtained by adding radioactive T_3/T_4 to plasma, then adding a hormone-binding resin. Any radioactive T_3/T_4 not bound to TBG is taken up by the resin. Free T_3/T_4 index is the product of the resin uptake and plasma T_3/T_4 levels.
  –plasma TSH: indicates the level of hypersecretion in hyperthyroidism (usually depressed, due to negative feedback by T_3 and T_4). High in primary hypothyroidism. May be measured after injection of TRH.
The gland also secretes calcitonin, important in **calcium** homeostasis, from parafollicular (C) cells.
  Anaesthetic considerations of thyroid surgery: as for hyperthyroidism.

Thyrotoxicosis, *see Hyperthyroidism; Thyroid crisis* ·

Tibial nerve block, *see Ankle, nerve blocks; Knee, nerve blocks*

Tidal volume. Volume of gas inspired and expired with each breath. Normally 7 ml/kg. Measured using **spirometers** or **respirometers**. 'Effective' tidal volume equals tidal volume minus **dead space** volume.

Time constant (τ). Expression used to describe an **exponential process**. Equals the time in which the process would be completed if the rate of change were maintained at its initial value. At 1 τ the process is 63% complete (i.e. 37% of the initial quantity remains), at 2 τ it is 86.5% complete, and at 3 τ it is 95% complete. After 6 τ the process is 99.75% complete.
  When used to refer to expiration of air from the lungs, τ equals **compliance** × **resistance**; thus stiff alveoli served by narrow airways empty at similar rates to compliant alveoli served by wide airways.
See also, Half-life

Time to sustained respiration. Time for adequate regular respiration to occur in the **neonate** after delivery, without stimulation. Related to **fetal wellbeing** and respiratory depression caused by drugs administered to the mother before delivery.
See also, Fetus, effects of anaesthetic drugs on; Obstetric analgesia and anaesthesia

TIVA, *see Total intravenous anaesthesia*

TMJ, *see Temporomandibular joint*

TNS, Transcutaneous nerve stimulation, *see Transcutaneous electrical nerve stimulation*

Tocainide hydrochloride. Class Ib **antiarrhythmic drug**. An analogue of **lignocaine**, but undergoes less **first-pass metabolism** when given orally, and with longer elimination **half-life** (10–12 hours). Reserved for life-threatening ventricular **arrhythmias** because of its toxicity.
● Dosage:
  –400–800 mg 8 hourly, orally.
  –500–750 mg iv over 30 minutes. Hypotension and bradycardia may occur.
● Side effects: as for lignocaine; also GIT disturbances, agranulocytosis, aplastic anaemia, thrombocytopenia, and a lupus erythematosus-like syndrome.

Tocolytic drugs. Used to inhibit uterine contractions when premature delivery of the fetus is threatened. Drugs most commonly used are β_2–**adrenergic receptor** agonists and include **salbutamol**, **terbutaline**, isoxsuprine and ritodrine. Side effects may persist after discontinuation of the infusion; these include tachycardia, arrhythmias, hypotension and occasionally **pulmonary oedema** (thought to be caused by increased pulmonary hydrostatic pressure). Arrhythmias may occur if **halothane** is subsequently used.
See also, Obstetric analgesia and anaesthesia

Tolazoline hydrochloride. α-Adrenergic **antagonist**, structurally related to **phentolamine**. Traditionally used by iv infusion to relieve arterial spasm following accidental intra-arterial injection of **thiopentone**. Also used to reduce **pulmonary vasular resistance**, e.g. in congenital **diaphragmatic hernia**.
● Dosage: 1 mg/kg.

Tolerance. Progressively decreasing response to repeated dosage of a drug. May result from altered number of receptors, altered response to receptor activation, altered **pharmacokinetics** (e.g. **enzyme induction**) or development of physiological compensatory mechanisms. Classically occurs with **morphine**.
See also, Tachyphylaxis

Tongue. Muscular organ attached to the hyoid bone and mandible. Covered by mucous membrane and divided into anterior ⅔ and posterior ⅓ by a V-shaped groove, the sulcus terminalis. At the latter's apex is a small depression, the foramen caecum. The lower surface is attached to the floor of the mouth by the frenulum.
● Muscles of the tongue:
  –genioglossus: fibres fan back from the superior genial spine of the mandible to the tip and whole length of the dorsum of the tongue. The lowest fibres attach to the hyoid bone.
  –hyoglossus: attached to the body and greater horns of the hyoid bone, passing upwards and forwards into the sides of the tongue.
  –palatoglossus and styloglossus: pass from the palate and styloid process respectively.
  –intrinsic muscles: include vertical, longitudinal and transverse fibres.
● Nerve supply:
  –sensory: glossopharyngeal nerve to the posterior ⅔ and facial nerve to the anterior ⅓.
  –motor: hypoglossal nerve.
The tone in genioglossus is important in preventing approximation of the tongue and posterior pharyngeal

wall which results in **airway obstruction**. Genioglossus tone varies with respiration and is maximal in inspiration. It also decreases during **sleep**; this may contribute to the development of **sleep apnoea**. Anaesthetic and sedative agents decrease this tone and thus predispose to obstruction, which may be relieved by elevating the jaw, placing the patient in the lateral position, and use of pharyngeal **airways**.

Macroglossia predisposes to respiratory obstruction and may hinder tracheal intubation, e.g. in **acromegaly** and **Down's syndrome**. It may also occur after posterior fossa **neurosurgery**.

Tongue forceps, *see Forceps*

Tonicity. Refers to the effective **osmotic pressure** of solutions in relation to that of **plasma**. Thus a urea solution may be isosmotic with plasma but its effective osmotic pressure (and thus tonicity) falls after infusion because urea distributes evenly across cell membranes. Similarly, 5% dextrose solution is isosmotic with plasma but hypotonic when infused since the dextrose is metabolized by red blood cells leaving water.
See also, Intravenous fluids

Tonometry, gastric, *see Gastric intramucosal pH*

Tonsil, bleeding. Haemorrhage usually occurs within a few hours postoperatively, but may be delayed.
● Problems include:
　–hidden blood loss if the patient (usually a child) swallows it; **hypovolaemia** may thus be severe before diagnosis is made.
　–risk of **aspiration of gastric contents** (mostly altered blood).
　–airway management and tracheal intubation may be difficult if bleeding is torrential.
　–significant amounts of the anaesthetic agents used previously may still be present.
　–possibility of an undiagnosed **coagulation disorder**.
● Management:
　–preoperative assessment of coagulation and cardiovascular status, with iv resuscitation. Nasogastric aspiration is controversial, since it may exacerbate bleeding.
　–experienced assistance is required. Each of the following techniques has its advocates:
　　–inhalational induction in the left lateral position (with suction available), using **halothane** in O$_2$, and tracheal intubation during spontaneous ventilation. The main advantage is the maintenance of spontaneous ventilation if intubation is difficult. However, induction may be prolonged and hindered by bleeding, gagging, etc., and the high concentrations of halothane required plus hypovolaemia may cause significant hypotension.
　　–rapid sequence induction using a small dose of iv agent, e.g. **thiopentone** followed by **suxamethonium** and intubation. Advantages of this technique include rapidity of intubation and the greater familiarity of most anaesthetists with it. However, it should only be attempted if intubation was easy at the initial operation. Hypotension may follow induction, and visualization of the larynx may be difficult in torrential haemorrhage.

–nasogastric aspiration is performed before extubation. This should be performed when the patient is awake and laryngeal reflexes have returned.
See also, Ear, nose and throat surgery; Induction, rapid sequence

Topical anaesthesia. Application of **local anaesthetic agent** to skin or mucous membranes to produce anaesthesia. Used on the skin, conjunctiva, nasal passages, larynx and pharynx, tracheobronchial tree, rectum and urethra. Local anaesthetic has also been instilled into the bladder, pleural cavity, peritoneal cavity and synovial fluid of joints.
Application may be via direct instillation, soaked swabs, pastes/ointments or sprays. Agents used include **cocaine**, **lignocaine**, **amethocaine** and benzocaine. Systemic absorption may be rapid and the maximal safe doses should not be exceeded.
See also, EMLA cream

Torr. Unit of **pressure**; 1 torr = $\frac{1}{760}$ atmosphere = 1 mmHg. [Evangelista Torricelli (1608–1647), Italian physicist]

Torsade de pointes. Atypical **VT** characterized by polymorphic **QRS complexes** with repeated fluctuations of QRS axis, the complexes appearing to twist about the baseline (Fig. 133). Often associated with a prolonged

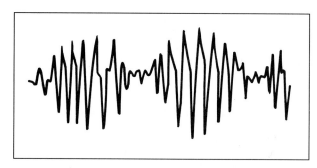

Figure 133 *Torsade de pointes*

Q–T interval. Initiated by a **ventricular ectopic beat** occurring during a prolonged pause after a previous ectopic.
● Causes include:
　–electrolyte abnormalities, e.g. **hypokalaemia**, **hypomagnesaemia**, **hypocalcaemia**.
　–drugs, e.g. class I **antiarrhythmic drugs**, **tricyclic antidepressant drugs**, **phenothiazines**.
　–heart disease.
● Treatment:
　–of predisposing condition.
　–**cardioversion**.
　–increasing the heart rate, e.g. **isoprenaline**, **cardiac pacing**.
Class I antiarrhythmic drugs should be avoided.
Alexander MG, Potgieter PD (1983) Anaesthesia; 38: 269–74

Total intravenous anaesthesia (TIVA). Anaesthetic technique employing iv agents alone, and avoiding the use of inhalational agents. Drugs are given usually by infusion to achieve hypnosis, analgesia and neuromuscular blockade (where required). The patient breathes O$_2$, air or a mixture of the two. The drugs chosen are usually of short action and **half-life** to reduce risk of accumulation and prolonged recovery. Examples include **propofol** or **methohexitone**, together with **alfentanil** or **fentanyl**. **Ketamine** has been used for its analgesic properties, e.g. together with **midazolam**. **Neuroleptanaesthesia** has also been used.

- Advantages:
  - avoids unwanted effects of **inhalational anaesthetic agents**.
  - avoids pollution by gases and vapours.
  - may be used without complex apparatus such as anaesthetic machines, cylinders, vaporizers, etc., e.g. in wars, etc.
- Disadvantages:
  - requires repeated injections or infusion devices, e.g. syringe pumps, etc.
  - prediction of plasma levels of anaesthetic agents is more difficult than with inhalational agents, because of the more complicated **pharmacokinetics**. Thus **awareness** or excessive dosage may occur unless one is familiar with the technique. Computer-assisted infusion has been employed to provide steady plasma levels according to pharmacokinetic data collected from hundreds of patients.
  - once a drug has been infused, it cannot be removed from the body other than by metabolism and excretion. Thus there is less control than with inhalational agents, which may be removed by ventilation.

Total lung capacity. Volume of gas in the lungs after maximal inspiration. Normally approximately 6 litres. Determined by helium dilution (does not measure gas in poorly ventilated regions) or with the **body plethysmograph**.
See also, Lung volumes

Total parenteral nutrition, *see Nutrition, total parenteral*

Tourniquets. Used to reduce bleeding during limb surgery, and to allow **IVRA**. Inflated following exsanguination of the limb, e.g. by raising it for 2–3 minutes with the artery compressed, or by using a rubber Esmarch bandage. The latter increases CVP and may provoke cardiac failure in susceptible patients. It may also dislodge emboli from **DVTs**.
- Measures suggested to reduce compression and ischaemic damage:
  - inflation pressures:
    - arm: systolic BP + 50 mmHg (+ 100 mmHg for IVRA).
    - leg: systolic BP × 2.
    Suggested values vary, and depend partly on age, weight, etc.
  - inflation time: 2 hours maximum is the most common recommendation, although 60 minutes for the arm and 90 minutes for the leg are often quoted. Periodic deflation and reinflation may allow longer use.
Equipment should be checked before use. Tourniquets should not be used in **sickle-cell anaemia** (avoidance in sickle trait has also been suggested). Careful padding is required under the tourniquet. Skin preparation solutions may cause chemical burns if allowed to soak into the padding.
[Johann FA von Esmarch (1823–1908), German surgeon]
Fletcher IR, Healy TEJ (1983) Ann Roy Coll Surg Engl; 65: 409–17

Toxic shock syndrome. Systemic illness associated with certain *Staphylococcus aureus* strains, thought to be caused by exotoxins (possibly with concurrent Gram-negative **endotoxin** production). Streptococci have also been implicated.

First described in 1978; the reported incidence increased around 1980, especially associated with menstruation and use of tampons. Features typically occur rapidly and include fever, hypotension, GIT upset, headache and myalgia. Generalized rash and/or oedema leads to desquamation 10–20 days later. Multiorgan failure may occur. Treatment is supportive, with **antibacterial drug** therapy.
Resnick S (1990) J Pediatrics; 116: 321–8

TPN, Total parenteral nutrition, *see Nutrition, total parenteral*

TPR, Total peripheral resistance, *see Systemic vascular resistance*

Trachea, *see Tracheobronchial tree*

Tracheal administration of drugs. Has been used when iv administration is not possible, e.g. **cardiac arrest**. Twice the iv dose is usually given, injected via a catheter placed through the tracheal tube. 2–3 manual hyperinflations aid dispersal of the drug. **Atropine**, **adrenaline** and **lignocaine** are the drugs most commonly administered in this way; **isoprenaline** and **naloxone** have also been given. Solutions which may cause local tissue damage should be avoided, e.g. **calcium**, **bicarbonate**. Many respiratory drugs are administered using inhalers and nebulizers.
Greenbaum R (1987) Anaesthesia; 42: 927–8

Tracheal intubation, *see Intubation, tracheal*

Tracheal tubes. Developed along with techniques for tracheal intubation. **O'Dwyer** described his intubating tube in 1885, although various tubes had been used previously, e.g. for **CPR**. The modern wide bore tracheal tube was developed by **Magill** and **Rowbotham** after World War I, following the use of thin gum-elastic tubes for **insufflation techniques**. Separate tubes were placed into the trachea for delivery and removal of gases; these were eventually replaced by a single rubber ('Magill') tube. Red rubber tracheal tubes have largely been replaced by sterile disposable polyvinyl chloride tubes, since the former deteriorate on repeated sterilization, are more costly to use, and are irritant to the respiratory mucosa. Plastic tubes soften as they warm, e.g. in the trachea; they may be softened in warm water, e.g. before nasal intubation.
- Features of 'typical' modern tracheal tubes (Fig. 134a):
  - marked with the following information:
    - size (internal diameter in mm; the external diameter may be marked in smaller lettering).
    - the letters IT or Z79–IT (for plastic tubes) denote that the material has been implantation tested in rabbit muscle for tissue compatibility, according to American National Standards Committee number Z79, formed in 1956.
    - the distance from the tip of the tube is marked at intervals along the tube's length. Most plastic tubes are longer than is usually required, and may be cut to size.

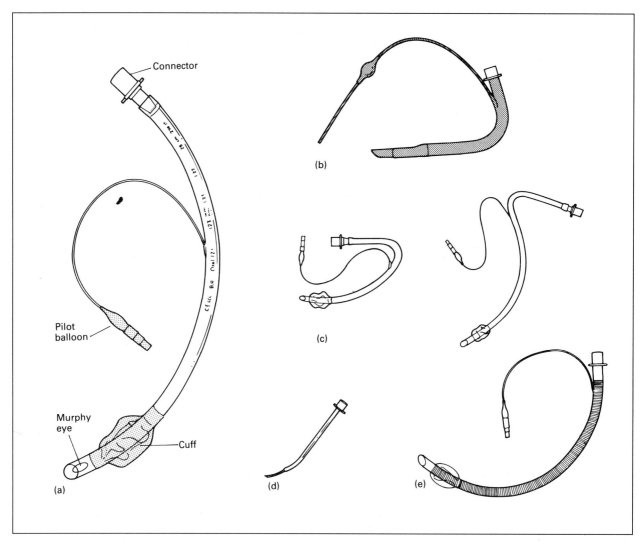

Figure 134 *Tracheal tubes: (a) 'typical'; (b) Oxford; (c) oral and nasal RAE; (d) Cole; (e) reinforced*

–other markings may refer to the manufacturer, the trade name of the type of tube, and whether it is intended for oral or nasal use.

A radio-opaque line is incorporated in most modern tubes, to aid detection on chest X-rays.

–curved with a left-facing bevel at the distal end. There may be a hole in the wall opposite the bevel (Murphy eye), to allow ventilation should the end become obstructed by the tracheal wall or mucus.

–attached to a tracheal tube **connector** at the proximal end.

–may bear a **cuff** near the distal end, with a pilot balloon running towards the proximal end.

• Other shapes and types of tubes (Fig. 134b–e):

–Oxford tube: conforms more closely with the shape of the mouth and pharynx, thus less liable to kink. The bevel faces posteriorly; insertion of the tube is aided by a gum-elastic bougie protruding a short distance from the distal end. Traditionally made of red rubber, they are thicker-walled than traditional red rubber tubes. Available with or without cuffs.

–RAE tube: plastic; designed to be even more 'anatomically' shaped than the Oxford tube. Nasal RAE tubes are also available, as are other manufacturers' versions. Available with or without cuffs.

–Cole tube: used in **neonates**. Shouldered, with thickened walls to prevent kinking. Designed to minimize **resistance** to **flow** of gas by virtue of their wide proximal portion; however, they increase resistance by causing turbulence at the junction with the narrow portion. They also may cause damage to the **larnyx** and trachea if the shoulder is forced too far distally. Their avoidance has therefore been repeatedly suggested.

–reinforced tubes: resemble standard tubes but contain a spiral of metal or nylon in the tube wall. Used where kinking of the tube may otherwise occur, e.g. **neurosurgery**, **faciomaxillary surgery**. Originally made of latex rubber, they are now commonly made of plastic. They cannot be cut to size. Available with or without cuffs.

Tubes may bear an extra channel for sampling of distal gases or for jet ventilation. A directional tube has also been described, in which traction on a ring at the proxi-

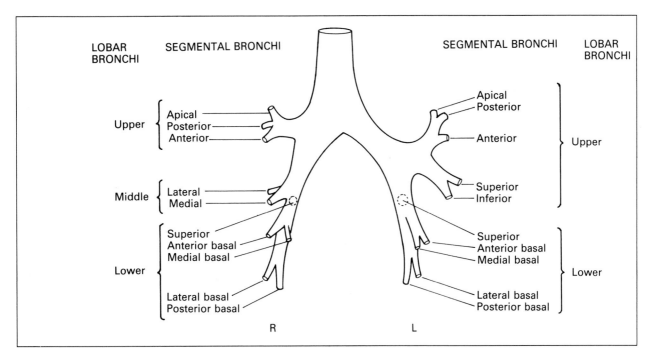

Figure 135 *Lobar and segmental bronchi*

mal end flexes the distal end, aiding placement during tracheal intubation. **Laser** protected tubes include tubes made totally out of metal and those coated with 'laser-proof' substances.

Size 9 mm and 8 mm tubes are usually employed for men and women respectively. Average suitable length is 22–25 cm for oral tubes, and 25–28 cm for nasal tubes (*for sizes of tubes for children, see Paediatric anaesthsia*).
[Frank J Murphy (described 1941), Detroit anaesthetist; Frank Cole (1918–1977), US anaesthetist; RAE: Wallace H Ring, John C Adair, Richard A Elwyn, Salt Lake City anaesthetists]
See also, Endobronchial tubes; Intubation, tracheal; Tracheostomy

Tracheobronchial tree. Branching system consisting of 23 generations of passages from trachea to alveoli, comprised of:
- conducting airways: make up anatomical **dead space**:
    - trachea (generation 0): 10 cm long and 2 cm wide in the adult. Descends from the **larynx** level with C6, passing through the neck and thorax to its bifurcation level with T4–5. Its walls are formed of fibrous tissue reinforced by 15–20 U-shaped cartilagenous rings (deficient posteriorly), united behind by fibrous tissue and smooth muscle. Lined with ciliated epithelium.
      Relations: lies anterior to the oesophagus, with the recurrent **laryngeal nerve** in the groove between them. In the neck (*see Fig. 97; Neck, cross-sectional anatomy*) it is crossed anteriorly by the isthmus of the **thyroid gland**. Laterally lie the lateral lobes of the thyroid, the inferior thyroid artery and carotid sheath (containing the internal **jugular vein**, common **carotid artery** and **vagus nerve**). In the thorax (*see Fig. 89b; Mediastinum*) it is crossed anteriorly by the brachiocephalic artery and vein. On the left lie the

common carotid and subclavian arteries above, and the aorta below. On the right lie the mediastinal pleura, right vagus nerve and azygous vein.
- right and left main bronchi (generation 1): arise at T4–5:
    - right: 3 cm long, and wider and more vertical than the left, and therefore likelier to receive foreign bodies. The right upper main bronchus arises about 2.5 cm from its origin.
      Relations: separated from the pericardium and superior vena cava by the right pulmonary artery. The azygous vein lies above.
    - left: about 5 cm long.
      Relations: separated from the left atrium by the left pulmonary artery. The aortic arch lies above, and the bronchial vessels posteriorly (separating it from the oesophagus and descending thoracic aorta).
- lobar and segmental bronchi (generations 2–4) (Fig. 135).
- small bronchi to terminal bronchioles (generations 5–16).
- respiratory airways:
    - respiratory bronchioles (generations 17–19): bear occasional alveoli.
    - alveolar ducts (generations 20–22): lined with alveoli.
    - alveoli (generation 23).
See also, Alveolus; Cilary activity; Lung

Tracheo-oesophageal fistula (TOF). Oesophageal atresia occurs in 1:3000 births, with TOF in 25% of cases. Different forms exist (Fig. 136). Babies may be premature and have other congenital abnormalities. TOF may present with choking during feeds, production of copious frothy mucus from the mouth, or repeated chest infections

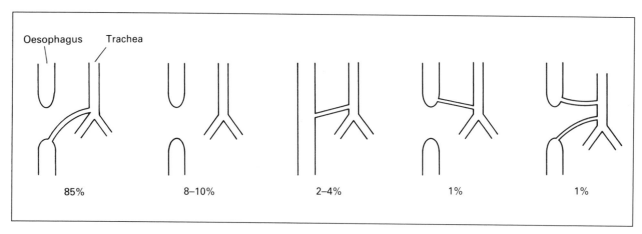

Oesophagus   Trachea

85%   8–10%   2–4%   1%   1%

Figure 136 *Different forms of tracheo-oesophageal fistulae and their incidence*

following pulmonary aspiration. It is diagnosed by passing a radio-opaque nasogastric tube into the blind pouch; contrast medium is avoided because of risk of aspiration. Treated by surgery, performed via right thoracotomy. Primary anastomosis of the oesophagus is performed if possible.

- Anaesthesia is as for **paediatric anaesthesia**. In particular:
    - preoperatively:
        - the baby is nursed head-up, with continuous suction to the blind pouch to prevent pulmonary aspiration.
        - correction of electrolyte imbalance may be required.
    - peroperatively:
        - traditionally, tracheal intubation is performed awake, avoiding IPPV by facepiece to prevent gastric inflation. Intubation of the fistula may occur; if this happens the tracheal tube may be withdrawn and reinserted with the bevel direction altered. Positioning of the tip of the tube distal to the fistula prevents gastric inflation; this may be achieved by deliberate endobronchial intubation, followed by careful withdrawal of the tracheal tube until breath sounds are heard on both sides of the chest.
        - classically, neuromuscular blockade and IPPV are avoided until the chest is open, to prevent gastric distension. Many paediatric anaesthetists use gentle manual IPPV, since gastric distension is rare.
        - surgical manipulation may cause sudden increases in airway pressures or reductions in cardiac output.
    - postoperatively: IPPV may be required.

After repair, a blind passage may remain at the site of the fistula, making subsequent tracheal intubation difficult. Tracheomalacia may also occur.

Tracheostomy. First performed in the 1700s for upper **airway obstruction**. Modern indications:

- prophylactic or therapeutic relief of airway obstruction.
- to protect the **tracheobronchial tree** against aspiration of food, saliva, etc. when pharyngeal and laryngeal reflexes are obtunded, e.g. neurological disease.

- to allow suction and removal of secretions.
- **IPPV** lasting longer than 2–3 weeks. Cited advantages over conventional tracheal intubation include easier nursing management, improved patient comfort, ability for oral nutrition and speech, and possibly assistance of **weaning** by a 30–50% reduction in **dead space**. However, the benefits of tracheostomy over prolonged conventional intubation are controversial, in view of its complications.

The procedure may be performed under general or local anaesthesia. The patient lies supine with the neck hyperextended, and a horizontal incision is made 1.5 cm below the level of the cricoid cartilage. After location of the trachea, a vertical incision is made through the 2nd, 3rd and 4th tracheal rings. A slit or circular opening is made in the trachea (creation of a tracheal flap has been implicated in causing tracheal stenosis). During general anaesthesia, ventilation with 100% O_2 should precede withdrawal of the tracheal tube (which is withdrawn into the larynx only, in case readvancement is required). The tracheostomy tube is then inserted. Stay sutures may be brought out on to the skin from the trachea, to aid subsequent tube reinsertion.

A percutaneous method has recently been described, in which successive stomal dilatations are made using a **Seldinger technique**. This method may be performed in the ICU and has fewer short-term complications than conventional tracheostomy, although the incidence of long-term complications is unknown.

- Tracheostomy tubes:
    - uncuffed: plastic or metal (usually silver). They may allow speech if a one-way valve is used; air is drawn into the lungs through the tracheostomy and exhaled through the larynx and mouth. A fenestration in the tube improves the strength of the voice.
    - cuffed: plastic, with low pressure, high volume **cuffs** to minimize tracheal mucosal damage. The cuff may be deflated and the tube occluded with a finger during expiration, to allow speech. Cuffed tubes may also be fenestrated. Some incorporate a separate catheter opening just above the cuff, through which O_2 may be diverted using a manual control to allow speech. The catheter may also be used for suction.
- Complications may be early or late:
    - early:

–haemorrhage, especially from branches of the anterior jugular veins or thyroid isthmus.

–displacement of the tube: extrusion or endo-bronchial intubation.

–blockage, e.g. by secretions, compression by the cuff or occlusion against the carina.

–subcutaneous emphysema.

–**pneumothorax**.

–late:

–infection, including superficial wound infection, tracheitis and chest infection.

–tracheal erosion and ulceration, e.g. into blood vessels, oesophagus, etc.

–tracheal stenosis; usually occurs level with the stoma or the tube's cuff, although subglottic stenosis may also occur. Surgical resection may be required.

–tracheal dilatation may occur.

• Tracheostomy care includes:

–**humidification**: vital to reduce risk of obstruction by viscous secretions.

–suction: sterile technique is mandatory. The suction catheter's diameter should not exceed half that of the tracheostomy tube. Suction is applied on withdrawal, not insertion, of the catheter.

–daily cleaning and dressing to reduce risk of infection.

–secure fixation, e.g. with double tapes.

–presence of tracheal dilators, spare tracheostomy tubes, and equipment for manual ventilation and tracheal intubation, in case of displacement.

–provision of a means of communication, e.g. pen and paper.

The initial tube is usually left *in situ* for at least a week, to allow formation of a tract. Changing may be assisted by removing and inserting tubes over a thin catheter. Once decannulated, the stoma usually closes spontaneously within a few days, but surgical closure may be required.

See also, Minitracheotomy

Train-of-four nerve stimulation, *see Neuromuscular blockade monitoring*

Tramadol hydrochloride. Opioid analgesic drug, available in Continental Europe but not in the UK. A weak agonist at all opioid receptors, it also inhibits **noradrenaline** uptake and **5-HT** release. Causes only slight respiratory depression.

• Dosage: 50 mg orally; 50–100 mg im/iv/sc/pr.

Tranexamic acid. Antifibrinolytic drug, used to reduce bleeding, e.g. in prostatectomy, menorrhagia or dental extraction in haemophiliacs; it has also been used in **streptokinase** overdose and **hereditary angioneurotic oedema**.

• Dosage:

–1–1.5 g 6–12 hourly, orally.

–1 g slowly iv, 8 hourly.

• Side effects: GIT disturbances, dizziness. Contraindicated in thromboembolic disease.

Transcutaneous electrical nerve stimulation (TENS). Stimulation of peripheral nerves via cutaneous electrodes, to relieve **pain**. Based on the **gate theory** of pain transmission; i.e. stimulation of Aβ fibres (by high frequency TENS) and Aδ fibres (by low frequency TENS) inhibits pain transmission by C fibres. Current is provided by a battery-powered pulse generator which typically delivers a range of currents (0–50 mA), frequencies (0–200 Hz) and pulse widths (0.1–0.5 ms). Rectangular pulses are usually employed. Surface electrodes are usually carbon-impregnated silicone rubber.

The electrodes are placed either side of the painful area or its supplying nerves, and the current increased until tingling is felt. Experimentation with timing and duration is usually required to achieve maximal effects.

Has been used successfully in acute pain (e.g. for fractured ribs, labour, postoperatively, etc.), but is usually employed for chronic **pain management** (peripheral nerve disorders, spinal cord and root disorders, muscle pain and joint pain). Efficacy is difficult to assess as there is significant placebo effect, but TENS may significantly reduce analgesic requirements.

Allergic dermatitis at electrode sites may occur. Contraindicated in patients with pacemakers.

Anon (1989) Drug Ther Bull; 27: 25–7

Transducers. Devices which convert one form of energy to another, usually to electricity in **monitoring** systems.

• May be:

–passive: involving changes in:

–**resistance**, e.g. strain gauge, thermistor, photoresistor.

–**inductance**, e.g. pressure transducers.

–**capacitance**, e.g. condenser microphone.

–active, i.e. involving generation of potentials:

–piezoelectric effect: generation of voltage across the faces of a quartz crystal when deformed.

–photoelectric cell.

–thermocouple.

–radiation counters.

–electrode potentials, e.g. pH electrode.

–electromagnetic induction.

See also, Arterial blood pressure measurement; Damping; pH measurement; Pressure measurement; Temperature measurement

Transfer factor, *see Diffusing capacity*

Transfusion, *see Blood transfusion*

Transplantation. Use of cadaveric or live donor tissues has increased with improved techniques and introduction of the **immunosuppressive drug** cyclosporin.

• Main points:

–identification of donors and matching with recipients. There may be underutilization of potential donor organs following **brainstem death** in some ICUs.

–**organ donation**.

–preoperative state of the recipient, surgical procedure and postoperative course.

–chronic physical and psychological effects of transplantation, drug therapy and possible organ rejection.

See also, Heart transplantation; Heart–lung transplantation; Liver transplantation; Renal transplantation

Transposition of the great arteries. Accounts for 5% of **congenital heart disease**. Caused by failure of the truncus arteriosus to rotate during embryological development. The aorta arises from the right ventricle and the pulmonary artery from the left ventricle. Thus the pulmonary and systemic circulations work independently, resulting in severe hypoxaemia. Survival is only possible if a connection exists between the two circulations, e.g. **ASD**, **VSD** or patent **ductus arteriosus**. Other malpositions of the great arteries may occur.

Features include cyanosis, early **cardiac failure** and right ventricular hypertrophy, with normal pulmonary and systemic pressures. 85–90% of infants die within a year without treatment.

- Treatment:
  –palliation: **shunt** procedures, e.g. creation of an ASD by balloon septostomy or surgery.
  –correction: use of baffles, e.g. Mustard procedure: redirection of vena caval flow into the left atrium, and pulmonary venous blood into the right atrium, using a pericardial patch. The right ventricle thus supplies the systemic circulation. Systemic venous obstruction and poor long-term right ventricular function have led to increased use of procedures which switch the pulmonary and systemic circulations, at ventricular or arterial levels.

[William T Mustard (1914–1987), Toronto surgeon]

Transurethral resection of the prostate (TURP). Cystoscopic procedure for the removal of hypertrophied prostatic tissue.

- Anaesthetic considerations:
  –**preoperative assessent**: most patients are elderly, with coexisting disease. Some may have prostatic **malignancy** with systemic manifestations; oestrogen therapy may cause fluid retention. Renal impairment may be present.
  –use of irrigating solution (usually glycine) may result in the **TURP syndrome**.
  –**positioning of the patient** in lithotomy position, with restricted ventilation and increased venous return. Venous pooling in the legs may occur when the legs are brought down at the end of the procedure, with possible hypotension.
  –blood loss may be major but is difficult to assess. Transfusion has been suggested if resection time exceeds one hour.
  –postoperative complications are common and include urinary and chest infections, sepsis and haemorrhage.

General or regional techniques may be used. Postoperative course is generally considered to be better with the latter (**spinal** or **extradural anaesthesia**), which also allow monitoring of CNS function during the procedure.

Hatch PD (1987) Anaesth Intensive Care; 15: 203–11

Trauma. Most common cause of death in young adults in the UK and USA, and the third commonest cause overall. Management has been consistently shown to be inadequate in many cases, exacerbated by poor coordination of resources. Care in some countries, e.g. USA, West Germany and Australia, is better organized than in the UK (e.g. 20% of deaths were considered preventable in the latest Royal College of Surgeons of England report). Hypoxia and missed diagnoses were common.

- Improved results are thought to require:
  –improved prehospital care and transport, e.g. involving helicopters (used in many countries); possibly doctors should accompany emergency vehicles. The debate concerning stabilization at the scene of the accident versus 'scoop and run' continues.
  –centralized trauma centres, with full facilities for **CPR**, imaging and surgery within one unit, to handle severe injuries. Patients would present directly from accidents or via referring hospitals, which would deal with less severe trauma cases. Emergency, anaesthetic, ICU, orthopaedic, neurosurgical, cardiothoracic and general surgical staff should be available at all times.
  –use of **trauma scales** and **triage** to facilitate appropriate management, especially in major **accidents**.

- Management of individual cases:
  –initial rapid assessment and CPR. O$_2$ administration and large iv cannulae are mandatory. Cervical spine injury should be assumed until proven otherwise, and the neck immobilized with a collar. Full stomach and **alcohol** intake are likely. **Antigravity suits** may be useful in severe blood loss, especially prior to hospital. Life-theatening conditions requiring immediate detection and treatment include:
    –**airway** obstruction.
    –tension or open **pneumothorax**, haemothorax.
    –**flail chest**.
    –**hypovolaemia**.
    –**cardiac tamponade**.
  –further assessment:
    –examination of the patient's face and head, spine, chest, abdomen and limbs, including the back (the patient should be unclothed).
    –type of injury is important, e.g.
      –penetrating injury: internal damage is likely, especially with high velocity missiles.
      –blunt injury: crushing, shearing damage and fractures may result. Speed of collision, height of fall, etc. are important.
    –**burns**/blast injury, etc.
    –trauma scales/triage.
  –specific management as for **haemorrhage**, **head injury**, **chest trauma**, **spinal cord injury**; coexistent conditions e.g **smoke inhalation**, **aspiration of gastric contents**, **hypothermia**, **eye injury** may be present. Intra-abdominal bleeding may be revealed by peritoneal lavage (instillation of 1 litre saline through a catheter, and observation for blood staining on drainage).
  –continuous monitoring of pulse, BP, **urine** output, neurological signs, **CVP, etc.** Pulse **oximetry** is particularly useful.
  –imaging, e.g. X-ray, CAT scanning, etc., as appropriate.
  –analgesia, e.g. **Entonox**, local blocks, iv opioids.
  –late problems:
    –**fat embolism**: classically occurs on the second day; its incidence may be reduced if fractures are fixed early.
    –**DVT**: classically during the second week.
    –wound infection: **tetanus** prophylaxis and antibiotics are given as appropriate; staphylococcal, streptococcal and anaerobic infections are most common.
    –**chest infection/ARDS**.
    –those associated with massive **blood transfusion**.
    –renal impairment, e.g. associated with hypotension, **crush syndrome**, etc.
    –**catabolism** may be marked after multiple trauma.

- Anaesthesia may be required for fixation of fractures, removal of foreign bodies, cleaning/debridement/suturing of wounds, evacuation of clot, control of internal haemorrhage, skin grafting, etc. Problems:

–nature of injury.

–alcohol or other drugs.

–**gastric emptying** is reduced by trauma; the time between last oral intake and injury is more important than the time between intake and surgery.

–hypovolaemia.

–risk of massive **hyperkalaemia** following **suxamethonium** administration; time of onset is related to the nature of injury.

Adequate resuscitation is required first unless surgery is life-saving; risks of delayed surgery are weighed against anaesthetic risks. Regional techniques may be useful if no contraindications exist. Sedation should be avoided in head injury. Postoperative care should be on ICU/HDU unless injury is minor.

See also, Emergency surgery

Trauma scales. Developed to aid the assessment of injury caused by **trauma**, the prediction of outcome and comparison between centres/countries, etc. Have also been used to aid **triage**.

- Examples:
  –Trauma Score (TS): 1–16 points are awarded according to respiratory rate and effort, systolic BP, capillary refilling and **Glasgow Coma Scale**. Survival at 8–9 points is 50%, with worse outcome at lower scores.
  –Injury Severity Score (ISS): Points are awarded for each of: respiratory, cardiovascular and central nervous systems, abdomen, extremities and skin. The highest three scores are squared and added; the maximum possible is 75 (worst outcome). Survival is 50% at 30–40 points depending on age.
  –others, e.g.:
    –TRISS: combination of TS, ISS and age.
    –CRAMS: circulation, respiration, abdomen, motor modalities and speech.
    –specific paediatric scales.
    –generalized **coma scales**.

Smith EJ, Ward AJ, Smith D (1990) Br J Hosp Med; 44: 114–8

See also, Audit; Mortality/survival prediction on intensive care unit

Traumatic neurotic syndrome. Psychological diagnosis applied to patients whose claims of **awareness** during anaesthesia were met with professional denial, before the possibility of awareness was fully appreciated by anaesthetists. Sharing features with a general post-traumatic stress disorder, it was characterized by recurrent nightmares, anxiety, irritability, preoccupation with death, and fear of insanity. An excellent prognosis was possible once the patient's experience was accepted by health workers.

Treacher Collins syndrome, *see Facial deformities, congenital*

Triage. Sorting of patients according to severity of injury in order to maximize total number of survivors. Usually refers to **trauma** cases in battles or major **accidents**, although similar approaches have been used in other fields of acute medicine, e.g. chest pain. First used during Napoleon's Russian campaign by **Larrey**, who scored soldiers according to their need for medical treatment, treating the most severely injured first. Modern triage systems give first priority to those patients who might survive only if treated, leaving until later those expected to die even if treated, and those expected to survive even without treatment.

- Many systems exist, but most divide survivors into:
  –1st priority: immediate treatment/transfer required.
  –2nd priority: treatment urgent, but with stabilization first.
  –3rd priority: minor injury, e.g. 'walking wounded'.
  –4th priority: expected to die, therefore low priority.

Triage is helped by using **trauma scales**, with sorting according to score. Attention is also paid to the mechanism of injury. Some systems include colour coded labels with details of injuries, treatments, etc., to be attached to patients. Triage may be repeated at different stages of retrieval and treatment, e.g. at the scene of accident, at the receiving hospital, on wards, etc.; thus patients may change priorities as circumstances change.

Trials, clinical, *see Clinical trials*

Tricarboxylic acid cycle (Citric acid cycle; Krebs cycle). Final common pathway for oxidation of **carbohydrate**, **fat** and some **amino acids** to CO_2 and water. Consists of a sequence of reactions which occur within mitochondria and require O_2. Acetyl-coenzyme A (containing two carbon atoms) enters the cycle, having been formed from fat **metabolism** or **glycolysis** via pyruvate (Fig. 137). At each step where a carbon atom is lost, CO_2 is produced. For each turn of the cycle, 15 ATP molecules are formed via transfer of hydrogen atoms to the **cytochrome oxidase system** or formation of guanosine triphosphate (including the two ATP molecules generated by conversion of pyruvate to acetylcoenzyme A).

[Hans A Krebs (1900–1981), German-born English biochemist]

Trichloroethylene. CCl_2CHCl. **Inhalational anaesthetic agent**, synthesized in 1864 and used clinically in 1935. Although extremely cheap, its use has declined over the last decade, leading to its withdrawal from commercial

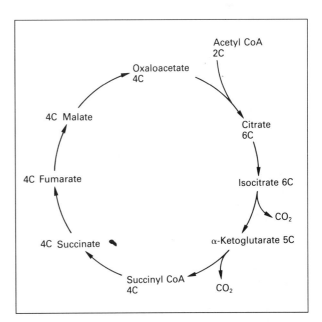

Figure 137 *Tricarboxylic acid cycle*

manufacture in the UK in 1988. Previously popular in obstetrics as an analgesic agent, and for providing analgesia during IPPV. Still used instead of N_2O by the Armed Forces (e.g. in the **triservice apparatus**).
- Properties:
  - colourless liquid, but coloured with waxoline blue to distinguish it from **chloroform**.
  - mw 131.4.
  - boiling point 87°C.
  - **SVP** at 20°C 8 kPa (60 mmHg).
  - **partition** coefficients:
    - blood/gas 9.
    - oil/gas 960.
  - **MAC** 0.17.
  - non-flammable at anaesthetic concentrations. Decomposed by light, and stabilized by **thymol** 0.01%. Adsorbed on to rubber.
  - interacts with **soda lime** to form dichloroacetylene (C_2Cl_2) at 60°C. The latter compound is a potent neurotoxin, and may cause temporary or permanent damage to the **cranial nerves**, especially V and VII.
- Effects:
  - CNS:
    - slow induction and recovery.
    - powerful analgesic properties.
  - RS:
    - markedly increases respiratory rate, partly via peripheral sensitization of pulmonary stretch receptors. Reduces tidal volume.
  - CVS:
    - maintains BP at low concentrations.
    - **arrhythmias** are common at high concentrations. Sensitizes the myocardium to **catecholamines**.
  - other:
    - dose dependent uterine relaxation.
    - nausea and vomiting are common postoperatively.
    - skeletal muscle relaxation is poor.

Undergoes extensive biotransformation, with formation of trichloroethanol and trichloracetic acid. **Chloral hydrate** is an intermediary metabolite. Hepatotoxicity has not been reported.

Tricuspid valve lesions. Tricuspid stenosis is usually associated with **mitral stenosis** and aortic valve disease resulting from **rheumatic fever**; may also coexist with pulmonary stenosis in the **carcinoid syndrome**. Isolated tricuspid stenosis is very rare.
- Features:
  - increased right atrial pressure with peripheral oedema and hepatomegaly.
  - prominent 'a' wave in the jugular **venous pulse**.
  - mid- and late diastolic **heart murmur**, heard best in inspiration at the left lower sternal edge.
  - right atrial enlargement may be shown on **chest X-ray** and **ECG**.

Tricuspid regurgitation usually results from right ventricular enlargement, e.g. in right-sided **cardiac failure**. Usually causes little clinical impairment.
- Features:
  - large systolic wave in the jugular venous pulse.
  - pansystolic murmur at the left lower sternal edge.

Anaesthetic considerations are related more to the accompanying mitral and aortic lesions than to the tricuspid lesion itself.

See also, Ebstein's anomaly

Tricyclic antidepressant drugs. Group of **antidepressant drugs**; the term includes several newer 1–, 2– and 4–ring structured drugs with similar actions. Competitively block reuptake of **noradrenaline** by postganglionic sympathetic nerve endings. Also have CNS anticholinergic properties. Used in depression and **pain management**; analgesic properties are thought to be associated with impairment of **5–HT** reuptake (e.g. especially by amitriptyline and clomipramine). Many cause sedation, e.g. amitriptyline, dothiepin, mianserin, trazodone and trimipramine. Sedation is less likely with clomipramine, nortriptyline, imipramine and desipramine.

2–4 weeks' therapy is required before their effect is apparent. **Half-lives** may be up to 48 hours. Metabolized in the liver and excreted renally.
- Anaesthetic considerations: increased sensitivity to **catecholamines** may result in hypertension and **arrhythmias** following administration of **sympathomimetic drugs**. Ventricular arrhythmias may occur with high concentrations of volatile anaesthetic agents, especially **halothane**. Account for about 10% of cases of poisoning. Features are those of anticholinergic poisoning: tachycardia, hypotension, urinary retention, blurred vision, pyrexia and coma. Hyperreflexia and convulsions may also occur. In addition, impaired myocardial contractility and conduction may cause **AF**, widening of the **QRS complex**, **heart block** and **VF**. ECG monitoring for at least 12–24 hours is required. Management is as for general **poisoning and overdoses**, including measures to prevent gastric absorption of drug. **Physostigmine** has been used to restore consciousness and slow heart rate. β-Adrenergic antagonists have been used in ventricular tachyarrhythmias; **cardiac pacing** may be required for bradyarrhythmias.

Trigeminal nerve blocks, see *Gasserian ganglion block; Mandibular nerve blocks; Maxillary nerve blocks; Nose; Ophthalmic nerve blocks*

Trigeminal neuralgia (Tic douloureux). Chronic **pain** state characterized by brief, severe lancinating pain involving the trigeminal nerve distribution. Usually involves the mandibular division; may also involve the glossopharyngeal nerve. Pain tends to be unilateral during the acute attack, which may be triggered by non-noxious stimulation of the ipsilateral nasal or perioral region (sometimes restricted to one specific zone). There is minimal or no sensory loss in the trigeminal distribution. Pain-free intervals typically separate attacks, which may be so severe as to cause suicide. Aetiology is uncertain although it may involve a structural abnormality in the trigeminal root adjacent to the pons.
- Treatment includes:
  - drugs, including **carbamazepine** (beneficial in 70% of cases), **phenytoin**, **clonazepam** and simple analgesics.
  - trigeminal nerve blocks.
  - surgical decompression of the trigeminal nerve.
  - destructive lesions, e.g. with alcohol injection, radiofrequency coagulation, or surgical destruction. **Anaesthesia dolorosa** may ensue.
  - acupuncture.

See also, Gasserian ganglion block

Trigger points. Areas in muscle or fascia; may be latent (tender when palpated) or active (painful at rest or on exertion or stretching). Mechanical stimulation may cause muscle weakness and/or local twitching. Pain is often referred, giving rise to **myofascial pain syndromes**. Examination may reveal tender nodules within taut bands of muscle, felt especially if the finger tips are moved perpendicular to the direction of muscle fibres. May be numerous, and may correspond to traditional **acupuncture** points. Local anaesthetic injection and acupuncture may relieve symptoms.

Trimeprazine tartrate. Phenothiazine-derived **antihistamine drug**, widely used for **premedication** in children. More sedative than other antihistamines. Has antiemetic properties.
- Dosage: 2–4 mg/kg orally 1–2 hours preoperatively. The maximal recommended dosage has recently been reduced by the manufacturers to 2 mg/kg.
- Side effects include dry mouth, circumoral pallor and dizziness. May cause postoperative restlessness due to **antanalgesia**. Has been implicated in causing prolonged respiratory depression on rare occasions.

Trimetaphan camsylate. Ganglion blocking drug, used to lower BP during **hypotensive anaesthesia**. Also has direct relaxant effects on venous and arterial vascular smooth muscle. May cause **histamine** release from **mast cells**, increasing its hypotensive effect. Acts within 3 minutes, with duration of action under 15 minutes; thus usually given by iv infusion. Compensatory tachycardia is common. **Tachyphylaxis** may occur. Does not cross the **blood–brain barrier**. Partially broken down by plasma **cholinesterase** and may have prolonged action in patients with decreased activity of this enzyme.
- Dosage: 10–50 µg/kg/min iv.
- Side effects include mydriasis, cycloplegia, ileus and urinary retention due to parasympathetic ganglion blockade.

Triservice apparatus. Anaesthetic apparatus adopted by the Armed Forces for battle use. Consists of (in order, starting at the patient):
- **facepiece** with **non-rebreathing valve** fitted.
- short length of ordinary tubing connected to a **self-inflating bag**.
- another length of tubing.
- two Oxford Minature **Vaporizers** in series.
- an O_2 cylinder may be attached, between the vaporizers and a further length of tubing which acts as a reservoir.

For spontaneous ventilation, a **draw-over technique** is employed. Controlled ventilation may be performed by squeezing the bag, or replacing it with a suitable ventilator. A variety of volatile agents may be used in the vaporizers, the calibration scales of which may be changed accordingly. They are specially adapted to contain more liquid (50 ml), and are fitted with extendable feet. **Halothane, enflurane** or **isoflurane** are traditionally used in the upstream vaporizer, and **trichloroethylene** (to compensate for the absence of N_2O) in the downstream one.

Trismus. Spasm of the masseter muscles, resulting in impaired mouth opening (lockjaw).
- Causes may be:
  - local:
    - abscess/infection around jaw, teeth, etc.
    - mandibular fractures.
    - parotitis.
    - **temporomandibular joint** disease.
  - systemic:
    - **tetanus**.
    - strychnine poisoning.
    - **phenothiazines**.
    - **CVA**.
    - hysteria.

May occur after administration of **suxamethonium** (e.g. **masseter spasm** or in **dystrophia myotonica**).

Anaesthesia in the presence of trismus is as for **airway obstruction** and difficult intubation. Injection of local anaesthetic into the masseter muscle may relieve the spasm.

See also, Intubation, difficult

Tropical diseases. Many diseases are restricted to tropical and subtropical regions. Several are considered 'tropical' because they have been largely eradicated in the West. Diseases may be imported by travellers. Anaesthetic involvement may be related to management of severe cases on ICU, or surgery related to, or incidental to, the disease concerned.
- Common diseases or those of particular anaesthetic interest may share **anaemia** and **malnutrition** as common features, and include:
  - **malaria**.
  - diarrhoeal illness (e.g. typhoid, giardiasis, amoebic dysentery, cholera): cause electrolyte imbalance and dehydration.
  - amoebiasis: may cause systemic illness, diarrhoea, bowel perforation and hepatic abscesses. Treatment may include surgery.
  - hydatid disease: parasites may form cysts, usually in the liver but occasionally in the lungs, heart, kidneys or brain. Spillage of hydatic fluid intraoperatively may cause allergic reactions.
  - leprosy: chronic infective granulomatous disease affecting peripheral nerves, skin and upper respiratory tract mucosa. Patients may be taking steroids. Areas of skin may be anaesthetic.
  - trypanosomiasis:
    - African (sleeping sickness): parasitic CNS invasion with confusion, coma and death. Myocarditis and hepatitis may occur.
    - American (Chagas' disease): meningoencephalitis, **hepatic failure**, **cardiomyopathy** and **achalasia** of the cardia may occur.
- Other diseases much more common in underdeveloped countries include:
  - **syphilis**.
  - **tetanus**.
  - **hepatitis**.
  - **TB**.
  - **poliomyelitis**.
  - **rabies**.

[Carlos Chagas (1879–1934), Brazilian physician]

TSR, *see Time to sustained respiration*

TT, Thrombin time, *see Coagulation studies*

Tuberculosis (TB). Infection with the acid- and alcohol-fast bacillus *Mycobacterium tuberculosis* which mainly affects the lungs and lymph nodes, although any tissues may be affected. Previously a common cause of death in the West, it is now mainly restricted to inhabitants of and migrants from underdeveloped countries, immunosuppressed patients and the homeless and destitute.

- Classified into:
  - primary TB: occurs in patients not previously infected (i.e. tuberculin-negative). Following a mild inflammatory reaction at the site of infection (e.g. lung or GIT), infection spreads to the regional lymph nodes. The lesions usually heal and calcify without further sequelae, but occasionally active organisms enter the bloodstream. This may cause 'haematogenous lesions' especially involving the lungs, bones, joints and kidneys. Rarely, a tuberculous focus ruptures into a vein causing acute dissemination (acute miliary TB).

    Patients may be asymptomatic, with evidence of infection provided by routine chest X-ray or conversion of the tuberculin test from negative to positive. Primary infection may be accompanied by a febrile illness. Occasionally primary TB is progressive and may cause pleurisy, pleural effusions and **meningitis**.
  - postprimary pulmonary TB: occurs in patients previously infected (i.e. tuberculin-positive). Usually affects the upper lobes. Reactivation (or reinfection) causes a brisk inflammatory response; resultant fibrosis tends to limit the spread of infection. Regional lymph node involvement is therefore unusual. Again the lesion usually heals, but it may rupture into a bronchus causing cavitation. It may then spread throughout the lung, or rarely via the bloodstream causing miliary TB.

    Usually insidious in onset, features include productive cough, haemoptysis (early) and dyspnoea (late). Pleuritic pain may be caused by pleurisy or **pneumothorax**.

Diagnosis includes history and examination (based on a high index of suspicion), chest X-ray, examination and culture of sputum for acid-fast bacilli (both may be negative), and tuberculin test (in primary TB).

- Management includes isolation, testing of contacts, and drug therapy which includes combinations of:
  - isoniazid: may cause peripheral neuropathy and rarely hepatitis.
  - rifampicin: may cause hepatic impairment, GIT disturbances, renal failure, dyspnoea, shock and thrombocytopenia.
  - pyrazinamide: may cause hepatic impairment.
  - ethambutol: may cause visual impairment.
  - streptomycin: may impair renal function and augment **non-depolarizing neuromuscular blockade**.

Patients may also be receiving **steroid therapy**.

Anaesthetic equipment used for patients with active TB should be cleaned and sterilized before reuse.

See also, Contamination of anaesthetic equipment

Tubocurarine chloride (D-tubocurarine chloride). Nondepolarizing **neuromuscular blocking drug**, isolated from **curare** in 1935. Its name is derived from the early classification of curare according to the means of storage ('tubes' refers to tubular bamboo canes). Initial dose is 0.3–0.5 mg/kg; this gives relaxation within 3–5 minutes, lasting for 30–50 minutes. Supplementary dose: 0.5–1 mg/kg. Commonly causes **histamine** release and ganglion blockade, causing vasodilatation and hypotension. Severe **anaphylactoid reactions** are rare. Excreted mainly in the urine, but 30% via the liver.

Tumour necrosis factor (TNF). Protein released by macrophages infiltrating tumour tissue; also released by the action of **endotoxin** on macrophages. Reduces fat anabolism causing cachexia and weight loss; also causes pyrexia and increased vascular permeability. Possibly acts via the cyclooxygenase pathway of **prostaglandin** synthesis. Thought to be central in the development of the features of sepsis, particularly **septic shock**. Antibodies to it, if given early enough, protect animals from death following endotoxin administration. TNF may also be involved in the development of **ARDS** in sepsis.

Abraham E (1989) Intensive Care Med; 17: 590–1

Turbulence, *see Flow*

Turner's syndrome (Gonadal dysgenesis). Congenital absence of the second X chromosome. Sufferers are female in appearance, but with primary amenorrhoea and immature genitalia. Other features include short stature, short webbed neck and high palate; thus tracheal intubation may be difficult. Renal abnormalities, **hypertension** and **coarctation of the aorta** may occur.

[Henry H Turner (1892–1970), US physician]

TURP, *see Transurethral resection of the prostate*

TURP syndrome. Syndrome following **TURP**, occurring in less than 10% of cases. Caused by absorption of irrigating fluid (usually hypotonic **glycine** 1.5%) through open prostatic vessels. Has also been reported following other procedures involving irrigation with electrolyte-free solutions, e.g. percutaneous lithotripsy.

Symptoms are caused by intravascular volume overload, dilutional **hyponatraemia** and intracellular oedema. Additional effects are caused by glycine and its metabolites, e.g. ammonia.

Features include bradycardia, hypotension (often preceded by hypertension), angina, dyspnoea, visual and mental changes, convulsions and coma. Severity depends on the volume of irrigant absorbed. Features may occur shortly after starting surgery, or postoperatively.

- Preventative measures:
  - limiting the height of the reservoir bag of irrigant to 60 cm.
  - limiting the volume of irrigant infused.
  - restriction of resection time to 60 minutes.
  - resection by experienced surgeons.
  - avoidance of hypotonic iv fluids.
- Measures to aid its detection:
  - use of **spinal** or **extradural anaesthesia**, allowing respiratory monitoring and detection of mental changes.
  - **CVP** measurement for patients at risk.
  - monitoring of plasma sodium concentration or **osmolality** gap.
  - monitoring of the volume of irrigant absorbed using tracer substances, e.g. ethanol (measured in the blood or breath).
- Management: as for hyponatraemia, convulsions, raised **ICP**, **acidosis**, etc. Diuretics, e.g. **frusemide** are usually advocated. Hypertonic saline solutions have been used.

Jensen V (1990) Can J Anaesth; 38: 90–7

Twilight sleep. Technique formerly popular in obstetrics as a means of easing labour pain and reducing subsequent recall. Injection of **morphine** and **hyoscine** was followed by hyoscine alone. Apart from causing maternal restlessness, it often caused neonatal respiratory depression. Now rarely used.

See also, Obstetric analgesia and anaesthesia

U

U wave. Low amplitude positive deflection following the **T wave** of the **ECG**, possibly representing slow repolarization of papillary muscle. Not always present. Made more prominent by **hypokalaemia**. Reversed polarity may indicate **myocardial ischaemia**.

U–D interval. During **Caesarean section**, the time between incision of the uterus and delivery of the baby. As the interval increases, so **fetal wellbeing** is compromised, probably due to disruption of placental blood flow. Fetal acidosis is thought to be unlikely at U–D intervals of 1.5–3 minutes.
See also, I–D interval

Ulnar artery. A terminal branch of the brachial artery, arising at the apex of the **antecubital fossa**. Lies superficial to flexor digitorum profundus and deep to the superficial flexors in the forearm. Then passes deep to flexor carpi ulnaris, lateral to the **ulnar nerve**. At the wrist, it lies between flexor carpi ulnaris and flexor digitorum profundus tendons. Passes anterior to the flexor retinaculum to end lateral to the pisiform bone. Branches supply the deep extensor and ulnar muscles of the forearm, the wrist and elbow joints, and the deep and superficial palmar arches. May be cannulated for **arterial BP measurement**.

Ulnar nerve (C7–T1). A terminal branch of the medial cord of the **brachial plexus**. Descends on the medial side of the upper arm, first in the anterior, and later in the posterior compartment. Passes behind the medial epicondyle to enter the forearm; descends on the medial side deep to flexor carpi ulnaris, medial to the **ulnar artery**. Divides into cutaneous branches 5 cm above the wrist. Dorsal and palmar cutaneous sensory branches supply the skin of the ulnar half of the hand and palm, and the medial 2.5 fingers. Also supplies the elbow joint, flexor carpi ulnaris and the ulnar side of flexor digitorum profundus. In the hand, it supplies the hypothenar muscles, interossei, third and fourth lumbricals and adductor pollicis.

The nerve may be damaged by stretcher poles hitting the elbow. Injury results in loss of cutaneous sensation on the ulnar 1.5 fingers and the ulnar side of the hand. Paralysis of the small muscles of the hand results in clawing.

May be blocked at various sites (*see Brachial plexus block; Elbow, nerve blocks; Wrist, nerve blocks*).

Ultrasound. Technique originally developed for use in industry, now established as a valuable tool for imaging soft tissues. Relies on the transmission of high frequency vibrations and the detection of echoes resulting from their reflection at tissue interfaces. The simplest system provides information concerning tissue depth (amplitude or A scan). If the vibrations are repeated rapidly, the echoes are capable of detecting movement at tissue interfaces (movement or M mode). If the direction of the ultrasound source is then varied, a two-dimensional tomogram may be produced (B mode).

Uses include diagnostic and fetal imaging, and assessment of cardiac function (**echocardiography**). It has also been used to localize the internal jugular vein prior to cannulation and to assess the depth of the **epidural space**.
See also, Doppler effect

Unconsciousness, *see Coma*

Units, SI. System of units (Système Internationale d'Unités) introduced in 1960 by the General Conference of Weights and Measures (Conférence Générale des Poids et Mesures) and based on the metric system. There are seven base units: **metre, second, kilogram, ampere, kelvin, candela** and **mole**. Derived units include the **newton, pascal, joule, watt** and **hertz**.
Powsner ER (1984) JAMA; 252: 1737–41

Universal gas constant. Constant (symbol R) in the **ideal gas law** equation $PV = RT$, where P = pressure, V = volume and T = temperature of a perfect gas. Equals 8.3144 J/K/mol (1.987 cal/K/mol).

Uraemia. Strictly, a plasma **urea** exceeding 7.0 mmol/l; the term was formerly used to describe the clinical picture in **renal failure**.

Urea. NH_2CONH_2; a product of hepatic **amino acid** breakdown to ammonia. Produced in the urea cycle from hydrolysis of arginine; ornithine is also produced and reacts with carbamoyl phosphate and then aspartate to reform arginine. Ammonia and CO_2 are introduced into the cycle by 'carrier' molecules. Freely filtered at the glomerulus of the **nephron**; about 50% is reabsorbed in the proximal tubule. Excretion in the **urine** accounts for ⅚ daily nitrogen excretion. Normal plasma levels: 2.5–7.0 mmol/l. Increased production (e.g. from increased **protein** intake or **catabolism**) may increase plasma urea slightly, but levels above 13 mmol/l usually represent impaired renal function. **Creatinine** measurement or **clearance** studies may aid diagnosis.
See also, Nitrogen balance

Urinalysis, *see Urine*

Urinary retention, postoperative. Most common after **spinal** or **extradural anaesthesia** (including use of **spinal opioids**), after abdominal or pelvic procedures, in elderly males with prostatic hypertrophy, and following administration of drugs with anticholinergic effects. May cause agitation and **confusion** postoperatively. Confirmed by abdominal palpation and percussion. Urinary catheterization may be required if encouragement (running taps, etc.) is unsuccessful.

See also, Oliguria

Urine. Liquid containing **urea** and other waste products, excreted by the **kidneys**. Normal output in temperate climates is 800–2500 ml/day. Coloured yellowish by the pigments urochrome and uroerythrin, it darkens on standing by oxidation of urobilinogen to urobilin. Coloured red by **haemoglobin** or **myoglobin**. **Specific gravity** is normally 1.002–1.035. **Osmolality** may range between 30 and 1400 mosmol/kg, depending on fluid and hormonal status. **pH** is usually below 5.3. Normally contains under 150 mg protein/24 hours. Abnormal constituents include **glucose**, ketones, bilirubin, erythrocytes, large numbers of leucocytes and casts.

Urinalysis is usually performed using reagent sticks; the reagents change colour according to the presence and amount of various normal and abnormal constituents in the sample. Specific gravity and pH can also be quantified.

Despite the kidneys' ability to concentrate the urine, a minimum of 500 ml/day is required to eliminate urea and other electrolytes. **Oliguria** is usually defined as less than 0.5 ml/kg/h and may indicate **hypovolaemia** or **renal failure**; anuria is complete cessation of urine flow and may indicate obstruction or urinary retention in addition. Polyuria occurs in **diabetes insipidus**, renal failure, diuretic therapy, **diabetes mellitus** (because of the osmotically active glucose load) and excessive water intake (**water diuresis**).

Urine output is often measured during major surgery, since it reflects the volume status of the circulation (assuming normal renal and cardiac function). Although renal blood flow is often reduced and circulating levels of **vasopressin** are high during surgery, urine output is usually maintained. Most anaesthetists will aim for an hourly output of at least 0.4–0.5 ml/h.

See also, Nephron

Urokinase, *see Fibrinolytic drugs*

Uterus. Pear-shaped pelvic organ, 7.5 cm long, 5 cm wide and 2.5 cm thick when non-gravid. Divided into the upper body and lower cervix, separated by the isthmus. Separated from the bladder anteriorly by the uterovesical pouch, and from the rectum posteriorly by the uterorectal pouch. The broad ligaments lie laterally.

Blood supply is from the uterine artery, a branch of the internal iliac artery. The uterine vein drains into the internal iliac vein.

● Nerve supply:
  –sympathetic motor preganglionic fibres from T1–L2 and parasympathetic motor preganglionic fibres from S2–4 via the paracervical plexus. Actions are variable, depending on the stage of the menstrual cycle and **pregnancy**.
  –sensory fibres via sympathetic pathways, emerging in the paracervical tissues and passing through the hypogastric plexus to T11–12, sometimes also to T10 and L1.

● Actions of drugs on the pregnant uterus:
  –**α-adrenergic receptor agonists**, e.g. **noradrenaline, methoxamine**: increase uterine tone and strength of contraction.
  –**β-adrenergic receptor agonists**, e.g. **adrenaline, salbutamol**: decrease uterine tone and strength of contraction. Agonists specific for β_2–receptors are used as **tocolytic drugs** to delay premature labour.
  –**oxytocin** and **ergometrine**: produce powerful contraction.
  –**prostaglandins** PGE_2 and $PGF_{2\alpha}$: stimulate uterine contraction.
  –volatile **inhalational anaesthetic agents**: cause dose-related reduction of uterine tone.
  –**iv anaesthetic agents**, sedative and analgesic drugs, **neuromuscular blocking drugs, acetylcholinesterase inhibitors**: no effect on uterine tone.
  –others: **acetylcholine**, bradykinin, **histamine** and **5-HT** increase contraction. Smooth muscle relaxants, e.g. amyl nitrite and **papaverine** cause cervical relaxation. **Alcohol** has a direct relaxant action and suppresses oxytocin secretion from the **pituitary gland**.

See also, Obstetric analgesia and anaesthesia

V

Vacuum insulated evaporator (VIE). Container for storage of liquid O_2 and maintenance of **piped gas supply**. An outer carbon steel shell is separated by a vacuum from an inner stainless steel shell which contains O_2. The inner temperature varies between –160 and –180°C. Gaseous O_2 is withdrawn and heated to ambient temperature (and thus expanded) as required (Fig. 138). If pressure within the container falls, liquid O_2 may be withdrawn, vaporized in an evaporator and returned to the system, restoring working pressure. If passage of heat across the insulation causes vaporization of liquid O_2 and a rise in pressure, gas is allowed to escape through a safety valve. The contents are indicated by a weighing device incorporated into the chamber's supports.

Howells RS (1980) Anaesthesia; 35: 676–98

Vagus nerve. Tenth **cranial nerve**. Arises in the medulla from the:
  –dorsal nucleus of the vagus (parasympathetic).
  –nucleus ambiguus (motor fibres to laryngeal, pharyngeal and palatal muscles).
  –nucleus of the tractus solitarius (sensory fibres from the **larynx**, **pharynx**, GIT, **heart** and **lungs**, including taste).

Leaves the medulla between the olive and inferior cerebellar peduncle, and passes through the jugular foramen of the **skull**. Descends in the neck within the carotid sheath between the internal **jugular vein** and internal/common **carotid arteries** (*see Fig. 97; Neck, cross-sectional anatomy, and Fig. 89a; Mediastinum*). Passes behind the root of the lung to form the pulmonary plexus, then on to the oesophagus to form the oesophageal plexus with the vagus from the other side. Both pass through the oesophageal opening of the **diaphragm** to supply the abdominal contents and GIT as far as the splenic flexure (*see Fig. 16; Autonomic nervous system*).
• Branches:
  –to the external auditory meatus and tympanic membrane.
  –to muscles of the pharynx and soft palate.
  –**laryngeal nerves**.
  –to cardiac, pulmonary and oesophageal plexuses.
  –to intra-abdominal organs.

The vagi form a major part of the **parasympathetic nervous** system. Vagal reflexes causing bradycardia, **laryngospasm** and **bronchospasm** may be troublesome during anaesthesia. Intense stimulation may result in partial or complete **heart block** or even **asystole**. This may follow traction on the extraocular muscles (**oculocardiac reflex**) and stimulation (e.g. surgical) of the rectum, mesentery, biliary tract, cervix, uterus, bladder, urethra, testes, larynx, glottis, bronchial tree and carotid sinus. Anal and cervical stretching are particularly intense stimuli (e.g. **Brewer– Luckhardt reflex**). Skin incision may also stimulate the vagus.

Anticholinergic drugs help prevent vagal reflexes during surgery. Should they occur, surgical activity should cease, and **atropine** administered if necessary.

Valence. Capacity of an atom or group of atoms to combine with others in definite proportions; compared with that of hydrogen (value of 1). Dependent on the number of electrons in the outer shell of the atom; covalent bonds are formed when electrons are shared between different atoms, e.g. water: H–O–H.

Valproate/valproic acid, *see Sodium valproate*

Valsalva manoeuvre. Forced expiration against a closed glottis after a full inspiration, originally described as a technique for expelling pus from the middle ear. In its standardized form, 40 mmHg pressure is held for 10 seconds.
• Direct arterial BP tracings in normal subjects show four phases (Fig. 139):
  –phase I: increase in intrathoracic pressure expels blood from thoracic vessels.
  –phase II: decrease in BP due to reduction of venous return; activation of the **baroreceptor reflex** causes tachycardia and vasoconstriction, raising BP towards normal.

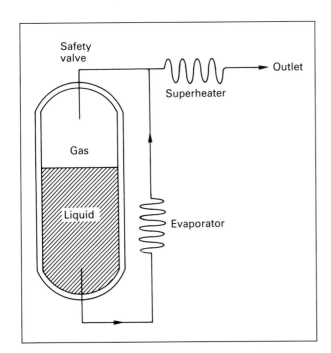

Figure 138 *Vacuum insulated evaporator*

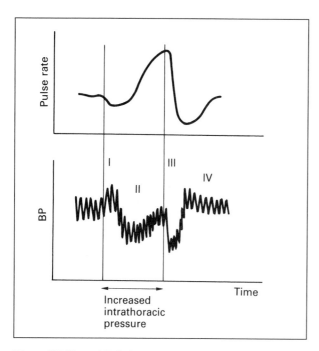

Figure 139 *Normal Valsalva response (see text)*

–phase III: further drop in BP as intrathoracic pressure suddenly drops, with pooling of blood in the pulmonary vessels.
–phase IV: overshoot, as compensatory mechanisms continue to operate with venous return restored. Increased BP causes bradycardia.
• Abnormal responses:
–'square wave' response, seen in **cardiac failure**, constrictive **pericarditis**, **cardiac tamponade** and valvular heart disease, when **CVP** is markedly raised. BP rises, remains high throughout the manoeuvre, and returns to its previous level at the end.
–autonomic dysfunction, e.g. **autonomic neuropathy**, drugs. BP falls and stays low until intrathoracic pressure is released. Pulse rate changes and overshoot are absent.
–an exaggerated reduction in BP may be seen in **hypovolaemia**, e.g. during **IPPV**.
Useful as a bedside test of autonomic function. Concurrent **ECG** tracing allows accurate measurement of changes in heart rate. The manoeuvre may be useful in evaluating **heart murmurs**, and may be successful in terminating **SVT** (because of increased vagal tone in phase IV).
[Antonio Valsalva (1666–1723), Italian anatomist]
Nishimura RA, Tajik AJ (1986) Mayo Clin Proc; 61: 211–7

Valtis–Kennedy effect. Shift to the left of the **oxyhaemoglobin dissociation curve** during **blood storage**, originally described for acid–citrate–dextrose storage. The shift reflects progressive depletion of **2,3–DPG**.
[DJ Valtis, Greek physician; Arthur C Kennedy, Glasgow physician]

Valveless anaesthetic breathing systems. Anaesthetic breathing systems designed to eliminate resistance which inevitably results from **adjustable pressure-limiting valves**.

In the Samson system, the valve is replaced by an adjustable orifice; in the Hafnia systems, expired gases pass through a port, assisted by an **ejector flowmeter**.
[Heyman H Samson, South African anaesthetist; *Hafnia*: Latin name for Copenhagen]

Valves, *see Adjustable pressure-limiting valves; Demand valves; Non-rebreathing valves*

Valvular heart disease. Causes, features and anaesthetic management: as for **congenital heart disease** and individual lesions. Valve replacement: as for **cardiac surgery**. Many prosthetic valves are available in different sizes, e.g. silastic ball-and-cage, metal flaps and porcine valves. Thrombosis may form on prostheses, hence the requirement for long-term anticoagulation. Patients with prosthetic valves also require prophylactic antibiotics as for congenital heart disease.

Van der Waals equation of state. Modification of the **ideal gas law**, accounting for the forces of attraction between gas molecules, and also the volume of the molecules:

$$RT = (P + a/V^2)\,(V - b)$$

where R = **universal gas constant**.
T = temperature.
P = pressure exerted by the gas.
V = molar volume of gas.
a and b = correction terms.
[Johannes van der Waals (1837–1923), Dutch physicist]

Van der Waals forces. Weak attractive forces between neutral molecules and atoms, caused by electric polarization of the particles induced by the presence of other particles.
See also, Van der Waals equation of state

Van Slyke apparatus. Device used to measure blood gas partial pressures. O_2 and CO_2 are released into a burette from the blood by addition of a liberating solution. Each gas in turn is converted to a non-gaseous substance by chemical reaction, and the pressure drop in the burette measured for each. The same reagents may be used as in the **Haldane apparatus**.
[Donald D van Slyke (1883–1971), US chemist]
See also, Carbon dioxide measurement; Gas analysis; Oxygen measurement

Vaporizers. Devices for delivering accurate and safe concentrations of volatile **inhalational anaesthetic agents** to the patient. In modern types, e.g. 'Tec' (temperature compensated) vaporizers, fresh gas is divided by the control dial into two streams, one of which enters the vaporization chamber, becomes fully saturated with agent, and rejoins the other stream at the outlet. The ratio of the two streams (**splitting ratio**) determines the final delivered concentration. In the 'copper kettle' type (now obsolete), a separate supply of O_2 is passed through the vaporizer, becoming fully saturated. It is then added to the main fresh gas flow, at a rate calculated according to desired final concentration and vaporizer temperature. The original design included a large mass of copper as a heat sink, hence its name.
• Factors affecting the delivered concentration:

–splitting ratio.

–**SVP** of the volatile agent: equals the partial pressure of the agent within the vaporizer. Agents with high SVP, e.g. **diethyl ether**, are easier to vaporize than those with low SVPs, e.g. **methoxyflurane**.

–temperature of the liquid: affects the SVP. As liquid vaporizes, **latent heat** of vaporization is lost, and temperature and thus SVP falls. Delivered concentration of agent would therefore fall if not for temperature compensation devices, e.g.:

–bimetallic strip at the outlet (Tec Mark 2) or inlet (subsequent Tec models) of the vaporization chamber.

–fluid-filled bellows at the gas outlet, e.g. EMO inhaler (see below); expands as temperature rises.

–longitudinally expanding metal rod at the gas outlet, e.g. Dräger models.

Temperature loss is reduced by providing heat sinks of metal (e.g. Tec) or water (EMO). Older vaporizers incorporated heating devices or thermometers.

–surface area of the gas/liquid interface: increased with:

–wicks and baffles, e.g. most plenum vaporizers (see below). Wicks maintain surface area despite gradual emptying of the vaporizer (level compensation).

–a cowl to direct gas flow on to or into the liquid (e.g. the original **Boyle's** bottle).

–production of many tiny bubbles with a sintered brass or glass diffuser, e.g. copper kettle type vaporizers.

–fresh gas flow: the output of older devices varied considerably with gas flow; modern vaporizers, with improved design, perform more consistently.

–**pumping effect**.

• Classified into:

–plenum vaporizers:

–gas passes through the vaporizer under pressure at the back bar of the **anaesthetic machine**.

–have high resistance.

–include the Tec series of vaporizers. Features of the Mark 4 over the Mark 3:

–flow of liquid agent into the delivery line is prevented if the vaporizer is inverted.

–interlock system prevents use of more than one vaporizer at a time, if mounted side by side.

–fitted with the **key filling system** (not fitted to all Mark 3 models).

Features of the Mark 5 over the Mark 4:

–increased capacity.

–improved filling system.

–draw-over vaporizers:

–gas is drawn into the vaporizing chamber by the patient's inspiratory effort.

–resistance must be low.

–may be suitable for use within **circle systems**, e.g. Goldman vaporizer, a small uncompensated device with a glass container. Delivered concentration depends on gas flow. Similar vaporizers were designed by **McKesson** and **Rowbotham**, the latter's containing a wire gauze wick.

–also used for **draw-over techniques**, e.g.:

–EMO (Epstein and Macintosh of Oxford) ether inhaler: large vaporizer, incorporating a large vaporization chamber, a water-jacket for a heat sink, and a temperature-compensating fluid-filled bellows at the outlet.

–OMV (Oxford miniature vaporizer): small uncompensated device, containing a water-filled heat sink (with antifreeze). Contains wire wicks; may thus be emptied of one agent, flushed and refilled with another. Different calibration scales may be fixed to the control valve for the various agents. A modified form is used in the **triservice apparatus**.

–obsolete types, used until recently for obstetric analgesia:

–Emotril (Epstein and Macintosh of Oxford/Trilene) **trichloroethylene** apparatus: incorporated within a metal box.

–Cardiff methoxyflurane inhaler: free-standing on a base.

For vaporizers in series: contamination of the second with vapour from the first may occur if both are turned on simultaneously. Although this cannot occur with modern vaporizers, for other types the one containing the less volatile agent (i.e. with lower SVP) should be placed upstream, because:

–it requires proportionally more of the fresh gas flow than the vaporizer containing the more volatile agent, and would thus receive more contaminant if placed downstream.

–the more volatile agent, being easier to vaporize, would attain higher (and thus potentially dangerous) concentrations than those set if it contaminated the vaporizer designed for a less volatile agent.

Some modern devices add volatile agent directly to the fresh gas stream, at a rate calculated automatically to produce the desired concentration. They may be incorporated into computerized anaesthetic machines.

Vaporizers have been associated with many hazards, and require regular servicing.

[Heinrich Dräger (1847–1917), German engineer; Victor Goldman, London anaesthetist; HG Epstein, Oxford physicist]

White DC (1985) Br J Anaesth; 57: 658–71

See also, Altitude, high

Vapour. Matter in the gaseous form below its **critical temperature**; i.e. its constituent particles may enter the liquid form. As liquid vaporizes, heat is required (**latent heat** of vaporization); as vapour condenses, an equal amount of heat is produced. These processes occur continuously above the surface of a liquid at equilibrium.

See also, Vapour pressure

Vapour pressure. Pressure exerted by molecules escaping from the surface of a liquid to enter the gaseous phase. When equilibrium is reached at any temperature, the number of molecules leaving the liquid phase equals the number entering it; the vapour pressure now equals **SVP**. Raising the temperature of the liquid increases the molecules' kinetic energy, allowing more of them to escape and raising the vapour pressure. When SVP equals atmospheric pressure, the liquid boils.

Variance. Standard deviation squared. Thus an indicator of spread of values within a **sample**.

See also, Statistics

Vascular resistance, *see Pulmonary vascular resistance; Systemic vascular resistance*

Vasoactive intestinal peptide (VIP). GIT hormone, also found in the **hypothalamus**, cortex, retina and bloodstream. Stimulates intestinal electrolyte and water secretion, and inhibits gastric acid secretion. Dilates peripheral blood vessels. Tumours secreting VIP (VIPomas) may cause severe diarrhoea and hypotension.

Vasoconstrictor drugs, *see Vasopressor drugs*

Vasodilator drugs. Drugs causing vasodilatation as their main effect (cf. **isoflurane, ganglion blocking drugs**). The term is sometimes reserved for drugs acting directly at vascular smooth muscle itself.
- May be divided according to their main site of action, although considerable overlap occurs:
  –venous system: **glyceryl trinitrate, isosorbide.**
  –arterial system: **hydralazine, calcium channel blocking drugs, salbutamol, diazoxide, minoxidil, adenosine.**
  –venous and arterial systems: **sodium nitroprusside, α-adrenergic receptor antagonists, angiotensin converting enzyme inhibitors.**
- Used to reduce **SVR** and thus:
  –systemic BP, e.g. in **hypotensive anaesthesia, hypertensive crisis, pre-eclampsia.** Their effect is somewhat offset by reflex tachycardia.
  –**afterload** and ventricular work, e.g. in **cardiac failure, shock.** Increase **stroke volume** and reduce myocardial O_2 demand. Also reduce **preload** via venous dilatation.

Also used to reduce **pulmonary vascular resistance** in **pulmonary hypertension**, although the systemic circulation is usually affected too.

Fyman PN, Cottrell JE, Kushins L, Casthely PA (1986) Can Anaesth Soc J; 33: 629–43
See also, Inotropic drugs

Vasomotor centre. Group of neurones in the ventrolateral medulla, involved in the control of **arterial BP.** Projects to sympathetic preganglionic neurones in the **spinal cord.** Normal continuous discharge causes partial contraction of vascular smooth muscle (vasomotor tone) and resting sympathetic stimulation of the heart.
- Discharge is increased by :
  –**chemoreceptor** discharge.
  –pain, emotion.
  –**hypoxia** (causes direct stimulation initially, but depression follows).
- Discharge is decreased by:
  –**baroreceptor** discharge.
  –lung inflation.
  –prolonged pain, emotion.

Thus responds to hypotension (reduced baroreceptor discharge) by increasing sympathetic activity.

Dorsal and medial neurones functionally constitute the **cardioinhibitory centre**, stimulation of which inhibits the vasomotor centre and increases vagal activity.

Vasopressin (Arginine vasopressin, AVP; Antidiuretic hormone, ADH). Neuropeptide synthesized in the cell bodies of the supraoptic and paraventricular nuclei. Transported down their axons to the posterior lobe of the **pituitary gland**, from which it is secreted.

- Effects:
  –water retention by the kidney, via increased adenylate cyclase activity and **cAMP** levels. Increases the permeability of renal collecting ducts, allowing water to pass back into the renal interstitium. Urine volume decreases; its concentration increases. Conversely, plasma volume increases; its concentration decreases.
  –vasoconstriction due to a direct effect on vascular smooth muscle; increases BP if given in high doses. Thought to have a minor role in BP regulation.
  –increased plasma levels of **coagulation** factor VIII.
- Release is increased by:
  –increased plasma **osmolality**; detected by **osmoreceptors** in the anterior **hypothalamus**.
  –decreased **ECF** volume (e.g. in **haemorrhage**); detected by **baroreceptors**.
  –pain, emotional and physical stress.
  –drugs, e.g. **morphine, barbiturates.**
  –angiotensin II.
- Release is inhibited by:
  –decreased plasma osmolality.
  –increased ECF volume.
  –drugs, e.g. **alcohol, butorphanol**.

Used therapeutically as argipressin, lypressin, terlipressin or **desmopressin** to treat **diabetes insipidus**, to increase factor VIII levels in **haemophilia** and **von Willebrand's disease**, and to control variceal bleeding due to portal hypertension. **Half-life** is about 20 minutes.
See also, Syndrome of inappropriate antidiuretic hormone secretion

Vasopressor drugs. Drugs causing vasoconstriction; used to increase arterial BP, e.g. during anaesthesia, intensive care or **CPR**, or to prolong the action of **local anaesthetic agents** by preventing their systemic absorption. Formerly used rather indiscriminately to increase BP, they are now reserved for situations where vasodilatation is a specific problem, e.g. **anaphylactic reaction, spinal anaesthesia**, etc.
- Mostly **sympathomimetic drugs:**
  –**catecholamines, e.g. adrenaline, noradrenaline, dopamine.**
  –non-catecholamines, e.g. **ephedrine, metaraminol, phenylephrine, methoxamine.**
- Directly-acting vasopressor hormones and their analogues have also been used, e.g.:
  –**vasopressin:** synthetic analogues **felypressin**, used in local anaesthesia, and argipressin, used for bleeding oesophageal varices.
  –angiotensin (*see Renin/angiotensin system*).

Smith LDR, Oldershaw PJ (1984) Br J Anaesth; 56: 767–80

Vasovagal syncope. Fainting, often caused by emotion. Vasodilatation in muscle (sympathetic discharge) and bradycardia (vagal discharge) cause hypotension and loss of consciousness, usually short-lived.

Sneddon JF, Camm AJ (1993) Br J Hosp Med; 49: 329–34

Vecuronium bromide. Non-depolarizing **neuromuscular blocking drug**, introduced in the UK in 1983. A monoquaternary aminosteroid, similar in structure to **pancuronium**. Initial dose is 80–100 µg/kg; good intubating conditions occur within 90 seconds. Relaxation lasts for 20–30 minutes; duration is increased to 50 minutes if 150 µg/kg is used, and 80 minutes if 250 µg/kg is used. Supplementary dose: 30–50 µg/kg. May also be given by infusion, at 50–80 µg/kg/h. Causes minimal **histamine** release, ganglion or vagal blockade even at several times the usual doses. Thus has minimal effects on BP and pulse, but may allow unopposed vagal stimulation to cause bradycardia. Excreted mainly in bile, but also in urine. Reversal of action is fast, and **acetylcholinesterase inhibitors** may not always be required. Cumulation is unlikely.

Venous admixture. Refers to lowering of arterial P_{O_2} from the 'ideal' level which would occur if there were no **shunt** or $\dot{V}/\dot{Q}$ **mismatch**, either of which may lower P_{O_2}. Defined as the amount of true shunt which alone would give the observed P_{O_2}. May be calculated from the **shunt equation**.

Venous drainage of arm. Deep veins accompany the arteries. Superficial veins on the back of the hand form the dorsal venous arch, from which the basilic and cephalic veins arise. Smaller veins arise from the anterior aspect of the arm (Fig. 140). The anatomy of the veins may vary considerably, especially that of the cephalic vein.

● Main veins of the forearm:
  –basilic vein: ascends on the posteromedial side of the forearm, passing to the anterior side below the elbow. Passes along the medial side of the biceps muscle and pierces the deep fascia. Becomes the axillary vein at the axilla.
  –cephalic vein: ascends on the lateral side of the forearm, passing anterior to the elbow. Runs on the lateral aspect of biceps, along the groove between deltoid and biceps, and pierces the clavipectoral fascia at the lower border of pectoralis major, to join the axillary vein. The angle at which the vessels meet, and the presence of valves at the junction, may cause difficulty in 'feeding' a catheter past this point.
See also, Antecubital fossa

Venous drainage of head and neck, *see Cerebral circulation; Jugular veins*

Venous drainage of leg. The main veins are superficial and deep:
  –the important superficial veins arise at the ankle (Fig. 141):
    –long (great) saphenous vein: passes anterior to the medial malleolus behind the saphenous nerve. Ascends behind the medial condyles of the tibia and femur, passing into the thigh and through the saphenous opening in the deep fascia to end in the femoral vein.
    –short (small) saphenous vein: passes behind the lateral malleolus, piercing the deep fascia to join the popliteal vein.
  –deep veins start as digital and metatarsal veins in the sole, forming the lateral and medial plantar veins. These form the posterior tibial veins. The anterior tibial veins pass through the interosseus membrane,

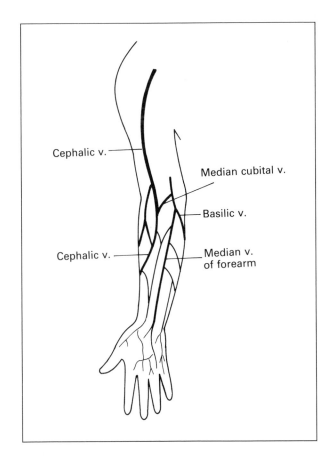

Figure 140 *Venous drainage of the arm*

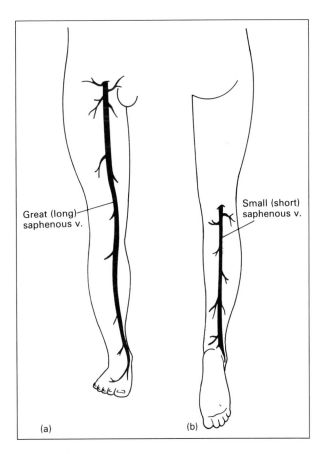

Figure 141 *Superficial veins of the leg: (a) anterior; (b) posterior*

joining the posterior tibial veins to form the popliteal vein. This ascends through the popliteal fossa to form the femoral vein, which becomes the external iliac vein deep to the inguinal ligament.

Venous pressure, *see Central venous pressure; Jugular venous pressure; Venous waveform*

Venous return. Refers to the volume of blood entering the right atrium per minute. A major determinant of **cardiac output** as described by **Starling's Law.**
- Depends on:
  - venous tone.
  - intrathoracic pressure.
  - blood volume.
  - right and left ventricular function.
  - muscular activity.
  - posture.
  - vasodilator/vasopressor drug therapy.

See also, Preload

Venous waveform. Obtained from the tracing of **CVP.** Can be seen but not felt in the neck as the **JVP.** Consists

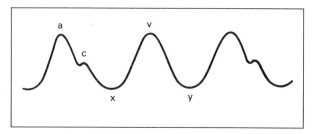

Figure 142 *Venous waveform*

of named waves and descents (Fig. 142):
- 'a' wave is due to atrial contraction.
- 'c' wave is thought to be due to transmitted pulsation from the carotid arteries, or to bulging of the tricuspid valve into the right atrium.
- 'v' wave is due to the rise in atrial pressure before tricuspid opening.
- 'x' descent is due to atrial relaxation.
- 'y' descent is due to atrial emptying as blood enters the ventricle.
- Abnormalities seen in the JVP wave may assist diagnosis of certain valve and rhythm disorders:
  - no 'a' wave: **AF.**
  - enlarged 'a' wave:
    - tricuspid stenosis.
    - stiff right ventricle, e.g. pulmonary stenosis, **pulmonary hypertension.**
  - enlarged 'v' wave: tricuspid regurgitation, e.g. due to **cardiac failure.**
  - cannon waves (large waves, not corresponding to 'a', 'v' or 'c' waves):
    - complete **heart block** (irregular).
    - **junctional arrhythmias** (regular).

A similar waveform is seen in the left atrial pressure tracing.

See also, Cardiac cycle

Ventilation, controlled, *see Airway pressure release ventilation; Assisted ventilation; High frequency ventila-*

tion; *Intermittent mandatory ventilation; Intermittent negative pressure ventilation; Intermittent positive pressure ventilation; Inverse ratio ventilation; Mandatory minute ventilation*

Ventilation, spontaneous, *see Breathing, control of; Breathing, work of; Respiratory muscles*

Ventilation/perfusion mismatch ($\dot{V}/\dot{Q}$ mismatch). Imbalance between **alveolar ventilation** ($\dot{V}$) and pulmonary capillary blood flow ($\dot{Q}$). In the ideal lung model, ventilation would be distributed uniformally to all parts of the lung and would be matched by uniform distribution of blood flow (i.e. $\dot{V}/\dot{Q} = 1$). However, even in a healthy 70 kg male, alveolar ventilation and blood flow are unequal (4 l/min and 5 l/min respectively), giving a $\dot{V}/\dot{Q}$ ratio of 0.8.

In addition, gravitational forces result in a gradient of $\dot{V}/\dot{Q}$ ratios in the lung as one travels from the apex to the base in the upright position. Both ventilation and perfusion increase from apex to base, but ventilation to a lesser extent than perfusion. Thus the $\dot{V}/\dot{Q}$ ratio is higher at the apex ($\dot{V}/\dot{Q}$ = 3.3) than at the base ($\dot{V}/\dot{Q}$ = 0.63). Similar but smaller changes occur across the lung in the supine position.

$\dot{V}/\dot{Q}$ mismatch may result in $\dot{V}/\dot{Q}$ ratios ranging from zero (perfusion but no ventilation; **shunt**) to infinity (ventilation but no perfusion; **dead space**). Its effects on gas exchange are those of shunt and dead space, and can be assessed by determining **venous admixture** and physiological dead space. $\dot{V}/\dot{Q}$ mismatch is a common cause of **hypoxaemia** in pulmonary disease, e.g. **COAD, asthma, chest infection, pulmonary oedema**, etc., and circulatory disorders, e.g. **PE.**

Mismatch may be measured using **radioisotope** scanning of ventilation and perfusion separately, e.g. with xenon and technetium.

See also, Pulmonary circulation

Ventilators. Mechanical devices for delivering ventilation to the lungs. First described in the early 1900s as an alternative to resuscitation equipment incorporating **bellows.** Many developments took place alongside those in **thoracic surgery** in the first half of the century; the polio epidemics in Denmark in the 1950s were a major impetus to the development of reliable positive pressure ventilators.
- Divided into:
  - negative pressure devices used for **intermittent negative pressure ventilation**: create a negative pressure around the thorax, causing chest expansion and drawing in air:
    - tank ventilators ('iron lungs'):
      - enclose the whole body (apart from the head and neck) within an airtight casing.
      - efficient, but access to the patient is very restricted.
    - cuirass ventilators:
      - enclose the thorax and upper abdomen. Inflatable jacket versions have been described.
      - less restrictive but less efficient.

Do not protect against **aspiration of gastric contents.** Their efficiency may be reduced by indrawing of the soft tissues of the upper airway during inspiration. **Tracheostomy** may be required if this occurs.
  - positive pressure devices used for **IPPV**: deliver positive pressure to the lungs via a **tracheal tube,**

tracheostomy, injector device or more recently, facemask or nasal mask (**nasal positive pressure ventilation**).

Positive pressure ventilators are widely used during anaesthesia and in ICU. They may be powered:
– electrically, e.g. employing a crankshaft (e.g. Cape ventilator) or solenoid (e.g. Siemens or Engström ventilators).
– by a separate supply of compressed air or O_2 employing **fluidics** or pneumatics (e.g. Penlon Nuffield ventilator).
– by anaesthetic gases (e.g. Manley ventilator). These type are 'minute volume dividers' (see below).

• Classification of positive pressure ventilators: many different classifications have been suggested. One simple classification according to the mechanism of action was described by Ward:
– 'mechanical thumbs': intermittent occlusion of the open limb of a T-piece, e.g. by a solenoid, e.g. the Sheffield infant ventilator. 'Intermittent blowers' may be used to achieve a similar effect by moving a column of driving gas forwards and backwards along a length of tubing connecting the ventilator with the T-piece, e.g. the Penlon Nuffield ventilator attached to the Bain **coaxial anaesthetic breathing system**. Anaesthetic gases are delivered separately through the other limb of the T-piece. A similar technique may be used with a **circle system**.
– 'minute volume dividers': supply only the minute volume of anaesthetic gas delivered to them, by dividing the preset minute volume into equally sized breaths. Delivered minute volume may be read directly from the **anaesthetic machine** flowmeters. Widely used for anaesthesia in the UK, they are cheap and simple to use, e.g. Manley ventilators.

The East–Freeman automatic vent is a small device containing a magnetized bobbin, and is placed at the patient end of an **anaesthetic breathing system** (e.g. **Magill** system) whose **adjustable pressure-limiting valve** is closed. The **reservoir bag** distends until the upstream pressure exceeds a certain limit, and gas is delivered to the patient. As upstream pressure falls, the bobbin closes the vent, and the cycle repeats. Such vents are usually reserved for emergency or temporary use only. Similar (now obsolete) devices include the Flowmasta and Minivent ventilators.
– 'bag-squeezers': employ mechanical or pneumatic force to compress the bag or bellows intermittently, e.g. Airshields ventilator, Oxford ventilator (pneumatic), Cape ventilator (mechanical). Widely used in the USA, they may be easily used with circle systems. Bellows which ascend during filling are preferable to those that descend during filling, since the former will not fill if there is a disconnection whereas the latter will still descend.
– 'intermittent blowers': produce intermittent flow from a high pressure source, e.g. **cylinders**. Include the Bird ventilators used on ICU, and small devices used for transportation of ventilated patients, e.g. Pneupac ventilator. The Penlon Nuffield ventilator is widely used in anaesthesia in the UK and is suitable for use with the Bain and circle systems; it may also be used for children (with a paediatric pressure release valve) using the T-piece.

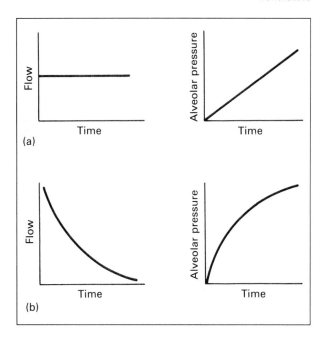

Figure 143 *Inspiratory characteristics of (a) constant flow and (b) constant pressure generators*

– jet ventilators: include those used for **injector techniques** and **high frequency ventilation**.

• Another widely used classification is that suggested by Mapleson in 1969, according to the characteristics during the inspiratory phase and inspiratory to expiratory (I to E) cycling:
– inspiratory characteristics:
– flow generators: produce a high generating pressure (e.g. 400 kPa) and are thus able to deliver flow which is unaffected by patient characteristics. The flow produced may be constant or non-constant (usually the former). Non-constant flow generators include the Cape ventilator, in which flow is sinusoidal because of the crank mechanism employed. These ventilators are able to produce the high inflation pressures required to achieve the preset flow in non-compliant lungs, e.g. in **bronchospasm**, and most ICU ventilators are therefore flow generators (Fig. 143a). **Barotrauma** may occur if high **airway pressures** are reached.
– pressure generators: produce low generating pressure (e.g. 1.5 kPa); thus the flow delivered is affected by patient characteristics (Fig. 143b). The pressure produced may be constant or non-constant (usually the former. Non-constant pressure generators include the East–Freeman automatic vent, in which the tension in the stretched reservoir bag falls as the reservoir bag empties). Since the airway pressure attainable is preset, the risk of barotrauma is reduced. However, the **tidal volume** delivered depends on the resistance of the tubing and the patient's respiratory mechanics, e.g. **compliance**, **airway resistance**, etc. Pressure generators are usually employed in **paediatric anaesthesia**, to reduce the risk of barotrauma. Examples of constant pressure generators are the Manley and East Radcliffe ventilators.

–I to E cycling:
- –time cycled: the duration of inspiration is preset, e.g. Manley MP2, Penlon Nuffield, Siemens Servo 900 series.
- –pressure cycled: expiration begins when a preset airway pressure is reached, e.g. Bird ventilator.
- –volume cycled: expiration begins when a preset tidal volume has been delivered, e.g. Manley Pulmovent ventilator.
- –flow cycled (pressure generators only): expiration begins when a preset inspiratory flow is reached, e.g. Bennett PR-2 ventilator. Rarely used as a method of cycling.

Many sophisticated ventilators may be employed as either flow generators or pressure generators, with a choice of cycling methods, e.g. Siemens Servo 900 series, Engström Emma. Thus they may be used for different clinical situations, e.g. on ICU.

The expiratory phase usually involves passive recoil of the lungs to atmospheric pressure. Many ventilators allow application of **PEEP** if required. **Negative end-expiratory pressure** is no longer used. The changeover from expiratory to inspiratory phases is usually time cycled, although it may be triggered by the patient in some modes.

The ideal ventilator for use on ICU should include flexibility in flow or pressure generation and cycling as above, allow PEEP and special modes to be used, e.g. for **weaning**, allow **humidification** and administration of nebulized drugs, be easy to sterilize and incorporate monitors and alarms.

[Ernst W von Siemens (1816–1892), German engineer; Carl-Gunnar Engström, Swedish physician; Roger EW Manley (1930–1991), UK anaesthetist and engineer; Crispian S Ward, Huddersfield anaesthetist; William W Mapleson, Cardiff physicist]
Smallwood RW (1988) Anaesth Intensive Care; 14: 251–7
See also, Monitoring

Ventile, *see Scavenging*

Ventricular ectopic beats

(VEs, VEBs; Premature ventricular contractions/beats, PVC/PCBs). Contraction of ventricular muscle caused by an ectopic focus instead of normal impulse conduction. The ventricles discharge early; the next sinus impulse finds the ventricular muscle refractory, causing a pause before the next beat. VEs typically appear as wide bizarre complexes on the **ECG** (Fig. 144); VEs arising from different sites (i.e. multifocal) may have different configurations.

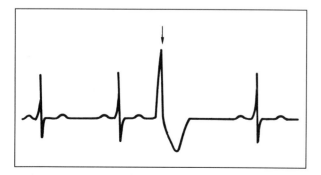

Figure 144 *Ventricular ectopic beat*

They may occur in normal hearts, but may also indicate organic heart disease. Other causes include drugs, e.g. **halothane** and **digoxin**, electrolyte and acid–base disturbances, **hypoxaemia**, **hypercapnia** and pain. Common during anaesthesia, especially with spontaneous ventilation with halothane. May occur at regular intervals, e.g. every 2nd or 3rd beat. Usually do not require treatment, apart from correction of the cause. **Antiarrhythmic drugs** (usually **lignocaine**) are usually recommended for VEs more common than 5 per minute, or if multifocal or close to the preceding **T wave** with risk of the **R on T phenomenon**.
See also, Arrhythmias

Ventricular fibrillation

(VF). Incoordinated and ineffective ventricular contraction caused by completely irregular ventricular depolarization. Usually follows the **R on T phenomenon**. Causes include **myocardial ischaemia**, **MI**, **hypoxaemia**, **electrocution**, electrolyte imbalance, **hypothermia** and drug toxicity (e.g. **adrenaline**, **digoxin**). There is no cardiac output; **asystole** therefore follows unless treated. VF is the most common cause of **cardiac arrest**. The **ECG** shows continuous random electrical activity without **QRS complexes** (Fig. 145).
Treated by **defibrillation**.

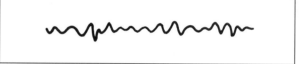

Figure 145 *Ventricular fibrillation*

Ventricular septal defect

(VSD). Accounts for 20–30% of **congenital heart disease**; may also follow **MI** or **trauma**. The commonest congenital form involves the membranous septum immediately below the tricuspid valve; bulbar or muscular septal involvement is rarer. Blood flows across the defect from left to right during systole. As right ventricular pressures decrease after birth, **shunt** increases. May cause **cardiac failure** in infancy. Small defects with normal **pulmonary artery pressures** are often asymptomatic (Maladie de Roger) and may close spontaneously. Large defects may lead to **pulmonary hypertension** and **Eisenmenger's syndrome**.
- Features:
  - –harsh pansystolic murmur, heard best in the left 4th intercostal space (louder with small defects). Splitting of the second **heart sound**.
  - –of Eisenmenger's syndrome if present.
  - –of left and right ventricular hypertrophy on **ECG** and **chest X-ray**.

  Up to 25% of patients may be affected by bacterial **endocarditis** at some time.
- Treated by surgery. Anaesthesia is as for congenital heart disease and **cardiac surgery**.

[Henri L Roger (1809–1891), French physician]

Ventricular stretch receptors, *see Baroreceptors*

Ventricular tachycardia

(VT). Rapid series of **ventricular ectopic beats** (usually defined as more than three in succession). The pulse rate usually lies between 130 and

250 beats/min. Normal atrial activity may continue independently, or the ventricular impulses may pass retrogradely to the atria.

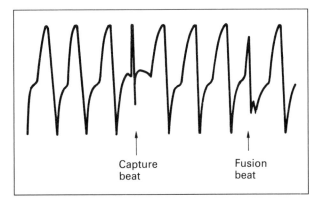

Figure 146 *Ventricular tachycardia, showing capture and fusion beats*

- Distinguished from **SVT** by the following features (Fig. 146):
    - **QRS complexes** are usually wide and bizzare.
    - retrograde conduction to the atria may result in inverted **P waves** (which may be hidden by the QRS complexes).
    - independent atrial activity may be suggested by:
        - occasional P waves.
        - capture beats (normal QRS complexes following occasional normal atrioventricular conduction).
        - fusion beats (with combined features of normal and ectopic QRS complexes, representing simultaneous atrially-conducted and ectopic ventricular activity).
    - marked left axis deviation, with all of the chest leads either negative or positive.
    Both VT and SVT may be regular, and associated with normotension or hypotension. Differentiation between broad-complex VT and SVT may be particularly difficult. The response to **adenosine** may aid diagnosis.
    Causes are as for ventricular ectopic beats.
- Treatment (following **CPR** if necessary):
    - **antiarrhythmic drugs**, e.g. **lignocaine** and related drugs, **amiodarone**.
    - cardioversion, especially if VT causes hypotension or drugs are contraindicated or ineffective.
    - **cardiac pacing** has also been used.
    - prophylaxis of recurrent VT includes antiarrhythmic drugs, surgical excision of the ectopic focus, and implantable defibrillators.

See also, Torsade de pointes

Venturi principle. Entrainment of a fluid through a side-arm into an area of low pressure caused by a constriction in a tube (**Bernouilli effect**). Entrainment depends on careful positioning of the side-arm, a suitably-shaped constriction, and the gradual increase in diameter of the limb distal to the constriction.
The principle is employed in gas mixing devices, **suction equipment**, **ejector flowmeters**, **scavenging** equipment, and devices used to circulate gases round breathing systems.
[Giovanni Venturi (1746–1822), Italian physicist]

Verapamil hydrochloride. Calcium channel blocking drug, mainly used as an **antiarrhythmic drug** to treat **SVT**. Acts by prolonging conduction through the atrioventricular node. Also used in angina and hypertension. Undergoes extensive **first-pass metabolism** when given orally. Excreted renally.
- Dosage:
    - 5 mg by slow iv injection, repeated up to 15–20 mg at 5 minute intervals.
    - 40–160 mg 8 hourly, orally.
May cause hypotension, bradycardia, complete heart block and asystole, especially if the patient has received **β-adrenergic receptor antagonists**. Its action may be potentiated by the commonly used **inhalational anaesthetic agents**, especially **halothane**.

Veratridine. Steroidal alkaloid, which binds specifically to open **sodium** channels and prevents them from closing. Has been used experimentally to block unmyelinated C fibres preferentially.

Vertebrae. Bony components of the vertebral column. The latter is about 70 cm long in the adult male and is flexed throughout its length in the fetus; after birth two secondary curves appear so that the cervical and lumbar regions are convex forwards and the thoracic and sacral regions are concave. There are 7 cervical vertebrae, 12 thoracic, 5 lumbar, 5 fused sacral and 3–5 fused coccygeal. Vertebral bodies of C2 to L5 are separated by fibrocartilagenous vertebral discs, accounting for about 25% of the spine's total length. Each has an outer fibrous annulus fibrosus, and the more fluid inner nucleus pulposus. The latter may prolapse through the former, impinging upon the spinal cord. Discs thin with age, resulting in reduced height. Vertebrae and discs are united by the **vertebral ligaments**.
- Structure of a typical vertebra:
    - body: short and cylindrical and lies anteriorly.
    - arch: encloses the **vertebral canal** and lies posteriorly. Composed of the rounded pedicles anteriorly and the flattened laminae posteriorly. The laminae are united in the midline by the spinous process. They also bear transverse processes and superior and inferior articular processes which bear facets for articulation with adjacent vertebrae.
- Regional differences:
    - cervical (Fig. 147a):
        - each has the foramen transversarium passing through its transverse processes, through which pass the **vertebral arteries**.
        - C1 (atlas):
            - has neither body nor spine.
            - articular facets superiorly articulate with the base of the skull.
            - facet on the anterior edge of the vertebral canal articulates with the odontoid peg.
        - C2 (axis): odontoid peg projects from the superior surface of the body, held against the body of the atlas by the transverse ligament. The gap between the peg and atlas is normally less than 3 mm on neck flexion (5 mm in children).
        - C2–6: bifid spinous processes.
        - C7 (vertebra prominens): non-bifid spine (the first easily palpable spine encountered, feeling from the skull downwards; T1 below it has a more prominent spine).

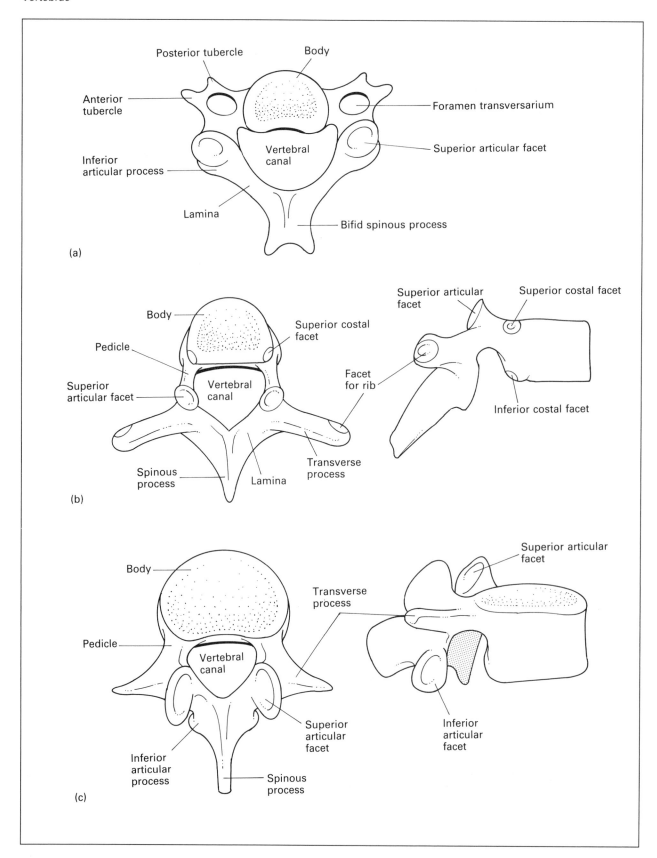

Figure 147 *'Typical' vertebrae: (a) cervical, superior view; (b) thoracic, superior and lateral views; (c) lumbar, superior and lateral views*

–thoracic (Fig. 147b):
  –body: heart-shaped, articulating with the **ribs** via superior and inferior costal facets at the rear of the body.
  –transverse processes: large, passing backwards and laterally, and bearing facets which articulate with the ribs' tubercles (except the last two thoracic vertebrae).
  –spines: long, inclined at about 60°C to the horizontal.
  –anatomical variations:
    –T1: has a longer upper facet for the 1st rib and a smaller lower facet for the 2nd rib.
    –T10–12: usually bear single costal facets on their bodies.
–lumbar (Fig. 147c):
  –body: kidney-shaped.
  –transverse processes: thick, passing laterally. Bear posteriorly the accessory processes at their bases.
  –spines: project horizontally backwards.
  –L5: short but massive transverse processes, arising from the sides of the body and pedicles. The body is deeper anteriorly than posteriorly.
–sacral: fused to form the sacrum, enclosing the **sacral canal**.
–coccygeal: fused to form the triangular coccyx, the base of which articulates with the sacrum.

Vertebral arteries. Arise from the subclavian arteries, passing upwards through the foramina transversaria of the upper six cervical **vertebrae** and passing medially behind the lateral mass of the atlas. They enter the **skull** through the foramen magnum, uniting to form the basilar artery after piercing the dura. Vertebrobasilar insufficiency typically results in dizziness, vertigo, diplopia and hemiparesis.

May be damaged or entered during **central venous cannulation** and **brachial plexus block**.

See also, Cerebral circulation

Vertebral canal. Triangular canal within the **vertebrae**, with its base posteriorly. Contains:
  –**extradural space** and contents.
  –**spinal cord** and **spinal nerves**/roots.

Vertebral ligaments. Individual **vertebrae** are linked by a number of ligaments (Fig. 148):
  –anterior longitudinal ligament: runs from C2 to the sacrum, attached to the anterior aspects of the vertebral bodies. Continues superiorly to form the anterior atlanto-occipital membrane.
  –posterior longitudinal ligament: as for the anterior, but attached to the posterior vertebral aspects. Continues superiorly to form the membrana tectoria between the axis and occiput.
  –ligamenta flava (yellow ligaments): run between the laminae of adjacent vertebrae. More developed in the lumbar than thoracic regions. Continue superiorly as the posterior atlanto-occipital membrane.
  –interspinous ligaments: run between the spines of adjacent vertebrae.
  –supraspinous ligament: runs from C7 to the sacrum, attached to the tips of the spines.
● Additional ligaments at the atlanto–occipito–axial complex:
  –transverse ligament of the atlas: runs between medial

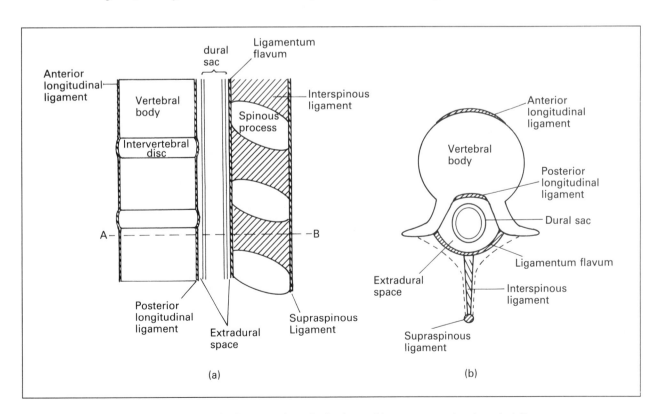

Figure 148 *Vertebral ligaments: (a) longitudinal section of vertebral column; (b) transverse section through A-B*

aspects of the atlas' lateral masses, securing the odontoid peg.
–alar ligaments: pass from the sides of the odontoid peg to the occipital condyles.
–apical ligament: thin band, connecting the odontoid's tip to the anterior aspect of the foramen magnum.
• Sacrococcygeal ligaments:
–posterior: overlies the sacral hiatus.
–anterior: passes over the anterior aspect of the sacrum and coccyx.
–lateral: joins the lateral angle of the sacrum to the transverse processes of the coccyx.

VF, *see Ventricular fibrillation*

Victoria, Queen (1819–1901). British monarch, given **chloroform** by **Snow** during the births of her eighth and ninth children: Prince Leopold in 1853, and Princess Beatrice in 1857 (on the latter occasion, Prince Albert administered chloroform himself prior to Snow's arrival). This gave respectability to pain relief during labour, which had been criticized as being against God's will.
[Leopold (1853–1884), Beatrice (1857–1944), Albert (1819–1861)]
See also, Obstetric analgesia and anaesthesia

VIE, *see Vacuum insulated evaporator*

VIP, *see Vasoactive intestinal peptide*

Viscosity (η). Tendency of **fluids** to resist **flow**. Measured in **poise**. Equal to shear **force** (force per unit surface area) divided by velocity gradient between adjacent fluid layers. Dependent on intermolecular attractive forces, e.g. **van der Waals forces**, and entanglement of bulky molecules. Decreased at high temperatures; particles have more kinetic energy and may escape from their neighbours more easily. Laminar **flow** is inversely proportional to viscosity.

Blood viscosity depends largely on **haematocrit** (increasing exponentially as haematocrit increases), red cell characteristics and blood protein concentration. It rises with age and smoking. It is increased slightly by volatile anaesthetic agents. Blood viscosity alters with different flow rates; i.e. blood is a non-newtonian fluid. At vessel diameters of less than 0.3 mm, it drops markedly, resulting in greater flow than with a newtonian fluid. The reason is unclear, but may involve 'plasma skimming' (the tendency of cellular components of blood to remain in the middle of vessels whilst plasma passes into branches arising from the vessel wall). Blood cell deformability may also be important. At very low **blood flow**, viscosity increases as the cells clump together.

Relative viscosity (compared with water) of normal plasma is 1.5; that of normal whole blood is 3.5.

Viscosity may be derived by measuring the time taken for a liquid to drain through a narrow tube. Alternatively, the torque on an inner drum may be measured when an outer drum is rotated, the specimen liquid filling the space between the drums.
[Sir Isaac Newton (1642–1727), English scientist]

Vishnevskiy technique (Transverse injection anaesthesia). Injection of local anaesthetic agent into a transverse 'slice' of a limb; originally described using **procaine**. Infil-

tration is performed from skin to bone, using large volumes of agent. Has been called the 'squirt and cut' technique.
[Aleksandr V Vishnevskiy (1874–1948), Russian surgeon]

Vital capacity. The largest volume of air that can be expired slowly after maximal inspiration; measured by a **spirometer**. Reduced in the supine position. Also reduced in the elderly, and in patients with restrictive lung disease, muscle weakness, abdominal swelling and pain.
See also, Forced vital capacity; Lung function tests; Lung volumes

Vitamin B$_{12}$ (Cobalamin). Water-soluble vitamin present in many animal tissues, especially eggs and liver. Exists as various related compounds, e.g. hydroxo- or cyanocobalamin. Combines with gastric intrinsic factor, enabling its absorption from the terminal ileum. Required for red blood cell maturation and as a cofactor by **methionine synthase**. Deficiency may be caused by failure of intrinsic factor production due to atrophic gastritis (pernicious anaemia) or gastric resection, or by disease/resection of the ileum. Dietary deficiency is rare. Inhibited by **N$_2$O**. Deficiency results in macrocytic megaloblastic **anaemia** and subacute combined degeneration of the cord.

Administered im 3 monthly as hydroxocobalamin; cyanocobalamin requires more frequent administration. It has been used in the treatment of **cyanide poisoning**.

Vitamin deficiency. May occur in:
–inadequate intake relative to requirements, e.g. **malnutrition** (including inadequate provision during **TPN**).
–malabsorption, e.g. due to gastric disease (**vitamin B$_{12}$**), pancreatic disease (fat-soluble vitamins: A, D, E and K).
–impaired metabolism of precursors, e.g. osteomalacia in renal failure.
–antagonism by drugs, e.g. **warfarin** (**vitamin K**), **N$_2$O** (folate and vitamin B$_{12}$).
• Specific deficiency states of possible anaesthetic importance:
–vitamin B$_1$ (thiamine): **peripheral neuropathy**, encephalopathy, **cardiomyopathy** (beriberi). May accompany chronic **alcohol** abuse.
–vitamin B$_2$ (riboflavin): **anaemia**, mouth lesions.
–vitamin B$_6$ (pyridoxine): **convulsions**, anaemia. May accompany chronic alcohol abuse.
–niacin: dermatitis, diarrhoea, dementia (pellagra).
–vitamin B$_{12}$: anaemia, subacute combined degeneration of the cord.
–vitamin C: generalized bleeding (especially gums), anaemia, weakness, poor wound healing (scurvy).
–vitamin D: **hypocalcaemia**, hyperphosphataemia, muscle weakness, rickets (in children), osteomalacia (in adults).
–vitamin E: **haemolysis**, oedema.
–vitamin K: bleeding tendency.

Vitamin K. Fat-soluble group of vitamins which catalyse the carboxylation of glutamic acid residues to activate **coagulation** factors II, VII, IX and X. Deficiency results in increased tendency to bleed and may result from:
–inadequate intake: rare in adults, common in the newborn.

–inadequate absorption, e.g. malabsorption syndromes, biliary obstruction.

–inadequate utilization, e.g. liver disease.

–drug therapy: especially **warfarin** and similar drugs which act as vitamin K antagonists.

May be given orally, iv or im to help correct deficiency; takes up to 12 hours to work. May cause several weeks' upset to coagulation control in patients on long-term warfarin therapy. Available as a synthetic analogue (menadiol sodium phosphate) or as phytomenadione (vitamin K₁).

- Dosage: 2.5–10 mg, repeated as necessary. Prothrombin time should be monitored.

Anaphylactoid reactions may follow rapid iv injection.

See also, Coagulation studies

Vocal cords, *see Larynx*

Volatile anaesthetic agents, *see Inhalational anaesthetic agents*

Volt. Unit of electrical potential. One volt is the potential difference between two points when 1 **joule** of **work** is done per **coulomb** of electricity passing from one point to the other.

[Alessandro Volta (1745–1827), Italian physicist]

Volume of distribution (V_d). Mathematical concept indicating the amount of a drug in the tissues; equal to the volume of water in which an injected dose would have to be diluted in order to give the measured plasma concentration. For a drug confined to plasma, V_d equals blood volume. For a drug distributed equally throughout the body, it equals total body water volume. For a drug concentrated in the tissues, V_d exceeds total body water volume. May be calculated from the graph of plasma drug concentration against time after iv injection:

$$V_d = \frac{dose}{concentration\ at\ time\ 0}$$

Examples:

–**digoxin**: V_d = 500 litres

–**propranolol**: V_d = 250 litres

–**lignocaine**: V_d = 120 litres

–**insulin**: V_d = 50 litres

–**aspirin**: V_d = 12 litres

–**warfarin**: V_d = 9 litres

(approximate values for a 70 kg man)

See also, Pharmacokinetics

Vomiting. Reflex involving retrograde passage of **gastric contents** through the mouth. The vomiting centre in the reticular formation of the medulla receives afferent impulses from the:

–GIT, abdominal organs and peritoneum via the vagus and sympathetic nerves.

–heart mainly via the vagus.

–vestibular apparatus.

–**chemoreceptor trigger zone** (CTZ).

–higher centres.

Chemical irritants, e.g. strong saline, stimulate the vomiting centre via receptors in the GIT. Drugs, e.g. **apomorphine**, stimulate the CTZ. Raised **ICP** is thought to cause vomiting via increased pressure on the floor of the fourth ventricle.

Motor impulses travel through **cranial nerves** V, VII, IX, X and XII to the upper GIT and through spinal nerves to the diaphragm and abdominal muscles.

- Sequence of events:

–salivation increases.

–breathing deepens.

–glottis closes.

–breath is held in midinspiration.

–abdominal muscles contract.

–oesophageal sphincters relax.

–gastric contents are expelled.

Incidence of postoperative vomiting has been found to vary from 15 to 90%. Usually distressing, but particularly undesirable in ear and **ophthalmic surgery**, and **neurosurgery**.

- Factors likely to increase postoperative vomiting:

–use of **opioid analgesic drugs**, including **premedication**.

–use of **diethyl ether**, **trichloroethylene**, **cyclopropane** and **etomidate**. **N₂O** has been implicated, acting via a direct central effect, GIT distension or expansion of middle ear cavities.

–gynaecological/abdominal surgery.

–**hypoxaemia/hypotension**.

–early postoperative eating and drinking.

–young age.

–female sex. Incidence increases during menstruation and decreases after the menopause, i.e. is presumably hormonally-mediated.

–anxiety, especially in patients who 'always vomit'. Increases in circulating **catecholamine** levels may be important.

–possibly prolonged anaesthesia and the use of **neostigmine**.

Reduced by avoidance of causative drugs where possible, and use of **antiemetic drugs** and others thought to be associated with low incidence of vomiting, e.g. **propofol**. **Acupuncture** has been used at the point P6 (Pericardium 6: 1–2 inches (2.5–5 cm) proximal to the distal wrist crease, between flexor carpi radialis and palmaris longus tendons): 5 minutes manual or electrical stimulation may reduce the incidence of vomiting.

- Effects of prolonged vomiting:

–loss of hydrogen, chloride, potassium and sodium ions, and water.

–renal bicarbonate loss to restore pH, causing alkaline urine.

–fall in sodium and ECF causing **aldosterone** release, which causes renal sodium and fluid retention, in exchange for potassium and hydrogen ions. If **hypokalaemia** is severe, hydrogen ion loss predominates, with paradoxical acid urine.

–thus **dehydration**, metabolic **alkalosis** and total body potassium depletion may occur.

Supplement (1992) Br J Anaesth; 69: 1S–68S

Von Recklinghausen's disease, *see Neurofibromatosis*

Von Willebrand's disease. Inherited **coagulation disorder**, first described in 1926, with autosomal dominant transmission. Deficiency of von Willebrand Factor, a protein involved in **platelet** adhesion and carriage of **coagulation** factor VIII, leads to factor VIII deficiency, abnormal platelet adhesiveness and abnormal vascular endothelium. Epistaxis and bruising are more common than haemarthrosis and haematoma.

- Investigations:
  - –platelet count: low or normal.
  - –prothrombin time: normal.
  - –partial thromboplastin time: prolonged.
  - –bleeding time: prolonged.

Fresh frozen plasma or cryoprecipitate may be given prior to surgery. **Desmopressin** administration may boost levels of factor VIII and von Willebrand factor, and may be used preoperatively (0.4 µg/kg iv). **Tranexamic acid** 1 g orally has also been advocated. **Antiplatelet drugs** must be avoided.

[Erik von Willebrand (1870–1949), Swedish physician]
Cameron CB, Kobrinsky N (1990) Can J Anaesth; 37: 341–7
See also, Blood products; Coagulation studies

V̇/Q̇ mismatch, *see Ventilation/perfusion mismatch*

VSD, *see Ventricular septal defect*

VT, *see Ventricular tachycardia*

W

Wakefulness, *see Awareness*

Wake-up test. Intraoperative awakening to allow assessment of spinal cord function during **spinal surgery**. Has also been used to assess cerebral function during basilar artery clipping.

Abott TR, Bentley G (1980) Anaesthesia; 35: 298–302.

Warfarin sodium. Oral **anticoagulant drug**, first synthesized in 1944. Rapidly absorbed by mouth and almost totally protein bound. Competes with **vitamin K** in the synthesis of **coagulation** factors II, VII, IX and X in the liver; therefore requires 1 to 2 days for its effect to develop. Metabolized in the liver and excreted in urine and faeces. **Half-life** is about 30 hours. Dosage is adjusted according to results of **coagulation studies**: the International Normalized Ratio (INR) is maintained at about 2–3 for prophylaxis and treatment of **DVT**, **PE** and transient ischaemic attacks; 3–4.5 for recurrent DVT/PE, cardiac and arterial prostheses. The usual maintenance dose is 3–9 mg/day.

Hepatic enzyme-inducing drugs, e.g. phenobarbitone and phenytoin, reduce its effect. If the second drug is withdrawn without reducing the dose of warfarin, haemorrhage may occur. Effects may be enhanced by drugs which displace it from protein binding sites, e.g. sulphonamides, NSAIDs.

- Guidelines for patients taking warfarin who present for surgery:
  –with heart valves: maintain warfarin therapy for short (under 30 minutes) surgery, with fresh frozen plasma available. Otherwise, stop warfarin 3 days preoperatively, and start **heparin** infusion 24 hours later (about 15 000 units/12 h), maintaining activated partial thromboplastin time (APPT) at 2–3 times normal. Stop heparin 6 hours preoperatively, and check INR and APTT 1 hour preoperatively. Surgery may be delayed, or plasma administered, if INR exceeds 1.5. Restart warfarin as soon as possible postoperatively, or heparin if nil by mouth for over 48 hours. Extra precautions have been suggested for prosthetic mitral valves, since the risk of emboli is greater than for other valves: **aspirin** 75 mg or **dipyridamole** 300 mg/day is started when warfarin is stopped. Heparin is restarted 6–12 hours postoperatively until able to take warfarin.
  –other conditions: stop warfarin for 48 hours before surgery. The INR should be less than 1.5. Heparin may be given perioperatively sc to reduce thromboembolism until warfarin is restarted, or iv infusion used postoperatively in high risk cases, e.g. recurrent PE.
  –emergency surgery: give vitamin K, and wait for synthesis of new clotting factors (about 12 hours); this may interfere with subsequent anticoagulation for weeks afterwards. Alternatively, fresh frozen plasma may be given. The INR is monitored throughout.

[**W**isconsin **A**lumni **R**esearch **F**oundation, where warfarin was developed]

Warren, John C (1778–1856). Professor of Surgery and Anatomy at Harvard Medical School. It was at Warren's invitation that **Wells** gave his demonstration of **N₂O** anaesthesia, which ended in failure. Later, at **Morton's** first public demonstration of **diethyl ether**, Warren performed the surgery.

Washout curves. Graphs displaying the exponential decline in concentration of a substance which is continuously being removed from a system. The substance may be 'washed out' by blood flow, in the case of dye **dilution techniques**, or by ventilation of the lungs, in the case of **nitrogen washout**. The term is sometimes used to describe any **exponential process**.

Water, *see Fluid balance; Fluids, body*

Water balance, *see Fluid balance*

Water diuresis. Diuresis occurring about 15 minutes after the intake of a large volume of hypotonic fluid. Absorption of the fluid is followed by inhibition of **vasopressin** secretion and by increased urinary water loss.

Water intoxication, *see Hyponatraemia*

Waters cannister, *see Carbon dioxide absorption in anaesthetic breathing systems*

Waters, Ralph Milton (1883–1979). US anaesthetist; became Assistant Professor of Surgery in charge of anaesthetics at University of Wisconsin, leading to his appointment as the first university Professor of Anaesthesia in the USA (1933). Was the first to establish a resident training programme in anaesthesia and the first to use **cyclopropane** clinically (1930). Re-examined **chloroform** toxicity, advocated the use of inflatable **cuffs** on tracheal tubes, and was involved in many aspects of anaesthesia, including the use of **thiopentone** and **endobronchial intubation**. Designed his 'to-and-fro' cannister for **CO₂ absorption in anaesthetic breathing systems**, and the Waters airway, a metal oropharyngeal airway with a side-arm for attachment to a gas supply.

Waterton, Charles (1783–1865). Squire of Walton Hall, Yorkshire; made his first voyage to South America in 1812. Described the preparation of **curare** and the blow pipes, darts, bows and arrows used by the Indians of the

Amazon and Orinoco basins. Experimented with the drug on his return to England, and maintained life in a paralysed donkey by employing artificial ventilation. Published details of his work and travels in *Wanderings in South America* (1825).

Watt. **Unit** of **power**. One watt (W) = 1 **joule** per second (J/s).
[James Watt (1736–1819), Scottish engineer]

Waveforms. Repetitive patterns plotted against time produce waveforms which may be complex, e.g. **ECG**, or simple, as in the sine wave. All waveforms may ultimately be broken down into component sine waves (**Fourier analysis**). For any sine wave, there is oscillation about a mean value, the maximal displacement from which is the amplitude. The number of complete oscillations per second is the frequency, and the distance between successive points at the same stage of the cycle, e.g. successive peaks, is the wavelength.

Weaning from ventilators. Usually presents no problems, but sometimes withdrawal of ventilatory support is difficult, especially if the period of **IPPV** has been prolonged.
- Criteria for beginning weaning are controversial; the following have been suggested:
  –absence of major organ or system failure, particularly CVS.
  –predisposing illness is successfully treated.
  –absence of severe infection or fever.
  –adequate **nutrition**.
  –absence of severe fluid, acid–base or electrolyte imbalance, e.g. of potassium, magnesium or phosphate.
  –minimal **sedation**.
  –respiratory function:
    –arterial blood gases are near premorbid values.
    –respiratory rate is under 35/min.
    –maximal negative inspiratory airway pressure attainable exceeds –25 cmH$_2$O.
    –**tidal volume** exceeds 5 ml/kg.
    –minute ventilation is under 10 litres.
    –**vital capacity** exceeds 15 ml/kg.
    –**FRC** exceeds 50% of predicted value.

After long-term ventilation, scoring systems have been proposed, reflecting F_1O_2 and level of **PEEP** required, lung **compliance**, work of breathing, temperature, pulse rate and arterial BP, etc.
- Techniques of weaning:
  –**humidification** of inspired air is important.
  –sitting the patient up increases **FRC** and diaphragmatic efficiency.
  –the lowest F_1O_2 necessary to maintain adequate oxygenation should be used, to decrease the risk of absorption **atelectasis**, and possibly promote **hypoxic pulmonary vasoconstriction**. High F_1O_2 must be avoided in patients with **COAD**.
  –a simple T-piece is often used. A 30 cm expiratory limb and fresh gas flow of twice minute volume will prevent indrawing of room air with lowering of F_1O_2, and rebreathing.
  –**CPAP** is often preferred, especially following PEEP, in **ARDS** and in left ventricular dysfunction.
  –ventilatory modes:

–**IMV** and variants: allows closer monitoring of recovery and reduces complications of IPPV.
- –**inspiratory pressure support**, **mandatory minute ventilation**, **high frequency ventilation** and variants, and **negative pressure ventilation** have also been used.
–overall time for completion of weaning may not be reduced by the above methods, but sedation and complications of IPPV may be reduced, and patient morale may benefit from 'coming off' the ventilator sooner. Assessment is also made easier.
–short periods of spontaneous or assisted ventilation may be introduced and gradually increased, with clinical monitoring and frequent arterial blood gas measurements. Tachypnoea, tachycardia, fatigue, restlessness and distress may precede worsening blood gas results. IPPV should be re-established should this occur.
–extubation may be performed when the patient is stable and able to guard the airway. Excessive secretions may be removed via **minitracheotomy**.

Work of breathing is increased by demand and expiratory valves, tubing, etc., especially using CPAP and IMV circuits through certain ventilators. Sophisticated modern ventilators generally provide circuits of low resistance, with minimal exertion required to open demand valves. Weaning may be impaired by **respiratory muscle fatigue**, especially of the diaphragm, e.g. due to electrolyte abnormalities, prolonged illness (particularly involving infection), acidosis and hypoxia.
Brown, DRG (1988) Hosp Update; 14: 1809–18 and 1898–1906

Wedge pressure, *see Pulmonary capillary wedge pressure*

Weight. The **force** a body exerts on anything which supports it. The weight of a body of **mass** 1 kilogram is 1 kilogram weight (kilogram force).

Wells, Horace (1815–1848). US dentist, present at **Colton's** demonstration of **N$_2$O** in Hartford, Connecticut on 10th December 1844. Noticing that a member of the audience (Samuel Cooley) had knocked his shin under the gas' influence and felt no pain, he suggested its use for dental extraction. Wells had one of his own teeth pulled out by John Riggs the following day, whilst breathing N$_2$O prepared by Colton. Performed successful painless extractions in several patients over subsequent days, before his ill-fated demonstration of N$_2$O before **Warren** at Harvard Medical School, Boston, at which the patient complained of pain and Wells was denounced as a fraud. Continued to practise dentistry, but became increasingly disillusioned as acceptance of N$_2$O was overshadowed by **Morton's** discovery of **diethyl ether**. Later a chloroform addict, he committed suicide by cutting his femoral artery whilst in prison.
[Samual Cooley, druggist's assistant; John Riggs (1810–85), US dentist]

Wenckebach phenomenon, *see Heart block*

Wheezing. During anaesthesia, may be caused by:
  –**bronchospasm** (e.g. caused by **asthma**, **aspiration of gastric contents**, **pulmonary oedema**).
  –**pneumothorax**.

–coughing or straining.

–inadvertent endobronchial intubation.

–mechanical **airway obstruction**, e.g. kinked **tracheal tube**, overinflated **cuff**, or placement of the tracheal tube's bevel against the posterior wall of the trachea.

–malfunction of directional or expiratory valves.

Bronchospasm should be diagnosed only when other causes have been excluded.

Whistle discriminator. Device used to confirm correct attachment of **N_2O** and **O_2** supplies to an **anaesthetic machine**. Placed at the fresh gas outlet; when O_2 passes through it, the whistle sounds at a higher pitch than with N_2O at the same flow rate, because O_2 has lower density.

Wilcoxon signed rank test, *see Statistical tests*

Willis, circle of, *see Cerebral circulation*

Wolff-Parkinson-White syndrome. Condition in which a congenital accessory connection between the atria and ventricles conducts more rapidly than the atrioventricular (AV) node, but has a longer refractory period. An atrial extrasystole finds the accessory bundle still refractory, but when the impulse passes via the AV node to the ventricles, the accessory bundle has recovered, and can conduct the impulse back to the atria. Circular conduction can continue with resultant **SVT**. **AF** and **atrial flutter** may also occur, but less commonly.

The **ECG** classically shows a short **P-R interval** and wide **QRS complexes** with δ waves (Fig. 149). A positive QRS complex in lead V_1 denotes type A (accessory bundle on the left side of the heart); if negative, type B (right side of heart).

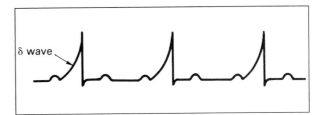

δ wave

Figure 149 *ECG showing δ waves*

Anaesthetic management should be directed at avoiding increased sympathetic activity, including due to anxiety. Drugs causing tachycardia (e.g. **atropine, ketamine, pancuronium**) should be avoided.

Treatment of perioperative arrhythmias follows standard measures. **Digoxin** may increase impulse conduction through accessory pathways by blocking conduction through the AV node.

[Sir John Parkinson (1885–1976), London cardiologist; Louis Wolff (1898–1972) and Paul White (1886–1973), US cardiologists]

Work. Product of **force** and distance. SI **unit** is the **joule**. Work is done whenever the point of application of a force moves in the direction of that force.

Work of breathing, *see Breathing, work of*

World Federation of Societies of Anaesthesiologists. Founded in 1955 at the first World Congress of Anaesthesiologists in The Hague, Holland, in order to promote anaesthetic education, research, training and safety

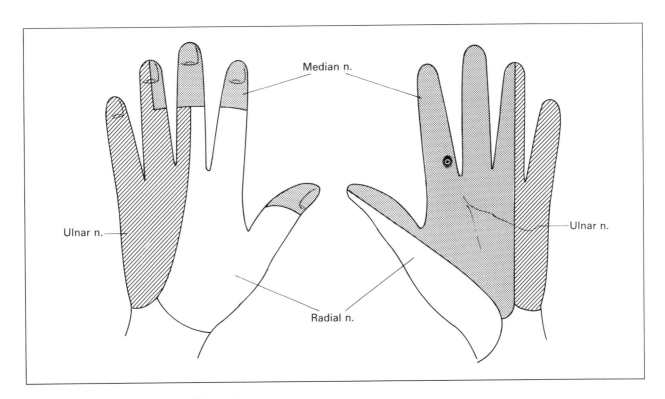

Median n.

Ulnar n.

Ulnar n.

Radial n.

Figure 150 *Cutaneous innervation of the hand*

standards throughout the world. World Congresses are held every 4 years (since 1960).

Wrist, nerve blocks. Used for minor surgery to the hand.
- The following nerves are blocked (Fig. 150):
  - **median nerve** (C6–T1): at the level of the proximal skin crease, it lies between flexor carpi radialis tendon laterally and palmaris longus tendon medially. With the wrist dorsiflexed, 2–5 ml **local anaesthetic agent** is injected just lateral to the palmaris longus tendon, at a depth of 0.5–1 cm.
  - **ulnar nerve** (C7–T1): lies under flexor carpi ulnaris tendon proximal to the pisiform bone, medial and deep to the ulnar artery. At the level of the ulnar styloid process, a needle is inserted between flexor carpi ulnaris tendon and the ulnar artery, and 2–5 ml solution injected. The two cutaneous branches of the nerve may be blocked by subcutaneous infiltration around the ulnar side of the wrist from the flexor carpi ulnaris tendon.
  - **radial nerve** (C5–T1): its branches pass along the radial and dorsal aspects of the wrist. At the level of the proximal skin crease, a needle is inserted lateral to the radial artery, and 3 ml solution injected. Infiltration around the radial border of the wrist blocks superficial branches.

X

Xamoterol fumarate. Orally active partial β_1-**adrenergic receptor agonist**, used to treat mild **cardiac failure**. Has inotropic effects at low resting sympathetic tone, increasing **myocardial contractility** and **cardiac output**. At high resting sympathetic tone, (e.g. moderate/severe **cardiac failure**), it has detrimental β-receptor antagonist effects and increases mortality.
- Dosage: 200 mg once-twice daily.

Xanthines (Methylxanthines). Derivatives of dioxypurine; they include **caffeine** and **theophylline**. **Phosphodiesterase inhibitors**, with wide spectra of activity including CNS stimulation, diuresis, increased **myocardial contractility** and smooth muscle relaxation. May also inhibit **adenosine** and reduce **noradrenaline** release.

Xenon. Inert gas, present in air in minute concentration. Shown to have anaesthetic properties (**MAC** 71), with little effect on cardiovascular stability. Its radioactive isotope ^{133}Xe is used in estimations of organ **blood flow**, and in analysis of pulmonary perfusion and ventilation.
Boomsma F, Rupreht J, Man In 't Veld AJ et al (1990) Anaesthesia; 45: 273–8

Y

Yates correction, *see Statistical tests*

Yohimbine. Alkaloid with similar structure to **reserpine**. A competitive α_2–**adrenergic receptor antagonist**; given iv it causes hypertension and tachycardia. Not used clinically.

Z

Zeolite. Hydrous silicate, used for ion- or molecule-trapping. An artificial zeolite is used in **O₂ concentrators**, to retain nitrogen from compressed air.

Zero, absolute. The lowest possible **temperature** that can be attained: 0 **kelvin** (corresponds to –273°C).

Zero-order kinetics, *see Pharmacokinetics*

Zidovudine, *see Antiviral drugs*

Zone of risk. Area of the operating room in which mixtures of anaesthetic agents may be explosive. Originally defined in the UK in 1956 as extending to a height of 4 ft 6 in above the floor, and 4 ft laterally from the anaesthetic equipment. Re-defined subsequently as extending 25 cm from any part of the apparatus or patient's airways that contains the anaesthetic mixture. Any flame or potential source of sparks should be placed outside this zone.
See also, Explosions and fires